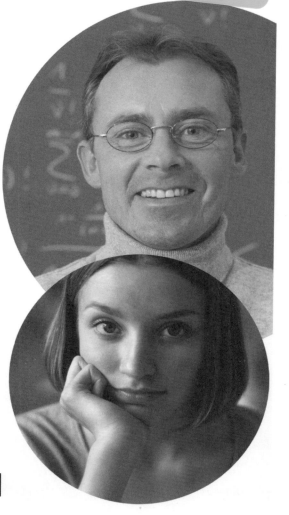
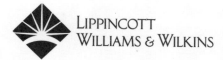

ACSM's Advanced Exercise Physiology

EDITORS

Editor
Charles M. Tipton, PhD, FACSM
Department of Physiology
University of Arizona
Tucson, Arizona

Section Editors
Michael N. Sawka, PhD, FACSM
U.S. Army Research Institute of Environmental Medicine
Thermal and Mountain Medicine Division
Natick, Massachusetts

Charlotte A. Tate, PhD, FACSM
Dean, Applied Health Sciences
University of Illinois—Chicago
Chicago, Illinois

Ronald L. Terjung, PhD, Drhc, FACSM
Department of Biomedical Sciences
University of Missouri
Columbia, Missouri

ACSM's Advanced Exercise Physiology

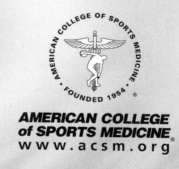

AMERICAN COLLEGE
of SPORTS MEDICINE
w w w . a c s m . o r g

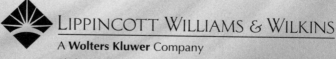

LIPPINCOTT WILLIAMS & WILKINS
A **Wolters Kluwer** Company

Philadelphia • Baltimore • New York • London
Buenos Aires • Hong Kong • Sydney • Tokyo

Acquisitions Editor: Emily Lupash
Managing Editor: Matthew J. Hauber
Marketing Manager: Christen DeMarco
Production Editor: Jennifer Glazer
Preproduction: Hearthside Publishing Services
Designer: Risa Clow
Compositor: Circle Graphics Inc.
Printer: Courier—Kendallville

ACSM's Publications Committee Chair: Jeffrey L. Roitman, EdD, FACSM
ACSM Group Publisher: D. Mark Robertson

Library of Congress Cataloging-in-Publication Data

ACSM's advanced exercise physiology / editor, Charles M. Tipton; section editors, Michael N. Sawka, Charlotte A. Tate, Ronald L. Terjung.
    p.; cm.
  Includes bibliographical references and index.
  ISBN 0-7817-4726-0
  1. Exercise–Physiological aspects. I. Title: Advanced exercise physiology. II. Tipton, Charles M., 1927- III. American College of Sports Medicine.
  [DNLM: 1. Exercise–physiology. WE 103 A187 2006]
QP309.A83 2006
612'.044—dc22

                    2005011768

The publishers have made every effort to trace the copyright holders for borrowed material. If they have inadvertently overlooked any, they will be pleased to make the necessary arrangements at the first opportunity.

06 07 08 09
2 3 4 5 6 7 8 9 10

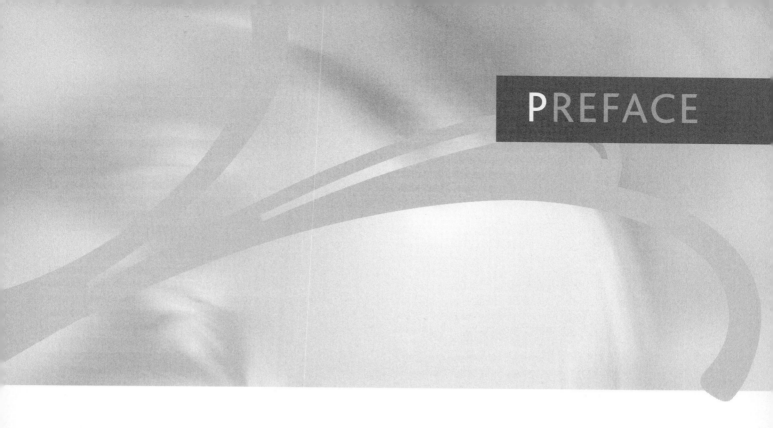

PREFACE

At the turn of the century, ACSM's publications committee concluded there was a need for an advanced textbook in exercise physiology and initiated publishing arrangements with Lippincott Williams & Wilkins while selecting individuals to serve as editors. The text was organized according to physiological systems that emphasized an integrated and quantitative approach to its content matter. Although this approach has elements of redundancy, we felt repetition was not a hindrance to learning. In addition, the chapters are presented as templates for lectures or discussions of topical matters within various systems. Believing that many undergraduate students in the exercise sciences have a limited understanding of the history of exercise physiology, the details of classical experiments, and the foundations for physiological genomics, the text contains chapters or sections devoted to these topics.

Authors of select chapters were invited because of their acknowledged expertise in the subject matter and their experience in teaching graduate classes. While most are members or fellows of the college, this was not a factor in their selection. Scientific expertise was also the primary factor for selection of reviewers, and each chapter was carefully evaluated and critiqued by experts chosen by the editors. In addition, we are indebted to Dr. Carl Foster, who served as the review editor for the publications committee's mandate that the content of all chapters receive an external review for appropriateness and to ensure they are presented in a format that is acceptable for advanced undergraduate and beginning graduate students. Obviously, we would appreciate receiving comments from the readership as to whether we achieved our objectives on both content and presentation.

To make faculty members' jobs easier when using this text, we have created Power Point slides and an image collection that are available at *http://connection.lww.com/go/acsmexphys*.

Our heartfelt gratitude and appreciation is extended to the following individuals who served as reviewers for this text: Drs. Robert B. Armstrong, Kenneth M. Baldwin, Kris Berg, Michael Berry, Jack W. Berryman, Susan Ann Bloomfield, Katarina T. Borer, Priscilla M. Clarkson, Victor A. Convertino, Edward F. Coyle, Craig G. Crandall, Allen Cymerman, J. Mark Davis, Roger M. Enoka, Karyn Esser, Peter A. Farrell, Hubert V. Forster, Patty Freedson, Phillip Gardiner, L. Bruce Gladden, John E. Greenleaf, Marc T. Hamilton, Christopher D. Hardin, William Herbert, Monica Hubal, Michael J. Joyner, Donna H. Korzick, G. Patrick Lambert, M. Harold Laughlin, Donald K. Layman, Kerry S. McDonald, Scott Montain, Steven R. Muza, David C. Nieman, James S. Pattison, David C. Poole, Peter B. Raven, Jeffrey L. Roitman, Don D. Sheriff, Espen Spangenburg, Michael J. Tipton, Lorraine P. Turcotte, and Charles E. Wade.

It is a pleasure to acknowledge the special leadership talents of Associate Editor Michael Sawka for finalizing the text for publication.

Lastly, we want to acknowledge the leadership contributions of W. Larry Kenney, Jeffrey L. Roitman, and D. Mark Robertson from the College and Pete Darcy and Matt Hauber from Lippincott Williams & Wilkins for bringing this important endeavor to fruition.

Charles Tipton, *Editor*

CONTRIBUTORS

Per Aagaard, PhD
Department of Neurophysiology
Institute of Medical Physiology
Bispebjerg Hospital
University of Copenhagen
Copenhagen, Denmark

Jens Bangsbo, PhD, DMSc, ScD
Copenhagen Muscle Research Centre
August Krogh Institute
University of Copenhagen
Copenhagen, Denmark

Shawn E. Bearden, PhD
Idaho State University
Pocatello, Idaho

Frank W. Booth, PhD, FACSM
Health Activity Center
University of Missouri
Columbia, Missouri

Vincent J. Caiozzo, PhD, FACSM
Department of Orthopaedics and
Department of Physiology and Biophysics
College of Medicine
University of California
Irvine, California

John R. Claybaugh, PhD
Department of Clinical Investigation
Tripler Army Medical Center
Honolulu, Hawaii

Victor A. Convertino, PhD, FACSM
U.S. Army Institute of Surgical Research
Fort Sam Houston
Houston, Texas

Jerome A. Dempsey, PhD, FACSM
Department of Population Health Sciences
John Rankin Laboratory of Pulmonary Medicine
University of Wisconsin
Madison, Wisconsin

V. Reggie Edgerton, PhD, FACSM
Department of Physiological Sciences
University of California at Los Angeles
Los Angeles, California

Robert Elsner, PhD
Institute of Marine Science
University of Alaska
Fairbanks, Alaska

Robert H. Fitts, PhD, FACSM
Department of Biological Sciences
Marquette University
Milwaukee, Wisconsin

Barry A. Franklin, PhD, FACSM
Preventive Cardiology
Beaumont Health Center
Royal Oak, Michigan

Charles S. Fulco, ScD
U.S. Army Research Institute of Environmental Medicine
Thermal and Mountain Medicine Division
Natick, Massachusetts

Mark Hargreaves, PhD, FACSM
Department of Physiology
The University of Melbourne
Melbourne, Australia

Laurie Hoffman-Goetz, PhD, MPH, FACSM
Department of Health Studies
University of Waterloo
Waterloo, Ontario, Canada

David A. Hood, PhD, FACSM
School of Kinesiology and Health Science
and Department of Biology
York University
Toronto, Ontario, Canada

Isabella Irrcher, MSc
School of Kinesiology and Health Science
and Department of Biology
York University
Toronto, Ontario, Canada

Jeremy M. LaMothe, PhD
Faculties of Kinesiology, Medicine, and Engineering
University of Calgary
Calgary, Alberta, Canada

Anne B. Loucks, PhD, FACSM
Department of Biological Sciences
Ohio University
Athens, Ohio

Gary W. Mack, PhD, FACSM
Department of Exercise Sciences
Brigham Young University
Provo, Utah

Robert S. Mazzeo, PhD, FACSM
Department of Integrative Physiology
University of Colorado at Boulder
Boulder, Colorado

Ronald A. Meyer, PhD
Departments of Physiology and Radiology
Michigan State University
East Lansing, Michigan

Jordan D. Miller, PhD
Department of Population Health Sciences
John Rankin Laboratory of Pulmonary Medicine
University of Wisconsin
Madison, Wisconsin

Russell L. Moore, PhD
Department of Integrative Physiology
University of Colorado at Boulder
Boulder, Colorado

Robert Murray, PhD, FACSM
Gatorade Sports Science Institute
Barrington, Illinois

P. Darrell Neufer, PhD
John B. Pierce Laboratory
Department of Cellular and Molecular Physiology
Yale University
New Haven, Connecticut

Donal S. O'Leary, PhD
Department of Physiology
Wayne State University
School of Medicine
Detroit, Michigan

Bente Klarlund Pedersen, MD, DSc
Department of Infectious Diseases
Rigshospital
Copenhagen, Denmark

Jeffrey T. Potts, PhD
Department of Physiology
School of Medicine
Wayne State University
Detroit, Michigan

Lee M. Romer, PhD
School of Sport and Education
Brunel University
West London, United Kingdom

Bryan Rourke, PhD
Department of Orthopaedics and Department of
Physiology and Biophysics
College of Medicine
University of California
Irvine, California

Roland R. Roy, PhD, FACSM
Brain Research Institute
University of California at Los Angeles
Los Angeles, California

Michael N. Sawka, PhD, FACSM
U.S. Army Research Institute of Environmental Medicine
Thermal and Mountain Medicine Division
Natick, Massachusetts

Suzanne M. Schneider, PhD
Department of Exercise Science
University of New Mexico
Albuquerque, New Mexico

Douglas R. Seals, PhD, FACSM
Department of Integrative Physiology
University of Colorado at Boulder
Boulder, Colorado

Steven S. Segal, PhD, FACSM
The John B. Pierce Laboratory & Department of Cellular
and Molecular Physiology
Yale University School of Medicine
New Haven, Connecticut

Xiaocai Shi, PhD, FACSM
Gatorade Sports Science Institute
Barrington, Illinois

Keizo Shiraki, MD, PhD
Department of Physiology
University of Occupational and Environmental Health
Kitakyushu, Japan

Lawrence L. Spriet, PhD, FACSM
Department of Human Biology and Nutritional Sciences
University of Guelph
Guelph, Ontario, Canada

Charles M. Tipton, PhD, FACSM
Department of Physiology
University of Arizona
Tucson, Arizona

Richard Tsika, PhD
Department of Biomedical Sciences
University of Missouri—Columbia
Columbia, Missouri

Anton J. M. Wagenmakers, PhD
Chair of Exercise Biochemistry
School of Sport and Exercise Sciences
University of Birmingham
Birmingham, United Kingdom

Peter D. Wagner, MD
Department of Medicine
University of California, San Diego
La Jolla, California

Robert W. Wiseman, PhD
Departments of Physiology and Radiology
Michigan State University
East Lansing, Michigan

Gregory R. Wohl, PhD
Faculties of Kinesiology, Medicine, and Engineering
University of Calgary
Calgary, Alberta, Canada

Andrew J. Young, PhD, FACSM
U.S. Army Research Institute of Environmental Medicine
Military Nutrition Division
Natick, Massachusetts

Edward J. Zambraski, PhD, FACSM
U.S. Army Institute of Environmental Medicine
Military Performance Division
Natick, Massachusetts

Ronald F. Zernicke, PhD, FACSM
Faculties of Kinesiology, Medicine, and Engineering
University of Calgary
Calgary, Alberta, Canada

CONTENTS

Introduction to Exercise Physiology

CHAPTER 1

The Language of Exercise

CHARLES M. TIPTON AND BARRY A. FRANKLIN

Introduction

Like education, the term *exercise* has different meanings for different people, resulting in unnecessary confusion and uncertainty when it is prescribed or its impact is being interpreted. To the etymologists, exercise is a noun of Middle English vintage with a Middle French origin (exercice) that evolved from the Latin terms exercitium and exercitius, and means "to drive forth" (1).

1. Galen of Pergamon (129–200 A.D.) identified exercise with "vigorous motion" (2).
2. Bouchard and Shephard at a Consensus Symposium defined exercise to be a form of "leisure-time physical activity that is usually performed on a repeated basis over an extended period of time (exercise training) with a specific external objective such as the improvement of fitness, physical performance, or health" (3).
3. We consider exercise to be a displacement of the homeostasis of rest elicited by muscle contractions resulting in movement and increased energy expenditure (4).

Exercise can occur in occupational, leisure, recreational, competitive, or noncompetitive environments using modalities that require select muscle contractions producing coordinated movements, such as walking, jogging, running, cycling, swimming, rowing, skiing, skating, climbing, throwing, lifting, pushing, pulling, carrying, squeezing, or combinations thereof. The purpose of this chapter is to clarify the meaning of the term *exercise;* to indicate how it is identified, classified, and used; to illustrate the components, value, and application of the exercise prescription; and to provide guidelines for maintaining and improving one's health and fitness status.

Acute Exercise And Its Description

Acute exercise is the physiological responses associated with the immediate effects of a single bout of physical activity regardless of the modality used or the exercise history or characteristics of the subject, human or animal (5). Over the years, physiologists have used a multitude of descriptive terms and synonyms to characterize acute exercise. Many have their origin with the movements produced by the muscle contractions being initiated. For example, dynamic exercise refers to bodily movements caused by concentric and eccentric muscle contractions, which produce work. (Originally it was associated with isotonic contractions, but the use of this term was discouraged because maintaining constant tension is unlikely with the movements of human performance [5].) *Static exercise* describes the physiological changes that result from isometric muscle contractions (5), while *isokinetic exercise* refers to movements produced by eccentric or concentric muscle contractions whose velocity (torque around a joint) is held constant by a special device so that the "resistance is in direct ratio to the varying force applied through the full course of a natural movement" (6). Acute exercise is also characterized by metabolic descriptors and aerobic exercise is an example (7). While this term is useful in indicating that aerobic metabolism is the primary energy source for the activity, it does not indicate the degree or magnitude of the aerobic involvement. In essence, it is more an approximation of steady state conditions over time because of the difficulty in securing precise measurements of the energy transformation process. Anaerobic exercise is frequently used to describe power activities whose energy demands of muscle require increased-velocity movements or elevated force or torque values that facilitate phosphagen and glycolytic transformations within cells and a metabolic profile shift to anaerobic metabolism (8). Like aerobic metabolism, the term does not indicate the degree of the transformation or change. Interestingly, Brooks and associates have recommended that anaerobic power tests be designated as high-intensity exercise tests because glycolysis occurs as a result of motor unit selectivity rather than for biochemical reasons per se (8).

Endurance is the ability to maintain an established intensity (usually moderate to heavy) over a long period; hence, the term endurance exercise (9). Since endurance exercises are prolonged and continuous, require a sustained and elevated somatic oxygen consumption, and usually necessitate rhythmical movements (9), we advocate using dynamic exercise as the inclusive term that encompasses the features of endurance as well as isotonic, aerobic, continuous, and rhythmical exercise (Table 1.1).

Moving animate or inanimate objects (as in combat or lifting stones, respectively) has been an integral component of human existence since prehistoric times. When related activities evolved into recreational or competitive events, some were incorporated into a sport, as was the case with wrestling and weightlifting. However, when the purpose was rehabilitation, as during World War II, lifting weights became known as progressive resistive exercise (10,11). This term is used to describe the process by which muscular forces or torques are increased to overcome the internal or external resistances imposed upon skeletal muscles. Because resistance activities can be performed by concentric, eccentric, and isometric muscle contractions, they can be classified as either dynamic or static resistance exercise (10). Cellular oxidative energy transformations are more time dependent than nonoxidative processes (8); hence, some investigators assume that isometric exercise and anaerobic exercise are synonymous terms. This is a tenuous assumption because this condition can only be achieved when the contractions are brief (8) or sufficiently intense to impede the blood flow to the contracting muscle groups. For example, a metabolic shift toward anaerobic metabolism can occur during sprinting exercises for runners, swimmers, skiers, skaters, and cyclists and with the power movements of weight lifters (7,8).

TABLE 1.1	Modified Classification of Exercise Intensities as Recommended for Healthy Adults by ACSM and the Surgeon General[a]								
	Relative Intensity of Dynamic Exercise					Absolute Intensity of Dynamic Exercise (MET) for Healthy Adults of Various Ages				
Intensity[b]	$\dot{V}O_2$ R (%)	$\dot{V}O_{2max}$ (%)	HR Reserve (%)	Maximal HR (%)	Rating PE	Young (20–39 yr)	Middle Aged (40–64 yr)	Old Age (65–79 yr)	Very Old Age (80+ yr)	Static Resistance Exercise % MVC
Very light	<20	<25	<20	<35	<10	<2.4	<2.0	<1.6	<1.0	<30
Light	20–39	25–44	20–39	35–54	10–11	2.4–4.7	2.0–3.9	1.6–3.1	1.1–1.9	30–49
Moderate	40–59	45–59	40–59	55–69	12–13	4.8–7.1	4.0–5.9	3.2–4.7	2.0–2.9	50–69
Heavy	60–84	60–84	60–84	70–89	14–16	7.2–10.1	6.0–8.4	4.8–6.7	3.0–4.24	70–84
Very heavy	≥85	≥85	≥85	≥90	17–19	≥10.2	≥8.5	≥6.8	≥4.25	≥85
Maximal	100	100	100	100	20	12	10.0	8.0	5.0	100

[a]Table foundation is for dynamic exercise lasting for 60 minutes (9).
[b]Contains consistent and historic terminology e.g. heavy for hard, very heavy for very hard
HR, heart rate; R, reserve; PE, perceived exertion; MET, metabolic equivalent; MVC, maximum voluntary contraction; RPE, Borg listings on a scale of 6–20 (20,32).
MET expressed in units of milliliters of oxygen per kilogram per minute, as 1 MET = 3.5 mL · kg^{-1} · min^{-1}. MET values are approximate means for men; women's means are 1 to 2 METs lower (9).
Permission to use the template for Table 1.1 was granted by Dr. William Haskell of Stanford University.
Modified from Table 2.4 of the Surgeon General Report by the U.S. Department of Human Services (9) and from Table 1 of the Position Stand on the Quantity and Quality of Exercise by ACSM (20).

Chronic Exercise and Its Description

The term *chronic exercise* refers to the repeated performance of acute exercise; it is better known as physical training or just training (4). Habitual physical exercise is also used by authors for the same purpose. To achieve a trained state or for a conditioning effect to exist, the process of chronic exercise must have produced one or more significant morphological or physiological changes from the status before training (4). Although there is no universal agreement among physiologists on the terminology describing these exercise-induced alterations with time, significant changes that occur within a week are considered brief or transient effects; those that result after several weeks or months are labeled short-term training effects; and those that appear or persist after a year or more are regarded as long-term training effects. Traditionally, exercise physiologists have used the term *adaptation* to describe the transitional changes that emerge with chronic or habitual exercise, and several of the contributing authors will use this terminology in their chapters. However, to be consistent with environmental and comparative physiologists, we advocate that only the long-term training effects be synonymous with adaptation.

The Prescription of Exercise

To interpret the physiological effects of exercise, it is essential to know the modality employed and how the exercise was prescribed. In the 1970s, the American Heart Association and the American College of Sports Medicine (ACSM) presented the concept of exercise testing and prescription to the medical community (12,13); however, the idea was not new to the athletic or sports community, as rudiments have been advocated since the eras of Herodotus (480–? B.C.), Hippocrates (460–370 B.C.), Galen (129–210 A.D.), and Philostratos (219–230 A.D.) with the "professional athletes" of Athens (14).

While the characteristics of the prescription and its benefits will vary depending on the age, gender, health status, fitness level, and goals of the individual (Fig. 1.1), the components will contain modality, frequency, intensity, duration, and rest intervals. The modality prescribed (e.g., running, cycling, swimming, lifting, hiking) is crucial because the short- and long-term effects of exercise will be influenced by this variable; for example, arm strength will not be increased by running. In fact, single or combined arm and leg training studies have shown only minor improvements, with submaximal or maximal exercise responses when the effects of limb-specific exercises are assessed (7,15–17). This concept, which incorporates the distinctive nature of the exercise stimuli and the unique motor unit recruitment profile, is known as the specificity of exercise (4), and it is an essential consideration when evaluating the effectiveness of various exercise regimens.

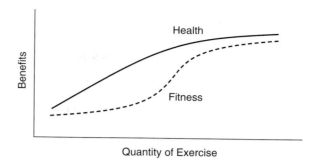

FIGURE 1.1   Conceptual relationship between chronic exercise and its health and fitness benefits. Health benefits can occur at lower intensities, durations, and frequencies that may not notably affect cardiorespiratory fitness. *(Reprinted with permission from Piscatella JC, Franklin BA. Take a Load off Your Heart. New York: Workman, 2003, p. 156).*

Frequency of Exercise

Frequency of exercise is a key component of any prescription if acute or chronic effects are to be achieved. Recommendations from ACSM (18), Centers for Disease Control and Prevention (19), and the Surgeon General (9) concerning the appropriate frequency of endurance-related activities (dynamic exercise) for adults advocate a minimum frequency of three times a week with an upper limit of 5 days. In fact, the Surgeon General's report favors moderate-intensity exercise "on most, if not all days of the week" (9). Recently the Institute of Medicine made a similar recommendation for frequency. In the 1998 ACSM position stand on the quantity and quality of exercise for developing cardiorespiratory and muscular fitness plus flexibility, the recommendation was 3 to 5 days a week (20). For resistance exercise, both the Surgeon General and ACSM advocate at least 2 days a week (9,10).

Intensity of Exercise

Intensity is an essential component of the prescription because of its importance in eliciting the acute while maintaining the chronic effects of exercise (21). It refers to the magnitude of the physiological disruption or stress caused by the activity. The terminology used to describe intensity evolved from the practice of early physiologists, who would *load* (add weights to) their muscle preparations; characterize their loads as being light, medium, or heavy for the muscle in question; and when appropriate, discuss the workload features of the experiment. Today, exercise physiologists use the terms *load* and *resistance* as synonyms for intensity (8) but generally confine their use to resistance exercise (10). For dynamic exercise, intensity is best characterized by a measure of energy expenditure, which may be expressed on an absolute or relative basis (7,20). To use a relative unit, it is necessary to directly measure maximal oxygen consumption ($\dot{V}O_{2max}$) (7) or the maximal oxygen uptake reserve ($\dot{V}O_2$ R) (20), which ACSM advocates as a more precise measure. This latter unit is the difference between resting and $\dot{V}O_{2max}$ (20). The percentage prescribed depends upon the purpose of the prescription. If the intent is to perform exercise for developing and maintaining cardiorespiratory fitness for health purposes (Fig. 1.1), the intensity level of dynamic exercise recommended for adults by ACSM is 40 or 50–85% of the $\dot{V}O_2$ R value (20). In 1995, the ACSM recommended an intensity corresponding to 40 to 85% $\dot{V}O_{2max}$, and this guideline continues to be followed by many centers throughout the United States (21).

As shown in Table 1.1, the percentages of $\dot{V}O_{2max}$ or $\dot{V}O_2$ R can range from 20 to 100%, depending upon the intensity level that is to be performed. To prescribe an absolute energy expenditure unit, the oxygen consumption value (mL $O_2 \cdot$ kg $\cdot$ min^{-1}) is converted into metabolic equivalents (METs) after dividing by a constant of 3.5 mL $O_2 \cdot$ kg $\cdot$ min^{-1} (which is representative of the average adult resting metabolic rate) and equal to 1 MET (12). Since oxygen consumption is affected by age, training, gender, environmental conditions, and health status, absolute values for prescription or evaluation purposes for healthy untrained adult populations are listed according to age ranges and are 1 to 2 METs lower for women (20) (Table 1.1). Also listed in Table 1.1 are MET values for progressive exercise intensities (i.e., very light to maximal) with specific reference to populations of different ages. Although relative and absolute approaches continue to be employed for prescriptive purposes, METs are recommended more for rehabilitation than for fitness purposes.

Measurement of maximal oxygen consumption is not feasible at all sites where exercise is prescribed. However, results from studies conducted by Robinson (22), the Astrands (5), and Pollock and associates (23) have demonstrated a linear relationship between oxygen consumption and heart rate during exercise until very heavy or maximal exercise is performed (5). This relationship enabled investigators indirectly to relate heart rate values to energy expenditure units and directly to use a percentage of the maximum heart rate (MHR) for prescription of exercise intensity (7,20,23). However, as shown in Figure 1.2, a given percentage of the maximum heart rate is not equal to the same percentage of the maximum oxygen consumption (23,24).

Ideally, the maximal heart rate should be obtained directly from exercise testing, but it can be predicted by using an equation to estimate a maximal heart rate for adult populations:

$$\text{MHR} = 220 \text{ heart beats per minute} - \text{age in years} \, (24)$$

The equation was developed for healthy untrained male adults but can be used with children and healthy untrained adult female populations (25). Recently, the validity of this

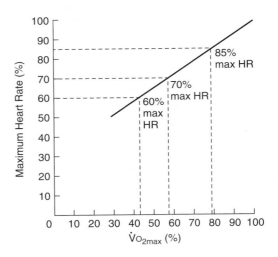

FIGURE 1.2 The linear relationship between maximum heart rate and percent $\dot{V}O_{2max}$. *(Reprinted with permission from Pollock ML, Wilmore JH, Fox SM III. Health and Fitness Through Physical Activity. Modified from American College of Sports Medicine Series. New York: Wiley, 1978, p. 123).*

time-honored equation was effectively challenged by Tanaka and associates (26) at the University of Colorado. These researchers developed a new one that predicts maximal heart rate without consideration of gender:

$$\text{MHR} = 208 - 0.7 \times \text{age in years} \, (26)$$

We think this equation has sufficient promise to warrant its use in the future with healthy populations. ACSM recommends that healthy adults perform regular dynamic exercise to develop and maintain cardiovascular fitness at an intensity level that is 55 or 65 to 90% of the MHR (20), while Table 1.1 denotes that light exercise is associated with MHR values of 35 to 54% (9). Karvonen and associates introduced the concept of the heart rate reserve (HRR) for purposes of the exercise prescription (27). This is calculated by subtracting the resting heart rate from the maximal heart rate. The difference is multiplied by a certain percentage or a range of percentages (e.g., 50–75%) for intensity purposes and added to the resting heart rate (25,27). To illustrate, ACSM advocates that normal healthy adults perform dynamic exercise at an intensity level that represents 40 or 50 to 85% of their heart rate reserve to improve and maintain cardiorespiratory fitness (20). According to Table 1.1, these percentages represent intensities ranging from moderate to very heavy exercise. Emerging from the heart rate reserve concept is the idea of *target heart rates*, which refers to the use of a percentage of the MHR or the HRR to identify the upper and lower limits of the exercise heart rate necessary to elicit training effects (25,27). Target heart rates are commonly displayed at commercial fitness centers for treadmill and cycle ergometer users and exhibit age-related estimates of the lower and upper limits of the training-sensitive heart rate zones (25). The use of heart rate to denote exercise intensity requires an awareness that the mode of exercise will affect maximal heart rate; namely, lower body (leg) exercise will elicit higher maximum heart rate values than upper body (arm) exercise (16,25). Although a large database is lacking, swimming is associated with mean maximal heart rates that are essentially 13 beats per minute lower than those recorded while running (25), whereas arm ergometer exercise is associated with mean maximal heart rates that are approximately 11 beats per minute lower than values recorded during leg exercise (16). Consequently, the guidelines used by Franklin are recommended; namely, the prescribed training heart rates followed for leg exercise should be reduced by 10 to 15 beats per minute for arm training programs (personal communication from Barry Franklin, December 12, 2002).

With resistance exercise, load rather than energy expenditure becomes the essential consideration. Before exercise prescription became an integral component of exercise and clinical sciences, the load prescribed was usually in absolute units for the purposes of increasing strength, endurance, and muscle mass and was restricted to the lifting of free weights. As noted previously, the formal use of resistance exercise (progressive resistance exercise) was promoted initially by DeLorme (11) for rehabilitation purposes during and after World War II. It continues to serve this function. Currently, the ACSM intensity recommendations for health and muscular fitness development and maintenance purposes for individuals starting an exercise program is a load that can be lifted successfully 8 to 12 times (repetitions and a set) with 8 to 10 different movements involving various muscle groups of the upper and lower body and trunk (10). However, for local muscular endurance training, the ACSM advocates a routine of light to moderate loads with an increase in repetitions (10,18) (Fig. 1.3).

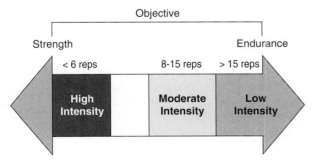

FIGURE 1.3 ACSM-recommended resistance exercise program to improve muscle strength and endurance, considering age and health status. *(Reprinted with permission from American College of Sports Medicine. ACSM's Guidelines for Exercise Testing and Prescription. 6th ed. Baltimore: Williams & Wilkins, 1995, p. 23).*

Because of the time required to exercise all the angles of joints, there are no general recommendations concerning the systematic performance of static resistance exercise, although the intensity can be characterized by the magnitude of the isometric contraction by using the percentage of the maximum voluntary contraction (MVC). For example, light exercise represents 30 to 49% of the MVC, whereas heavy exercise would correspond to 70 to 84% of the measured MVC (Table 1.1) (7,20).

With training, the foundation for the intensity being prescribed for dynamic exercise with healthy adults is the repetition maximum, which refers to the heaviest load that can be lifted or moved once (1-RM) (10,28,29). Depending upon the specific purposes of the training program, such as to produce muscular strength, endurance, power, or mass (hypertrophy) and the status of the healthy population (e.g., sedentary, athletic, elderly), the load or loads, 1-RM, repetitions, or sets being prescribed will vary, and detailed guidelines are available for such purposes (10,30). Research has shown that a stimulus of 45 to 60% of the 1-RM will increase strength in untrained and novice subjects (10), whereas higher percentages (80–100% of the 1-RM) may be required for more experienced lifters and athletes (10). An ACSM-suggested prescription for a healthy sedentary adult who is beginning to train is to perform one set of dynamic resistance exercises at a load equal to 60 to 80% of 1-RM with 8 to 12 repetitions (10).

In contrast to the dynamic resistance exercise guidelines for general health and fitness purposes, there are none that pertain to the performance of static exercises. Approximately 5 decades ago, the concept was advanced that a single isometric contraction maintained at a load that represented 67% of the MVC for 6 seconds would produce weekly strength gains that approximated 5% of the original strength measure (25). While this concept was not substantiated by additional research and the gains in strength were demonstrated to be largely angle specific, some authorities have suggested that maintaining a nearly maximal contraction for longer durations (~20 seconds) will increase muscular strength. Although numerous training studies have been conducted with the load established at varied MCV values, there are no universally available static exercise training programs being prescribed for untrained healthy subjects.

In 1962, Gunnar Borg introduced the rating of perceived exertion (RPE) to the exercise science community as a psychological indicator for the degree of physical strain (31). Subsequent research has demonstrated that RPE is significantly correlated with heart rate, oxygen consumption, pulmonary ventilation, and lactate concentrations to validate its use for the prescription and monitoring of exercise intensity (25,32). The RPE scale (Table 1.1) ranges from 6 to 20, with 15 numerical levels that contain descriptive effort ratings at progressive intensity levels (7,20).

Duration of Exercise

In 1975, ACSM recommended that normal healthy individuals perform physical activity for 20 to 30 minutes a day without specifying how much time should be devoted to resistance exercise (21). Currently it recommends 20 to 60 minutes of continuous or intermittent dynamic exercise per day (minimum of 10-minute bouts accumulated throughout the day) (18,20). Because the duration of exercise required to elicit a significant training effect varies inversely with the intensity, the guidelines recommend individuals performing at the lower intensity levels continue to exercise for 30 minutes or more, whereas those performing at higher intensities should strive to complete 20 minutes or more (20). Although the recommendations do not specify the duration, the 20- to 60-minute period should be more than adequate to perform one set of 8 to 10 different resistance exercises.

Rest Intervals and Exercise

The subject of rest or rest intervals is seldom listed as a characteristic of the exercise prescription. However, when considered in regard to the exercise–rest interval cycle, it is an important component of the interval training programs followed by swimmers and runners (7,28); the resistance training programs advocated for weight lifters, football players, wrestlers, etc. (10); and the circuit training programs promoted for nonathletes, athletes, or physically active populations, such as firemen (33). A physiological rationale for rest periods is the time profile (seconds to minutes) associated with the energy transformations of the adenosine triphosphate (ATP), phosphocreatine (PCr), and glycolytic systems that occur with different types of activities, maintaining an emphasis on the concentration of lactic acid being formed (see previous section on acute exercise). By using information for high-intensity exercise that includes one's best performance time, a recommended pace, designated distance (e.g., 110 yards) for the primary activation of a specific energy system (ATP and PCr), a given number of repetitions (e.g., 20), and an established rest period (e.g., 10 seconds), it is possible to increase the amount of exercise being performed within a given workout, enhance the intramuscular ATP and PCr system, improve anaerobic glycolysis, enhance the shuttle of pyruvate to the Krebs cycle, facilitate lactate transporters, and delay the sensation of fatigue while elevating the capacity of skeletal muscles for aerobic glycolysis (7,25,29). According to Brooks and associates, rest periods are essential for training adaptations to occur (8).

Rest with resistance exercise is advocated for hormonal and metabolic reasons. Short rest periods (1–2 minutes) with moderate to high-intensity exercise elicit greater increases in anabolic hormones when contrasted to longer durations of rest (10,29,34), whereas extended rest periods replenish ATP and PCr stores and minimize the effects of anaerobic glycolysis on fatigue and performance (30). Recently, ACSM recommended that 1- to 2-minute rest periods be used in novice and intermediate training programs, whereas individuals in advanced training programs should consider using 1- to 2-minute rest periods with moderate resistance exercise and 2- to 3-minute intervals when heavy resistance exercise is performed (10). In essence, the ACSM recommendations of 2 days a week of resistance exercise for general health and fitness purposes has an inherent rest component because it allows the various muscle groups to recover from the metabolic and anatomical effect of the previous exercise session (10). The same logic applies to the periodization training cycles (3 days/week) that are followed by weight lifters (10,29,34). When resistance circuit training programs are followed (~6–8 stations), a 1-minute rest period is recommended (10,29). Whether this duration is appropriate for the objectives of the program has yet to be determined.

Progression and Exercise

Progression is seldom included in the exercise prescription unless training is involved. Although an important consideration in designing training programs, it has failed to receive the critical research attention received by other components. Consequently, the opinions of experts and the practices of successful coaches and athletes are generally the rule rather than the exception. Wilmore and Costill have defined the principle of progressive overload which states that all training programs must include overload and progression (7). Holly and Shaffrath address the issue of progression with dynamic exercise by noting that the functional capacity, medical and health status, age, goals, and exercise preferences of the individual must be considered before initiating a three-stage prescription (33). In accordance with ACSM recommendations (18), the initial stage consists of moderate-intensity exercise (40–60% of the HRR) 3 days a week with a duration that starts at 15 minutes a day and proceeds to 30 minutes while causing a minimum of muscle soreness and discomfort. This prescription lasts approximately 4 weeks. Next is the improvement stage, which is associated with increases in intensity from moderate to very heavy exercise corresponding to HRR values of 50 to 85% (Table 1.1), which are expected to last for an additional 4 or 5 months. While intensity is progressively elevated from moderate to heavy to very heavy exercise, duration is consistently increased every 2 to 3 weeks until the individual is capable of sustaining 35 to 40 minutes of exercise. How the individual adjusts to these alterations is the primary determinant of when to implement these serial increases. When the prescription has achieved these objectives, it means for most individuals that the training program has entered the maintenance stage (18,33).

With resistance training, progression is associated with different approaches. If resistance exercise is being performed, progression occurs when a specific number of repetitions of moving a designated load has been achieved. Specifically, if untrained individuals can effectively complete

8 to 12 repetitions of a given load (e.g., 60% of a 1-RM), they progress to a load that is 2 to 10% higher, depending upon the muscle group involved and whether single or multiple joint movements are undertaken (10).

One or more training cycles a year can occur with advanced lifters following a periodization training program (29,34). For them, progression can proceed from a preparation phase (~6 weeks of 3–5 sets, 8–12 repetitions, 50–80% of 1-RM), to a first transition phase (~6 weeks of 3–5 sets, 5–6 repetitions, 80–90% of 1-RM), to a competitive phase (~6 weeks of 3–5 sets, 2–4 repetitions, 90–95% of 1-RM). This is followed by a second transition phase that includes about 2 weeks of recreational activities with various modalities and lower-intensity resistance exercises (25). As noted by Kraemer and Ratamess, rapidly increasing evidence demonstrates that periodized training is superior to "constant load and set" training for producing improvements in strength (35).

Implicit and Explicit Features of the Exercise Prescription

Most exercise prescriptions advocated by various professional groups are intended for a nondiseased and predominantly sedentary adult population with the intent of promoting health and fitness. It is apparent that age is a major consideration with exercise performance, and Table 1.1 reflects that concern with dynamic exercise. Physiological reasons for such a concern will be addressed by authors of subsequent chapters. With resistance exercise by healthy individuals, the demarcations are less well defined, and being over or under age 50 is currently the reference point in determining the number of repetitions to prescribe (10). ACSM has no prescription recommendations for adults of any age for a minimum load or a percentage of a minimal load to develop and maintain muscular fitness. Because of the complexities of growth and development on cardiorespiratory and metabolic systems, it is understandable that "authorities" start at 20 years of age when listing prescriptions (Table 1.1).

When METs are employed, gender must be considered, because at any given intensity level, females are generally exercising at a higher percentage of their aerobic capacity than their male counterparts. Hence, at an absolute level the values are lower (Table 1.1). This difference is attributed to females having less muscle mass and a lower aerobic capacity than males. This is partially explained by lower blood volumes, hemoglobin concentrations, and stroke volumes (7). Research has shown that the stage of the menstrual cycle at the time of testing has little or no impact on the subsequent prescription (7). In the ACSM recommendations to develop and maintain muscular fitness, gender is not an issue, as the emphasis is on a standard number of repetitions (8–12) that an adult can perform using the major muscle groups of the body (20).

Inherent in the use of the cardiovascular (HR), energy expenditure (oxygen consumption), force (1-RM) or psy-chological (RPE) data for predictive purposes is that they were obtained under standardized resting, exercise, environmental, and "stress-free" conditions. The same assumption applies when referring to tables that identify various intensity levels (e.g., Table 1.1). However, when field testing occurs (e.g., track, football field, swimming pool) away from the laboratory, the investigator must be cognizant of potentially confounding variables, including previous activity, environmental temperature or humidity, changes in air pollutants, elevations in noise, appearance of onlookers, and organizational distractions that could impact the results and necessitate caution in the interpretation and use of the collected information.

SUMMARY

Exercise is displacement of the homeostasis of rest elicited by muscle contractions which result in movement and an increase in energy expenditure; it can be either acute or chronic. Acute exercise has been characterized by its metabolic effects (aerobic, anaerobic), muscle contraction types (isotonic, either concentric and eccentric or isometric), muscle contractions being controlled (isokinetic), muscle contraction movement profiles (dynamic or static), duration (endurance, short-term, or long-term), movement characteristics (plyometric), movement sequence (continuous, intermittent, or rhythmical), or by the load that muscle contractions must overcome (resistance). We advocate the use of *dynamic exercise* as the inclusive term for aerobic, isotonic, endurance, continuous, and rhythmical physical activity that is associated with cardiorespiratory fitness and advocate use of the term *dynamic resistance exercise* when movements occur because of concentric and eccentric contractions of skeletal muscles. When isometric contractions are initiated and the force of the MVC determined, we advocate using *static resistance exercise* to describe the process. Although anaerobic responses are an important but not exclusive metabolic effect of resistance exercise, the results of the activity and not the type of exercise (dynamic or resistance) should to be used to describe the exercise. Regardless of the purpose of exercise—recreational, competitive, rehabilitation, health maintenance, fitness enhancement, or leisure time pursuit—it is performed (knowingly or unknowingly) with regard to the components of the exercise prescription: mode, frequency, intensity, duration, rest, and progression. All are involved in eliciting changes and improvement and are essential for understanding and interpreting acute and chronic exercise responses. Of these components, intensity is the most important. Because of the practices of early muscle physiologists, load became synonymous with intensity and provided the rationale for characterizing intensity as being light, moderate, heavy, very heavy, or maximal. We favor continuation of the practice, although descriptors as easy, hard, very hard, low, high, intense, strenuous, and exhaustive have been advocated and found in the published literature (and disappointingly, in subsequent chapters of this book). Inherent in the prescription is that the exercise must be individualized for the participant and be implemented with regard for the specificity of the response.

ACKNOWLEDGMENT

It is a pleasure to acknowledge the insightful advice and counsel of Dr. William Kramer of the University of Connecticut in the preparation of this manuscript.

REFERENCES

1. Oxford English Dictionary. Available at <http://dictionary.oed.com/framesok/logo.dlt>. Accessed January 5, 2002.

2. Green RM. A translation of Galen's Hygiene (De sanitate tuenda). Springfield: Charles C. Thomas, 1951.

3. Bouchard C, Shephard RJ. Physical activity, fitness, and health: the model and key concepts. In Bouchard C, Shepherd RJ, Stephens T, eds. Physical Activity, Fitness and Health. Champaign, IL: Human Kinetics, 1994;77–97.

4. Scheuer J, Tipton CM. Cardiovascular adaptations to physical training. Ann Rev Physiol 1977;39:221–251.

5. Astrand PO, Rodahl K. Textbook of Work Physiology. 3rd ed. New York: McGraw Hill, 1986.

6. Thistle HG, Hislop HJ, Moffroid M, et al. Isokinetic contraction: a new concept of resistive exercise. Arch Phys Med Rehab 1967;48:279–282.

7. Willmore JH, Costill DI. Physiology of Sport and Exercise. 2nd ed. Champaign, IL: Human Kinetics, 1999.

8. Brooks GA, Fahey TD, White TP, et al. Exercise Physiology. 3rd ed. Mountain View, CA: Mayfield, 2000.

9. U.S. Department of Health and Human Services. Physical activity and health: a report of the Surgeon General. Atlanta: HHS, Centers for Disease Control and Prevention, National Center for Chronic Disease Prevention and Health Promotion, 1996.

10. American College of Sports Medicine. Position stand: progression models in resistance training for healthy adults. Med Sci Sports Exerc 2002;34:364–380.

11. DeLorme TL, Watkins AL. Progressive Resistance Exercise. New York: Appleton–Century Crofts, 1951.

12. American College of Sports Medicine. Guidelines for Graded Exercise Testing and Exercise Prescription. Philadelphia: Lea & Febiger, 1975.

13. American Heart Association. Exercise Testing and Training of Apparently Healthy Individuals: Handbook for Physicians. Dallas: American Heart Association, 1972.

14. Berryman JW. Exercise and the medical tradition from Hippocrates through antebellum America: a review essay. In Berryman JW, Parks RJ, eds. Sport and Exercise Science. Urbana: University of Illinois, 1992;1–56.

15. Rasmussen B, Klausen K, Clausen JP, et al. Pulmonary ventilation, blood gases, blood pH after training of the arms or the legs. J Appl Physiol 1975;38:250–256.

16. Franklin BA. Exercise testing, training and arm ergometry. Sports Med 1985;2:100–119.

17. Magel JR, Folgia GD, McArdle WD, et al. Specificity of swim training on maximal oxygen uptake. J Appl Physiol 1975;38: 151–155.

18. American College of Sports Medicine. ACSM's Guidelines for Exercise Testing and Prescription. 6th ed. Baltimore: Lippincott Williams & Wilkins, 2000.

19. Pate RR, Pratt M, Blair SN, et al. Physical activity and public health: a recommendation from the Centers for Disease Control and Prevention and the American College of Sports Medicine. JAMA 1995;273:402–407.

20. American College of Sports Medicine. Position stand: the recommended quantity and quality of exercise for developing and maintaining cardiorespiratory and muscular fitness, and flexibility in healthy adults. Med Sci Sports Exerc 1998;30:975–991.

21. American College of Sports Medicine. ACSM's guidelines for exercise testing and prescription. 5th ed. Baltimore: Williams & Wilkins, 1995.

22. Robinson S. Experimental studies of physical fitness in relation to age. Arbeitsphysiologie 1938;10:251–323.

23. Pollock ML, Wilmore JH, Fox III SM. Health and Fitness Through Physical Activity. American College of Sports Medicine Series. New York: Wiley, 1978.

24. Fox SM, Naughton JP, Haskell WL. Physical activity and the prevention of coronary heart disease. Ann Clin Res 1971;3: 404–432.

25. McArdle WD, Katch FI, Katch VL. Exercise Physiology. 5th ed. Philadelphia: Lippincott Williams & Wilkins, 2001.

26. Tanaka H, Monhan KD, Seals DG. Age-predicted maximal heart rate revisited. Am Coll Cardiol 2001;37:153–156.

27. Karvonen M, Kentela K, Mustala O. The effects of training heart rate: a longitudinal study. Ann Med Exp Biol Fenn 1957;35:307–315.

28. Fox EI, Mathews DK. Interval Training. Philadelphia: Saunders, 1974.

29. Kraemer WJ, Fleck SJ. Resistance training: exercise prescription. Phys Sportsmed. 1988;18:69–81.

30. Fleck SJ, Kraemer WJ. Designing Resistance Training Programs. 2nd ed. Champaign, IL: Human Kinetics, 1997.

31. Borg GA. Physical performance and perceived exertion. Studia Psychologica Et Paedogica Investigations 1962;11:5–64.

32. Borg GA. Psychophysical bases of perceived exertion. Med Sci Sports Exerc 1982;14:377–381.

33. Holly RG, Shaffraath JD. Cardiorespiratory endurance. In Roitman JF, ed. ACSM's Resource Manual for Guidelines for Exercise Testing and Prescription. 4th ed. Philadelphia: Lippincott Williams & Wilkins, 2001;449–459.

34. Kraemer WJ, Bush JA. Factors affecting the acute neuromuscular responses to resistance exercise. In Roitman JF, ed. ACSM's Resource Manual for Guidelines for Exercise Testing and Prescription. 4th ed. Philadelphia: Lippincott Williams & Wilkins, 2001, 167–175.

35. Kraemer MJ, Ratamess NA. Physiology of resistance training. Orthop Physical Ther Clin North Am 2000;9:467–513.

CHAPTER 2

Historical Perspective: Origin to Recognition

CHARLES M. TIPTON

Introduction

In prehistoric times, exercise was a way of life and essential for existence. However, this role changed when humans became "civilized" and began to develop the various cultures within different geographical regions of the world. Regardless of the culture involved, two important reasons for a "role change" were the incidence of diseases and an evolving concept of health.

In 1542, the French physician and astronomer Jean Fernel (1497–1558) introduced the term *physiology* to explain bodily function (1), and more than 300 years later the words *physiology* and *exercise* were first included in a scientific publication by William H. Byford (2). While this information indicates that physiology is a sixteenth-century addition to our scientific vocabulary and that exercise physiology was identified in the middle of the nineteenth century as a potential scientific discipline, it ignores the perspective used by both Hippocrates and Galen in that the Greek word *Physis* means a natural state or the functioning of an organism as a whole (3). Inherent with the use of the term *Physis* by early Greek physicians was the concept that a living organism, under natural conditions, acted primarily as a whole, whereas the actions of its parts were subordinate to a supreme function. Hence, the more an organism functioned as a whole, the healthier it became. However, the more the parts of the organism began to function independently of a supreme function, the more unhealthy the organism became (3).

Thus an important linkage of exercise physiology with antiquity was an ancient belief that regular exercise would promote and improve one's health status while preventing or avoiding disease. This view has persisted throughout the ages regardless of how health or disease is perceived or defined. Readers are encouraged to examine position stands of various professional organizations pertaining to health, diseases, and disorders and notice the frequency with which exercise is advocated to promote and to enhance one's health status—and in several documents, to prevent certain diseases and disorders. On the matter of disease, Hippocrates states in IX in the *Nature of Man,* "Those due to exercise are caused by rest, and those due to idleness are cured by exercise" (4, p. 25).

The purposes of this chapter are to provide a historical background for the idea that exercise is important for one's health status and to identify the beliefs, observations, and findings of ancient and early investigators on the acute and chronic effects of exercise. These findings were related to the evolvement of functional concepts associated with the various physiological systems that were occurring with the emergence and recognition of exercise physiology as a scientific discipline during the early twentieth century. Keep in mind that for a discipline to be recognized, a critical body of knowledge and subject matter must be available and sufficiently well organized to be presented as a formal course of learning in an educational environment (5). In addition, an acknowledged reference text must be available (6).

Exercise and Its Relationship to Health

In ancient cultures, it was common to revere gods responsible for health (Ninurta in Babylonia and Assyria; Thorth in Egypt, and Hygeia in ancient Greece). Hence, the idea that regular exercise will promote and improve health is not new. Moreover, exercise has been advocated even when health was not effectively defined or left to the appeasement of the gods. Medical historians Lyons and Petrucelli (7) infer that as early as 2600 B.C., exercise was promoted for health purposes when the medical compendium *Nei Ching* was formulated (7). Since it is known that Buddhism, yoga, and aspects of Indian medicine came to China from India, these historians suggest that the well-characterized Chinese breathing exercises were prescribed for health purposes before the era of Hippocrates (460–370 B.C.) (Fig. 2.1).

Actually, it was before the time of the Greek physician Herodicus (480 B.C.–?) of Cnidus, who wrote on dietetics while functioning as a wrestling and boxing instructor in the gymnasiums of that era (8). He believed that exercise would be beneficial in protecting an individual against disease. According to Berryman, most historians are in agreement that Herodicus influenced Hippocrates to promote the healthful benefits of diet and exercise (8). However, Hippocrates' interest in exercise and his proclamations about its practices and effects were related to his concept of the human body

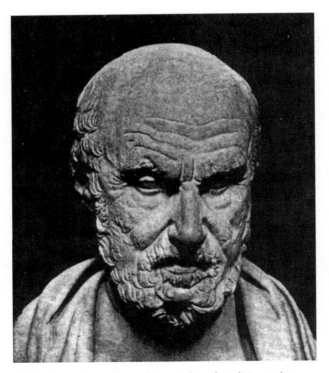

FIGURE 2.1   Hippocrates of Cos. Father of medicine and author of the humoral theory for which exercise was advocated to maintain its homeostatic balance. *(From Singer S. Greek Biology and Greek Medicine. Oxford, UK: Oxford University, 1922;91.)*

and to its four humors with their respective qualities and elements (4,9,10). Specifically, blood was hot and moist and representative of the element air; phlegm was cold and moist and representative of the element water; yellow bile was hot and representative of the element fire, while black bile was cold and dry and representative of the element earth. Thus, to develop and maintain health, these respective humors and their opposing qualities and elements had to be in equilibrium ("harmonious state or balance"). Moreover, any disruption of the equilibrium between these humors led to sickness and disease (4). Since select diseases were attributed to bodily changes in heat, cold, dryness, and moisture, moderate exercise was advocated to restore the equilibrium between the various humors and to improve the health status of the individual.

The essence of the humoral theory and its relationship to health appears to have been accepted and promoted by Plato (429–347 B.C.), Aristotle (384–322 B.C.), Diocles of Carystus (ca. 350 B.C.), Praxagoras of Cos (ca. 300 B.C.), and Herophilus of Chalcedon (335–280 B.C.) before it was included in the medical theory that was promoted by Claudius Galenus, or Galen (129–200 A.D.), of Roman Asia Minor (11–13). However Erasistratus of Ceos (310–250 B.C.), considered by some historians as the founder of physiology, discarded the humoral theory and championed the concept that diseases originated from the tissues and blood vessels of the body (an idea with similarities to one held by Egyptians between 2200 and 1550 B.C.) (14). However, these views had minimal impact on acceptance of the humoral doctrine by subsequent generations.

The significance of the Galenic medical theory as it pertains to the advocacy of exercise for health purposes was that it was accepted and practiced throughout the world for approximately 1500 years! The essence and relevance of the theory is best described by Berryman (8, pp. 2, 3):

> Galen, who borrowed much from Hippocrates, structured his "theory" around the naturals (of or with nature—physiology), the non-naturals (things not innate—hygiene), and the contra-naturals (against nature—pathology). Central to this theory were the six non-naturals:
>
> 1. Air
> 2. Food and drink
> 3. Motion and rest
> 4. Sleep and wake
> 5. Excretions and retentions
> 6. Passions of the mind
>
> The non-naturals needed to be utilized in moderation as to quantity, quality, time, and order; for if taken in excess or put into an imbalance, disease would result. Regulation of the six non-naturals could also influence the naturals, especially the qualities (hot, cold, moist, and dry) and the humors (blood—hot and moist; yellow bile—hot and dry; and black bile—cold

and dry. Therefore, along with drugs and surgery, the non-naturals were critical therapy for a variety of disease states. Exercise then, as part of motion and rest in the non-national traditional, was incorporated in much of the early regimen, hygiene, and preventive medicine literature, and to a lesser extent, the literature of therapeutic medicine.

—Claudius Galenus

While Galen regarded exercise as a component of hygiene and hygiene to be part of the science of medicine, his impact on the prescription of exercise for healthful reasons must be viewed within the context of the six non-naturals. Moreover, even without or after the Galenic influence, when health was considered solely to be the absence of disease or illness was a manifestation of the violation of God's laws, exercise continued to be advocated for health purposes.

Observations by Ancient and Early Investigators Concerning Physiology, the Acute and Chronic Effects of Exercise, and Exercise Prescriptions

Ancient Period: The Greek Influence

Few would dispute that through the ages, heart rate has been the single most recorded measure to characterize an exercise response. Yet there is no evidence in the Ebers Papyrus of 1550 B.C. or in the pulse chart of Pien Ch'iao of China (600 B.C.–500 B.C.) to indicate that exercise was considered or being described (7). Although Herophilus (335–280 B.C.) used a water clock (clepsydra) to assess pulse rate of aged individuals of various health states (believed arteries were connected to the heart and contained air or pneuma plus blood and had the properties of contraction and dilation), all pulse recordings were from resting individuals (13).

Since pneuma (air-inhaling spirit that is outside the body) was essential for life, there is reason to believe that Hippocrates recognized that respiration increased with exercise. In fact, he states (4, p. 355), "running in a circle dissolves flesh least, but reduces and contracts the belly most, because as it causes the most rapid respiration, it is the quickest to draw moisture to itself." Because rapid breathing was a means to cool the "innate heat" of life, which originated in the heart, increased respiration was not regarded as a health liability. As heat was one quality of the elements whose excess could alter humoral equilibrium, temperature regulation was an important consideration to Greek physicians. Hippocrates acknowledged that body temperature would increase with exercise. For example, he notes in "Regimen II" with LXII concerning walking (4, p. 351), "the properties of the several kinds of walking are as follows. . . . As the body moves and grows warm, the . . ."

Later with LXIII he adds (p. 353), "of running exercises, such as are not double and long, if increased gradually, have the power to heat, concoct and dissolve the flesh: they digest the power of the food that is in the flesh" (the Greek word for flesh can also mean muscle). Moreover, Hippocratic physicians knew that exercise would produce and increase sweating: "it makes the body more moist" (4, p. 353). This observation was related to the Greek dogma that the condensation of water vapors rising from within a heated body or from a warmed skin would form bile, urine, phlegm, or sweat (15). However, if "immoderate exercise" should cause a fever that could be associated with "hot sweat," blood-restorative procedures were to be implemented. These included bathing in warm water, drinking soft wine, eating a hearty meal, resting, walking, vomiting, and sleeping (4). Diocles (~350 B.C.; the "younger Hippocrates") disagreed with Hippocrates on the merits of sweating. He believed that "sweating is against nature" and that the perspiration associated with vigorous exercise should be avoided (12). Hippocratic physicians proclaimed that all living things were nourished by solids, liquids, and air. Moreover, diet alone did not produce health, and provisions must be made in the regimen for exercise, which would require food consumption.

Although it is unclear whether Hippocrates had an insight on "quantitative metabolism," as suggested by some scientists, it is evident he had definitive ideas on digestion (10). Moreover, food became the refined nutrient of blood by the process of concoction (digestive process from innate heat), which was absorbed into and distributed, along with pneuma, by the arteries. According to Asclepiades, digestion was aided by exercise, although this view was not shared by Diocles (12).

Hippocrates recognized that acute exercise would result in the "pain of fatigue," which was due in part to the untrained state, or in his words, "men out of training suffer these pains" (4, p. 359). In "Regimen II" (4) he recommended undertaking regular exercise, defined as accustomed, natural, or moderate, whereas violent exercise should be sparingly used, and only when necessary with the primary purposes to warm, thin, and purge the humors via sweat and breath (4). While discouraging the use of violent exercise to achieve a trained state, he acknowledged that individuals who trained would experience less muscle pain while increasing muscle mass, tone ("hardness"), strength, and endurance. However, Hippocrates had a low regard for athletes because physical perfection did not allow for improvement, which meant that any bodily change was for the worse. He states in the First Section of *Aphorisms* (4, pp. 99–101), "In athletics a perfect condition that is at its highest pitch is treacherous. Such conditions cannot remain the same or be at rest, and change for the better is impossible, the only possible change is for the worse." This belief, coupled with concern for the fever that occurred when intensity was increased and prolonged, may explain why Hippocrates was against encouraging strenuous exercise for his countrymen and why he criticized Herodikos of Selymbria for prescribing strenuous exercise to his subjects (16). Despite his disdain for the athletic state, Hippocrates advised athletes in training to wrestle and run in the winter and decondition in the summer by increased walking with reduced wrestling activities. To become refreshed (they would warm the body as well), fatigued wrestlers should practice running, while fatigued runners should wrestle.

Ancient Period: Galen and Roman Influences

As mentioned, Claudius Galenus, or Galen, was from Pergamon in Asia Minor. He studied medicine at Alexandria, settled in Rome in 162, and 7 years later became the personal physician to the emperor Marcus Aurelius. An admirer of Hippocrates, he incorporated many Hippocratic concepts within his own texts. Because his writings influenced physiological thinking and medical practices for numerous centuries, we should consider his definition of exercise, how it was classified, and his guidelines for prescribing exercise for others (Fig. 2.2).

According to Galen, movement had to be vigorous, with increased respiration, to be called exercise. Work and exercise appeared to be equivalent terms, but he was receptive to different organizational approaches if others wished to pursue the point. In fact, activities such as shadow boxing, leaping, discus throwing, small or large ball activities, and climbing ropes were regarded as exercise, whereas digging, rowing, plowing, reaping, riding, fighting, walking, hunting, etc., were considered to be work or exercise. Exercises were classified as either being swift or slow, vigorous or atony, violent or gentle. Running and ball exercises were examples of swift exercises; lifting a heavy weight, climbing a slope, and digging were cited for vigorous exercise, while discus throwing and continuous jumping were regarded as violent exercises (17). (After the various translations of the writings of Hippocrates and Galen, the terms violent and excessive exercise have been interpreted to be the equivalent of very heavy or maximal exercise.)

Galen believed blood was produced in the liver, carried by the vena cava into the right heart, and distributed through the lungs and interventricular septum into the left ventricle,

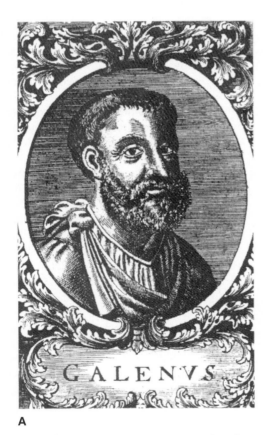

A

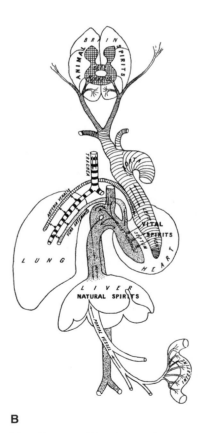

B

FIGURE 2.2   A. Claudius Galenus, or Galen of Pergamon. Considered by many historians as the most important figure in medicine and physiology since Hippocrates. The only individual known to directly influence physiological thinking and practices for 1200 years. **B.** Galen's view of physiology.
(Reprinted with permission from West JB. Respiratory Physiology: People and Ideas. New York: Oxford University, 2003;76, 141.)

where it was ejected (pulsations), containing air and heat, into the periphery. However, the blood was propelled not only by the contraction of the ventricle but by the contraction of the arteries as well. Thus the pulse rate changes recorded by previous cultures was a result of an active dilation of the arteries that was initiated by cardiac contraction. Moreover, Galen appears to be the first to record that pulse rate is increased with exercise (but without providing data). In *The Pulse for Beginners* (18) he notes that moderate exercise "renders the pulse vigorous, large, quick and frequent." Also mentioned was that if vigorous movement did not cause an increase in respiration, it should not be labeled as exercise.

Other statements associate exercise with "accelerated movements of respiration" (17). These statements must be placed in this physiological context: Galen considered air or pneuma to be essential for life, absorbed by the lungs, carried by the left heart to all organs, and the object of respiration; but not the principle responsible for specific respiratory movements (19). He commented that an increase in inspiration would nourish the "vital spirit" and the "vaporization of the humors" that originated in the heart and arteries (20). His views were similar but not identical to those of Aristotle, Galen thought the increased respiration would cool the heart and elevate body temperature. Unlike Aristotle, he believed the increased respiration would increase combustion within the left ventricle (19).

Galen and Acute Exercise, Training, and Athletes

In his description of the uses and values of exercise, Galen (17) referred to a "readier metabolism." One physiological interpretation of this observation is that he was referring to the combustion of substrates that occurred essentially in the left ventricle and led to the liberation of heat (19). As noted earlier, this process would also elevate body temperature. Acute exercise also increased the digestive process, which involved the heat of digestion transforming the substrate (food) into lymph and then into humors. Subsequently, the humors would provide the materials for the tissues of the body. In Book 1 of Galen's *Hygiene* (*De Sanitate Tuenda*) it is evident that the increased evacuation of excrement was considered to be an acute effect of exercise. Moreover, if the excrement was retarded with problems of constituency, one possible cause was the "insufficiency of warmth" (heat for dissolving purposes) which occurred because of the lack of exercise (17). He also proclaimed that some of the fluid consumed would become urine, with components being passed "off as sweat or insensible perspiration" with sweating occurring with the "violence of exercise." However, when exercise was excessive and an overproduction of heat had occurred (immoderation of the heat), fever would result (17). In most circumstances, Galen regarded fever as a disease and usually treated it with an application of cold to the body. Acute exercise was also associated with fatigue. He states (17, p. 143) in Book II, "the art of exercise is no small part of hygienic sci-

ence, and avoiding fatigue is no small part of the art of exercise," while noting that fatigue without exercise is a symptom of disease (he identified several types of fatigue). Exercise physiologists who relate the fatigue of muscular exercise to the presence of lactic acid should realize that Galen wrote in Book II that excessive exercise with faulty secretions would result in "an acidity of the thin and warm fluids, which erode and prick and sting the body" (17, pp. 145–146). Besides the sensations of pain, fatigue was associated with reduced strength, a disinclination to movement, arrhythmias of the pulse, and an impaired power of the mind.

Galen considered trained individuals to possess the "peak" condition of health while exhibiting elevated muscle tone (hardness of the organ), accelerated respiration, increased muscle strength, "readier metabolism," an elevated "intrinsic warmth," better nutrition and diffusion of all substances, with enhanced elimination of excrements (17). Despite his responsibilities with gladiators, he had a low regard for athletes, especially wrestlers, and the individuals who trained them. As did Hippocrates, Galen viewed athletes as "the extremes of good conditions" and as such, in a "dangerous state." On the other hand, if they were in good condition, the humors were in equilibrium and the blood would be well-distributed throughout the body. As for wrestlers, he felt they were overfed and overtrained, which produced an unhealthy body type (unequal distribution of fat and muscle) and humoral imbalance. However, Galen recognized that the energy demands of boxers and wrestlers in training required a diet of pork and "special" breads because the traditional diet of vegetables and "ordinary" bread would be disastrous for the athlete (17).

Despite Hippocrates' and Galen's negative opinions of athletes, athletes and their training were an integral component of the Greek and Roman cultures. Insights on their practices were provided by Flavios Philostratos (170–244), a teacher of rhetoric, philosophy, and fine living, who traveled between Athens and Rome and wrote *Concerning Gymnastics* (20). He extensively commented on Galen's view that trainers were inadequately prepared for their responsibilities or were unable to provide meaningful advice on how to train. He also argued against the rigid tetrad system of training that was being implemented in select gymnasiums because the "whole of gymnastics has been ruined" (20). With this 4-day training schedule, the first day was devoted to preparing the athlete; the second was scheduled so the athlete was "intensively engaged"; the third was allocated for recreation; and on the fourth day the athlete was "moderately exerted." Philostratos felt the system made no allowances for individualized training programs ("they deprive their science of intelligent understanding in respect to the condition of the athlete to be trained"). In addition, athletes must better integrate exercise and diet in their training programs. However, he did note that distance runners (light exercise) were running 8 to 10 laps in their training programs; sprint runners (stade-race = furlong) had trained by running against hares and horses, and the athletes in the heavy exercise category (wrestlers and boxers) were lifting and carrying heavy burdens, bending or straightening out thick iron plates, pulling yokes with oxen, or even wrestling (actually fighting) with bulls and lions! While his observations contained limited physiological insights or explanations, he reported that moderately hard exercise by individuals who consumed too much wine would produce secretions of sweat that could be harmful to the blood. Consequently, he recommended milder exercise and massages, which would keep the pores open and drain off the stale liquid (20).

Training and the Roman Legions

During this era, the Roman legions acquired much fame and recognition for their physical performance associated with the conquest of other lands. However, there are few documents pertaining to the physiology of exercise, and it is assumed that the beliefs of Galen were followed. While the opinion in military circles was that daily exercise by the legions contributed more to the health of the soldiers than the advice provided by their physicians, it does appear that the leaders of Caesar's legions were following various training principles in the conditioning of their troops.

For example, in the general rules of war (21, p. 109), Vegetius states, "An army is improved by work, enfeebled by inactivity." Additionally (22), marches were increased in duration to promote fatigue ("the march was made longer than usual to wear out those who straggled"). Exercise was performed at the same intensity as one was expected to perform ("but every day each soldier exercises with as much intensity as he would in war"). The army used a tetrad system that provided for a rest or recovery period in the training of the infantry which included marching on the first day. ("He bade them on the first day do a run of nearly 4 miles in full kit, on the second to rub down . . . on the next day to rest and do nothing: and on the following, some men to fight with wooden swords . . . others to throw javelin . . . on the fifth day to revert to the marching they had done on the first"). It also (21) promoted an increase in strength by using overload conditions ("to launch spear-shafts of heavier weights than the real javelins. . . . For by this exercise the arms gain in strength").

The Medieval Period to the Renaissance

The medieval period encompassed the Eastern barbarian invasion of the West that started with the Christian era, the anti-Hellenist practices of the Christian church toward Greek and Roman writings, and the establishment of Islam in the seventh century in Arabia and its spread to Greece, Africa, Spain, and some regions of France. It was an era when new medical schools in Italy, France, England, and the Netherlands were formed; Vesalius (1514–1564) dismissed Galen's views on anatomy and physiology; and the Swiss chemist Theophrastus

Bombastus von Hohenheim, or Paracelsus (1493–1541), "revolted" against Galen and his concepts (7,23).

As emphasized by Berryman (11), the Hippocratic and Galenic concepts pertaining to medical practice were dominating influences during most of this period. Their influence was first demonstrated in the Islamic world and later in the Christian sphere because of the Arabic and Latin translations of their texts. When exercise was discussed, it was generally within the context of the non-naturals advocated by Galen and explained by his complex system of physiology, which included the humors, elements, qualities, members, facilities, operations, and spirits. However, within the Arabic world and much of Europe, the prevailing influence was the writings of abu-Alial al-Husayn ibn-Sina, or Avicenna (980–1037), a Persian physician and author of more than 100 books, of which his most renowned was the *Canon of Medicine* (24,25). Osler considered this book to be the most famous medical textbook ever written, and the text was described by Rothschuh (19) as a "thorough systemization of all the medical knowledge available since antiquity." To the physiologist, Avicenna incorporated the galenic concepts of humors, elements, qualities, members, facilities, operations, and spirits into a complex system of principal members (heart, brain, liver), with each member having a controlling influence on the functions of other organs. Inherent in each separate system were virtues (actions), operations (functions), and faculties (selected characteristics of organs). There were three virtues (vital, animal, natural) associated with "spiritus" for distribution throughout the body. The most relevant was the vital virtue, the source of innate heat. It was found in the heart and blood, was responsible for heart rate and respiration, contained the "spiritus" (vital spirit) that Hippocrates labeled as pneuma, and was distributed by the arteries (24).

With regard to Avicenna's writings and the exercise concepts of Galen, Avicenna promoted and reinforced the idea that moderate exercise was beneficial (a necessary factor with rest) for living because it (25, p. 24) "balances the body by expelling residues and impurities and are factors of good nutrition for adults and of happy growth for the young." He also noted that moderate exercise (walking) "would repel the bad humors." He indicated that exercise effects were dependent upon the degree (intensity), amount (frequency and duration), and rest taken, cautioning his readers that excessive exercise could adversely affect the innate heat and lead to a state "akin to death" (25). Avicenna's focal point was the production and consequences of innate heat, which he considered responsible for the large and strong pulse with exercise. In addition, he emphasized that exercise was associated with elevated body temperatures (would make the body "very hot"), that perspiration occurred with physical exhaustion, and that exercise should cease when sweating stops because an abundant sweat was "a symptom of moist illnesses." Chronic exercise was recommended for weak and undeveloped limbs, and he appears among the first to acquaint Western culture with the ancient Hindu practice of breathing exercises for individuals with respiratory weakness (25). For individuals in geographical areas that were not receptive to or influenced by the writings of Avicenna, the non-natural concepts of Galen were followed on matters that pertained to exercise and its effects.

In 1553, a Spanish physician, Cristobal Mendez (1500–1561), published in Latin the *Book of Bodily Exercise* (26). In translation the text consisted of 82 pages containing 40 distinctive chapters that were organized in accordance with four treatises:

1. Exercise and its benefits
2. The division of exercise
3. Common exercises and which ones are the best
4. The time convenient for exercise and its value

The contents were essentially Greek and Roman concepts concerning exercise with an emphasis on its importance to health. To be beneficial, moderate exercise must be frequent, enjoyable, and continuous (intermittent exercise will fail to consume and dissipate the humor, causing it to leave by the pores opened by the heat of movement), and associated with shortness of breath (caused by the increased heat within the heart and the need for more air via elevated ventilation). Besides extolling the health virtues of exercise and the need to avoid overexercising, he devoted several chapters to the heat produced by exercise and its consequences. While noting that movement per se will increase body heat, he mentions that with movement caused by exercise, the "blood rubs very much with the parts as do the spirits and bile, causing subtlety and lightness, and showing heat in them" (p. 19). Although the text has historical significance, it had a limited circulation and a minimal impact on the medical profession.

The Seventeenth Century

The seventeenth century has been characterized in the history of science as the Age of the Scientific Revolution because it was a time when the emphasis was on how (not why) things happen, speculation changed to experimentation, interpretation became mechanistic, mathematics entered into the language of science, and measurements began in medicine. Moreover, it was when the philosophies of René Descartes (1596–1650) and Sir Francis Bacon significantly contributed to these transitions and when Jon Baptista van Helmont of Belgium (1577–1644) reported that disease did not have to originate within the body, that the body contained "ferments" (enzymes) which aided digestion, and that fever had no relationship to the putrefaction of the humors (7). The German Franz de le Boe (1614–1672), or Franciscus Sylvius, ignored the humoral theory and related health to the interactions between bodily acids, bases, and their neutralization. However for exercise physiology, it was a time of reformulation of ideas and association, because the prevailing concepts of Galen had been rejected and the ones based upon physiological investigations were evolving as they were discovered. Of the individuals who

did promote exercise for health purposes during this time, they followed the non-naturals approach of Galen (8).

Early Investigations Pertaining to the Cardiovascular, Respiratory, and Neuromuscular Systems

The single most important scientific event during this time (7) was the discovery in 1628 of the continuous circulation of the blood by William Harvey (1578–1657) in England (27). His discovery was "completed" in 1661 by Marcello Malpighi (1628–1649), who identified in the lung the existence of capillaries (19). Harvey's epic investigation established that cardiac output and its distribution to the periphery had the capacity to increase, was dependent upon the "strength of the pulse," and indicated that "the heart makes more than a thousand beats in a half hour, in some two, three, or even four thousand" (27). While at Oxford University, Richard Lower (1631–1693) championed the findings of Harvey and declared in his 1669 publication (28) the heart to be a muscle (as had Harvey, Stensen, and Leonardo da Vinci). He notes in Chapter 1 of his publication that the heart is "more carefully fashioned than all other Muscles of the Body. For its work is more necessary and continuous than that of all other muscles, and hence it was particularly appropriate that it should also far surpass them in the elegance of its structure."

According to Lower, the heart was not the source of heat production by the body; the movement of the heart was dependent upon the inflow of spirits through the nerves. Moreover, with violent exercise (likely maximal in intensity), the movement of the heart was accelerated in proportion to the blood that was "driven and poured into its ventricles in great abundance as a result of the movement of muscles" (p. 122). He also has been reported as indicating that exercise would enhance blood flow to the brain and that exercise and movements of the body were an aid to health (29). As for the effects of training, Harvey appears to be the first to indicate that a history of physical activity by animals, and likely humans, would be associated with cardiac enlargement ("have a more thick, powerful, and muscular heart" (27).

During the time of Harvey, van Helmont reported that air was composed of different gases, and Robert Boyle (1627–1691) in Oxford proved air was necessary for life and formulated the gas laws which bear his name (30). Sir Michael Foster, a famous English physiologist, described these experiments of Boyle as being the most fundamental in the physiology of respiration (31). Later, Giovanni Borelli (1608–1679), an ardent Italian physicist and iatrophysicist, began and reported on his studies on the mechanics of respiration (31). Robert Hooke, who was associated with the Oxford physiologists, knew that air and breathing were essential for life but felt that neither lung movements or blood flow were the most important aspect of breathing; rather, it was the air in the lungs that caused the color change within the venous blood (29). John Mayow (1643–1679), an Oxford contemporary of both Boyle and Hooke, published in 1674 a text entitled *Medico-Physical Works* (32) in which he clarified the findings of Borelli on the mechanics of breathing and emphasized that the lungs passively followed the movements of the thorax. Furthermore, respiration had no relationship to the cooling of the blood or to the promotion of blood flow. But the inspiration of air was essential for the transfer of some elastic nitrous particles, the *spiritus nitroaereus,* from the air into the blood. To Mayow, breathing facilitated the contact between air and blood, enabling the transfer of the niter particles to the blood, which subsequently reacted with sulfurous and combustible particles, resulting in elevated body and blood temperatures and a change in the color of the blood. He was also of the opinion that violent exercise would increase the frequency of breathing and create an intense heat within the body because of the greater effervescence caused by the increased number and presence of nitro-aerial particles (19,29,32).

Early Neuromuscular Investigations

As noted earlier, during the early decades of the seventeenth century, a prevailing concept was that nerves conveyed "spirits" to muscles, which initiated contraction. Thomas Willis (1621–1675) of Oxford, teacher of Robert Hooke, John Locke, and Richard Lower (33), was a major proponent of the idea that animal spirits from the brain traveled down nerve fibers to muscles, where they met nitrous and sulfurous particles which caused an "explosion" resulting in inflated muscles when they contracted (33). Giovanni Borelli (1608–1679) of Pisa, Italy, stated that a spirituous juice (*succus nerveus*) was carried by nerves to the brain to cause sensations or to the muscles which interacted with the blood to produce an effervescence (reaction between fermentation and ebullition) causing inflation and contraction of muscles, which resulted in limb movements (19,31). Later, a Cambridge physician, Francis Glisson (1597–1677), challenged the concept that nerves conveyed a "spirit" to muscles which inflated them during contraction. He proved his point by demonstrating that no water displacement took place when a forceful underwater contractile effort was made. In addition, he reported that muscle fibers had the property of irritability, which was later "rediscovered" and made famous by Albrecht Haller (19). A Danish physician, Niels Stensen (1638–1686), noted that skeletal muscle fibers contract in a geometric manner, which decreased their length while increasing their width (19). In 1694, the Swiss mathematician Johann Bernoulli (1667–1748) published a dissertation entitled *On the Mechanics and Movement of the Muscles* (34) in which he described muscles as small machines, used differential calculus to explain their functions, and described (p. 139) the contraction process as follows: "When the mind wishes that a limb of the body moves, some agitation of animal spirits occurs in the brain so that, by twitching the origin of some nerve, they shake the spirituous juice contained inside over its whole length and, because of the irritation of the origin of the nerve, the last droplet of nervous

juice is driven out by the slight vibration at the other orifice." According to Bernoulli, muscular strength was related to the availability of the spirituous juice being released, while muscular fatigue (tiredness) was dependent upon the quantity of consumed spirits. In fact, he states (p. 135), "I also assume that carrying same weight at the same height during the same time consumes the same quantity of spirits."

According to William Croone, an English physician (1633–1684), violent exercise was associated with painful and stiff muscles caused by a combination of an inadequate blood flow, sweating, and the removal of "spirits." In addition, he was of the opinion that the presence of sweat on muscles was associated with the swelling and contraction of skeletal muscles (35).

Early Metabolic and Thermal Investigations

Beginning in the sixteenth century and continuing through the early eighteenth century, contemporary scholars made a concerted effort to use mathematical and physical principles to address medical and biological questions. One prominent individual in this movement was an Italian physician and professor at Venice and later Padua, Santorio Santorio (1561–1636), who developed accurate instruments to measure changes in heart rate, body temperature, and body weight (balance chair). These instruments were used to measure changes with sitting, sleeping, after exercise, meal consumption, excretion, etc., which became the forerunner of metabolic balance studies (19,36). Santorio also conducted studies pertaining to changes in sensible and insensible perspiration. His aphorisms indicated (#19) that violent exercise of both mind and body would result in a lighter body weight, while hastening old age and the threat of untimely and early death. To maintain a youthful face, individuals should avoid sweating or perspiring too much in the heat (#36). Another aphorism pertaining to temperature regulation stated that the fluid evacuated by violent exercise was sweat that originated from unconcocted (unheated) juices (#1) and that if sound bodies did not perspire, this condition could be corrected by exercise (#34).

It is apparent that few seventeenth century scientists advocated strenuous or violent exercise because they, like Hippocrates and Galen, continued to believe it was unhealthy. This belief was prevalent with iatrophysicists and iatromechanicists. The extreme was to relate a specific organ to a machine (7). These individuals felt that heavy or maximal activity (e.g., running, dancing) and especially singing, which markedly increased lung movements, could lead to disorders including asthma, hemoptysis (blood-stained sputum), and phthisis (tuberculosis of the lung) (37).

The Eighteenth Century: The Era of Enlightenment

The eighteenth century has been labeled by both Berryman and Rothschuh as the Enlightenment because it was a time of emergence and implementation of several new and important philosophies: John Locke (1632–1704) of England argued that all knowledge had to be based on experience. Jean le Rond d'Alembert (1717–1783) and Denis Diderot (1713–1784) of France advocated replacing the era of theology and faith with science. Gottfried W. Leibniz (1646–1716) of Germany strove to reconcile existing and opposing views on matter and spirit, mechanism and teleology, experience and knowledge, freedom and necessity, religion and philosophy. Finally, the German Immanuel Kant (1724–1804) advocated that individuals use their intelligence without being guided by another person (7,11,19). Interestingly, there were few physiological investigations or discoveries during the first half of the eighteenth century. The individuals of note were physicians or "systematists" who devoted their efforts in arranging and organizing the existing body of physiological knowledge that had relevance to medicine.

The Influences of Hoffman and Stahl

One systematist of note was Friedrich Hoffmann (1660–1742) of Germany, an inspiring teacher and a productive author whose lectures and writings had a profound effect on students and practitioners at home and in France and England. To Hoffmann, motion was essential for life, and all vital actions had to be explained on a mechanical basis. For this to occur, particles were required. Muscle contraction occurred because of a nervous fluid ("nervous ether") that originated from the blood to the nerves, where it circulated before causing muscles to dilate and shorten in the process. Cardiac contraction resulted when particles in the blood at the level of the lungs entered cardiac nerves and vessels while diastole occurred when the intrinsic elasticity of cardiac tissue returned to its resting level. The blood particles that were constantly in motion were responsible for the heat (animal heat) that ensued. His view was that vesicular and elastic particles in the air entered the body, not by the lungs, but by food and through pores. However, once within the blood and at the level of the lungs, the events of respiration occurred (7,19,38).

Another systematist was Georg Ernst Stahl (1660–1734) of Germany, who rejected the concept of Descartes that man was a machine and postulated the existence of "anima sensitiva," a vital force in controlling man's activities, motion, and health. Stahl, as described by Foster (31, p. 167), "maintained the view that all the chemical events of the living body, even though they might superficially resemble, were at the bottom wholly different from the chemical changes taking place in the laboratory, since in the living body all chemical changes were directly governed by the sensitive soul, anima sensitiva, which pervaded all parts and presided over all events." A competent chemist, Stahl proposed that during the combustion or calcination of metals and in the process of respiration and fermentation, a combustible element named *phlogiston* escaped. Although the theory was

wrong, his prominence delayed the discovery and role of oxygen for decades (7).

The Influences of Boerhaave and Haller

Hermann Boerhaave (1668–1738) was a Dutch professor from Leyden who is recognized because of his scholarship and the mentoring of Albrecht von Haller (1708–1777), who rediscovered the irritability of muscle. During the first half of the century Boerhaave's influence prevailed because of his publications, a reputation in Europe as a "master teacher," and for having "institutes of medicine" become the means by which physiology was taught in medical schools. Boerhaave was a scholar with competence in botany, mathematics, physics, and philosophy and was knowledgeable about the views of Stahl, Boyle, Hooke, Borelli, Stensen, and others of his era. His perspective of containing human body (19, p. 117), was that "the human body was truly a machine whose solid parts were primarily composed of vessels. These vascular structures contained, directed, modified, divided and secreted the body's fluids, while the other structures acted like a mechanical instrument which could support or determine certain motions according to their own form and composition." Intrinsic to this perspective was that fluids had the mechanical property of coherence and elasticity, while the blood contained various particles. To Boerhaave, the motion, obstruction, and stagnation of these fluids was a "matter of life or death, health or disease." He rejected Stahl's concept of "anima spiritus" and perpetrated the idea that nerve fibers were hollow to transmit the fluid or spirit from the brain into skeletal muscles so that contraction could occur (19).

During the latter half of the century, Haller's writings and lectures made him famous in Europe. This image was enhanced by the 1786 publication of his text *First Lines of Physiology* (39). Haller extended the views of his former teacher and introduced the concepts of sensibility and irritability after stimulus-response experiments in which he found that only certain tissues (nerves) were associated with pain or had sensibility, whereas other tissues without this characteristic (skeletal muscle, cardiac tissue) exhibited contraction (irritability) when stimulated via mechanical, chemical, or electrical means. Thus, when stimulated (irritated), skeletal muscles would shorten, exhibit great feats of strength ("they will raife a weight equal to, or much greater than, that of the whole human body itself," p. 238) and "grow ftrong with exercife" (f is the long s [ʃ] that survives in mathematics) while their "brawny" parts become thicker (p. 243).

Haller felt that the heart was the most irritable organ of the body and that cardiac nerves had no role in heart rate, as the pulse originated when blood was ejected from the heart and distended the arterial walls. Subsequent arterial filling initiated vessel contraction, which sent the blood to the periphery. Although Stephen Hales of England had by 1733 published *Statical Essays: Containing Haemastaticks*, in which he recorded the direct blood pressure of a resting mare (40),

Haller failed to grasp the significance of this finding. However, he taught Harvey's views on the circulation of the blood and considered respiration to be essentially a mechanical process caused by "dilation" (widening) of the thorax, with the lungs assuming a passive role in the process (39). The idea that blood would absorb air at the level of the lung was ignored, and he considered Mayow's hypothesis on the absorption of niter particles to be incorrect. He stated that the blood was cooled in the lungs and proclaimed the beliefs of the iatromechanicists (as did Boerhaave) that blood temperature and its increases were the result of friction between blood and vessel walls. However, he did not address the issue of body temperature or aspects relevant to metabolism. Digestion was regarded as requiring the presence of saliva, gastric, pancreatic, and intestinal juices, the involvement of bile, the breakdown of food, and an absorption process that included mesenteric vessels and lymphatic channels (19,39).

Finally, Haller taught his students that the kidney separated water and salts from the blood by forcing these components out during flow through the smaller renal vessels while the larger components, cells and fibrin, remained with the blood (19,39).

Respiratory, Metabolic, and Circulatory Observations During This Era

Near the end of the eighteenth century, Karl W. Scheele (1742–1786) of Sweden discovered oxygen ("fiery air") and Joseph Priestly of England (1733–1804) proclaimed the existence of "dephlogisticated air." About the same time, the brilliant French chemist Antoine L. Lavoisier (1743–1794) conducted experiments that destroyed the phlogiston theory of Stahl and established the chemical foundations for respiration, metabolism, and animal heat (19). Of the systematists mentioned during this time, all promoted exercise for health reasons, as did other physicians whose texts were not concerned with physiological thinking or advancement. In such instances, exercise was usually discussed in the Galenic context of the non-naturals (8). However, the most significant respiratory and metabolic studies of the century were conducted by Lavoisier and the French chemist Armand Seguin (1776–1835). They measured the oxygen consumption (of Seguin) that occurred with resting, fasting, digestion, and when performing work (foot moving a treadle); the work is detailed later, in the Milestone of Discovery section (41). From prior studies that included animals, they knew the carbon within the body underwent "combustion" to produce heat, water, and carbonic acid (carbon dioxide reacting with water). However, he thought the heat was generated by combustion in the lungs of a substance found in blood.

During this century insights into the circulation came early, from the extensive studies of the English physician John Floyer (1649–1734). Floyer developed an accurate pulse watch in 1707 and used its readings to classify people into different humoral states and identify certain disorders

and diseases (42). For example, a pulse of 75 to 80 was listed as being Hot in the first degree, associated with a choleric disposition and caused by hot seasons, hot air, exercise, passions, cards, study, hot medicines, hot baths, hot diet, and retained excrements. A rate between 65 and 60 was Cold in the second degree and identified with melancholic individuals, occurring in the spleen, and caused by hydropic tumors and cachexias. The normal value was 70 to 75 beats per minute, and a value of 140 beats per minute could be associated with death! It was Floyer's belief that changes in blood temperature, spirits, and humoral rarefaction caused by exercise were responsible for the changes in pulse rate. Moreover, if the rate was higher than 140 beats per minute and if death did not occur, it was difficult to count. When serving as the subject, he reported that a half-hour of moderate walking caused his pulse to increase to 112 beats per minute; also, his pulse was 76 before he rode on a horse and 90 beats per minute after an hour's ride. He also measured respiratory frequency and related it to the pulse rate, but there was no evidence that he measured both during exercise. He did regard respiration as an aid to circulation in the movement of blood (29).

Several decades later, an Irish physician and researcher named Byran Robinson (1680–1746) published an important but frequently overlooked text, *A Treatise of the Animal Oeconomy* (43). He wrote that an individual in the recumbent position had a pulse rate of 64 beats per minute, which would change to 68 beats per minute when sitting, to 78 beats per minute with standing, to 100 beats per minute after walking 4 miles in 1 hour, and to 140 to 150 beats per minute after running as hard as possible (43). At this time Seguin and Lavoisier had recognized that the amount of oxygen consumed was related to the frequency of heart rate multiplied by the number of inspirations, and Stephen Hales had noted that exercise was associated with a brisk circulation, an increased number of systoles, an improved blood flow to dilated and agitated lungs, the stomach, and the gut (intestines). Lastly, Robinson observed that muscle blood flow was related to the force created by the contracting muscles.

Neuromuscular, Digestion, Temperature, and General Observations During This Era

Robinson also felt the forces that caused limb movements were controlled by the will, which acted on nerves. To him, nerves were "the principal instruments of sensation and motion" (43, p. 91). He advocated moderate exercise to increase muscle strength and size and acknowledged that laboring (trained) individuals had larger and stronger muscles than inactive sedentary individuals. During this time, James Keill (1673–1719), an English physician, made the observation that muscle strength was related to the number of fibers present (44). Around 1760, John Theophilus Desaguliers (1683–1744), an English priest, curator, and admirer of strongmen, helped to develop a dynamometer that could accurately measure muscular strength (45,46). In a text pertaining to the benefits of therapeutic exercise, the Paris physician Joseph-Clement Tissot (1747–1826) indicated that motion (exercise) would increase muscle size and strength (47).

The idea that exercise would enhance digestion was repeated by both Hales and Tissot, as was the concept that it would aid the descent and evacuation of bowel contents. Tissot stated that exercise would increase sweating while removing the "sour salts" and "heterogenous parts" from the blood, which would avoid the possibility of "spoiling" the blood (47). Robinson indicated that exercise should give a "glowing warmth" to the skin as long as it caused a "fever." He also described experiments in which individuals traveled 2 miles in 30 minutes, producing 8 and 9 ounces of sweat, or eight times the amount they produced when not exercising in the summer heat (43). Robinson examined the relationship between sweating and urine production during exercise and observed that both processes were about equal at the beginning of exercise, but as the exercise continued, urine production decreased until it became less than recorded at the start. When expressed on a ratio basis, it changed from 6:1 to 16:1 when the skin exhibited a "glowing warmth" (43). Before Lavoisier reported that an essential function of insensible perspiration was to control the magnitude of the body heat (e.g., temperature regulation), Black determined the latent heat of the evaporation of water and Blagden reported a cooling effect from the evaporation of sweat (15). However, there are no reports that Lavoisier conducted exercise experiments with Seguin on this subject.

Tissot's text was published in French in 1780 but was not translated into English until 1964 (47). Since it was associated with therapeutic exercise, these two aspects discouraged citation of it in many of the early publications. This was unfortunate, because numerous pages were devoted to the effects of motion on nondiseased individuals and to the principles of the exercise prescription. The most notable was his third rule of gymnastics, which pertained to the intensity and duration of exercise according to the season and the age, sex, and temperament of the patient. He described moderate exercise as the condition which "just leads to perspiration, or lassitude or fatigue." His position on strenuous or violent exercise is unclear, but he does state (47, p. 20) that "whether the motion is moderate or violent, as long as its duration is in the proper ratio to the strength of person exercising and conforms to the therapeutic indication for which it was proposed"; namely, "it always produces most of the good effects of which we have spoken."

The Nineteenth Century to the Time of Byford (1855)

The medical historians Lyons and Pertrucelli (7) described the nineteenth century as "the beginnings of modern medicine," while Rothschuh, the physiology historian (19), labeled this era as "the beginnings." To Berryman, the exercise historian (11), it was a time when "exercise was receiving more attention from physicians because of its traditionally important role in the maintenance of health." It is my viewpoint that the beginning of exercise physiology started after Byford, when formal instruction in exercise physiology occurred in established educational institutions by qualified individuals, during the latter quarter of the nineteenth century. The first decades of the nineteenth century were a continuation of the era of Enlightenment, or an "analysis of the laws of nature, history and religion with the help of reason . . . leading to the development of liberalism, individualism and democracy at the social level." The natural sciences, notably physiology and chemistry, "marched from discovery to discovery . . . and established a series of general laws" while providing the foundations of knowledge on which most twentieth-century technological achievements were based (7).

Early Nineteenth Century Physiological Observations From France, Germany, England, and Canada

At this time, France was the leader of the scientific world and the champion of vitalism (the idea that all essential biological actions in tissues were the effects of vital forces) (19). Sensibility and contractile effects were responsible for circulation, absorption, nutrition, digestion, secretion, and excretion. Empirical physiology was the practice of the times (empirical rationales, unbiased observations, practical experimentation) with a fascination for the function of the nervous system that equaled the seventeenth-century interest in the circulatory system (7,19). Two French physiologists deserving of mention were Claude Bernard (1813–1878) and Charles Edouard Brown-Seguard (1817–1894). Bernard is regarded as the founder of experimental physiology and the single most important individual in changing empirical physiology to experimental physiology. He is considered the father of homeostasis and was highly regarded as a teacher and as a mentor; American physiologists such as Silas Mitchell, John Dalton, and Austin Flint came to study in his laboratory (19). Because of his investigations of the liver and pancreas, he and Brown-Seguard—who reported that the adrenals, thyroid, pancreas, liver, spleen, and kidneys had secretions (later called hormones) which entered the bloodstream and were carried to other parts of the body—have been associated with the establishment of the field of endocrinology (7).

Germany soon emerged as a scientific center, and the brilliant chemist Justus Liebig (1803–1873) of Munich published *Animal Chemistry* in 1842. This book had a profound influence on establishing metabolic dogma and promoting metabolic investigations. Without experimental evidence, he indicated that proteins were the substrates for muscular activity. Several years later, Emil H. du Bois-Reymond (1818–1896) of Bonn confirmed Galen's observation that muscles became acidic with exercise and related the finding to the 1807 report of his fellow countryman, Jons Jacob Berzelius (1779–1848), who found elevated lactic acid concentrations in muscle from stags (48).

In England, few physiologists had an interest in exercise. However, there was a heightened interest in sports, and before 1810 the Earl of Caithness, John Sinclair, published texts that addressed aspects of training for humans and animals (49). An interesting aspect of his views was that they were formulated from observations reported by Herodicus, Asclepiades, Celsus, Galen, Sir Francis Bacon, and Byran Robinson plus opinions of renowned trainers from that era. The composite conclusion was that training would reduce extraneous fat, increase muscle mass, make bones harder and less likely to be injured, increase perspiration, improve the wind (lungs), prolong breath-holding time, and reduce recovery time. With animals, trained horses exhibited less fatigue and would not wear out sooner than their untrained counterparts. Considering the times and the educational background of the trainers, it is no surprise that Sinclair did not propose to change the "core of all training regimens," namely, purging, puking, sweating, diet, and exercise (50).

In 1833, William Beaumont (1785–1853) attracted the attention of physiologists outside of the United States with his observations of Alexis St. Martin of Canada, who survived a gunshot wound resulting in a gastric fistula. Beaumont conducted more than 70 experiments, including exercise, with the interior of St. Martin's stomach (51). He concluded that moderate exercise was conducive to rapid and healthy digestion, whereas severe and fatiguing exercise would retard the process. In addition, he stated (p. 94) that "Exercise, sufficient to produce moderate perspiration, increases the secretions from the gastric cavity and produces an accumulation of a limpid fluid, within the stomach, slightly acid, and possessing the solvent properties of the gastric juice in an inferior degree. This is probably a mixed fluid, a small proportion of which is gastric juice."

Exercise Physiology According to Combe, Dunglison, and Byford

Beginning in 1834, an Edinburgh physician named Andrew Combe (1787–1847) wrote a textbook on physiology applied to health and physical and mental education that contained 9 chapters and had 16 printings in the United States by 1854 (52). In his text, exercise was advocated for its health benefits because of the effects of movement on bones, muscles, heart, lungs, the digestive system, and the central nervous system. While moderate and progressive exercise was prescribed, the need for rest intervals was noted. Moreover, lack of exercise was associated with muscle weakness, and in the case of the lungs, the potential for diseases. Concerning muscles, he indicated that exercise increased their blood flow; that they were proportional in size and structure to the effort required of them; that when used frequently, muscles would increase in thickness and possibly with greater

force; and that increased power was associated with increased activity of the nervous system (52).

Although Beaumont ignored his advice concerning functioning of the digestive system, Robley Dunglison's (1798–1869) views on medicine and physiology, published in 1835, were highly regarded because he had authored prominent textbooks on both subjects. While a faculty member of the hygiene department at the University of Maryland, his text (53) was the first book on preventive medicine for medical students (8). The book contained an 18-page chapter devoted to exercise. Dunglison emphasized that exercise was important for one's health and that "inglorious inactivity" would cause an individual to "suffer" because of a loss of function of the nervous, muscular, circulatory, digestive, secretory, and excretory systems and that the loss could lead to "hypochondriasis, hysteria, and the whole train of nervous diseases," and for many grave "bodily ailments" (53, p. 442). He classified exercise as active or passive and emphasized the importance of traveling exercises, which meant covering long distances in unfamiliar outdoor environments for improved digestive and mental functions. Exercise in moderation was advocated for its beneficial and tonic influences on the body, whereas violent exercises, such as running, dancing, and wrestling, were discouraged because they caused air to contain less oxygen and more carbon dioxide and led to respiratory turmoil leading to suffocation, cardiac dilations, aneurysms of large vessels, hemorrhages from the lungs and nose, body shocks, hernias, dislocations, and more muscle sprains and lacerations. Besides the physiological effect of enhancing digestion, moderate exercise increased the action of the heart and the connected respiratory movements; promoted blood flow to the capillaries and its functions (nutrition and secretion); increased muscle firmness, elasticity, and bulk; and promoted loss of fat around the muscles (53).

The first time a publication included the words and addressed the subject of the physiology of exercise was 1855 (2). The author was William H. Byford, a physician and professor at Rush Medical College in Chicago who had a history of conducting exercise experiments with animals and humans pertaining to heat, circulation, breathing, and secretion. Byford was aware of the health benefits of exercise and concerned that the medical profession appeared indifferent to the subject. Hence, his article was an attempt to inform and to educate others on its importance while encouraging them to initiate related research. Byford defined exercise as "voluntary discharge of any or all the animal functions, as intellect, sensation, locomotion and voice" and described the phenomena of exercise as "vascular excitement, increased heat, redness of the surface and augmented secretion and excretion" (2, p. 33). However, he neglected to mention the types or intensity levels being advocated. Since blood was the foundation from which all organs received their nutrients to discharge their functions, it was essential that the supply of blood increase in proportion to the elevated demands of the organ, which was, in turn, dependent upon increased muscle activity. As nutritive material was removed from blood and the effete matter it contained, the exchange within the capillaries was also enhanced by muscle contractions. He described the exchange process as the capillary force of the circulation and noted that when the muscles were contracting quickly and frequently, they would attract a large amount of blood from the capillaries and pass it on to the veins and to the heart. Moreover, it was an exchange that was accomplished by the mechanical action of muscles upon the veins. He acknowledged that this explanation was incomplete because it ignored cerebral influences and the important role of capillary circulation. Besides involving circulatory and muscular systems, the excitement of exercise included emotions and possible atomic or molecular changes occurring in nervous centers as well as organic functions associated with perspiration and urinary excretions. When vascular excitement was specifically mentioned, it referred to the distribution of blood and its nutrients to all of the vital organs and tissues. This role gave importance to exercise because it enhanced organ development and functions of which muscles were deemed the most important. He noted that blood contained high levels of albuminous or protein compounds which provided the structure for other organs and served the exclusive functions of muscle (he thought more than half of the albumin found in blood would likely be consumed by the muscles) (2). Byford then proceeded to discuss the role of albumin in disease states and the value of physical activity in the process. Exercise was important for increasing the warmth of the body and the temperature of the blood because this change enhanced nutrient disintegration. In addition, the digestive process was facilitated. He stated (2, p. 40), "It is this beautiful mutual dependence and reciprocal stimulation, by affording the material ready prepared as it were to each other, both in a physiological and physical sense, that the health, efficiency, and even integrity of the animal and organic are preserved in their proper condition for the support of the whole system." Secretions from the skin, kidney, and liver were also facilitated by exercise. However, physiological consequences arose when organs associated with these secretions were unable to perform their functions, in part because of a lack of muscular activity.

After Byford to the Establishment of Formal Courses In Exercise Physiology

Byford's article did not stimulate American physiologists to conduct exercise-related research or to consider including exercise physiology in the medical school curriculum. However, after the Civil War, there was a heightened interest by the American public in personal and public health, gymnastics, calisthenics, physical training, physical education, outdoor recreation, and competitive athletics (50). Moreover, this interest remained intense well into the twentieth century and led to the establishment of secondary school and college physical education programs and professional organizations. Included in their objectives were the promotion of hygiene or bodily health and educational development. Intrinsic to the hygienic goal was the dissemination of information related to the physiology of the circulatory, respiratory, muscular, digestive, and excretory systems (50). One example of a program designed to prepare their graduates for positions in schools, athletic clubs, agencies such as the YMCA, gymnasiums and the like was the Lawrence Scientific School and its department of anatomy, physiology, and physical training at Harvard University in Massachusetts (54). Although the Lawrence Scientific School was established in 1847, it was not until 1892 that a 4-year scientific program in anatomy, physiology, and physical training was initiated to prepare individuals to be responsible for gymnasiums or to enter the second year of medical school. Physiology of exercise was taught in the fourth year as a theory class by George Wells Fitz, MD. This course required a laboratory experience that was the first of its kind in the United States. The program, which had nine graduates, ended in 1899 for financial, philosophical, leadership, and political reasons. It remains unknown whether a text was required or what subject matter was taught (54). Before the turn of the twentieth century, other institutions established degree programs that required formal instruction in exercise physiology. Examples include Oberlin College in Ohio (Delphine Hanna, MD); International Young Men's Christian College (now known as Springfield College) in Massachusetts (Luther Halsey Gulik, MD, and later James H. McCurdy, MD); Stanford University in California (Thomas Denison Wood, MD); and the one at Harvard University that involved Fitz. The significance of these course offerings is that they highlight an important requirement of a emerging scientific discipline.

Select Publications After Byford That Contributed to the Recognition of Exercise Physiology

Byford's 1855 article identified the discipline, provided a tepid template for its continuance, and loudly proclaimed the need for supportive research. Soon afterward in England (1863), a pedestrian champion named Charles Westhall published a book on physical training that is notable because it contained advice relative to current views on exercise prescription, the specificity of training, and the possibility of overtraining and its problems (55). This was followed by a text on exercise and training by an English physician, Robert Lee, who defined the physiology of exercise (p. 9) as the "mechanical effects which muscular contraction produces on the structures of the body." It also provided insights on fatigue, the observation that muscle power can be estimated from size, and a daily schedule for rowers to follow (56). The individual after Byford whose publications noticeably promoted exercise physiology was a physician, Austin Flint, Jr. (1853–1915).

Frequently Flint failed to identify his Junior status as his father was an accomplished physician and author (1812–1886), so his publications have authorship problems. After graduation, he studied with Bernard in France, served as a professor at the Medical School in Buffalo, and became renowned while serving on the physiology faculty at Bellevue Hospital Medical College in New York. His 1875 publication *A Textbook of Human Physiology*, which had four editions, was likely the most influential because of its extended use within medical schools, which were responsible for most course instructors and investigators in exercise physiology during these times (57). In this text, Flint discussed the effect of exercise on the heart and cited the data of Byran Robinson. He emphasized the changes in blood pressure, mentioned the blood flow data of Chauveau, and noted that muscular contractions enhanced venous return. When discussing metabolism, he included the exercise results of Seguin and Lavoisier (see Milestone of Discovery) concerning oxygen consumption changes, the ventilatory increases noted by Vierordt, and the carbon dioxide results of Edward Smith. Furthermore, he mentioned that with conditions of great fatigue and exhaustion, the carbon dioxide content of the expired air was decreased (hyperventilation). At the time of the first edition, Flint was engaged in a controversy as to whether nitrogen was excreted with muscular exercise (argument was associated with the issue of whether proteins were the prime substrate for muscle function). In 1870, Flint carefully studied the urinary nitrogen excretion of an individual who walked about 318 miles in 5 days and found that for every 100 parts of nitrogen ingested, 154 parts of nitrogen were excreted. Thus he felt that "violent" exercise would cause tissue breakdown which would be reflected with an increased loss of body proteins (58). In the textbook, muscle action or effort was generally discussed with regard to the responses of frog muscles to electrical stimulation. He did note that muscles increased in size and power with frequent exercise. In addition, he felt that repeated exercise would increase the size but not the number of the fasciculi. While muscle fluid (or juice) was slightly alkaline at rest, moderate exercise would cause it to become more neutral, whereas with strenuous exercise, it would become acidic because of the presence of lactic acid.

The effect of exercise on body temperature was emphasized. and an upper limit of 104°F (40°C) was listed with "violent, muscular exercise," which in turn would increase sweating. The fact that muscle activity could increase muscle temperature was verified by inserting a thermoelectric needle into the biceps of an individual sawing wood and observing a rise of 2°F. Lastly, Flint felt that exercise would enhance the development of bones and suggested that it would prolong life (57).

In 1878, Flint published *On the source of Muscular Power*, in which he details the experiments of Liebig, Lehmann, Fick and Wislicenus, Parkes, Pavy and those he conducted with Weston (59). Not surprisingly, the topic was the effect of exercise on nitrogen balance. Significant conclusions were as follows (pp. 94–96):

> V. *Experiments show that excessive and prolonged muscular exercise may increase the waste or wear of certain of the constituents of the body to such a degree that this wear is not repaired by food. Under these conditions, there is an increased discharge of nitrogen, particularly in the urine. . . .*
>
> VII. *By systemic exercise of the general muscular system or of particular muscles, with proper intervals of repose for repair and growth, muscles may be developed in size, hardness, power and endurance. The only reasonable theory that can be offered in explanation of the process is the following: While exercise increase the activity of dissimulation of the muscular substance, a necessary accompaniment of this is an increased activity in the circulation of the muscles, for the purpose of removing the products of their physiological wear. This increased activity of circulation is attended with an increased activity of the nutritive processes, provided the supply of nutriment be sufficient, and provided, also, that the exercise be succeeded by proper periods of rest. It is in this way only that we can comprehend the process of development of muscles by training; the conditions in training being exercise, rest following the exercise, and appropriate alimentation, the food furnishing nitrogenized matter to supply the waste of the nitrogenized parts of the tissues. . . .*
>
> VIII. *All that is known with regard to the nutrition and disassimilation of muscles during ordinary or extraordinary work teaches that such work is always attended with destruction of muscular substance, which may not be completely repaired by food, according to the amount of work performed and the quantity and kind of alimentation.*

In 1886, Edward M. Hartwell, PhD, MD, of Johns Hopkins University, addressed a convention of the American Association for the Advancement of Physical Education. The title of his presentation was "On the Physiology of Exercise." The speech was subsequently published in two parts in the *Boston Medical and Surgical Journal* (60,61). He spoke on this topic because "the fundamental and essential characteristics of exercise are generally misstated and its proper effects so frequently overlooked, that I have chosen the physiology of exercise as my theme" (60, p. 297). After using du Bois-Reymond's definition of exercise ("the frequent repetition of a more or less complicated action of the body with the co-operation of the mind, or an action of the mind alone, for the purpose of being able to perform it better"), he discussed the anatomical and contractile characteristics of muscle tissue and its response to neural stimuli before it "begins working." The importance of an increased blood flow to working skeletal muscles was emphasized. He mentioned that the blood entering muscle was bright red, rich in oxygen, and low in carbonic acid, whereas it was dark blue, had a higher temperature, and contained waste products and "poorer" oxygen when it left to return to the heart. If these conditions could not be reversed, muscle irritability became less and a stronger stimulus was required. He proposed that if muscles received adequate food, oxygen, and rest, they would increase in size and weight because fibers number and sizes would increase. Repeated exercise would make the muscles larger, harder, and stronger. He noted that muscles were "more perfect power-machines" than are steam engines and rifled cannons because of the energy transformations within the tissue ("the potential energy of organized material is transformed into the work which we see manifested in motion, animal heat, and the chemical actions involved in nutritive, secretory, and excretory processes" (60, p. 301). Exercise was important for achieving a healthy state, and failure to exercise could be associated with incomplete oxidation of food, the accumulation of effete products, disordered digestion, an enfeebled nervous system, flabby muscles, impaired secretions, an onset of ill health, and the occurrence of diseases (p. 301). He concluded that to achieve a healthy state, an average individual should walk 8 or 9 miles daily.

Hartwell also focused on the growth and development of individuals from various segments of English society. It was apparent to Hartwell that young individuals from "well-to-do parents" and environments had stature and weight measures that were superior to those from working parents. He inferred that this difference was due in part to inadequate play activity and the failure to receive sufficient exercise. In the final segments of his presentation, he addressed the effect of exercise on the nervous system with an emphasis on the brain. After mentioning the effect of use and disuse on the muscular system, he indicated that use and disuse had "similar effects in the case of nerve cells and fibres, both sensory and motor." Hartwell compared the nervous system of a blacksmith with that of a 5-year-old male and attributed the size, branching, and connections of the motor nerves and the cells within the motor area to be larger and more numerous in the motor area in the blacksmith, in part because of the effect of chronic exercise during the critical phase of growth and development. He then discussed aspects of human inheritance and stated that "muscular exercise deserves more attention than is usually given it, and that, when properly chosen, regulated and guided, it not only does a man good, but makes him better; at least, it may make him a better man, in many respects, than his father was, and enable him to transmit to his progeny a veritable aptitude for better thoughts and actions" (61, p. 324). However, he provided no evidence to support his statements.

In 1893, the accomplished German sportsman and physician George Kolb had his book the *Physiology of Sport* translated and published in English (62). The text contains results and opinions from his case studies with the members of the "Berliner-Ruder-Club" with a focus on the maximal exertion and training of sportsmen (predominately rowers). He began his text with a discussion of the fatigue with maximum exertion which is first experienced by the skeletal muscles but is related to the insufficiencies of the circulation of the blood, the respiratory system, the nervous system, and possibly to the fact that the athlete is overtrained. Besides indicating that skeletal muscles were important for sporting activities and associated with "sportsman fatigue," they must be strengthened in "every way." For rowers, this meant daily practice (3 minutes) for the arms and legs with dumbbells weighing 4 to 5 pounds each and deep knee bends for the extensors of the upper thigh. Several chapters were devoted to the responses of the cardiovascular system, with many pages devoted to pulse wave tracings recorded with a sphygmograph (p. 33). He reported that maximal effort in rowers was associated with heart rates of 230 to 350? beats per minute and radial artery pressures around 185 mm Hg. After several months of training, heart rates would be reduced by 16 beats per minute, while blood pressure was lowered by 20 mm Hg.

From his analysis of the sphygmographic results, he concluded that maximal exertion would increase the rate and work of the heart, alter cardiac dilation, elevate the velocity of blood flow, and cause muscle and cardiac hypertrophy. The term "cardiac dullness" was invoked to describe dilation or enlargement of the heart. He indicated that there were pathological conditions in which cardiac dullness was increased, but this condition was not a characteristic in trained rowers. Kolb elaborated on the respiratory changes of rowers and reported that respiratory rates could increase from 12 to 60 per minute and be maintained with heavy exertion. Actually, he reported frequency values as high as 140 before muscle failure occurred (?). Vital capacity values were decreased after rowing events, presumably because of the increased volume of blood within the lungs. Using himself as a subject in rowing races that lasted 1 to 9 minutes, he found the percentage of carbon dioxide in expired air to increase from 4.3% to 6% and to 9.0% once the event had ended. He calculated that in an 8-minute race he had a gaseous exchange of 600 L of air in the lungs, of which approximately 39 L was carbon dioxide. He felt that dyspnea occurred because of the combined influence of an oxygen lack and an increase in carbon dioxide acting on the respiratory center. In addition, he attributed the fatigue of rowers to the respiratory system because muscles were unable to counteract the increased "development of carbonic acid." Trained rowers were characterized as having lower resting and exercise respiratory frequencies while possessing stronger and hypertrophied respiratory muscles (assumed from force measurements). Kolb felt it was necessary to "exercise the lungs" and recommended a daily short and fast run of 3 minutes.

He reported that rowing frequently increased rectal temperatures to 104°F with no apparent harm to the individual, although cold-water douching after practice or competition was a routine procedure with most clubs. Although the energy cost of rowing was calculated to be 33,000 kg·m⁻¹ per second, he acknowledged that it was more an approximation than factual. The textbook contains a chapter on urinalysis in which the importance of being hydrated is emphasized, while minimal concern is shown about the increases in urea and albumin with exercise. In the chapter on nervous insufficiency, he attempted to explain how it could be a cause of muscular fatigue and used sphygmographic tracings to support his assumptions and position. In essence, he described it as a depressed state associated with overtraining whose cause was related to "the increased outflow from the arterial system depending on the chronic dilation of the capillaries in the muscles chronically hypertrophied" (62, p. 163).

In 1890, the French textbook of the physician Fernand LaGrange, *Physiology of Bodily Exercise,* was translated into English and made available to instructors of exercise physiology (63). It contained 395 pages in 38 chapters containing six parts that listed titles such as muscular work, fatigue, habituation to work, different exercises, results of exercise, office of the brain in exercise, and 20 citations. Since its publication the book has been surrounded with controversy, initially by George Fitz for its incomplete and unscholarly presentation and its limited comprehension of the subject matter (64) and recently by McArdle, Katch, and Katch, who challenged Berryman's designation that it was the first textbook in exercise physiology (65). Tipton agrees with the Fitz's assessment but disagrees with his distinguished colleagues because a poorly written text with inadequate documentation and incomplete explanations doesn't change its intent, presentation, or date of publication. Using the criteria of McArdle, Katch, and Katch, his choice would be the 1919 edition of *The Physiology of Muscular Activity* by F. A. Bainbridge, published by Longmans, Green & Company (6), which was selected as the authoritative reference text to denote recognition.

In 1910, while at the University of Pennsylvania as director of physical education, the renowned sculptor of sport, R. Tait McKenzie, MD, published the first of several editions of *Exercise in Education and Medicine* (66). The text was addressed (p. 9) to "students and practitioners of physical training; to teachers of the youth; to students of medicine and to its practitioners, with the purpose to give a comprehensive view of the space exercise should hold in a complete scheme of education and in the treatment of abnormal or diseased conditions." After defining exercise and sorting it into active and passive categories, McKenzie discussed exercises of effort, skill, and endurance while indicating that endurance exercises were associated with different types of fatigue. The emphasis on the physiology of exercise was predominately limited to changes associated with the muscular, respiratory, and cardiovascular systems, with minimal details on metabolic, hemopoietic, and excretory systems. Little, if any, of the information mentioned by Robinson, Seguin and Lavoisier, Byford, Hartwell, Flint, or Kolb was included, although the views mentioned by Lagrange were noted.

Select Studies After Byford That Were Associated With the Recognition of Exercise Physiology

Pertaining to the Central, Peripheral, and Autonomic Nervous Systems

The last decades of the nineteenth century as well as the early years of the twentieth century saw heightened activity in the structures and functions of the central, peripheral, and autonomic nervous systems. In 1888, when German physiology was dominating Europe and Nathan Zuntz (1847–1920) in Berlin was achieving recognition for his exercise studies, it was accepted that activation of the nervous system would result in locomotion. During this year, Geppert and Zuntz conducted a hyperpnea experiment which advanced the ideas that neural and autonomic systems were involved; exercise caused the release of a substance into the blood that acted directly on the respiratory center within the brain, and neural receptors within exercising muscle would directly elicit increased respiratory responses (67). Several years later in Stockholm, Jons Erik Johansson showed that passive leg exercise with a rabbit resulted in an increase in heart rate that appeared to be related to activation of neural centers in the brain (68).

After the turn of the century, August Krogh (1862–1949, Nobel laureate in 1920) and Johannes Lindhard (1870–1947) of Denmark (Fig. 2.3) investigated the cardiorespiratory effects of light and heavy exercise and observed that various responses that were likely due to a "neural mechanism" occurred in "less than a second" (69). They associated their results with an "irradiation of impulses from the motor cortex rather than a reflex from the muscles" (69, p. 122). Little did they realize that their observations would become the foundation for the concept of a central command with exercise!

To assess autonomic influences, measurement of heart rate changes were made. In 1895, Henrich Ewald Herring (1886–1948) of Prague exercised rabbits and explained the increase via an elevation in accelerator nerve activity and a decrease in vagal (parasympathetic) influences (70). Using exercising subjects at the University of Michigan, Wilbur Bowen in 1904 measured the latency periods after the initial heart rate cycle and indicated that the increase could be from a decrease in the restraining influence of the inhibitory center (vagal activity) because of the motor cortex and/or nerve endings of muscles (71, p. 243). Ten years later, Herbert Gasser and Walter Meek at the University of Wisconsin studied exercising dogs that had been subjected to a muscarinic receptor blocker (atropine), vagal sectioning, and adrenalectomy. They concluded that inhibition of vagal impulses (vagal withdrawal) was the "most economical means" by which an increase in heart rate could occur (72).

The idea that the sympathetic nervous system would be active during exercise can be attributed to Walter B. Cannon

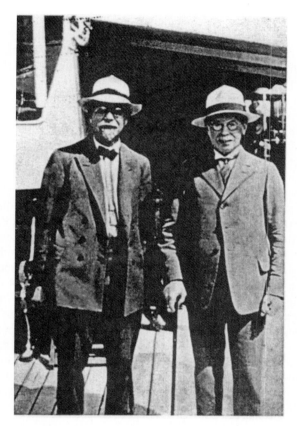

FIGURE 2.3 August Krogh and Johannes Lindhard of Copenhagen. These distinguished investigators conducted seminal exercise studies in respiration, circulation, and metabolism that helped gain recognition for the discipline of exercise physiology. Krogh was awarded the Nobel Prize in Physiology and Medicine in 1920. *(Reprinted with permission from McArdle WA, Katch FI, Katch VL. Exercise Physiology, 5th ed. Philadelphia: Lippincott Williams & Wilkins, 2001.)*

(1871–1945) of Harvard University, who became interested in an extract from the adrenal gland whose physiological effects were similar to those of the substance released by the adrenal gland with stimulation of the splanchnic nerve. During these times, Cannon regarded epinephrine more as an endocrine product than as a neurotransmitter and considered its actions in raising glucose concentrations useful for the muscle power and redistribution of blood flow needed to fight or to run (73). In a subsequent chapter (Chapter 9) on the autonomic nervous system, Seals will elaborate in more detail on the roles of the sympathetic and parasympathetic systems during an exercise response.

The Muscular System

With the development and perfection of dynamometers after the middle of the nineteenth century, the assessment and attainment of strength acquired a new importance that extended for many decades. The subject was of sufficient importance to the Union Army during the 1860s that strength data were collected on soldiers before the practice was extended to student populations at Amherst College or the YMCA International College in Massachusetts (65). Since the time of Milo of Croton or even before, it had been accepted that for an increase in strength to occur, the load or resistance had to be increased. Improvements in coordination and an increase in mass were the most frequent explanation to explain the changes. Park describes the years between 1870 and 1914 as a time when physiologists, physicians, and physical educators in many countries sought to extend scientific understanding of the severe effects of muscle exertion on the body (74). By 1892, Angelo Mosso (1846–1910) at the University of Turin in Italy had developed the first ergograph and was recording work performance and quantifying the process of muscular fatigue (75). Because fatigued muscles would respond to external electrical stimulation, Mosso was a proponent of "central fatigue," an idea attributed to August Waller (1816–1870) in London (76). Although not frequently acknowledged, Mosso had evidence for "peripheral fatigue," which in voluntary exercise includes the events of neuromuscular transmission (transmission fatigue) and the process of muscular contraction (contraction fatigue) (75). Using an ergograph to assess fatigue, Theodore Hough at Massachusetts Institute of Technology after the turn of century reported the presence of muscle soreness and attributed its existence to diffusible waste products and to possible tissue ruptures (77). In a related investigation concerned with neuromuscular fatigue, he concluded that nerve cells fatigued more rapidly than muscle fibers (78). The association between muscle fatigue and lactic acid levels in humans was increased when Ryffel in 1910 found running 12 laps in 2 minutes and 45 seconds increased blood levels to 71 mg $\cdot$ 100 mL^{-1} and urine levels to 2.3 g $\cdot$ mL^{-1} (79). However, isolated muscle preparations had to be developed and experiments conducted before it was possible to investigate muscle mechanics in exercising humans. Although Heidenhaim and Fick preceded him, A. V. Hill by 1913 had carefully developed and effectively perfected an *in vitro* muscle preparation that enabled him to quantify work performed and the mechanical efficiency of the responses. In fact, he reported for frog muscle that it could be as high as 50%, although it was usually between 25% and 30% (80). Later, he measured the heat being produced and used the preparation to experimentally develop the essential relationships for the force-velocity equation emphasized in Chapter 5.

Morpurgo in 1897 at the University of Siena in Italy reported that the histological changes in the sartorius muscles of two dogs before and after a 2-month period of wheel running resulted in a 54% increase in cross-sectional areas because of increases in fiber diameter without changes in numbers of fibers or nuclei. Although he was uncertain of the role of spindles, which were measured, their numbers did not increase as well. He concluded that the hypertrophy was due to an increase in sarcoplasm (81). Using the Johansson ergograph to determine the effects of training, Hedvall reported in 1915 that forearm training increased muscular endurance by 819% (82).

The Cardiovascular System

From the time of John Floyer (~1707) to the era of Wilbur Bowen (~1904), heart rates were recorded by palpations of the pulse, palpations of the heart, auscultation of heart sounds, or by graphic records of the pulse. The most accurate and reliable for exercise purposes was the placement of a tambour without button or membrane over the carotid artery, which allowed the pulsations of the artery to be transmitted to a recording drum. Using this approach, Bowen in 1904 reported rates while subjects rode a stationary bicycle for various durations. The highest heart rate achieved was 150 beats per minute (71). Several years later, Lowsley reported heart rates of individuals who participated in a 100-yard dash at about 140 beats per minute or a 20-mile run at about 125–100 beats per minute (83). Besides vagal withdrawal, nervous impulses stimulating the accelerator center, elevated blood temperature, waste products within the heart, and increased muscle metabolites were the explanations for the higher values.

Stephen Hales used the horse to make the first measurement of blood pressure, and during 1863 Etienne Marey (1830–1904) in France used the same animal to record the pressure response with exercise. In England during 1898, while using a Hill-Barnard sphygmomanometer, Leonard Hill (1866–1952) had a subject run 400 yards before recording an arterial pressure of 130 mm Hg (84). He was likely the first to report that postexercise blood pressures were lower than normal resting values after "severe muscular work." While at the International YMCA College in Massachusetts, McCurdy was among the first to record blood pressure from humans during exercise. In 1901 he recorded blood pressures (with a Hill and Riva-Rocci sphygmomanometer) of students performing maximum back and leg lifts and noted that the average values increased from 111 to 180 mm Hg (highest was 210 mm Hg). He attributed the increase to an elevation in intrapulmonary and intra-abdominal pressures, which were also measured (85). Several years later, Bowen measured blood pressure of subjects performing light exercise on a bicycle (~400 kg · m · min^{-1}) and felt the elevations (60–70 mm Hg) were a result of the increase in the output of the heart plus the augmented intra-pulmonary and intra-abdominal pressures (71). In the subsequent Lowsley study, the subjects training for a marathon ran 5 to 9 miles and exhibited increases in systolic pressure of 32.5 mm Hg and diastolic pressure of 20.6 mm Hg. As with Hill's findings, there was a decrease in the average postexercise pressures (83). In 1911 Hooker measured the effect of "violent" cycling exercise on the venous blood pressures of six subjects and observed mean increases of 9.5 cm of water, which were due in part to local vasodilation and the vasoconstriction of the splanchnic bed (86).

Once Harvey explained the existence of circulation, several centuries passed before the theory and methodology of its measurement occurred. The theory was the conservation of mass (e.g., oxygen leaving and entering the lungs), and the methodology was either the direct or indirect Fick (measuring mixed venous blood from the pulmonary artery and arterial blood from a systemic artery or the dilution effect of rebreathing foreign gases, using dyes or isotope clearance procedures) (87). In 1898 Zuntz and Hagerman used the direct Fick method with horses exercising on a treadmill and found the expected increases (88). Using the nitrous oxide rebreathing procedure with humans exercising on a bicycle, Johannes Lindhard of Copenhagen during 1915 found that cardiac output could increase from 4.9 to 28.6 L · min^{-1}, with heart rates changing from 70 to 166 beats per minute (89). Lindhard's data suggested that stroke volume would be increased with exercise and enhanced by training. Since Peterson, Piper, and Ernest H. Starling (1886–1927) of England in 1914 conducted the research (nonexercise design) in 1914 leading to Starling's "law of the heart," Bainbridge was the first to offer an explanation, which over the years continues to create discussions among physiologists. He stated (6, p. 54) that "the powerful heart of the athlete, while obeying the law of the heart, is able to respond to a moderate increase of venous inflow by a much larger output per beat."

The effect of exercise on the size of the heart has intrigued men of science since the time of Harvey. Soon after the discovery of x-rays in 1895 by the German Wilhelm C. Röntgen (1845–1923), Nobel laureate in 1901, numerous individuals have measured heart size before and after exercise. In a 1915 study by C. S. Williamson that carefully considered the phase of respiration when the photographs (teleroentgens) were taken immediately after the cessation of "severe exercise" (running up and down stairs), 88% of the subjects exhibited decreases (90). While increased cardiac contractility was mentioned, the results were appropriately criticized because they were not obtained during exercise. Many decades passed before methodology would be available for accurate measurement during exercise. These aspects will be covered in subsequent chapters.

Not unexpectedly, the first insights on changes in blood flow with movement came from the horse. In France during 1887, J. B. Auguste Chauveau (1837–1917) and Kaufman found chewing caused a fivefold increase in flow to the levator labii superioris (levator muscle of upper lip) (91). In studies on capillaries which culminated in a Nobel Prize for physiology and medicine in 1920, Krogh found that simulated work (electrical stimulation of muscles in guinea pigs and frogs) resulted in marked increases, from 10- to 30-fold, in the number of capillaries per millimeter of cross-sectional area being observed (92).

Because of the popularity of rowing and uncertainty as to its healthful effects, the Harvard University athletic committee in 1899 had Eugene Darling conduct physiological tests on the eight- and four-man varsity crew members during the strenuous component of the competitive season (93). The cardiovascular investigations were concerned with the size of the heart (determined by percussion, the occurrence of abnormal sounds, and the character of the pulse). Cardiac hypertrophy was considered to be a sign of strength and power, while cardiac dilation was evidence of cardiac fatigue. The measurements indicated that cardiac enlargement did occur, but Darling could not differentiate the hypertrophy from the dilation. He was unable to demonstrate that the heart was "overtrained" but felt some of changes were "unpleasantly near to pathological conditions" and advocated constant supervision and observations when crew members were in training. None of the heart sound results had significance, while the pulse results showed they were "invariably of high tension after unusual effort." Two years later (94), Darling reported on the effects of training and its aftereffects as they pertained to members of the crew and football team. Cardiac hypertrophy was a consistent finding for both groups, but it was not considered to be pathological. He summarized his findings by noting (94, p. 559) "that no ill effects, which could reasonably be attributed to training, were to be discovered 9 months after stopping the training."

The Respiratory System

During the time of Byford, the English penal system was using scheduled walking on massive treadwheels for punishment and ostensibly for health reasons. In London from 1856 to 1859, a physician and social activist with an interest in respiration, Edward Smith (1818–1874) (Fig 2.4) conducted systematic respiratory studies on the effects of exercise that included himself and prisoners (95).

Using a mask, a gasometer for inspiratory volumes, an absorption chamber with potassium hydrate, and a dehumidifier chamber, he reported mean values for liters of inspired volumes, respiratory rates, and heart rates with activities including swimming, rowing, walking 4 mph, walking 3 mph while carrying 50.9 kg, and walking on the treadwheel, which had 43 steps and covered 8.73 meters per minute. The inspired volumes ranged from 23.1 to 39.1 L per minute; the respiratory rates from 20 to 30 breaths per minute, and the heart rates from 114 to 189 beats per minute (96). When he measured the amount of carbonic acid formed during exercise, he found walking at 2 mph expired about 18 grains, or 1.15 g; 3 mph yielded 26 grains, or 1.66 g; treadwheel walking resulted in 48 grains, or 3.07 g (97). While it is uncertain whether his results significantly changed penal procedures or laws, they provided a foundation for subsequent respiratory and metabolic research in the late nineteenth and early twentieth centuries while demonstrating that the production of carbon dioxide was linearly related to the intensity of exercise (95).

Recall that it was hyperpnea experiments by Geppert and Zuntz during 1888 that led to the idea that an exercise stimu-

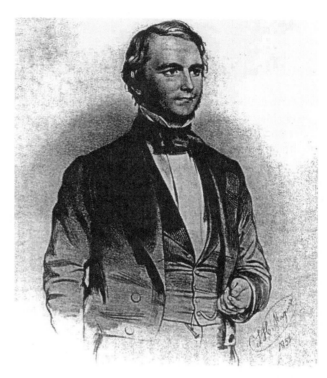

FIGURE 2.4   Edward Smith of Coldbath Fields Prison fame in England. He has been described by Carleton Chapman as a physiologist, ecologist, and reformer. His seminal investigations on the respiratory responses during exercise have become a foundation for the recognition of exercise physiology. *(Reprinted with permission from McArdle WA, Katch FI, Katch VL. Exercise Physiology. 5th ed. Philadelphia: Lippincott Williams & Wilkins, 2001.)*

lus from the brain or from metabolites affecting muscle would activate the respiratory center (67). The rapid pulmonary ventilatory responses observed by Krogh and Lindhard in 1913 conclusively demonstrated that the onset of exercise increased the excitability of the center (69). They also suggested that hydrogen was primarily responsible for the rapid increase in ventilation, and this concept has stimulated much research and will be discussed in some detail in Chapter 10. The linear relationships between work performed (0– ~1500 kg · M^{-1}), oxygen consumption (~0.4–3.3 L · min^{-1}) and pulmonary ventilation (~15–65 L · min^{-1}) was best demonstrated by the 1915 investigation of Lindhard in Denmark (89). C. Gordon Douglas (1822–1963) and John S. Haldane (1860–1936) in England found that intense exertion elevated alveolar carbon dioxide pressure by about 10 mm Hg before it decreased (98). This research was followed by Hough, who noted that running at 4 mph increased both oxygen and carbon dioxide tension, but as the intensity increased and if the run was "hard," carbon dioxide could fall 11 mm Hg, while oxygen values could rise to 112 to 125 mm Hg (99). He attributed these changes to overventilation of the lungs and to the entrance into the blood of a "muscular katabolite."

Douglas and Haldane demonstrated that respiratory dead space increased approximately threefold with exercise (100) during the time of the Copenhagen debate between Christian Bohr (1855–1911) and Krogh concerning whether oxygen reached the blood by secretion or diffusion. Krogh showed that diffusion was the responsible mechanism, while his wife, Marie, reported in 1915 that oxygen diffusion with moderate to heavy exercise was associated with increases ranging from 31 to 66% (101).

The Oxygen Transport System and Maximal Oxygen Uptake

After the Smith experiments with prisoners during the 1850s (95), new apparatus and methods became available for the collection and analysis of expiratory gases. Around the turn of the twentieth century, Zuntz (Fig. 2.5) developed a treadmill that was used mainly for animals. He also had access to the portable Zuntz-Geppert "breathing machine" for metabolic studies with laboratory, sporting, hiking, and high-altitude activities (19).

During the early decades of the twentieth century, Frances G. Benedict (1870–1957) of Wesleyan University in Connecticut, who had been associated with "metabolic lead-

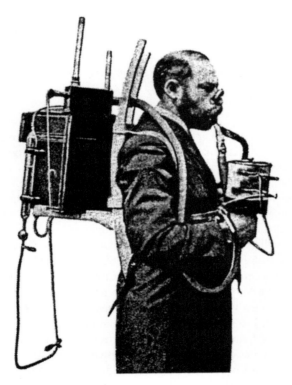

FIGURE 2.5 Nathan Zuntz of Germany. A distinguished investigator whose metabolic and hemopoietic studies have a foundation for the establishment of exercise physiology. *(Reprinted with permission from McArdle WA, Katch FI, Katch VL. Exercise Physiology. 5th ed. Philadelphia: Lippincott Williams & Wilkins, 2001.)*

ers" such as Voit and Wilbur O. Atwater (1844–1907), conducted careful and comprehensible metabolic studies with exercising subjects and noted systematic elevations as intensity progressively increased, with 3.06 L · min⁻¹ being the highest value being recorded (102). In the bicycle ergometer study conducted by Lindhard (89), when cardiac output (28.6 L · min⁻¹) was measured by an improved nitrous oxide method, the oxygen consumption value was 2.8 L · min⁻¹. However, more than 3 decades would elapse before careful measurements of systemic arteriovenous oxygen differences were used to assess maximal oxygen uptake.

The number of circulating erythrocytes, the concentration of hemoglobin, and the magnitude of the blood volume are important factors for obtaining a maximal response, and select aspects will be mentioned in the discussion on the hemopoietic system. As noted previously, by 1915 Marie Krogh had measured the diffusion of oxygen from the alveolus to the blood during dynamic exercise; this value later was estimated to be 4.0 to 6.0 L · min⁻¹.

Metabolic Systems and Their Substrates

Between the Seguin and Lavoisier experiments in the 1790s and the research activities of Edward Smith during the 1850s, the principle leading to the law of the conservation energy was independently proposed by J. Mayer and Hermann von Helmholtz (1821–1894) of Germany (confirmed in 1894 by an energy balance study by Max Rubner). Early investigators after Smith, like Max von Pettenkofer and Carl von Voit, used carbon dioxide production, measured the work performed (foot lathe) with and without fasting, and calculated the oxygen being consumed. With Nathan Zuntz leading the entry into the twentieth century, accurate treadmills for energy transformation studies with animals and humans were constructed (bicycles as well); spirometers, calorimeters, and a portable (Zuntz-Geppert) apparatus were developed; and the 1888 Geppert-Zuntz equation for the determination of "true oxygen" was in use (67). According to Benedict and Cathcart (102), the first metabolic studies concerned with muscular work using either the treadmill or the bicycle were performed in the Zuntz laboratory. However, the most comprehensive and careful were the ones they reported in 1913 pertaining to the metabolic transformations (oxygen consumption, work performed, heat produced, mechanical efficiency) that occurred with subjects walking and running while fasting or consuming diets high and low in carbohydrates (102).

During these formative times, von Pettehhofer and von Voit indicated that Liebig was wrong concerning whether proteins were the substrate of choice for muscular activity. In 1891, George Katzenstein in Zuntz's laboratory reported RER values (but as respiratory quotients) that were 0.80 at rest, 0.80 while walking, and 0.80 while climbing (103). Five years later, Chauveau of France cited RQ results of 0.75 at rest, 0.84, 0.87, 0.97, and 0.87 with 70 minutes of stair climbing that became 0.84 after 60 minutes of rest (104). He interpreted the increases with exercise as indicating that carbohydrates were being used and the declines as representing conversions of fats into carbohydrates before oxidation occurred. Immediately, Zuntz and Chauveau became involved in a controversy concerning which substrates were being preferentially used during exercise. It was Zuntz's view that muscles, whether resting or active, would use fat and carbohydrates in the proportion they were presented to the tissues.

In 1913 Benedict and Cathcart observed that muscular activity caused a small increase in the RQ regardless of whether the diet was high or low in carbohydrates (102). When a high-carbohydrate diet was consumed with exercise, the RQ changed from 0.85 to 0.90 before decreasing to 0.78, whereas with a low-carbohydrate diet the RQ increased from 0.79 to 0.82 before returning to 0.75. Their key conclusion was that the energy for muscular work was primarily derived from carbohydrates (102).

Intrinsic to metabolic transformation studies with exercise are calculations concerning mechanical efficiency. Using the recorded data and making various assumptions, Benedict and Cathcart estimated that the foot treadle experiments of Seguin and Lavoisier had a net mechanical efficiency of 7.7% (102). Hermann von Helmholtz (1821–1894) of Germany used the heat data from Edward Smith's walking studies and computed a gross efficiency value of 20.0%. In the first bicycle experiment involving Leo Zuntz in 1899, the net efficiency was 28.0%. Between 1900 and 1915, the most extensive and detailed studies concerning the mechanical efficiency of cycling, walking, and running in a variety of circumstances were conducted by Benedict with Carpenter or with Cathcart. They reported net efficiency values ranging from a low of 9.9% to a high of 25.2%, with most in the low twenties (102).

The Hemopoietic System

The concept that acute exercise would increase the number of erythrocytes and the concentration of hemoglobin began in 1894 with J. Mitchell in Philadelphia, when he observed higher red blood cell counts in subjects who ran before participating in a massage experiment (105). After the turn of the century, Zuntz and Schumberg made measurement of soldiers before and after 7-hour marches while covering 18 to 25 km and carrying packs of 22 to 31 kg. They found an average increase of 9% in the number of red blood cells (106). Hawk in 1904 at the University of Pennsylvania had 22 subjects perform exercise experiments that included walking, sprinting, short-distance runs, long-distance runs, jumping, and bicycling. In all experiments they found mean increases in erythrocytes that ranged from 10 to 23% (107). Eleven years later Edward Schneider and Havens at Colorado College measured the influences of sprints, 2-mile runs, and a composite of running and sprints and found increases in red blood cell counts ranging from 3 to 23% depending upon the event (108). They also measured hemoglobin in their subjects and found increases ranging from 4 to 10%. Hawk explained the elevations

as being the result of new corpuscles, release of corpuscles from storage sites, copious sweating, loss of fluids from the lungs, and movement of fluid into muscle (107). These investigators attributed the hemoconcentration effect of exercise to the passage of a protein-poor fluid from the vascular system into the interstitial space. Schneider and Havens studied the effect of 3 months of training for the 2-mile run by three members of the track team and reported two exhibited increases in erythrocyte numbers (5% and 18%) and hemoglobin concentration (4% and 9%) (108). Boothby and Berry had subjects exercise on a bicycle ergometer and found increases in red blood cells of 0 to 25% and 7 to 11% for hemoglobin (109). Rather than relate their results to work performed, they concluded that increases would result if sweating occurred because of the withdrawal of water from the cells.

In 1903, Christian Bohr (1855–1911) in Copenhagen demonstrated the S-shaped oxygen dissociation curve and a year later with Hasselbalch and Krogh showed that the curve was displaced by the carbon dioxide content of the blood (110). Joseph Barcroft in England during 1910 found that the addition of acid to solutions of hemoglobin caused a shift in the curve similar to what was exhibited when carbon dioxide content was elevated (111). Two years later, Barcroft and associates used a 1910 equation determined by A. V. Hill to show that "severe" exercise (climbing 1000 feet in the mountains in 20 minutes) shifted the dissociation curve in the direction of greater acidity (to the right), whereas normal exercise (climbing 1000 feet in 45 minutes) had no noticeable effect on the curve (111). Although Barcroft showed in 1914 that temperature changes would also alter the curve in a manner found with increased levels of acidity (110), several decades would elapse before Barcroft and Rodolfo Margaria (1901–1983) would conduct the definitive studies associated with dynamic exercise. As to the effects of training on these measures, including blood volume, several decades would pass before they effectively addressed.

Body Fluids and Temperature Regulatory Systems

Because before 1919 no techniques to accurately measure plasma volume; intracellular, interstitial, and extracellular fluid volumes; or total body water were available, changes in hemoconcentration, weight loss, sweat production, and urine formation were used to assess the effects of exercise. Not unexpectedly, weight loss was the method of choice. Perspiration was also assessed by the collection of sweat. Recall that in 1734 Byran Robinson collected and weighed samples while his subjects continued to exercise (43). Sweat glands were first identified in 1664 by Steno, who reported that insensible perspiration and sweat "passed out" of them (112). By 1887 it was accepted that the evaporation of sweat would have a cooling effect on the body and serve an important role in thermal regulation (15), an idea advanced a century earlier by Lavoisier. The concept that individuals exposed to exercise and heat should consume body fluids was advocated as early as 1866 for sportsmen by the trainer Archibald Maclaren (113), although the need to maintain fluid balance was promoted in 1912 by E. H. Hunt (114).

During the 1850s, it was considered prudent to exercise to the point when body temperature was increased, the skin was moist with sweat, and the cheeks were red; but not to the signs of fever. However, that perspective changed when the emphasis changed to learning of the effects with maximal exertion (50). In 1898 Pembrey and Nicol recognized the unreliability of recordings of oral temperatures during dynamic exercise and recommended securing either rectal temperatures or urine temperatures after micturition. Rectal temperatures of exercising individuals produced values from 38.3 to 40°C (100 to 104°F) (115). Interestingly, they provided little information on "surface" temperatures. Soon researchers in Europe and the United States were assessing body temperature changes (mostly rectal, but several insisted on oral) associated with marching soldiers, mountain climbers, cyclists, runners, skiers, and individuals performing various exercises. Since external environmental conditions will affect internal temperature measurements, efforts were made to study rectal temperature changes under standardized ambient conditions. At the turn of the century, Lagrange indicated that a rise in body temperature during exercise would increase the mechanical efficiency of muscle and recommended a "preliminary canter" for warming up (63). Investigations on the rectal temperature changes in 1904 Olympic marathon runners showed increases ranging from 1.15 to 1.9°C, with the highest value being 38°C (100.4°F) with a runner showing no distress (116). Benedict and Cathcart in 1913 (102) were among the first to carefully control external conditions and to measure the heat produced with exercise. They demonstrated that "severe" exercise on a bicycle ergometer was associated with a rapid rise in body temperature (before peaking at 37.7°C and falling to a plateau of 37.4°C). They felt the rise in temperature during exercise was proportional to the intensity of the work performed and would be associated with an enhanced muscle blood flow (100).

The Renal System

Beginning in the Dark Ages, health status was assessed by examination of the urine for color, turbidity, sediments, smell, and taste (7). This practice persisted for centuries and partly explains why most of the early exercise literature on kidney function consists of uroscopy reports.

One of the first to analyze urine for functional insights was August Flint Jr. As mentioned previously, he collected urine from a pedestrian (Edward Weston) who was capable of walking 100 miles in less than 22 hours (58). Of interest was an increase in urinary water, nitrogenous products, sulfates, and phosphates, with no meaningful changes in chlorides. Because of the nature of the diet and types of fluids

consumed, uncertainty existed on the importance of his findings. Eight years later in Germany, Justus von Leube (1803–1873) observed the presence of albumin in urine from soldiers after a strenuous march but felt it was a physiological process (filtration through the pores of the glomerular membrane) (117). When the urinary results from a march of 100 km were analyzed, 40% of the soldiers had elevated protein levels. In fact, the urinary profile (protein, blood cells, and casts) was similar to that associated with a disease condition, acute parenchymatous nephritis. This resemblance gave rise to the concept that prolonged exercise was associated with "pathological urine" (118). Urinalysis results were also used to assess the effects of the marathon on kidney function, and all of the Olympic runners tested exhibited evidence of albumin, and most had casts, red blood cells, and acetone bodies. None had evidence of glucose being filtered (116). Not surprisingly, these results continued to fuel the controversy as to whether prolonged heavy exercise had a pathological effect on the kidneys.

This concern was one factor that impelled the Athletic Committee at Harvard University to have Darling include kidney function in his assessment of the acute and chronic effects of competitive rowing. He found notable increases in urinary specific gravity, urea, albumin, and casts and concluded, "Finally, this investigation has demonstrated that the physiological effects of training, on the heart and kidneys in particular, may approach unpleasantly near to pathological conditions, and that there should be some competent supervision to insure that the safe limits, when those are determined, shall not be passed" (93, p. 233). Two years later (1901) he published a followup study on these same crew members in which he included minimal information on kidney changes (94). His summary stated (94, p. 559), "It may be said that no ill effects, which can reasonably be attributed to training, were to be discovered nine months after stopping the training."

Gastrointestinal System

Digestion was included in the Harvard crew study initiated by Darling. The concern was weak stomachs and the prostration caused by diarrhea. However, after repeated observations, he concluded that the issue was one of nutrition and eating habits rather than exertion (93). Other than infrequent episodes of indigestion after the cessation of training, there was no information or conclusion on this subject.

At the turn of the century, Walter Cannon (1871–1945) of Harvard University began his illustrious research career by studying the functioning of the gastrointestinal system. His interest in gastric hunger contractions motivated Anton J. Carlson (1875–1956) at the University of Chicago to study the effects of exercise on this phenomenon. In humans he found little change when subjects were standing or walking, while running had an inhibitory effect (119). When he placed gastric fistulas in dogs and ran them on a treadmill at progressive speeds, the results were similar to what he had reported for humans.

The Endocrine System

At the time of the Byford manuscript, castration was known to affect the sexual characteristics and functions of males; Claude Barnard had shown that the liver released glucose into the blood as an "internal secretion"; and Thomas Addison of Guy's Hospital and Medical School in London had characterized a syndrome associated with the destruction of the adrenal cortex. Thus, any implication of an endocrine influence of exercise related to a vestige of the humoral doctrine of Hippocrates. Around the turn of the century, William Bayliss (1860–1924) and Ernst Starling (1866–1927) in London contributed to the birth of endocrinology when they reported that a chemical substance from intestinal tissue called secretin was responsible for stimulation the secretion of fluids from the pancreatic gland (7).

Endocrinology evolved primarily because of animal experiments. In 1892 Jacobj of Germany demonstrated that the electrical stimulation of the splanchnic nerves supplying the adrenal glands released a substance that altered the amplitude of contractile tissue (120). Three years later, Oliver and Schafer discovered an adrenal extract that was similar to the one found after stimulating the splanchnic nerves (121). Cannon used this knowledge in planning his experiment with de la Paz and showed that the blood of cats excited by barking dogs contained epinephrine and increased concentrations of glucose (73). This information led to the splanchnic nerve experiment with Nice (122) demonstrating that stimulated fatigued tibialis anterior muscles increased their force production and contributed to the fight-or-flight concept associated with Cannon because he believed the increased epinephrine would enhance muscle power and blood flow in the process. When Cannon was conducting these experiments, others had shown with isolated preparations that epinephrine would increase heart rate, oxygen consumption, cardiac contractility, and coronary vasodilation; thus, it would appear during the recognition years that physiologists were advocating a key role for epinephrine in augmenting an exercise response. Surprisingly, that was not the case with Bainbridge. He considered the uncertainty and variability found with such measurements too great. In fact, he states (6, p. 132), "It is very doubtful, therefore, whether the suprarenal glands, as regards the secretion of adrenalin, take any share in bringing about the circulatory and other changes occurring during exercise under ordinary conditions."

Because of the astute observations of Thomas Addison (1793–1860) in the middle of the nineteenth century, an association existed between the adrenal gland (cortex) and muscular weakness and fatigue. In fact, Charles Edouard Brown-Seguard (1817–1894) of London in 1856 proposed that the adrenal cortex detoxified the metabolites of muscular activity (123). However, almost 80 years would elapse before experimental exercise studies were undertaken with adrenalectomized animals and adrenal cortical extracts to investigate the basis of Addison's observations. In addition, it was well after the recognition years that exercise studies involving the pituitary, thyroid, and pancreatic glands were studied.

The Immune System

In ancient Rome, the term *immunity* described an exemption of service or duty to the state. When defined medically, it meant protection against infectious diseases. However, before it was defined, it was recognized and accepted that the first attack of a disease provided protection against a second incident. As the germ theory of disease was being accepted, immunology was born in the French laboratory of Louis Pasteur (1822–1895). In the 1880s, his acquired immunity results with chicken cholera and sheep anthrax were soon known by the scientific and medical community (14). Although the field was evolving, with discoveries related to the presence and actions of antigens and antibodies or the existence of cellular and autoimmunity, little interest or concern pertained to how exercise would alter immune responses. Of the attention given, most pertained to infections and the role of leukocytes in the process.

One of first studies on the effects of exercise on leukocytes (in 1835 physiology texts they were known as white globules) was conducted by Zuntz and Schumburg in 1901 with soldiers (106). Their post march results showed elevations in leukocyte counts, which were attributed to increases in neutrophils and lymphocytes. In the 1904 Hawk investigation on the effects of various athletic activities (N = 13) on blood constituents, leucocytes increased in all events by an average of 57% (107).

Compared to nonathletic subjects of that era, the athletes in the Hawk study had resting values (8,000 leucocytes per milliliter) that were noticeably higher (~11%). Schneider and Havens, in their study of track athletes, also found increases in leucocytes after running events that ranged from 3 to 23%. When they performed differential white cell counts, the polymorphonuclear cells increased by 9 to 45%, whereas the mononuclear cells exhibited decreases ranging from 14 to 55% (108). Collectively, these changes were attributed to the redistribution of cells and fluids with exercise, and no attempt was made to relate them to the responses associated with infections. (However, some investigators who followed have made such an assertion.)

The interest in the relationship between physical fitness status and immunity against infectious diseases is in part related to a post–World War I observation by Professor Hans Zinsser in Boston, that athletic men serving in the American Overseas Expeditionary Force (AEF) experienced a high incidence of influenza and death (presumably higher than found with nonathletic soldiers (124). Although this observation remained unresolved, modern-day insights on the relationship are presented in Chapter 23.

A description of the study (in French and English) and a listing of the results can be found in Benedict and Cathart (100, p. 6) and in Flint (58, p. 138). From his previous studies, including those on animals, Lavoisier knew that respirable air (he later named it *oxygine*) would enter the lung and leave it as chalky aeriform acids (carbon dioxide) in almost equal volumes. In addition, the respirable portion of the air had the property to combine with blood and to change its color to red. These studies led him to conclude that respiration was a slow combustion process between carbon and hydrogen that required oxygen and resulted in the formation of heat that dispersed throughout the body (he thought the combustion process occurred in the lungs). Therefore, to determine the effects on respiration of resting, food consumption, and exercise, he had the chemist Armand Seguin wear a copper mask to breath oxygen provided via a trough and to perform work using a foot treadle (nearby table). His wife, Marie-Anne Lavoisier (Fig. 2.6) served as a recorder, and a physician was present to assess the health status of Seguin (heart sounds and heart rate). The copper mask was held in place by wax or a cementlike substance.

The experiment had five phases. The first two were to measure resting oxygen consumption and carbon dioxide production in the fasting state at two external temperatures, about 26 and 12°C. Then Seguin performed work with a foot treadle that lifted a 7.343-kg weight to a height of 613 pieds, or about 200 m, in a 15-minute period. After he consumed a meal (believed to be his breakfast), resting measurements were repeated as was the work experiment. However, after the meal, Seguin lifted the same weight to an equivalent of 650 pieds, or about 211 m, in the allotted time. Oxygen consumption was recorded in pounces (1000 pounces = 19.8363 L) and expressed on an hourly basis. The results were as follows.

Condition	Cubic Pounces per Hour	Liters per Hour	Liters per Minute	Work performed, Kilograms per Minute
Resting, 26°C, fasting	1210	24.002	0.400	
Resting, 12°C, fasting	1344	26.660	0.444	
Resting after food	1800–1900	37.689	0.628	
Work, fasting	3200	63.477	1.058	1469
Work after food	4600	91.428	1.524	1549

Ignoring the obvious problems in design and methodology (values are an approximation), Seguin and Lavoisier demonstrated for the first time in humans the transformations of energy with specific reference to the effects of external temperature, digestion, and exercise. By measuring oxygen consumption and having a physician record heart rates during the experiment (data not shown), they revealed an awareness of a relationship between the circulatory and metabolic systems well in advance of nineteenth-century investigators. To the exercise physiologist of today, oxygen consumption is the gold standard to assess and prescribe exercise; thus, we should not forget that it started with Lavoisier more than 200 years ago!

Seguin A, Lavoisier A. Premier Memoire sur la Respiration des Animaux. Mem Acad R Sci 1789;566–584.

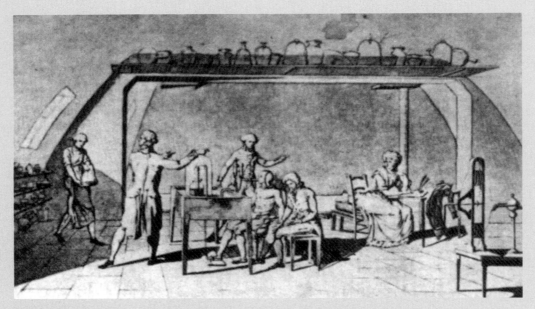

FIGURE 2.6   Sketch by Marie-Anne Lavoisier, one of two depicting the experiment by Lavoisier and Seguin. *(From McKie D. Antoine Lavoisier, Scientist, Economist, Social Reformer. New York: Henry Schuman, 1952;353.)*

SUMMARY

With ancient humans, exercise was a way of life and a means of survival. However, this relationship changed with the dawn of civilization and the establishment of cultures, as moderate exercise was perceived to enhance one's health and to facilitate avoidance of disease. Although the Greek and Roman physicians explained this relationship by the humoral theory of Hippocrates, historians have yet to explain why similar perceptions concerning exercise existed prior to its formulation. Because of the association between elevated body temperatures and the fever of diseases, "violent" (heavy and maximal exercise) exercise was discouraged by physicians until the beginning of the nineteenth century. Hippocrates and Galen were advocates of regular exercise, but they had little respect for professional athletes. Since Galen's influence lasted 1200 years or more, this aspect may help to explain the long historical disdain for heavy exercise.

Physiology is an experimental science whose foundations are based on measurement, and the same is true for exercise physiology. Thus the physiological effects of exercise from the time of Hippocrates to the seventeenth century were confined to observations and reports that were usually explained by health rather than by physiology. While understandable, these observations pertained to the circulatory (pulse rates, pulse "force"), respiratory (breathing rates), muscular (mass, strength, endurance, tone), thermoregulatory (sweating, fever), and digestive systems (bowel movements, indigestion). The seventeenth century was identified as the demarcation point because during that time measurements relevant to exercise physiology were made by Glisson, Borelli, Stensen, Santorio, Harvey, and Bernoulli.

Described as the Era of Enlightenment, the eighteenth century could be remembered as the era of Lavoisier, Floyer, Robinson, and Tissot. Lavoisier is recognized for providing the chemical foundation for respiration, metabolism, and body temperature while measuring oxygen consumption during exercise; Floyer for being the first to record the effects of exercise on heart rate; Robinson for his experiments and ideas pertaining to heart rate, muscle strength, blood flow, and temperature regulation; and Tissot because he provided a template for the exercise prescription.

The nineteenth century has been described as the beginning for both physiology and medicine. For exercise physiology, it was after Byford, in the later portion of the century, when formal instruction occurred in established educational institutions. While its beginnings were not as auspicious or noteworthy as those of physiology or medicine, it was a start. The early decades of the twentieth century were identified as the recognition years, as a sufficient number of investigations in the United States and in Europe were concerned with the circulatory, respiratory, nervous, metabolic, muscular, and thermoregulatory systems to indicate that exercise physiology was being recognized as a emerging scientific discipline.

ACKNOWLEDGMENT

It is a pleasure to acknowledge Jack W. Berryman, PhD, of the School of Medicine at the University of Washington, whose scholarship on the history of exercise was a major contributor to this chapter.

REFERENCES

1. Sherrington C. Man on His Nature. New York: Macmillan, 1941;6–8.
2. Byford WH. On the Physiology of Exercise. Am J Med Sci 1855;30:32–42.
3. Brock AJ. Greek Medicine. London: Dent & Sons, 1929.
4. Hippocrates. With an English translation by WHS Jones. Vol. 4. Cambridge, MA: Harvard University, 1939.
5. Tipton CM. Contemporary exercise physiology: fifty years after the closure of the Harvard Fatigue Laboratory. Exerc Sport Sci Rev 1998;26:315–339.
6. Bainbridge FA. The Physiology of Muscular Exercise. London: Longmans, Green, 1919.
7. Lyons AS, Petrucelli RJ. Medicine: An Illustrated History. New York: Harry Abrams, 1978.
8. Berryman JW. Exercise and the medical tradition from Hippocrates through antebellum America: a review essay. In Berryman JW, Park RJ, eds. Sport and Exercise Sciences: Essays in the History of Sport Medicine. Urbana: University of Illinois, 1992;1–57.
9. Gordon BL. Medicine Through Antiquity. Philadelphia: FA Davis, 1949.
10. Hippocrates. With an English translation by WHS Jones. Vol. 1. London: William Heinemann, 1923.
11. Berryman JW. Ancient and early influences. In Tipton CM, ed. Exercise Physiology: People and Ideas. New York: Oxford University Press, 2003;1–38.
12. Van Der Eijk PJ. Diocles of Carystus. Leiden, Netherlands: Koninkiylke Brill, 2001.
13. Von Staten H. Herophilus: The art of medicine in early Alexandria. Cambridge, UK: Cambridge University Press, 1989.
14. Paul WE. Fundamental Immunology. 3rd ed. New York: Raven Press, 1993.
15. Renbourn ET. The natural history of insensible perspiration: a forgotten doctrine of health and disease. Med History 1960;4:135–152.
16. Craik EM. Hippocrates, Places in Man. New York: Oxford University, 1998.
17. Green RM. A Translation of Galen's Hygiene (De sanitate tuenda). Springfield, MO: Charles C. Thomas, 1951.
18. Galen. The pulse for beginners. In Galen: Selected Works. New York: Oxford University Press, 1997;325–344.
19. Rothschuh KE. History of physiology. Huntington, New York: Robert E. Krieger, 1973.
20. Woody T. Philostratus: Concerning gymnastics. Res Quart 1936;7:3–26.
21. Vegetius. Epitome of Military Science. Milner NP, trans., notes and introduction. Liverpool: Liverpool University Press, 1993.

22. Keppie L. The Making of the Roman Army. London: Batsford, 1984.

23. Prioreschi P. History of Medicine, vol 1. 2nd ed. Omaha: Horatius Press, 1995.

24. Grunner OC. A Treatise on the Canon of Medicine of Avicenna, Incorporating a Translation of the First Book. New York: Augustus M. Kelley, 1970.

25. Krueger HC. Avicenna's Poem on Medicine. Springfield, MO: Charles C. Thomas, 1963.

26. Mendez C. Book of Bodily Exercise (1553). Copyright Elizabeth Licht. Baltimore: Waverly Press, 1960.

27. Harvey W. Exercitatio Anatomica De Motu Cordis et Sanguinis in Animalibus. 3rd ed. Presented by Leake CD. Springfield, IL: Charles C. Thomas, 1941.

28. Lower R. A treatise on the heart on the movement and colour of the blood and on the passage of the chyle in the blood. London: Printed by John Redmayne for James Allestry at the sign of the Rose and Crown in the street commonly called Duck Lane. 1669. In Gunther RT, Early Science in Oxford. Oxford: Printed for the Subscribers, 1932.

29. Frank RG Jr. Harvey and the Oxford Physiologists. Berkeley: University of California Press, 1980.

30. Boyle RA. Defense of the doctrine touching the spring and weight of the air. London: Printed by F.G. for Thomas Robinson Bookseller in Oxon, 1662.

31. Foster M. Lectures on the History of Physiology During the Sixteenth, Seventeenth, and Eighteenth Centuries. London, New York: Dover Publications, 1970.

32. Mayow J. Medico-physical Works, Being a Translation of Tractatus Quinque Medico Physici. Edinburgh: Printed for James Thin, 1674, republished by the Alembic Club in London by Simpkin, Marshall, Hamilton, Kent, 1907.

33. Isler H. Thomas Willis, 1621–1675, Doctor and Scientist. New York: Hafner, 1968.

34. Bernoulli J. Dissertations on the Mechanics of Effervescence and Fermentation and on the Mechanics of the Movement of the Muscles by Johann Bernoulli. Philadelphia: American Philosophical Society, 1997.

35. Wilson LG. William Croone's theory of muscular contraction: Notes and records. Royal Society of London 1961;16:158–178.

36. Santorio S. Medicina statica, or, Rules of Health in Eight Sections of Aphorisms. London: Printed for John Starkey, 1676.

37. Finney G. Fear of exercising the lungs related to iatro-mechanics 1675–1750. Bull Hist Med 1971;45:341–366.

38. Hoffmann FH. Fundamental Medicinae. Translation and an introduction by King LS. New York: American Elsevier, 1971.

39. Haller A. First lines of physiology. the sources of science. Vol. 1, 2. New York: Johnson Reprint, 1966.

40. Hales S. Statical Essays: Containing Haemastaticks. New York: Hafner, 1964.

41. Seguin A, Lavoisier A. Premier Memoire sur las Respiration des Animaux. Mem Acad R Sci 1789;566–584.

42. Floyer SJ. the Physician's Pulse-Watch; or, An Essay to Explain the Old Art of Feeling the Pulse, and to Improve it by the Help of a Pulse Watch. London: Printed for Sam Smith and Benj. Walford, 1707.

43. Robinson BA. A treatise of the Animal Oeconomy. 2nd ed. Dublin: Printed by S. Powell for George Ewing and William Smith, 1734.

44. Keill J. An Account of Animal Secretion, the Quantity of Blood in the Humane Body, and Muscular Motion. London: Printed for George Strahan, 1708.

45. Hall AR. John Theophilus Desaguliers, 1663–1744. In Gillispie CC, ed. Dictionary of Scientific Biography, Vol V. New York: Charles Scribner & Sons, 1971, 43–46.

46. Pearn J. Two early dynamometers: an historical account of the earliest measurements to study human muscular strength. J Neurobiol Sci 1978;37:127–134.

47. Tissot J-C. Gymnastique Médicinale et Chirurgicale. Licht E, Licht S, trans. New Haven: Elizabeth Licht, 1964.

48. Berzelius JJ. Jahres-bericht über die Fortschritte der physischen Wissenschaften. In Needham DM. Machina Carnis, the Biochemistry of Muscular Contraction in its Historical Development. Translated from the Swedish by Wohler F in 1836. Cambridge: University Press, 1971;41.

49. Sinclair J. The Code of Health and Longevity; or, A Concise View of the Principles Calculated for the Preservation of Health and the Attainment of Long Life. Edinburgh: Arch, Constable and Co., 1807.

50. Park RJ. Athletes and their training in Britain and America, 1800–1914. In Berryman JW, Park RJ, eds. Sport and Exercise Science. Urbana: University of Illinois, 1992.

51. Beaumont W. Experiments and Observations on the Gastric Juice and the Physiology of Digestion. In Osler W. A pioneer American physiologist (facsimile of the original edition of 1833 with a biographical essay). New York: Dover Publications, 1959.

52. Combe A. The Principles of Physiology Applied to the Preservation of Health, and to the Improvement of Physical and Mental Education. New York: Harper, 1836.

53. Dunglison R. On the Influence of Atmosphere and Locality; Change of Air and Climate; Seasons; Food; Clothing; Bathing; Exercise; Sleep; Corporeal and Intellectual Pursuits, etc. etc. on Human Health; Constituting Elements of Hygiene. Philadelphia: Carey, Lea & Blanchard, 1835.

54. Park RJ. The rise and demise of Harvard's B.S. program in anatomy, physiology, and physical training: a case of conflicts of interest and scarce resources. Res Quart Exerc Sport 1992;63:246–260.

55. Westhall C. The Modern Method of Training for Running, Walking, Rowing and Boxing. Including Hints on Exercise, Diet, Clothing, and Advise to Trainers. 7th ed. London: Ward, Lock, and Tyler, 1863.

56. Lee RJ. Exercise and Training, Their Effects on Health. London: Smith, Elder and Co., 1873.

57. Flint A. A Textbook of Physiology. 4th ed. New York: Appleton, 1896.

58. Flint A Jr. On the Physiological Effects of Severe and Protracted Muscular Exercise: With Special Reference to Its Influence Upon the Excretion of Nitrogen. New York: Appleton- Century-Crofts, 1871.

59. Flint A Jr. On the Source of Muscular Power. New York: Appleton, 1878.

60. Hartwell EM. On the physiology of exercise (part 1). Boston Med Surg J 1887;116:297–302.

61. Hartwell EM. On the physiology of exercise (part 2). Boston Med Surg J 1887;116:321–324.

62. Kolb G. Physiology of Sport. 2nd ed. London: Krohne & Sesemann, 1893.

63. Lagrange F. Physiology of bodily exercise. New York: Appleton, 1890.

64. Fitz GW. American Physical Education Review. 2:56, 1897. In McArdle WA, Katch FI, Katch VL, Exercise Physiology. 5th ed. Philadelphia: Lippincott Williams & Wilkins, 2001.

65. McArdle WA, Katch FI, Katch VL. Exercise physiology. 5th ed. Philadelphia: Lippincott Williams & Wilkins, 2001.

66. McKenzie RT. Exercise in Education and Medicine. Philadelphia: Saunders, 1910.

67. Geppert J, Zuntz N. Über die Regulation der Atmung. Arch Ges Physiol 1888;42:189–244.

68. Johansson JE. Über die Einwirkung der Muskelthatigkeit auf die Athmung und die Herzthatigkeit. Skan Arch Physiol 1893;5:20–66.

69. Krogh A, Lindhard J. The regulation of respiration and circulation during the initial stages of muscular work. J Physiol (Lond) 1904;31:112–133.

70. Herring HE. Über die Beziehung der extracardialen Herznerven zur Steigerung der Herzchlagzahl dei Muskelthatigkeit. Pflugers Arch Ges Physiol 1895;40:429–492.

71. Bowen WP. Changes in heart-rate, blood pressure, and duration of systole resulting from bicycling. Am J Physiol 1904;11:59–77.

72. Gasser HS, Meek WJ. A study of the mechanisms by which muscular exercise produces acceleration of the heart. Am J Physiol 1914;34:48–71.

73. Cannon WB, de la Paz D. Emotional stimulation of adrenal secretion. Am J Physiol 1911;28:64–70.

74. Park RJ. Physiologists, physicians, and physical educators: Nineteenth century biology and exercise, hygienic and educative. J Sport Hist 1987;14:28–60.

75. Mosso A. Fatigue. Drummond M, Drummond WB, trans. London: George Allen & Unwin; New York: Putnam's Sons, 1915.

76. Waller A. The sense of effort: an objective study. Brain 1891;14:179–249.

77. Hough T. Ergographic studies in muscular soreness. Am J Physiol 1902;7:76–92.

78. Hough T. Ergographic studies in neuromuscular fatigue. Am J Physiol 1901;5:240–265.

79. Ryffel JH. Experiment on lactic acid formation in man. J Physiol (Lond) 1910;39:XXIX–XXXII.

80. Hill AV. The absolute mechanical efficiency of the contraction of an isolated muscle. J Physiol (Lond) 1913;46:435–469.

81. Morpurgo B. Über Activitats-Hypertrophie der wikurlichen Muskeln. Virchows Arch 1897;150:522–544.

82. Hedvall B. Fatigue and training. Skan Arch Physiol 1915;32:115.

83. Lowsley OS. The effects of various forms of exercise on systolic, diastolic and pulse pressures, and pulse rate. Am J Physiol 1911;27:446–466.

84. Hill L. Arterial pressure in man while sleeping, resting, working, bathing. J Physiol (Lond) 1898;22:XXVI–XXX.

85. McCurdy JH. The effect of maximum muscular effort on blood-pressure. Am J Physiol 1901;5:95–103.

86. Hooker DR. The effect of exercise on venous blood pressure. Am J Physiol 1911;28:235–247.

87. Rowell LB. The cardiovascular system. In Tipton CM, ed. Exercise Physiology: People and Ideas. New York: Oxford University, 2003;98–137.

88. Zuntz N, Hagermann O. Untersuchungen über den Stoffwechsel des Pferdes bei Ruhe und Arbeit. Landw Jb 1898;27(Erganz Bd 3):371–412.

89. Lindhard J. Über das Minutenvolumen des Herzens bei Ruhe und bei Muskelarbeit. Pflugers Arch 1915;161:233–383.

90. Williamson CS. The effects of exercise on the normal and pathological heart: based on the study of one hundred cases. Am J Med Sci 1915;149:492–503.

91. Chauveau A, Kaufman M. Expériences pour la détermination du coefficient de l'activité nutritive et respiratoirs des muscles en repos et en travail. C R Acad Sci (Paris) 1887;104:1126.

92. Krogh A. The supply of oxygen to the tissues and the regulation of the capillary circulation. J Physiol (Lond) 1919;52:457–474.

93. Darling E. The effects of training: a study of the Harvard University crew. Boston Med Surg J 1899;141:229–233.

94. Darling E. The effects of training: second paper. Boston Med Surg J 1901;144:550–559.

95. Chapman CB. Edward Smith (? 1818–1874) physiologist, human ecologist, reformer. J Hist Med Allied Sci 1967;22:1–26.

96. Smith E. Inquires into the quantity of air inspired throughout the day and night and under the influence of exercise, food, medicine, temperature, &c. Proc Royal Soc 1857;8:451–454.

97. Smith E. Experimental inquiries into the chemical and other phenomena of respiration, and their modifications by various physical agencies. Phil Trans 1859;149:681–714.

98. Douglas CG, Haldane JS. The capacity of the air passages under varying physiological conditions. J Physiol (Lond) 1912;45:235–238.

99. Hough T. The influence of muscular activity upon the alveolar tensions of oxygen and carbon dioxide. Am J Physiol 1912;30:18–36.

100. Douglas CG, Haldane JS. The regulation of breathing. J Physiol (Lond) 1908;38:420–440.

101. Krogh M. The diffusion of gases through the lungs of man. J Physiol (Lond) 1915;49:271–300.

102. Benedict FG, Cathart EF. Muscular Work. Washington: Carnegie Institute of Washington, 1913.

103. Katzenstein G. Über die Einwirkung der Muskelthatigkeit auf den Stoffverbrauch des Menschen. Pflugers Arch Ges Physiol 1891;49:330–404.

104. Chauveau A. Source et nature du potentiel directment utilisé dans le travail musculaire, d'après les échanges respiratoires, chez l'homme en état d'abstinence. C R Acad Sci (Paris) 1896;122:1163–1221.

105. Mitchell JK. The effect of massage on the number and hemoglobin value of red blood cells. Am J Med Sci 1894;107:502–515.

106. Zuntz N, Schumberg W. Studien zu einer Physiologie des Marsches. Berlin: Hirschwald, 1901.

107. Hawk PB. On the morphological changes in the blood after muscular exercise. Am J Physiol 1904;10:384–400.

108. Schneider EC, Havens LC. Changes in the blood after muscular activity and during training. Am J Physiol 1915;36:239–259.

109. Boothby W, Berry FB. the effect of work on the percentage of haemoglobin and numbers of red corpuscles in the blood. Am J Physiol 1915;37:378–382.

110. Astrup P, Severinghaus JW. Blood gas transport and analysis. In West JB, ed. Respiratory Physiology: People and Ideas. New York: Oxford University Press, 1996;75–107.

111. Barcroft J, Peters RA, Roberts FF, et al. The effect of exercise on the dissociation curve of blood. J Physiol (Lond) 1912;45:XIV.

112. Renbourn ET. The history of sweat and the sweat rash from the earliest times to the end of the 18th century. J Hist Med Allied Sci 1959;14:202–227.

113. Maclaren A. Training in Theory and Practice. London: Macmillan, 1866.

114. Hunt EH. The regulation of body temperature in extremes of dry heat. J Hygiene 1912;12:479–488.

115. Pembry MS, Nicol BA. Observations upon the deep and surface temperature of the human body. J Physiol (Lond) 1898;23:386–406.

116. Barauch JH. Physiological and pathological effects of severe exertion (the marathon race). Am Phys Ed Rev 1912;16:1–11, 144–150, 200–205, 262–268, 325–334.

117. Von Leube W. Über die ausscheidung von eiweiss im harn ges gesunden Menschen. Virchow Archiv Pathol Anat Physiol Klin Med 1878;72:145–157.

118. Baldes, Heishelheim, Metzger. Untersuchungen über den einfluss grosser koperanstrengungen auf zirkulationapparat, nieren und nervensystem. Muenchen Med Wschr 1906;53:1865–1866.

119. Carlson AJ. The control of hunger in health and disease. Chicago: University of Chicago, 1916.

120. Jacobj C. Beitrage zur physiologischen und pharmakologischen Kenntniss der Darmbewegungen mit besonder Berucksichtigung der Beziehung der Nebenniere zu denselben. Arch Exp Pathol Pharmak 1892;29:71–211.

121. Oliver G, Schafer EA. The physiological effects of extracts of the suprarenal capsules. J Physiol (Lond) 1895;18:230–276.

122. Cannon WB, Nice LB. The effect of adrenal secretion on muscular fatigue. Am J Physiol 1913;32:44–60.

123. Brown-Sequard CE. Recherches expérimentales sur la physiologie et la pathologie des capsules surrenals. C R Acad Sci 1856;43:422–425.

124. Jokl E. Physiology of Exercise. Springfield, Il: Charles C. Thomas, 1964.

Exercise and Responses
of Biological Systems

CHAPTER 3

The Nervous System and Movement

V. REGGIE EDGERTON AND ROLAND R. ROY

Introduction

The first portion of this chapter is focused on how the nervous system controls and generates movement, with emphasis on posture and locomotion. In the second portion, neural adaptations to locomotion and other forms of exercise are discussed. Both of these topics are important in understanding the role of the nervous system in modulating the response of the body to single and repetitive movements. Since this is the only chapter in this textbook focusing on the nervous system, most of the topics addressed are necessarily brief. Two strategies are used in selecting the topics to address. Some topics were selected because they seemed to be the most relevant from an exercise physiology perspective, and these are discussed in some detail. Other selections were based on our perception of their particular interest and importance for further study. These topics are highlighted but not discussed in depth. We hope these topics will stimulate you to examine them more thoroughly.

One could easily argue that the nervous system is more important than the muscular system from the standpoint of defining motor performance and understanding how the body generates, responds to, and adapts to movement. In the study of any of the physiological systems, the nervous system largely defines the quality and degree of perfection of a movement as well as how it adapts to repetitive movements and training.

How Is Movement Generated?

The maximum force generated by a single muscle fiber is proportional to the number of cross-bridges that are arranged in parallel in one-half of a sarcomere and that are in the force-generating phase of cross-bridge cycling at that instant. Essentially the force generated by a muscle is directly related to the number of muscle fibers arranged in parallel that are activated by the nervous system. The maximum force potential of a muscle is determined by the maximum number of fibers in parallel that the nervous system can activate at the same time. Larger muscles usually have the potential to generate higher forces because they have more fibers in parallel. Of course, muscles also can increase their force potential when individual fibers become larger in cross-sectional area, that is, when the fibers hypertrophy. This increased force potential results from the larger fibers having more cross-bridges in parallel that can be in a force-generating phase at any instant.

The Force-Generating Capability of a Muscle: A Function of Its Physiological Cross-Sectional Area

Factors other than the number and size of fibers affect the force potential of a muscle. For example, the angle of attachment of the fibers relative to the line of pull on the muscle tendon can have some impact on the force-generating capacity of the muscle. Muscle fibers can be arranged in series, and these fibers also add to the mass and the displacement potential, but not the force-generating potential, of the muscle (Fig. 3.1).

One can calculate the physiological cross-sectional area (PCSA) of a muscle, which is directly proportional to maximum force potential, using the following formula:

$$PCSA = (\text{muscle mass})(\text{cosine of the angle of pinnation})$$
$$\div (\text{fiber length})(\text{muscle density})$$

Thus the mass of a muscle can contribute to its force and displacement and therefore to its velocity potential. In some muscles, most of the fibers are arranged *in parallel,* whereas in other muscles most fibers are arranged *in series.* Almost all muscles have fibers that are arranged in both manners. Thus the relative force and displacement potential of a muscle of a given size is a function of the relative proportion of sarcomeres arranged *in parallel* or *in series.* Details of these structure–function relationships can be found elsewhere (1,2).

Relationship Between PCSA and Size of Muscle Fibers

Theoretically, an increase in PCSA can be accomplished by adding sarcomeres *in parallel* within existing fibers (hyper-

trophy) or by adding new fibers *in parallel* (hyperplasia). The former case is analogous to existing muscle fibers becoming larger in diameter or circumference. However, factors other than PCSA, for example the efficacy of each cross-bridge in generating force and general changes in cross-bridge dynamics, define the force output potential of a muscle.

Skeletal muscles in large animals, such as humans, have very complex designs. In most muscles, as noted earlier, muscle fibers are not arranged strictly either in *parallel* or in *series.* The maximum force and displacement potential of a muscle, however, rarely have real functional relevance. This is because almost all movements are generated by the nervous system recruiting a relatively small percentage of fibers in any given muscle. From a neural perspective, the force and displacement generated by a given muscle are functions of the number of fibers recruited within the muscle that are in *series* or in *parallel*, respectively.

How the Nervous System Decides How Many and Which Motor Units to Activate for Each Movement

Motor unit activation is determined automatically by the neural control mechanisms, discussed later. The force generated is modulated by recruiting muscle fibers in increments of motor units. A motor unit consists of an α-motor

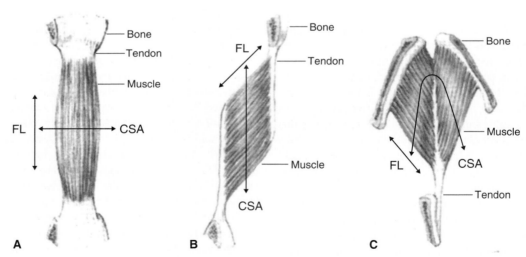

FIGURE 3.1 Examples of whole-muscle architecture demonstrating various muscle fiber arrangements. Muscle contraction velocity is proportional to FL, whereas contraction force is proportional to CSA. **A.** Longitudinal architecture designed to provide high contraction velocity. **B.** Pinnate architecture with fibers at a fixed angle relative to the axis of force generation to provide high contractile force while conserving space. This muscle generates more force and contracts more slowly than the muscle shown in A. **C.** Pinnate architecture with the fibers at varying angles relative to the axis of force generation. This muscle generates more force than the muscles in either A or B. All three muscles appear to be of similar size, but normalization of force or velocity to gross muscle size is misleading. FL, average fiber length; CSA, average fiber cross-sectional area. *(Reprinted with permission from Lieber RL. Skeletal muscle adaptability. I: Review of basic properties. Dev Med Child Neurol 1986;28:390–397.)*

neuron and all of the extrafusal muscle fibers that it innervates. The amount of force generated by a muscle at any particular instant is largely a function of the following:

1. Number of motor units activated
2. Frequency at which those motor units are activated
3. The total cross-sectional area of all of the muscle fibers controlled by those motor units

The total cross-sectional area of a given motor unit is determined primarily by the number of fibers in that motor unit. The size of the individual fibers also affects the total cross-sectional area, but this variable probably contributes less than 10% of the variance in the maximum force generated among motor units within a given motor pool (Fig. 3.2). When a regression line is plotted among fast and slow units, a smaller slope is seen among the slow units than among the fast units. This difference in the slopes is a reflection of the production of only a modestly smaller amount of force per cross-sectional area for slow than fast motor units.

Similarly, the phenotype of the muscle fibers of a given motor unit contributes to only a few percentage points of the range in forces generated among the motor units of a single muscle. All α-motor neurons that project to a given muscle collectively are called a motor pool. Each motor pool innervates different combinations of muscle fiber phenotypes, but each motor unit usually innervates only one fiber phenotype (Fig. 3.3). As noted earlier, the wide difference in the force-generating capability is attributable largely to the difference in the number of fibers innervated by the motor neuron.

Bodine-Fowler and associates (3) observed that within a muscle the cross-sectional area occupied by an individual motor unit, that is, the motor unit cross-sectional territory, in the predominantly fast tibialis anterior of the cat was about 10

to 25% of the total muscle cross-section, with the slow motor units generally having the smallest territories (Fig. 3.4). Similar calculations for the homogeneously slow cat soleus muscle yielded motor unit territories that are somewhat larger, ranging between 40 and 75% of the muscle cross-section.

Motor Unit Types

The concept of muscle fiber phenotypes is widely recognized (see Chapters 5–8), but the concept of motor unit phenotypes is less well recognized (Fig. 3.3). This is in part due to the absence of observations that specific molecular features of motor neuron phenotypes have been linked to specific molecular features of the muscle fibers of a motor unit, that is, the muscle unit. These phenotypic features of motor units depend largely on the properties of the muscle unit. There is, however, a long list of electrophysiological and morphological features that differentiate motor neuron types (Table 3.1). Unlike the muscle unit phenotypes that can be classified by specific profiles of protein isoforms, differences among motor neurons are largely linked to characteristics that fall on a continuous scale, such as cell body size, number of dendrites, total surface area, input resistance, threshold for depolarization, and so on.

Given the many features of motor neurons and the muscle fibers that they innervate, most motor units from a wide variety of animal species, including humans, fall within a general profile of one of three categories. These motor unit types have been identified according to their isometric contractile twitch speed and fatigability as fast fatigable, fast fatigue–resistant, and slow fatigue–resistant (4) (Fig. 3.3). A fourth category of motor units has been identified as fast intermediate, but in our view it does not represent a qualitatively unique fast type (4). An alternative nomenclature combines a physiological and a biochemical property, that is, fast glycolytic, fast oxidative, glycolytic, and slow oxidative (5). A simpler and more commonly used nomenclature relative to muscle fiber properties has been based only on the myosin phenotype, that is, slow (type I) or fast (type II) (see Chapter 5).

Linked tightly to the force-generating properties of motor unit types are the speed-related properties. In fact, this is implied in the nomenclature noted earlier. One of the explanations for these differences in velocities among different fiber types is the myosin isoform that is prominent among muscle fibers innervated by a given motor neuron (Fig. 3.3). However, it is also apparent that other factors within muscle fibers define their speed of shortening, such as different combinations of myosin light chains and C-protein.

Motor Unit Types and Recruitment

At this point it should begin to be clear why the concept of motor unit types plays a central role in understanding how muscle force is modulated. Thus, an understanding of how different types of motor units are recruited in normal movements is key to understanding how movements are controlled

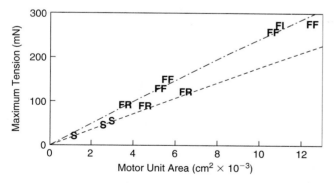

FIGURE 3.2 Relationship between the maximum tension and the total cross-sectional area of 11 glycogen-depleted motor units from the cat tibialis anterior identified as slow fatigue resistant (S), fast fatigue resistant (FR), fast fatigue intermediate (FI) and fast fatigable (FF). Regression lines represent the slow (- - -) and the fast (— · —) motor units. The correlations were 0.97 and 0.99 for the fast and slow motor units, respectively. *(Modified from Bodine SC, Roy RR, Eldred E, et al. Maximal force as a function of anatomical features of motor units in the cat tibialis anterior. J Neurophysiol 1987;57:1730–1745.)*

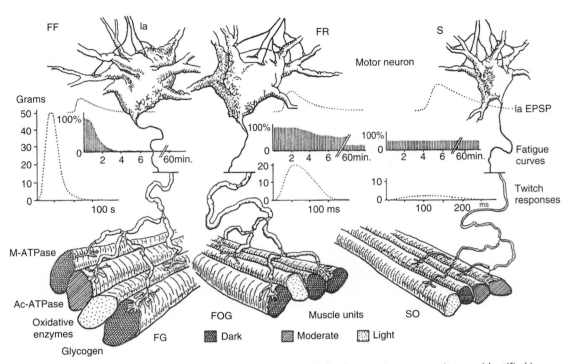

FIGURE 3.3 The most important features of the organization of the three major motor unit types identified in a typical predominantly fast mammalian muscle: FF, fast fatigable; FR, fast fatigue resistant; and S, slow fatigue resistant. The size of the motor neurons, axons, and muscle fibers are scaled appropriately for each motor unit type based on observations from a population of motor neurons. The density of Ia terminals and size of Ia excitatory postsynaptic potentials (EPSPs) are S > FR > FF, whereas the number of Ia terminals per motor neuron are approximately the same for each motor unit type. The shading of the muscle fibers denotes the relative staining intensity for each of the histochemical reactions identified in the fibers of the FF motor unit: M-ATPase, myofibrillar adenosinetriphosphatase, alkaline preincubation; AcATPase, myofibrillar ATPase, acid preincubation; oxidative, a representative marker of oxidative metabolic capacity; and glycolytic, a representative marker of glycolytic metabolic capacity. The M-ATPase staining is closely linked to the expression of specific myosin isoforms identified immuno-histochemically. The fatigue resistance to repetitive stimulation and the isometric twitch contraction time are S > FR > FF. The neurons with the largest cell bodies also have the largest dendritic trees and axons. The largest axons have the fastest conduction velocities. The larger axons also branch intramuscularly more times and innervate more muscle fibers than the smaller axons. FG, fast glycolytic fiber; FOG, fast oxidative glycolytic fiber; S slow oxidative fiber. (*Adapted with permission from Edington D, Edgerton V. The Biology of Physical Activity. Boston: Houghton Mifflin, 1976, p. 53*)

and why there is a link between the intensity of an exercise and the duration that this intensity can be sustained. This comprehension is fundamentally important in studying mechanisms related to exercise performance capacity and adaptability to a given type of exercise.

One of the most commonly used techniques to study how motor units are recruited is to identify the specific muscle fibers that have been depleted of glycogen following activation. An example of the range of staining levels for glycogen among fibers of a typical mixed, predominantly fast muscle, that is, the tibialis anterior of an adult cat, after repetitive stimulation of a single motor unit is shown in Figure 3.5. Fibers belonging to the same motor unit can be depleted of glycogen (no staining) by isolating the motor neuron or its axon and then repeatedly electrically stimulating it. Note

that there is a range of glycogen (staining) levels even among the muscle fibers that were not stimulated. In an animal with a diet containing sufficient carbohydrates, the lighter-staining (for glycogen) fibers are typically slow, whereas the darker-staining fibers are typically fast; that is, with the fast fatigue–resistant muscle units having the highest levels of glycogen. Note also the wide range in fiber size among the glycogen-depleted fibers, all of which are innervated by the same motor neuron. This variation in fiber size reflects the facts that most fibers in the cat tibialis anterior taper to a smaller size over a substantial length of the fiber and that the size of a fiber within a motor unit differs no matter where along its length it is sectioned (6). Also note that the glycogen-depleted fibers are spatially arranged within the cross-section of the muscle such that there are few adjacent

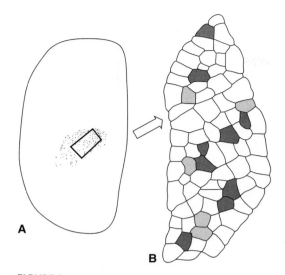

FIGURE 3.4 **A.** Distribution of depleted muscle fibers (dots) belonging to a single motor unit within a single muscle cross-section. The outlined region represents the area within the motor unit territory that was selected for analysis. **B.** A single fascicle within the selected area of the motor unit. All fibers were classified as being depleted or not depleted on the basis of periodic acid-Schiff staining and slow or fast on the basis of myosin ATPase (alkaline preincubation) staining. Muscle fibers in the fascicle are identified as depleted motor unit fibers (shaded), slow undepleted fibers (dark), or fast undepleted fibers (white) *(Modified from Bodine SC, Garfinkel A, Roy RR, et al. Spatial distribution of motor unit fibers in the cat soleus and tibialis anterior muscles: local interactions. J Neurosci 1988;8:2142–2152.)*

depleted fibers. There seems to be some mechanism during development to prevent adjacent fibers from being innervated by the same motor neuron (7). The tissue section in Figure 3.5 shows only a small proportion of the muscle fibers that were depleted and thus innervated by the same motor neuron. Figure 3.4 shows the cross-section of a muscle along with the total region of the muscle cross-section that was occupied by a single motor unit, that is, the motor unit territory. Although the physiological significance of the spatial distribution of muscle fibers and the cross-sectional territory of a muscle unit are unknown, these probably reflect important features that the nervous system must take into account in modulation of continuously changing forces during a movement.

Relationship Between Motor Unit Architecture and Physiological Properties

There is some clear clinical relevance to the spatial distribution of muscle fibers of a single motor unit. For example, if one suspects damage to the peripheral nerves, which occurs in some chronic overuse syndromes, the clinician may study the activation properties of single motor units using an indwelling recording electrode. In such a case, if the electrode is inserted to the middle of the region of this motor unit, the highest-amplitude action potential will be recorded (highest density of fibers generating action potentials simultaneously). If the recording tip of the electrode is outside this region, an action potential is recorded, but its amplitude is smaller (lower density of activated fibers and more distance from the recording electrodes). All muscle fibers of the motor unit will generate an action potential at essentially the same time. Thus, there will be a single action potential shape recorded for all muscle fibers for each activation signal generated by a given motor neuron. The importance of re-

Property	Slow	Fast Fatigue Resistant	Fast Fatigable
Soma diameter (micrometers)	49	53	53.0
Total membrane area (micrometers)	249	323	369.0
Stem dendrite number	12	12.6	10.0
Input resistance (megaohms)	1.6–2.6	0.9–1.0	0.6
Rheobase (nanoamperes)	5	12	21.3
Threshold depolarization (millivolts)	14.4	18.5	20.1
Afterhyperpolarization duration (milliseconds)	161	78	65.0
Minimum firing frequency (impulses per second)*	10	1.4	22.0
Maximum firing frequency (impulses per second)*	20	+++	70.0
Current/frequency slope (impulses per second per nanoampere)	1.4	53.0	1.4
Late adaptation	+	369.0	+++
Membrane bistability	++	10.0	+

TABLE 3.1 Morphological and Electrophysiological Properties of Cat Motor Neurons Innervating Various Motor Unit Types

*Primary range of firing.

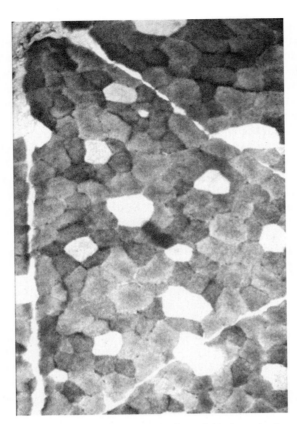

FIGURE 3.5 Contrast between the staining intensity for the periodic acid-Schiff reaction (glycogen content) in depleted and surrounding undepleted fibers of a motor unit in the cat tibialis anterior. The motor unit fibers were depleted of glycogen by ventral root teasing of a single axon innervating the muscle and repetitive stimulation of the ventral root in a preparation in situ. Among the undepleted fibers, the fast fibers typically stain darker than the slow fibers. *(Unpublished micrograph.)*

cording these action potentials that represent the electrical properties of a single motor neuron is that it provides one of the most readily available sites from which neurons from the nervous system can be observed *in vivo*.

Motor Pools

As noted previously, all of the motor neurons that innervate fibers within the same muscle constitute a motor pool. A motor pool is usually distributed over several contiguous spinal cord segments. Within this cluster or pool the size and type of motor neurons seem to be spatially distributed in a random fashion (8). For example, a motor neuron of a given type is as likely to occur in one region of the pool as another. A similar randomness of location within a motor pool seems to be true for the smaller α-motor neurons that innervate the intrafusal muscle fibers of a primary sensory organ within the muscle, that is, the muscle spindles (discussed later).

All motor pools are located in the ventral horn of the gray matter of the spinal cord. The axonal projections of these motor neurons exit the spinal cord as a ventral root. This ventral root contains thousands of axons from multiple motor pools. As these axonal projections from several spinal ventral roots extend peripherally, they merge to form large peripheral nerves that project further peripherally and begin to subdivide into muscle nerves as they reach a given muscle. At the point that the single axon of each motor neuron reaches the muscle, the axon will divide into as many branches as necessary to innervate all of the muscle fibers of a given muscle unit. For example if a motor neuron innervates 300 muscle fibers, it will have at least 300 branches. If it innervates only two muscle fibers, the axon will branch only once (as occurs in some extraocular muscle units).

The nerve trunks formed by the merging of ventral roots also contain sensory axons that project from the periphery toward the spinal cord via dorsal roots. The peripheral nerves, on the other hand, are mixed in the sense that they have axons projecting action potentials both distally (peripherally) to the muscles (motor) and centrally (sensory) to the spinal cord.

The spinal cord can be readily divided into white and gray matter. The white matter contains few cell bodies and is composed primarily of ascending and descending axons. In general the gray matter of the spinal cord contains cell bodies along with some axons and dendrites. The dorsal horn of the gray matter contains neurons that receive input from multiple sources, including the brain, higher segmental levels within the cord itself, and from the sensory input from the periphery. An anatomical depiction of the complexity and orientation of the axonal projections along a coronal slice within the spinal gray matter is shown in Figure 3.6. In general, input from the brain and periphery will travel from the dorsal edge of the dorsal horn toward the ventral horn, eventually reaching a motor neuron within a given motor pool.

Size Principle of Recruitment Within a Motor Pool

Among all of the attempts to understand how the nervous system controls movement, the efforts that resulted in the formulation of the size principle of motor unit recruitment have been the most significant. As noted previously, the motor neurons within a motor pool are generally distributed spatially within an elongated, core-shaped volume in a very predictable position within the gray matter of the ventral horn of the spinal cord. Although the motor neurons within this confined region are randomly distributed with respect to the type and size, there is an impressive consistency in the order of the sequence of activation of these motor neurons within each pool. The size principle states that within a single motor pool the motor neurons will be recruited in order of ascending size, the smallest first and the largest last, regardless of the type of effort (9,10).

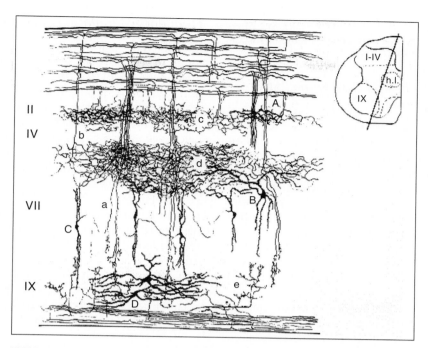

FIGURE 3.6 Slightly oblique sagittal section through the cat spinal cord at L6 showing the complexity and orientation of the axonal projections. Much of the supraspinal and peripheral input travels from the dorsum to activate interneurons and eventually the motoneurons located in the gray matter. A: Gelatinosa cell; B: Cell at interface between intermediate nucleus of Cajal, d, whose axonal neuropile is longitudinally oriented, and the underlying lamina VII, where the neuropile is essentially dorsoventrally oriented, as exemplified by the dendrite orientation of interneuron C; D: Motoneurons of the ventral flexor pool; a, terminal components of a small microbundle of primary afferent collaterals; b, individual primary afferent apparently breaking up in the intermediate nuclear pool; c, gelatinosa neuropile; e, terminal collaterals from anterior funiculus. Inset diagram shows plane and postistion of the section and identifies the location of the spinal cord laminae. Rapid Golgi modification, X155. *(Modified from Scheibel M, Scheibel A. A structural analysis of spinal interneurons and Renshaw cells. In Brazier MAB, ed. UCLA Forum in Medical Science: The Interneuron. Los Angeles: University of California Press, 1969, p. 177.)*

Defining the Size of a Motor Unit

An obvious question is which features of a motor unit best reflect its size. This has been the topic of numerous experiments, and although there is not complete agreement among scientists studying this issue, there is a consensus. The data presented in Table 3.1 show that the smallest motor neurons have the smallest soma membrane surface area and the fewest dendrites and branches, and they innervate the fewest muscle fibers. The smallest motor units also generate the smallest amount of force, since the number of muscle fibers determines, in large part, the amount of force generated by a given motor unit. The opposite is true for the largest motor neurons. Thus, although a large number of parameters are highly correlated with motor unit recruitment order, the amount of force that a motor unit can generate is one of the most consistent to date (11) (Fig. 3.3).

How the Size of the Motor Neuron Determines Order of Recruitment

The most basic explanation for the size principle is that the net excitatory current needed to reach the activation threshold of a motor neuron is inversely related to the total surface area of the membrane of the motor neuron (12). Since it appears that all sources of input to a given motor pool are more or less evenly distributed among the motor neurons, the smaller the motor neuron, the more likely that it will be excited when the motor pool is presented with a given level of depolarizing current from all of its synapses. As noted earlier, the amount of input from a given source is generally evenly distributed among the motor neurons of a given motor pool. An analogy would be water spouts releasing water at the same rate placed over buckets differing in size: the smallest bucket would always be filled first; that is, its threshold would be reached first. As noted earlier, the amount of input from a given source is generally evenly distributed among the motor neurons of a given motor pool.

Identifying Motor Units and Their Firing Patterns Using Electromyography

The order of recruitment within a motor pool can be readily observed by recording the action potentials from muscles using electromyography (EMG). The firing patterns of single motor units can be recorded from electrodes placed on the skin overlying a specific muscle (surface EMG) or more readily from needle or fine wire electrodes placed in the muscle. Action potentials from single motor units can be discerned more easily when the active recording sites of the electrodes are very small and there is a small distance between electrodes. It is also easier to identify action potentials from a single motor unit when small forces are produced, that is, when a small number of motor units are recruited (Fig. 3.7).

Action potentials belonging to the same motor unit can be identified by the similarity in their amplitude and shape. The uniqueness of the amplitude and shape for a given motor unit action potential is a function of the location of the active electrode recording site relative to the fibers within the motor unit. As the force exerted increases, motor units with larger action potentials, that is the larger motor units, will be recruited, as dictated by the size principle. Generally, the larger motor units generate a higher-amplitude action potential because the signal is derived from more muscle fibers than for the smaller motor units. Therefore, in general, under controlld isometric condition there is a direct relationship between the force and EMG amplitude during motor unit recruitment (Fig. 3.7). Often the force threshold for derecruitment is lower than that for recruitment (Fig. 3.8). There is no clear explanation for this hysteresis effect.

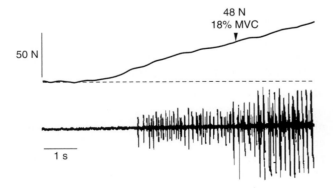

FIGURE 3.7 Recording of motor unit potentials in a human subject during a ramp force generated by the plantarflexors. Larger action potentials appear at selected levels of torque, representing the force threshold for that motor unit. Each action potential generated by a given motor unit will have a similar amplitude and shape. Only the amplitudes can be differentiated in this graph because of the slow time scale in plotting the graph. (*Unpublished observation, V.R. Edgerton*)

Frequency Modulation of Motor Units

In addition to the recruitment of more motor units, muscle force can be modulated by the frequency of activation of the motor units (Fig. 3.9). There have been a number of studies to determine the relative importance of these two mechanisms in modulating force, but there is no consensus on this issue. There seems to be a difference in their relative importance from muscle to muscle (13) and in the amount of force being exerted within a muscle. At the lower forces, recruitment seems to be the more important, whereas at the higher force levels, frequency modulation may become more important. For example, if there are 100 motor units in a motor pool, motor unit 5 in the recruitment order would probably have its frequency modulated during a contraction force requiring only 10% of the maximum force potential. If the muscle force required was at 80% of maximum, however, unit 5 would have already been activated at its maximum frequency. Most of the frequency modulation is likely to occur among the motor units that have been most recently recruited or derecruited as the force is increasing or decreasing, respectively.

Another feature associated with frequency modulation is that motor units seem to have an initial (minimum) firing frequency of 5 to 10 Hz, that is, action potentials per second. The maximum frequencies vary among motor units, with the higher-threshold units generating the higher frequencies within a burst of potentials, mostly in the range of 25 to 35 Hz. Single individual interspike intervals, however, can be as long as 200 Hz.

The amount and rate of current presented to a motor neuron will define its frequency response. Once the current reaches a certain level, there will be no further frequency modulation of that unit. As more excitatory input is presented to the motor pool, however, additional motor units will be recruited. Figure 3.10 shows the relationship between frequency of excitation and the amount of force generated by a slow and a fast muscle. The curve for the fast muscle is shifted to the right compared to the curve for the slow muscle. This reflects the greater speed of force development and relaxation in the fast muscle and therefore the necessity for a higher frequency to reach the same relative force as a slow muscle.

An example of both recruitment and frequency modulation of motor units from a human muscle is shown in Figure 3.11.

Several additional features of frequency modulation of motor unit activation have important implications for the generation of force and control of movement. For example, the catch principle can be described as follows (14): the interval between two consecutive action potentials within a motor unit and the previous history of this interval duration within a given burst of action potentials can be critically important in defining the force generated by a motor unit. In Figure 3.12, a motor unit is stimulated with a consistent frequency to serve as a control. When there is a prolonged inter-

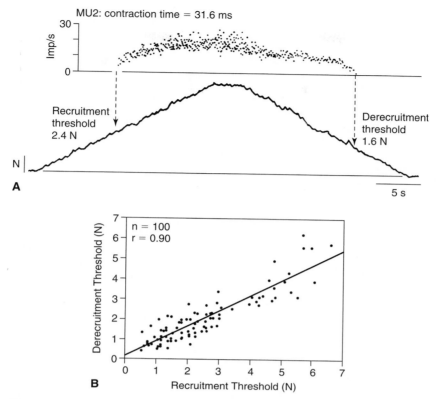

FIGURE 3.8 **A.** Recruitment and derecruitment of a motor unit in the extensor carpi radialis of human subjects during isometric imposed-ramp contraction and relaxation. Derecruitment threshold is lower than recruitment threshold. **B.** Relationship between recruitment and derecruitment thresholds for 20 extensor carpi radialis motor units. Again, the derecruitment threshold is systematically lower than the recruitment threshold. *(Modified from Romaiguere P, Vedel JP, Pagni S. Comparison of fluctuations of motor unit recruitment and de-recruitment thresholds in man. Exp Brain Res 1993;95:517–522.)*

pulse interval in the middle of a train of impulses, the tension will drop significantly and continue at this lower level even though subsequent pulses are identical to those of the control condition. The significance of this observation is that this catch property provides a mechanism by which the nervous system can provide remarkably subtle changes in the excitation pattern to produce a significant modulation of force (15).

Ballistic-type resistance training (involving maximal intentional rate of force development) markedly increases the incidence of doublets, that is, two successive action potentials with an unusually short interspike interval. Training with dynamic contractions results in more synchronous firing of motor units at the start of a brisk contraction (16). Although there are clear examples of short interpulse intervals occurring early in a burst, when the force ramp is very rapid, it remains unclear to what extent the nervous system can and does use this mechanism.

To understand how the central nervous system (CNS) modulates the force, it is convenient to think of the relative and absolute forces generated by a motor pool relative to the percent of the motor neurons activated within that motor pool. As discussed previously, motor units generally are assumed to be recruited according to the size principle. If all motor units were the same size, the relationship between the number of motor units recruited and the cumulative force from the active units would be linear. The forces generated during walking or even running are small relative to the maximum force that can be generated by the motor pool. Although only about 20% of the maximum force potential of the muscle may be required during running, more than 50% of the motor units in the motor pool are recruited (Fig. 3.13). There also is a high probability that the smaller motor units are the slow type, the fast fatigue–resistant units are moderate size, and the fast fatigable units are the largest units and recruited last (Fig. 3.3). This is not to mean, however, that this order and type relationship is rigid. Although the same level of detail for human motor units is not available, there is indirect evidence that the same principles apply (17).

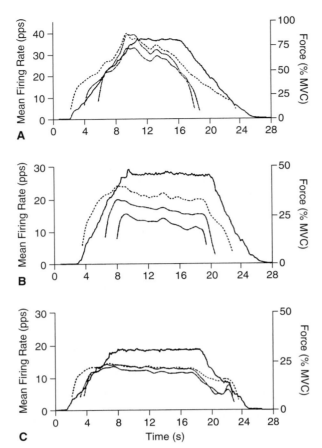

FIGURE 3.9 Examples of firing rates of motor units in tibialis anterior during isometric dorsiflexion of the ankle at (**A**) 80%, (**B**) 50%, and (**C**) 30% of maximum voluntary contraction (MVC). The force record (showing plateau) is the thick line. The other three lines show mean firing rates of detected motor units. Firing rates decrease throughout the constant-force interval at all force levels. *(Reprinted with permission from de Luca CJ, Foley PJ, Erim Z. Motor unit control properties in constant-force isometric contractions. J Neurophysiol 1996;76:1503–1516.)*

It is also useful to recognize that not all motor pools and muscles have the same proportion of motor unit types. There even is remarkable variability for any given muscle from individual to individual. Figure 3.14 illustrates the range in tetanic forces, isometric twitch times, and fatigability among a population of motor units within the cat medial gastrocnemius motor pool.

Changes in Recruitment Order

Even though the size principle seems to explain many features of motor unit recruitment, in some situations other neural control factors are operating. It appears that in some physiological states the usual order of recruitment of motor units within a pool can be altered. For example, electrical stimulation of the skin over the index finger in humans can change the order of recruitment of motor units within the

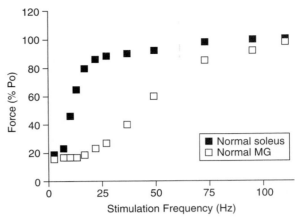

FIGURE 3.10 Relationships of relative force (percent of maximum tetanic tension, Po) and frequency of stimulation for a typical fast (medial gastrocnemius [MG]) and a typical slow (soleus) rat hindlimb muscle. A higher frequency of stimulation is necessary to produce the same relative force in a fast than a slow muscle. The same relationship exists at the motor unit level. *(Modified from Roy RR, Baldwin KM, Martin TP, et al. Biochemical and physiological changes in overloaded rat fast- and slow-twitch ankle extensors. J Appl Physiol 1985;59:639–646.)*

first dorsal interosseous muscle during isometric contractions (18). Changes in recruitment order also have been reported in very rapid contractions compared to very slowly increasing the force in an isometric contraction (19). A more significant change in recruitment order seems to occur when a muscle is activated in a rapid eccentric compared to a slow isometric contraction (20). It appears that in the eccentric mode there is some selection of fast motor units in preference

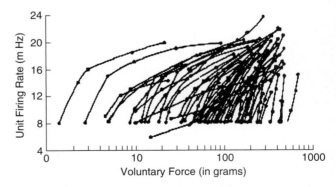

FIGURE 3.11 Firing frequencies of individual motor units in human extensor digitorum communis muscle. All units discharge in approximately the same frequency range but for different ranges of voluntary force. The frequency for the smaller, lower-threshold motor units has peaked before many of the larger, high-threshold motor units are recruited initially. *(Modified from Stuart DG, Enoka RM. Motoneurons, motor units, and the size principle. New York: Churchill Livingstone, 1983, p. 486.)*

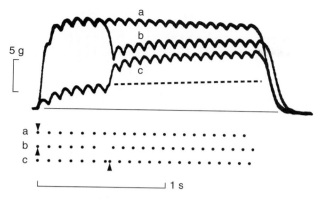

FIGURE 3.12 Tension responses of a slow medial gastrocnemius motor unit to three trains of 22 stimuli each at a basic rate of 12.2 pps (interpulse interval, 82 ms). In each train, one or two stimulus intervals were altered. The tension traces are labeled *a* to *c*, and the corresponding pulse sequences are similarly designated. The arrows at the first pulses in *a* and *b* indicate double stimulation with an interpulse interval of 10 ms. The arrow in *c* denotes a single pulse following the previous pulse with an interval shorter than that in the basic train but longer (about 26 ms) than the double stimuli in *a* and *b*. In trace *b*, the tension drops to a new level when one interval in the train was lengthened to about 117 ms. This sensitivity to single interspike intervals in the generation of force illustrates that it is critical to control single intervals in generating and maintaining a given force level and that a short interval at the beginning can have a lasting effect on a train of impulses. This phenomenon is referred to as the "catch property." *(Modified from Burke RE, Rudomin P, Zajac FE 3rd. Catch property in single mammalian motor units. Science 1970;168:122–124.)*

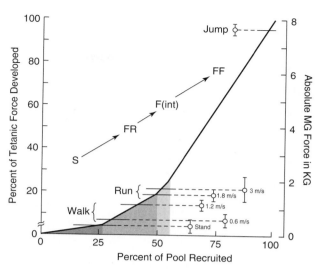

FIGURE 3.13 Recruitment model for medial gastrocnemius (MG) motor unit pool based on distributions of motor unit types and of maximum tetanic tension for individual motor units. The heavy solid curve indicates estimated percentage of maximum (fused tetanus) MG force (left ordinate) as a function of percentage MG pool recruited (abscissa). (See original reference for assumptions.) Intensity of shading beneath the curve denotes relative fatigue resistance of the motor unit groups in MG (types S > FR > F(int) > FF). The assumption for generating the cumulative force is that all motor units are recruited in order of increasing size. The labeled circles and brackets indicate means ± SD MG forces during standing, locomotion at various speeds, and 120-cm jumps, all referred to right ordinate scaled in kilogram weight. There is no clear line of demarcation of motor units of a certain size being of the same type. It is more accurate to view the graph as a progressively changing probability, with the smaller motor units probably being slow and the largest motor units probably being fast fatigable units. *(Modified from Walmsley B, Hodgson JA, Burke RE. Forces produced by medial gastrocnemius and soleus muscles during locomotion in freely moving cats. J Neurophysiol 1978;41:1203–1216.)*

to the usually more excitable smaller slow motor units. Another apparent exception can be seen in a paw shake compared to locomotion in cats in the relative recruitment of the slow soleus and the fast medial gastrocnemius (21). However, this is a reversal of recruitment order of motor neurons across rather within a motor pool.

There also is evidence of an alternation (rotation) in motor unit recruitment in repetitive and prolonged movements (22). For example, Tamaki and associates (23) reported a rotation in the activation of the triceps surae muscles during low-level contractions, indicating that there were sudden and frequent changes in the combinations of motor units and motor pools being recruited during these prolonged efforts.

There are some exceptions to the size principle, and several important questions relate their significance and to how they should be interpreted. In very rapid contractions the order of the action potentials of a pair of motor units is probably trivial in terms of the functional consequences. There is always the question of how far apart in excitability are the thresholds of the motor units showing a change in recruitment order. If they have very similar thresholds, they will readily rotate in order. Another fundamental issue relates to the definition of a motor pool. Many muscles are divided anatomically,

and to some extent physiologically, into neuromuscular compartments (2,24). For example, the cat lateral gastrocnemius muscle has four anatomically distinct compartments that can be independently recruited during locomotion, as reflected by EMG recordings from each compartment (25). In humans, superficial and deep compartments in the tibialis anterior can be controlled somewhat independently; this is assumed to be reflected by the activation of different regions of the cerebral cortex when recruiting these two compartments (26). These anatomical and physiological properties both neurally and muscularly suggest that there is likely to be some degree of flexibility on the order of recruitment within a single muscle.

There have been many disputes about the consistency of the size principle. It is our view that with some exceptions, in most cases the order of recruitment is remarkably constant. In terms of a neural control strategy, this would seem

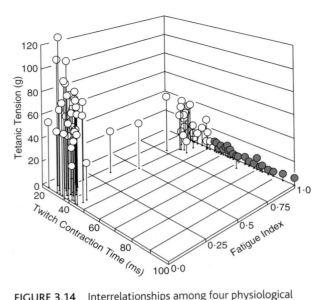

FIGURE 3.14 Interrelationships among four physiological properties of 81 medial gastrocnemius muscle units in a representative sample pooled from three animals. Open circles denote units with sag in unfused tetani (types FF and FR); stippled circles, those without sag (type S). Clustering of unit groups in different regions of the multidimensional space is defined by the four parameters. (*Modified from Burke RE, Levine DN, Tsairis P, et al. Physiological types and histochemical profiles in motor units of the cat gastrocnemius. J Physiol (Lond) 1973;234:723–748.*)

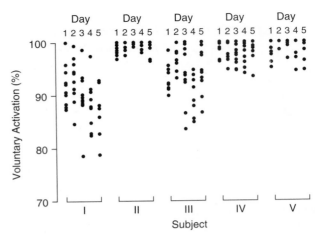

FIGURE 3.15 Ability to activate elbow flexors maximally during a MVC varies among trials on the same day among subjects. Five subjects were given ten trials on each of five days. Voluntary activation was calculated as (1 − superimposed twitch in response to electrical stimulation during MVC/twitch at rest) × 100, a technique called twitch interpolation. (*Modified from Allen GM, Gandevia SC, McKenzie DK. Reliability of measurements of muscle strength and voluntary activation using twitch interpolation. Muscle Nerve 1995;18:593–600.*)

to greatly simplify the control. It seems logical, given the predictability of the type and kind of work that the neuromotor system routinely performs, that a relatively fixed order can be a very significant advantage in survivability.

Limitations in the Ability to Maximally Recruit All Motor Units Within a Motor Pool

Can an individual recruit all motor units within a motor pool? Intuitively one may assume that the nervous system can routinely recruit even the highest-threshold motor units within a motor pool. However, this does not seem to be the case (Fig. 3.15). For example, when five subjects were asked to generate a maximum voluntary plantarflexion on multiple occasions within a single day and over a period of 5 days, the maximum torque that could be generated was estimated to vary between 78 and 100%. This assessment was based on a technique called "twitch interpolation," whereby the muscle is electrically stimulated with a single maximum pulse during the maximum voluntary contraction. If the twitch adds force to the maximum voluntary effort, the contraction is interpreted as a submaximal effort. None of the subjects could produce a maximal effort on every occasion during a maximum voluntary effort. In fact, one subject could recruit all motor units on only one occasion of several attempts. However, some studies use a short tetanus rather than a twitch

and report that a twitch may not be enough to ensure a maximum contraction. The relative ability to recruit all motor units within a motor pool also does not seem to be closely related to the level of training of the individual. Although some improvement can be observed with practice, there still remains a high incidence of some submaximal efforts when one is attempting to generate the maximum force.

Size Principle Across Motor Pools

There is some evidence for a size recruitment principle that operates across motor pools (27). For example, the recruitment order would be independent of the pools but dependent on the size within the combined motor pools. But this observation still does not address what are the neural mechanisms for selecting different portions of multiple pools to be recruited for a given movement or task. A movement may require 10, 50, and 80% of the motor units recruited from three motor pools. The nervous system then may select 15, 45, and 80% of the motor units from these same motor pools to generate a slightly different movement. There is little insight as to how the nervous system matches an intention to make a precise movement with the precise combination of motor units that are recruited during a movement.

Relative Levels of Recruitment of Motor Unit Types During Routine Movements

To identify the stimuli that may be responsible for inducing metabolic adaptations to exercise, it is important to understand some fundamental features of the strategy used by the CNS to execute movements varying in force, velocity, and duration. What neural control strategies allow an individual to run faster or run uphill, or to bicycle at a fast pedaling rate on the flat versus on a 5° incline?

Differential Activation of Extensors and Flexors

During treadmill locomotion in intact quadrupeds (28) a hyperbolic relationship exists between the step cycle duration and the speed of locomotion (Fig. 3.16). Furthermore, as the speed of locomotion increases, the duration of the support phase of each step cycle decreases more than the swing phase (29). These relationships also have been observed in low thoracic, chronically spinalized cats during assisted treadmill locomotion and in the individual legs of decerebrate cats walking on a split treadmill when each belt moved at different speeds (28,30).

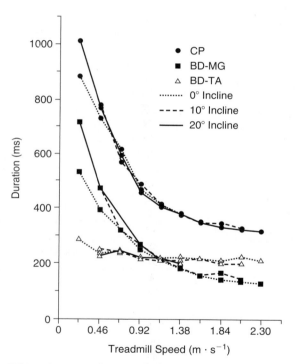

FIGURE 3.16   Cycle period (CP) and burst durations (BD) of an ankle extensor, the medial gastrocnemius (MG), and an ankle flexor, the tibialis anterior (TA), plotted against treadmill speed and incline for one cat. The duration of the MG is consistently about 200 ms shorter than the cycle period, while the duration of the TA remains constant. As the animal runs faster, the CP becomes shorter, with most of the reduction in cycle duration due to a shortening of extensor muscle BD, with little change in the TA BD. (Modified from Pierotti DJ, Roy RR, Gregor RJ, et al. Electromyographic activity of cat hindlimb flexors and extensors during locomotion at varying speeds and inclines. Brain Res 1989;481:57–66.)

In accordance with the assumption that the size principle is a predominant factor in determining the order of recruitment within a motor pool, the high threshold, fast-contracting fibers that can produce the highest tensions will be activated when the demands on the work rate are increased (Figs. 3.11 and 3.13). At higher speeds and/or inclines, the fast muscles can provide most of the additional power necessary to complete the work in the time available per step. Because of the greater rise of the animal's center of gravity, the extensor musculature must complete more work per step when the incline is increased. When speed is increased along with incline, more work—that is, more power—must be produced in shorter periods. EMG recordings indicate that the excitability of motor units of different types, sizes, and thresholds holds true, at least to some degree, across motor pools, as it does within a motor pool (9). Changes in the duration of the swing phase of a step cycle are small, and the inertial forces imposed on the leg are relatively constant over a range of speeds.

In adult cats, the horizontal distance that the hip travels during the support phase increases from about 16 to almost 30 cm over a range of speeds of locomotion from 0.1 to 0.9 m · s⁻¹ on the flat (30). However, it also has been reported that the cat's joint angles at the hip, knee, and ankle remain relatively constant during a walk and a trot (31). These observations demonstrate that the strategy to control extensor muscles must differ from those of the flexor musculature, particularly during load-bearing locomotion. The presence of these common features in activation among flexor and extensor motor pools in such a variety of species and conditions demonstrates a fundamental neural strategy in the control of locomotion at varying speeds and intensities. It remains unclear what features of which neural circuitry are responsible for the asymmetrical modulation of extensors and flexors as one runs faster.

A fundamental variable to control speed of locomotion at a given incline is the activation level of extensor motor pools. The levels of excitation of the extensor and flexor motor pools are important with respect to the time and the distance the animal travels. These time–distance factors also have metabolic consequences. Hoyt and Taylor (32) demonstrated that the rate of energy consumption in horses at a given gait increases linearly with stride frequency. Indeed, the integrated EMG per minute of the fast extensors increased linearly with speed. The additional effort required for locomotion at increased speeds and inclines seems to be supplied primarily by the fast extensor muscles. While the mean EMG per minute of predominantly fast muscles increases with speed and incline, it actually decreases in the slower soleus. This results in a higher power output of type II fast muscles and a relative decrease in the power output of the type I slow soleus (33). Gregor and associates (34) reported a 20% decrease in soleus and a 40% increase in medial gastrocnemius *in vivo* tendon peak forces at comparable speeds and inclines. It appears that the soleus may be at a mechanical disadvantage in the latter stages of the stance phase, when the velocity of shortening required to produce force is at its highest. Additionally, the soleus could become slightly unloaded due to a greater amount of force contributed by its major synergists.

Type of Contraction and Energy Cost

Whether a movement involves principally isometric, shortening, or lengthening contractions also has a significant effect on the fatigue properties and the neural control strategies. For example, the neural control strategies used by subjects differed significantly when they were asked to make repetitive maximum contractions at the knee in a concentric versus an eccentric mode (35). The level of activation progressively increased with repeated concentric contractions, whereas the activation level remained relatively constant with repeated eccentric contractions (Fig. 3.17). This differential neural response is linked to the fact that energy expenditure is much lower during lengthening than concentric contractions (36). These features are likely related to the fundamentally different mechanical dynamics with respect to the metabolic cost per cross-bridge cycle and the duration of the force-generating stage of the cross-bridge interactions between these two contractile modes.

The significance of the size principle and the consistency of the control of different joints is that the neural control is closely linked to the metabolic properties of the skeletal muscle via motor unit types. Therefore, the nature of the movement will have a very predictable consequence with respect to fatigue, energy consumption, and even the type of substrates that are used in a given type of effort.

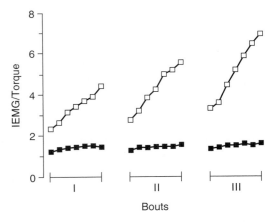

FIGURE 3.17 Integrated (I) EMG/torque ratio during concentric (CON) (*open squares*) and eccentric (ECC) (*solid squares*) bouts of exercise. IEMG for the vastus lateralis and rectus femoris muscles were combined and averaged. The progressive increase in the ratio during CON is progressive, but ECC contractions from bouts I to III are not. There was a higher IEMG during the maximum CON than ECC contractions. *(Modified from Tesch PA, Dudley GA, Duvoisin MR, et al. Force and EMG signal patterns during repeated bouts of concentric or eccentric muscle actions. Acta Physiol Scand 1990;138:263–271.)*

The Pattern of Glycogen Loss in Skeletal Muscle Fibers: Consistent With the Size Principle of Recruitment

As shown in Figure 3.5, the amount of glycogen in a skeletal muscle fiber can be semiquantitatively assessed using a dye that binds to glycogen, that is, the histochemical periodic acid-Schiff (PAS) reaction. The amount of glycogen in a muscle fiber is determined by the rate of glycogen degradation (largely a function of the level of contractile activity and the metabolic profile of the muscle fiber) and the rate of glycogen synthesis (37).

Taking these variables into account, one can gain considerable insight into the interactions among the metabolic properties of muscle fibers, muscle fiber phenotypes, and the recruitment strategies used by the nervous system. For example, in Figure 3.18 the changes in the level of glycogen in four fiber phenotypes in response to different intensity levels of exercise performed over 60 to 80 minutes reflect a combination of metabolic and phenotypic properties along with recruitment strategies. When subjects exercised at 43% of maximum oxygen uptake for 60 minutes, there was a gradual loss of glycogen only in the type I fibers. At this low intensity of exercise, type II fibers were recruited minimally, and although they have a relatively low oxidative capacity, little glycogen loss was observed. When the subjects exercised at a slightly higher percentage (61%) of their maximum, some glycogen was lost from the type IIa fibers, and according to the size principle, these fibers' motor units would be expected to be recruited after the type 1 fibers. At the highest power output (91% of maximum), all fiber types were recruited to a significant degree. However, there still was slightly less glycogen loss in type II than type I fibers. Two points should be highlighted. First, these data are consistent with the orderly recruitment of motor units according to the size principle, even at very high power outputs. Second, although all fiber types lost glycogen at the highest power output, because of the glycogen-sparing effect of the high oxidative capacity of the type I fibers, one cannot conclude that type II fibers were recruited as often as type I fibers.

In another variation of this experiment, subjects worked intermittently to exhaustion at 75% of their maximum oxygen uptake (38). The level of glycogen depletion was consistent with the expected recruitment levels among fiber phenotypes; that is, the least depletion was observed in the fast type IIb (largest and least recruited) fibers, and the most depletion in slow type I fibers. Although the subjects exercised to exhaustion, the type IIb and IIa fibers still had approximately half of their normal glycogen content. This indicates that considerable glycogen can remain in some muscle fibers even at exhaustion. It is extremely difficult to deplete all of the glycogen in all of the muscle fibers by exercising, and a significant level of glycogen depletion in most of the fibers occurs only when the exercise is about 75 to 85% of maximum. If the exercise

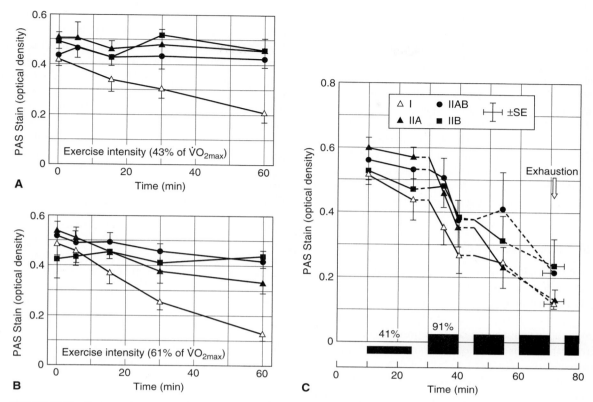

FIGURE 3.18   Decrease in average glycogen content (measured by periodic acid-Schiff staining intensity) of individual fiber types in the vastus lateralis during bicycle ergometer exercise at several intensities: (**A**) 43%, (**B**) 61%, and (**C**) 91% of maximal oxygen consumption. The higher the work rate, the higher the proportion of glycogen depletion in the larger motor units, that is, those that require more excitatory input to reach their excitation threshold. *(Modified from Vollestad NK, Blom PC. Effect of varying exercise intensity on glycogen depletion in human muscle fibres. Acta Physiol Scand 1985;125:395–405.)*

intensity is greater, most fibers will not be depleted of glycogen unless the high-intensity exercise is repeated a number of times. In other words, glycogen depletion as a factor in fatigue is likely to be important only in a limited number of exercise scenarios. In general, the results shown in Figure 3.18 are consistent with a combination of two factors:

1. The relative probability of recruitment of a given muscle fiber phenotype.
2. The relative differences in the oxidative capacity and glycogen-sparing properties of the muscle fiber phenotypes.

Spinal Control of Posture and Locomotion

Historically the level of control that the spinal cord can have in performing postural and locomotor tasks has been substantially underestimated. Some new insight is now being gained into the properties of the spinal cord that enable it to

execute these tasks largely without supraspinal control. Some of the reflexes commonly used to test motor function will be examined, with a focus on the phenomenon of central pattern generation (CPG) within the spinal cord. Emphasis is on the concept of spinal automaticity, that is, the ability of the neural circuitry of the spinal cord to interpret complex sensory information and to make appropriate decisions to generate successful postural and locomotor tasks (39). Much of our understanding of how the spinal cord can control locomotion is based on studies of a wide range of the vertebrates (28).

The mechanical and electrical events during locomotion are so closely linked that when the locomotion is being performed in a constant environment, the knowledge of the EMG activity of only one muscle provides extensive predictability of the activity patterns and the kinematic patterns of the limbs during locomotion. These observations suggest that individual muscles and joints are controlled by the nervous system not as individual components but as a highly interactive system with all of its components highly interdependent. The implications to locomotion are that the control system can essentially vary a single parameter to achieve locomotion over a range of speeds. This greatly simplifies the neural control by reducing the degrees of freedom that must be controlled to execute very complex but largely stereotypical movements, at least in a constant environment. It is this type of control that has led to the evolution of the concept of automaticity or the automatism of stepping.

Although there is remarkable consistency in the overall activation patterns, an important point about the neural control mechanisms of locomotion is that the activity patterns of the muscles vary much more than the kinematic patterns. This means that the nervous system can generate multiple patterns of activity and still accomplish basically the same mechanical effects.

Central Pattern Generation

CPG is a physiological phenomenon in which an oscillatory motor output is generated in the absence of any oscillatory input (28). In mammalian systems, CPG represents an important component of the neural circuitry in the lumbosacral spinal cord that generates and controls posture and locomotion. There are other examples of CPGs in biological systems, such as those associated with breathing and chewing. Considerable progress has been made in understanding the circuitry that can generate CPGs by using relatively simple vertebrate systems, such as the lamprey (40). This has been helpful to understanding neural control in humans because in the evolution of the neural control of movement, conservation of the circuitry and the neurotransmitters of the circuitry is remarkable. In this chapter, we focus on CPG in mammalian systems associated with locomotion.

A major challenge for biologists has been to identify the mechanisms for CPG. One general hypothesis is that the oscillatory output is generated by specific neurons that behave similarly to the pacemaker of the heart, which generates the heartbeat. An alternative hypothesis is that the oscillatory behavior is a manifestation of the properties of a network of neurons (41). It seems reasonably clear that even in invertebrate systems multiple neurons are necessary to generate sustained oscillatory motor outputs.

Methods of Studying Central Pattern Generation

The importance of CPG can be illustrated under a range of experimental conditions. A method commonly used over the last 30 years has been to record from muscle nerves of a decerebrated (to avoid the effects of anesthesia) and completely spinalized (low thoracic, to avoid any supraspinal influences on the spinal circuitry) cat whose peripheral nerves have been severed and/or the muscles paralyzed (for example, with curare) to prevent any modulation from movement-related sensations. When this animal is given an appropriate pharmacological stimulus, such as L-dopa, combined with an inhibitor of dopamine reuptake (for example, monoamine oxidase), oscillatory efferent output can be sustained for

hours (Fig. 3.19). The efferent output is highly coordinated, and there is alternating ipsilateral as well as contralateral flexion and extension activity. Both motor neurons and interneurons are active throughout all layers of the gray matter of the spinal cord and over all of the lumbosacral segments in a steplike pattern (42). A highly significant point with respect to CPG is that a highly coordinated oscillatory pattern (resembling that observed during locomotion) can be generated by the circuitry within the spinal cord in the absence of input from the brain or the periphery.

Importance of Sensory Input to Spinal Neural Circuits That Can Generate CPG

Without sensory input to provide cues associated with the environment, the functional significance of the CPG by itself is limited. If, on the other hand, the spinal cord has access to sensory information from peripheral receptors, then a wide range of useful and highly adaptable motor tasks can be performed without input from the brain (Fig. 3.20). For example, an adult completely spinalized (low thoracic level) cat can generate full weight-bearing stepping and readily adjust the stepping pattern to the speed of a moving treadmill belt (43). It is apparent that this stepping ability results from a combination of the processing of the sensory input and the CPG itself.

The Spinal Cord Is Smart

The circuitry responsible for CPG receives and interprets the sensory information in a highly dynamic way. That is, whether a group of muscles is excited or inhibited by a given afferent from a mechanoreceptor during locomotion often will depend on the stage of the step cycle. For example, a stimulus applied to the dorsum of a cat's paw (as in a stumbling response) will excite the flexor muscles of the ipsilateral limb when applied during the swing phase, whereas the same stimulus will excite the extensor muscles when applied during the stance phase of the step cycle (44). This observation and a series of other experiments demonstrating qualitatively similar capabilities of the spinal cord has led to the concept that the spinal cord is smart (45,46). That is, the spinal cord receives sensory information and makes a decision as to the appropriate response at that time. In this context, it is logical to think of the spinal cord as interpreting the total ensemble of afferent information at any given time, as opposed to receiving input from each sensory receptor and responding to each receptor in a stereotypically reflexive manner. An analogy is the way we interpret a visual image. When we are observing an artistic painting, it is the total visual field of the painting that our brain interprets as opposed to processing each individual "pixel" of information independently and then deriving a final image. At any given instant in time, the spinal cord is receiving information from all receptors throughout the body and then "deciding" which neurons to excite.

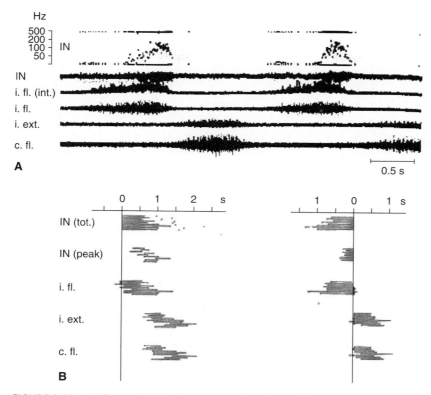

FIGURE 3.19 **A.** The equivalent of two step cycles showing fictive locomotion, whereby oscillating efferent (motor) output from peripheral nerves leading to flexor and extensor muscles is generated by the spinal cord without any input from the brain (complete low thoracic spinal cord transection) or from the periphery (all muscle nerves are cut and the animal is paralyzed with curare). IN, activity (frequency of action potentials) from a single interneuron in the lumbar spinal cord during the two cycles. Note the similarity in the timing and frequency modulation of the IN for both cycles and the similar timing relationship to the activity from an ipsilateral flexor (integrated and raw signal), ipsilateral extensor, and contralateral flexor muscle nerve. **B.** The relative timing of the IN and the muscles for nine consecutive cycles, with the onset of IN firing as a common reference point for each cycle. The dot after each line illustrating IN activity marks the end of each cycle. Note the variation in the absolute times for the activities; regardless of this variation, the relationships between the on and off times are remarkably consistent. *(Modified from Edgerton V, Grillner S, Sjostrom A, et al. Central Generation of Locomotion in Vertebrates. In Herman RM, Stein PSG, Stuart DG, eds. Neural control of locomotion. New York: Plenum, 1976;439–464.)*

The smart and integrative features of CPGs provide a basis for the automaticity in the neural control of posture and locomotion. For example, in the completely spinalized animal, the CPG neurons can predict the next logical sequence of neurons to activate based on the specific groups of neurons that were activated immediately prior to that point. The importance of CPG is not that it can continuously generate repetitive cycles but that these networks can receive and interpret sensory input and then predict the next logical sequences of action. It is perhaps useful to think of the neurons that produce CPG as basically modulating the probability of a given set of neurons being active at any given time, while the peripheral sensory input modulates the probability of completing each component of a motor task successfully. The degree of detail in motor output that can be generated by the spinal cord in combination with the information from the periphery can be appreciated by comparing the EMG and force signals from a battery of muscles from a cat before and after a complete spinal cord transection at a low thoracic level (Fig. 3.21). Although there are some differences in the EMG signals in chronically spinalized cats during bipedal stepping relative to that in intact controls, these are relatively minor and may be associated with only slight differences in the biomechanics of the hindquarters.

Sources of Peripheral Sensory Information

Overview

In this section we will discuss principally mechanoreceptors that provide sensory information to the spinal cord about the

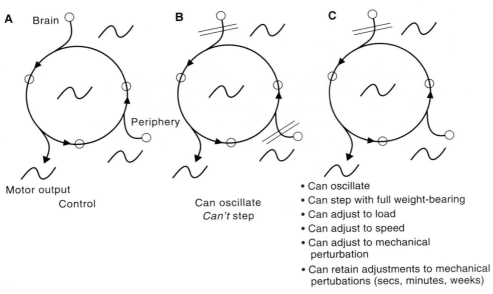

FIGURE 3.20   The motor output capabilities of the spinal cord under three conditions. *Left.* The control situation: the spinal cord is able to receive normal input from the brain and peripheral nerves transmitting proprioceptive input largely from mechanoreceptors. Movement capability is normal. *Center.* Output potential when both brain and peripheral input are eliminated. As in Figure 3.19, the spinal cord can generate oscillating efferent patterns that approximate the properties observed during actual locomotion. *Right.* The motor capacity of the spinal cord without input from the brain but with the peripheral input preserved has a greatly enhanced capability, including the ability to step over a range of speeds and loads, and can even make adjustments when the legs are tripped. The spinal cord also can learn motor tasks. *(Unpublished observation, J.R. Edgerton and R.R. Roy)*

physiological and mechanical environment associated with the control of movement. All modes of sensory information in some way may feed into the motor system and thus can initiate, modulate, and control to varying degrees the execution of a motor task. The following section addresses the sensory information associated with the mechanical (mechanoreceptors) and chemical (chemoreceptors) events associated with muscular activity. The different types of receptors probably provide ensembles or patterns of activity from specific receptors at specific locations and within a specific temporal characterization that have meaning to the spinal cord and the brain. With respect to proprioception, the mechanoreceptors, spindles, and Golgi tendon organs provide an abundance of sensory input for the spinal cord to integrate and interpret. An important component of the neural control of movement lies within the skeletal muscles, tendons, and joints, where a wide range of mechanoreceptors provides the CNS with the kinematic and kinetic state of the movement.

The classic physiologist Arthur Steinhaus often stated that the muscles are the largest sensory organs in the human body. The brain and spinal cord constantly receive sensory input throughout one's life, and it is readily apparent that the patterns and modes of input influence the immediate re-

sponses in the brain. It can be approximated that a single afferent from the hindlimbs of a cat can generate action potentials at an average rate of 80 per second and that there are about 10,000 large afferents in the hindlimb musculature. Thus during one second of locomotion, about 800,000 action potentials are conducted centrally. These action potentials diverge to conduct excitatory potentials to virtually all homonymous motor neurons and to many motor neurons innervating synergistic muscles. One could approximate that a conservative number of neurons receiving excitatory potentials would be about 10,000. Therefore, some 8 billion excitatory postsynaptic potentials could be generated per second from a single large afferent.

Not only are the brain and spinal cord receiving and integrating information continuously, they are receiving very complex patterns from sensory receptors, for example, vision, audition, smell, taste, touch, and proprioception. Based on the number of sensory axons in peripheral nerves to all of the skeletal muscles and joints, more than one-half of the axons in muscle nerves are sensory, and most of the body mass is composed of muscle. Thus, if one considers only the muscle nerves, one must expect that exercise and motor training can play a significant role in shaping how the CNS functions. Among these sensory axons are a number of types

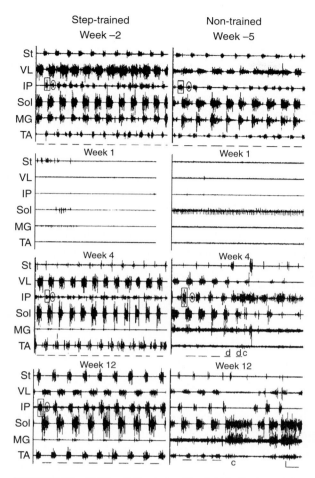

Step-trained
Week –2

Non-trained
Week –5

St VL IP Sol MG TA

Week 1 — Week 1

Week 4 — Week 4

Week 12 — Week 12

FIGURE 3.21 EMG activity during bipedal hindlimb stepping in a step-trained and an untrained cat before (–2 or –5 weeks) and 1, 4, and 12 weeks after a complete low thoracic spinal cord transection. Raw EMG was recorded from selected hindlimb muscles during stepping at a treadmill speed of 0.4 m/second. Stance phase during full weight-bearing step cycles is indicated by the horizontal lines below the EMG records. Open box, IP bursts during swing (IPsw); open circle, stance (IPst) in one step cycle; c, a step failure (collapse); d, contact of dorsal surface of paw on treadmill belt (toes curled). Horizontal calibration, 1 s, and vertical calibration, 1.0 mV for all muscles except for the Sol (2.0 mV). St, semitendinosus; VL, vastus lateralis; IP, iliopsoas; Sol, soleus; MG, medial gastrocnemius; TA, tibialis anterior. *(Reprinted with permission from de Leon RD, Hodgson JA, Roy RR, et al. Locomotor capacity attributable to step training versus spontaneous recovery after spinalization in adult cats. J Neurophysiol 1998;79:1329–1340.)*

of mechanoreceptors that are capable of detecting changes in muscle length, force, and pressure. In addition, some nerve branches are essentially all or predominantly sensory, and they project to tendons, joints, and skin. One of the most studied mechanoreceptors is the skeletal muscle spindle that provides proprioceptive information to the CNS (47). During exercise the brain also receives input from

axons that convey touch, sound, vision, smell, and taste, and these sources of information influence the physiology of the CNS. There are many examples of ways these sensory systems affect our motor performance, reflecting the fact that each of these sensory modes has input to the motor system. A loud sound can increase voluntary strength. Cutaneous cues shape our reactions in maintaining posture and in the kinematics of locomotion. Vision is a major source of input for guiding virtually all movements. Sound can direct our posture and head position. Even olfactory input can initiate locomotor movements.

Muscle Spindles

A muscle spindle consists of about four to six small muscle fibers surrounded by a collagenous sheath. The maximum diameter of the collagenous sheath usually approximates the size of the intrafusal muscle fibers. The muscle fibers within the capsule are striated, similar to the extrafusal muscle fibers; these are intrafusal muscle fibers. The ends of these intrafusal fibers commonly project beyond the clearly defined spindle capsule. The intrafusal fibers are innervated by γ-motor neurons, and each intrafusal muscle fiber is surrounded by several sensory axons called primary and secondary spindle afferents (Fig. 3.22). These sensory axons generate action potentials when the length of the intrafusal fiber changes. Stretch of the intrafusal fibers can be caused by two events: (a) activation of the γ-motor neurons, which will cause shortening of the distal ends of the intrafusal fibers and therefore stretch the center where the annulospiral sensory nerve endings are; and (b) passively lengthening or shortening the intrafusal fibers, since they lie parallel and are physically attached indirectly to the extrafusal muscle fibers. Very small changes in length can stimulate the primary (also referred to as Ia afferents) and secondary sensory fibers from the spindle. In general, the primary afferents from the muscles spindles demonstrate a more dynamic response, whereas the secondary fibers have a more static response to changes in length. The primary Ia fibers are the main afferents responding to a tendon tap and vibration (48).

Afferents During Locomotion

Some specific examples of how Ia fibers from muscle spindles in the ankle extensors (plantarflexors) of the cat function during locomotion are shown in Figure 3.23. In Figure 3.23A the spindle was firing throughout the step cycle with the frequency being modestly higher during stance, that is, E1 through E3. The E1 phase is the extension of the limb at the end of the swing phase prior to paw contact. The E2 phase begins at paw contact and extends to the end of the yield phase of stance. The E3 phase continues throughout the remainder of the stance phase. In B, again the spindle Ia is activated throughout the step cycle, but at a higher firing rate during E2 and E3. Also, the level of activation of the extensor muscle was higher in B than in A. In early E1 in B a

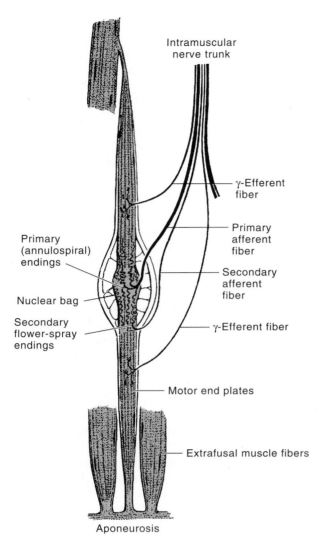

Intramuscular
nerve trunk

γ-Efferent
fiber

Primary
afferent
fiber

Secondary
afferent
fiber

Primary
(annulospiral)
endings

γ-Efferent fiber

Nuclear bag

Secondary
flower-spray
endings

Motor end plates

Extrafusal muscle fibers

Aponeurosis

FIGURE 3.22 A muscle spindle attaches at its ends to connective tissues within a muscle. Sometimes two or even three spindles are interconnected in series. A connective tissue capsule surrounds three to eight intrafusal fibers within each spindle. Motor end plates at the ends of each intrafusal fiber form the junction of the γ-motor neuron with the intrafusal muscle fiber and provide a mechanism for inducing the intrafusal fiber to shorten or place tension on the center of the muscle fiber. This increased tension triggers action potentials in the sensory endings, that is, annulospiral (primary) and flower spray (secondary) afferent fibers. These endings also can be activated by passively stretching the muscle and therefore the spindles. The afferent input projects to the spinal cord, making synaptic contact on most motor neurons that project to that muscle. This input also projects to some motor neurons that innervate synergistic muscles and to interneurons that inhibit motor neurons innervating antagonistic muscles. *(Modified from Ross M, Romrell L, Kaye G. Histology: A Text and Atlas. 3rd ed. New York: Harper and Row, 1995, p. 227.)*

few pulses with a very short interpulse interval can be seen. *C* shows a similar pattern to that in *A* and *B*, but in the first step cycle shown the highest firing frequency occurred at mid E3, whereas in the next step, it occurred at mid E1. This emphasizes the variation in the details of the activation patterns of γ- and α-motor neurons, not only among different afferent fibers but even from step to step for the same afferent. This step-to-step variability is a steadfast feature of locomotor networks even under the most controlled conditions possible. All three of these examples illustrate the likelihood that the γ-motor neuron innervating the intrafusal muscle fibers were sufficiently active during all phases of the step cycle to sustain some sensitivity of the spindle to the intramuscular mechanical events (48).

One of the most common ways to demonstrate the responsiveness of muscle spindles to stretch is to tap the tendon to trigger a muscle contraction. Tapping the tendon induces a monosynaptic reflex by activating the spindle afferents that project to the dendrites of the motor neurons associated with the same muscle containing the spindle. Each spindle afferent sends axonal branches to nearly every motor neuron within that motor pool and to a significant proportion of the motor neurons that innervate synergistic muscles (49). In addition, the same Ia afferent from the spindle projects to interneurons that inhibit the motor neurons innervating antagonistic muscles (Fig. 3.24).

One can vibrate a muscle-tendon unit with a wide range of cycle frequencies such that the peak-to-peak change in length is less than 1 mm. This stretch will activate the Ia afferents, which in turn will excite motor neurons innervating that muscle and thus enhance its force generation even when the muscle is fatiguing during a maximal voluntary contraction (Fig. 3.25).

The density of muscle spindles varies widely among muscles. Muscles or muscle regions having a high percentage of slow fibers usually have a relatively high incidence of spindles and thus are highly sensitive to length changes (50). The intrinsic muscles of the hip, for example, have a high spindle density, are extremely sensitive to length changes, and provide very important information for modulating the motor output during routine motor tasks such as stepping (51). These length sensors provide important cues as to when the stance and swing phases of a step should begin and terminate and when the body weight is being shifted from one leg to the other while standing.

Other Mechanoreceptors

Another mechanoreceptor within the muscle tendon unit is the Golgi tendon organ (GTO). In spite of the name, most GTOs are within the muscle. They are able to detect small changes in force generated within the muscle. The high level of sensitivity to force of the GTOs contrasts with the traditional concept that they are activated only by high forces and that their function is to prevent tendon injury by inhibiting

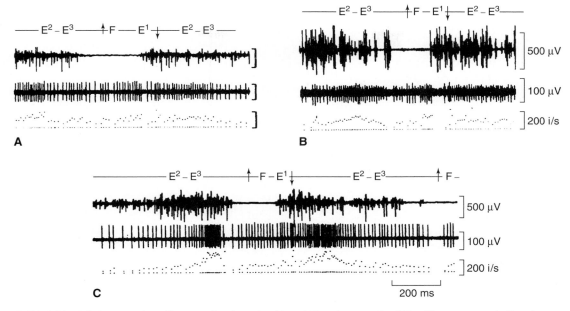

FIGURE 3.23 Discharge trains of intermediately active (**A** and **B**) and very active (**C**) ankle extensor spindle primary afferents during step cycles. Upper traces: lateral gastrocnemius EMG; lower traces: afferent discharges and their instantaneous firing rate. All three afferents show slightly different firing patterns, but each has a higher firing rate during stance. **C** represents the most extreme degree of presumed α-γ coactivation, since the afferents were active during the phase of the cycle when the muscle was shortening. There is no correspondence between primary afferent firing rate and EMG amplitude. *(Reprinted with permission from Prochazka A, Westerman RA, Ziccone SP. Discharges of single hindlimb afferents in the freely moving cat. J Neurophysiol 1976;39:1090–1104.)*

the muscle from generating excessive forces (47,52). The sensory information generated by GTOs will excite some muscles and inhibit others, with these effects being highly state dependent. For example, the specific neurons that are excited or inhibited can change with the phase of a step cycle and probably other physiological conditions. A third type of muscle mechanoreceptor is referred to as free nerve endings because there is no remarkable specialization at the ends of these axons. These free endings generate action potentials when excited by mechanical as well as biochemical (metabolic) stimuli. Free nerve endings actually constitute most of the sensory endings from muscle. Their function is not well understood, although they are thought to be actively involved in muscle spasticity in individuals with spinal cord injury.

From the perspective of the systems level all of the muscle spindle afferents, GTOs, and free nerve endings serve as mechanoreceptors that provide important information associated with proprioception. Proprioception is a broad term often used to convey the idea that there are sensory receptors that provide precise information to the spinal cord and brain regarding the exact biomechanical state of the musculoskeletal system at any given time. As noted earlier, mechanoreceptors seem to have specialized in the periphery, which enables them to provide detailed information about the kinematics of a movement from a micro and macro perspective and also from a dynamic and static perspective. The combined effect of all of these mechanoreceptors projecting to the spinal circuits is to provide an ensemble of sensory information that provides the instructions needed for the spinal cord to control and modulate the kinematics of the movements in a very predictable way, thus minimizing the necessity for supraspinal (conscious) control of routine movements.

As noted previously, an important basic neurophysiological concept with respect to proprioceptive input from the mechanoreceptors, as well as cutaneous receptors, is that their synaptic functional connectivity to the spinal circuitry is highly dynamic. The connectivity between these mechanoreceptors and specific interneuronal populations within the spinal cord vary according to the physiological state. Even the efficacy of the monosynaptic input from muscle spindles to the motor neuron changes readily from one portion of the step cycle to another and according to whether a subject is running or walking (53,54).

Smart Responses in the Spinal Cord of Humans

Another excellent example of the ability of the spinal cord to receive complex proprioceptive input and to use this information in a functional way was shown by Harkema and colleagues (55) (Fig. 3.26). These authors demonstrated that the level of activation of an extensor muscle, the soleus, is modulated according to the amount of load that is placed

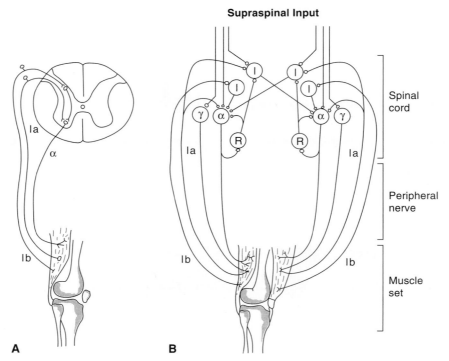

Supraspinal Input

A   **B**

FIGURE 3.24 Spinal connections between sensory receptors in muscle and α-motor neurons. The Ia axon conveys afferent information from the muscle spindle to the CNS. The Ib axon represents a similar connection but from the tendon organ. **A.** Homonymous relationships: muscle spindles and tendon organs in a muscle connect with the α-motor neurons that activate the same muscle. Afferent and efferent axons that service muscles on the right side of the body enter and exit the spinal cord on the right side, and vice versa. **B.** The same connections for an agonist-antagonist muscle set (for example, the hamstrings and quadriceps for the right leg) emphasizing the complexity of the interneuronal connections. Also note the input from the brain to the same interneurons that receive peripheral afferent input from the muscles. Open circles, excitatory connections; filled circles, inhibitory effects; α, α-motor neuron; γ, γ-motor neurons; I, Ia inhibitory interneuron; 1a, muscle spindle afferent; 1b, tendon organ afferent; R, Renshaw cell. *(Modified from Enoka R. Neuromechanical basis of kinesiology. Champaign, IL: Human Kinetics, 1988, p. 139.)*

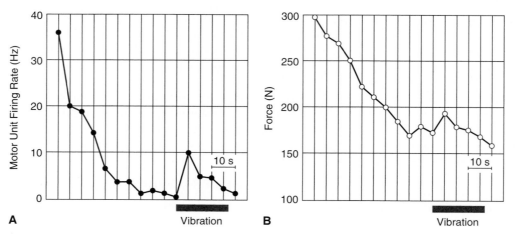

A   **B**

FIGURE 3.25 Vibration of the tibialis anterior temporarily counteracts (**A**) the decline in motor unit firing rates and (**B**) muscle force during a maximum voluntary contraction of foot dorsiflexors. *(Modified from Bongiovanni LG, Hagbarth KE. Tonic vibration reflexes elicited during fatigue from maximal voluntary contractions in man. J Physiol (Lond) 1990;423:1–14.)*

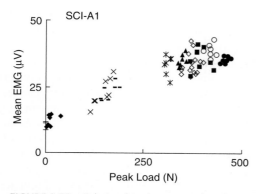
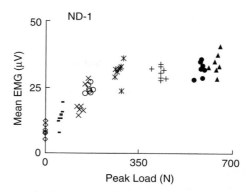

FIGURE 3.26   Relationships between soleus EMG mean amplitude (mV) and limb peak load (N) for an ASIA A spinal cord–injured (SCI-A1) and A now disabled (ND-1) subject stepping on a treadmill with a harness suspended from overhead to provide a range of loading conditions. An ASIA A SCI subject is one commonly called complete, that is, there is no clinical evidence of any motor control below the lesion site or sensory information from below the lesion. Each data point represents one step, and each symbol represents a series of consecutive steps at one level of body weight support. As the subjects bear more body weight, the EMG amplitude increases similarly in both the SCI and ND subjects. *(Adapted with permission from Harkema SJ, Hurley SL, Patel UK, et al. Human lumbosacral spinal cord interprets loading during stepping. J Neurophysiol 1997;77:797–811.)*

on the lower limbs of a human subject. In the example on the left of the figure the increase in the level of activation, as illustrated by the EMG amplitude, is directly related to the load imposed on the limb. The results of a similar experiment on a subject who has a complete spinal cord injury (no voluntary control of any muscles below the lesion and no sensation from tissues below the lesion) are shown on the right.

The similarity of the relationship between the level of loading and the level of activation of the motor pool (EMG amplitude) in the uninjured subjects and those with complete spinal cord injuries demonstrates that the spinal cord circuitry is able to sense the level of load and activate the soleus and other motor pools accordingly. Two of several interpretations of how the spinal cord senses load on-line are as follows:

1. Sensory receptors in the limbs (e.g., soles of the feet, tendons, muscles, joints) specifically sense load.
2. An ensemble of many types of sensory receptors at multiple locations within the limbs generate a highly recognizable image to inform the spinal circuitry of the biomechanical status of the weight bearing.

The second interpretation is the one we favor. It is consistent with the concept that has been alluded to many times previously; that is, it is the ensemble of sensory input that has meaning and can be interpreted by the spinal cord circuitry so that an appropriate motor pattern can be generated (56,57). These data also demonstrate that the spinal cord can activate the motor pools in a precise and highly coordinated manner. Thus, contrary to a pervasive perception, the spinal cord is not hardwired. Rather, the combination of the intrinsic activity and the sensory input to the spinal circuitry lets the spinal cord readily adjust to parameters such as the speed of

stepping, the level of load imposed on the stepping, and a wide range of unpredictable patterns of sensory anomalies (58). This plasticity and adaptability can occur over milliseconds to months.

Some of the key points related to sensory processing by the spinal cord:

1. Within the musculoskeletal and cutaneous tissues is an extensive network of mechanoreceptors and metaboreceptors that continuously update the spinal cord on the physiological state of the peripheral tissue.
2. These mechanoreceptors provide highly integrated and perceptually meaningful information as well as an ensemble of this information to the spinal cord.
3. The spinal cord is smart enough to interpret and appropriately respond to the highly complex but meaningful sensory ensembles.
4. The human spinal cord also demonstrates this smartness and automaticity.

Supraspinal Control of Posture and Locomotion

Overview

In general, the functional organization of the neural control of locomotion in humans and quadrupeds is similar. Although the spinal cord has neuronal systems that alternate the activation patterns of the musculature to produce stance and swing phases during locomotion, the brain also has neuronal systems that can accomplish these tasks. These supraspinal neuronal networks are highly responsive to sensory information from the periphery. A hypothesis presented by Orlovsky, Deliagina, and Grillner (59) is that each limb is modulated from supraspinal input via groups of spinal neurons called controllers. These controllers respond to a simple tonic drive from the brain by generating a relatively complex rhythmic pattern that activates the limb musculature in a coordinated pattern to generate locomotion. It is not clear what these controllers anatomically are or how many there are, but one can imagine a number of such controllers that could interact in very predictable ways to control the individual joints in each limb. Shik and Orlovsky (29) proposed a two-level automatism control system for locomotion. One level provides nonspecific tonic input that determines the intensity of locomotion (speed and grade). The second level is responsible for making fine adjustments in the control of the limbs, including maintaining equilibrium. This

level of the control system normally interacts with sources of sensory information, such as visual and proprioceptive inputs, to execute fine adjustments in the locomotor pattern (Fig. 3.27).

Locomotion seems to be initiated by supraspinal centers that activate these limb controllers, with the reticulospinal neurons and the mesencephalic locomotor region (MLR) playing important roles. There are differences in opinion regarding the relationship of the neural control of posture to that of locomotion. One hypothesis is that the control systems are rather distinct. An alternative hypothesis is that the neural programs for posture and locomotion are highly integrated and share extensively in the control of standing and stepping.

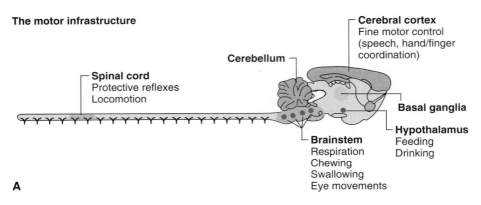

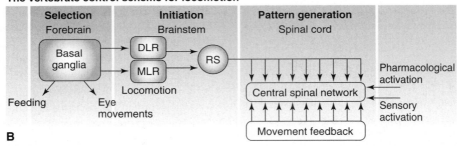

FIGURE 3.27   The motor infrastructure. **A.** Location of various networks (central pattern generators [CPGs]) that coordinate various motor patterns in vertebrates. These areas can coordinate the activation of different CPGs in a behaviorally relevant order. For instance, if the fluid intake area is activated, an animal will look for water, walk toward it, position itself, and start drinking. The cerebral cortex is important in particular for fine motor coordination involving hands and fingers and for speech. **B.** General control strategy for vertebrate locomotion. Locomotion is initiated by activity in reticulospinal neurons of the brainstem locomotor center, which produces the locomotor pattern in close interaction with sensory feedback. With increased activation of the locomotor center, the speed of locomotion increases and interlimb coordination can change (e.g., from a walk to a gallop). The basal ganglia exert a tonic inhibitory influence on motor centers that is released when a motor pattern is selected. Locomotion can also be elicited by administration of excitatory amino acid agonists and by sensory input. RS, reticulospinal neuron; DLR, diencephalic locomotor area; MLR, mesopontine locomotor area. *(Modified from Grillner S. The motor infrastructure: from ion channels to neuronal networks. Nat Rev Neurosci 2003;4:573–586.)*

Descending Pathways for Controlling Locomotion

The primary anatomical descending pathways for initiating locomotion are the corticospinal, reticulospinal, vestibulospinal, and rubrospinal tracts. The motor cortex gives rise to the corticospinal tract, which decussates and influences the spinal circuitry associated with the contralateral limbs. Some of these neurons have rhythmic firing patterns during locomotion. This rhythm seems to be generated by the spinal circuitry driven by CPG as well as by sensory feedback. In quadrupeds, the motor cortex has a minimal role in generating the basic locomotor pattern, but it appears to be involved in corrective actions and in making adjustments to weight-bearing levels (60). However, the motor cortex does play an important role in executing more skilled movements that are not repetitive and in adjusting the basic activation patterns during locomotion in a more variable environment. Although corticospinal neurons may provide instruction for refining or modifying locomotor movements, it is clear that the basic locomotor patterns can be relatively normal without corticospinal input (Fig. 3.28).

In primates, including humans, lesions of the motor cortex or spinal cord may produce a greater disruption of the basic locomotor patterns than in lower mammalian species (61). Most of the dysfunction occurs in the distal musculature that controls the wrist, ankle, and digits.

The medial reticular formation of the pons and medulla gives rise to neurons that form the reticulospinal tract. These axons descend within the ventrolateral funiculi of the spinal cord, and a single neuron can project to multiple levels of the spinal cord. The neurons that form the reticulospinal tract receive input from the brainstem, including the MLR, and from the cerebellum. The MLR, just rostral to the medial reticular formation (Fig. 3.29), provides input to the neurons that form the reticulospinal tract. Stimulation of the MLR (a 1-mm-long strip of cells in the nucleus cuneiformis) can elicit locomotion.

Stimulation of the MLR region activates reticulospinal neurons that in turn can stimulate the spinal centers producing locomotion. Reticulospinal neurons become more active during locomotion than when the animal is at rest. The reticulospinal tract in cats is necessary to elicit locomo-

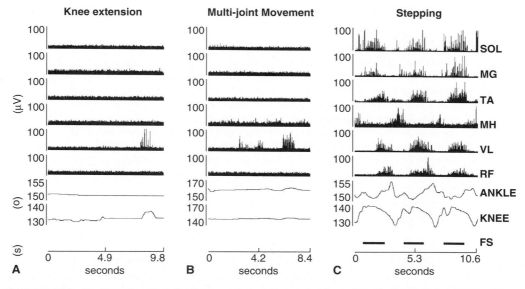

FIGURE 3.28 Single and multiple joint movements and stepping by a clinically incomplete but severely injured SCI subject. When the subject is asked to extend the knee, little movement occurred (lower left of A) and EMG was recorded from one muscle. The subject was slightly more successful when instructed to move the limbs in a cycling motion. EMG activity (µV) from the soleus (SOL), medial gastrocnemius (MG), tibialis anterior (TA), medial hamstrings (MH), vastus lateralis (VL), and rectus femoris (RF); knee and ankle angles (o); and foot switches (black bars indicate stance phase) during an attempted single-joint movement (A), multiple joint movement (B), and during weight-bearing stepping at 0.28 m/second with 56% body weight support (C). Minimal EMG was observed only in the VL during attempted knee extension (A), and only the MH became more active (although no clear EMG burst) during multiple-joint effort (B). Minimal movement of the knee or ankle occurred. This EMG pattern contrasts with the alternating bursts in each muscle during stepping (C). These results emphasize the fact that voluntary control from the brain is not essential to generate stepping. The TA was largely synchronized with the SOL and MG, while the MH EMG was reciprocal to that in the VL and RF and with ankle muscles. *(Modified from Maegele M, Muller S, Wernig A, et al. Recruitment of spinal motor pools during voluntary movements versus stepping after human spinal cord injury. J Neurotrauma 2002;19:1217–1229.)*

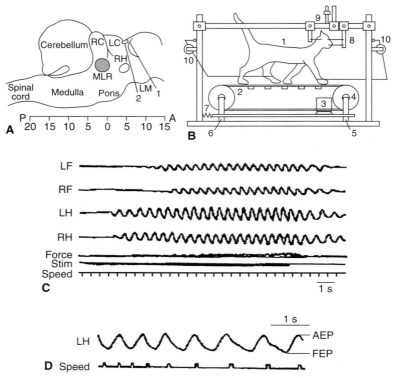

FIGURE 3.29 Shik developed a preparation that consisted of a decerebrated (**A**) animal placed in a frame over a treadmill belt (**B**). When the brainstem is sliced so that the superior colliculus and red nucleus lie just caudal to the slice, the animal can generate full weight-bearing stepping (**C**). Movements of the limbs are recorded by levers attached to the ankles (**C**). The timing of the brainstem stimulation is indicated by the thick horizontal line. Stepping begins several seconds after the stimulation is initiated and continues for a number of seconds after the tonic stimulation is terminated. An adjustment in stepping cycle rate accommodates the changing speed of the treadmill belt (**D**). In A: MLR, mesencephalic locomotor region; LM, corpus mammillare; LC, superior colliculus; RC, inferior colliculus; RH, red nucleus. In C: LF, left forelimb; RF, right forelimb; LH, left hindlimb; RH, right hindlimb. In D: AEP, anterior extreme position; FEP, posterior extreme position. (*Modified from Orlovsky G, Deliagina T, Grillner S. Neuronal Control of Locomotion: From Mollusc to Man. Oxford: Oxford University Press, 1999, p. 166.*)

tion during stimulation of the MLR. Also, if the ventrolateral funiculi of the spinal cord are cut, a coordinated locomotor pattern cannot be initiated. A second area in the brainstem that can initiate locomotion and that also projects to reticulospinal neurons is the subthalamic locomotor region (59).

The exact manner in which these neurons induce locomotion is not known. However, activity of neurons in the MLR increases during locomotion. There is some evidence that MLR region is controlled by inhibition and that initiation of stepping may be induced by disinhibition (59). Neurons that form the reticulospinal, vestibulospinal, and rubrospinal tracts are rhythmically active during locomotion. Most of the vestibulospinal neurons are active at the beginning of stance. Most of the neurons forming the rubrospinal and reticulospinal tracts are maximally active during the swing phase of

a step cycle. Thus, the vestibulospinal tract seems to facilitate extensor motor neurons, whereas the reticulospinal tract mainly facilitates flexor and inhibits extensor motor neurons. The rubrospinal and corticospinal tracts mainly facilitate flexor motor neurons (59).

Activity in these neurons seems to have a modulatory effect on the motor neurons only during specific phases of the step cycle, as noted previously. Furthermore, the rhythm and firing of these descending tracts are due in large part to the influences from ascending input derived from the spinal cord circuitry. This phasic input (cyclic input associated with stepping) can occur independently of the afferent input from the periphery. For example, in paralyzed and decerebrated cats in which phasic afferent inflow from the periphery is precluded, phasic descending and ascending activity between the spinal cord and supraspinal centers is still present during spontaneous motor activity. Thus, it appears that the rhythmic drive intrinsic to the spinal circuits is sufficient to induce rhythmic drive of descending neurons that provide the excitatory input to the appropriate motor pools during locomotion.

It appears that supraspinal centers such as the MLR can increase or decrease the force or velocity of contraction of a muscle by changing the level of excitatory and/or inhibitory input to the motor neuronal pools (28). However, if treadmill speed is kept constant, increased input to the midbrain in a decerebrate cat has no effect on the duration of the stance phase or step frequency (62). This suggests that the cycle duration is influenced by mechanical factors, such as the position or the placement of the hindlimb, and therefore is mediated at least in part by proprioceptive signals.

Role of Cerebellum in Locomotion

The cerebellum also plays an important role in motor control. A major function of the cerebellum is to assist in the control of limb movements by modulating supraspinal motor centers, as noted previously. It mediates sensory feedback from the spinal cord and modifies the motor output accordingly. The cerebellum also receives information from CPGs of the limbs to modulate the motor output. In addition, the cerebellum compares different inputs and based on these comparisons provides a means of correcting intended movements (59).

Automaticity in Posture and Locomotion

This section addresses the relative importance of different supraspinal nuclei in initiating and controlling locomotion. It is apparent that these different centers can differentially control different muscle groups, such as extensors versus flexors. Each of these control centers has a strong gating function whereby its input is timed closely with the phase of the step cycle. Clearly, specific regions within the brainstem can initiate and control very complex motor behaviors, apparently with little or no necessity for conscious control, resulting in the generation of largely automatic responses.

It is often assumed that the initiation of a movement, even the more automatic ones, such as stepping, is triggered by a conscious event in the motor cortex. Even a superficial examination of this assumption raises the question of what is consciousness. Actually, there seems to be a continuum of consciousness ranging from a totally simple reflex without any conscious awareness or capability of control to modulation of a task in which one is fully and continuously aware of every aspect of the movement. What is the level of consciousness when one begins to step compared to the level of automaticity during a simple monosynaptic reflex? Even the monosynaptic efficacy can be modulated by conscious con-

trol by a rat, monkey, or human. A human with a spinal cord injury and with no supraspinal control below a low thoracic lesion can learn to stand and initiate steps using sensory information associated with unilaterally bearing weight and manipulating the hip position (63). This spinal stepping can be initiated consciously and voluntarily, although the subject initiates the process "reflexively" in that the subject manipulates the afferent inflow by controlling critical biomechanical and neurophysiological signals by manipulating other parts of the body (64).

A variety of approaches have been used to identify how one initiates a movement. Functional magnetic resonance imaging (fMRI) is being used to examine where the decision is made to initiate a movement. A number of studies suggest that the urge to move precedes the actual initiation of movement by about 200 ms. Thus, there seems to be a readiness potential that precedes the subjective decisions. Functional MRI shows elevated blood flow in the dorsal prefrontal cortex, intraparietal sulcus, and supplementary motor area in preparation for a movement (65).

Automaticity Derived From the Brainstem to Control Locomotion

There is a strong element of automaticity in the neural control of most movements, from both the brain and spinal cord (59,66). For example, once the decision to walk across a room is made, very little conscious effort is required to perform the details of that task. It seems that the CNS is designed so that much of the intricate decision making associated with posture and locomotion occurs automatically. Both supraspinal and spinal sources contribute to the pathways responsible for this automaticity. For example, a subthalamic cat, decerebrated just rostral to the mammillary bodies, can walk in response to exteroceptive stimulation and can sometimes walk spontaneously. A cat decerebrated at the caudal border of the mammillary bodies cannot walk under either condition. Therefore, subthalamic locomotor region lies between these two transection levels. When the subthalamic locomotor region is destroyed, the animal can walk by itself, go to a plate of food, and even kill and eat a mouse.

Automaticity and Autonomic Function During Locomotion

Automaticity also is evident in coordination of the neural control of locomotion with that of respiration and cardiovascular function. For example, not only does the stimulation of the MLR generate remarkably normal locomotion, it also leads to a modulation of cardiovascular and respiratory function that is appropriate for locomotion. When the MLR of a mesencephalic cat is stimulated and the limbs are stepping on a treadmill, a 20 to 35% higher arterial blood pressure, a 70 to 90% greater cardiac output, and an increase of 15 to 20% in heart rate relative to the resting condition has been observed (67). In addition, pulmonary ventilation can increase threefold as a result of increased tidal volume and frequency of breathing. These observations demonstrate the highly integrated and automated nature of the neural system to control locomotion with some assurance that the cardiovascular and inspiratory systems will be modulated accordingly. It would be interesting, however, to perform experiments whereby the MLR was stimulated in a paralyzed preparation to exclude the involvement of mechanisms directly linked to activation of the muscle tissue and the consequential metabolic impact of muscular contractions.

Levels of Automaticity

Clearly there are a number of levels of automaticity (absence of conscious detailed control) of the neural control of posture and stepping. For example, decerebrate cats can run without hitting obstacles and jump over obstacles. When the MLR is stimulated, the decerebrate cat can generate locomotion along with spatial orientation. In animals with a chronic lesion (several weeks) in the subthalamic locomotor region, locomotor behavior is nearly normal.

Spinal automaticity remains in the absence of supraspinal input, as occurs after a complete transection of the spinal cord. A large body of data demonstrates that the spinal cord is much more than a static conduit for communication between the brain and muscles. It was known in the mid 1970s that kittens whose spinal cord was transected at a neonatal age can be trained to take steps on all four limbs (28,30). A significant level of automaticity also was evident when it was learned that stimulating the dorsum of the lumbosacral spinal cord in a tonic pattern will generate stepping motions in paraplegic mammals (42,68), including humans (69). Also, rhythmic locomotor patterns can be induced by the spinal cord when selected regions of the brainstem are stimulated tonically, even in the absence of sensory feedback from the spinal cord. The spinal cord also can generate patterns resembling locomotion in the absence of sensory feedback when the spinal cord is stimulated pharmacologically, as with L-dopa.

After a complete transection at the midthoracic level of the spinal cord, the automaticity generated from the lumbosacral spinal cord is attributable to two primary processes:

1. CPG (70).
2. Sensory input to the spinal cord from the periphery (56,70a).

When sensory input from cutaneous and proprioceptive sources is combined with CPG, the spinal circuitry is capable of executing a much wider range of complex motor tasks than when the output is generated by the spinal circuitry alone. How does the automaticity of posture and locomotion emerge from the interactions between the sensory inputs and the spinal circuits that generate CPG? For these two systems to work in synergy, each system must have intrinsic activation and inhibition patterns that are orderly, sequential, and coordinated. For example, the sequence of activation patterns associated with a step cycle can occur only with a critical level of synergy between the sources and modes of peripheral input and the cyclic events from CPG. The patterns of afferent information must interface with the CPG circuitry, as do two pieces of a jigsaw puzzle, at any given time bin, or segment of time, within a step cycle:

1. To inform the CPG of the current state of the step cycle.
2. To make the circuitry aware of which bin or bins preceded that instant.
3. To predict which bin or bins should occur next.

In this scenario a bin consists of the afferent input and stage of activation-inhibition of the neurons that generate the CPG output at that instant. Again, the temporal patterns of ensembles of peripheral inputs must be matched at some critical level with that of the CPG for locomotion to continue effectively.

Automaticity and the Spinal Cord

In subjects with an injured spinal cord, the level of automaticity manifested is quite striking. Even with no input from the brain, the spinal cord is highly capable of interpreting and responding to sensory information from the periphery. From a systems standpoint, the specific combination of recruited motor pools and the net level of activation of this combination of motor pools at any given time within a step cycle must be highly precise if the subject is to step successfully. Equilibrium and balance must be sustained under highly dynamic conditions, that is, avoid falling when faced with a perturbation. Even when the precision of the activation patterns is not impressive at the individual motor pool level, the net effect can be remarkably consistent at the systems level.

Spinal Learning

While spinal cord plasticity can be modulated to alter its motor capacity after a complete spinal cord injury, one may argue that this behavior requires long periods of motor training and formation of new neuronal connections in the spinal cord. However, the state-dependent property of the spinal circuitry, which permits highly functional and integrated responses, also can occur in acute, novel situations. For example, when an object is placed in front of a spinal cat stepping on a treadmill or during the swing phase of one hindlimb, that limb will exhibit a greater degree of flexion during the following steps to avoid the perturbation (44). Hyperflexion induced by a stumbling stimulus during the swing phase of a step will persist for several steps even after the removal of the perturbation (46), suggesting that a learning and memory type of phenomenon may be taking place (Fig. 3.30).

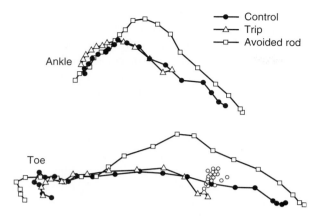

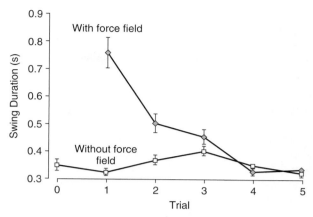

FIGURE 3.30 Swing trajectories of the foot (lower traces) and ankle (upper traces) of a spinal cat responding to the placement of a 1–cm-diameter bar in the path of the foot during the swing phase of the step cycle. The control trace shows the trajectory before placement of the bar. The trip trace shows the trajectory of the ankle and toe when the cat hit the bar. The remaining trace shows the trajectory when the foot cleared the bar. The bar position for each frame of the digitized video is shown by an open circle. Although the trajectory of only one tripping sequence is shown, the multiple open circles represent the position of the tripping bar during a series of tripping sequences. Note the increased elevation of the foot well before it encountered the bar in the step and following the first step when the trip occurred. The rod was avoided in the first step after the tripping episode. *(Adapted with permission from Hodgson JA, Roy RR, de Leon RB, et al. Can the mammalian lumbar spinal cord learn a motor task? Med Sci Sports Exerc 1994;26:1491–1497.)*

FIGURE 3.31 The changes in swing duration over five trials with and without an imposed perturbation (upward force field) for one representative rat. The swing duration is elevated more than twofold during the first perturbation and then quickly returns to levels observed without any perturbation. Swing durations were consistent across trials when the stepping was performed without any force field. Bars are SEM. *(Modified from de Leon RD, Reinkensmeyer DJ, Timoszyk WK, et al. Use of robotics in assessing the adaptive capacity of the rat lumbar spinal cord. In McKerracher L, Doucet G, Rossignol S, eds. Progress in brain research. Amsterdam: Elsevier Science, 2002, 141–149.)*

The persistent hyperreflexive action must be considered as more than a momentary adaptation, because a memory trace is shown behaviorally in a number of these studies, even after the perturbation requiring adaptation is removed.

More recent evidence of the smartness of the spinal cord was demonstrated when a robotic device was used to apply specific forces to rat hindlimbs during certain phases of a step cycle. In one experiment a downward force proportional to the velocity of stepping was applied unilaterally or bilaterally to one or more ankles of spinal rats. Step timing and kinematics were altered within a few minutes to allow locomotion to continue (71). In a separate but similar set of experiments, a robotically induced upward force proportional to the forward velocity of the swing (swing-phase force field, or SWPFF) was exerted at the ankle of one limb during the swing phase, resulting in a visually obvious kinematic disturbance. After as few as 20 steps, the limb adjusted its output to become kinematically similar to that observed prior to the perturbation, although with different EMG patterns (72). Furthermore, with repetitive trials of about 20 steps followed by 20 steps off of the SWPFF paradigm, the average swing duration dur-

ing the force-field-on period decreased to force-field-off levels by the fourth bout (Fig. 3.31).

The results of these studies show that in essence the spinal cord is solving problems in real time based on the continually changing state of incoming peripheral information to elicit a nearly constant behavior, even though the means to the end point differs.

The implication of these studies is that spinal learning takes place in a very short period, and a type of memory trace allows for quicker adaptation upon repeated exposure to a given perturbation. Although the underlying cellular mechanisms are unknown, some of the molecules and processes involved in spinal learning are similar to those involved in hippocampal learning. Whether this phenomenon continues for longer periods (hours to days) is unknown. Indeed, the spinal cord can exhibit long-term potentiation (LTP) and depression (LTD) (synaptic changes that are recognized as vital in hippocampal learning) in dorsal horn neurons in the spinal cord in response to nociceptive stimuli (73). Whether spinal learning occurs via similar processes as occurs in the hippocampus remains to be determined.

From a teleological perspective one can question the concept of automaticity with respect to how useful these autonomic responses are. All sensory and motor systems, however, have evolved so that they can function within this known environment. Similar sensory and motor components among a wide range of animals with vastly different musculoskeletal structures have evolved in a manner that enables many postural and locomotor tasks to occur quite automatically within the Earth's gravitational fields (56). The automaticity aspect of these functions reflects the successful evolution that enables postural and locomotor responses to occur without relying on more complicated, and probably more unpredictable, delayed decision making by higher neural centers. A greater reliance on the brain would require additional time and would impose disadvantages in the execution of a variety of postural and locomotor tasks, particularly when the response time is critical for survival. In this sense, evolutionary learning has played a key role in the automaticity of neural control during the execution of motor tasks. Thus the nervous system, even without conscious control, not only demonstrates a sophisticated level of automaticity but also is smart and highly adaptable or plastic. This plasticity includes the ability to learn motor tasks that are practiced.

Central Nervous System and Fatigue

What is the nature of central fatigue? Although this subject is discussed in more detail in Chapter 8, we consider central fatigue in the performance of a motor task as the failure to maintain the required or expected force or power output when these specific deficits cannot reasonably be explained by dysfunction within the muscle itself. The site for this fatigue can be in the brain, spinal cord, or even neuromuscular junction. In some conditions there undoubtedly can be failing elements within the autonomic nervous system. Furthermore, the fatiguing components may lie within sensory pathways, at interneuronal synapses, or at the level of the motor neuron. CNS fatigue of sensorimotor function can be demonstrated during maximum voluntary contractions using the twitch or tetanic interpolation technique; that is, the force produced during a maximum voluntary contraction can be enhanced by a single maximum stimulus or a brief train of electrical stimulation, as described previously. Clearly a state dependence of the excitability of neurons is associated with motor control.

Motor Cortex and Motor Fatigue

Changes in neuronal excitability are found in the human motor cortex in response to a fatiguing effort. The threshold for excitation and inhibition in the motor cortex declines after a few seconds of a maximal voluntary effort and recovers within 15 seconds, even if the muscle is maintained in an ischemic state. A brief facilitation occurs immediately after fatiguing exercise, but this is usually followed by a depression in the EMG responses to cortical stimulation lasting several minutes. Although the frequency discharge of motor neurons

during a fatiguing contraction decreases, this does not seem to be due a decline of corticospinal input, since stimulation of the cortex during a fatiguing contraction results in a decline in motor unit frequency discharge rates (74).

Evidence that the reduced excitability of the motor cortex to transcranial stimulation associated with fatigue is physiologically relevant is indicated by the fact that cortical stimulation of a rested muscle does not generate a force that exceeds the normal maximum voluntary contraction. After fatigue, however, cortical stimulation routinely generates a force that exceeds what can be produced voluntarily. In addition, after a fatiguing exercise transcranial magnetic stimulation can activate only a portion of the spinal motor neurons, suggesting a higher threshold for either the cortical neurons or the interneurons that project to a given motor pool (75). Most evidence suggests that fatiguing contractions do not change the threshold for excitation of corticospinal neurons. It is interesting to note that fatigue is more pronounced when the subjects are concentrating on their performance than when they are distracted or when performing with the eyes closed as opposed to open (76). Impaired motor performance is usually associated with increased perceived effort as well as the actual failure to produce the desired force. Each of these observations demonstrates that a significant element of neural fatigue can be at the conscious level. Clearly, our perception and cognition of performing a task under fatiguing conditions can affect the level to which we can activate a given motor pool (76a).

Why might there be a reduction in corticospinal drive to the motor neurons as a result of performing a repetitive task? This may be due to a reduction in corticospinal impulses reaching the motor neurons and/or an inhibition of motor neuron excitability by neurally mediated afferent feedback from the muscles. The latter is referred to as the sensory feedback hypothesis (77). Specifically, this hypothesis states that feedback from mechanoreceptors inhibits motor neurons and reduces their firing rates. These mechanoreceptors may be group III and IV free nerve endings, which are sensitive to muscle metabolites that accumulate during fatigue. Sedentary and dynamically exercised subjects performed fatiguing isometric plantarflexion contractions (30% maximum voluntary contraction [MVC] initially, and considered fatigued when there was a 30% decline in torque) (78). Surprisingly, at the end of the fatiguing task, the H-reflex amplitude had declined by 47% in the sedentary subjects and 67% in the trained subjects. Only a small change occurred in M-wave amplitude, indicating that the H-reflex decline was not due to neuromuscular propagation failure. The possible reasons for the different response:

1. The trained subjects required less central drive to maintain the relatively simple task at 30% MVC, especially at the early time points.
2. The trained subjects were able to relax more than the sedentary subjects when at rest. Thus, the endurance-

trained subjects could maintain a submaximal contraction with a level of reflex inhibition that was greater than in sedentary subjects. It appears that this fatigue-related multifaceted reflex inhibition cannot be explained solely by small-diameter afferents (group III and IV) responding to the byproducts of muscle contraction.

Motor Unit Rotation

In some way, the neural control system continuously adapts to changing physiological conditions by alternating different combinations of motor units that are active. When subjects are asked to maintain a low constant plantar flexor load (10% MVC) for longer than 3 hours, surface EMG recordings show alternating periods of high and low activity in the three major plantar flexors (soleus and medial and lateral heads of the gastrocnemius) (23). These synergistic muscles rotate in a complementary manner to maintain a nearly constant torque. The number of alternating instances is more frequent as the duration of the effort increases, that is, when motor unit fatigue would be expected to be occurring. Similar alternating motor unit patterns during prolonged elbow flexion at 10% MVC have been observed (22). Combined, these results are consistent with the view that one recruitment strategy to maintain low-level contractions for long periods is to alternate the activation levels among synergists in a pattern that is not stereotypical.

Adaptation Strategies of the CNS During Fatigue

The adaptive strategy of the nervous system during repetitive, fatiguing contractions differs with the type of movement. For example, while repetitive maximum knee extensions in a concentric mode result in a significant loss of torque, repetitive eccentric contractions not only result in a significantly higher torque, but the maximum torques do not decline. The neural control differs for these conditions in that the vastus lateralis and rectus femoris activation levels are 25 to 40% higher during concentric than eccentric maximal efforts. Furthermore, the EMG levels relative to the amount of torque increases as fatigue progresses during concentric but not eccentric contractions (Fig. 3.17). These data show clear differences in the neural control properties of muscles, depending on whether they are lengthening or shortening in a maximally activated state.

Role of Neurotransmitter Modulation in Fatigue

Underlying all of these physiological changes are many biochemical changes that are tightly linked in ways that we understand very little at a systems level. Some examples of these changes readily demonstrate the complexity of the biochemical changes that modify motor performance during the onset of fatigue.

Most areas of the brain have elevated levels of norepinephrine (NE) and serotonin (5-HT) after training on a treadmill, and a single bout of exercise increases the release of NE (79,80). Elevated levels of 5-HT within the CNS are associated with fatigue. One mechanism to counter fatigue could be to decrease the release of serotonin (79). For example, a reduction in the sensitivity to serotonin after 6 weeks of treadmill training in rats has been observed, perhaps due to a reduction in 5-HT1A receptors. Also, when 5-HT reuptake is inhibited pharmacologically, which increases the levels of 5-HT, there is increased fatigability and impaired cognition in humans. It also is interesting that when blood glucose levels in the brain are elevated, the levels of 5-HT decrease, most likely because of a decrease in its release. On the other hand, running increases the rate of synthesis of 5-HT in the brain, which in turn could contribute to fatigability. These and other results in general suggest that the levels of activity within a neural circuit may affect the efficacy of the synapses within that circuit by modulating the amount and duration of availability of neurotransmitters and/or the number of receptors that can bind to that neurotransmitter (79).

During locomotion 5-HT is an important neurotransmitter in the spinal cord, as it is in the brain. The cell bodies of these serotonergic spinal projections are in the brainstem. When rats were run on a treadmill for 60 minutes up a 5% slope, the peak levels of 5-HT in the ventral funiculus of the spinal cord increased about fourfold, whereas these levels slightly decreased in the ventral horn (gray matter) (81). There also is some evidence that training may decrease the sensitivity to 5-HT release by reducing the receptor density (82). Since 5-HT has been associated with fatigue, this reduced sensitivity to 5-HT may be a mechanism by which training could lead to greater resistance to fatigue (83). However, clear evidence for a training-induced reduction in sensitivity to 5-HT in humans has not been reported. The modulation of 5-HT receptors in response to exercise training also has been examined. Although 7 weeks of training on a treadmill had no effect on 5-HT1B receptor mRNA in the striatum or hippocampus, the levels in the frontal cortex and cerebellum were reduced (84). It was observed that the sensitivity to 5-HT1B receptors was reduced or eliminated in the hippocampus by the exercise training. Exercise training at a moderate intensity has been reported to increase the level of 5-HT transporters and the 5-HT2A receptors in isolated platelet membranes. Platelet membranes were studied because they seem to serve as a convenient indicator of neuronal effects. Heavy exercise training, on the other hand, actually decreased the 5-HT2A receptors in the platelet membranes (83).

Norepinephrine and Exercise

NE levels increase in the whole brain in response to running and swimming. As expected, the increase in the brain is highly region specific. For example, 8 weeks of training results in a significant increase in NE and its metabolites in the pons, medulla, and spinal cord but not in the frontal cortex and hippocampus of rats (80). More than half of the NE in the brain is in the pons and medulla. Several days of a running exercise increased tyrosine hydroxylase activity (a measurement of catecholamine activity) in the locus ceruleus and ventral tegmental area of the rat brain (85).

It is speculated that the reduction in depression reported in response to exercise training is related to the modulation in NE levels. Chronic dynamic exercise (wheel running) of rats also has been reported to prevent the depletion of NE that occurs when exposed to foot shock. In addition, exercise reduced the latency before responding to a foot shock, consistent with there being a NE-mediated modulation of the behavior (80). Changes in NE metabolism and function in response to training is also of interest because of its potential role in regulating cardiovascular function. Rats that are trained on a treadmill have a reduced affinity for and density of α_2-adrenergic receptor binding sites in the nucleus tractus solitarii. In addition, there is an increase in affinity of vasopressin receptors in the nucleus tractus solitarii. Both of these adaptations are important in the neural control of cardiovascular function (86).

Dynamic Exercise Training and the CNS

There is a surge in interest in the ways exercise affects the nervous system. Some of the reasons for this surge include the evidence accumulating that dynamic exercise can

1. Enhance the recovery from neurotraumatic injuries.
2. Enhance learning.
3. Even stimulate neurogenesis.

As a result of this surging interest, a large number of published papers report results that do not yet form a logical or consistent basis for formulating useful generalizations of their scientific or clinical significance. However, the results of many of these studies are interesting and intriguing and warrant continuing study. There is substantial evidence that the rate of axoplasmic transport in neurons is elevated in rats trained on a treadmill. The peak and average transport velocities, as well as the total amount of protein-bound radioactivity, for fast axonal transport in the sciatic nerve is higher in trained than untrained rats (87). The effects are most likely chronic adaptations in fast axonal transport, since the measurements were made 21 or 22 days after the last exercise bout. The responses varied among different motor pools, with the increase apparently being related to the amount of overload imposed on the motor pool. In rats that were run on a treadmill with increasing intensity over 8 weeks (88) axonal transport of acetylcholinesterase was enhanced in the rat sciatic nerve. However, swim training did not have this effect. Despite the controversial nature of the swimming of rats for training purposes, these findings raise the question as to the significance of training in maintaining normal neural control of movement.

Each of these observations showing changes in neurotransmitters and their receptors with dynamic exercise and training demonstrate that the brain is adapting to different levels and kinds of activity in many and complex ways. The studies to date have not led to any fundamentally new concepts regarding exercise or how the brain functions. They do show, as would be expected, that many if not most areas of the brain and spinal cord are very dynamically involved in most movements. How the changes noted earlier relate to changes in functional capacity and in the perception of the quality of performance is a subject for further investigations as we learn more about how the CNS accommodates movement.

Muscle Atrophy and Movement Control

To execute fine motor control, the brain and spinal cord must generate a series of action potentials that will reach a very specific number and kind of motor neurons in a very specific sequence. In addition, the brain and spinal cord must know rather precisely the mechanical consequences of activation of a given set of motor neurons. Therefore, the brain and spinal cord assume the force- and speed-generating properties of the muscle fibers that are activated. During the performance of normal daily activities, there are continuous opportunities for the nervous and muscular systems to become familiarized with or update one another so that the nervous system can accurately predict the mechanical consequences of muscle hypertrophy or atrophy. Our understanding of how the adjustments or resynchronization of neural and muscular elements occurs, however, remains incomplete.

When the mechanical output is an error of consequence during the performance of a routine task, the nervous system assumed that a different mechanical output had occurred. For example, if the nervous system is predicting a 10g force from a motor unit but the muscle fibers have atrophied, the force and power will be less than expected. When this mismatching occurs, the nervous system can readily adjust by recruiting more motor units or by increasing the frequency of excitation of the active motor units. Since muscle atrophy often occurs gradually, as observed with aging and some neuromuscular diseases, these adjustments can be made more readily. There must be numerous neural and musculoskeletal mechanisms through which this compensation can occur.

Another indirect consequence of the muscle atrophy on motor unit recruitment and movement performance is an increase in fatigability (Fig. 3.32).

Often it is assumed that increased fatigability of a muscle can be attributed to a decrease in the metabolic potential of the individual muscle fibers. The loss of fatigue resistance attributable to these intrinsic properties of the muscle fibers,

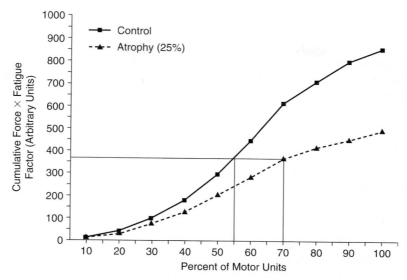

FIGURE 3.32 Impact of muscle atrophy without any further pathology on the functional output potential of that motor pool when performing a task lasting for several minutes. Two factors limit the performance in this case. There is the obvious deficit due to the 25% muscle loss and the proportional loss in force. Thus, to accomplish a given motor task, more motor units must be recruited. The higher in the recruitment order within a motor pool, the more fatigable the larger units are, so the combined loss of force and the increased fatigability of the additional units that must be recruited to complete a task result in the individual fatiguing more rapidly even if there is no loss in the fatigability of the individual units. With atrophy 70% of the motor pool would have to be recruited to perform the same task as 55% of the motor pool in the absence of atrophy. (*Unpublished figure, J.R. Edgerton and R.R. Roy*)

however, is often rather small, even after prolonged periods of decreased activity or inactivity (89).

The more dramatic effect of muscle atrophy on fatigability may be attributed to the fact that more motor units must be recruited and at a higher frequency of excitation for an atrophied muscle to perform a given motor task. The overall fatigability will be greater because the additional motor units recruited—those with the higher threshold levels and lower fatigue resistance—will be more fatigable. Consequently, muscle fiber atrophy imposes several critical adjustments in the totally integrated neural control of the motor system: altered sensory feedback, additional recruitment of motor units, and increased fatigability.

Long-Term Neuronal Influences on Motor Unit Properties and Fatigability

Multiple factors regulate fatigability. A fundamental but partially unresolved issue is what factors determine the fatigability of each motor unit. Fatigue resistance clearly is directly related to the mitochondrial content of the muscle unit, that is, the fibers of the motor unit (90). The mitochondrial content of a fiber is determined to a large extent by neural factors independent of activity. Mitochondrial content of any given motor unit, however, can be modulated upward with greater neuromuscular activity, as occurs with prolonged endurance-type exercise. High activity levels of enzymes linked to oxidative phosphorylation are inversely related to the fatigability of the muscle, motor unit, or muscle fiber (91). Many other factors also affect the fatigability of a motor unit. For example, the rate at which adenosine triphosphate (ATP) is hydrolyzed to adenosine diphosphate (ADP) and inorganic phosphate (Pi) is determined in part by the myosin phenotype. For example, if a fiber has slow myosin, it will have a slow maximum rate of ATP hydrolysis, and the fiber will be more resistant to fatigue. With respect to maintaining homeostasis, a general concept would be that the ratio of oxidative phosphorylation to ATP hydrolysis potential is directly related to the resistance to fatigue of a muscle, motor unit, or muscle fiber (also see Chapter 8).

The fatigue resistance of the soleus muscle and its motor units is largely maintained after cross-reinnervation with a nerve that normally innervates a fatigable muscle (92), after spinal cord transection (93), after spinal cord isolation (94), and after chronic hindlimb unloading (95). These results indicate that the fatigue properties of type I (slow) muscle fibers can be relatively independent of the amount of activation and loading and of phenotypic changes. Following spinal cord injury in humans the fatigue resistance of the soleus muscle is maintained for about 6 weeks, but it becomes more fatigable after about a year of complete paralysis (96).

Normal *in Vivo* Neuromuscular Activity Patterns

As alluded to several times earlier in this chapter, the nervous system not only controls specific movements; it also determines to a very large extent the properties of a muscle, such as size, speed, and fatigability. So what is it about the activation patterns generated by the CNS that defines the muscle properties? There is an interactive effect between the daily activation and loading characteristics of a muscle in determining its mechanical and phenotypic properties. Also, the

relationship between the total daily activity of a muscle and its mass is highly nonlinear (Fig. 3.33).

For example, the soleus muscle of a normal adult cat is active about 14 to 23% of the day during routine cage activity (97,98). When the muscle is made chronically inactive (<1% of normal activity) via spinal cord isolation, the mass is reduced to about one-third of normal (94). Therefore, one-third of the mass of this predominantly slow muscle is independent of its electrical activity and passive mechanical events. However only approximately 9 minutes of high-resistance isometric, shortening, or lengthening electrically evoked contractions per day (0.62% of the day) results in the maintenance of about 64, 55, and 55% of the mass of the otherwise inactive soleus muscle, respectively. In chronic complete low thoracic spinal cord transected cats the soleus is active about 8% of the day (115 minutes) during routine cage activity, and 56% of its mass is maintained (97). Note the similarity in the preservation of muscle mass in the spinal cord transected (about 56%) and spinal cord isolated plus electromechanically stimulated (~55–64%) cats despite daily activation durations of 115 compared to 9 minutes. This comparison highlights the role of the loading dynamics in maintaining muscle mass. When electrically and me-

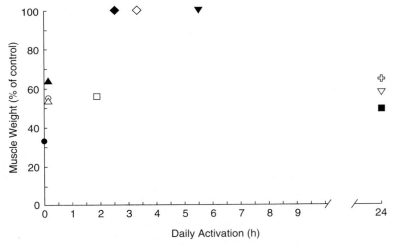

FIGURE 3.33   Relationship between muscle weight (relative to control) and the daily activation level of the muscle. Control soleus: cat (◊) and Rhesus monkey (▼). Four month spinal cord isolated (SI) cat soleus: SI only (●); SI plus shortening contractions (△); SI plus lengthening contractions (○); SI plus isometric contractions (▲). Six month spinal cord transected cat soleus: (□). Chronically electrically stimulated: rabbit tibialis anterior (TA) for 2 weeks at 10 Hz (+); rabbit TA for 6 weeks at 10 Hz (▽), and rabbit TA for 12 weeks at 10 HZ or rat TA for 8 weeks at 10 to 20 Hz (■). Note that as little as 9 min of contractions in the otherwise silent cat soleus muscle maintained a similar relative weight as continuous stimulation of the rabbit or rat TA for 2 to 12 weeks. These data suggest that there is an optimal amount of activation-load that will preserve the size of muscle fibers. *(Modified from Roy RR, Zhong H, Hodgson JA, et al. Influences of electromechanical events in defining skeletal muscle properties. Muscle Nerve 2002;26:238–251.)*

chanically silenced muscles are stimulated electrically with the same duration and pattern but under isometric, shortening, or lengthening conditions, the relative preservation of the muscle mass is: isometric > lengthening > shortening (99). These results demonstrate that the mechanical events as well as the electrical events play a role in defining the mass of the muscle.

Daily EMG activity levels of selected hindlimb muscles also have been assessed in Rhesus monkeys during normal cage activity (100). The soleus is a highly active muscle relative to the medial gastrocnemius, tibialis anterior, and vastus lateralis, regardless of how the activity is expressed or normalized (Fig. 3.34).

However, as with the cat, one of the most active muscles, the soleus, is inactive for a large proportion of the day. Similar trends are observed when comparing the soleus and medial gastrocnemius activity in humans (101). However, when one looks at the details, there is no close link between how active a muscle is and its predominant phenotype.

Plasticity of the Nervous System in Response to Activity: A Neural Darwinian Process

How does the nervous system continuously adapt to changing demands throughout life? Edelman (102) theorized that the brain is dynamically organized into cellular populations containing individually varied networks, the structure and function of which are selected by different means during development and behavior. The cellular populations are proposed to be collections of hundreds to thousands of strongly interconnected neurons acting as a functional unit. The key functional elements of this concept of neuronal group selection areas follows: (a) There is continuous spatial temporal representation of an object and a mechanism for continuous updating of the selection of neuronal groups that can generate a given motor synergy or pattern. (b) These neuronal groups that generate a movement pattern can degenerate by selectively matching sensory and motor processes. This concept also assumes that different neuronal groups can accomplish the same function. From a Neural Darwinian perspective, the adaptive nature of these functional units reflects neural projections that formed either during development (primary repertoire) or as a result of experience and via changing synaptic efficacy (secondary repertoire) (Fig. 3.35)

The concept of neuronal group selection, a key component of Neural Darwinism, can play a dominating role in the execution of motor patterns controlled by the lumbosacral spinal cord. The neuronal group selection theory, although originally considered a supraspinal phenomenon, is as relevant to the circuitry within the spinal cord as it is to the brain. For example, the human spinal cord can generate motor synergies

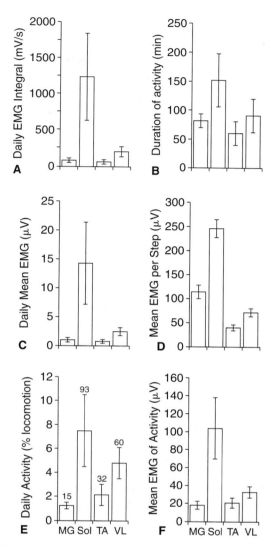

FIGURE 3.34 A summary of the daily activity for 5 monkeys housed in colony cages. **A.** The daily integral is the integral of EMG for the entire day. **B.** The duration of activity is the total time that EMG activity was detected in the muscle. **C.** The daily mean EMG is the daily integral divided by 24 hours (86,400 seconds). **D.** Mean EMG per step is the mean EMG amplitude calculated over the entire step. It was calculated from 5 steps of treadmill locomotion at 1.33 m/second. **E.** Daily activity (percent locomotion) is the percentage of the day that the Rhesus would have to spend walking at 1.33 m/second to generate the daily EMG integral equivalent for each muscle, assuming that it participated in no other activity. The duration of the locomotion in minutes is shown above the bar for each muscle. **F.** The mean EMG of activity is the total daily activity divided by the duration of activity (A/B). MG, medial gastrocnemius; Sol, soleus; TA, tibialis anterior; VL, vastus lateralis. Bars, SEM. (*Modified from Hodgson JA, Wichayanuparp S, Recktenwald MR, et al. Circadian force and EMG activity in hindlimb muscles of rhesus monkeys. J Neurophysiol 2001;86:1430–1444.*)

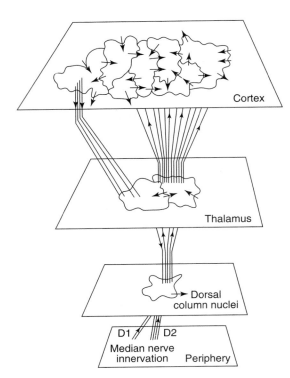

FIGURE 3.35 Dynamic vertical and horizontal reentrant connectivity across a linked system of laminae and nuclei. Changes in any one level must result in readjustment of all linked levels. The concept is that different functional groups of neurons are forming throughout life and that this reorganization is activity dependent. These functional groups form during development (primary) and in the adult (secondary). *(Modified from Edelman GM. Neural Darwinism: The Theory of Neuronal Group Selection. New York: Basic Books, 1987, p. 173.)*

that can be categorized as being primary (formulated during development) and secondary (formulated from experience and learning) repertoires (Fig. 3.36).

Experiments have demonstrated that the human lumbosacral spinal cord can match complex proprioceptive information with predictable motor repertoires, such as stepping, standing, and limb flexion, even after severe muscle atrophy and neural impairment. The execution of these motor tasks in subjects with spinal cord injuries and with no supraspinal input demonstrate that dynamically organized cellular populations can generate synergies that are not confined to the brain. Furthermore, it appears that secondary repertoires can occur in the human spinal cord, since the synaptic efficacy of the networks that generate stepping and standing can be markedly improved with repetitive movements in which the sensory ensemble is appropriately matched, that is, context dependent. In addition, these data are consistent with the neuronal group

selection theory in that the motor tasks studied can be performed by functionally, but not morphologically, equivalent networks.

Spinal Learning With Motor Training

Neuromotor training is a primary intervention that consistently improves the ability to step and stand even after the spinal cord is isolated from the brain (45,58). There is strong evidence that training of complete spinal humans on a treadmill belt using a weight-supporting device combined with overground training can increase the levels of motor pool activation, improve coordination of motor pool recruitment (Fig. 3.36), and reduce muscle atrophy (63). However, these improvements occur slowly, that is, after weeks or even months of training. Neuromotor training provides a means by which the sensory system can become synchronized with the spinal circuitry and with the motor pools that are linked to this circuitry.

A Simple Model of Spinal Learning: Flexor Withdrawal Response

Early evidence that spinal circuits respond to neuromotor training came from studies of simple hindlimb motor reflexes in animals with complete spinal cord transection. Simple hindlimb reflexes, for example the hindlimb withdrawal reflex, can be modulated via classical (103) or operant (104) conditioning techniques. An example of operant conditioning of the spinal cord is the prolonged dorsiflexion that occurs in a spinal rat after a series of electrical stimuli are presented to the paw. In this paradigm, when the paw drops below a threshold position, a stimulus is delivered to the leg. Over 5 to 20 minutes a completely spinalized rat can be conditioned to avoid the stimuli by maintaining a more dorsiflexed position, even though there can be no conscious perception of the shock (105). In contrast, no conditioning occurs in yoked spinal rats that get shocked in a manner that is not associated with a specific foot position. All of these findings are consistent with the conclusion that spinal circuits can be trained to perform relatively simple hindlimb motor tasks in the absence of any connection between the spinal cord and the brain.

Learning of More Complex Motor Tasks in the Spinal Cord

The works of Nesmeyanova (106) and Shurrager and Culler (107) were the first to suggest that complex postural and locomotor tasks can be improved after some training paradigm. It is now clear that hindlimb stepping in spinal cats can be improved with daily practice of walking on a treadmill. Several laboratories (43,108,109) have demonstrated that adult spinal cats performed full weight-bearing hindlimb

SCI-C1

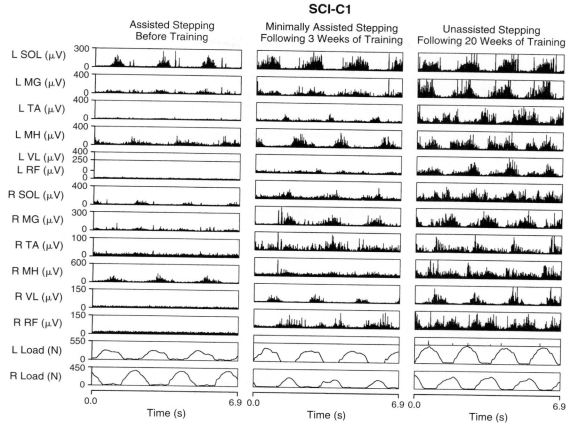

FIGURE 3.36 Development of new functional neuronal groups, probably in the spinal cord, of a severely injured spinal cord subject. The facts that more motor pools can be activated with locomotor training and that shifts in the timing of the bursts can occur illustrate the formation of secondary neuronal groups (Fig. 3.35). L, left; R, right; SOL, soleus; MG, medial gastrocnemius; TA, tibialis anterior; MH, medial hamstrings; VL, vastus lateralis; RF, rectus femoris; μV, micro voltage. *(Compliments of Susan Harkema, University of California, Los Angeles.)*

stepping on a treadmill after as little as 2 to 3 weeks of loco-motor training (Fig. 3.37).

These data provided the most compelling behavioral evidence that the circuitry within the lumbosacral spinal cord that generates hindlimb stepping can be modified by the sensorimotor experience. With training, there is a steady increase in the maximum treadmill speed achieved with full weight bearing and by the number of plantar surface steps performed (110). In addition, locomotor training tended to normalize the characteristics of the locomotion based on similarities in EMG and kinematic patterns of trained spinal and intact cats. Normal flexor and extensor muscle activation relationships, EMG burst waveform shapes, and adjustments in EMG burst durations across speeds of locomotion are preserved in trained spinal cats. With step training, the overall patterns of joint angle excursions during a step cycle, the sequence of flexion and extension movements in hindlimb joints, and the force levels in the soleus muscle are

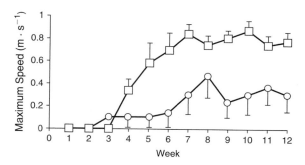

FIGURE 3.37 Bipedal hindlimb stepping on a treadmill after a complete transection of the spinal cord at a low thoracic level in step-trained and untrained cats. Average maximum speeds for 6 step-trained (□) and 6 untrained (○) cats are shown 1 to 12 weeks after spinal cord transection. The difference between the two lines represents the effects of training versus spontaneous recovery. Bars, SEM. *(Modified from de Leon RD, Hodgson JA, Roy RR, et al. Locomotor capacity attributable to step training versus spontaneous recovery after spinalization in adult cats. J Neurophysiol 1998;79: 1329–1340.)*

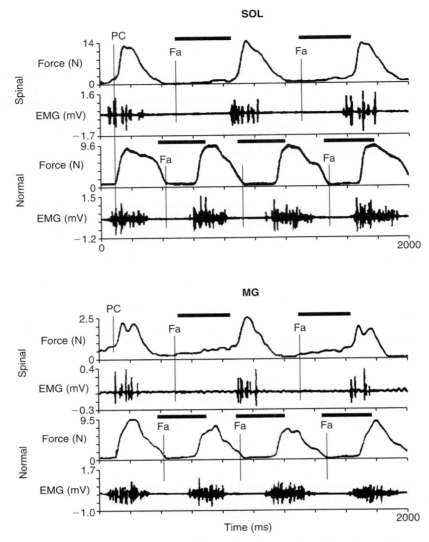

FIGURE 3.38 Force and EMG records from the soleus and medial gastrocnemius muscles of a spinal (complete transection at T12) and a control cat stepping on a treadmill belt moving at a moderate speed. The force was recorded using implanted strain gauges on the tendons of the muscles. The timing of the EMG and force patterns are similar for the spinal and control cats. However, there are some obvious differences. For example, the force pattern in the soleus is shorter in the spinal cat. Also, although the peak force levels are similar in the soleus, the peak force in the medial gastrocnemius (MG) of the spinal cat is much less than in the control. This reflects a limitation in the level of recruitment of the motor pools consisting of the larger, less excitable motor units. This is also indicated in the intensity of the EMG signals of the MG of the spinal versus the control cat. PC, time of paw contact, Fa, point of ankle flexion. The thick horizontal line indicates time for stance in the contralateral limb. *(Modified from Lovely RG, Gregor RJ, Roy RR, et al. Weight-bearing hindlimb stepping in treadmill-exercised adult spinal cats. Brain Res 1990;514:206–218.)*

similar, but not identical, during stepping in intact and spinal cats (Fig. 3.38).

The fact that the activity in neural networks of the lumbar spinal cord is to a large extent determined by the pattern of activity in the hindlimbs is further demonstrated by the ef-

fect of stand training in spinal cats. Spinal cats can be trained to perform full weight-bearing extension (maintaining posture) for long periods (111). However, most stand-trained spinal cats cannot generate even a few successful weight-supported steps. Thus, the spinal cord learns the specific motor task presented during the training sessions. Furthermore, when the step training is stopped for 12 weeks, the stepping ability is as poor as it was prior to any training; that is, the spinal cord appears to forget the specific motor task if it is not practiced (Fig. 3.39).

Although it is possible that these learned behaviors can occur only in the injured spinal cord, a more logical interpretation is that some aspects of these repetitive motor responses can be learned by neural networks in the spinal cord of uninjured individuals as well.

Supraspinally Induced Plasticity of the Spinal Monosynaptic Reflex

Several studies showing an increase in both the firing threshold potential and the amplitude of the afterhyperpolarization potential of motor neurons after an H-reflex conditioning protocol provide evidence that the efficacy of the monosynaptic synapse can be modulated via some activity-dependent mechanisms. These studies show functional as well as morphological changes associated with the Ia fiber terminals on motor neurons as a result of supraspinal modulation of the excitability of these afferent synapses over weeks or even months. The changes in the monosynaptic efficacy in the spinal cord observed after several weeks persisted immediately after a complete midthoracic spinal cord transection (112). In addition, Beaumont and Gardiner (113) reported that slow-type motor neurons of 12-week treadmill-trained rats had greater afterhyperpolarizations than control rats. Thus, there are adaptations in the intrinsic properties of motor neurons as well as the synapses that modulate motor neuron excitability associated with motor learning and training.

Understanding the synaptic plasticity that underlies more complex motor tasks, however, is a very difficult challenge. Our general interpretation of the findings about spinal learning is that the lumbar spinal circuitry can learn to step with exposure to repetitive step training. In the absence of any training, the patterns of motor output are generated in response to the stimuli associated with the movement of the treadmill. However, the probability that the correct patterns, that is, synchronization of ipsilateral and contralateral events, will be generated in untrained animals over a series of consecutive step cycles is low. The effect of training, therefore, is to repetitively activate the appropriate extensor and flexor networks in a specific temporal and spatial pattern so that the probability of generating successful responses will be improved.

A Continuously Adapting Synaptic Milieu for Motor Control

A fundamental property of the neuromotor control system is its intrinsic variability in the circuitry that is activated during

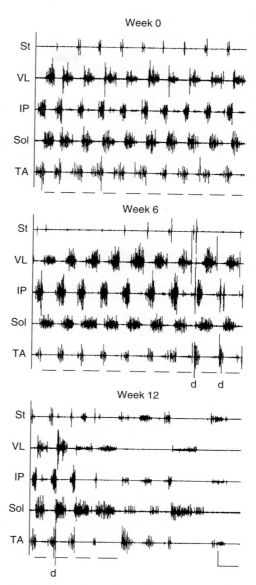

FIGURE 3.39   Raw EMG recorded from selected hindlimb muscles of one spinal cat during tests of stepping at a treadmill speed of 0.4 m · s⁻¹ after step training (week 0) and after the cessation of step training (weeks 6 and 12). St, semitendinosus; VL, vastus lateralis; IP, iliopsoas; Sol, soleus; TA, tibialis anterior. Lines drawn under the EMG records indicate the stance phases in which full weight-bearing occurred on the plantar surface of the paw. Horizontal calibration, 1 s; vertical calibration 1 mV for all muscles except for the Sol, 2 mV. Note that only after a 12-week absence of motor training was there a significant degradation in the coordination of the lower limb motor pools. *(Modified from de Leon RD, Hodgson JA, Roy RR, et al. Retention of hindlimb stepping ability in adult spinal cats after the cessation of step training. J Neurophysiol 1999;81:85–94.)*

a motor task (114) (Fig. 3.23). Even when one is completely rested and there is little or no likelihood of fatigue, there will be variation in the motor task from one effort to the next. After years of practicing to make a free throw in basketball, one is rarely successful 95% of the time. In most cases, the percentage is about 75% even for professional athletes. In addition to this baseline level of variability under the most optimal and constant conditions, further variations are imposed by continuously changing physiological states. The term *physiological states* as used here encompasses a time scale ranging from milliseconds to years. In this sense the nervous system is changing constantly, at least physiologically, and some features change more rapidly than others. These continuously fluctuating properties reflect changing probabilities of excitation and inhibition of neuronal synapses between multiple supraspinal centers and the neuromuscular junctions. Given that millions of synaptic events shape every instant of a motor task, some variation in the pattern of activation of the net ensemble of motor neurons activated from effort to effort is to be expected. Although some of the changes in the efficacy of excitation of some synapses might be viewed from a perspective of fatigue, this seems unlikely unless one's definition of fatigue includes any activity or state-dependent phenomenon. The key point is that the history of the synaptic effects plays a role in defining the probabilities of excitation at some point thereafter.

Examples will be used to illustrate these general concepts. These examples represent synaptic plasticity ranging from the cerebral cortex to the neuromuscular junction. Two of the most studied synapses in mammalian physiology have been the neuromuscular junction and the monosynaptic stretch reflex. The reason for focusing on these synapses is their accessibility for experimentation. However, implications of changing synaptic efficacy of other synapses often can be implied by indirect methods and with clever experimental designs. In most cases it is difficult to ascertain which synapses are responsible for the experimental observations, particularly in models *in vivo*. Although there may be a scientific urge to pinpoint the synapse to which a change in performance *in vivo* can be attributed, it is likely that the changes reflect highly interactive dynamics involving synaptic efficacy at multiple levels (115).

Effects of Mental Practice and Cross-Education on Motor Performance

One can mentally rehearse a motor task so that maximum strength and motor skill will improve (116). Although synaptic efficacy at supraspinal sites may be important to these changes in performance, some effects may be at the spinal cord level. For example, there is an elevated level of excitation of the relevant motor pools to the extent that both motor units and mechanoreceptors are activated in muscles during mental practice. Even when there is no apparent activation of motor units during mental practice, however, there tends to be an elevated level of excitability of the motor pools associated with the mentally practiced motor task. But even when there is some activity in a muscle during mental practice, the synaptic events needed to excite a large number or even all motor units within a pool do not occur. It appears that with mental practice there is a sufficient level of net excitatory input to a population of motor neurons and interneurons, although at a subliminal or subthreshold level, such that a lingering memory trace can be formed (116).

Cross-Education Training

Another example of training-induced synaptic adaptation is improvement in strength in an untrained limb when the contralateral limb is trained. Although some of this cross-education effect may occur at a supraspinal level, the improvement in strength in both limbs brought about by voluntarily activating the muscles of only one limb also may be due to changes in the spinal cord. The presence of this cross-education effect has been demonstrated in a variety of muscles, and in response to isometric, concentric, and eccentric training (117–119). The primary contralateral muscles that are affected are the homologous muscles. The magnitude of the effect has varied considerably among the many experiments studying this phenomenon. These cross-education effects appear to be highly specific for the mode of training and testing. In response to training by voluntary isometric or concentric contractions, the gains in strength in the contralateral limb vary from about 5 to 25% (119). Training eccentrically results in greater contralateral effects, with the gains being as high as 75% of the ipsilateral effect (117). Electrical stimulation has an even greater contralateral effect when tested in the same mode as used during the training (118).

In most of the studies of contralateral training effects, it seems reasonably clear that the activity level in the untrained muscles during training is relatively low and no muscle hypertrophy is usually observed. It also appears that both supraspinal and spinal circuits contribute to these cross-education effects. Obviously, not all of the motor neurons of the motor pools that actually execute a movement need be activated to improve the performance of that movement. Perhaps it is necessary only to activate neural circuits that set up the execution of a movement, and the activation of these planning circuits can improve the performance of an intended task.

Adaptations of Muscle Afferents

Short- and Long-Term Changes in the H-Reflex

Many of the properties of the sensory input from the neuromuscular system are activity dependent. The excitability of the monosynaptic stretch reflex or its electrical analog, the H-reflex, can change from millisecond to millisecond, and it can adapt over weeks or months by either increasing or decreasing its sensitivity to stretch. The H-reflex is a measure of the efficacy of the transmission of Ia afferent to homonymous motor neurons. Testing monosynaptic efficacy by electrically stimulating the peripheral nerve enables one to control the excitatory signals (the number of sensory axons excited) more accurately than by actually controlling it mechanically using a muscle-tendon tap.

Modulation of the H-Reflex Within a Step Cycle

The clearest example of the acute plasticity of the monosynaptic reflex is its modulation during a single step. For example, during walking the H-reflex rises during the stance phase, falls during the onset of the swing phase, and then gradually rises during the latter portion of the swing phase of each step. During running, the H-reflex falls during the stance phase at the interval between the end of stance and beginning of the swing phase. However, the H-reflex increases to its highest level at the end of the swing and the beginning of stance (54) (Fig. 3.40).

In these experiments using the H-reflex as an indicator of the excitability of monosynaptic reflexes under different conditions or at different times, it is essential that the same number of sensory axons be stimulated for the conditions being compared. Given this assumption, how many motor neurons reach the threshold for excitation for a given number of sensory axons stimulated? Since the number of motor neurons activated differs over the course of a step cycle, the synaptic efficacy of the sensory projections is also changing. This is due to the modulation of other synaptic inputs directly onto the Ia terminals. These synaptic inputs can increase or decrease the efficacy of the monosynaptic reflex, and this input can come from supraspinal or spinal neurons. Since the H-reflex is modulated during stepping in humans with a complete spinal cord injury, it is apparent that the H-reflex can be mediated by the spinal circuits in the absence of supraspinal input. This does not mean, however, that there is no supraspinal modulation, as the work of Wolpaw and colleagues (112) shows.

Changes in the H-Reflex Due to Repetition and Training

The stretch reflex gain (greater response per stimulus input) is elevated during and after fatiguing contractions. In response to resistance training and an increase in strength, the H-reflex excitability is elevated during a maximal voluntary contraction (120). The H-reflex also is elevated in humans following jump, resistance, or endurance training

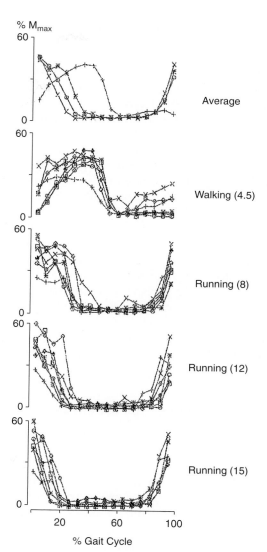

FIGURE 3.40 H reflex modulations. In the top tracings, the modulation of the soleus H reflex is shown as the average from seven subjects during walking at 4.5 km · h⁻¹ (+), running at 8 km · h⁻¹ (*), running at 12 km · h⁻¹ (−) and running at 15 km · h⁻¹ (×). Each tracing shows data for each subject and for each velocity investigated. Each of the seven subjects is represented by a specific symbol. All data are expressed as a percentage of M_{max}, which is the maximum amplitude of the EMG response when stimulating the nerve. The gait cycle was divided into 16 time slices and normalized with heel strike at 0 and 100%. Each cycle starts at foot contact. In all cases the H reflex amplitude rises rapidly just prior to foot contact and is suppressed during the swing phase. Walking differs from running in that the facilitation state persists for almost half of the cycle compared to a shorter duration of facilitation at the fastest running speeds (see average plots). Also, during walking there tends to be less facilitation prior to foot contact than with running. These data are consistent with the view that the stretch reflex contributes significantly to the dynamics of stepping, perhaps by taking advantage of the considerable amount of elastic energy that can be stored in muscle-tendon units. *(Modified from Simonsen EB, Dyhre-Poulsen P. Amplitude of the human soleus H reflex during walking and running. J Physiol 1999;515:929–939.)*

(120). This elevated H-reflex may be due to greater presynaptic excitatory drive from higher centers to the monosynaptic synapses, although smaller H-reflexes have been reported in athletes trained for explosive power, such as volleyball players, sprinters, and ballet dancers (121). These results should be viewed cautiously, since the H-reflex amplitudes are a function of the percentage of the motor unit types. Since athletes tend to migrate to events that take advantage of their predominance of fiber types, this may also be accompanied by basic differences, as in the H-reflex. For example, is it the training or the selection of certain phenotypes that explains a given athlete's physiological properties?

Interestingly, chronic exposure to microgravity reduces the threshold for excitation of the monosynaptic reflex and raises the gain of this reflex. These studies demonstrate that the efficacy of the monosynaptic reflex is routinely and easily modulated in response to neuromuscular activity levels. However, observations to date leave it unclear what the mechanisms following different activity paradigms may be. Also, the eventual functional significance of these modulations in controlling a motor task remains unclear.

Modulation of Other Spinal Reflexes

Other spinal reflexes also can be modulated by input that changes the excitability of a synaptic circuit. Extremely acute changes in smaller muscle afferents (types III and IV) occur with the onset of fatigue. Type III and IV afferents fire at higher rates during fatiguing contractions, and modulation of these afferents may contribute to changes in blood pressure and heart rate. For example, when the ulnar nerve of human subjects is stimulated to generate isometric forces, blood pressure rises and is directly and closely linked to a decrease in isometric force. The sensitivity of the muscle afferents to the force-generating status is further illustrated when the hand is elevated. Under these conditions, the muscle force declines more and the blood pressure increases proportionally more than with the hand not elevated. An important point here is the highly integrative nature of the muscle afferents: not only do they sense changing kinematics and kinetics, they also induce a correspondingly appropriate compensatory action in the cardiovascular system (122).

Firing Patterns of Afferents From Muscle Spindles During Locomotion

Recordings from spindle primary afferents (group Ia fibers) during locomotion demonstrate a range of firing behaviors. These afferents are large and have a low threshold for activation when the axons are electrically stimulated. Examples of these are shown in Figure 3.23.

The slightly smaller group Ib fibers have their receptors (GTOs) toward the end of the muscle fascicles and near aponeuroses and tendons. These mechanoreceptors are activated during low-force contractions as well as at high forces, similar to the group Ia fibers. It is a common misconception that the group Ib fibers associated with the GTOs are very insensitive to modest forces and that their function is to detect very high forces and in response provide a strong inhibition of the motor neurons to that muscle to prevent excessive forces. It appears, however, that the GTOs represent another mechanoreceptor that provides unique input to the spinal cord and brain about the routine modulation of forces in the musculotendinous structures (50).

The even smaller group III and IV afferent fibers also seem to provide important information about the environment of the muscle. It is well known that these small afferents mediate reflexes from the muscle that can modulate heart rate, blood pressure, myocardial contractility, and ventilation. For example, when muscles in an anesthetized animal are stimulated via the ventral root, arterial pressure, heart rate, and ventilation will increase. However, this response is eliminated if the dorsal roots, which carry the sensory information from the muscle to the spinal cord and brain, are cut (123). Subsequent experiments have demonstrated that the large afferents, that is, group I and II afferents, play little or no role in these cardiovascular and ventilatory responses and that the reflex component can be attributed largely to the group III and IV afferents (124). Furthermore, it appears that the group III and IV afferents differ in their sensitivity to mechanical perturbations. Most group III fibers (almost 80% in the cat) respond vigorously within a second after a contraction of the triceps surae muscle complex, whereas about 40% of the group IV fibers respond to a similar stimulus. Perhaps more important is that almost all of the group III fibers slowed or terminated their response as the tension declined, but the response tended to increase in group IV fibers as the contraction continued. Also, group IV afferent excitation is not closely linked to the oscillations in force generation after the first few contractions of a longer series of contractions.

These observations led to the hypothesis that group III and particularly group IV afferents were sensors of the metabolic status of the muscle, that is, metaboreceptors. Muscle ischemia alone resulted in an increase in afferent activity in almost 50% of the group IV compared to about 10% of the group III fibers (125). It appears that infusion of lactic or arachidonic acid (without an adjustment in pH) will increase excitation of group III and IV afferents (126).

In effect, muscles are exquisite sensors of mechanical and chemical events. There are thousands of mechanoreceptors and metaboreceptors in each muscle. About half of most peripheral nerves are sensory and half motor. Furthermore, combinations of sensors can provide precise information about the levels and locations of forces and displacements. Many of these mechanoreceptors and metaboreceptors combined, both within and among muscles, provide extensive detail about the functional state of the whole body.

Regions of the Brain Activated During Dynamic Exercise

Since the motor system receives input from so many sensory sources, one would expect that most of the areas of the brain become activated during exercise. This is the case, but to date a consistent pattern of activation relative to resting conditions has not emerged. Vissing, Andersen, and Diemer (127) reported 40% increases in the total radiolabeled glucose uptake in the rat brain during running at 28 m · min^{-1}. The greatest increase was observed in the cerebellum (110%), while the motor cortex (39%), basal ganglia (30%), and substantia nigra (37%) also had significant increases. All of these areas of the brain are linked to the coordination of motor functions. The auditory and visual cortex had increases of 32 and 42%, respectively, suggesting enhanced neuronal activity associated with the sound of the treadmill and the constant visual input associated with running on a treadmill belt in a relatively confined cubicle. Other areas of the brain, including those associated with autonomic function—subthalamic nuclei (47%), posterior hypothalamic nuclei (74%), and hippocampus (29%)—had substantial increases in glucose uptake. The major point is that significant increases in the metabolic properties occur in many areas of the brain during most motor tasks, in this case locomotion.

In spite of the limitations in techniques to gain insight to how the CNS controls motor function, it is apparent that most of the brain participates in these fundamental tasks. A major advantage of the glucose uptake approach is that *in vivo* experiments can be performed. But information about the changes in glucose uptake only gives clues to which areas of the brain are involved. It provides no insight to how the physiological properties of these areas are changing. Advances in molecular biology have led to a number of techniques that permit one to ask what cellular events underlie changes in behavior. With new *in vivo* imaging technologies, it is now possible to repetitively monitor specific mRNA expressions *in vivo* over weeks using microPET (micro positron emission tomography). In this technology the energy emitted from radioligands can be detected and localized. These radioligands are designed to have short half-lives and are relatively expensive to generate. Future studies are likely to provide extremely valuable information on how the CNS functions as a totally integrated system during exercise.

Because most of the known cell-to-cell interactions in the brain and spinal cord in the form of action potentials are generated by neurons, most of the emphasis in trying to understand neural function during exercise has focused on these cells. However, another population of cells in the CNS plays important supportive roles that largely remain unclear. These cells are called glia, meaning glue. They have been described as cells that provide the medium within which the neurons rest. Most of the cells in the brain are glial cells, not neurons. These glial cells probably play a major role in defining the patterns of glucose uptake and the general physiological state of its surrounding neurons. It is generally assumed (without good evidence to support it) that changes in the glucose uptake of the glia will occur primarily in the areas where the neurons are electrically active. Glia also may play an important role in the modulation of neurotrophic factors during exercise.

Changes in Neural Control Properties After Dynamic and Resistive Training

Changes in Cortical Function With Training

Neural adaptations can contribute to strength increments and efficiency of motion simply by improving muscular coordination. Resistance training of the fingers increases muscular strength and the stability of sensorimotor coordination during a difficult motor task; that is, the muscles are recruited in a more consistent manner (the variation in the timing, amplitude, and duration of muscle activity being lower) after than before training (128). It is not clear at all, however, where the neural adaptations occur. Synaptic effectiveness of neural connections between areas within the primary cortex can be modified through physical activity (129). It also appears that motor learning may be associated with physiological adaptations in the primary cortex, contributing to more efficient execution of the learned movements. Use-dependent changes occur in the movement representations in the primary motor cortex of squirrel monkeys (130). Also there are changes in the activity levels in secondary motor areas when a motor task involving sequential movements is learned (131). Training for a specific motor task also may improve performance in related tasks (positive transfer) by reducing the extent of cortical activation and thus the activation of the neural elements that may interfere with or are not necessary for the optimal execution of the movement. Dettmers and associates (132) reported that neural activity increases in the primary motor cortex and caudal supplementary motor area as greater levels of isometric force are produced.

When resistance training produces muscle hypertrophy, fewer motor units are needed to generate a given level of torque. This could reduce the level of activation of the motor areas and improve performance. A reduction in activity at several supraspinal sites (e.g., dorsal premotor area, parietal cortex, and lateral cerebellum) may occur with the acquisition of a motor skill (133).

Resistance training can induce relatively long-lasting changes in the functional properties of the corticospinal pathway in humans. The magnitude of the compound EMG, commonly called motor-evoked potentials (MEP), in response to transcranial magnetic stimulation (TMS) is smaller after resistance training. The magnitude of muscular responses to TMS reflects the level of transsynaptic excitation of the corticospinal cells. The peak MEP also occurs at a lower percentage of maximum voluntary contraction following resistance training, suggesting that the level of contraction at which the entire population of motor units receiving the transcranial volley was recruited was lower after training.

Changes in the Areas of Activation in the Brain With Resistance Training

It has been demonstrated that as a subject changes the level of force exerted, unique regions of the brain are activated (134). There is growing interest in the possibilities of associating the performance of specific motor tasks with the activation of specific regions of the brain and spinal cord. Functional MRI studies have shown that the area of the primary cortex activated during a specific sequence of finger movements increases after 3 weeks of daily practice (135) and the size of the hand area in the motor cortex increases after 2 hours of piano practice for 5 days (136). Elite racquet players show heightened excitability of the cortical projection to the hand (137). Patten and Kamen (138) used a dorsiflexion force modulation training regimen (a motor learning paradigm) to improve force accuracy and surprisingly found an increase in maximum voluntary force in young individuals. The increase in strength is related to a lower force threshold for motor unit recruitment and higher motor unit discharge rates, indicative of adaptations at the spinal segmental level (increased excitability of the agonist motor neuron pools) and thus a more complete recruitment of available motor units (139). Also these results are consistent with observations that the volume of muscle activated can increase within 2 weeks of resistance training (140). We now know that motor neuron excitability can increase in a range of muscles, including the extensor digitorum brevis, soleus, brachioradialis and hypothenar, after weeks and months of strength training (141).

The greater excitability of motor neurons after training theoretically should result in higher levels of motor pool activation, as reflected in the whole-muscle EMG signal. The activation levels of motor pools as measured using integrated EMG increases after strength training involving weight lifting, isometric contractions, isokinetic eccentric contractions, and explosive jumping. Therefore, with strength training subjects can more fully activate their prime movers during maximum voluntary contractions. Reflex potentiation has been observed to increase after strength training and also to be enhanced in weight lifters (142) and elite sprinters (143). All of these results are consistent with significant adaptations in the motor cortex resulting from training, activity, and learning.

Changes in Motor Unit Synchronization With Training

Motor unit synchronization, a measure of the correlation between the discharge times of action potentials by two or more motor units, is another sign of neural adaptation with training. Motor unit synchronization increases during the performance of attention-demanding tasks (144). The amount of synchronization of low-threshold motor units varies with the type of contraction. Semmler and colleagues (145) demonstrated a striking difference between the level of synchronization of motor units in the first dorsal interosseous during shortening and lengthening contractions. They observed a 50% higher level of synchronization in eccentric than in concentric contractions and thus considerably more common input on the motor neurons during eccentric than concentric contractions. Synchronization of motor units is more evident in the hand muscles of weightlifters (146), increases with strength training (142), but is less in some musicians (146).

Training the dorsiflexors with rapid dynamic contractions at 30 to 40% of maximum for 12 weeks also increases the force of motor units in the tibialis anterior distributed across the entire pool (based on spike-triggered averaging), without a change in recruitment order (16). Training also increased the average instantaneous discharge rate from 69 to 90 Hz, and there was an increase in the number of doublets. Thus, the increase in strength (MVC) and speed could be linked to an increased motor unit initial discharge rate. Synchronization may increase the rate of force development but does not necessarily influence the maximum force capability (147). This increase in synchronization may result from (a) an increase in the number or strength of common presynaptic inputs onto populations of motor neurons and/ or (b) descending corticospinal tract neurons with branched-stem axons (148). In summary, typical interpulse intervals of motor units can change with training. Recall that changing a single interpulse interval can significantly improve the force generated by a motor unit, that is, the catch property. In addition, there is evidence that the interaction of motor units can become more synchronized with training and that this level of synchronization is a function of the type of muscular effort.

Dynamic Exercise, Nerve Growth Factors, and Learning

Activity Levels, Brain-Derived Neurotrophic Factor Expression, and Learning

There is substantial evidence that dynamic exercise can facilitate learning a hippocampal spatial task in rats. Similar evidence has been reported in comparisons of the ability to learn and recall in humans who are physically active versus those who are inactive. Some understanding of the possible mechanisms for the exercise-induced facilitation of learning is emerging. Rats that are allowed to run at will in a wheel connected to their cage have significantly higher brain-derived neurotrophic factor (BDNF) protein levels in the hippocampus and spinal cord within 3 days than those of rats that are housed in a standard cage without access to running wheels (149,150). BDNF mRNA also is elevated in the hippocampus and spinal cord in these voluntarily exercising rats.

BDNF plays a critical role in the cascade of biochemical reactions thought to be important for LTP. LTP and LTD are thought to be important in many forms of learning, although there is some evidence that they are not essential. BDNF also is associated with many of the cellular events associated with synaptic plasticity in general. For example, synapsin 1, a member of a family of nerve terminal–specific phosphoproteins that are associated with synaptic vesicle turnover, and growth-associated protein (GAP-43), which is related to synaptic reorganization, are linked to BDNF, and both are up-regulated in the hippocampus and spinal cord in response to exercise (Fig. 3.41).

Dynamic Exercise, BDNF Expression, and Neurogenesis

In addition, several genes linked to BDNF are up-regulated in animals that have access to a running wheel compared to those that do not. Animals that are exercised in a running wheel or housed in an enriched environment can learn a water maze task more quickly than animals housed in a standard sedentary cage. The number of new neurons, that is, those labeled with BrdU, in the dentate gyrus can double in response to wheel running exercise, compared to those of mice that swim for the same period. An increase in the number of surviving BrdU neurons also was observed in mice that trained in a Morris water maze four times a day for 4 days compared to rats that did not train (151). There is some evidence that the exercise-induced neurogenesis and improved learning depend on the N-methyl D-aspartate (NMDA) receptors (152). Also consistent with these observations is that BDNF and its TrkB receptor are reduced in the hippocampus when rats are deprived of habitual running. In summary, there appears to be a general positive effect of exercise on learning and memory of motor tasks. Although it remains to be demonstrated, BDNF may be a key mediator of these general effects on learning.

There is also evidence that 12 weeks of dynamic exercise (forced running) may reduce neural damage (reduce the size of a neural infarct) following an injury via a neurotrophic mechanism (153). Dynamic exercise training also increases the nerve growth factor (NGF) receptor, p75. It is known that the septohippocampal axis is activated with exercise (154) and that wheel running in rodents evokes hippocampal theta activity (activation of medial septum GABAergic afferents during running could contribute to BDNF gene up-regulation). NE and 5-HT levels also may play an important role in the exercise-induced modulation of BDNF in the hippocampus (155). Thus it appears that an enriched environment that includes exercise increases hippocampal BDNF mRNA and protein that is regulated by neuronal activity and neurotransmitter input.

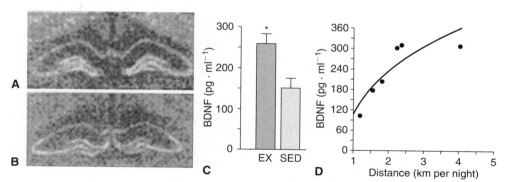

FIGURE 3.41 Effects of exercise on hippocampal brain-derived neurotrophic factor (BDNF) mRNA and protein levels. In situ hybridization shows that the expression of BDNF mRNA in the rat dentate gyrus, hilus, CA1 to CA3 regions, and cortex is greater following exercise (7 days of voluntary wheel running) (**A**) than in sedentary animals (**B**). **C.** ELISA quantification of BDNF protein levels in the hippocampus in sedentary (SED) and exercising (EX) animals after 5 days of wheel-running (*$P < .05$). **D.** Rats and mice acclimate rapidly to the running wheel and progressively increase their extent of daily running. BDNF protein levels correlate with running distance (average over 14 days running; $R^2 = 0.771$). *(Reprinted with permission from Cotman CW, Berchtold NC. Exercise: a behavioral intervention to enhance brain health and plasticity. Trends Neurosci 2002;25:295–301.)*

...riments also have been designed to determine ...ether there is a more specific interaction between neuronal circuits that are involved in performing more precise motor skills and the ability to perform the skill itself. Rats that live in an enriched environment as opposed to a standard caging environment develop more astrocytes, but no neurons or oligodendrocytes, in the cerebral cortex. New neurons, however, were formed in the hippocampus. There is some evidence that insulin-like growth factor-I plays a role in mediating this neurogenesis. Rats trained for a specific motor skill for a month have more synapses per Purkinje cell from both parallel fibers and climbing fibers in the cerebellum than rats that have been exercised in a wheel or sedentary rats (156). More mitochondria were observed in Purkinje cells following motor skill training. Rats that lived in a cage with a running wheel for a month had more capillary growth in the motor areas of the cerebral cortex than sedentary rats, and they had a higher blood flow rate in the same area when they exercised. Other experiments have attempted to differentiate the neural adaptations associated with exercise in general from those associated with actually learning a specific motor task. For example, rats that learned a task showed greater synaptogenesis than rats that were more active but did not learn the task (157).

Pharmacological treatments were used to remove either serotonergic or noradrenergic input, and then the rats were allowed to run in voluntary cages for 7 days (86). Systemic deletion of the NE system eliminated the exercise increase in BDNF mRNA in all hippocampal subfields except one and in the dentate gyrus, whereas a 5-HT lesion did not alter the BDNF mRNA response to dynamic exercise.

Dynamic Exercise–Induced Changes in Growth Factors in the Spinal Cord

BDNF levels also are increased in the spinal cord as well when rats or mice are allowed to run in a wheel. In a number of examples the BDNF and neurotrophin (NT-3) differ in their response to exercise. For example, after running in a wheel for 7 days, the NT-3 levels in the hippocampus are reduced. NT-3 levels in the spinal cord, cerebellum, and hippocampus are less responsive to exercise than is BDNF (149).

Fibroblast Growth Factor and Dynamic Exercise

Fibroblast growth factor (FGF-2) mRNA and protein (immuno) levels also increase in the hippocampus (but not the striatum or cerebral cortex) after 4 nights of running and then return to control levels after 7 nights of running (158). The time course suggests that exercise could be beneficial at the early stages of a training program. The point is that the hippocampus is important for cognitive function (trophic factor involvement in cognition). FGF, a known angiogenic factor, also may be involved with the angiogenesis associated with exercise (159). In many cases growth factors are likely to be mediators for the positive effects of exercise on the brain.

Plasticity of Motor Neurons to Varying Levels of Neuromuscular Activity

The motor neuron is the final common pathway for the motor system (160). Exercise involves a substantial increase in the number of action potentials generated by at least some of the motor neurons innervating the musculature, and with resistance training the target size of individual motor neurons increases, that is, muscle fiber hypertrophy ensues. Thus, it may be expected that motor neurons adapt their size and/or metabolic properties to reflect the increase in the volume and/or oxidative capacity of their target cells and the increase in their activation levels. However, some motor neuron properties are generally resistant to chronic adaptations in neuromuscular activity levels. For example, motor neuron size and metabolic properties have been reported to be generally unaffected in response to hindlimb unloading, space flight, nerve block via tetrodotoxin administration, functional overload, and muscle nerve stimulation (161,162). After endurance training, small adaptations have been observed in mitochondrial enzyme activities in motor pools that are innervating muscles composed primarily of fibers of the slow phenotype (163). In other studies, there were no or only small changes in oxidative phosphorylation enzyme activity and soma size of motor neurons of slow and fast motor pools in response to endurance training or functional overload (164–166).

More substantial changes seem to occur in the physiological properties of motor neurons in response to changes in neuromuscular activity levels. In rats that were allowed to run spontaneously for 12 weeks in wheels the mean resting membrane potential became more hyperpolarized, the spike trigger voltage decreased, and the mean amplitude of the afterhyperpolarization increased in slow but not fast motor neurons (113). Munson and associates (167) also reported that motor neurons innervating the medial gastrocnemius are more excitable (lower rheobase) and have higher input resistance (smaller) and longer duration of afterhyperpolarization after 6 months of chronic electrical stimulation—also reflecting that the motor neurons were becoming slower.

Chronic spinal cord injury in cats, which reduces the activity levels of soleus motor neurons by 75% (97), results in a shortening of the afterhyperpolarization and an elevation of rheobase, consistent with the motor neurons changing toward a fast type. Also, some muscle fibers change to a fast phenotype after a complete spinal cord transection (168). Therefore, it seems that some activity-linked mechanisms may induce some slow motor units to become faster in their physiological and biochemical properties (93). Trophic factors, such as calcitonin gene-related peptide (CGRP) (169) and BDNF (169) also increase in response to exercise in a running wheel. Also chronic infusion of BDNF into the gastrocnemius in the rat decreases motor neuronal rheobase after 5 days (170), which suggests that trophic substances from the active muscles influence the motor neuron properties.

Adaptation of the Neuromuscular Junction to Changing Levels of Dynamic and Resistive Exercises

The neuromuscular junction for many years has served as a useful model for understanding synaptic function and adaptability in the peripheral nervous system (Fig. 3.42). It continues to be useful in efforts to understand use-dependent synaptic plasticity and adaptability. Although it is generally recognized that there is a significant margin for the amount of neurotransmitter that can be released from the neuromuscular junction, it appears that repetitive activation can induce significant changes in function and morphology. Resistance training, that is, climbing up a grid with attached weights for 7 weeks, produced a number of adaptations in the neuromuscular junctions in the soleus muscle (171). For example, end plate perimeter length and area increase, and the membrane area containing the acetylcholine receptors within the end plate region is enlarged, even when there is no change in muscle fiber size or type. Dynamic exercise training of an endurance nature also increases neurotransmitter release at the neuromuscular junction (172–174). Crocket and associates (175) found that moderate endurance exercise increased the acetylcholinesterase-positive staining area at the end plates of the white vastus muscle in rats. Also, the muscles of endurance-trained rats have larger and more complicated neuromuscular junctions, that is, more nerve terminal sprouts and growth configurations, than controls (172,176). Voluntary wheel running markedly up-regulates the total acetylcholinesterase mRNA and protein at the neuromuscular junction of the rat extensor digitorum longus, with a lesser increase in the soleus (177).

A single bout (30 minutes) of running downhill can result in an increase in the numbers of CGRP-positive motor neurons of selected motor pools, such as the triceps surae (178). However, other motor pools, including the anterior crural, did not change with the same exercise paradigm. It is not clear how the duration, intensity, and kind of neuromuscular activity relate to the induction of a CGRP response in motor neurons. The function of CGRP in the 3motor system appears to include establishing and maintaining the neuromuscular junction, and it is present when there is axonal sprouting (179). These data are consistent with the sprouting at the motor terminals in the soleus muscle after a single 9-hour bout of voluntary wheel running in mice (180). However, the reverse may not be true; that is, CGRP may not always be a positive indicator of axonal sprouting.

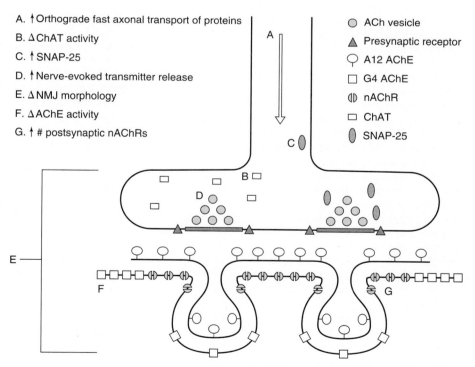

FIGURE 3.42 A summary of endurance exercise training–induced adaptations at the mammalian neuromuscular junction (NMJ). Each letter in the schematic of the NMJ (A–G) corresponds to an adaptation described in the upper left of the figure. The symbols at the upper right represent the various proteins and components found at the NMJ. *(Modified from Gardiner P. Neuromuscular aspects of physical activity. Champaign, IL: Human Kinetics, 2001, p. 132.)*

The Size Principle of Motor Unit Recruitment

It was clear when these three classic papers were published that there was an important link between the specific motor pool and the type of muscle that it normally innervated. It was also known that there were slow and fast muscles in all mammals and probably all animals. Earlier, Wuerker and Henneman (181) suggested that muscle fibers were homogeneous within a motor unit and alluded to the findings of Buller and associates (182,183) showing a neural effect on muscle properties. These researchers transected the nerves to the slow soleus muscle and the fast flexor digitorum longus muscle and then crossed the nerves so that they would reinnervate the opposite muscle. About 1 to 6 months after cross-reinnervation, they examined whether there was any evidence of plasticity in the spinal cord. Some of the personal details of the situation surrounding this initial experiment, which is a classic one of its own, are interesting, to say the least. Based on my (VRE) personal conversations with Buller, the story goes like this. Sir John Eccles, who was at the Australian National University in Canberra at that time, was one of the most famous physiologists in the world. He received the Nobel Prize in Physiology several years later (1963) for his work on the electrophysiology of spinal neurons. Buller, who had just completed his PhD in England and was considered to be among the most outstanding young physiologists in England, was given the opportunity to study with Eccles. So he boarded a freighter heading for Australia. After about a 2-week journey, Eccles met him and took him directly to the laboratory where the first cross-reinnervation experiments were being performed.

Part of the irony is that the experiments were done to examine the plasticity of the synapses of the spinal cord, not the muscle. The original intent was to determine whether the afferent projections to a given motor pool would realign as a result of the nerves innervating a foreign muscle. The way that Buller describes that first night goes like this. The cat had been prepared for the experiment and electrodes had been placed on the muscle nerves. When the normally slow soleus muscle was stimulated, it visibly had a fast twitch. (A standard procedure in studying motor neurons is to stimulate the peripheral nerve, record the antidromic spikes, and thus identify which muscle the motor neurons innervated.) Eccles immediately became excited by this observation. Realize that one can readily see the difference in the twitch properties of a predominantly slow versus a predominantly fast muscle in a cat, and certainly Eccles had had plenty of experience. At this point in the experiment Eccles elected to take a quick nap before proceeding with the experiments. This was commonly done during very long experimental procedures. Before he began his nap, however, he instructed young Buller to find a force transducer and record the muscle properties. But Buller did not know what a force transducer looked like. He began going through the laboratory drawers to find one but eventually swallowed his pride and awakened Eccles to ask what a force transducer looked like.

As history has shown, in effect these observations of the muscle properties after cross-reinnervation defined, at least to a very large extent, that the motor neurons in some way controlled the gene expression of thousands of myonuclei within each muscle unit. Although it remains today somewhat unclear as to how this neural dominance on muscle gene expression is accomplished, it is clear that this modulation or control is mediated by both activity-dependent and activity-independent factors. At this time slow and fast myosins had been isolated, and a direct relationship between myosin ATPase and muscle speed was often assumed.

With respect to the size principle, these researchers' observation provided the backdrop for the idea that the specific motor neuron–muscle fiber linkage was very important in ways other than being a way to activate the muscle. The papers by Henneman and coworkers concluded that slow motor units tended to be small (generating low force) and fast units tended to generate the highest forces. This range in forces among motor units within a motor pool was linked to the size of the axons as measured by conduction velocity as well as the input resistance to current. Finally, the crucial observation was that the order in which these motor units became excited when stimulating via afferent inputs was constant and was directly related to the size of the unit. They also demonstrated in this series of papers that the size was a determining factor regardless of the source of the excitation (using excitatory reflexes). These studies also showed a constant relationship between size and the level of inhibitory input; that is, the larger the unit, the more susceptible it was to inhibition.

Thousands of papers have challenged this principle. Although some exceptions have been noted over many years, these many challenges have contributed to its robustness, importance, and significance rather than the reverse. For a number of years, our laboratory performed experiments designed to determine whether in some types of efforts the order of recruitment of motor units within a motor pool could be altered. But in the end, Henneman and coworkers were much more right than wrong. In essence, the design of a system whereby decisions as to which motor units and how many to activate for every movement would require an enormously large and complex neural control system. As it turns out, having many degrees of freedom in choosing which motor units are activated is neither feasible nor necessary.

Subsequent to the initial papers on the size principle, a number of other papers further clarified many details of the motor neuron–muscle fiber relationship, most of which demonstrate the centrality of the size principle. The concept of the size principle set the plate for a series of observations. The Henneman papers make this motor neuron–fiber type linkage obvious. Histochemical, biochemical, and physiological analyses of slow and fast muscles; the size principle; and cross-reinnervation experiments made it clear that the muscle fiber biochemical and physiological properties are determined in large part by the motor neuron. It also became clear that the fast muscles could be divided into a fatigable and non-fatigable population and that the observed electrophysiological properties of motor neurons were consistent with this subdivision. But still there was no direct link of a muscle fiber type to a specific motor neuron type until the technique of glycogen depletion came on the scene. At almost the same time, Kugelberg and Edstrom (184) and our laboratory (185) reported that glycogen depletion (or phosphorylase depletion) could be observed in individual muscle fibers following repetitive stimulation. Kugelberg and Edstrom electrically stimulated muscle nerves *in situ* and found that the larger fast and low oxidative fibers were preferentially depleted of glycogen. This work showed the feasibility of using glycogen depletion to identify muscle fibers that had been active. Given the ease with which the large, low-oxidative fibers were depleted of glycogen and phosphorylase with stimulation, they suggested that these fibers must be used sparingly over short periods and thus would be innervated by motor neurons with very high thresholds. Thus, these motor units would be recruited only during strong, quick contractions and innervated by phasically discharging motor neurons. In fact, when we exercised rodents on a treadmill, the slow, high-oxidative fibers were selectively depleted, as might be expected according to the size principle.

These two results are actually what we would expect, in that electrical stimulation of a muscle nerve will selectively activate the larger, faster axons. But more important, when the stimulus is maximal (activates all axons) the large, low-oxidative fibers are more susceptible to glycogen depletion and therefore will be depleted more quickly than the high-oxidative fibers (as long as blood flow is adequate). The crucial experiment that confirmed a close relationship among the size of a motor unit, the physiological properties of the muscle, and the biochemical properties of the muscle fibers was performed by Burke and colleagues (186) when they linked the motor neuron properties and the muscle unit properties of the same motor neurons using glycogen depletion techniques. In this case, they depleted the muscle fibers by individual motor neurons and definitively linked the electrophysiology of motor neurons with the physiology and biochemistry of the muscle unit.

Henneman E, Somjenn G, Carpenter DO. *Functional significance of cell size in spinal neurons. J Neurophysiol 1965;28:560–580.*

Henneman E, Olson CB. *Relations between structure and function in the design of skeletal muscles. J Neurophysiol 1965;28:581–598.*

Henneman E, Somjen G, Carpenter DO. *Excitability and irritability of motor neurons of different sizes. J Neurophysiol 1965:28:599–620.*

SUMMARY

Movements are produced by modulating the activation of specific combinations of motor pools and by controlling the level of activation within each of these motor pools. The "final common pathway" is the motor unit, i.e., a motoneuron and all of the muscle fibers that it innervates. The order of recruitment of motor units within each motor pool is defined largely by the size principle, i.e., the recruitment order within and across synergistic motor pools is normally from the smallest to the largest units. The size of a motor unit is directly related to the size of the motoneuron, dendritic tree, axons; the number of muscle fibers innervated by the motoneuron; and the force generated by the motor unit. Modulation of the forces derived from a motor pool are determined by the number of motor units that are recruited and the frequency of excitation of those motor units, with the frequency modulation being sensitive to a single inter-spike interval (catch-property).

The motor units that are the most excitable are likely to be slow fatigue resistant (S), those that are moderately excitable are likely to be fast fatigue resistant (FR), and those that are the least excitable are likely to be predominantly fast fatigable (FF) motor units. Therefore, indirectly but to a major degree, the size principle defines the metabolic and physiological responses to an exercise of a given duration and intensity. For example, according to the size principle, the patterns of glycogen depletion during an exercise will reflect the recruitment of motor units.

The three primary components of the nervous system that regulate posture and locomotion can be conveniently categorized into those neuronal systems a) within the brain, b) within the spinal cord that are associated with CPG, and c) involved with providing sensory input to the nervous system. The primary descending systems from the brain that control posture and locomotion are the reticulospinal, rubrospinal, vestibulospinal, and corticospinal tracts. There are several areas in the brainstem that receive information associated with locomotion and posture that can generate stepping and standing when stimulated tonically. One of the primary areas that can generate these motor tasks is referred to as the MLR.

There is an extensive level of automation in generating posture and locomotion. Central pattern generation of locomotion refers to the generation of alternating patters of flexion and extension that mimic those patterns that occur during locomotion, but without any alternating or rhythmic input from either the brain or the periphery. This alternating output from CPG is referred to as fictive locomotion.

In preparations that eliminate supraspinal input, the spinal cord can interpret sensory information derived from the limbs as an ensemble that provides a precise "picture" of the position of the limbs at any given time during posture or locomotion. Therefore, the spinal cord can respond to these ensembles of input without assistance from the brain, and generate effective weight-bearing locomotion and standing posture. In addition, the spinal nerual networks that generate standing and locomotion can learn to produce these tasks more effectively when they are trained to perform that specific task. The sensory information provided to the spinal cord is derived in large part from a variety of mechanoreceptors located in muscles, tendons, ligaments, and skin.

Fatigue while performing a motor task can have a central, as well as muscular, origin. Central fatigue refers to the failure to maintain the required or expected force or power output when these deficits cannot be explained by a muscle dysfunction. The site for this fatigue can be in the brain, spinal cord, or neuromuscular junction. Exercise training can induce adaptations of any of these sites to enhance performance.

The neuromotor system is in a constant state of adaptation, similar to what is conceptually described as Neural Darwinism. There is extensive modulation of synaptic efficacy throughout the nervous system as a result of varying levels of physical activity, and there seems to be a "specificity" of the exercise effect. Neurotrophic growth factors most likely play a major role in the adaptive process of the nervous system to exercise.

REFERENCES

1. Lieber RL. Skeletal muscle structure and function. Baltimore: Williams & Wilkins, 1992;303.
2. Roy RR, Edgerton VR. Skeletal muscle architecture and performance. In Komi PV, ed. Strength and Power in Sport: Encyclopedia of Sports Medicine. Oxford: Blackwell Scientific, 1992;115–129.
3. Bodine-Fowler S, Garfinkel A, Roy RR, et al. Spatial distribution of muscle fibers within the territory of a motor unit. Muscle Nerve 1990;13:1133–1145.
4. Burke RE, Levine DN, Tsairis P, et al. Physiological types and histochemical profiles in motor units of the cat gastrocnemius. J Physiol (Lond) 1973;234:723–748.
5. Peter JB, Barnard RJ, Edgerton VR, et al. Metabolic profiles of three fiber types of skeletal muscle in guinea pigs and rabbits. Biochemistry 1972;11:2627–2633.
6. Ounjian M, Roy RR, Eldred E, et al. Physiological and developmental implications of motor unit anatomy. J Neurobiol 1991;22:547–559.
7. Bodine SC, Garfinkel A, Roy RR, et al. Spatial distribution of motor unit fibers in the cat soleus and tibialis anterior muscles: local interactions. J Neurosci 1988;8:2142–2152.
8. Ishihara A, Roy RR, Edgerton VR. Succinate dehydrogenase activity and soma size of motoneurons innervating different portions of the rat tibialis anterior. Neuroscience 1995;68:813–822.
9. Henneman E, Mendell LM. Functional organization of motoneuron pool and its input. In Brookhart JM, Mountcastle VB, eds. Handbook of physiology. Section 1, vol 2: The Nervous System, Motor Control, Part 1. Bethesda: American Physiological Society, 1981, 423–507.
10. Henneman E, Olson CB. Relations between structure and function in the design of skeletal muscles. J Neurophysiol 1965;28:581–598.
11. Cope TC, Clark BD. Motor-unit recruitment in the decerebrate cat: several unit properties are equally good predictors of order. J Neurophysiol 1991;66:1127–1138.
12. Pinter MJ, Curtis RL, Hosko MJ. Voltage threshold and excitability among variously sized cat hindlimb motoneurons. J Neurophysiol 1983;50:644–657.
13. Kukulka CG, Clamann HP. Comparison of the recruitment and discharge properties of motor units in human brachial biceps and adductor pollicis during isometric contractions. Brain Res 1981;219:45–55.
14. Burke RE, Rudomin P, Zajac FE 3rd. Catch property in single mammalian motor units. Science 1970;168:122–124.
15. Burke RE, Rudomin P, Zajac 3rd FE. The effect of activation history on tension production by individual muscle units. Brain Res 1976;109:515–529.
16. Van Cutsem M, Duchateau J, Hainaut K. Changes in single motor unit behaviour contribute to the increase in contraction speed after dynamic training in humans. J Physiol (Lond) 1998;513:295–305.
17. Enoka RM, Fuglevand AJ. Motor unit physiology: some unresolved issues. Muscle Nerve 2001;24:4–17.
18. Stephens JA, Garnett R, Buller NP. Reversal of recruitment order of single motor units produced by cutaneous stimulation during voluntary muscle contraction in man. Nature 1978;272:362–364.
19. Desmedt JE, Godaux E. Fast motor units are not preferentially activated in rapid voluntary contractions in man. Nature 1977;267:717–719.
20. Nardone A, Romano C, Schieppati M. Selective recruitment of high-threshold human motor units during voluntary isotonic lengthening of active muscles. J Physiol (Lond) 1989;409:451–471.
21. Smith JL, Betts B, Edgerton VR, et al. Rapid ankle extension during paw shakes: selective recruitment of fast ankle extensors. J Neurophysiol 1980;43:612–620.
22. Fallentin N, Jorgensen K, Simonsen EB. Motor unit recruitment during prolonged isometric contractions. Eur J Appl Physiol 1993;67:335–341.
23. Tamaki H, Kitada K, Akamine T, et al. Alternate activity in the synergistic muscles during prolonged low-level contractions. J Appl Physiol 1998;84:1943–1951.
24. Bodine SC, Roy RR, Meadows DA, et al. Architectural, histochemical, and contractile characteristics of a unique biarticular muscle: the cat semitendinosus. J Neurophysiol 1982;48:192–201.
25. English AW. An electromyographic analysis of compartments in cat lateral gastrocnemius muscle during unrestrained locomotion. J Neurophysiol 1984;52:114–125.
26. Akima H, Ito M, Yoshikawa H, et al. Recruitment plasticity of neuromuscular compartments in exercised tibialis anterior using echo-planar magnetic resonance imaging in humans. Neurosci Lett 2000;296:133–136.
27. Cope TC, Sokoloff AJ. Orderly recruitment among motoneurons supplying different muscles. J Physiol (Paris) 1999;93:81–85.
28. Grillner S. Control of locomotion in bipeds, tetrapods, and fish. In Brookhart JM, Mountcastle VB, eds. Handbook of physiology. Section 1, vol. 2: The Nervous System, Motor Control, part 1. Bethesda: American Physiological Society, 1981;1179–1236.
29. Shik ML, Orlovsky GN. Neurophysiology of locomotor automatism. Physiol Rev 1976;56:465–501.
30. Halbertsma JM. The stride cycle of the cat: the modelling of locomotion by computerized analysis of automatic recordings. Acta Physiol Scand Suppl 1983;521:1–75.

31. Goslow Jr GE, Reinking RM, Stuart DG. The cat step cycle: hind limb joint angles and muscle lengths during unrestrained locomotion. J Morphol 1973;141:1–41.

32. Hoyt D, Taylor R. Gait and the energetics of locomotion in horses. Nature 1981;292:239–240.

33. Whiting WC, Gregor RJ, Roy RR, et al. A technique for estimating mechanical work of individual muscles in the cat during treadmill locomotion. J Biomech 1984;17:685–694.

34. Gregor RJ, Roy RR, Whiting WC, et al. Mechanical output of the cat soleus during treadmill locomotion: in vivo vs in situ characteristics. J Biomech 1988;21:721–732.

35. Tesch PA, Dudley GA, Duvoisin MR, et al. Force and EMG signal patterns during repeated bouts of concentric or eccentric muscle actions. Acta Physiol Scand 1990;138:263–271.

36. Ryschon TW, Fowler MD, Wysong RE, et al. Efficiency of human skeletal muscle in vivo: comparison of isometric, concentric, and eccentric muscle action. J Appl Physiol 1997;83:867–874.

37. Vollestad NK, Vaage O, Hermansen L. Muscle glycogen depletion patterns in type I and subgroups of type II fibres during prolonged severe exercise in man. Acta Physiol Scand 1984;122:433–441.

38. Vollestad NK, Blom PC. Effect of varying exercise intensity on glycogen depletion in human muscle fibres. Acta Physiol Scand 1985;125:395–405.

39. Edgerton VR, Tillakaratne N, Bigbee A, de Leon R, Roy RR. Plasticity of spinal circuitry after injury. Ann Rev Neurosci 2004;27:145–167.

40. Parker D, Grillner S. Neuronal mechanisms of synaptic and network plasticity in the lamprey spinal cord. Prog Brain Res 2000;125:381–398.

41. Feldman JL, Mitchell GS, Nattie EE. Breathing: rhythmicity, plasticity, chemosensitivity. Annu Rev Neurosci 2003;26:239–266.

42. Edgerton V, Grillner S, Sjostrom A, et al. Central generation of locomotion in vertebrates. In Herman RM, Stein PSG, Stuart DG, eds. Neural Control of Locomotion. New York: Plenum, 1976;439–464.

43. Lovely RG, Gregor RJ, Roy RR, et al. Effects of training on the recovery of full-weight-bearing stepping in the adult spinal cat. Exp Neurol 1986;92:421–435.

44. Forssberg H. Stumbling corrective reaction: a phase-dependent compensatory reaction during locomotion. J Neurophysiol 1979;42:936–953.

45. Edgerton VR, de Leon RD, Harkema SJ, et al. Retraining the injured spinal cord. J Physiol (Lond) 2001;533:15–22.

46. Hodgson JA, Roy RR, de Leon RB, et al. Can the mammalian lumbar spinal cord learn a motor task? Med Sci Sports Exerc 1994;26:1491–1497.

47. Hutton RS, Atwater SW. Acute and chronic adaptations of muscle proprioceptors in response to increased use. Sports Med 1992;14:406–421.

48. Prochazka A. Proprioceptive feedback and movement regulation. New York: Oxford University, 1996;89–127.

49. Nelson SG, Mendell LM. Projection of single knee flexor Ia fibers to homonymous and heteronymous motoneurons. J Neurophysiol 1978;41:778–787.

50. Botterman B, Binder M, Stuart D. Functional anatomy of the association between motor units and muscle receptors. Am Zool 1978;18:135–152.

51. Andersson O, Forssberg H, Grillner S, et al. Phasic gain control of the transmission in cutaneous reflex pathways to motoneurones during "fictive" locomotion. Brain Res 1978;149:503–507.

52. Nichols TR. Receptor mechanisms underlying heterogenic reflexes among the triceps surae muscles of the cat. J Neurophysiol 1999;81:467–478.

53. Capaday C. The special nature of human walking and its neural control. Trends Neurosci 2002;25:370–376.

54. Simonsen EB, Dyhre-Poulsen P. Amplitude of the human soleus H reflex during walking and running. J Physiol (Lond) 1999;515:929–939.

55. Harkema SJ, Hurley SL, Patel UK, et al. Human lumbosacral spinal cord interprets loading during stepping. J Neurophysiol 1997;77:797–811.

56. Edgerton VR, Roy RR, de Leon RD. Neural Darwinism in the mammalian spinal cord. In Patterson MM, Grau JW, eds. Spinal Cord Plasticity: Alterations in Reflex Function. Boston: Kluwer, 2001;185–206.

57. Prochazka A, Gorassini M. Ensemble firing of muscle afferents recorded during normal locomotion in cats. J Physiol (Lond) 1998;507: 293–304.

58. Edgerton VR, de Guzman CP, Gregor RJ, et al. Trainability of the spinal cord to generate hindlimb stepping patterns in adult spinalized cats. In Shimamura M, Grillner S, Edgerton VR, eds. Neurobiological basis of human locomotion. Tokyo: Japan Scientific Societies, 1991;411–423.

59. Orlovsky G, Deliagina T, Grillner S. Neuronal control of locomotion: from mollusc to man. Oxford, UK: Oxford University, 1999.

60. Grillner S. The motor infrastructure: from ion channels to neuronal networks. Nat Rev Neurosci 2003;4:573–586.

61. Vilensky JA, Moore AM, Eidelberg E, et al. Recovery of locomotion in monkeys with spinal cord lesions. J Mot Behav 1992;24:288–296.

62. Shik ML, Orlovskii GN, Severin FV. [Organization of locomotor synergism]. Biofizika 1966;11:879–886.

63. Harkema SJ. Neural plasticity after human spinal cord injury: application of locomotor training to the rehabilitation of walking. Neuroscientist 2001;7:455–468.

64. Wernig A, Muller S. Laufband locomotion with body weight support improved walking in persons with severe spinal cord injuries. Paraplegia 1992;30:229–238.

65. Eagleman DM. Neuroscience: the where and when of intention. Science 2004;303:1144–1146.

66. Baev K. Biological neural networks: the hierarchical concept of brain function. Boston: Birkhauser, 1998.

67. Sirota MG, Shik ML. The cat locomotion elicited through the electrode implanted in the mid-brain. Sechenov Physiol J USSR 1973;59:1314–1321.

68. Gerasimenko YP, Avelev VD, Nikitin OA, et al. Initiation of locomotor activity in spinal cats by epidural stimulation of the spinal cord. Neurosci Behav Physiol 2003;33:247–254.

69. Dimitrijevic MR, Gerasimenko Y, Pinter MM. Evidence for a spinal central pattern generator in humans. Ann N Y Acad Sci 1998;860:360–376.

70. Grillner S, Ekelberg O, El Manira A, et al. Intrinsic function of a neural network—a vertebrate central pattern generator. Brain Res Rev 1998;26:184–187.

70a. Prochazka A, Gritsenko V, Yakovenko S. Sensory control of locomotion: reflexes versus higher-level control. Adv Exp Med Biol 2002;508:357–367.

71. Timoszyk WK, De Leon RD, London N, et al. The rat lumbosacral spinal cord adapts to robotic loading applied during stance. J Neurophysiol 2002;88:3108–3117.

72. de Leon RD, Reinkensmeyer DJ, Timoszyk WK, et al. Use of robotics in assessing the adaptive capacity of the rat lumbar spinal cord. In McKerracher L, Doucet G, Rossignol S, eds. Progress in Brain Research. Netherlands: Elsevier Science, 2002;141–149.

73. Garraway SM, Hochman S. Serotonin increases the incidence of primary afferent-evoked long-term depression in rat deep dorsal horn neurons. J Neurophysiol 2001;85:1864–1872.

74. Gandevia SC, Petersen N, Butler JE, et al. Impaired response of human motoneurones to corticospinal stimulation after voluntary exercise. J Physiol (Lond) 1999;521:749–759.

75. Andersen B, Westlund B, Krarup C. Failure of activation of spinal motoneurones after muscle fatigue in healthy subjects studied by transcranial magnetic stimulation. J Physiol (Lond) 2003;551:345–356.

76. Asmussen E, Mazin B. Recuperation after muscular fatigue "diverting activities." Eur J Appl Physiol 1978;38:1–7.

76a. Todd G, Taylor JL, Gandevia SC. Measurement of voluntary activation of fresh and fatigued human muscles using transcranial magnetic stimulation. J Physiol (Lond) 2003;551:661–671.

77. Enoka RM, Stuart DG. Neurobiology of muscle fatigue. J Appl Physiol 1992;72:1631–1648.

78. Garland SJ. Role of small diameter afferents in reflex inhibition during human muscle fatigue. J Physiol (Lond) 1991;435:547–558.

79. Davis JM, Bailey SP. Possible mechanisms of central nervous system fatigue during exercise. Med Sci Sports Exerc 1997;29:45–57.

80. Dishman RK. Brain monoamines, exercise, and behavioral stress: animal models. Med Sci Sports Exerc 1997;29:63–74.

81. Gerin C, Becquet D, Privat A. Direct evidence for the link between monoaminergic descending pathways and motor activity: I. A study with microdialysis probes implanted in the ventral funiculus of the spinal cord. Brain Res 1995;704:191–201.

82. Dwyer D, Browning J. Endurance training in Wistar rats decreases receptor sensitivity to a serotonin agonist. Acta Physiol Scand 2000;170:211–216.

83. Weicker H, Struder HK. Influence of exercise on serotonergic neuromodulation in the brain. Amino Acids 2001;20:35–47.

84. Chennaoui M, Drogou C, Gomez-Merino D, et al. Endurance training effects on 5–HT(1B) receptors mRNA expression in cerebellum, striatum, frontal cortex and hippocampus of rats. Neurosci Lett 2001;307:33–36.

85. Tumer N, Demirel HA, Serova L, et al. Gene expression of catecholamine biosynthetic enzymes following exercise: modulation by age. Neuroscience 2001;103:703–711.

86. De Souza CG, Michelini LC, Fior-Chadi DR. Receptor changes in the nucleus tractus solitarii of the rat after exercise training. Med Sci Sports Exerc 2001;33:1471–1476.

87. Jasmin BJ, Lavoie PA, Gardiner PF. Fast axonal transport of labeled proteins in motoneurons of exercise-trained rats. Am J Physiol 1988;255:C731–C736.

88. Jasmin BJ, Lavoie PA, Gardiner PF. Fast axonal transport of acetylcholinesterase in rat sciatic motoneurons is enhanced following prolonged daily running, but not following swimming. Neurosci Lett 1987;78:156–160.

89. Roy RR, Baldwin KM, Edgerton VR. The plasticity of skeletal muscle: effects of neuromuscular activity. Exerc Sports Sci Rev 1991;19:269–312.

90. Martin TP, Bodine-Fowler S, Roy RR, et al. Metabolic and fiber size properties of cat tibialis anterior motor units. Am J Physiol 1988;255:C43–C50.

91. Burke RE, Edgerton VR. Motor unit properties and selective involvement in movement. Exerc Sport Sci Rev 1975;3:31–81.

92. Edgerton VR, Goslow Jr GE, Rasmussen SA, et al. Is resistance of a muscle to fatigue controlled by its motoneurones? Nature 1980;285:589–590.

93. Cope TC, Bodine SC, Fournier M, et al. Soleus motor units in chronic spinal transected cats: physiological and morphological alterations. J Neurophysiol 1986;55:1202–1220.

94. Roy RR, Zhong H, Hodgson JA, et al. Influences of electromechanical events in defining skeletal muscle properties. Muscle Nerve 2002;26:238–251.

95. Winiarski AM, Roy RR, Alford EK, et al. Mechanical properties of rat skeletal muscle after hind limb suspension. Exp Neurol 1987;96:650–660.

96. Shields RK. Fatigability, relaxation properties, and electromyographic responses of the human paralyzed soleus muscle. J Neurophysiol 1995;73:2195–2206.

97. Alaimo MA, Smith JL, Roy RR, et al. EMG activity of slow and fast ankle extensors following spinal cord transection. J Appl Physiol 1984;56:1608–1613.

98. Hensbergen E, Kernell D. Daily durations of spontaneous activity in cat's ankle muscles. Exp Brain Res 1997;115:325–332.

99. Roy RR, Zhong H, Monti RJ, et al. Mechanical properties of the electrically silent adult rat soleus muscle. Muscle Nerve 2002;26:404–412.

100. Hodgson JA, Wichayanuparp S, Recktenwald MR, et al. Circadian force and EMG activity in hindlimb muscles of rhesus monkeys. J Neurophysiol 2001;86:1430–1444.

101. Edgerton VR, McCall GE, Hodgson JA, et al. Sensorimotor adaptations to microgravity in humans. J Exp Biol 2001;204:3217–3224.

102. Edelman GM. Neural Darwinism: The theory of neuronal group selection. New York: Basic Books, 1987.

103. Durkovic RG, Damianopoulos EN. Forward and backward classical conditioning of the flexion reflex in the spinal cat. J Neurosci 1986;6:2921–2925.

104. Buerger AA, Fennessy A. Learning of leg position in chronic spinal rats. Nature 1970;225:751–752.

105. Grau J, Joynes RL. Pavlovian and instrumental conditioning within the spinal cord: methodological issues. In Patterson MM, Grau JW, eds. Spinal Cord Plasticity: Alterations in Reflex Function. Boston: Kluwer, 2001;13–54.

106. Nesmeyanova T. Experimental studies in regeneration of spinal neurons. New York: Wiley, 1977.

107. Shurrager P, Culler E. Conditioning in the spinal dog. J Exp Psychol 1940;26:133–159.

108. Barbeau H, Rossignol S. Recovery of locomotion after chronic spinalization in the adult cat. Brain Res 1987;412:84–95.

109. Lovely RG, Gregor RJ, Roy RR, et al. Weight-bearing hindlimb stepping in treadmill-exercised adult spinal cats. Brain Res 1990;514:206–218.

110. de Leon RD, Hodgson JA, Roy RR, et al. Locomotor capacity attributable to step training versus spontaneous recov-

ery after spinalization in adult cats. J Neurophysiol 1998;79:1329–1340.

111. de Leon RD, Hodgson JA, Roy RR, et al. Full weight-bearing hindlimb standing following stand training in the adult spinal cat. J Neurophysiol 1998;80:83–91.

112. Wolpaw JR, Tennissen AM. Activity-dependent spinal cord plasticity in health and disease. Annu Rev Neurosci 2001;24:807–843.

113. Beaumont E, Gardiner P. Effects of daily spontaneous running on the electrophysiological properties of hindlimb motoneurones in rats. J Physiol (Lond) 2002;540:129–138.

114. Kording KP, Wolpert DM. Bayesian integration in sensorimotor learning. Nature 2004;427:244–247.

115. Scheidt RA, Dingwell JB, Mussa-Ivaldi FA. Learning to move amid uncertainty. J Neurophysiol 2001;86:971–985.

116. Yue G, Cole KJ. Strength increases from the motor program: comparison of training with maximal voluntary and imagined muscle contractions. J Neurophysiol 1992;67:1114–1123.

117. Hortobagyi T, Lambert NJ, Hill JP. Greater cross-education following training with muscle lengthening than shortening. Med Sci Sports Exerc 1997;29:107–112.

118. Hortobagyi T, Scott K, Lambert J, et al. Cross-education of muscle strength is greater with stimulated than voluntary contractions. Motor Control 1999;3:205–219.

119. Zhou S. Chronic neural adaptations to unilateral exercise: mechanisms of cross education. Exerc Sport Sci Rev 2000;28:177–184.

120. Aagaard P. Training-induced changes in neural function. Exerc Sport Sci Rev 2003;31:61–67.

121. Casabona A, Polizzi MC, Perciavalle V. Differences in H-reflex between athletes trained for explosive contractions and non-trained subjects. Eur J Appl Physiol 1990;61:26–32.

122. Gandevia SC. Mind, muscles and motoneurones. J Sci Med Sport 1999;2:167–180.

123. Coote JH, Hilton SM, Perez-Gonzalez JF. The reflex nature of the pressor response to muscular exercise. J Physiol (Lond) 1971;215:789–804.

124. McCloskey DI, Mitchell JH. Reflex cardiovascular and respiratory responses originating in exercising muscle. J Physiol (Lond) 1972;224:173–186.

125. Kaufman MP, Rybicki KJ. Discharge properties of group III and IV muscle afferents: their responses to mechanical and metabolic stimuli. Circ Res 1987;61:I60–65.

126. Rotto DM, Kaufman MP. Effect of metabolic products of muscular contraction on discharge of group III and IV afferents. J Appl Physiol 1988;64:2306–2313.

127. Vissing J, Andersen M, Diemer NH. Exercise-induced changes in local cerebral glucose utilization in the rat. J Cereb Blood Flow Metab 1996;16:729–736.

128. Carroll TJ, Barry B, Riek S, et al. Resistance training enhances the stability of sensorimotor coordination. Proc R Soc Lond B Biol Sci 2001;268:221–227.

129. Cohen LG, Ziemann U, Chen R, et al. Studies of neuroplasticity with transcranial magnetic stimulation. J Clin Neurophysiol 1998;15:305–324.

130. Nudo RJ, Milliken GW, Jenkins WM, et al. Use-dependent alterations of movement representations in primary motor cortex of adult squirrel monkeys. J Neurosci 1996;16:785–807.

131. Jenkins IH, Brooks DJ, Nixon PD, et al. Motor sequence learning: a study with positron emission tomography. J Neurosci 1994;14:3775–3790.

132. Dettmers C, Ridding MC, Stephan KM, et al. Comparison of regional cerebral blood flow with transcranial magnetic stimulation at different forces. J Appl Physiol 19;9681:596–603.

133. van Mier H, Tempel LW, Perlmutter JS, et al. Changes in brain activity during motor learning measured with PET: effects of hand of performance and practice. J Neurophysiol 1998;80:2177–2199.

134. Cramer SC, Weisskoff RM, Schaechter JD, et al. Motor cortex activation is related to force of squeezing. Hum Brain Mapp 2002;16:197–205.

135. Karni A, Meyer G, Jezzard P, et al. Functional MRI evidence for adult motor cortex plasticity during motor skill learning. Nature 1995;377:155–158.

136. Pascual-Leone A, Nguyet D, Cohen LG, et al. Modulation of muscle responses evoked by transcranial magnetic stimulation during the acquisition of new fine motor skills. J Neurophysiol 1995;74:1037–1045.

137. Pearce AJ, Thickbroom GW, Byrnes ML, et al. Functional reorganisation of the corticomotor projection to the hand in skilled racquet players. Exp Brain Res 2000;130:238–243.

138. Patten C, Kamen G. Adaptations in motor unit discharge activity with force control training in young and older human adults. Eur J Appl Physiol 2000;83:128–143.

139. Suzuki S, Hayami A, Suzuki M, S. et al. Reductions in recruitment force thresholds in human single motor units by successive voluntary contractions. Exp Brain Res 1990;82:227–230.

140. Akima H, Takahashi H, Kuno SY, et al. Early phase adaptations of muscle use and strength to isokinetic training. Med Sci Sports Exerc 1999;31:588–594.

141. Sale DG. Neural adaptation to resistance training. Med Sci Sports Exerc 1988;20:S135–S145.

142. Milner-Brown HS, Stein RB, Lee RG. Synchronization of human motor units: possible roles of exercise and supraspinal reflexes. Electroencephalogr Clin Neurophysiol 1975;38:245–254.

143. Upton A, Radford P. Motoneuron excitability in elite sprinters. In Komi PV, ed. Biomechanics. Baltimore: University Park, 1975;82–87.

144. Schmied A, Pagni S, Sturm H, et al. Selective enhancement of motoneurone short-term synchrony during an attention-demanding task. Exp Brain Res 2000;133:377–390.

145. Semmler JG, Kornatz KW, Dinenno DV, et al. Motor unit synchronisation is enhanced during slow lengthening contractions of a hand muscle. J Physiol (Lond) 2002;545:681–695.

146. Semmler JG, Nordstrom MA. Motor unit discharge and force tremor in skill- and strength-trained individuals. Exp Brain Res 1998;119:27–38.

147. Taylor AM, Steege JW, Enoka RM. Motor-unit synchronization alters spike-triggered average force in simulated contractions. J Neurophysiol 2002;88:265–276.

148. Farmer SF, Bremner FD, Halliday DM, et al. The frequency content of common synaptic inputs to motoneurones studied during voluntary isometric contraction in man. J Physiol (Lond) 1993;470:127–155.

149. Gomez-Pinilla F, Ying Z, Opazo P, et al. Differential regulation by exercise of BDNF and NT-3 in rat spinal cord and skeletal muscle. Eur J Neurosci 2001;13:1078–1084.

150. Neeper SA, Gomez-Pinilla F, Choi J, et al. Exercise and brain neurotrophins. Nature 1995;373:109.

151. van Praag H, Kempermann G, Gage FH. Running increases cell proliferation and neurogenesis in the adult mouse dentate gyrus. Nat Neurosci 1999;2:266–270.

152. Kitamura T, Mishina M, Sugiyama H. Enhancement of neurogenesis by running wheel exercises is suppressed in mice lacking NMDA receptor epsilon 1 subunit. Neurosci Res 2003;47:55–63.

153. Cotman CW, Berchtold NC. Exercise: a behavioral intervention to enhance brain health and plasticity. Trends Neurosci 2002;25:295–301.

154. Lee TH, Jang MH, Shin MC, et al. Dependence of rat hippocampal c-Fos expression on intensity and duration of exercise. Life Sci 2003;72:1421–1436.

155. Ivy AS, Rodriguez FG, Garcia C, et al. Noradrenergic and serotonergic blockade inhibits BDNF mRNA activation following exercise and antidepressant. Pharmacol Biochem Behav 2003;75:81–88.

156. Anderson BJ, Alcantara AA, Greenough WT. Motor-skill learning: changes in synaptic organization of the rat cerebellar cortex. Neurobiol Learn Mem 1996;66:221–229.

157. Swain RA, Harris AB, Wiener EC, et al. Prolonged exercise induces angiogenesis and increases cerebral blood volume in primary motor cortex of the rat. Neuroscience 2003;117:1037–1046.

158. Gomez-Pinilla F, Dao L, So V. Physical exercise induces FGF-2 and its mRNA in the hippocampus. Brain Res 1997;764:1–8.

159. Black JE, Isaacs KR, Anderson BJ, A. et al. Learning causes synaptogenesis, whereas motor activity causes angiogenesis, in cerebellar cortex of adult rats. Proc Natl Acad Sci USA 1990;87:5568–5572.

160. Sherrington C. The integrative action of the nervous system. New Haven: Yale University, 1906.

161. Edgerton VR, Bodine-Fowler S, Roy RR, et al. Neuromuscular adaptation. In Rowell LB, Shepherd JT, eds. Handbook of physiology. Section 12: Exercise: Regulation and Integration of Multiple Systems. New York: Oxford University, 1996;54–88.

162. Roy R, Edgerton V, Ishihara A. Influence of endurance training and detraining on motoneurone and sensory neurone morphology and metabolism. In Shepherd RJ, Astrand PO, eds. Endurance in sport, encyclopaedia of sports medicine. Oxford: Blackwell Scientific, 2000;136–157.

163. Nakano H, Masuda K, Sasaki S, et al. Oxidative enzyme activity and soma size in motoneurons innervating the rat slow-twitch and fast-twitch muscles after chronic activity. Brain Res Bull 1997;43:149–154.

164. Chalmers GR, Roy RR, Edgerton VR. Motoneuron and muscle fiber succinate dehydrogenase activity in control and overloaded plantaris. J Appl Physiol 1991;71:1589–1592.

165. Gerchman LB, Edgerton VR, Carrow RE. Effects of physical training on the histochemistry and morphology of ventral motor neurons. Exp Neurol 1975;49:790–801.

166. Seburn K, Coicou C, Gardiner P. Effects of altered muscle activation on oxidative enzyme activity in rat alpha-motoneurons. J Appl Physiol 1994;77:2269–2274.

167. Munson JB, Foehring RC, Mendell LM, et al. Fast-to-slow conversion following chronic low-frequency activation of medial gastrocnemius muscle in cats: II. Motoneuron properties. J Neurophysiol 1997;77:2605–2615.

168. Roy RR, Talmadge RJ, Hodgson JA, et al. Training effects on soleus of cats spinal cord transected (T12–13) as adults. Muscle Nerve 1998;21:63–71.

169. Gharakhanlou R, Chadan S, Gardiner P. Increased activity in the form of endurance training increases calcitonin gene-related peptide content in lumbar motoneuron cell bodies and in sciatic nerve in the rat. Neuroscience 1999;89:1229–1239.

170. Gonzalez M, Collins WF 3rd. Modulation of motoneuron excitability by brain-derived neurotrophic factor. J Neurophysiol 1997;77:502–506.

171. Deschenes MR, Judelson DA, Kraemer WJ, et al. Effects of resistance training on neuromuscular junction morphology. Muscle Nerve 2000;23:1576–1581.

172. Andonian MH, Fahim MA. Endurance exercise alters the morphology of fast- and slow-twitch rat neuromuscular junctions. Int J Sports Med 1988;9:218–223.

173. Deschenes MR, Maresh CM, Crivello JF, et al. The effects of exercise training of different intensities on neuromuscular junction morphology. J Neurocytol 1993;22:603–615.

174. Waerhaug O, Dahl HA, Kardel K. Different effects of physical training on the morphology of motor nerve terminals in the rat extensor digitorum longus and soleus muscles. Anat Embryol (Berl) 1992;186:125–128.

175. Crockett JL, Edgerton VR, Max SR, et al. The neuromuscular junction in response to endurance training. Exp Neurol 1976;51:207–215.

176. Stebbins CL, Schultz E, Smith RT, et al. Effects of chronic exercise during aging on muscle and end-plate morphology in rats. J Appl Physiol 1985;58:45–51.

177. Sveistrup H, Chan RY, Jasmin BJ. Chronic enhancement of neuromuscular activity increases acetylcholinesterase gene expression in skeletal muscle. Am J Physiol 1995;269:C856–C862.

178. Homonko DA, Theriault E. Calcitonin gene-related peptide is increased in hindlimb motoneurons after exercise. Int J Sports Med 1997;18:503–509.

179. Sala C, Andreose JS, Fumagalli G, et al. Calcitonin gene-related peptide: possible role in formation and maintenance of neuromuscular junctions. J Neurosci 1995;15:520–528.

180. Wernig A, Salvini TF, Irintchev A. Axonal sprouting and changes in fibre types after running-induced muscle damage. J Neurocytol 1991;20:903–913.

181. Wuerker RB, Henneman E. Reflex regulation of primary (annulospiral) stretch receptors via gamma motoneurons in the cat. J Neurophysiol 1963;26:539–550.

182. Buller AJ, Eccles JC, Eccles RM. Differentiation of fast and slow muscles in the cat hind limb. J Physiol (Lond) 1960;150:399–416.

183. Buller AJ, Eccles JC, Eccles RM. Interactions between motoneurones and muscles in respect of the characteristic speeds of their responses. J Physiol (Lond) 1960;150:417–439.

184. Kugelberg E, Edstrom L. Differential histochemical effects of muscle contractions on phosphorylase and glycogen in various types of fibres: relation to fatigue. J Neurol Neurosurg Psychiatry 1968;31:415–423.

185. Edgerton VR, Simpson D, Barnard RJ, et al. Phosphorylase activity in acutely exercised muscle. Nature 1970;225:866–867.

186. Burke RE, Levine DN, Zajac 3rd FE. Mammalian motor units: physiological-histochemical correlation in three types in cat gastrocnemius. Science 1971;174:709–712.

CHAPTER 4

The Skeletal–Articular System

Ronald F. Zernicke, Gregory R. Wohl, and Jeremy M. LaMothe

Introduction

The skeletal–articular system comprises connective tissues that serve primarily mechanical roles in locomotion and in protection of vital organs. Bones provide support for movement as levers and pivots for muscle-driven motion; and ligaments, tendons, and menisci at the joints blend muscular forces into controlled skeletal motions. Normally, these musculoskeletal tissues function at loads well below their mechanical limits, while possessing safety factors seven- to tenfold greater than normal physiological use to minimize the likelihood of failure and sustain normal function. Although generally perceived as inert tissues, skeletal–articular tissues are patently dynamic and adapt to changes in their physiological environment, such as exercise.

The turnover (replacement of old tissue with new tissue) of musculoskeletal tissues can be influenced by dynamic and resistance exercises. In particular, exercise can substantially influence bone morphology. Although the precise nature of the exercise stimuli that orchestrate adaptive responses remains elusive, it is generally accepted that tissue strain (change in dimension of a loaded tissue normalized to the original dimension of the tissue) influences tissue adaptation. Specifically strain magnitude, frequency, rate, and gradients all influence adaptive responses. Potentially, cells in skeletal–articular connective tissues sense stimuli arising from exercise via cell deformations, or indirectly via exercise-induced tissue fluid flow, and orchestrate adaptive responses. Of the skeletal–articular tissues, bone is by far the most studied. Bone loss (e.g., osteoporosis) in aging individuals has significant implications for quality of life and mobility in individuals and for cost of health care to society. A significant amount of skeletal–articular research focuses on the effects of exercise on bone adaptation. Physical activity can dramatically enhance bone mass. Consequently, the effects of exercise on bone mass have significant clinical implications, and understanding the precise nature of the stimuli influencing bone may allow identification of exercise regimens that more effectively counter age-related bone loss.

In this chapter, we describe the basic structure and biochemistry of bone, ligament, tendon, and meniscus and the response of these connective tissues to exercise stimuli. To examine the effects of exercise on the skeletal–articular tissues, first we present the effects of mechanical stimuli on connective tissue adaptation, and second we present mechanisms by which connective tissues adapt to their mechanical environment. Included in the exposition are explanations of how components of loading (e.g., strain magnitude, rate, frequency, and gradients) influence skeletal–articular tissue adaptation, and further, how the cells interpret their mechanical milieu through different means of mechanical transduction. Understanding how physical forces interact with skeletal–articular tissues may lead to a clearer view of how skeletal–articular structure and function can be optimized for normal function and for prevention of tissue damage. It also may help to develop effective nonpharmacological treatments to combat skeletal–articular pathologies characterized by low bone mass.

Skeletal–Articular Physiology

The biochemical composition of the skeletal–articular tissues complements their mechanical roles in the body. Ligaments and tendons are collagenous bands central to the transduction of muscular forces into controlled movements. Ligaments tether bones across a joint (Fig. 4.1) and—in tandem with articular geometry—control the relative motion of the joint.

Tendons connect muscles to bones and transmit muscular forces to the bones. Menisci are fibrocartilage structures that help maintain joint components in appropriate position, reduce joint stress by bearing load, and enhance rotation in synovial joints. In the knee, for example, menisci are avascular crescent-shaped and triangular structures (Fig. 4.2). Menisci are firmly attached to the tibiae with ligaments.

Compared to other organ systems, skeletal–articular tissues have low cellularity, and extracellular matrix constitutes most tissue volume. The extracellular matrix of the soft connective tissues is 70–75% water, and collagen is 60–70% of the dry mass. In ligaments and tendons, the quintessential collagen molecule is tropocollagen. Five parallel tropocollagen molecules tightly stagger together to form microfibrils (Fig. 4.3).

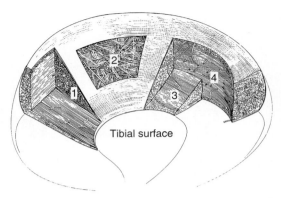

FIGURE 4.2   Reconstruction of the fiber pattern of the meniscus. At the tibial surface (*1*), collagen fibers predominantly lie radial. Tangential to the femoral meniscal surface, fibers are predominantly woven together (*2*). Fibers are predominantly organized circumferentially through the center of the meniscus (*3*). Through the thickness of the meniscus parallel to its edge, fibers are predominantly radial (*4*). Collagen bundles from the radial fibers curl up into the body of the meniscus. *(Modified from Bullough PG, Munuera L, Murphy J, et al. The strength of the menisci of the knee as it relates to their fine structure. J Bone Joint Surg Br 1970;52:564–567.)*

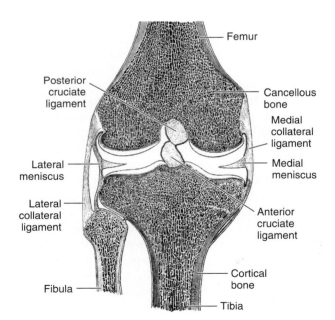

FIGURE 4.1   Frontal section of the knee, including ligaments, bones, and menisci. *(Modified from Platzer W, ed. Volume II: Thorax, Abdomen, and Extremities. Baltimore: Urban & Schwarzenberg, 1989.)*

Sequentially, microfibrils collate to form subfibrils, which aggregate to form fibrils and finally fibers; fibers aggregate to form fiber bundles (1). Fiber bundles are collated into fascicles. A tendon (ligament) is a collection of fascicles grouped by a sheath, the paratenon (or epiligament). Water plays a significant role in the mechanical behavior of the ligaments and tendons. Noncollagenous proteins called proteoglycans bind the water in the matrix, creating a gel-like matrix about the tightly packed collagen fibers. The glycosaminoglycans and collagenous network resist fluid flow during loading, contributing to the viscoelastic mechanical behavior of the tissues.

Similar to ligaments and tendons, the meniscal extracellular matrix is 70 to 75% water. In menisci there are two distinct zones, the outer superficial layer, and the deep inner zone (2). Type I collagen predominates in menisci. In the deep zone, collagen fibers are aligned circumferentially to resist stresses engendered during compressive loading in the knee, while the collagen fibers in the superficial layer are more randomly aligned (Fig. 4.2). Proteoglycans also bind water in the meniscus, but the avascular inner two-thirds produces more proteoglycan than the vascularized outer third.

In addition to mechanical support, bones are a center for hematopoiesis and are the body's largest calcium reservoir, which can be mobilized via bone resorption when serum calcium drops. Bone has unique tissue properties that are dependent on the interactions among an organic phase (about 25% by mass), inorganic phase (about 70%), and water (about 5%). As with ligaments and tendons, the

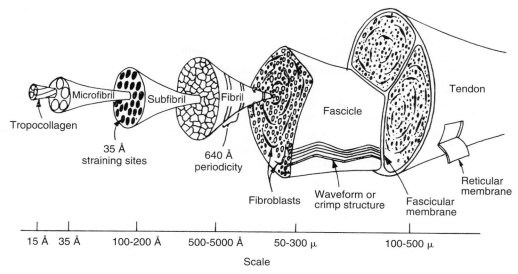

FIGURE 4.3 Structural hierarchy of tendon organization. *(Modified from Kastelic J, Galeski A, Baer E. The multicomposite structure of tendon. Connect Tissue Res 1978;6:11–23.)*

organic phase comprises mostly type I collagen, the mechanical function of which is to resist tensile forces, and numerous noncollagenous proteins (e.g., glycosaminoglycans) (3). Also like the other connective tissues, bone cells constitute a minor portion of the organic component. Bone is unique in that the compressive forces are principally supported by the inorganic mineral component of bone. Platelike calcium hydroxyapatite crystals, $Ca_{10}(PO_4)_6(OH)_2$, precipitate in the unmineralized organic matrix (osteoid) within and between the collagen fibrils. Collagen fibril organization and size and the presence of some noncollagenous proteins can regulate the size and timing of crystal growth. Water is present in spaces between hydroxyapatite crystals.

There are many levels of bone porosity. On a gross structural level bone can be highly porous, with large pores between bone fragments (called trabeculae) visible to the naked eye, or relatively compact, with small pores not visible to the naked eye. Highly porous bone, called trabecular, or cancellous, is found in flat bones (e.g., skull), in cuboidal bones (e.g., vertebrae), occasionally under ligament insertions, and at the end of long bones (Fig. 4.1). Bone marrow pervades the spaces between trabeculae, and trabecular bone is sheathed by a layer of more compact bone. The more compact bone is called cortical, or compact, bone. Cortical bone has small pores associated with vascularity (e.g., Haversian canals; about 10 μm); osteocyte lacunae and the canaliculi housing the osteocytes and their processes, respectively (about 200 nm); and pores associated with gaps in the mineral structure (about 10 nm). As with the soft connective tissues, on a gross structural level bone fluid saturates all levels of porosity, which adds to bone's viscoelastic behavior and likely is important in adaptation to exercise.

Skeletal–Articular Tissue Turnover

Cell populations in connective tissues maintain a fine balance of extracellular matrix components, turning over damaged matrix and repairing or building new matrix in response to injuries or mechanical stimuli. In ligaments and tendons, **fibroblasts** are the primary cell population, aligned in a columnar arrangement along the long axis of the tissue. In menisci, there are morphologically two distinct cell populations. Cells in the superficial layer are ovoid or fusiform, while cells in the deeper zones are round or polygonal. Regardless of their morphological characterization, it is unclear whether meniscal cells are chondrocytes or fibroblasts, and they have been called **fibrochondrocytes.**

The soft fibrous connective tissues are relatively avascular. Ligament and tendon vascular elements are limited mainly to the outer surface. Similarly, vascularity in mature menisci is limited to the outer third of the crescent. The low cellularity and vascularity have mechanical and biological implications. Biologically, low vascularity restricts the metabolic capacity of the fibroblasts and fibrochondrocytes during matrix turnover, and the adaptive response of these soft connective tissues to stimuli is less vigorous than in bone. Furthermore, ligaments, tendons, and menisci respond poorly to injury; the repaired tissue rarely achieves normal structure or function and commonly degenerates. Mechanically, cells and blood vessels create holes that weaken the tissue structure. Minimizing these "structural defects" improves mechanical efficiency for tissue size. Thus, fibrous connective tissues are optimized for mechanical function, and tissue turnover during normal activity is generally sufficient to maintain healthy tissues over a lifetime.

In contrast to the fibrous soft tissues, bone is the most dynamic of the skeletal–articular tissues and can completely turn over in as little as 3 years, depending on location in the body. Bone is formed and maintained by cells of two different origins (3). **Osteoblasts,** mononuclear cells of stromal origin, secrete unmineralized matrix as the first phase of bone formation and are responsible for bone formation. Occasionally osteoblasts become quiescent on the bone surface after matrix secretion and are called **bone-lining cells,** or they become encased in matrix and are called **osteocytes.** Osteocytes maintain connections with adjacent osteocytes throughout the bone matrix via cellular processes in interconnecting bony tunnels called canaliculi. Giant multinuclear cells of hematogenic origin called **osteoclasts** degrade and remove bone by first adhering to a bone surface. To dissolve the inorganic and organic components of bone mineral, protons and proteolytic enzymes are secreted across the osteoclast cell membrane adjacent to sites of adhesion to the bone matrix.

Turnover of the bone tissue occurs through two main processes—**modeling** and **remodeling** (Fig. 4.4). In the process of modeling, osteoblasts and osteoclasts can work in-

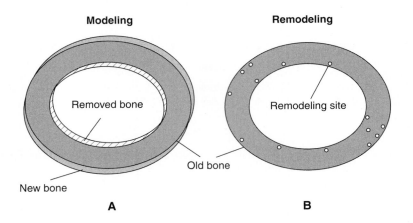

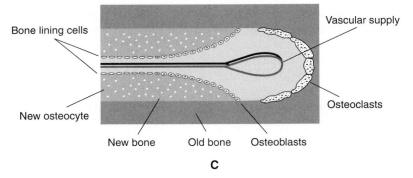

FIGURE 4.4 Modeling and remodeling in a bone diaphyseal cross-section (original bone shown as dark gray). **A.** During modeling, bone is removed from one surface (e.g., the endosteum—hatch mark), and by a separately regulated process, formed on another surface (e.g., the periosteum—light gray). Modeling can change the size or shape of the bone. **B.** During remodeling, osteoclasts remove existing bone (white circles within cortex), and the resorption is normally coupled immediately with subsequent bone formation. **C.** In cortical bone remodeling, the osteoclasts tunnel through the cortex, forming Haversian canals. A vascular supply is closely associated with the remodeling, as the process requires a significant amount of energy, nutrients, and waste removal. The osteoblasts follow, creating new osteoid matrix, and many of the osteoblasts become embedded in the matrix as osteocytes or remain on the surface as bone-lining cells. In the remodeling of trabecular bone, osteoclasts form pits (Howship's lacunae) on the surface of the trabeculae. As with cortical remodeling, that is typically coupled with subsequent bone formation.

dependently of each other on both the periosteal surface (i.e., outer surface of bone, apposed to the periosteum) and the endocortical surface (i.e., inner surface of bone, bordering the marrow cavity). This process involves cellular activation and bone formation and/or resorption, is most common during growth, and changes the size and shape of bones. Remodeling follows a more locally coupled process of activation, resorption, and formation in which osteoclasts are activated and resorb bone in focal regions (about 200 μm in diameter), and resorption is immediately coupled with the activation of osteoblasts to fill in the cavity with newly synthesized organic matrix that later mineralizes.

Factors in Tissue Adaptation

The structure of musculoskeletal tissues is determined by an intricate blend of genetic constraints and epigenetic conditions. Genetics can influence up to 80% of peak bone mineral density (BMD), and the remaining influences are a summation of environmental conditions. In humans, bone strength is typically approximated using bone mass, density, size, and geometry. Dual energy x-ray absorptiometry (DXA) and quantitative computed tomography (QCT) are used to measure bone mineral content, apparent areal (DXA) and volumetric (QCT) bone density, and cross-sectional area of bone (QCT). DXA or QCT (indirect measures), however, do not give the full picture of the quality and quantity of bone, as the microarchitecture of cancellous and cortical bone also influences bone strength. DXA is further limited in that bone cross-sectional area and shape influence bone strength. Systemic factors, such as diet and hormones, can interact with local factors (e.g., mechanical environment) and collectively affect the ability of bone to adapt to exercise.

Tissue Response to Mechanical Stimuli

Genetics plays a significant role in the shape and size of the musculoskeletal tissues, but the structure of connective tissues is also determined in part by mechanical environment. Chronic exercise can lead to bone hypertrophy. Conversely, chronic immobilization may lead to bone atrophy, which can manifest as shape alterations (such as a loss of long bone curvature) and decreased density. The sensitivity of the skeleton to these mechanical stimuli is a function of particular characteristics of the mechanical stimuli itself and can also be influenced by a host of variables, including genetic, dietary, hormonal, and ontogenetically related considerations.

Ligament and Tendon

Although studies describing the mechanical and biochemical properties of ligaments and tendons are extensive, there are few details of how these collagenous structures respond to exercise and immobilization. These deficiencies can partly be explained by reports as recent as a few decades ago suggesting that ligaments and tendons were essentially inert and unresponsive to exercise (4). It has become obvious, however, that ligaments and tendons can respond to exercise, although most adaptation data pertain to ligament rather than tendon.

Catabolic Stimuli

Joint immobilization can cause significant changes in ligament, which can lead to substantial decrements in ligament stiffness and strength (5,6). Histologically and biochemically, immobilization can induce notable changes (7–10). Immobilization decreases the number of small-diameter collagen fibrils and the mean collagen fibril density, meanwhile increasing the number of large-diameter collagen fibrils. Immobilization disrupts the parallel orientation of the collagen fibrils in ligament and tendons, decreases glycosaminoglycan and water content, and increases collagen cross-linking. Furthermore, collagen turnover increases and the whole collagen mass decreases.

As with ligament, immobilization increases the overall collagen turnover in tendon (11). Reports indicate, however, that the relative quantity of tendon components and overall tendon mass do not change (11–13). Despite the lack of substantial biochemical change, immobilization can significantly decrease tendon stiffness, failure load, and ultimate strength (12,13). The loss of tendon and bone mechanical integrity during immobilization demonstrates the dramatic interplay between the tissues in response to altered loading. After 4 weeks of immobilization, Achilles tendon failure typically happens at the insertion into bone, whereas at 8 weeks, failure typically occurs by means of calcaneal fracture (13). If the Achilles tendon is severed (simulated injury), the glycosaminoglycan content, fibroblast number, and number of small collagen fibers increase, and these changes are minimal if the tendon is sutured (14). Thus, tensile load appears to be necessary to maintain tendon biochemical and biomechanical properties.

Anabolic Stimuli

Normal daily activity (without training) is sufficient to maintain 80 to 90% of a ligament's mechanical potential, and thus exercise or training can enhance the mechanical potential by 10 to 20% (5). Following chronic exercise, significant increases occurred in the strength and stiffness of the anterior cruciate ligaments in exercised rats; those increases were greater when endurance exercises were conducted more frequently and for a shorter duration (15). Biochemically, exercise can increase collagen concentration, glycosaminoglycan content, collagen turnover, and collagen irreducible cross-links (16). Furthermore, ligaments in exercised rats have more small-diameter collagen fibers than in rats that have not been exercised (17). Together, these biochemical alterations may account for the observed increase in stiffness and load-bearing capabilities of exercised ligaments. Although the effects of training on ligaments can be moderate, injured ligaments that have been exercised consistently have improved biochemical and mechanical properties relative to injured ligaments that have not been exercised.

Similar to ligament, tendon can exhibit adaptive responses to exercise. Exercise can increase the number of active fibroblasts (18) and collagen synthesis in growing tendon (19). Mice exercised on a treadmill for 1 week showed increases in the number and size of the collagen fibrils and in the total cross-sectional area of the digital flexor tendons (20). Following 7 weeks of exercise training, the average collagen fibril diameter was smaller than in sedentary controls, and that reduction appeared to be caused by a splitting of the collagen fibrils. By 10 weeks of training, the flexor tendons' cross-sectional areas were similar to control values. In another long-term exercise experiment immature swine were exercised at a moderate level for 1 year, after which there were no significant differences in tendon biomechanical properties or cross-sectional areas between exercisers and controls (21). Other models reported enhanced biomechanical properties following chronic exercise training. A long-term exercise regimen resulted in increased tendon stiffness in guinea fowl (22). Chronic exposure to repetitive loading can produce tendon hypertrophy. Runners who trained at least 80 km per week had significantly larger Achilles tendon cross-sectional area than did age-matched controls who did not run (23). Conversely, in a randomized control trial, an exercise intervention (about 9 months of running) did not alter the mechanical properties of the triceps–surae aponeurosis complex or the cross-sectional area of the Achilles tendon (24). Thus, while some reports suggest that exercise does not influence tendon geometrical or mechanical properties, other reports indicate that tendon, like other musculoskeletal tissues, adapts its geometrical or mechanical properties to mechanical stimuli.

Meniscus

Meniscal adaptation to exercise is poorly understood. Until the 1970s, menisci were thought to have no functional role in the knee, and meniscectomy was advocated for meniscal injury. Damage or removal of the menisci can lead to joint degradation. Partial meniscectomy is the gold standard treatment for meniscal bucket-handle tears, but it can lead to articular cartilage degradation and osteoarthritis (25). Despite the importance of menisci in proper joint function, there is a paucity of data about their adaptive responses to disuse and training.

Catabolic Stimuli

Immobilization can be a potent catabolic stimulus for the musculoskeletal system. Reports of the specific responses of menisci, however, are sparse. After immobilization for 8 weeks, significant atrophy of periarticular bone in dogs

was reported, but there was no atrophy of the menisci (26). Biochemically, however, significant changes were reported. Aggrecan is one of the major proteoglycans of the meniscus and is largely responsible for giving the meniscus its viscoelastic compressive properties. Aggrecan gene expression decreased and water content increased when beagles were immobilized for 4 weeks (27). Data suggest that the amount of nutrient delivery to the tissue is strongly related to the degree of tissue surface exposed to synovial fluid (28), and cyclic loading during exercise may improve nutrient delivery to the tissue. Thus, immobilization may impair cell function via starvation. Ochi and colleagues examined the penetration of a tracer with immobilization and remobilization (29). They injected horseradish peroxidase into the knee joints and immobilized the rabbit's leg with a cast. In joints that were not immobilized, the tracer pervaded the entire meniscus. After 8 weeks of immobilization, however, the tracer was restricted to the superficial layer, and degenerative changes were seen in the deep layer of the meniscus as early as 6 weeks. Meniscal permeability was recovered with remobilization, but the degenerative changes remained, even after 4 weeks of remobilization. Immobilization can also impair the normal healing process. With meniscal injury, blood flow to the meniscus significantly increases, and immobilization during recovery prevents blood flow enhancement (30).

Anabolic Stimuli

The effects of exercise on meniscal biomechanics and biochemistry are not as well documented as the effects of exercise on other skeletal articular tissues. Anabolic and catabolic changes have been reported for exercise, with the nature of the change likely related to exercise intensity. Strenuous exercise can delay the formation of collagen pyridinoline crosslinks in menisci in skeletally immature chickens and cause premature decrements in dermatan sulphate proteoglycans (31). Nitric oxide affects matrix metabolism in various intraarticular tissues, and its production can increase in lateral and medial porcine meniscal explants when dynamically compressed (32). In one of the more prominent studies detailing the adaptive response of menisci to exercise (33), rats were trained to run on a motor-driven treadmill 5 days a week for 12 weeks. The potential for the exercise to elicit an adaptive response was apparent: there was a 65% increase in gastrocnemius succinate dehydrogenase. In response, the posterior lateral horn of the meniscus, which likely received principally compressive stress during locomotion, had significantly greater concentrations of collagen, proteoglycans, and calcium. Increases in collagen and proteoglycan would augment the meniscus's ability to bear mechanical loading (34). Although collagen fiber orientation was not measured, it likely also is relevant to a meniscus's load-bearing capabilities. Longitudinal collagen fibers ensure tension resistance in the meniscus, while the transverse fiber bundles unite the longitudinal fibers and thus retain the shape of the meniscus (35).

Bone

The salutary effects of exercise on bone are well known, but more dramatic examples of bone mechanosensitivity are exemplified when mechanical stimuli are removed. The Space Studies Board of the American National Research Council has stated that along with radiation exposure, the most significant obstacle to long space missions remains the osteopenia associated with microgravity (36). In space flight, bone loss has been reported to approach 1.6% per month in regions such as spine, femoral neck, and long-bone metaphyses (37). The implications of significant increases in fracture risk during long missions in space are apparent, especially upon reexposure to earth's gravitational field. As with microgravity, prolonged bed rest or immobilization can dramatically impair bone formation rates and increase resorption, with a net loss in BMD. A more extensive account of the potent effects of microgravity is provided in Chapter 29.

Positive Effects of Exercise

Bone formation in response to dynamic and resistance exercises can lead to an increase in bone cross-sectional area. Thus, the forces generated by exercising will be applied over a greater area of bone, and that will lead to a reduction in bone mechanical stresses (stress is force per unit area). Wolff's law ostensibly describes the ability of bone to alter its morphology in accordance with the prevailing mechanical milieu. The originator of that concept, however, was actually von Roux, and it is simpler and more appropriate to refer to the *functional adaptation* of bone. Long-term chronic exercise can augment BMD and increase bone strength. Larger, stronger bones can decrease bone stresses generated during normal physiological activities. Thus, exercise-induced adaptations may enhance the safety factor of the bone (difference between typical peak load and load at which bone fractures).

Bone formed in response to exercise can be adaptive at two levels, structural and material. Structurally, bone accretion through modeling will alter geometry. If exogenous loads differ in direction from the loads normally applied to the bone, the cross-sectional shape of the bone may be altered to optimize the mechanical properties of the bone in response to this new loading regimen. Cross-sectional geometry can be altered by a modeling phenomenon termed a *modeling drift*. Bone added to the periosteal surface, farther from the cross-sectional neutral axis or centroid, renders the bone more resistant, respectively, to bending or torsion. Cross-sectional moment of inertia numerically represents the distribution of material about the neutral axis of bending and how this material resists bending. Polar moment of inertia numerically represents the distribution of material

about the centroid axis and how the material resists torsion. Such a functional adaptation appears to occur during aging, even in the absence of specified exercise regimens. Though BMD and mineral content decrease with age, the cross-sectional moments of inertia in long bones increase by endocortical resorption and periosteal apposition, which effectively preserves bone strength.

At the material level, newly accreted bone may have different properties from those of older, existing bone. Initially, there is a lag of about 1 to 2 weeks from when the osteoid is first laid down to about 65% of its complete mineralization. Recently formed bone is less mineralized than older bone. Over the next few months the bone tissue, normally will become completely mineralized. Evidence suggests that following complete mineralization, the material properties of newer bone do not differ from those of preexisting bone (38). Nevertheless, the degree of active remodeling can affect the amount of bone incompletely mineralized at any given time and hence the net bone mineral content.

Numerous studies report the relations between exercise and bone mass (Fig. 4.5). Cross-sectional studies and longitudinal studies generally show that exercise significantly increases BMD. Cross-sectional studies, however, can be riddled with confounding variables. On average, cross-sectional studies contain younger subjects of whom a higher proportion are male than longitudinal studies. Furthermore, it remains unclear how much of a role genetics plays in the differences between exercise and sedentary population groups; subjects in cross-sectional studies may be self-selected for sports and vigorous physical activity. While genetics may be responsible

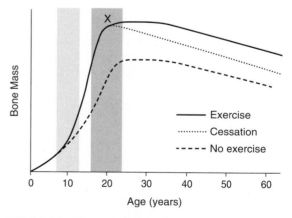

FIGURE 4.5 Theoretical relation between exercise and bone mass. The velocity of bone mass accrual increases during peripuberty (light gray rectangle) and decreases when peak bone mass is achieved (dark gray rectangle). Commencement of exercise is associated with enhanced peak bone mass. Cessation of exercise (**X**) is associated with a more rapid loss of bone with aging. *(Modified from Modlesky CM, Lewis RD. Does exercise during growth have a long-term effect on bone health? Exerc Sport Sci Rev 2002;30:171–176.)*

for up to 70 to 80% of an individual's bone mass, mechanical loads associated with exercise and physical activity are key to a healthy skeleton. Unilateral loading studies (e.g., of athletes in racquet sports) are useful in that use of the lesser active appendage as an internal control eliminates genetic and lifestyle effects. Many studies have shown that racquet sports significantly augment bone growth in the playing limb compared to the contralateral limb (39).

In human studies, bone gains in response to exercise are commonly assessed with DXA, which uses the principle of x-ray beams being differently attenuated by tissues of varying densities. The differential attentuations allow tissues to be separated into bone and soft tissue. DXA is fast and relatively precise, and it exposes patients to only low radiation doses (40). Bone strength is determined by the bone material characteristics and geometry, but DXA is unable to quantify the latter. DXA is two-dimensional and cannot resolve three-dimensional bone geometry. Furthermore, DXA may not be able to resolve small amounts of bone accretion in response to exercise. Small quantities of new bone, if placed correctly, can dramatically increase biomechanical properties. A DXA-measured BMD increase of 5.4% corresponded to a 64% increase in ultimate force and a 94% increase in the energy to failure of the rat ulna (41).

Small amounts of new bone can significantly increase resistance to bending, because stress in a loaded beam is inversely proportional to the cross-sectional moment of inertia. The cross-sectional moment of inertia is proportional to the radius of the section to the fourth power. Thus, small increments of bone accreted on the outer (periosteal) surface can translate into large increases in mechanical properties. QCT has the benefit of being able to discern alterations in bone geometry due to bone accretion in addition to changes in BMD.

The relation between chronic exercise and bone adaptation is complex. In designing an exercise regimen for increasing bone mass, five training principles are classically considered (42):

1. Specificity
2. Overload
3. Reversibility
4. Initial values
5. Diminishing returns

Bone adaptation is a site-specific phenomenon, and therefore, exercise regimens should *specifically* target the bone of interest. Jumping exercises will stimulate gains in hip but not wrist BMD. In contrast to cardiovascular and muscular systems, bone has a "lazy zone" of imposed loading (via exercise) within which bone mass is maintained but no osteogenic activity is stimulated (43). Loading stimuli arising from exercise modes such as cycling may lie within this range, whereas stimuli from impact loading can *overload* (exceed) the upper threshold of this range and stimulate osteogenic adaptation. Accordingly, adaptive osteogenesis

varies with exercise mode. Generally, weightlifters have greater bone strength than marathon runners, though confounding factors such as diet may also play a role in the relatively poor bone mass of runners. As Borelli noted in the late seventeenth century, muscle insertions often lie close to the center of joint rotation, and thus muscles work at an incredible mechanical disadvantage. Because of that disadvantage, large local forces are transmitted to bones. Joint reaction forces during postural maintenance and during physical activity routinely exceed several multiples of body weight. Thus, excluding trauma, forces due to muscles are among the largest forces that weightbearing bones experience. Bone can adapt in response to such forces.

Adaptive gains in bone mass from exercises may be *reversible;* cessation of exercise can be coupled with a loss of exercise-induced gains in bone mass (42). That further supports the need for exercise to *maintain* bone mass, particularly in aging populations. The osteogenic potential of an exercise regimen also depends on the *initial* bone mass; there is an inverse relation between initial bone mass and the osteogenic potential of a specific exercise regimen. Thus, those with low bone mass have the most to gain through exercise. Osteogenesis in response to elevated mechanical loading is greater in the initial stages than in later stages. That is the phenomenon of *diminishing returns*. Adaptation in immature rat tibiae in response to jumping was seen after 5 jumps per day and did not substantially increase when rats jumped up to 40 times per day (44). As with muscles, a few brief bouts of exercise over a given duration can be more osteogenic than one long exercise bout. If the daily duration of physical activity is to be decreased, the duration of each exercise bout should be shortened, but eliminating exercise bouts diminishes the osteogenic potential of the exercise (45).

Systemic effects arising from exercise can modify exercise-induced changes in bone structure. Although the data regarding bone blood flow in response to exercise are sparse, acute exercise can increase bone blood flow. Vascular flow in lower appendages has been inversely correlated with the rate of bone loss at the hip and calcaneus in older women, which may be linked to reduced physical activity and osteoporosis (46).

Acute dynamic exercise alters intestinal and renal calcium absorption and secretion (see Chapter 25). Additional calcium is absorbed through the small intestine in response to exercise, and that calcium is required for new bone growth and replenishes the ions excreted in sweat.

An increase in bone mass in response to exercise may underpin the development of nonpharmacological treatments for osteoporosis. Osteoporosis adversely affects quality of life and burdens the health care system. In the 1990s osteoporosis-related fractures cost the United States health care system nearly $14 billion annually (47). Of those fractures, 90% of hip fractures and 50% of spine fractures resulted from unexpected falls (43). With an increase in global life expectancy, osteoporosis-related fractures have the potential to become a significantly greater problem. Exercise-induced bone formation may mitigate significant morbidity and mortality related to osteoporosis by four mechanisms:

1. Exercise in growing individuals could increase peak bone mass; younger bones have a greater adaptive response to exercise.
2. Exercise in adulthood may slow age-associated bone loss.
3. Exercise-induced bone accrual throughout adulthood and old age may counterbalance age-associated bone loss and result in net gains.
4. Exercise can significantly improve musculoskeletal coordination, thereby reducing the risk of unexpected falls.

Negative Effects of Exercise

Traumatic injury aside, exercise is not always beneficial to bone. Extremely intense exercise can adversely affect the skeletal system. Prolonged bouts of extremely intense exercise can produce microdamage (i.e., microscopic cracks within bone matrix). Each load cycle by itself may be too small to cause microdamage, but the cumulative effect of some thousands of load cycles can lead to microdamage accumulation within bone in what is termed a *stress reaction* or *stress fracture*. A stress reaction is a site of increased cellular activity, while a stress fracture is a crack that propagates in bone. Stress fractures are painful, may or may not be evident in radiographs, and are a significant medical concern. Up to 73% of United States Marine recruits undergo stress fractures (48).

Females involved in extremely intense exercise can develop the *female athlete triad:* one or more eating disorders, amenorrhea, and osteoporosis (see Milestone of Discovery). When energy availability (total energy intake minus total energy expenditure) falls below 20 to 30 kcal $\cdot$ kg^{-1} lean body mass per day, reproductive dysfunction (amenorrhea) can result (49). Prolonged hormonal disruptions can lead to reduction in BMD, termed osteopenia, which in turn elevates the risk of developing osteoporosis years later (50). Weakened bones are especially dangerous for competitive athletes, as active competition elevates the risk of fracture above that in sedentary women.

Up to 26% of total adult skeletal calcium is accumulated through 2 years of peak skeletal growth during adolescence (51). Peak skeletal growth precedes peak height growth velocity and occurs earlier for girls (12.5 years) than boys (14 years) (52). Mineral accrual can be substantially altered with exercise during growth. Reportedly, there is a 9 and 17% increase in total body BMC for active boys and girls, respectively, relative to inactive children (53). However, extremely strenuous exercise during periods of rapid adolescent growth could interrupt normal growth, and as a result, body stature may be stunted.

Interactions With Exercise

The potential for exercise to increase bone mass is related to more than the nature of the mechanical stimuli. The requisite genetic, dietary, hormonal, and developmental conditions must be satisfied for exercise to mount a positive adaptive response. In some cases, if these conditions are unsatisfied, exercise that would normally exert positive effects can have negligible or negative effects.

Genetics

Heritability is deemed the most important determinant of BMD, as up to 80% of peak bone mass is typically attributed to genetics. Some of the genes controlling peak BMD have been revealed. Osteocalcin (most abundant noncollagenous protein in bone) and vitamin D receptor gene polymorphisms have been linked BMD differences among individuals (54,55). Evidence suggests that genes controlling BMD may interact with exercise to augment or attenuate its effects on bone adaptation. It has recently been shown that vitamin D receptor and interleukin-6 gene polymorphisms affect skeletal adaptation to exercise (56,57).

Diet

Some of the key dietary factors in bone health include minerals (most notably calcium), vitamin D, protein, and fat. Though diet and exercise can influence bone independently, a poor diet reduces the available nutritional building blocks and can diminish positive exercise-related effects on bone. The data about the relation between calcium intake and exercise, however, are equivocal and poorly understood. Analysis of exercise intervention trials that included information on dietary calcium intake reveal that exercise produces increases in BMD only when calcium intake exceeds 1000 mg daily, with this effect more pronounced in the lumbar spine, than in the radius (58). It is generally accepted that chronic exercise and dietary calcium can improve bone mass to a greater extent than calcium intake alone. The body uses calcium in numerous biological processes and functions, and it is imperative to maintain appropriate serum calcium balance. Bone's dual mechanical and biological roles can sometimes be in opposition, particularly if dietary calcium is low; bone will be resorbed to elevate serum calcium levels.

Vitamin D increases intestinal absorption of calcium, and thus diets rich in vitamin D may also augment bone formation in response to exercise. Protein is also important as a tissue building block, and diets high in protein have augmented the osteogenic effect of strenuous exercise in young growing rats (59). Dietary fatty acids can influence bone at both local and systemic levels. Saturated fatty acid triglycerides form soaps with calcium in the intestine and can reduce intestinal absorption of dietary calcium (60). At the bone tissue level, prostaglandins, involved in bone remodeling processes, are formed from n-6 fatty acid precursors in the cells. Diets high in saturated fatty acids alter the fatty acid profile of cells in the bone and may alter the bone's ability to respond to mechanical stimuli.

Hormones

Studies of male and female osteoporoses consistently show a close relation between hormones (e.g., growth hormone and estrogen) and BMD. However, the interaction between hormones and exercise and their effects on BMD remain largely equivocal. The loss of sex steroids in men and women with old age is coupled with substantial bone losses. Recently, it was shown that osteoblasts require estrogen receptor alpha (ER-α) to mount an effective osteogenic response to mechanical loading (61). ER-α expression is positively correlated with serum estrogen concentration, and therefore, age-related decrements in sex steroid concentrations could decrease the expression of ER-α and hence mechanical sensitivity. Hormone replacement therapy (HRT) can increase BMD following menopause but has been linked with a number of comorbidities, such as heart disease, breast cancer, and stroke. Exercise has been suggested to be a nonpharmacological method to augment BMD in postmenopausal women. However, there is no widespread agreement that absolute gains in BMD can be achieved by exercise alone in estrogen-deficient women. Some studies report that exercise and HRT can interact to bring about a synergistic increase in BMD, and it has been suggested that the synergistic increases in BMD in response to HRT and exercise is due to decreased bone turnover (62).

Development and Aging

Skeletons of all ages are sensitive to exercise, but responsiveness to exercise changes with age. Throughout growth (adolescence in particular), it is generally accepted that the adaptability of the skeleton is much greater than after maturity. In female squash players, significant differences in BMD between the playing and contralateral arm were greater if training was started before menarche (39). Emerging data (63,64) suggest that the critical period for exercise to be most efficacious during growth is just before puberty, but that remains a wide range within the context of growth. Thus, the exact timing of the bone response to exercise and differentially in the axial and appendicular skeleton and on bone surfaces should be characterized more specifically. Exemplifying that, two DXA studies have intervened with a single program of exercise in girls at different stages of maturity. They showed a significant advantage post training for premenarchal (all maturity groups within premenarche pooled) but not postmenarchal girls (65) and for early pubertal but not prepubertal girls (66). Together, those studies indicate that exercise is most effective in stimulating bone growth if initiated some time before or during early puberty

rather than after puberty. Differences in skeletal adaptability with age likely stem from the differing bone cell activities with age. During skeletal growth osteoblasts covering the periosteal surface act to expand bone size (considered periosteal expansion), whereas osteoclasts cover and act primarily at the endocortical surface, resorbing bone and enlarging the marrow cavity (considered endocortical expansion). Changes in bone shape that arise from osteoblasts and osteoclasts acting independently of each other are termed *modeling*. During puberty, both of these surfaces may be undergoing bone apposition. After peak BMD is reached at skeletal maturity (20 to 30 years of age), skeletal maintenance is dominated by *remodeling*, which typically does not alter skeletal shape. Presumably, it is easier to stimulate existing modeling bone cells to alter bone shape than to recruit a new population of bone cells, as would have to be done in mature bones. During growth, humoral factors necessary for proper skeletal development (e.g., insulin-like growth-factor 1) are abundant. With age, physiologically active concentrations of growth factors decline, potentially blunting exercise-induced osteogenesis.

Aging beyond skeletal maturity is associated with a loss of BMD. Cortical bone thinning is caused by an imbalance between endocortical expansion and periosteal apposition, where expansion is favored. Cortical thinning is less apparent in males than females because the difference between periosteal apposition and endocortical expansion rates is less in males. Cortical bone becomes heavily remodeled, trabeculae become less numerous, and trabeculae thin with age. The increased fracture risk due to compromised bone structure is compounded by diminished muscular coordination, which can lead to an increased risk of falling; hence, age is associated with a dramatic increase in risk of fracture.

Mechanisms of Bone Adaptation

Exercise and many other factors can modulate bone adaptation. The mechanisms regulating adaptation, however, remain elusive. Bone cells may respond directly to mechanical deformation or to other stimuli generated by mechanical load or exercise (e.g., pressure-driven fluid flow; see "Mechanical Transduction"), but either way, strain magnitude, frequency, rate, and gradients can all influence bone adaptation.

Proposed Strain Components

In vivo, there is considerable interaction among strain (change in length or original length) components, and the probability of synergistic effects modulating adaptation is high. For clarity, however, the following discussion assumes that all other parameters are held constant, with the parameter of interest varied.

Magnitude

Bone adaptation is roughly proportional to the magnitude of strain induced during loading. Accordingly, exercises with large ground reaction forces (e.g., gymnastics) have greater potential for osteogenic adaptation (63). Newly formed bone can be positioned effectively to minimize large strain magnitudes (i.e., periosteal surfaces). It has been proposed that strain magnitudes must be within a specified range to maintain healthy bone tissue. If strain magnitudes decline below that range, disuse adaptation ensues (bone loss, osteopenia). If strain magnitudes rise above that range, adaptation to increased loading ensues (bone gain). For a given strain magnitude to stimulate bone growth, a threshold number of daily load cycles must be reached (Fig. 4.6).

Frequency

Generally, bone adaptation is also proportional to frequency of loading stimulation. Daily, bones undergo thousands of small strains ($<10 \mu\varepsilon$) and only a few larger strains ($>1000 \mu\varepsilon$ [67]). Sustained muscular contractions, such as during postural regulation, subject bone to high-frequency (e.g., 30 Hz), low-magnitude vibrations. As the frequency of stimulation increases, the daily number of loading cycles also increases, and so high-frequency stimuli require only low-magnitude strains to surpass the threshold for osteogenesis (Fig. 4.6). Recently, it was shown in animal models that brief exposure (less than 1 hour) to high-frequency vibrations (about 30 Hz) produced an osteogenic response (68).

Rate

Static stimuli (strains held at a constant level; strain rate = 0) are not osteogenic. Dynamic stimuli are necessary for osteo-genesis; that is, strains must change with respect to time (strain rate > 0). Impact exercises are more osteogenic than other exercises. In addition to the larger-magnitude strains present with impact, impact exercises are also characterized by higher strain rates. Larger strain rates cause intracortical bone fluid to flow with greater velocities. Fluid velocity could positively correlate with the adaptive potential of transduction mechanisms, including fluid shear stresses and streaming potentials (see "Transduction Mechanisms").

Gradients

With exercise, bone is primarily deformed by a combination of axial loading and bending. As a result, strains differ spatially throughout bone. Strain gradient is the change in strain magnitude as a function of position on the bone. In the absence of large intramedullary pressures, intracortical strain gradients are proportional to pressure gradients (69). Intracortical fluid flow would be greatest where strain gradients are greatest.

Current hypotheses suggest that fluid flow within bone mediates bone adaptation (see "Transduction Mechanisms"). In avian models, strain gradients are correlated with sites of exercise-induced bone formation, supporting the view that fluid flow may mediate bone adaptation (69,70). Furthermore, strain gradients produce electrokinetic potentials across the bone, which may also influence bone adaptation (71).

Mechanical Transduction

Four steps in *mechanotransduction* must be completed for exercise to stimulate bone adaptation (72): (*a*) In *mechanocoupling* biophysical forces are converted to cellular vernacular. Once mechanical signals are comprehensible to cells, biological responses (e.g., release of autocrine and paracrine mediators) emanate in (*b*) *biochemical coupling*. Because bone cells do not exist in isolation, (*c*) *cell-to-cell signaling* is a prerequisite for coordinated function. Finally, individual cell biological responses are orchestrated into (*d*) an *effector response*, which results in bone homeostasis, bone formation, or bone resorption.

Cell Populations: Signal Pathways

For mechanotransduction to occur, physical stimuli must be perceived by biological entities. In the case of bone, four groups of cells (osteoclasts, osteoblasts, bone-lining cells, and osteocytes) conceivably could be linked by mechanocoupling to physical stimuli. Osteoblasts and osteoclasts are transient, as they are present when actively forming or resorbing bone, respectively. In mechanotransduction, bone formation by osteoblasts and resorption by osteoclasts occurs in response to perception of biophysical stimuli. Thus, it is unlikely that osteoblasts and osteoclasts are the cells responsible for biophysical stimuli perception. Osteoclasts

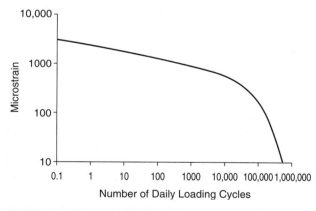

FIGURE 4.6 Strain threshold required for osteogenesis as a function of the number of daily loading cycles. Stimuli above the line are osteogenic. *(Modified from Qin YX, Rubin CT, McLeod KJ. Nonlinear dependence of loading intensity and cycle number in the maintenance of bone mass and morphology. J Orthop Res 1998;16:482–489.)*

eventually undergo apoptosis. Unlike osteoclasts, the fate of an osteoblast is tripartite. Osteoblasts can undergo apoptosis, become entombed in bone matrix (osteocytes), or lie quiescently on the bone surface as bone-lining cells. Osteocytes and bone-lining cells make up 95% of bone cells. In addition to their abundance and long-lived existence, osteocytes and bone-lining cells are ideally situated to perceive mechanical stimuli. Both bone-lining cells and osteocytes subsist throughout the entire cortex. When osteoblasts terminally differentiate into osteocytes, long, slender processes appear and extend through microscopic pores (canaliculi) in the bone matrix. Processes from osteocytes and bone-lining cells maintain connection with one another via gap junctions. Hence, cellular connections are maintained throughout the entire bone cortex. Two extensive communication systems exist between cells (73): *intercellular communication* via gap junctions, which create a syncytium of mechanosensory cells, and *extracellular communications,* which are mediated by fluid filing the spaces between osteocytes, their processes, and the adjacent bone matrix. Thus, osteocytes are ideally situated to perceive exercise-induced physical phenomena. Furthermore, because osteocytes maintain connections with the marrow and periosteal surface, augmented osteoblast recruitment is easily envisaged (Fig. 4.7). This is critical because osteogenic adaptation is marked by an increase in osteoblastic activity or osteoblast differentiation. Since osteocytes neither secrete bone matrix nor differentiate into osteoblasts, they must signal effector cells such as osteoblasts and preosteoblasts.

Transduction Mechanisms

Osteocytes may perceive and transduce biophysical stimuli via a number of mechanisms, none of which are mutually exclusive.

BONE CELL "STRAIN/STRETCH" RECEPTORS AND CYTO-SKELETON
Perturbations in cell shape may regulate cellular processes including growth, differentiation, and mechanotransduction. Regulation of these processes is mediated through the cytoskeleton, in which an interconnected network of microfilaments (tensile bearing), microtubules (compressive bearing), and intermediate filaments can link cell surface proteins to the nucleus (74). Cell surface proteins mediating mechanotransduction may include integrins, mechanosensitive ion channels, or humoral receptors. Signals from stimulation of these proteins could be transferred to the nucleus to influence cellular processes.

In vivo, deformations of bone during maximal exercise rarely exceed 3000 $\mu\epsilon$ (0.3% strain). However, *in vitro* studies typically demonstrate that bone cells, as do many other cell types (75), require strains considerably larger than 0.3% to elicit an adaptive response. Thus, it is questionable whether *in vivo* strains and deformations of bone cells caused by exercise are large enough to mediate bone cell mechano-

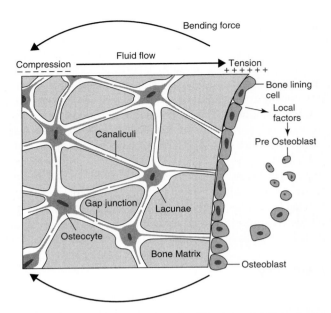

FIGURE 4.7 A section of bone in bending. Bone fluid in regions of compressive stress develops high hydrostatic pressures, and bone fluid in regions of tensile stress develops low hydrostatic pressures. To equalize this pressure differential, bone fluid flows from regions of high to low pressures. Fluid can flow through the lacunocanalicular system, aiding in nutrient transport and waste removal. Furthermore, the fluid flow can exert fluid shear stresses and streaming potentials on osteocytic membranes, which may cause them to initiate an adaptive response. Mechanotransductive signals are transmitted throughout the network of osteocytes via cell processes connected by gap junctions. Those connections terminate on bone-lining cells. Bone lining cells can subsequently release local factors (e.g., IGF-1) that stimulate the differentiation of preosteoblasts into osteoblasts, which can form new bone matrix.

transduction. Furthermore, it is questionable whether *in vitro* observations demonstrating bone cell responsiveness to direct deformation are specific to bone mechanotransduction or simply representative of the innate ability of all cells to respond to deformation.

PIEZOELECTRICITY
Piezoelectricity, a direct result of matrix deformation, refers to the ability of a range of materials to convert mechanical deformations into electric fields. Fukada and Yasuda discovered that bone is piezoelectric and concluded that bone piezoelectricity was due to collagen, as they observed similar piezoelectric effects in tendon (76). Bone collagen molecules consist of three interwoven tropocollagen polypeptide chains. Polypeptide chains aggregate into microfibrils, which aggregate into fibrils with a diameter of 0.2 μm and a length of several micrometers. During fibril formation, bone mineral is incorporated in fibril structure, and most of the bone mineral resides there. That arrangement yields an asymmetrical positive and negative charge, with the arrangement producing a net dipole moment aligned paral-

lel to bone's long axis (77). As the deformation of a piezoelectric material increases, so does the asymmetrical charge arrangement. Thus, net dipoles are exacerbated in a linear fashion with magnitude of deformation. Because electromagnetic fields can affect bone cell dynamics and fracture healing, alterations in the mechanical milieu of bone cells via piezoelectric fields may induce adaptive responses.

FLUID FLOW   Pressure-driven fluid flow, an indirect stimulus resulting from bone matrix deformation, is increasingly recognized as a critical stimulant effecting bone adaptation. As bones are deformed, hydrostatic and dynamic pressure gradients develop. Bone fluid flows from regions of high hydrostatic pressure (compression) to regions of low hydrostatic pressure (tension). Fluid flow generates three distinct signals, all of which may be perceived by bone cells: shear flow, ion flow, and nutrient flow.

Shear Flow   As fluid flows through bone pores, fluid shear stresses are imposed on both the matrix wall and cell membranes. With canaliculi of 6 to 7 nm in diameter, wall shear stresses have a magnitude of 0.8 to 3.0 Pa (77); shear stresses are tangential forces generated by velocity gradients (or shear rate) in fluid flow. Equations describing hemodynamic wall shear stresses in blood vessels are extendable to the flow of bone extracellular fluid within bone:

$$\tau_w = \mu \cdot \left(du/dy\right)_w \qquad \text{[Equation 4.1]}$$

where τ_w is the fluid-imposed wall shear stress, μ is the blood viscosity coefficient, u is the velocity component of the fluid flow parallel to the longitudinal direction of the wall, y is the perpendicular distance from the wall, and $(du/dy)_w$ represents the velocity gradient of blood flow at the wall. Fluid shear stresses stimulate an adaptive response in endothelial cells (78,79). Vascular endothelial cells release vasoactive substances in response to hemodynamic forces (79). Shear stresses as small as 0.2 to 0.5 Pa can initiate endothelial cell responses that control local blood pressure. Sensor cells in the endothelium produce paracrine signaling factors in response to changes in wall shear stresses. Signaling factors travel to the effector cell (vascular smooth muscle cell) and result in vasodilation or vasoconstriction (72). Cerebral pressure is regulated in that manner. As arterial pressure builds, shear stresses increase and vessels are stimulated to vasoconstrict. That helps maintain constant cerebral blood flow over a wide range of arterial pressures (79). Given the variety of cells that sense shear stresses, it is not surprising bone cells are sensitive to fluid shear stresses. Both osteoblasts and osteocytes produce signaling factors such as nitric oxide and prostaglandin E_2 (PGE_2) in response to 1 Pa fluid shear stress (80).

Ion Flow   When ionic solutions flow across charged surfaces, electric potentials emanate. These potentials are governed by the Helmholtz-Smoluchowski equation, which describes the electric potential in a capillary tube filled with an ion containing fluid. Equation 4.2 for streaming potentials in bone has been derived from that relation (81):

$$V_{SGP} = \left\{ \zeta \varepsilon / (4\pi\sigma\eta) \right\} P_{eff} \qquad \text{[Equation 4.2]}$$

where V_{SGP} is the streaming potential, ζ is the zeta potential, ε is the dielectric permitivity of the bulk fluid, η is the viscosity of the bulk fluid, σ is the conductivity of the bulk fluid, and P_{eff} is the effective driving pressure due to mechanical deformation. Fixed negative charges in bone matrix electrostatically attract bone extracellular fluid cations toward the solid–fluid interface. With an effective driving pressure parallel to the pore longitudinal axis, fluid flows parallel with the driving pressure (81). That produces a streaming current that develops a nonzero potential between the two ends of the bone pore. In response to this nonzero potential, an electrical field originates in 180° opposition to the streaming current. Because of the electrical field, ions flow opposite to the direction of the pressure-driven streaming current. Thus, the streaming current ion movement is countered, and a steady state is achieved. In that steady state, the potential difference between the two ends of the pore is referred to as the *streaming potential*. Streaming potentials can alter a bone cell's electrical environment. The electrical milieu of a bone cell may influence its cellular activities, thereby regulating adaptive response.

Nutrient Flow   Convective mixing of the media surrounding bone cells (bone extracellular fluid) displaces essential nutrients and wastes. Presumably, altering metabolite concentrations will affect cell activities and thereby provide a mechanism by which local adaptation can be coordinated. Experimentally, Knothe Tate and colleagues (82) demonstrated that diffusive transport is sufficient to transport small molecules (molecular weight 300–400 Da), such as amino acids, to osteocytes in the mid cortex within minutes. Diffusion alone, however, may not be sufficient to transport larger molecules (molecular weight 1800 Da) evenly throughout the cortex. Convective transport mediated by pressure-driven fluid flow may by necessary to supply osteocytes with proteins to prevent osteocyte starvation and regulate adaptive processes. Convective transport increases with higher loading magnitude and decreases with higher loading frequency.

SUMMARY

Skeletal-articular tissues allow our body to produce movements. Ligaments tether bones together; tendons transmit muscular forces to bones; menisci guide joints in their proper orientation and attenuate joint stresses; and bones support motion by acting as a system of rigid pivots and levers. The complex properties of skeletal articular tissues emerge from an intricate interaction of water, organic, and mineral (bone) phases. These properties, in conjunction with the organization of these tissues into functional units, enable them to serve unique biological, physical, and anthropological roles. Biologically, bone is a center for hematopoiesis and serves as the largest calcium reservoir in the body—a reservoir that is sensitively adjusted to metabolic demands. Physically, skeletal tissues coordinate motion, and bones also provide protection for vital organs. The biological and physical roles of bone can be at odds, but bone's role in calcium metabolism will supersede its mechanical role. The mineral content of bone that contributes substantially to its physical role also heightens the preservation of bone in the fossil record, thus providing anthropologists insight into processes of evolution.

Although skeletal articular tissues can appear static on gross morphological scales, they are highly dynamic and adapt their metabolism in response to the prevailing mechanical environment. Bone is by far the most dynamic and most studied of the skeletal articular tissues. Bone is consistently maintained by a highly dynamic group of cells. Osteoclasts degrade and osteoblasts deposit bone matrix. Occasionally osteoblasts are buried in their matrix, where they survive as osteocytes, likely key links in the mechanosensory chain. Bone cell activities can be modulated by exercise. Mechanical loading through dynamic resistance exercise can significantly influence bone morphology. Chronic exercise generally will lead to bone accretion. Disuse or lack of mechanical loading also has a profound and negative effect on bone morphology, leading to decrements in bone density, alterations in bone shape, and reduced mechanical integrity. Different exercise modalities can influence bone differently, the net result of the exercise stimulus is a complex blend of cellular and systemic interactions with local mechanical loading. Although the effects of physical activity on ligament, tendon, and meniscus are not as well documented as the effects on bone, the principle that physical activity and exercise have potent effects on the skeletal system is supported in all skeletal-articular tissues.

The precise nature of the stimuli underlying adaptation to exercise remains elusive, but experimental data reveal that magnitude, frequency, rate, and gradients of strain can all influence bone adaptation. Osteocytes likely perceive these stimuli via direct and indirect routes, with the prime candidates for mechanotransduction being bone fluid flow and shear stress effects on cytoskeletal conformation, piezoelectric fields, and streaming potentials. Understanding how skeletal tissues perceive and respond to physical stimuli may lead to the development of physical loading or exercise regimens that are effective alternatives to pharmacological therapies to combat low bone mass.

A MILESTONE OF DISCOVERY

Low estrogen levels, as found with postmenopause and amenorrhea, are linked to low bone mineral density (BMD). Physical activity can inhibit or potentially reverse bone loss in postmenopausal women, but as late as 1984, the interrelation between exercise and amenorrhea remained clouded. Amenorrhea (low estrogen level and an abnormally low number of menstrual cycles) has a greater prevalence in athletes, particularly at the elite level, than in the general population. The training regimens for endurance amenorrheic athletes far exceed the intensity of those effective for an osteogenic response in postmenopausal women. Prior to this pioneering study by Drinkwater and her colleagues, it was generally accepted that the intense physical activity of endurance amenorrheic athletes would exert a protective effect against bone loss. Their findings dismissed that prevailing view.

In their study, amenorrhea was defined as having had no more than one menstrual flow in the past 12 months. The researchers enrolled 14 amenorrheic athletes and from a large cohort selected 14 matched eumenorrheic (normal menstrual cycle) athletes. In order of priority, matches were based on sport, age, weight, height, and the frequency and duration of daily exercise. Women with a history of eating disorders were eliminated from the study. The experimental design maximized the potential for amenorrhea to be secondary to the athlete's physical exercise (athletic amenorrhea). Venous blood samples were assayed for estradiol, progesterone, testosterone, and prolactin. Distal radius and lumbar spine BMD was determined by photon absorptiometry. Dietary journals and questionnaires chronicled dietary information, menstrual history, and athletic activities.

The physical characteristics, training regimens, and diets were not significantly different between amenorrheic and eumenorrheic women—with one exception: amenorrheic women ran significantly greater distances than eumenorrheic women (table). Of greatest importance, however, was that the average BMD in the lumbar vertebrae of amenorrheic athletes was nearly 14% lower than that of matched eumenorrheic athletes (table), equivalent to that of women 51.2 years of age. As BMD is related to bone strength, decrements in bone density and mass may have substantial implications for fracture risk, especially in elite athletes. Furthermore, the bone losses in amenorrheic athletes may not be fully recoverable even upon resumption of normal menses.

This significant study revealed the first quantitative link between "athletic amenorrhea" and low bone density. That linkage was central to characterizing the *female athlete triad*, which comprises disordered eating behavior, amenorrhea, and low bone density. With the discovery of those three interrelated factors, scientists, physicians, coaches, and athletes began to realize the very significant clinical and performance consequences of the female athlete triad.

A MILESTONE OF DISCOVERY

Characteristics of Amenorrheic and Eumenorrheic Athletes

Traits of Athletes	Amenorrheic	Eumenorrheic	*P* Value
Age (yr)	24.9 ± 1.3	25.5 ± 1.5	NS
Length of participation in sport (yr)	7.0 ± 1.6	6.6 ± 1.1	NS
Miles run per week	41.8 ± 5.2	24.9 ± 3.0	<0.01
Vertebral BMD (g · cm^{-2})	1.12 ± 0.04	1.30 ± 0.03	<0.01
Mean estradiol (pg · mL^{-1})	38.58 ± 7.03	106.99 ± 9.80	<0.01
Peak estradiol (pg · mL^{-1})	67.75 ± 13.77	205.39 ± 20.6	<0.01

Drinkwater BL, Nilson K, Chesnut CH 3d, et al. Bone mineral content of amenorrheic and eumenorrheic athletes. N Engl J Med 1984;311:277–281.

ACKNOWLEDGMENTS

The development of this chapter has been supported in part by the Canadian Institutes for Health Research, the Natural Sciences and Engineering Research Council of Canada, the Alberta Heritage Foundation for Medical Research, Alberta Provincial CIHR Training Program in Bone and Joint Health, and the Wood Professorship in Joint Injury Research.

REFERENCES

1. Kastelic J, Galeski A, Baer E. The multicomposite structure of tendon. Connect Tissue Res 1978;6:11–23.
2. Sweigart MA, Athanasiou KA. Toward tissue engineering of the knee meniscus. Tissue Eng 2001;7:111–129.
3. Jee WSS. Integrated bone tissue physiology: anatomy and physiology. In Cowin SC, ed. Bone Mechanics Handbook. Boca Raton: CRC, 2001;1–53.
4. Butler DL, Grood ES, Noyes FR, et al. Biomechanics of ligaments and tendons. Exerc Sport Sci Rev 1978;6:125–181.
5. Frank CB. Ligament injuries. In Zachazewski JE, Magee DJ, Quillen WS, eds. Athletic Injuries and Rehabilitation. Philadelphia: Saunders, 1996;9–26.
6. Tipton CM, Matthes RD, Sandage DS. In situ measurement of junction strength and ligament elongation in rats. J Appl Physiol 1974;37:758–761.
7. Akeson WH. An experimental study of joint stiffness. Am J Orthop 1961;43-A:1022–1034.
8. Akeson WH, Amiel D, LaViolette D. The connective-tissue response to immobility: a study of the chondroitin-4 and 6-sulfate and dermatan sulfate changes in periarticular connective tissue of control and immobilized knees of dogs. Clin Orthop 1967;51:183–197.
9. Amiel D, Woo SL, Harwood FL, et al. The effect of immobilization on collagen turnover in connective tissue: a biochemical-biomechanical correlation. Acta Orthop Scand 1982;53:325–332.
10. Woo SL, Matthews JV, Akeson WH, et al. Connective tissue response to immobility. Correlative study of biomechanical and biochemical measurements of normal and immobilized rabbit knees. Arthritis Rheum 1975;18:257–264.
11. Klein L, Dawson MH, Heiple KG. Turnover of collagen in the adult rat after denervation. J Bone Joint Surg Am 1977;59:1065–1067.
12. Loitz BJ, Zernicke RF, Vailas AC, et al. Effects of short-term immobilization versus continuous passive motion on the biomechanical and biochemical properties of the rabbit tendon. Clin Orthop 1989;224:265–271.
13. Matsumoto F, Trudel G, Uhthoff HK, et al. Mechanical effects of immobilization on the Achilles' tendon. Arch Phys Med Rehabil 2003;84:662–667.
14. Flint M. Interrelationships of mucopolysaccharides and collagen in connective tissue remodelling. J Embryol Exp Morph 1982;27:481–495.
15. Cabaud HE, Chatty A, Gildengorin V, et al. Exercise effects on the strength of the rat anterior cruciate ligament. Am J Sports Med 1980;8:79–86.
16. Tipton CM, James SL, Mergner W, et al. Influence of exercise on strength of medial collateral knee ligaments of dogs. Am J Physiol 1970;218:894–902.
17. Binkley JM, Peat M. The effects of immobilization on the ultrastructure and mechanical properties of the medial collateral ligament of rats. Clin Orthop Relat Res 1986;203:301–308.
18. Zamora AJ, Marini JF. Tendon and myo-tendinous junction in an overloaded skeletal muscle of the rat. Anat Embryol (Berl) 1988;179:89–96.
19. Curwin SL, Vailas AC, Wood J. Immature tendon adaptation to strenuous exercise. J Appl Physiol 1988;65:2297–2301.

20. Michna H. Morphometric analysis of loading-induced changes in collagen-fibril populations in young tendons. Cell Tissue Res 1984;236:465–470.

21. Woo SL, Ritter MA, Amiel D, et al. The biomechanical and biochemical properties of swine tendons: long term effects of exercise on the digital extensors. Connect Tissue Res 1980;7:177–183.

22. Buchanan CI, Marsh RL. Effects of long-term exercise on the biomechanical properties of the Achilles tendon of guinea fowl. J Appl Physiol 2001;90:164–171.

23. Rosager S, Aagaard P, Dyhre-Poulsen P, et al. Load-displacement properties of the human triceps surae aponeurosis and tendon in runners and non-runners. Scand J Med Sci Sports 2002;12:90–98.

24. Hansen P, Aagaard P, Kjaer M, et al. The effect of habitual running on human Achilles tendon load-deformation properties and cross-sectional area. J Appl Physiol 2003;95:2375–2380.

25. Cox JS, Nye CE, Schaefer WW, et al. The degenerative effects of partial and total resection of the medial meniscus in dogs' knees. Clin Orthop 1975;109:178–183.

26. Klein L, Heiple KG, Torzilli PA, et al. Prevention of ligament and meniscus atrophy by active joint motion in a non-weight-bearing model. J Orthop Res 1989;7:80–85.

27. Djurasovic M, Aldridge JW, Grumbles R, et al. Knee joint immobilization decreases aggrecan gene expression in the meniscus. Am J Sports Med 1998;26:460–466.

28. Amiel D, Abel MF, Akeson WH. Nutrient delivery in the di-arthrial joint: an analysis of synovial fluid transport in the rabbit knee. Trans Ors 1985;10:196.

29. Ochi M, Kanda T, Sumen Y, et al. Changes in the permeability and histologic findings of rabbit menisci after immobilization. Clin Orthop 1997;334:305–315.

30. Bray RC, Smith JA, Eng MK, et al. Vascular response of the meniscus to injury: effects of immobilization. J Orthop Res 2001;19:384–390.

31. Pedrini-Mille A, Pedrini VA, Maynard JA, et al. Response of immature chicken meniscus to strenuous exercise: biochemical studies of proteoglycan and collagen. J Orthop Res 1988;6:196–204.

32. Fink C, Fermor B, Weinberg JB, et al. The effect of dynamic mechanical compression on nitric oxide production in the meniscus. Osteoarthritis Cartilage 2001;9:481–487.

33. Vailas AC, Zernicke RF, Matsuda J, et al. Adaptation of rat knee meniscus to prolonged exercise. J Appl Physiol 1986;60:1031–1034.

34. Mow VC, Holmes MH, Lai WM. Fluid transport and mechanical properties of articular cartilage: a review. J Biomech 1984;17:377–394.

35. Egner E. Knee joint meniscal degeneration as it relates to tissue fiber structure and mechanical resistance. Pathol Res Pract 1982;173:310–324.

36. Osborn MA. Strategy for research in space biology and medicine in the new century. Washington: National Academy, 1998.

37. Vico L, Collet P, Guignandon A, et al. Effects of long-term microgravity exposure on cancellous and cortical weight-bearing bones of cosmonauts. Lancet 2000;355:1607–1611.

38. Woo SL, Kuei SC, Amiel D, et al. The effect of prolonged physical training on the properties of long bone: a study of Wolff's Law. J Bone Joint Surg Am 1981;63:780–787.

39. Haapasalo H, Kannus P, Sievanen H, et al. Long-term unilateral loading and bone mineral density and content in female squash players. Calcif Tissue Int 1994;54:249–255.

40. Genant HK. Current state of bone densitometry for osteoporosis. Radiographics 1998;18:913–918.

41. Robling AG, Hinant FM, Burr DB, et al. Improved bone structure and strength after long-term mechanical loading is greatest if loading is separated into short bouts. J Bone Miner Res 2002;17:1545–1554.

42. Drinkwater BL. 1994 CH McCloy research lecture: Does physical activity play a role in preventing osteoporosis? Res Q Exerc Sport 1994;65:197–206.

43. Beck BR, Snow CM. Bone health across the lifespan—exercising our options. Exerc Sport Sci Rev 2003;31:117–122.

44. Umemura Y, Ishiko T, Yamauchi T, et al. Five jumps per day increase bone mass and breaking force in rats. J Bone Miner Res 1997;12:1480–1485.

45. Turner CH, Robling AG. Designing exercise regimens to increase bone strength. Exerc Sport Sci Rev 2003;31:45–50.

46. Vogt MT, Cauley JA, Kuller LH, et al. Bone mineral density and blood flow to the lower extremities: the study of osteoporotic fractures. J Bone Miner Res 1997;12:283–289.

47. Ray NF, Chan JK, Thamer M, et al. Medical expenditures for the treatment of osteoporotic fractures in the United States in 1995: report from the National Osteoporosis Foundation. J Bone Miner Res 1997;12:24–35.

48. Greaney RB, Gerber FH, Laughlin RL, et al. Distribution and natural history of stress fractures in US Marine recruits. Radiology 1983;146:339–346.

49. Loucks AB. Energy availability, not body fatness, regulates reproductive function in women. Exerc Sport Sci Rev 2003;31:144–148.

50. Khan KM, Liu-Ambrose T, Sran MM, et al. New criteria for female athlete triad syndrome? As osteoporosis is rare, should osteopenia be among the criteria for defining the female athlete triad syndrome? B J Sports Med 2002;36:10–13.

51. Bailey DA, Martin AD, McKay HA, et al. Calcium accretion in girls and boys during puberty: a longitudinal analysis. J Bone Miner Res 2000;15:2245–2250.

52. Martin AD, Bailey DA, McKay HA, Whiting S. Bone mineral and calcium accretion during puberty. Am J Clin Nutr 1997;66:611–615.

53. Bailey DA, HA McKay, Mirwald RL, et al. A six-year longitudinal study of the relationship of physical activity to bone mineral accrual in growing children: the university of Saskatchewan bone mineral accrual study. J Bone Miner Res 1999;14:1672–1679.

54. Gustavsson A, Nordstrom P, Lorentzon R, et al. Osteocalcin gene polymorphism is related to bone density in healthy adolescent females. Osteoporos Int 2000;11:847–851.

55. Morrison NA, Qi JC, Tokita A, et al. Prediction of bone density from vitamin D receptor alleles. Nature 1994;367:284–287.

56. Dhamrait SS, James L, Brull DJ, et al. Cortical bone resorption during exercise is interleukin-6 genotype-dependent. Eur J Appl Physiol 2003;89:21–25.

57. Nakamura O, Ishii T, Ando Y, et al. Potential role of vitamin D receptor gene polymorphism in determining bone phenotype in young male athletes. J Appl Physiol 2002;93:1973–1979.

58. Specker BL. Evidence for an interaction between calcium intake and physical activity on changes in bone mineral density. J Bone Miner Res 11:1539–1544, 1996.

59. Zernicke RF, Salem GJ, Barnard RJ, et al. Adaptations of immature trabecular bone to exercise and augmented dietary protein. Med Sci Sports Exerc 1995;27:1486–1493.

60. Atteh JO, Leeson S. Effects of dietary saturated or unsaturated fatty acids and calcium levels on performance and mineral metabolism of broiler chicks. Poult Sci 1984;63:2252–2260.

61. Lee K, Jessop H, Suswillo R, et al. Endocrinology: bone adaptation requires oestrogen receptor-alpha. Nature 2003;424:389.

62. Kohrt WM, Snead DB, Slatopolsky E, et al. Additive effects of weight-bearing exercise and estrogen on bone mineral density in older women. J Bone Miner Res 1995;10:1303–1311.

63. Khan K, McKay HA, Haapasalo H, et al. Does childhood and adolescence provide a unique opportunity for exercise to strengthen the skeleton? J Sci Med Sports 2000;3: 150–164.

64. Petit MA, McKay HA, MacKelvie KJ, et al. A randomized school-based jumping intervention confers site and maturity-specific benefits on bone structural properties in girls: a hip structural analysis study. J Bone Miner Res 2002;17: 363–372.

65. Heinonen A, Sievanen H, Kannus P, et al. High-impact exercise and bones of growing girls: a 9–month controlled trial. Osteoporos Int 2000;11:1010–1017.

66. Mackelvie KJ, McKay HA, Khan KM, et al. A school-based exercise intervention augments bone mineral accrual in early pubertal girls. J Pediatr 2001;139:501–508.

67. Fritton SP, McLeod KJ, Rubin CT. Quantifying the strain history of bone: spatial uniformity and self-similarity of low-magnitude strains. J Biomech 2000;33:317–325.

68. Rubin C, Turner AS, Mallinckrodt C, et al. Mechanical strain, induced noninvasively in the high-frequency domain, is anabolic to cancellous bone, but not cortical bone. Bone 2002;30:445–452.

69. Gross TS, Edwards JL, McLeod KJ, et al. Strain gradients correlate with sites of periosteal bone formation. J Bone Miner Res 1997;12:982–988.

70. Judex S, Gross TS, Zernicke RF. Strain gradients correlate with sites of exercise-induced bone-forming surfaces in the adult skeleton. J Bone Miner Res 1997;12:1737–1745.

71. Otter MW, Palmieri VR, Wu DD, et al. A comparative analysis of streaming potentials in vivo and in vitro. J Orthop Res 1992;10:710–719.

72. Duncan RL, Turner CH. Mechanotransduction and the functional response of bone to mechanical strain. Calcif Tissue Int 1995;57:344–358.

73. Burger EH, Klein-Nulend J, van der Plas A, et al. Function of osteocytes in bone: their role in mechanotransduction. J Nutr 1995;125:2020S–2023S.

74. Wang N, Naruse K, Stamenovic D, et al. Mechanical behavior in living cells consistent with the tensegrity model. Proc Natl Acad Sci USA 2001;98:7765–7770.

75. Smalt R, Mitchell FT, Howard RL, et al. Mechanotransduction in bone cells: induction of nitric oxide and prostaglandin synthesis by fluid shear stress, but not by mechanical strain. Adv Exp Med Biol 1997;433:311–314.

76. Martin RB, Burr DB. Structure, function, and adaptation of compact bone. New York: Raven, 1989.

77. Weinbaum S, Cowin SC, Zeng Y. A model for the excitation of osteocytes by mechanical loading-induced bone fluid shear stresses. J Biomech 1994;27:339–360.

78. Barakat AI, Davies PF. Mechanisms of shear stress transmission and transduction in endothelial cells. Chest 1998;114:58S–63S.

79. Lansman JB. Endothelial mechanosensors. Going with the flow. Nature 1988;331:481–482.

80. McAllister TN, Du T, Frangos JA. Fluid shear stress stimulates prostaglandin and nitric oxide release in bone marrow-derived preosteoclast-like cells. Biochem Biophys Res Commun 2000;270:643–648.

81. Kowalchuk RM, Pollack SR. Stress-generated potentials in bone: effects of bone fluid composition and kinetics. J Orthop Res 1993;11:874–883.

82. Knothe Tate ML, Niederer P, Knothe U. In vivo tracer transport through the lacunocanalicular system of rat bone in an environment devoid of mechanical loading. Bone 1998;22:107–117.

CHAPTER 5

The Muscular System: Structural and Functional Plasticity

VINCENT J. CAIOZZO AND BRYAN ROURKE

Introduction

The field of physiology has a number of principles. Some of these key principles are:

1. Homeostasis
2. The linkage between gene expression and physiology
3. Structure–function relationships

This last principle forms the foundation of this chapter. The concept of structure–function relationships extends across the organismal-to-molecular spectrum. At the organismal level, one can think about a number of examples. For instance, the structural relationship between the glenoid fossa and the head of the humerus gives the shoulder 6° of motion, a motion that is uncommon among other joints. At the molecular level, one can think about the structure of myosin heavy chains and how this translates into certain functional properties, such as the force–velocity relationship.

Exercise physiology is a subdiscipline or extension of physiology, and so its principles are essentially the same except that they are examined typically when physical activity has been altered. In this context, during the past 30 to 35 years a great deal of interest has been given to understanding the effects of both activity and inactivity on the structural and functional properties of skeletal muscle.

Of any cell or tissue type, skeletal muscle certainly exhibits some of the clearest structure–function relationships.

Given this perspective, one of the key objectives of this chapter is to provide a backdrop for some of the more detailed discussions in succeeding chapters. This chapter is organized into three sections. The first provides an overview of some of the key structural properties of skeletal muscle (macroscopic to molecular anatomy). The second part of the chapter addresses the linkage between structure–function and skeletal muscle plasticity as influenced by altered physical activity. The final section examines issues of muscle plasticity from a comparative perspective and introduces the concept of symmorphosis, a concept related to the optimality of design.

The Macroscopic and Molecular Anatomy of Skeletal Muscle

Overview

This section provides a brief overview of some of the key anatomical and structural features of skeletal muscle as shown in Figures 5.1–5.3. For the purposes of this chapter, however, the main story is illustrated in Figure 5.2, since three fundamental processes are ultimately responsible for determining the amount of work and power that can be produced across a broad spectrum of activities.

These are the three fundamental processes:

1. Ca^{++} cycling
2. Crossbridge cycling
3. Cellular respiration

From a temporal perspective, only the first of these two processes is important during activities that are relatively short in duration. However, as the duration of physical activity begins to extend beyond several minutes, cellular respiration becomes progressively more important in meeting the energy demands of both crossbridge cycling and Ca^{++} cycling. Therefore, extensive structural information about each of these three processes is included in Figure 5.2.

The Macroscopic Anatomy of Skeletal Muscle

As with most tissues, the structural anatomy of skeletal muscle is quite complex. However, the degree of structural organization in skeletal muscle is unsurpassed by any other tissue. This complexity is illustrated in Figures 5.1 and 5.2, which provide a macroscopic to microscopic perspective. Skeletal muscles are composed of individual cells also known as muscle fibers. The numbers and sizes of these fibers can differ significantly from one muscle to another. Skeletal muscles that are typically responsible for generating large forces contain thousands of individual muscle fibers, whereas muscles that are involved in fine motor control typically have far fewer fibers. Muscle fibers are packaged into small bundles (about 10–40 fibers per bundle) known as fascicles, and these fascicles are encased in a connective tissue sheath known as the endomysium.

From an architectural perspective, muscles are often classified on the basis of the orientation of the muscle fibers' longitudinal axes relative to that of the entire muscle. For instance, longitudinal muscles are composed of muscle fibers whose longitudinal axis runs parallel to that of the whole muscle. Good examples of this type of architecture are the rectus abdominis and the sartorius muscles. In fusiform muscles, the fibers run parallel to the longitudinal axis throughout most of the muscle but taper at its ends. The soleus and brachioradialis muscles are typical of this architecture. Muscles can also exhibit a so-called pennate (unipennate, bipennate) architecture wherein the longitudinal axis of the individual muscle fibers runs diagonal to that of the whole muscle. A good example of a bipennate muscle is the gastrocnemius. The muscle fibers of angular or fan-shaped muscles radiate from a narrow attachment at one end and fan out, resulting in a broad attachment at the other end, as is seen in the pectoralis major.

As noted earlier, the primary theme of this chapter is related to structure–function relationships, and in this context, muscle architecture can be an important determinant of muscle function. For instance, muscles with fusiform architecture have muscle fibers that are typically longer than those found in bipennate muscles. The functional consequence of such an architectural design is that the fusiform muscle can shorten and lengthen to a greater degree than the bipennate muscle, and assuming similar crossbridge cycling rates, can generate much higher shortening velocities. Conversely, the structural advantage of the bipennate design is that it optimizes the physiological cross-sectional area of the muscle, meaning that there are a greater number of muscle fibers and sarcomeres in parallel. Therefore, the bipennate design is better for the production of force than high shortening velocities.

Molecular Anatomy of the Myofibril

Figures 5.1 and 5.2 show that the structure of skeletal muscle at the molecular level is quite complex. Each muscle fiber is made up of thousands of so-called myofibrils that are arranged parallel to one another. Each myofibril has a cross-sectional area of approximately 1 to 2 μm^2; therefore, a muscle fiber with a cross-sectional area of about 1000 μm^2 would contain about 1000 myofibrils (for simplicity the relative volumes of the sarcoplasmic reticulum (SR) and mitochondria are not included in this estimate).

Typically, the cross-sectional area of a muscle fiber can range from about 1000 to 7000 μm^2. Each myofibril, which runs the entire length of a muscle fiber, consists of a repeating series of striations that are due to the arrangement of so-called sarcomeres in series. Sarcomeres are often referred to as the contractile units of skeletal muscle, and each sarcomere is approximately 2.5 μm in length. In a muscle fiber that is 100 mm long (as in the human brachioradialis muscle), each myofibril consists of about 40,000 sarcomeres in series. If it assumed that each myofibril has a cross-sectional area of 1 μm^2 and that the muscle fiber has a cross-sectional area of 5000 μm^2, then the muscle fiber contains about 200 million sarcomeres.

From a very basic perspective, sarcomeres consist of Z-lines, thin filaments, and thick filaments. The interdigitation of thick and thin filaments along with the presence of Z-lines is responsible for the striation pattern of skeletal muscle. As shown in Figure 5.1, the Z-lines are dense, thin structures found in the middle of the so-called I-band. In reality, each Z-line represents an anchor point to which thin filaments are attached. The I-band represents a region where there is no overlap of the thin filaments by thick filaments, which yields a relatively light band. The A-band is composed of the thick filament and is strongly birefringent, producing a dark band upon microscopic inspection. The length of the A-band is equivalent to the length of the thick filament. Normally there is a partial overlap between the thick and thin filaments, and as a result there is a lighter region in the middle of the A-band known as the H-zone.

Changes in sarcomere length and hence muscle fiber length are due to the sliding of the thick and thin filaments relative to one another. In its most simplistic sense, this model states that contraction takes place not because of changes in the individual lengths of thick and thin filaments but rather by the sliding of thin filaments past thick filaments.

Key Features

Muscle

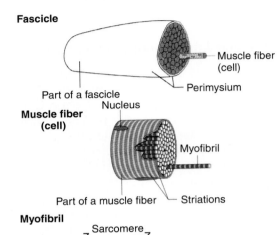

Epimysium Fascicle Muscle Tendon

Muscles are really a tissue, composed of many different cell types. Some of these include muscle fibers (cells), vascular cells, fibroblasts, and satellite cells.

Fascicle

Muscle fiber (cell)

Perimysium

Part of a fascicle

Skeletal muscle fibers (cells) are organized into bundles known as fascicles. Each bundle contains tens of fibers.

Muscle fiber (cell)

Nucleus

Myofibril

Part of a muscle fiber — Striations

Each skeletal muscle fiber is an individual cell, and they are primarily composed of a large number of cylinders known as myofibrils. Human muscle fibers have cross-sectional areas that range from ~3000–6000 μm^2. The majority of the cell volume is occupied by myofibrils, with the SR and mitochondrial volumes accounting for ~10% of the cell volume.

Myofibril

Z Sarcomere Z

Myofibril

H zone A band I band

Each myofibril runs the entire length of the fiber, and they are made up of repeating contractile units known as sarcomeres that are in series with one another. Each myofibril has a cross-sectional area of ~1–2 μm^2. Therefore, there are ~5000 myofibrils in a muscle with a cross-sectional area of 5000 μm^2. Myofibrils make-up ~85 – 90% of the total cell volume.

Sarcomere

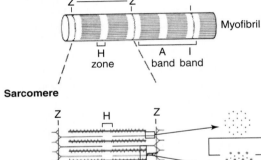

Z H Z

Sarcomeres are building blocks used to assemble myofibrils. Sarcomeres are sometimes referred to as contractile units of skeletal muscle. Number of sarcomeres in parallel determines the maximal force, whereas the number in series determines length excursion and shortening velocity. Typical sarcomere is 2.5 μm long, and there are ~40,000 in series in a muscle fiber 100 mm in length.

Filaments

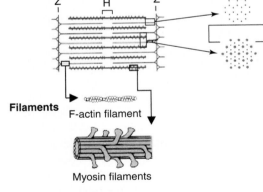

F-actin filament

Myosin filaments

Myosin molecule

The major filaments associated with the sarcomere are the thick and thin filaments. Each thin filament is composed of an actin filament and its associated regulatory contractile proteins (Tm, TnT, TnI, and TnC). Each thick filament is primarily composed of ~300 native myosin molecules.

FIGURE 5.1 Macroscopic-to-microscopic anatomy of skeletal muscle

This model of contraction is known as the sliding-filament hypothesis (1).

Molecular Anatomy of the Sarcomere

The so-called ultrastructure of the sarcomere is quite complex (Figs. 5.1 and 5.2), and the numbers of thick and thin filaments found within a given sarcomere illustrates this point. Each Z-line has a cross-sectional area of about 1 to 2 μm^2, and attached to each Z-line are about 3000 to 6000 individual thin filaments (thin filament density of about 3000/μm^2). In turn, there are approximately about 1000 to 2000 thick filaments (thick filament density of about 1000/μm^2) associated with the larger number of thin fila-

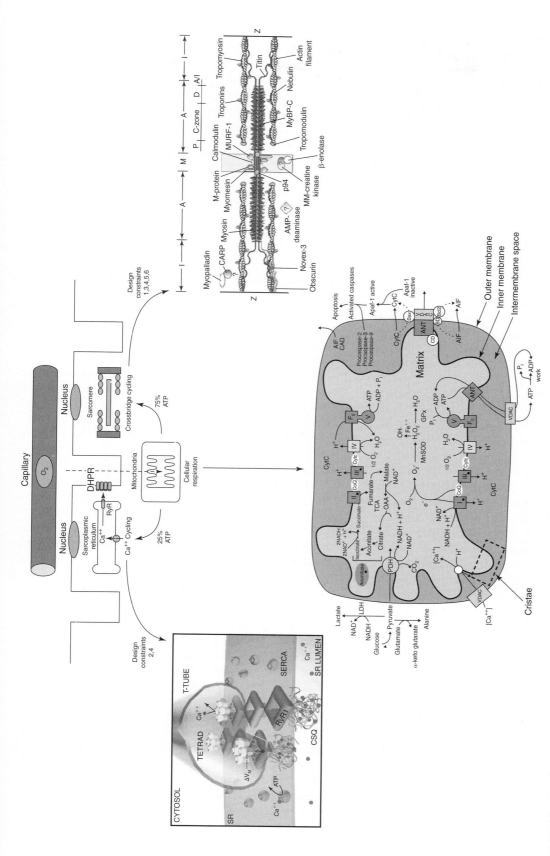

FIGURE 5.2 The three essential components that determine muscle function: Ca²⁺ cycling, crossbridge cycling, and cellular respiration (see inserts). Six key design constraints affect the ability of skeletal muscle to produce mechanical work and power. Constraints 1, 3, 4, 5, and 6 are properties of the sarcomere. In contrast, constraints 2 and 4 are largely determined by the SR. Abbreviations = RyR, ryanodine receptor; SERCA, sarcoplasmic reticulum calcium ATPase; CSQ, calsequestrin; SR, sarcoplasmic reticulum; CARP, cardiac Adriamycin responsive protein; MURF-1, muscle specific RING finger-1; MyBP-C, myosin binding protein-C; p94, calcium-activated protease-3 or calpain-3; cyt-c, cytochrome-c; NAD, nicotinamide adenine dinucleotide; LDH, lactate dehydrogenase; PDH, pyruvate dehydrogenase; OAA, oxaloacetate; TCA, tricarboxylic acid (TCA) cycle; VDAC, voltage-dependent anion channel; ANT, adenine nucleotide translocator; CD, cyclophilin D; MnSOD, manganese superoxide dismutase. (*Insert showing part of the sarcoplasmic reticulum is reprinted with permission from Fill M, Copello JA. Ryanodine receptor calcium release channels. Physiol Rev 2002;82:893–922. Insert of the mitochondria is reprinted with permission from Wallace DC. Mitochondrial diseases in man and mouse. Science 1999;283:1482–1488. Insert of the sarcomere is modified from Clark KA, McElhinny AS, Beckerle MC, et al. Striated muscle cytoarchitecture: an intricate web of form and function. Annu Rev Cell Dev Biol 2002;18:637–706.*)

ments. This yields a thin-to-thick filament ratio of 3:1. When one begins to consider the factors that are responsible for keeping sarcomeres in register, maintaining the organization of the sarcomere during force production and load bearing, and regulating the necessary pool of proteins, it is clear that the sarcomere is incredibly complex.

For many years, the numbers of proteins thought to be associated with the sarcomere were relatively few. However, over the course of the past 10 years, the list of proteins associated with the sarcomere has grown significantly (Fig. 5.2, Table 5.1). For a better appreciation of this, the reader is referred to the excellent article by Clark et al. (2). From a fundamental perspective, the proteins associated with the sarcomere can be categorized into three groups: (a) contractile proteins, (b) regulatory contractile proteins, and (c) structural and costameric proteins.

Actin and myosin are often referred to as contractile proteins, given their central role in the contractile process. Individual monomers of actin (globular form of actin; G-actin) bind to one another to form actin filaments (F-actin). The thick filament is composed primarily of myosin heavy chain molecules packed in an antiparallel arrangement. A more detailed description of myosin is provided later, in the section "Anatomy of Molecular Motor."

Regulatory contractile proteins are defined as those that turn the contractile apparatus on and off and those that can modulate the activity of the myosin heavy chain. In skeletal muscle, the regulatory contractile proteins involved in turning the contractile apparatus on and off are associated exclusively with the actin filament, and these proteins include the regulatory contractile proteins tropomyosin, troponin-T, troponin-I, and troponin-C. Collectively, the thin filament is composed of the actin filament and these regulatory contractile proteins. The myosin light chains (MLCs) are also classified as regulatory contractile proteins, and they are associated with the lever arm of the myosin heavy chain (see "Anatomy of Molecular Motor," later in the chapter). Although there is some debate over the precise role of MLCs in skeletal muscle, several studies have shown that they can modulate the kinetics of crossbridge cycling (3,4).

Structural and costameric proteins play several essential roles. Electron micrographs demonstrate that sarcomeres are organized in a very orderly fashion, such that the Z-lines of adjoining sarcomeres appear to be in register with one another. Intermediate filaments like desmin and vimentin are believed to play key roles in aligning the Z-line of adjacent sarcomeres. Other proteins, such as synemin, are also thought to be involved in the alignment of sarcomeres. Structural proteins also play a key role in developing a mechanical linkage between sarcomeres and the extracellular matrix. These sites of connectivity between the sarcomere–cell membrane–extracellular matrix have been referred to as costameres, and there is a growing list of proteins associated with these complexes (Table 5.1). Some of these proteins include dystrophin and the integrins.

The Anatomy of the Molecular Motor

The term *myosin molecule* is used commonly in conjunction with descriptions of the molecular motor. As has been documented in a number of publications (5–7), the myosin molecule is really in reference to the so-called native molecule, which is a hexameric complex composed of six proteins. The primary nomenclature used to describe each of these six proteins is based on their molecular weights. Two of the six proteins that make up the native myosin molecule are known as myosin heavy chains (MHCs) because they have the heaviest molecular weights (about 200 kDa) of any of the proteins making up the native myosin molecule. Each MHC is associated with one essential MLC, MLC_1 or MLC_3, and one regulatory MLC, MLC_2. Each MHC is made up of (a) a long rod region, (b) subfragment-2 (S2), and (c) a globular head (also known as subfragment-1 (S1). The rod region of the MHC is important from a structural perspective because it determines the packing of MHCs within the thick filament, with each thick filament composed of about 300 individual MHCs. In contrast, the globular head is directly involved in binding to actin and generating force and/or length steps. The globular head consists of three domains known as (a) the catalytic domain, (b) the converter domain, and (c) the lever arm. The catalytic domain contains sites involved with binding actin, binding adenosine triphosphate (ATP), and hydrolyzing ATP. The converter region is thought to be involved with the transduction of energy, while the lever arm transports the load. Mutations within the globular head are believed to play a key role in serious cardiomyopathies such as familial hypertrophic cardiomyopathy. Each MHC has one essential and one regulatory light chain bound to the S1 fragment. Finally, consider that within a single fiber from a human brachioradialis muscle there are about 200 million sarcomeres, that each sarcomere consists of about 1000 thick filaments, and that each thick filament consists of about 300 individual MHCs. The dimensions of the system reflect its complexity: about 10^{13} to 10^{14} individual MHCs molecules per single fiber.

The diversity of the native myosin molecule is further complicated by the presence of isoforms for both the MHC and MLCs. From a mechanical perspective, it has been known for quite some time that muscles could be categorized as slow and fast. During the course of the past 20 years, it has been shown at various levels that the speed-related properties of skeletal muscle are due primarily to the existence of different MHC isoforms and that the kinetics of crossbridge cycling can be secondarily modulated by MLC isoforms (3,4). The various MHC isoforms identified to date are shown in Table 5.1. As shown in this table, the main nomenclature used to classify fiber types is linked to the MHC isoform composition of that fiber. This seems quite appropriate, given that the ultimate design constraint of skeletal muscle is the force–velocity relationship and that the shape of this relationship depends on the kinetics

TABLE 5.1 Overview of Key Proteins Involved With the Sarcomere and Cytoskeletal–Extracellular Matrix Interactions in Skeletal Muscle

Classes and Types of Sarcomeric Proteins	Molecular Wt (kDa)	Isoforms	Location	Function
Contractile Proteins				
Myosin heavy chain	~200	~9	Thick filament	Molecular motor; binds to actin; generates force and length change
Embryonic				
Neonatal				
Slow Type Iβ cardiac				
Slow Type Iα cardiac				
Fast Type IIA				
Fast Type IIX				
Fast Type IIB				
Extraocular/type IIL				
Superfast type IIM				
Actin	~42		Thin filament	Binds myosin and translates force and/or length changes
Regulatory contractile proteins				
Tropomyosin	~37	>3	Thin filament	Regulates interaction between actin and myosin; stabilizes thin filament
Troponin-T	~30	>6	Thin filament	Couples troponin complex to actin?
Troponin-I	~22	2	Thin filament	Influences position of tropomyosin
Troponin-C	~18	2	Thin filament	Binds Ca^{++}; influences position of tropomyosin
Cardiac/slow TnC				
Fast TnC				
Myosin light chain-1	~22	2	Thick filament	Influences V_{max}?
Slow MLC1				
Fast MLC1				
Myosin light chain-2	~20	2	Thick filament	Influences tension-pCa^{++} relationship
Slow MLC2				
Fast MLC2				
Myosin light chain-3	~18	1	Thick filament	Influences V_{max}
Fast MLC3				
Structural proteins associated with thin filament				
CapZ-α, CapZ-β	~36, ~32	2	Z-line	Caps free end of actin, regulates actin filament length; binds to α-actinin
Tropomodulin	~40	2	Thin filament	Caps pointed end of actin filament
Nebulin	~600–900	+2	I-band	Anchors actin to Z-line; molecular ruler of actin filament length?
Associated with thick filament				
Myosin binding protein-C	~140	2	Thick filament	Binds to lever arm and rod region; titin binding site
Myomesin	~185	2	M-line	Binds to myosin and titin; may play role in linking myosin and titin
MurF-1	~40		M-line	May play key role in degradation
Calpain-3; p94		2	M-line	Binds to titin
Titin	~3000–4000	+2	Spans A-I bands	Molecular spring? Sarcomere template?

(continued)

TABLE 5.1   Overview of Key Proteins Involved With the Sarcomere and Cytoskeletal–Extracellular Matrix Interactions in Skeletal Muscle (*Continued*)

Classes and Types of Sarcomeric Proteins	Molecular Wt (kDa)	Isoforms	Location	Function
Associated with Z-line				
α-Actinin	~97	2	Z-line	Major protein of Z-line
LIM	~23	+2	Z-line	Binds α-actinin, zyxin, β-spectrin
FATZ	~32		Z-line	Binds calcineurin to Z-line
Intermediate filaments				
Desmin	~53		Z-line	Longitudinal and lateral alignment of sarcomeres
Skelemin	~200		M-band	M-line integrity
Vimentin	~53		Z-line	Periodicity of Z-lines
Costamere proteins				
Ankyrin	17–440	Many	Costamere	Localization
α-Dystrobrevin	~87	2	Costamere	Membrane stabilization; transmembrane signaling Involved with NOS
α/β-Dystroglycan	~156, 43	2	Costamere	Prevents injury to sarcolemma
Dystrophin	427		Costamere	Stabilizes cytoskeleton and sarcolemma
α-Fodrin	85		Costamere	Attachment of cytoskeleton to ECM; signaling
Integrins	~90 and 150	Many	Costamere	Stabilization of cytoskeleton
α-Sarcoglycan	~240		Costamere	Binds dystrophin and α-dystrobrevin; associated with NOS
α/β-Spectrin	~250	+2	Costamere	Stabilization of sarcomere
Syntrophins	~57–60	3	Costamere	NOS?
Talin	~235	3	Costamere-MT]	Role in stabilizing link between muscle fiber and tendon fibrils?
Vinculin	116	3	Costamere, MT]	Role in stabilizing link between muscle fiber and tendon fibrils?

NOS, nitric oxide synthase; ECM, extracellular matrix.

of crossbridge cycling. In small adult mammals, the primary MHC isoforms found throughout most of the body are known, in order of their ATPase activity, as the slow type I, fast type IIA, fast type IIX, and fast type IIB. It is thought that in humans only the first three MHC isoforms are expressed. The absence of the fastest MHC isoform (type IIB) in adult human skeletal muscle seems to be consistent with some allometric (scaling) considerations that might govern the speed of limb movement. Other adult MHC isoforms have been found in muscles associated with the larynx (EO/type IIL), mastication (superfast type IIM), and movement of the eyes (EO). Two developmental MHC isoforms have been found in mammalian skeletal muscle, and these are referred to as the embryonic (E) and neonatal (NEO) MHC isoforms. Finally, the hearts of both small mammals and humans are known to express two cardiac MHC isoforms, the β- and α-cardiac MHC isoforms. The β-cardiac MHC isoform is also known as the slow type I MHC isoform. Collectively, a total of eight or nine MHC isoforms have been reported in skeletal muscle.

Several nomenclatures have been developed for describing the various MLCs. The most prevalent terminology is based simply on electrophoretic migration of the MLCs, giving rise to the terms MLC_1, MLC_2, and MLC_3. Both MLC_1 and MLC_3 can also be categorized as so-called essential light chains, implying that their presence is essential for myosin ATPase activity. In reality, the term is a misnomer in skeletal muscle because the absence of these MLCs does not inhibit the ability to hydrolyze ATP. From a historical perspective, MLC_2 was initially classified as a regulatory light chain, meaning that its phosphorylation influenced or regulated crossbridge cycling. Clearly, in smooth muscle, the phosphorylation of MLC_2 is critical; however, in skeletal muscle it appears to be relatively unimportant. As with the MHCs, there are MLC isoforms. There are both slow and fast isoforms of MLC_1 ($sMLC_1$; $fMLC_1$) and MLC_2 ($sMLC_2$, $fMLC_2$), whereas only one type (a fast isoform) of MLC_3 ($fMLC_3$) isoform has been identified.

In thinking about the various types of MHC and MLC isoforms and how they might be arranged within a native myosin molecule, it becomes obvious that there are many possible combinations, as Pette and Staron discussed in some detail (6). Also, there are fast and slow isoforms of other sarcomeric contractile proteins, such as tropomyosin, troponin-T, troponin-I, and troponin-C (Table 5.1). Hence, one quickly appreciates the complexity that can arise in the design of sarcomeres on mixing and matching these contractile and regulatory contractile protein isoforms (see section "Muscle Fiber Types and Polymorphism").

The sequence of a crossbridge cycle is shown in Figure 5.3. In the first frame, myosin is detached from actin. Subsequently, the head of the myosin heavy chain is attached to actin and releases Pi, leading to the power stroke (change in position of head between view C and view D). Following completion of the power stroke, adenosine diphos-

phate (ADP) is released, and subsequently ATP binds to the nucleotide-binding site (Figure 5.3E). The hydrolysis of ATP ultimately leads to the globular head of the myosin heavy chain returning to its original position. The magnitude of crossbridge cycling that occurs during a single contraction is enormous; it can approach rates equivalent to 10^{17} to 10^{18} crossbridge cycles per gram of muscle per second, quite an astonishing number.

Molecular Anatomy of the Sarcoplasmic Reticulum

The ability of skeletal muscle to perform repetitive shortening and lengthening contractions involves four fundamental processes:

1. Excitation
2. Coupling
3. Contraction
4. Relaxation

Of these four processes, the second and fourth are governed by the structure–function properties of the SR that are involved in Ca^{++} cycling.

As illustrated in Figure 5.2, the calcium release channels of the SR lie close to the t-tubule, and this region of the SR is often referred to as the terminal cisternae. Collectively, one t-tubule and the terminal cisternae on both sides of the t-tubule are referred to as a triad. The calcium release channels of the SR are also known as ryanodine receptors (RyR) because they selectively bind the plant alkaloid ryanodine.

The conformational state of the RyR in skeletal muscle is regulated by the voltage-gated Ca^{++} channels in the membrane of the t-tubule. These voltage-gated Ca^{++} channels are also known as dihydropyridine receptors (DHPRs) because they selectively bind a class of drugs with this name. The exact mechanism by which the DHPRs regulate the conformational state of the RyRs is unknown, but it is thought that there is some type of physical contact between the two proteins. As illustrated in Figure 5.2, the physical arrangement between the DHPRs and RyRs appears to be quite complex. The DHPRs are arranged in tetrads within the membrane of the t-tubule, and every other RyR is associated with a tetrad in fast skeletal muscle. Depolarization of the t-tubule membrane is thought to produce a conformational change in the DHPR, which then acts via direct physical contact on the RyR. The connection between the DHPR and RyR may be mediated by a cytoplasmic loop of the DHPR. One of the important features of this form of communication between the tetrad and RyR is speed, allowing Ca^{++} to be released almost immediately following depolarization.

Following repolarization of the sarcolemma, the calcium-release channels (RyRs) of the SR close, and Ca^{++} is sequestered via calcium ATPase pumps in the SR, otherwise known as SERCAs. The SERCAs lie primarily along the longitudinal region of the SR. As with many proteins associated

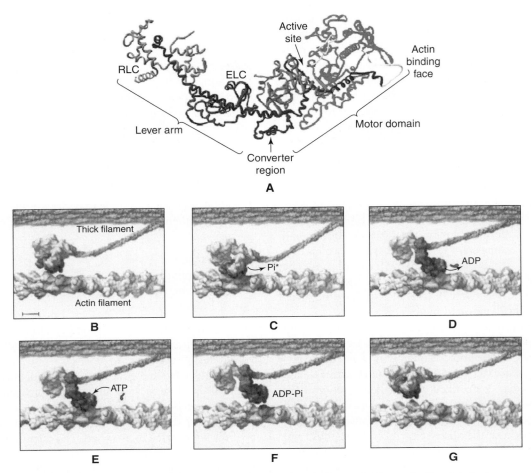

FIGURE 5.3 Ribbon diagram (**A**) and stop-motion movie (**B–G**) of a crossbridge cycle. The globular head of the MHC (**A**) consists of three key regions, the motor domain, converter region, and lever arm. The motor domain has also been referred to as the catalytic domain, given that it is involved in the hydrolysis of ATP. Abbreviations = ELC, essential light chain; RLC, regulatory light chain. *(Modified from Vale RD, Milligan RA. The way things move: looking under the hood of molecular motor proteins. Science 2000;288:88–95.)*

with the sarcomere, there are isoforms of the SERCAs, with SERCA2a found in slow skeletal muscle and SERCA1 found in fast skeletal muscle (see section "Muscle Fiber Types" for discussion of functional differences).

Molecular Anatomy of the Mitochondria

From a hierarchical perspective that simply revolves around the mechanical activity of skeletal muscle, one might think of the mitochondria as slaves to the energetic needs of the contractile apparatus and the SR. In reality, the mitochondria are involved in many other processes, some of which include the production of reactive oxygen species (ROS) and the initiation of apoptosis (programmed cell death). Both of these processes may be important in mediating muscle fiber size. Figure 5.2 illustrates some of the key features involved in these three processes (ATP production, production of ROS, and initiation of apoptosis).

The main morphological features of the mitochondria are:

1. Outer membrane
2. Inner membrane
3. Intermembrane space, between the outer and inner membranes
4. Cristae, the folds of the inner membrane that help to maximize inner membrane surface area
5. Matrix

As the length of physical activity increases beyond a few seconds, so does the demand on the mitochondria to provide ATP to the contractile apparatus and the SR. The production of ATP by the mitochondria involves an extensive set of biochemical and biophysical events that ultimately includes the transfer of energy from electrons to ATP. From a biochemical perspective, the Krebs cycle enzyme system (matrix) plays a key role in providing to the electron transport chain (within the inner membrane) electrons that are in a high-energy state. The electron transport chain consists of four complexes (Fig. 5.2) that are known simply as complexes I to IV, and these participate in a set of biophysical events:

1. Moving electrons from one metal ion to another
2. Reducing the energy levels of electrons, transferring (remember the first law of thermodynamics) that energy into a proton gradient across the inner membrane.

The large electrochemical H^+ gradient then causes H^+ to move from the intermembrane space into the matrix via ATP synthase. The ATP synthase is composed of two major subunits, F_o and F_1. The F_o subunit functions as a proton channel (Fig. 5.2), allowing H^+ to move along the electrochemical gradient and back into the matrix. The energy stored in the proton gradient is then used to drive the synthesis of ATP via the F_1/V_1 subunit of the ATP synthase (Fig. 5.2). The newly synthesized ATP is exported (in exchange for ADP and inorganic phosphate) out of the mitochondria and into the sarcoplasm via the adenine nucleotide transporter (ANT) (Fig. 5.2). Ultimately, this process depends on the presence of oxygen, given that it plays the central role in maintaining electron transport via the oxidation of cytochrome-a_3.

Collectively, these steps are referred to as oxidative phosphorylation, and the two major sources of fuel involved in providing electrons to the electron transport chain are pyruvate (derived from carbohydrate breakdown) and free fatty acids (FFAs). Both pyruvate and FFA are derived from exogenous and endogenous sources. With respect to pyruvate, the major exogenous sources of carbohydrates are the circulating levels of glucose in the blood and the glycogen stored in the liver. Glycogen is also stored in muscle fibers themselves, representing a large endogenous source of carbohydrates. With respect to FFA, most is found in the adipose fat stores of the body (i.e., there is a large exogenous source of FFAs). However, evidence is accumulating that an important source of FFA is triglyceride stores maintained within the muscle fibers themselves.

The mitochondria in skeletal muscle are primarily located between myofibrils, and these mitochondria are typically referred to as interfibrillar or core mitochondria. These mitochondria appear to be strategically located so that there is virtually no diffusional limitation regarding the supply of ATP to the contractile apparatus. Other mitochondria are also located just below the sarcolemma, and these are typically referred to as subsarcolemmal mitochondria. The functional significance of their location is unknown.

Since the mitochondria are one of the more plastic organelle systems in skeletal muscle fibers, there has been a great deal of interest in identifying a single index that can be used as a measure of cellular respiration. Some have used various biochemical markers, such as succinate dehydrogenase or citrate synthase activity. Others have quantified key electron transport proteins, such as cytochrome-c. Finally, some have applied morphometric measurements of mitochondrial volume density, an expression of mitochondrial volume per unit of cell volume.

Muscle Fiber Types and Polymorphism

Historical Perspective on Muscle Fiber Type Nomenclature

Many of the classic articles on muscle fiber types were written in the late 1960s and early 1970s. Some of the most frequently cited of these articles were those by Brooke and Kaiser (8) and Barnard et al. (9). Brooke and Kaiser (8) employed histochemical techniques that differentiated muscle fibers on the basis of the pH lability of the myofibrillar ATPase activity of myosin. Using this approach, these investigators identified fibers as slow type I, fast type IIA, and fast type IIB. Subsequently, this nomenclature was applied to the classification of MHC isoforms, and it is the dominant nomenclature currently used. This seems reasonable given that (a) the force–velocity relationship defines the maximum boundary of all forms of physical activity and (b) the shape of the force–velocity relationship is determined primarily by the MHC isoform composition. During the early 1990s, the nomenclature developed by Brook and Kaiser (8) was expanded to include the presence of fast type IIX fibers, which evolved from the discovery of the fast type IIX MHC isoform (7,10). The approach employed by Barnard et al. (9) attempted to develop acronyms that were more descriptive, incorporating information about both the mechanical and biochemical properties of the muscle fiber. This approach gave rise to the terms slow oxidative, fast oxidative glycolytic, and fast glycolytic.

Fiber Type Differences

Some of the key differences between fiber types can be found in a classic publication by Saltin and Gollnick (11), and these are summarized in Table 5.2. The brief discussion that follows addresses these differences with respect to the following:

1. Contractile proteins
2. Ca^{++} cycling and the SR
3. The mitochondria

Myosin is the molecular motor of skeletal muscle, and so the two main functions of myosin are to generate force and/or length changes. The forces and the rate of length change (velocity) are determined by the manner in which sarcomeres are arranged (i.e., numbers in parallel and in series) and the type of myosin. The numbers of sarcomeres in parallel determines to a large extent the maximal force that a muscle fiber can generate, whereas the numbers of sarcomeres in series is a key factor that determines both excursion and the maximal shortening velocity of a muscle fiber. A broad survey of human skeletal muscles suggests that fast

TABLE 5.2	Key Properties of Fiber Types With Emphasis on Human Skeletal Muscle		
Structural or Functional Property	**Slow Type I**	**Fast Type IIA**	**Fast Type IIX**
Speed-related contractile properties			
TPT	Slow	Fast	Fastest
$1/2$ RT	Slow	Fast	Fastest
K_{TR}	Slow	Fast	Fastest
V_{max}	Slow	Fast	Fastest
V_o	Slow	Fast	Fastest
Force-related contractile properties			
P_o	Same?	Same?	Same?
E	?	?	?
Tension-pCa^{++} relationship	Left	Right	Right
Pca$^{++}_{50}$	High	Low	Low
Fatigue-related contractile properties	Fatigue resistant	Moderately fatigable	Highly fatigable
Contractile-related proteins			
MHC isoform	Slow type I	Fast Type IIA	Fast Type IIX
Essential MLC isoform	sMLC1	fMLC1	fMLC3
Regulatory MLC isoform	sMLC2	fMLC2	fMLC2
Myosin ATPase activity	Lowest	Intermediate	Highest
TnC isoform	cTnC	fTnC	fTnC
TnT isoform	sTnT	fTnT	fTnT
TnI isoform	sTnI	fTnI	fTnI
Tropomyosin	β-TM	α-TM	α-TM
SR-related proteins			
Ca^{++} release channel isoform (RyR)	RyR1	RyR1	RyR1
Ca^{++} release channel number	Lowest	High	High
SERCA isoform	SERCA2a	SERCA1	SERCA1
SERCA number	Lowest	High	High
Phospholamban	Present	Absent	Absent
Parvalbumin	Low	High	High
Mitochondrial-related systems			
Respiratory capacity			
Per-unit muscle mass	Highest	Intermediate	Lowest
Per-unit mitochondrial mass	Same?	Same?	Same?
Proton conductance			
Per-unit mitochondrial mass	Same	Same	Same
Per-unit of surface area	Low	High	High
Capacity to handle reactive oxygen species			
MnSOD activity	Highest	Intermediate	Lowest
GPx activity	Highest	Intermediate	Lowest
Apoptosis	Unknown	Unknown	Unknown
Morphometric-related properties			
Cross-sectional area	Same	Same	Same
Myofibrillar volume density	Same	Same	Same
SR volume density	Lowest	Intermediate	Largest
Mitochondrial volume density	Largest	Intermediate	Smallest
Substrate-related properties			
Triglyceride	Highest	Intermediate	Lowest
Glycogen	Lowest	Intermediate	Highest
ATP	Same	Same	Same
CP	Lowest	Higher	Higher

(continued)

TABLE 5.2	Key Properties of Fiber Types With Emphasis on Human Skeletal Muscle (*Continued*)		
Structural or Functional Property	**Slow** **Type I**	**Fast** **Type IIA**	**Fast** **Type IIX**
Enzymatic activity properties			
Phosphorylase	Lowest	Intermediate	Highest
PFK	Lowest	Intermediate	Highest
LDH	Lowest	Intermediate	Highest
Triosephosphate dehydrogenase	Lowest	Intermediate	Highest
SDH	Highest	Intermediate	Lowest
CS	Highest	Intermediate	Lowest
Blood flow–related properties			
Capillary density	Highest	Intermediate	Lowest
Capillary length density per cell volume	Highest	Intermediate	Lowest
Krogh cylinder volume	Smallest	Intermediate	Highest
Mitochondrial volume:capillary volume	Same?	Same?	Same?
Myoglobin	Highest	Intermediate	Lowest

In some instances animal data have been included, since it is difficult to perform some of these analyses on human skeletal muscle. TPT, time peak tension; $\frac{1}{2}$ RT, one-half relaxation time; K_{TR}, time constant for the redevelopment of tension; V_{max}, maximal shortening velocity; V_o, maximal unloaded shortening velocity; P_t, twitch tension; P_0, maximal isometric tension; *E*, elastic modulus; ATP, adenosine triphosphate; CP, creatine phosphate; PFK, phosphofructokinase; LDH, lactate dehydrogenase; SDH, succinate dehydrogenase; CS, citrate synthase; MHC, myosin heavy chain; MLC, myosin light chain; TnC, troponin-C; TnT, troponin-T; TnI, troponin-I; RyR, ryanodine receptor; SERCA, sarcoplasmic reticulum Ca^{++} ATPase pump.

and slow muscle fibers do not differ markedly from one another with respect to cross-sectional area (an indirect measure of the number of sarcomeres in parallel) (11). In contrast, fast muscle fibers in rodents are usually much larger than slow fibers (the soleus muscle appears to be an exception to this rule). Importantly, the myofibrillar volume density appears to be very similar in both slow and fast human skeletal muscle. This basically means that slow and fast skeletal muscle fibers have the same number of sarcomeres per unit of cross-sectional area and as a consequence should be capable of producing the same amount of force when normalized to cross-sectional area (i.e., specific tension). Stated simply, the intrinsic ability to generate force should not be strongly dependent on fiber type. Interestingly, some single fiber studies have reported fiber type differences regarding specific tension. However, no attempt has been made to correlate such findings with whole muscle mechanics. In contrast to specific tension, the shortening velocity of skeletal muscle is highly dependent on fiber type owing to the presence of slow and fast MHC isoforms, and the existence of these isoforms is responsible for approximately a threefold to fivefold difference in maximal shortening velocity.

The ability to rapidly release and sequester Ca^{++} depends primarily on the properties of the SR. Therefore, the SR plays a central role in determining the rates of activation, relaxation, and hence the maximal frequency of oscillatory work that can be achieved. In human skeletal muscle, the SR accounts for about 2 to 6% of the cell volume, and the volume is the greatest in the fast type II fibers (about 5–6% cell

volume). This finding is consistent with the more rapid relaxation rates found in fast fibers.

The release of Ca^{++} from the SR is determined by the properties and types of RyRs. A number of RyRs have been identified and classified as RyR1, RyR2, and RyR3. The dominant form found in both slow and fast skeletal muscle is RyR1. RyR2 plays the central role in cardiac muscle, and RyR3 appears to be ubiquitously distributed in a number of tissues and cell types. Unlike the other two isoforms, RyR1 plays a fundamental role in excitation–contraction coupling in the absence of extracellular Ca^{++}, and this has been referred to as skeletal-type EC coupling. The greater release rate found in fast skeletal muscle (compared to slow) is primarily due to differences in the numbers of RyR1 receptors, with fast skeletal muscle having up to a tenfold difference. This results from (*a*) a twofold to threefold difference in SR volume density and (*b*) a twofold to threefold difference in the numbers of RyR1 per unit of SR.

As mentioned earlier, both fast (SERCA1) and slow (SERCA2a) SERCA isoforms are found in skeletal muscle. Given this observation, the question arises whether the rapid relaxation rates found in fast skeletal muscle are simply due to a greater SR volume density and/or the presence of a faster Ca^{++}-ATPase pump (i.e., SERCA). Current findings suggest that SERCA1 and SERCA2a have similar enzymatic properties, and this has given rise to the concept that the relaxation rate of skeletal muscle is highly correlated with SR volume density. However, the activity of SERCA2a can be modified by the presence of phospholamban (PLB). In a dephosphorylated state, PLB acts to inhibit the Ca^{++}-ATPase activity of

SERCA2a, whereas dephosphorylation of PLB causes it to dissociate from SERCA2a, allowing the Ca^{++}-ATPase activity of SERCA2a to increase.

The mitochondrial volume density in humans is about twofold to threefold different between slow type I and fast type II fibers. Mitochondrial volume density in human slow type I fibers is typically about 6%, whereas it only is about 2 to 3% in fast type II fibers. There are also corresponding differences in key enzymes. For instance, activity of succinate dehydrogenase (the only membrane-bound enzyme of the Krebs cycle) is about 1.5 and 3 times as high in slow type I fibers as in fast type IIA and fast type IIX fibers, respectively. Citrate synthase activity also follows a similar pattern. Interestingly, in rodent skeletal muscle, fast type IIA fibers (fast oxidative glycolytic) have a higher oxidative capacity than slow type I (slow oxidative) fibers.

Polymorphism

For many years it was believed that muscle fibers expressed only one type of MHC isoform. This helped to keep the concept of a muscle fiber type simple. One of the most significant concepts to evolve during the past 10 to 15 years has been the recognition that there can be an extensive proportion of hybrid or polymorphic fibers in both human and nonhuman species. Pette and Staron (10) were at the forefront of this issue, and it is now known that muscle fibers can express anywhere from one to four adult MHC isoforms in smaller mammals and one to three in larger mammals, such as humans (10,12,13). If muscle fibers are classified strictly on the basis of the MHC isoforms expressed in a given fiber, there are 15 possible combinations in the muscle fibers of small mammals (where four adult isoforms are expressed) and 7 combinations in human (where three adult isoforms can be found). If one considers muscles such as the posterior cricoarytenoid muscle of the larynx, which also expresses the EO/type IIL MHC isoform, the number of potential combinations of MHC isoforms increases to 31. The theoretical number of molecular motors is quite impressive when the possible combinations of MHC isoform are coupled with those for MLC proteins. If all of the individual components involved with Ca^{++} cycling, crossbridge cycling, and cellular respiration are considered, it is surprising that nature has been kind enough to allow us to think that there are discrete fiber types.

Muscle Fiber Type Plasticity and the I ⇄ IIA ⇄ IIX ⇄ IIB Transition Model

Each muscle appears to have its own unique pattern of muscle fibers that can vary by

1. Type
2. Region
3. Degree of polymorphism

Studies during the past 20 years have shown that the adaptation of muscle fiber composition to altered physiological states is muscle dependent. For instance, some muscles, like the plantar flexors of the ankle, appear to be more inclined to undergo atrophy and MHC isoform transitions than the dorsiflexors of the ankle. This concept has been refined further to indicate that adaptation is specific to fiber type. As with most generalizations, however, such rules do not always apply, and the same fiber types within a given muscle can respond differently to the same stimulus. As an example, it appears that there are different populations of slow type I fibers in the rat soleus muscle that differ in their sensitivity to mechanical unloading and thyroid state (14).

One area of muscle plasticity that merits further attention is related to the fiber type dependence of plasticity. In rats, the plasticity of MHC isoform expression is much greater in slow type I fibers than in fast type II fibers. For instance, it has been shown that most slow type I fibers in the soleus muscle can be converted into fast muscle fibers, whereas it is very difficult to perturb most fast fibers in rat muscles to become heavily biased in the slow direction.

As mentioned earlier, Pette and Staron (10) performed a series of studies examining transitions in single-fiber MHC isoform expression via electrophoretic techniques. As a result of these studies, they proposed that muscle fibers were obligated to follow a transition scheme that can be described as follows: I ⇄ IIA ⇄ IIX ⇄ IIB. According to this scheme, a muscle fiber undergoing a transition from a slow type I to fast type IIX phenotype would be obligated first to express the fast type IIA MHC isoform. More recently, however, other studies (12–14) found various combinations of MHC isoforms that are not consistent with this obligatory transition scheme. For instance, Caiozzo et al. (14) found pools of I/IIB and I/IIX/IIB fibers in muscles that were manipulated via mechanical unloading and hyperthyroidism. Additionally, it has recently been reported that muscles such as the diaphragm can contain pools of I/IIX fibers (12). These types of observations are further supported by those of Talmadge and colleagues (13,15) who observed significant pools of I/IIX fibers following hindlimb suspension or spinal cord transection. Thus, skeletal muscle fibers clearly have the ability to undergo MHC isoform transitions that do not adhere to the "obligatory" scheme. The question is whether such asynchronous transitions are an exception or the rule. This obviously requires much more investigation, especially at the myonuclear level (see the following section for further comment).

Myonuclear Plasticity

One of the remarkable features of skeletal muscle is the extensive multinucleation in each muscle fiber. A typical skeletal muscle fiber has 100 to 200 myonuclei per millimeter of length. Therefore, in small mammals like rats, there are about 3000 to 6000 nuclei per fiber in a muscle like the soleus. This is quite a remarkable number. Imagine how many myonuclei there are in a skeletal muscle fiber of the human brachioradialis muscle, where the fibers are longer than 100 mm (10,000–20,000?). One of the great challenges ahead is to understand the degree of coordination between individual myonuclei. Do all myonuclei have exactly the same gene expression program, or are there slight to large variations from one myonucleus to another? Does polymorphism arise because all myonuclei coexpress exactly the same set of sarcomeric protein isoforms, or is it possible that polymorphism exists because one myonucleus may express a set of sarcomeric protein isoforms that differs from its neighboring myonucleus? Several observations suggest that the gene expression programs of myonuclei can vary along the length of the fiber. For instance, it is known that the myonuclei associated with the neuromuscular junction express genes responsible for the localization of acetylcholine receptors (16). Additionally, Peuker and Pette (17) reported the existence of segmental variations in the MHC mRNA isoform expression, and consistent with this observation Edman and associates (18) found segmental differences in ATPase activity. If segmental variation does occur along the length of muscle fibers, this finding will surely excite and confuse us further regarding our concept of a fiber type. Ultimately, however, it will allow us to determine definitively whether there truly is an I $\rightleftarrows$ IIA $\rightleftarrows$ IIX $\rightleftarrows$ IIB transition scheme.

The observation that skeletal muscle fibers are capable of exhibiting a wide repertoire of MHC polymorphism gives rise to some interesting functional issues. These are addressed later, in the section "The Force–Velocity Relationship in the Shortening Domain."

Linking Structure to Function

Overview

When skeletal muscles are excited, they convert chemical energy to mechanical energy. The forces and/or length changes a muscle produces are determined by a number of key factors, and from a conceptual perspective investigators including Rome and Linstedt (19) and Josephson (20) referred to these various factors as "design constraints" or "primary/secondary determinants." Four primary design constraints determine the performance of skeletal muscle fibers under isometric and shortening conditions (Fig. 5.4).

These four factors are 1. the length–tension relationship, 2. the degree and rate of activation, 3. the force–velocity relationship in the shortening domain, and 4. the degree and rate of relaxation. During lengthening contractions, the mechanical properties of skeletal muscle are not only determined by the extent of activation but also by 5. the force–velocity relationship in the lengthening domain and 6. the passive stiffness of skeletal muscle (Fig. 5.4).

As will be noted throughout much of this section, m. of the processes associated with factors 2–5 are highly m. leable. With respect to this point, Booth and Baldwin (21) published an extensive review examining the effects of altered contractile activity on the mRNA levels of various contractile and metabolic genes (see Table 24.4 from their publication).

This section of the chapter is organized into three distinct sections. The first section will introduce the reader to "Muscle Mechanics 101" and will focus on mechanical measurements that illustrate the importance of (a) the degree of activation, (b) sarcomere length, and (c) the loading conditions imposed on the muscle. The second section addresses the plasticity of the force–velocity relationship both in the shortening and lengthening domains. The underlying basis for the emphasis on the force–velocity relationship is that it reflects the intrinsic properties of the molecular motor, and so sets the theoretical limits for muscle performance under all conditions. The third section introduces the work loop concept. Work loops offer an interesting perspective because the performance of skeletal muscle during a work loop (oscillatory length change) depends on the integration of all six design criteria. In this last section on work loops, special attention will be given to the importance of activation, relaxation, and passive stiffness.

Muscle Mechanics 101: The Relationship Between Activation, Stimulation Frequency, and Force Production

The term *activation* is typically used to describe the degree to which the contractile apparatus has been activated, or turned on. In reality, the degree of activation reflects the number of attached crossbridges, and in turn this depends primarily on the binding of Ca^{++} to troponin-C (TnC).

When a single muscle fiber receives a single brief stimulus, the muscle fiber produces a mechanical event known as a twitch. A twitch generates a relatively small amount of force (typically 15–25% of P_o) as a result of a complex interplay between Ca^{++} cycling, force production, and stretching of the series elastic component. Since a twitch results from a single stimulus, its duration is brief, and in this context, the duration of a twitch sets the theoretical limits regarding the oscillatory frequencies at which a muscle can operate (see "The Concept of Work Loops," later in the chapter). Twitch measurements are usually made while muscle length is held constant (i.e., isometric conditions), and this simplifies the potential complexity of making such measurements, especially since measures of twitch tension and relaxation depend on muscle length and shortening velocity.

Typically, three measurements are made from an isometric twitch (Table 5.3), and these include measures of

1. Twitch tension (P_t)
2. Time to peak tension (TPT)
3. One-half relaxation time ($\frac{1}{2}$ RT)

(*text continues on page 132*)

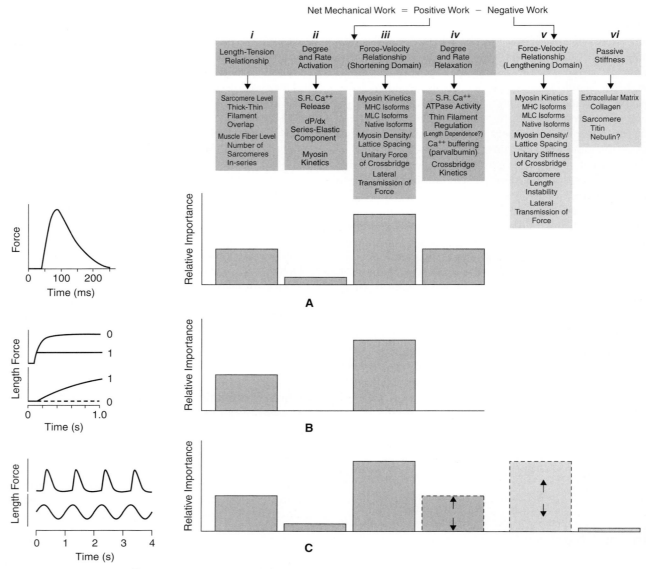

FIGURE 5.4 The six key design constraints that determine the amount of force, work, and power that can be produced under any contractile condition: (*i*) the length–tension relationship, (*ii*) the rate and extent of activation, (*iii*) the force–velocity relationship in the shortening domain, (*iv*) the rate of relaxation, (*v*) the force–velocity relationship in the lengthening domain, and (*vi*) the passive stiffness of skeletal muscle. Bar graphs illustrate the importance of each of these factors under different contractile conditions. **A.** An isometric twitch. The four factors that determine the kinetics of the twitch are factors *i to iv*, with factor *iii* dominant. **B.** Two examples of isotonic contractions used to determine the force–velocity relationship. Typically, the muscle is fully activated when these types of measurements are made, and relaxation kinetics are irrelevant to such measures. Hence, factors *i* and *iii* are critical to determining the shape of the force–velocity relationship. **C.** The length and force records during a work loop experiment. The work loop provides a more realistic measure of work and power that a muscle can produce than do similar measures made from force–velocity curves (Table 5.3). Each design criterion plays a role during work loops. The force–velocity relationship sets the theoretical limits of muscle performance under all conditions, so it always has the greatest importance. The arrows in the bars for factors *iv* and *v* indicate that the importance of these two factors can vary significantly with the length, which influences relaxation kinetics in slow skeletal muscle, and activation pattern, which might affect the amount of negative work required to relengthen the muscle.

TABLE 5.3 **Muscle Mechanics**

Name of Mechanical Measurement	Mechanical Measurements	Functional Significance	Key Structures	Malleability
Isometric twitch		TPT is often used as an index of the speed characteristics of a muscle. Reflects activation of contractile apparatus as well as cross-bridge kinetics. $\frac{1}{2}$ RT is used as an index of relaxation. Reflects sequestration of Ca^{++} by SR	Whole muscle Ca^{++} release by SR MHC isoforms Ca^{++} uptake by SR (SERCA isoforms) Single fiber Same as for whole muscle.	Both TPT and $\frac{1}{2}$ RT can be significantly altered, and this is true especially for slow muscles undergoing slow-to-fast transition. $\frac{1}{2}$ RT is probably more sensitive to altered physiological conditions than is TPT. Additionally, $\frac{1}{2}$ RT is sensitive to muscle/fiber length, *while TPT is relatively insensitive.*
Force–frequency relationship		This represents the relationship between stimulation frequency and force production. Stimulation frequency controls pCa^{++} and modulates force via the tension-pCa^{++} relationship.	Whole muscle SR Ca^{++} release SR Ca^{++} uptake TnC isoform Skinned single fiber TnC isoform	Whole muscle Shape of force–frequency relationship in slow skeletal muscle can be manipulated by producing a slow-to-fast transition via mechanical unloading or altered thyroid state. This results in a curve shifted to the right and reflects an increase in the kinetics of the SERCA. As noted in numerous places throughout the text, it is difficult to produce a fast-to-slow transition that results in a significant shift in the force–frequency relationship.
Tension-pCa^{++} relationship				Skinned single fiber The tension–pCa^{++} curve primarily reflects the binding of Ca^{++} to troponin-C. The cardiac or slow form of TnC (cTnC) has two binding sites for Ca^{++}. One of these is a high affinity site and always has Ca^{++} bound to it. The second site has a low affinity for Ca^{++}, and it is this site that regulates the actions of TnC. Muscles that undergo a cTnC → fTnC transition will exhibit a right shift in the tension–pCa^{++} relationship, because the fast form of TnC has two high- and two low-affinity binding sites. *(continued)*

TABLE 5.3   Muscle Mechanics (Continued)

Name of Mechanical Measurement	Mechanical Measurements	Functional Significance	Key Structures	Malleability
Afterload technique for determination of force–velocity relationship		Force–velocity relationship describes the force that a muscle can generate at any given shortening velocity. The top panel illustrates various afterloads, while the middle panel shows the corresponding length–time records. A given velocity is simply the slope of a given length–time record. The resultant force–velocity relationship is shown in the bottom panel. The force–velocity relationship sets the theoretical boundary for muscle performance. Muscles can work on or below this relationship, but they cannot operate above it.	Whole muscle Muscle architecture MHC isoforms MLC isoforms Lattice spacing Single fiber Same except for architecture	The force–velocity relationship is quite malleable. A decrease in physical activity will result in a loss of sarcomeres in parallel (atrophy). This will lead to a loss of force production. Typically, a slow-to-fast MHC isoform transition occurs concomitantly with muscle atrophy. The net result is an increase in V_{max}. The increase in V_{max} partially offsets the reduction in force production such that loss in maximal power is partially attenuated. Resistance training produces an increase in the number of sarcomeres in parallel, and as a consequence the muscle will be able to produce more force. It has been shown in both rodents and humans that resistance training also produces a faster-to-fast transition (e.g., IIX → IIA). Such shifts, however, do not result in large changes in V_{max}. (continued)

TABLE 5.3 Muscle Mechanics *(Continued)*

Name of Mechanical Measurement	Mechanical Measurements	Functional Significance	Key Structures	Malleability
Slack test		Provides measure of maximal un-loaded shortening velocity (V_o). Ratio of V_o:V_{max} in whole muscle may reflect heterogeneity of MHC isoform composition among individual fibers. In muscles where most fibers are slow (e.g., soleus muscle), the V_o:V_{max} will be high. In fast muscles, the V_o:V_{max} ratio will be lower.	Whole muscle MHC isoforms MLC isoforms Lattice structure Muscle architecture Single fiber MHC isoforms MLC isoforms Lattice structure	The V_o of fibers undergoing slow-to-fast transition will exhibit large in-creases in V_o. The V_o of fast fibers is difficult to alter given an apparent inability to make significant fast-to-slow transi-tions in MHC isoform composition.

(continued)

TABLE 5.3	Muscle Mechanics *(Continued)*			
Name of Mechanical Measurement	Mechanical Measurements	Functional Significance	Key Structures	Malleability
Ramp stretch or isovelocity lengthening contraction	$SRS = \Delta P/\Delta L$ or $E = \sigma/\delta$	The mechanical properties during lengthening contractions have not been extensively studied, especially under altered physiological conditions.	Whole muscle Muscle architecture Number of functional crossbridges Unitary stiffness of individual crossbridges	Stiffness: Stiffness is simply the slope of the relationship between force and length. Hence, it is dependent on cross-sectional area and muscle length. Disuse of skeletal muscle typically produces a loss of sarcomeres in parallel and as a consequence, cross-sectional area. This results in a decrease in isometric tension and a loss of stiffness. Resistance training, in contrast, increases the number of sarcomeres in parallel and the isometric tension of a muscle or muscle fiber. As a result, the muscle is stiffer when activated and lengthened.
		Stiffness of skeletal muscle may play an important role in joint stability.	Single fiber Dimensions of fiber Number of functional crossbridges Unitary stiffness of individual crossbridges	Additionally, atrophy seems to produce alterations in the lattice structure that appear to reduce the unitary stiffness of individual crossbridges. This reflects a so-called material property known as elastic modulus, which attempts to normalize stiffness to the geometric properties of a muscle.
		Modulus represents the slope of the relationship between stress and strain. Hence, it is normalized to the dimensions of the muscle.		
		Yield strain may be an important parameter with respect to protection of joints and joint ligaments to injury.		

(continued)

TABLE 5.3	Muscle Mechanics (Continued)			
Name of Mechanical Measurement	**Mechanical Measurements**	**Functional Significance**	**Key Structures**	**Malleability**
Work loop		The work loop technique provides a more realistic approach for studying the capacity of skeletal muscle to produce mechanical work and power during cyclical changes in length as might occur during locomotion. Comparing the theoretical work loop with the real work loop makes it possible to determine which factors impose the greatest limitations on the capacity of skeletal muscle.	Whole muscle Muscle architecture SR Ca^{++} release SEC MHC isoforms MLC isoforms Lattice spacing SR Ca^{++} uptake Length-dependent regulation of thin filament Connective tissue Single fiber Same except for connective tissue	Virtually every one of the key structures is malleable. This is true especially for factors controlling the shape of the force–velocity relationship and relaxation kinetics. Key structural features that determine the shape of the force–velocity relationship include architectural features such as the number of sarcomeres in parallel. The types of MHC and MLC isoforms are also critical in determining the shape of the force–velocity relationship. Relaxation kinetics are also very important in determining the amount of mechanical work that can be realized. Hence, the SR is a key structural feature.

Measures of P_t provide insight regarding the force that a muscle or muscle fiber can produce; however, P_t is a submaximal measure. With respect to Figure 5.4, a key determinant of P_t is the number of sarcomeres in parallel (factor a). In contrast to P_t, both TPT and $\frac{1}{2}$ RT are often referred to as speed-related properties. Time to peak tension reflects processes involved with activation (factor b) and the rate of crossbridge cycling (factor c). Time to peak tension will be very short in muscles and muscle fibers when Ca^{++} is rapidly released from the SR and crossbridge cycling is fast. Also, $\frac{1}{2}$ RT depends primarily on the kinetics of the sarcoplasmic reticulum Ca^{++} ATPase pumps and their numbers (factor d).

Mechanical unloading of slow skeletal muscle produces a slow → fast transition that influences the numbers of RyRs, myosin isoform composition, and SERCA isoform composition. As a consequence, this causes significant reductions in both TPT and $\frac{1}{2}$ RT.

The response of skeletal muscle to repetitive stimuli is much more complex than for a twitch, and it depends on the stimulation frequency. If the frequency is such that the muscle or muscle fiber completely relaxes between individual stimuli, the muscle or muscle fiber will generate a series of individual twitches, and peak tension will be approximately equal to P_t. If the frequency of stimulation is increased so that relaxation is not complete prior to the onset of the succeeding stimulus, the force generated during the second stimulus will add to the residual force from the preceding contraction, leading to a summation in force. This type of response is an unfused tetanus, or partial relaxation between individual stimuli. If stimulation frequency is increased further, so that there is no relaxation between individual stimuli, this will result in fused tetanus (no relaxation between individual stimuli). It is under these conditions that the muscle is fully activated and generates maximal isometric tension (P_o). The relationship between stimulation frequency and force reflects a complex set of events that involves the release of Ca^{++} from the SR, the binding of Ca^{++} to TnC, crossbridge cycling, and stretch of the series elastic component. As shown in Table 5.3, the force–frequency relationship has a sigmoidal shape, and fast muscles and muscle fibers have force–frequency relationships that are shifted to the right of those for slow muscles and muscle fibers. Altered physiological conditions (e.g., disuse or inactivity) that produce slow-to-fast transitions will typically produce a rightward shift in this relationship. Functionally, this means that the central nervous system will have to provide greater neural drive (i.e., higher stimulation frequency) to produce the same relative force.

The force–frequency relationship indirectly reflects the Ca^{++} bound to TnC, and this is determined by a complex set of events involved with Ca^{++} cycling (i.e., Ca^{++} release and Ca^{++} sequestration) and the binding of Ca^{++} to TnC. The Ca^{++} binding properties of TnC are often described by plotting the relationship between tension and [Ca^{++}], and the [Ca^{++}] is described using an inverse log plot analogous to that used to describe pH. A pCa^{++} of 7.0 is equivalent to a 0.0000001 (1 10-millionth) M concentration of Ca^{++}. TnC has both high- and low-affinity binding sites for Ca^{++}, and the numbers of these depend on the isoform of TnC. The slow or cardiac isoform of TnC (cTnC) has one high- and one low-affinity binding site for Ca^{++}. In contrast, the fast isoform of TnC (fTnC) has two high- and two low-affinity Ca^{++} binding sites. During rest, the high-affinity sites are saturated with Ca^{++}, while Mg^{++} is bound to the low-affinity sites. Immediately following excitation, Ca^{++} is quickly released from the SR, causing the concentration of free Ca^{++} to rise rapidly. The Ca^{++} then displaces Mg^{++} from the low-affinity sites and causes tropomyosin to undergo a conformational change such that the myosin binding sites on actin become exposed, allowing myosin to bind and generate force. Since the cardiac isoform of TnC has only one low-affinity binding site for Ca^{++}, the tension–pCa^{++} relationship of slow type I fibers is shifted to the left of that for fast type II fibers. The pCa^{++}_{50} is defined as the [Ca^{++}] required to produce 50% of P_o, and it reflects the binding properties of TnC. Hence, the pCa^{++}_{50} of slow type I fibers is greater than that of fast type II fibers, since less Ca^{++} is required to saturate the low-affinity sites of the cTnC isoform. Given this perspective, altered physiological conditions that produce transitions in TnC isoforms will produce corresponding shifts in the tension–pCa^{++} relationship and pCa^{++}_{50}.

Muscle Mechanics 101: The Length–Tension Relationship (Factor 1)

It has been known for more than 100 years that the force a muscle or muscle fiber can generate depends on its length. The length–tension relationship is shown in Figure 5.5.

Ultrastructural studies of mammalian skeletal muscle have shown that each thin filament is about 1 µm in length, whereas each thick filament has a length of about 1.6 to 1.7 µm. According to the sliding filament hypothesis, the force that a sarcomere can produce depends on the overlap between thick and thin filaments. For instance, at a sarcomere length of about 3.6 µm, there is no overlap between the thick and thin filaments, and as a consequence, there is no ability to produce force. At a sarcomere length of 2.2 µm, in contrast, the overlap between the thick and thin filaments is optimal, and force production is maximized.

Typically, three regions of the length–tension relationship are described. The ascending limb extends from a sarcomere length of approximately 1.3 to 2.0 µm. In this region, the amount of isometric tension increases in direct proportion to the increase in sarcomere length. The plateau region extends from about 2.0 to 2.5 µm in mammalian fibers, and in this range there is an optimal overlap between the thick and thin filaments. Beyond a sarcomere length of 2.5 µm, the isometric force that can be produced decreases as a linear function of sarcomere length, reflecting a progressive decrease in overlap between the thick and thin

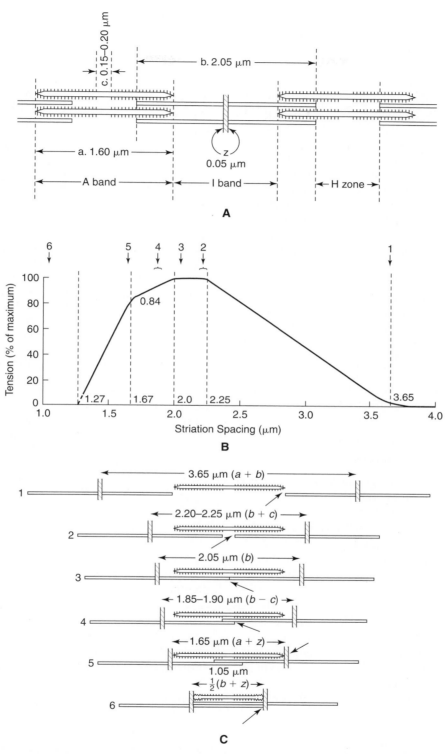

FIGURE 5.5   Classic length–tension relationship. *(Modified from Gordon AM, Huxley AF, Julian FJ. The variation in isometric tension with sarcomere length in vertebrate muscle fibres. J Physiol (Lond) 1966;184:170–192.)*

filaments. The changes in striation patterns during shortening contractions played a central role in developing the sliding filament hypothesis. Table 5.4 summarizes the changes in the striation pattern that occur during isometric, shortening, and lengthening contractions.

The length–tension relationship of the sarcomere is thought to be a static design criterion (19), implying that it does not change with various types of interventions, such as mechanical unloading. However, spastic conditions may alter some aspects of the length–tension relationship. In contrast to the length–tension relationship of a sarcomere, that of individual muscle fibers is quite malleable. For instance, it is well known that muscles immobilized in a lengthened position will increase the number of sarcomeres in series, leading to the longitudinal growth of the fiber. Conversely, immobilization in a shortened position will reduce the number of sarcomeres in series and result in a shorter muscle fiber. As a consequence, such manipulations have the potential to influence the overall length–tension relationships of muscle fibers and whole muscles. Normal types of physical activity and inactivity probably have little impact on the length–tension relationships of sarcomeres, muscle fibers, or whole muscles. In some abnormal states, such as those seen with contractures, however, there may be significant alterations in the length–tension relationship at all three levels (i.e., sarcomere, muscle fiber, muscle) (22,23).

Muscle Mechanics 101: The Force–Velocity Relationship (Factors 3 and 5)

A fully activated muscle will shorten at a slow velocity when it contracts against a heavy load (Table 5.3). In contrast, the shortening velocity will be much greater when this same muscle contracts against a light load. This inverse relationship between force and shortening velocity is simply known as the force–velocity relationship, and when the muscle shortens during the contraction, this relationship is hyperbolic (Fig. 5.6).

Fully activated muscles can also be forcibly lengthened by imposing on the muscle a force that exceeds P_o. These types of contractions are often called eccentric contractions. However, in this chapter they are called lengthening contractions. The shape of the force–velocity relationship in the lengthening domain is often represented as shown in Figure 5.6. However, as noted later, the mechanics in the lengthen-

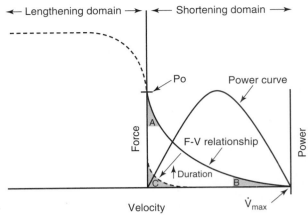

FIGURE 5.6 Illustration of the shortening and lengthening domains of the force–velocity relationship. Three areas of activity have been identified in the shortening domain. Activities performed in region A require the muscle to produce contractions that generate high forces and slow velocities of shortening. Contractions in region B produce high shortening velocities and low forces. From a temporal perspective, muscle activity in either region can only be supported for short periods of time. Hence, when the duration of activity increases, the forces and velocities that a muscle generates will move onto submaximal force–velocity curves as shown in region C. The force–velocity relationship in the lengthening domain is typically represented as shown in this figure. However, as noted in the text, the force–velocity relationship in the lengthening domain is much more complicated and is three-dimension in nature, having axes of force, velocity, and time. Although muscle fiber type plays an important role in determining the shape of the force–velocity relationship in the shortening domain, it is unclear how important muscle fiber type is in determining the shape of this relationship in the lengthening domain.

ing domain are determined by three variables, force, velocity, and time, and therefore, the shape of the force–velocity relationship in the lengthening domain is three-dimensional.

The force–velocity relationship accounts for two of the six design constraints noted earlier, and of any of these six, the force–velocity relationship sets the theoretical limit of muscle performance. Muscles can operate either on or below the force–velocity relationship, but they cannot operate above it. Hence, the other design constraints are really modulators of muscle performance. The force–velocity relationship is im-

TABLE 5.4	Effect of Types of Contractions on the Lengths of Various Bands, Zones, and Lines					
Type of Contraction	Z-line	I-band	A-band	H-zone	M-line	Sarcomere Length
Isometric	↔	↔	↔	↔	↔	↔
Shortening (Isotonic)	↔	↓	↔	↓	↔	↓
Lengthening (Eccentric)	↔	↑	↔	↑	↔	↑

↔, No change in length; ↑, increase in length; ↓, decrease in length.

portant not just because it describes the relationship between force and velocity. Rather, this relationship is also important because (a) it reflects the complexity of crossbridge cycling; (b) it determines the work and power that can be produced under any contractile condition; and (c) it determines the metabolic cost and mechanical efficiency of contractile activity.

One important feature of the force–velocity relationship that cannot be overemphasized is that it is a functional measurement that reflects important structural information. For instance, in the high-force region of the force–velocity relationship (Fig. 5.6, region A), the maximal isometric force (P_o) that a muscle can produce is (a) dependent on the number of sarcomeres that are in parallel with one another and (b) independent of myosin isoform composition. At the other end of the force–velocity spectrum (Fig. 5.6, region B), maximal shortening velocity (V_{max}) is determined by the myosin isoform composition and not the number of sarcomeres in parallel.

Plasticity of the Force–Velocity Relationship in the Shortening Domain (Factor 3)

The shape of the force–velocity relationship of **single fibers** really depends on a complex distribution of crossbridges whereby a crossbridge can act as either a positive or negative force generator. Huxley developed a model describing this complexity in 1957 (1). This model proposes that at slow velocities, crossbridges attach and act as positive force generators, detaching before they are swept into the region where they act as negative force generators. At higher shortening velocities, however, a greater proportion of the crossbridges that initially attach and generate a positive force will be swept into the negative force–generating region before they can detach, causing a reduction in net force production by the muscle fiber. Shifts in isoforms induced by altered neural, mechanical, or hormonal conditions can alter the MHC isoform composition of a muscle fiber and by doing so, influence the proportion of crossbridges acting as positive or negative force generators at any given velocity of contraction. This in turn alters the shape of the force–velocity relationship of the **single fiber.**

At the **whole muscle level,** the shape of the force–velocity relationship is a composite of the force–velocity relationships of each individual muscle fiber. In *First and Last Experiments in Muscle Mechanics* (24), Hill developed a statistical model that provided a mathematical approach to understanding the complexity of the force–velocity relationship. In his model, Hill used 82 fibers that were distributed in a manner consistent with a probability curve, yielding 10 pools of fibers. The Hill equation of the force–velocity relationship states:

$$(P+a)(V+b)=b(P_o+a) \qquad \text{[Equation 5.1]}$$

where P_o is maximal isometric tension, P is isotonic tension, V is shortening velocity, and a and b are constants with

dimensions of force and velocity, respectively. The curvature of the force–velocity relationship is represented by a/P_o. Equation 5.1 can be normalized to P_o and V_{max} as follows (25):

$$\left(P/P_o + a/P_o\right)\left(V/V_{max} + b/V_{max}\right) = b/V_{max}\left(1 + a/P_o\right) \qquad \text{[Equation 5.2]}$$

Equation 5.2 can be rewritten using the substitutions of $P/P_o = P'$, $V/V_{max} = V'$, and $a/P_o = b/V_{max} = 1/G$ such that

$$P' = \left(1 - V'\right)/\left(1 + VG\right) \qquad \text{[Equation 5.3]}$$

This equation can be used as shown in Table 5.5 to determine the force–velocity of any individual pool of fibers by (a) determining the relative shortening velocity for that pool of fibers and using this to solve Equation 5.3 and (b) determining the relative overall force and adjusting for the proportion of fibers in that pool. The V' for any pool of fibers (V'_{fiber}) is determined by dividing the maximal shortening velocity of that group of fibers ($V_{o, fiber}$) by the shortening velocity of the whole muscle (V_{muscle}). In the example in Table 5.5A, the whole-muscle shortening velocity is equivalent to 0.05 fiber lengths per second ($FL \cdot s^{-1}$). In this example, all of the fibers have a $V_{o, fiber}$ that exceeds this shortening velocity, and hence each fiber can contribute to overall force production. In contrast, when the muscle is shortening at a velocity equivalent to 1.10 $FL \cdot s^{-1}$ (Table 5.5B), the three slowest pools of fibers are unable to contribute to overall force production.

One of the utilities of Hill's 82-fiber statistical model is that it can be used to predict alterations in the force–velocity relationship of whole muscle based on changes in (a) cross-sectional area as is associated with hypertrophy and atrophy and (b) myosin isoform composition. A slow-to-fast myosin isoform transition can be modeled, for instance, by altering the distribution of the 82 fibers so that they are distributed in the four slowest pools of fibers. The predicted effect is quite evident: a reduction in the V_{max} of the muscle. The effects of hypertrophy or atrophy can be described by multiplying P'_{fiber} by a constant. For example, if a muscle atrophied by 50%, each P'_{fiber} value would be reduced by this proportion.

The application of Hill's approach has been extended (a) to model differences in the force–velocity relationships of hindlimb muscles in the rat (12) and (b) to explain the effects of myosin isoform transitions (26). The requirements for modeling the whole muscle force–velocity relationship in this fashion depend on (a) a statistical model, (b) knowledge about the distribution of myosin isoforms at the single fiber level, and (c) some assumptions regarding the maximal shortening velocity of slow type I, fast type IIA, fast type IIX, and fast type IIB fibers. The first requirement (a statistical model) involves the application of a model like Hill's or that described by Josephson and Edman (27). The second requirement (knowledge about single fiber myosin isoform composition) entails a large number of electrophoretic single

| TABLE 5.5 | Application of Hill's 82-Fiber Model | | | | |

n	p_{fiber}	$V_{o,fiber}$	V_{muscle}	V'_{fiber}	P'_{fiber}
1	0.012	2.4	0.05	0.0208	0.0110
3	0.037	2.2	0.05	0.0227	0.0328
7	0.085	2.0	0.05	0.0250	0.0757
13	0.159	1.8	0.05	0.0278	0.1387
17	0.207	1.6	0.05	0.0313	0.1785
17	0.207	1.4	0.05	0.0357	0.1749
13	0.159	1.2	0.05	0.0417	0.1302
7	0.085	1.0	0.05	0.0500	0.0676
3	0.037	0.8	0.05	0.0625	0.0274
1	0.012	0.6	0.05	0.0833	0.0084
					$\Sigma = 0.8453$

Panel A

n	p_{fiber}	$V_{o,fiber}$	V_{muscle}	V'_{fiber}	P'_{fiber}
1	0.012	2.4	1.10	0.4583	0.0023
3	0.037	2.2	1.10	0.5000	0.0061
7	0.085	2.0	1.10	0.5500	0.012
13	0.159	1.8	1.10	0.6111	0.0179
17	0.207	1.6	1.10	0.6875	0.0173
17	0.207	1.4	1.10	0.7857	0.0107
13	0.159	1.2	1.10	0.9167	0.0028
7	0.085	1.0	1.10	>1	0.000
3	0.037	0.8	1.10	>1	0.000
1	0.012	0.6	1.10	>1	0.000
					$\Sigma = 0.0692$

Panel B

Calculations are shown for whole muscle shortening velocities (V_{muscle}) of 0.05 (panel A) and 1.10 (panel B) FL/s.

n, Number of fibers in a given pool; p_{fiber}, number in the pool divided by the number of fibers ($n = 82$); $V_{o,fiber}$, maximal unloaded shortening velocity of fibers; V_{muscle}, shortening velocity of muscle; V'_{fiber}, relative shortening velocity for a given pool of fibers, defined as $V_{o,fiber}$ divided by V_{muscle}; P'_{fiber}, relative amount of force produced by a given pool of fibers, expressed as P divided by P_o. The amount of force produced by the whole muscle is the sum of the individual values for P'_{fiber}.

Example calculation for the fastest pool of fibers, given $p_{fiber} = 0.012$; $V_{o,fiber} = 2.4$ FL/s; $V_{muscle} = 0.05$ FL/s; $a/P_o = 0.25$; $G = 4$.

$$P'_{fiber} = \left[\left(1 - V'_{fiber}\right)/\left(1 + V'_{fiber} \times G\right)\right] \times p_{fiber}$$

$$P'_{fiber} = \left[\left(1 - 0.0208\right)/\left(1 + 0.0208 \times 4\right)\right] \times 0.012 = 0.0110$$

fiber analyses. These can be performed at the native MHC and/or MLC level. The third requirement (regarding V_{max}) can be met by actually making such measurements or by using published data, as Caiozzo and associates (12) did. The publications of Reiser and associates (28), Bottinelli (3), Bottinelli and associates (29), Larsen and Moss (30), and Edman and associates (18) have been pivotal in establishing the relationships between MCH and MLC isoforms and maximal shortening velocity as defined by V_{max} or V_o.

With respect to modeling the force–velocity relationships of various muscles in the rat, there are few true slow muscles like the soleus. Rather, most muscles are composed of various pools of monomorphic and polymorphic fast fibers. This is true even for so-called red regions of mus-

cles like the medial gastrocnemius. The modeling of force–velocity relationships of rodent hindlimb muscle suggests that there is a high degree of convergence, meaning that the differences in force–velocity relationships are subtle, not dramatic (12).

Hill's model has also been used to examine transitions in MHC isoform composition. Mechanical overload (e.g., compensatory overload; resistance training) has been shown to produce a fast-to-slow transition in myosin isoform phenotype in both humans and nonhuman species. Compensatory overload of the rat plantaris muscle typically produces a large increase in the percentage of fibers expressing the slow type I MHC isoform. On this basis, one might predict that V_{max} would be reduced in accordance with the increased percentage of fibers expressing the slow type I MHC isoform. Single-fiber electrophoretic analyses reveal, however, that there is no large increase in fibers that exclusively express the slow type I MHC isoform. Rather, the up-regulation of the slow type I MHC isoform results in polymorphic fibers that are typically dominated by a large proportion of fast MHC isoforms. In one study (26), the modeling of the force–velocity relationship using Hill's approach suggested that V_{max} of the whole muscle should be decreased mildly (about 10–15%) by compensatory overload, and this was close to the actual 14% decrease that was observed. Whether by design or coincidence, MHC isoform shifts that produce polymorphism (rather than monomorphic changes) seem to minimize the functional consequences of MHC isoform transitions (26).

Factors such as mechanical unloading (e.g., as accompanies cast immobilization) and altered thyroid hormone status will produce shifts in the contractile and regulatory contractile protein isoform profiles such that muscles and muscle fibers will become faster. For instance, cast immobilization may lead to a transition from the slow type I to the fast type IIX MHC isoform. From a functional perspective, this will lead to an increase in V_{max}. While it is commonly thought that strength training is an effective tool for increasing sprint speed, this appears to produce fast-to-slow transitions in MHC isoform expression.

V_o: A Measure of Maximal Unloaded Shortening Velocity

The maximal shortening velocity of a skeletal muscle or muscle fiber can be measured using any of several approaches. One method is extrapolation of the force–velocity relationship to where it intersects the Y-axis (Table 5.3, Fig. 5.6). This predicted maximal shortening velocity is typically referred to as V_{max}. Often, however, V_{max} does not provide an accurate estimate of a muscle's true maximal shortening velocity. There are several reasons for this. First, the force–velocity relationship is a composite that reflects the individual force–velocity relationships of all of the fibers. Hence, the shape of a muscle's force–velocity relationship can be biased by the slowest fibers such that V_{max} underestimates the true maximal shortening velocity (26). Additionally, the force–velocity relationship is typically modeled as though it perfectly fits a rectangular hyperbola, which it does not. Indeed, Hill noted that the force–velocity relationship deviated from a rectangular hyperbola in the low-force region (12). The degree to which V_{max} underestimates the true maximal shortening velocity depends on the muscle fiber composition of a muscle, and the underestimation will be the greatest in muscle with a large proportion of slow fibers and a small pool of fast fibers.

Another approach that is commonly used to measure maximal shortening velocity is the slack test (Table 5.3). Using this approach, the muscle is fully activated and allowed to rise to its isometric plateau. A rapid decrease in muscle length is then imposed on the muscle such that the velocity of the length step greatly exceeds the maximal shortening velocity of the muscle. This maneuver imposes a slack in the muscle and allows the muscle to contract against zero external load until the slack is taken up. The time required to take up the slack is defined as the interval between the onset of the length step and the reappearance of force. Performing a series of quick releases that vary in the length steps allows for plotting the relationship between length step amplitude and the time required to take up slack (Table 5.3). The slope of this relationship then defines maximal unloaded shortening velocity (V_o).

Changes in Maximal Shortening Velocity Without Concomitant Changes in MHC Isoform Expression

Key studies (3,4,28) have clearly established a relationship between MHC isoform expression and maximal shortening velocity. However, McDonald and colleagues (31) have consistently observed that mechanical unloading of slow type I fibers produces an increase in maximal shortening velocity (as defined by either V_{max} or V_o) without a concomitant slow-to-fast transition in MHC isoform expression. There are several possible explanations for these findings. First, unloading may produce an isoform transition that cannot be identified by current methods. Second, mechanical unloading of skeletal muscle produces significant alterations in the ultrastructure of skeletal muscle. For instance, it appears as though mechanical unloading may selectively reduce the density of thin filaments. The altered lattice structure that accompanies mechanical unloading may affect the interaction between actin and myosin such that it influences crossbridge cycling and increases maximal shortening velocity.

The Plasticity of the Force–Velocity Relationship in the Lengthening Domain (Factor 5)

While a great deal of attention has been given to the mechanical properties of skeletal muscle under isometric and shortening conditions, much less has been directed toward understanding the mechanical properties of skeletal muscles while actively lengthened. This is true especially with respect to conditions where the physiological conditions have been altered (e.g., altered loading state).

The force–velocity relationship in the lengthening domain is often represented as shown in Figure 5.6. However, the response of activated skeletal muscle to a lengthening contraction is much more complex than that shown in this figure, as is evident in Table 5.3. In the example of a ramp stretch shown in Table 5.3, the muscle is fully activated and allowed to rise onto its isometric plateau. When a ramp stretch equivalent to a strain rate of about 0.6 muscle lengths (ML) per second is imposed on the muscle, there is a very rapid rise in force above the isometric baseline. After a strain of approximately 1 to 2%, there is a dramatic yield in the force record such that force continues to rise but more slowly. This single example illustrates several key points. First, during the initial phase of stretch, tension rises even though the lengthening velocity is constant. This response is quite different from that seen under shortening conditions, and it indicates that in the lengthening domain the force–velocity relationship cannot simply be described by a planar curve, as it is in the shortening domain. Rather, in the lengthening domain, the force–velocity relationship is three-dimensional, with axes of lengthening velocity, force, and time. Second, a further complication in understanding the force–velocity relationship in the lengthening domain is the yield that occurs after a strain of approximately 1 to 2%. This yield may occur because (a) there is a rapid detachment of crossbridges and/or (b) so-called weaker sarcomeres pop. It is not clear which mechanism accounts for this yield.

In performing ramp stretches like those shown in Table 5.3, a number of mechanical measurements can be made. Some of these include stiffness (k) and elastic modulus (E). Stiffness (k) is simply the slope of the relationship between force and length ($\Delta P/\Delta L$), and the initial slope of this relationship during a ramp stretch has been defined as short-range stiffness (SRS). Since the force a muscle fiber can generate depends on the number of sarcomeres in parallel, stiffness is a function of structural properties such as cross-sectional area. Therefore, a muscle with a physiological cross-sectional area twice that of another muscle will have SRS that is also twice as great. In contrast to stiffness, E is an expression of stiffness that is normalized relative to the architecture and geometry of the muscle. In other words, E is the slope of stress (force per cross-sectional area, or σ) versus strain (relative change in length, or $\Delta L/L_0$; ε) relationship, and E is thought to represent a material property, meaning that it represents an intrinsic property of the material. Given this example, the muscle with twice the physiological cross-sectional area will have an E that is the same as that of the smaller muscle.

To date, few studies have attempted to examine the importance of muscle fiber type on the shape of the force–velocity relationship in the lengthening domain. As noted earlier, such studies are complicated, given that this relationship in the lengthening domain is three-dimensional and there appears to be a yield in the force record after a strain of about 1 to 2%. With focus on the force record before yield (for simplicity), it is not clear whether there should be a dependence on fiber type. It could be argued that the slower crossbridge cycling rate found in slow type I fibers will cause these slower crossbridges to be strained to a greater extent (at any given velocity) prior to detachment and that this will result in a more rapid rise in force during the initial phase of stretch (the phase before yield). Alternatively, while faster crossbridges may detach faster, they will also reattach faster, thereby offsetting or minimizing any potential influence of fiber type dependence. Obviously, more studies are needed to clarify whether the lengthening domain of the force–velocity relationship depends on fiber type.

Muscles constantly undergo cyclic activity during which they are loaded in the lengthening phase. In some instances, activation during the lengthening phase is necessary for motor control, and in others, the forcible lengthening of skeletal muscle may play an important role in protecting joints from ligamentous injury. Ligaments are often referred to as static joint stabilizers, whereas muscles are thought to function as dynamic joint stabilizers. Hypothetically, muscles that undergo atrophy and as a consequence have a reduction in stiffness presumably will act as poorer joint stabilizers and place the involved joint at greater risk for injury. Alternatively, muscles that hypertrophy in response to resistance training will have a greater stiffness and provide the involved joint with greater protection. It has been postulated that the higher incidence of knee ligament injuries in women may be due to weaker quadriceps that act as poorer joint stabilizers (32).

To date, few studies have examined the effects of mechanical unloading (as might result from cast immobilization) on SRS, E, and the force–velocity relationship in the lengthening domain. Stiffness is thought to be a structural property, as noted earlier, but in reality it depends not only on the physiological cross-sectional area but also on the E. It might be presumed that mechanical unloading simply affects stiffness by reducing the number of sarcomeres in parallel. This, however, is not the case, as E also appears to be influenced by such perturbed physiological conditions. The effects of mechanical unloading on E can be quite substantial, reducing E by 50% or more. The possible mechanisms responsible for such a large loss in E may include (a) a decrease in unitary crossbridge stiffness and/or (b) a reduction in the density of attached crossbridges. With respect to this second mechanism, a number of alterations may be responsible for the loss in E. First, there may be a number of dysfunctional myofibrils undergoing degeneration and/or disarray due to protein degradation. Second, thin filaments may have been altered so that their lengths are short or they are not attached to the Z-line. Third, there may be selective thin filament loss as reported by Riley and associates (33).

The Concept of Work Loops

The mechanical measurements described thus far result from experimental conditions in which the muscle produces single submaximal (twitch, force–frequency, tension–pCa++) or maximal contractions (force–velocity relationship). The ability of skeletal muscle to produce mechanical work and power can be calculated from the force–velocity relationship, but these are measures of so-called instantaneous mechanical work and power (Fig. 5.6). Typically, force–velocity and power curves are derived from conditions in which the contractile apparatus is fully activated. Hence, such measures of instantaneous mechanical work and power do not take into account issues related to activation and relaxation that must occur during cyclic activity. In this framework, the work loop technique popularized by Josephson (20) represents an approach for studying the mechanical properties of skeletal muscle during cyclic shortening and lengthening contractions.

An example of a work loop is shown in Table 5.3. In this example, the muscle undergoes a series of cyclic changes in length. The net mechanical work produced during a work loop can be calculated as

$$\text{Net mechanical work} = \underset{\begin{pmatrix} \text{shortening domain} \end{pmatrix}}{\overset{\text{work}}{\text{positive mechanical}}} - \underset{\begin{pmatrix} \text{lengthening domain} \end{pmatrix}}{\overset{\text{work}}{\text{negative mechanical}}}$$

[Equation 5.5]

While this formula is very basic, the factors that dictate the amount of positive and negative mechanical work produced during single or repetitive contractions are numerous and quite complex. This complexity, illustrated in Figure 5.4, involves the integration of all six design criteria noted earlier. If activation and relaxation were instantaneous events, the mechanical work and power a muscle could produce under any work loop condition would simply be defined by the theoretical work loop. A theoretical work loop can be developed by (a) determining the force–velocity relationship and (b) using this information to predict the force developed at any given velocity throughout the shortening phase of the work loop. Since neither activation nor relaxation is instantaneous, however, the amount of mechanical work and power that can be realized will always be less than predicted from the theoretical work loop. Given this backdrop, the question is, how important are the rates of activation and relaxation in limiting the production of mechanical work and power during cyclic activity?

The Rate of Activation (Factor 2)

Activation is a term applied to turning on the contractile apparatus, and the speed with which it occurs can be defined by measures such as dP/dt. As indicated in Figure 5.2, this involves a complex set of events that primarily includes (a) the release of Ca^{++} from the SR and the binding of Ca^{++} to TnC and (b) the rate of crossbridge cycling. From a temporal perspective, the release of Ca^{++} from the SR occurs quite rapidly, so that the rise in tension substantially lags behind the rise in Ca^{++}.

The limitations that activation and relaxation can impose on the production of mechanical work and power during cyclic activity depend on the frequency of length change. At a low frequency, 0.5 Hz for example, the shortening phase (1000 ms) is sufficiently long that the rate of neither activation nor relaxation imposes significant limitations. However, at a higher frequency, 4 Hz, the shortening phase becomes temporally compressed (125 ms in this example) such that processes involved in turning the contractile apparatus on (activation) and off (relaxation) may impose significant limitations.

In looking at the time course of a twitch in skeletal muscle fibers (especially slow type I fibers), TPT is often

much shorter than for complete relaxation. Such observations suggest that the rate of relaxation may impose a greater limitation on the production of mechanical work than the rate of activation. Consistent with this perspective, it appears as though factors controlling the rate of activation account for a relatively small amount of unrealized work (about 5 to 10%) in slow muscles like the soleus. Hence, even in slow skeletal muscles, the rate of activation does not impose a large limitation in producing mechanical work.

The Rate of Relaxation (Factor 4)

The rate of relaxation can be studied from a variety of perspectives. For instance, it can be described using measurements like $\frac{1}{2}$ RT. Alternatively, the rate of relaxation has also been studied using measures of −dP/dt. The main factors responsible for controlling the rate of relaxation are shown in Figure 5.4, and it is known that most (if not all) of these can be influenced by changes in neural, mechanical, and hormonal status.

Typically, the rate of relaxation is measured under isometric conditions, and so the true physiological relevance of such measurements is not clear. As noted earlier, we have used the work loop approach to provide an alternative perspective regarding the importance or relaxation kinetics, and our findings suggest that under some conditions the rate of relaxation may limit the production of mechanical work and power by about 50%. It has also been shown that this modulatory influence of relaxation kinetics can be dramatically altered by interventions such as mechanical unloading and hyperthyroidism. Each of these interventions significantly increases the rate of relaxation, such that a muscle can produce much more work under certain work loop conditions (5).

The rate of relaxation also appears to be length dependent in slow muscles and muscle fibers such that at lengths beyond L_o, $\frac{1}{2}$ RT increases substantially. This length dependence of relaxation may be due to the presence of the cTnC isoform.

Physiological perturbations such as mechanical unloading are known to increase the rate of relaxation in slow skeletal muscles and muscle fibers. For instance, Schulte and associates (34) observed that 28 days of hindlimb unloading produced a large increase in the fast SERCA isoform at both the protein and mRNA levels, and this led to a 170% increase in Ca^{++} ATPase activity.

Conditions such as immobilization and mechanical unloading produce significant amounts of atrophy and hence markedly reduce the ability of skeletal muscle to produce mechanical work and power. However, the mechanical unloading of slow skeletal muscle fibers produces compensatory effects that are manifested in (a) a slow $\rightarrow$ fast MHC isoform transition and (b) an increased rate of Ca^{++} sequestration. The first effect, via its influence on the force–velocity relationship, partially minimizes the loss of peak power predicted to occur from a reduction in the ability to produce force. The second effect (increased rate of Ca^{++}) means that the muscle can effectively operate and produce mechanical work at higher than normal cycling frequencies.

The Passive Stiffness of Skeletal Muscle (Factor 6)

During cyclic locomotor activity, the work required to lengthen a muscle depends on (a) the degree of activation, (b) the force–velocity relationship in the lengthening domain, and (c) the passive stiffness of the muscle. If the muscle is completely relaxed, the first two factors can be ignored and the work required to lengthen the muscle simply depends on the passive stiffness of the muscle. The passive stiffness of skeletal muscle can be measured by several means. One of these involves performing cyclic sinusoidal length changes with the muscle or muscle fiber in a passive state. This type of approach provides a more realistic and instantaneous measure of passive stiffness than other techniques like the stretch–release technique, with which measurements of passive stiffness are made under static conditions. The stretch–release approach involves small stepwise increments or decrements in stretch, and typically a step change in length is held for several minutes to allow for stress relaxation. The slope of the force–deformation curve represents stiffness, and if it is normalized to cross-sectional area and length, then E under passive conditions can be determined.

The passive stiffness and E of skeletal muscle are thought to be due to (a) the connective tissue content of skeletal muscle and (b) the presence of sarcomeric proteins like titin. Titin is sometimes referred to as a molecular spring, and it is a giant molecule (27,000 amino acids) with a molecular weight of about 3 Mda. Titin extends from the Z-line into the M-line, and it is the I-band segment of titin that is thought to possess the properties of a molecular spring. In this region three key segments have been identified as the (a) PEVK region, (b) the immunoglobulin (Ig) segments that flank the PEVK region, and (c) N2A segments. A number of titin isoforms have been identified, and these are believed to be partially responsible for differences in the passive properties of various types of muscles (slow, fast, cardiac).

Few studies to date have examined the effects of altered mechanical loading on the passive properties and titin content of single fibers. In one of the few studies in this area, Toursel et al. (35) reported that mechanical unloading of the soleus muscle actually produced a decrease in E under passive conditions. With respect to titin, this might occur as a result of transitions in titin isoforms or a reduction in the amount of titin per unit volume. Toursel et al. (35) observed that the reduction in E occurred in the absence of titin isoform transitions. Interestingly, there was a reduction in the titin–MHC ratio, and this finding is consistent with the hypothesis that the reduction in the passive E may have been partially or entirely due to a selective loss of titin per unit volume.

Structure–Function Relationships: Lessons Learned From Comparative Physiology

Overview

Comparative physiology, given its interest in organismal function, shares many interests with exercise physiology and provides a potentially beneficial perspective for thinking about structure–function relationships and their plasticity. In this section, design constraints are considered further, but from a comparative approach. When combined with earlier sections, this provides an important backdrop for discussing symmorphosis and the concept of optimality. One of the attractive features of the comparative approach is that it provides a broader survey of structure–function relationships and so may provide better insight into the actual rules of muscle plasticity.

As stated earlier, the briefest mechanical event that a muscle can produce is an isometric twitch, and this is simply the response to a single stimulus. The amplitude and time course of a twitch are defined by factors i to iv shown in Figure 5.5. The duration of a twitch can be quite short in some vertebrates, whereas in others it can be much longer. For instance, in sonic muscles of some fish (used for mating), the total twitch is very short (about 10–20 ms) and the muscles can operate at frequencies of 100 to 200 Hz. Similarly, the shaker muscles of rattlesnakes also have short twitches and can operate at frequencies of about 90 Hz. Human skeletal muscle fibers, in contrast, have much longer (about 250 ms) isometric twitches, and as a consequence are confined to operate at low frequencies (about 2–5 Hz).

As eloquently addressed by Rome and Linstedt (36), the simple contrast between sonic and shaker muscles brings forth some important design considerations that can be summarized as follows: ultimately the performance of a muscle largely depends on the distribution of SR, myofibrillar, and mitochondrial volumes. These general design considerations can be illustrated using the following examples. Muscles that operate at high frequencies are obligated to have fast Ca^{++} cycling kinetics, and as a result, a relatively large proportion of cell volume must be dedicated to the SR (in some instances more than 25% of the cell volume). If such muscles are active for long periods, a significant amount of the cell volume must also be dedicated to the mitochondria. In such muscles, the myofibrillar volume is relatively small and the muscles cannot generate large forces when normalized to cross-sectional area. Alternatively, if the muscles are active for only short durations, a much greater proportion of the cell volume can be occupied by myofibrils, allowing the muscle to generate moderate to large forces. The myofibrillar volume density is greatest in muscles optimized to produce force, but the tradeoff is that these muscles cannot operate at high oscillatory frequencies or support high levels of metabolic activity. Finally, muscles that are required to support high metabolic levels for long periods (like flight muscles) must have large mitochondrial volumes (e.g., 35% of the total cell volume), and this will correspondingly impose limitations on the SR and myofibrillar volumes and the functions they support. Given this perspective, most human skeletal muscles appear to be optimized for myofibrillar volume, suggesting that the generation of force may have been a prime factor in the evolution of human muscles.

Herein lies one of the unique aspects of contractile protein isoforms given the three-compartment model (SR, myofibril, mitochondria). The presence of contractile protein isoforms confirms a level of functional plasticity that can occur in the absence of changes in compartment volumes.

Symmorphosis and the Concept of Optimality

Collectively, the tradeoffs for space were referred to by Rome and Linstedt (36) as the "zero sum game." Some might extend this concept to state that muscles and muscle fibers are perfectly adapted to the physiological tasks that they perform. In this context, Weibel and associates proposed the concept of optimality of design in physiological structures: the concept of symmorphosis (37). This was defined as the perfect matching of structure to functional need, such that no excess capacity was maintained. In terms of energetic efficiency, the metabolic cost of building and maintaining structures superfluous to maximal performance should be prohibitive. Given the perspective described earlier relative to the three-compartment model, the concept of symmorphosis would postulate, for instance, that mitochondrial volume density is perfectly matched to the energetic requirements of the SR and myofibrils. Certainly the adjustment of muscle structure to higher functional demands (training) and the reverse when training ceases suggests a cost-to-benefit relationship may help shape "optimization" of muscle.

The notion of economical design in animals is not a recent one, but the formulation of symmorphosis has been a stimulus to much interesting research. It is an appealing and seemingly intuitive concept of design, and the discussion of the applicability of economy of structural costs to the evolution of organisms is a very fruitful area of investigation. However, as Diamond and Hammond (38) remarked, "The concept is worth posing not because we believe it to be literally true, but because only by posing [it] . . . can one hope to detect where it breaks down, and to identify the interesting reason for its breakdown."

SUMMARY

One of the tenets of biology is that structure determines function. Perhaps one of the best examples of this principle, at the cellular level, is found within skeletal muscle

fibers. Most notably, the structure of the sarcome contractile unit of both skeletal and cardiac muscle, mines many functional properties. Other key struc components of skeletal muscle include the SR and the mitochondria. During the past 30 years, it has become clear that skeletal muscle possesses a remarkable degree of plasticity as defined by structural changes in sarcomeres, the SR, and mitochondria. Such changes result in distinct functional consequences.

The objectives of this chapter are threefold. The first objective is to provide a brief overview of the macroscopic and microscopic structural design features of skeletal muscle. In presenting this overview, a specific emphasis is placed on describing the enormous numbers of sarcomeres and myosin molecules typically found within an individual muscle fiber. It is hoped that such examples illustrate both the complexity and the beauty of skeletal muscle design. Beyond such consideration, however, many of the so-called sarcomeric proteins exist as isoforms. For instance, in human skeletal muscle there are three protein isoforms of the adult MHC. Importantly, the presence of contractile protein isoforms confirms a level of functional plasticity that can occur in the absence of changes in the compartmental volumes (e.g., the myofibril), and as such, this represents a very important design consideration. The second objective of this chapter is to introduce both simple and complex mechanical measurements and to describe some of the underlying structural basis for key mechanical properties. This section of the chapter provides a detailed description of the force–velocity relationship and its plasticity. The basis for this emphasis is the observation that the force–velocity relationship represents a theoretical limit to muscle performance under all loading conditions and levels of excitation. Furthermore, very little is known about the shape, fiber type dependence, and plasticity of the force–velocity relationship in the lengthening domain. Importantly, this region of the force–velocity relationship is much different from that found in the shortening domain, and perhaps more complex as well. The third and final objective of this chapter is to introduce the potential power of the comparative physiology paradigm. One of the attractive features of the comparative approach is that it provides a broader survey of structure–function relationships, and so may provide better insight into the actual rule of muscle plasticity. A general but very important rule that evolved from this type of approach is that the performance of a muscle largely depends on the distribution of SR, myofibrillar, and mitochondrial volumes. Typically, the myofibrillar volume represents approximately 85 to 90% of the total volume of a human skeletal muscle fiber. The relative myofibrillar volume changes little with altered physical activity. The same observation also applies to the SR and mitochondrial volumes, but even small changes in the relative proportions of either of these two fractions may result in relatively large functional changes.

It is widely recognized that the structural and functional properties of skeletal muscles are under the influence of neural, mechanical, and hormonal factors. Although the specific rules of muscle plasticity remain to be completely elucidated, significant strides have been made on a number of fronts. Much of what has evolved emanated from landmark studies like that of Buller, Eccles, and Eccles. In this classic study, these investigators used a cross-innervation or cross-union paradigm whereby the slow soleus muscle of cat was reinnervated with the motor nerve of the fast flexor digitorum longus (FDL) muscle, and the FDL was reinnervated with the motor nerve from the soleus muscle. On the contralateral side, the motor nerves innervating a given muscle were simply cut and the ends sutured together. By contrasting the cross-innervated group with the reinnervated group, Buller, Eccles, and Eccles were able to account for changes induced by cross-innervation (Fig. 5.7).

Remarkably, these investigators observed that the cross-innervated slow soleus muscle adopted the functional properties of a fast muscle, while the cross-innervated fast FDL developed slower contractile properties. This occurred without any corresponding changes in the properties of the motor neurons. On the surface, these findings appear to agree with the frequency hypothesis, which simply states that the low firing frequency of motor neurons innervating the soleus muscle would cause the FDL to become a slower muscle, and the converse would be true of the high firing frequency of the motor neurons innervating the FDL. Interestingly, Buller, Eccles, and Eccles did not interpret these findings to support the frequency hypothesis. Rather, they reasoned that if the frequency hypothesis were correct, the complete cessa-

tion of stimulation should produce an even slower phenotype, which it did not. Their reasoning was apparently based on directional changes in firing frequency (i.e., progressively lower firing frequencies produce progressively slower phenotypes and vice versa).

Buller, Eccles, and Eccles also tested the aggregate hypothesis, which stipulated that the slow tonic firing pattern of the soleus motor nerve would result in a greater aggregate of impulses and hence a slower phenotype, whereas the phasic firing pattern of the fast motor nerve would produce a smaller aggregate and thereby faster contractile properties. The cross-innervation findings were certainly consistent with this hypothesis. However, Buller, Eccles, and Eccles observed that a complete lack of activation (as studied by spinal isolation) actually caused a fast muscle to become slower and not faster, as predicted by the aggregate hypothesis. Having rejected both the frequency and aggregate hypotheses, these investigators proposed the chemical hypothesis, which stated that motor neurons control the contractile properties of skeletal muscle by releasing a chemical (later referred to as trophic) substance that traverses the neuromuscular junction and then spreads along the length of the muscle fiber. Some 45 years later it is still unclear whether a trophic substance is produced by motor neurons. However, it is clear that this landmark study shaped several generations of scientific investigation and provided critical evidence to demonstrate that skeletal muscle possessed a plasticity that was previously unrecognized.

Buller AJ, Eccles JC, Eccles RM. Interaction between motoneurones and muscles in respect of the characteristic speeds of their responses. J Physiol (Lond) 1960;150:417–439.

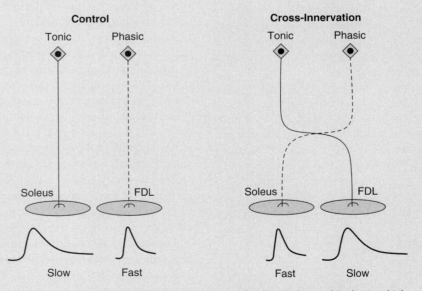

FIGURE 5.7 The cross-innervation experiment of Buller, Eccles, and Eccles in which the motor nerve to the flexor digitorum longus muscle (FDL) was changed to innervate the soleus muscle, whereas the motor nerve to the soleus muscle was altered so that it would innervate the FDL muscle.

ACKNOWLEDGMENTS

We appreciate the insight and comments of Dr. Kenneth M. Baldwin. This work was supported in part by NIH AR 46856 (VJC) and NIH F32 AR47749 (BCR).

REFERENCES

1. Huxley AF. Muscle structure and theories of contraction. Prog Biophys Chem 1957;7:255–318.
2. Clark KA, McElhinny AS, Beckerle MC, et al. Striated muscle cytoarchitecture: an intricate web of form and function. Annu Rev Cell Dev Biol 2002;18:637–706.
3. Bottinelli R. Functional heterogeneity of mammalian single muscle fibres: do myosin isoforms tell the whole story? Pflüger's Arch 2001;443:6–17.
4. Bottinelli R, Betto R, Schiaffino S, et al. Unloaded shortening velocity and myosin heavy chain and alkali light chain isoform composition in rat skeletal muscle fibres. J Physiol (Lond) 1994;478:341–349.
5. Caiozzo VJ. Plasticity of skeletal muscle phenotype: mechanical consequences. Muscle Nerve 2002;26:740–768.
6. Pette D, Staron RS. Cellular and molecular diversities of mammalian skeletal muscle fibers. Rev Physiol Biochem Pharmacol 1990;116:1–76.
7. Schiaffino S, Reggiani C. Myosin isoforms in mammalian skeletal muscle. J Appl Physiol 1994;77:493–501.
8. Brooke MH, Kaiser KK. Muscle fiber types: how many and what kind? Arch Neurol 1970;23:369–379.
9. Barnard RJ, Edgerton VR, Furukawa T, et al. Histochemical, biochemical, and contractile properties of red, white, and intermediate fibers. Am J Physiol 1971;220:410–414.
10. Pette D, Staron RS. Transitions of muscle fiber phenotypic profiles. Histochem Cell Biol 2001;115:359–372.
11. Saltin B, Gollnick PD. Skeletal muscle adaptability: significance for metabolism and performance. In Peachey L, ed. Handbook of Physiology. Bethesda: American Physiological Society, 555–631.
12. Caiozzo VJ, Baker MJ, Huang K, et al. Single-fiber myosin heavy chain polymorphism: how many patterns and what proportions? Am J Physiol 2003;285:R570–580.
13. Talmadge RJ, Roy RR, Edgerton VR. Persistence of hybrid fibers in rat soleus after spinal cord transection. Anat Rec 1999;255:188–201.
14. Caiozzo VJ, Baker MJ, Baldwin KM. Novel transitions in MHC isoforms: separate and combined effects of thyroid hormone and mechanical unloading. J Appl Physiol 1998;85(6):2237–2248.
15. Talmadge RJ, Roy RR, Edgerton VR. Distribution of myosin heavy chain isoforms in non-weight-bearing rat soleus muscle fibers. J Appl Physiol 1996;81:2540–2546.
16. Hall ZW, Ralson E. Nuclear domains in muscle cells. Cell 1989;59:771–772.
17. Peuker H, Pette D. Quantitative analyses of myosin heavy-chain mRNA and protein isoforms in single fibers reveal a pronounced fiber heterogeneity in normal rabbit muscles. Eur J Biochem 1997;247:30–36.
18. Edman KA, Reggiani C, Schiaffino S, et al. Maximum velocity of shortening related to myosin isoform composition in frog skeletal muscle fibres. J Physiol (Lond) 1988;395:679–694.
19. Rome LC, Linstedt SI. Mechanical and metabolic design of the muscular system in vertebrates. In Dantzler WH ed. Comparative Physiology. New York: Oxford University, 1997;1587–1651.
20. Josephson RK. Dissecting muscle power output. J Exp Biol 1999;202(pt 23):3369–3375.
21. Booth FW, Baldwin KM. Muscle plasticity: energy demand and supply processes. In Rowell LB, Shepard JT, eds. Exercise: Regulation and Integration of Multiple Systems. New York: Oxford University, 1996;1075–1123.
22. Friden J, Lieber RL. Spastic muscle cells are shorter and stiffer than normal cells. Muscle Nerve 2003;27:157–164.
23. Lieber RL, Friden J. Spasticity causes a fundamental rearrangement of muscle-joint interaction. Muscle Nerve 2002;25:265–270.
24. Hill AV. First and Last Experiments in Muscle Mechanics. New York: Cambridge University, 1970.
25. Woledge RC, Curtin NA, Homsher E. Energetic aspects of muscle contraction. New York: Academic Press, 1985;357.
26. Caiozzo VJ, Haddad F, Baker M, et al. MHC polymorphism in rodent plantaris muscle: effects of mechanical overload and hypothyroidism. Am J Physiol 2000;278:C709–C717.
27. Josephson RK, Edman KA. The consequences of fibre heterogeneity on the force-velocity relation of skeletal muscle. Acta Physiol Scand 1988;132:341–352.
28. Reiser PJ, Kasper CE, Moss RL. Myosin subunits and contractile properties of single fibers from hypokinetic rat muscles. J Appl Physiol 1987;63:2293–2300.
29. Bottinelli R, Schiaffino S, Reggiani C. Force-velocity relations and myosin heavy chain isoform compositions of skinned fibres from rat skeletal muscle. J Physiol (Lond) 1991;437:655–672.
30. Larsson L, Moss RL. Maximum velocity of shortening in relation to myosin isoform composition in single fibres from human skeletal muscles. J Physiol (Lond) 1993;472:595–614.
31. McDonald KS, Blaser CA, Fitts RH. Force-velocity and power characteristics of rat soleus muscle fibers after hindlimb suspension. J Appl Physiol 1994;77:1609–1616.
32. Wojtys EM, Huston LJ, Schock HJ, et al. Gender differences in muscular protection of the knee in torsion in size-matched athletes. J Bone Joint Surg Am 2003;85-A:782–789.
33. Riley DA, Bain JL, Thompson JL, et al. Decreased thin filament density and length in human atrophic soleus muscle fibers after spaceflight. J Appl Physiol 2000;88:567–572.
34. Schulte LM, Navarro J, Kandarian SC. Regulation of sarcoplasmic reticulum calcium pump gene expression by hindlimb unweighting. Am J Physiol 1993;264:C1308–C1315.
35. Toursel T, Stevens L, Granzier H, et al. Passive tension of rat skeletal soleus muscle fibers: effects of unloading conditions. J Appl Physiol 2002;92:1465–1472.
36. Rome LC, Linstedt SI. The quest for speed: muscles built for high-frequency contractions. NIPS 1998;13:261–268.
37. Weibel ER, Taylor CR, Hoppeler H. The concept of symmorphosis: a testable hypothesis of structure-function relationship. Proc Natl Acad Sci USA 1991;88:10357–10361.
38. Diamond J, Hammond K. The matches, achieved by natural selection, between biological capacities and their natural loads. Experientia 1992;48:551–557.

CHAPTER 6

The Muscular System: Design, Function, and Performance Relationships

PER AAGAARD AND JENS BANGSBO

Introduction

The muscular system consists of a multitude of components, which have important influence on the mechanical and metabolic behavior of the muscle (Fig. 6.1). Muscle morphology and architecture, along with myosin isoform composition, play a major role in the contractile strength characteristics of the muscle, evaluated as maximal isometric, concentric, and eccentric contraction force and maximal rate of force development and power generation. Glycolytic muscle enzyme levels and ionic transport systems are the major determinants of anaerobic muscle performance, when expressed either as anaerobic power or as anaerobic capacity. Likewise, mitochondrial enzyme levels and capillary density exert a strong influence on aerobic muscle performance. In turn these factors affect the force development and maximal power output of human skeletal muscle and influence the endurance performance of the muscle fibers.

This chapter describes the influence of muscle morphology, muscle architecture, myosin isoform composition, glycolytic and mitochondrial enzyme levels, ionic transport systems, and capillary density on the contractile strength characteristics, energy production, fatigue behavior, and endurance performance of human skeletal muscle *in vivo*. Further, the chapter addresses the adaptive plasticity of these factors seen with training and inactivity.

Basic Mechanical Properties of Skeletal Muscle: Functional Implications

As described in detail for the first time by Hill in 1938, there is a reciprocal relationship between contractile muscle force and shortening speed, and it relies on the inherent mechanical properties of the muscle (1) (see Milestone of Discovery). More specifically, contraction force varies with the velocity of shortening in an inverse hyperbolic manner, as initially observed for isolated muscle *in vitro* (1) (Fig. 6.2). Similar hyperbolic force–velocity relationships may be observed during maximal voluntary contraction of human skeletal muscle *in vivo*, although force–velocity patterns that were distinctly not hyperbolic have been reported (Fig. 6.3). At the microscopic level, however, isolated single muscle fibers, including human skeletal muscle fibers, appear to follow a hyperbolic force–velocity relationship that closely resembles the one observed for whole muscle *in vitro*.

The maximal contractile strength (joint torque) generated by human skeletal muscle *in vivo* has been investigated in well-controlled experimental conditions by use of isokinetic dynamometers. Isokinetic dynamometry is particularly useful to evaluate the expression of maximal volitional muscle strength both during controlled lengthening (eccentric) and shortening (concentric) muscle contraction

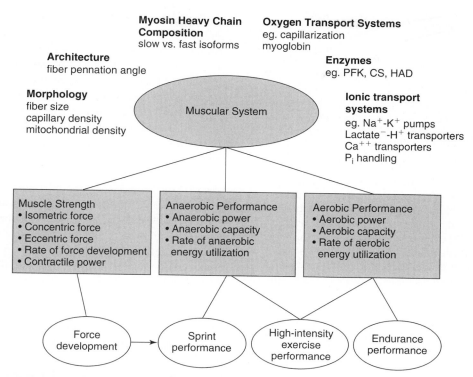

FIGURE 6.1   The muscular system consists of a multitude of components with important influence on the mechanical and metabolic behavior of the muscle. Muscle morphology, muscle architecture, and myosin isoform composition play a major role in the contractile strength characteristics of the muscle, which *in vivo* is modulated by the central nervous system. Glycolytic enzyme levels and ion transport systems are the major determinants of anaerobic muscle performance, while mitochondrial enzyme levels and capillary density exert a strong influence on aerobic muscle performance.

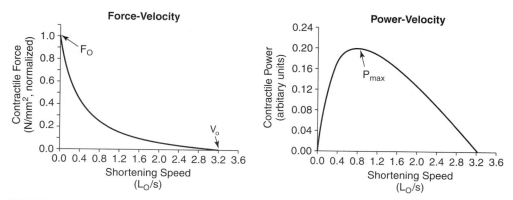

FIGURE 6.2   In isolated muscle preparations and in single muscle fibers, an inverse hyperbolic relationship is observed between muscle contraction force and velocity of shortening (*left*). Contractile power is generated by multiplying force and velocity at any given shortening velocity (*right*). Maximal isometric contraction force (F_o), unloaded shortening speed (V_o), and maximal contractile power (P_{max}) are shown. Equation is discussed in Box 6.1.

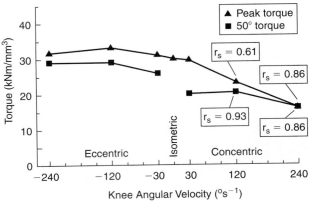

FIGURE 6.3 Maximal concentric and eccentric muscle strength (quadriceps femoris) measured *in vivo* by use of iso-kinetic dynamometry. Maximal muscle strength was obtained both as peak torque and constant-angle torque generated at 50° knee joint angle (0° = full knee extension). Negative knee joint angular velocities denote eccentric muscle contraction, while positive velocities denote concentric muscle contraction. Zero velocity denotes maximal isometric quadriceps strength, obtained at 70° knee joint angle. Boxes show the relationship (Spearman's Rho, r_s) between maximal concentric contraction strength (knee extension torque relative to muscle volume) and the proportion of fast type II MHC isoforms in the vastus lateralis muscle. During concentric contraction significant relationships were observed at medium to fast contraction speeds, characterized by very short contraction times (~100–300 ms), with which a high intrinsic rate of force development becomes particularly important. *(Modified from Aagaard P, Andersen JL. Correlation between contractile strength and myosin heavy chain isoform composition in human skeletal muscle. Med Sci Sports Exerc 1998;30:1217–1222.)*

(Fig. 6.3). In addition, human contractile muscle function has been assessed in single-joint or two-joint movements by use of flywheel methodology and during more complex movements using force plate analysis. Perhaps the most important feature of modern isokinetic dynamometry is to enable a standardized and reproducible evaluation of eccentric contraction strength. As discussed in more detail later, this aspect of *in vivo* muscle function deserves special attention, since eccentric muscle contraction not only appears to comprise unique mechanisms of neuromuscular activation but also is important for providing dynamic joint stabilization.

The Force–Velocity Relation: Influence of Neural Activation Pattern

When isolated skeletal muscle is activated *in vitro,* maximal eccentric contraction force exceeds maximal isometric and concentric muscle force by 40 to 60% (2). In contrast, maximal eccentric contraction strength is about equal to or only slightly greater than maximal isometric strength and slow

concentric strength when recorded *in vivo* for untrained human skeletal muscle during contraction of maximal voluntary effort (Fig. 6.3). Indications of a deficit in neuromuscular activation during maximal eccentric quadriceps contraction have been observed by superimposing brief tetanic electrical stimulation onto maximal voluntary muscle contraction (3) (Fig. 6.4). This deficiency in eccentric activation is observed only in sedentary subjects and is not present in strength athletes, which suggests that the underlying neural mechanisms can be modulated by training. Reduced levels of neuromuscular activation appear to be reason for the apparent deficit in maximum eccentric muscle strength *in vivo.* Further, maximal eccentric muscle strength has consistently been shown to increase (20–40%) in response to heavy-resistance strength training (3). This training-induced enhancement in maximal eccentric muscle strength may be explained by a removal of the suppression in neural activation (3). In turn, this specific type of neural adaptation has important functional benefits. In everyday life, eccentric muscle actions are mostly involved with the deceleration or damping of specific limb movements, for example in downhill running, descending stairs, or landing from a jump. However, certain types of movements, particularly those encountered in sports and exercise, can involve maximal or near-maximal eccentric muscle forces (i.e., maximal vertical or horizontal jumping). Also, a high level of eccentric contraction strength of the involved antagonist muscle or muscles is important to ensure an optimal joint function *in vivo,* as this allows active deceleration of fast limb movement at the end range of motion, thereby providing protection to ligaments and capsular joint structures during rapid and forceful limb movements. Consequently, an increase in maximal eccentric antagonist muscle strength (induced by resistance training) results in an enhanced capacity for dynamic joint stabilization.

Contractile Rate of Force Development: Implications for Rapid Movements

During many types of human movement the time available for muscle contraction is highly limited. For example, ground contact times or muscle contraction times of 75 to 200 ms can be observed in activities such as sprint running, long jump, karate, and boxing. In human skeletal muscle, however, it typically takes 300 to 400 ms to reach the level of maximal force generation relative to the instant of force onset. Consequently, the rate of force rise (so-called rate of force development: RFD = Δforce/Δtime) in the initial phase of muscle contraction (Fig. 6.5), rather than maximal muscle force, is the main determinant of the contractile force, power, and impulse (hence speed) that can be achieved during fast limb movements (4). In such rapid movements, therefore, it is more important to exert a high contractile RFD in the initial phase of contraction (0–200 ms relative to force onset), rather than reaching a high level of maximal

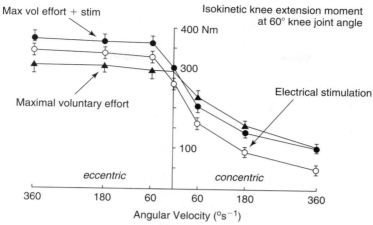

FIGURE 6.4 Maximal concentric, eccentric, and isometric *in vivo* muscle strength obtained in untrained subjects during maximal voluntary activation of the quadriceps femoris muscle (triangles), with percutaneous electrical stimulation applied to the resting muscle (*open circles*), and when electrical stimulation was applied to ongoing maximal voluntary contraction (*solid circles*). Eccentric muscle strength was about 30% greater than isometric strength when the muscle was electrically activated. In contrast, during maximal voluntary activation, eccentric muscle strength was only 5% elevated, suggesting the existence of a neural inhibitory pathway during voluntary eccentric muscle contraction. (*Modified from Westing SH, Seger JY, Thorstensson A. Effects of electrical stimulation on eccentric and concentric torque-velocity relationships during knee extension in man. Acta Physiol Scand 1990;140:17–22.*)

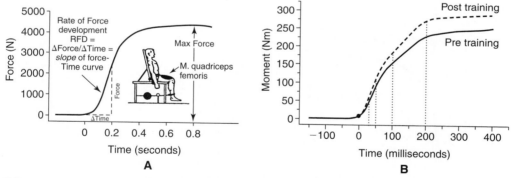

FIGURE 6.5 **A.** Contractile rate of force development (RFD) is defined by the slope of the force-time curve (or the moment-time curve) during maximal isometric muscle contraction. RFD can be calculated as the peak slope as well as the average slope within predefined time intervals, that is, from onset of contraction (time 0) to 200 ms after contraction onset. Contractile RFD is the main determinant of muscle force that can be exerted during rapid muscle contractions (<300 ms) and is as such more important than maximal muscle strength in situations of restricted contraction time. **B.** Group mean force (moment)–time curves obtained in the quadriceps femoris muscle before and after 14 weeks of heavy-resistance strength training (n = 15). Following training, steeper slopes (greater RFD) were observed at time intervals 0 to 30, 50, 100 and 200 ms (dotted vertical lines). (*Modified from Aagaard P, Simonsen EB, Magnusson SP, et al. Increased rate of force development and neural drive of human skeletal muscle following resistance training. J Appl Physiol 2002;93:1318–1326.*)

muscle force later in the contraction phase. For example, to avoid fall accidents caused by transient loss of postural balance, the elderly person may often rely on the ability to exert a rapid rise in contractile force generation within fractions of a second. Notably, RFD has consistently been demonstrated to increase in response to resistance training, in both elderly and young subjects (Fig. 6.5B).

The contractile RFD, also denoted by explosive muscle strength or rapid muscle strength, is positively influenced by

1. The magnitude of efferent neural drive to the muscle fibers, including muscle fiber innervation rate (MU firing frequency)
2. Muscle cross-sectional area (CSA)
3. Muscle fiber type and myosin heavy chain (MHC) isoform composition

Contractile RFD is particularly influenced by muscle fiber innervation rate, as a marked increase in RFD is observed when motor neuron firing frequency is increased (Fig. 6.6A).

When individual motor units are stimulated in animal preparations, RFD continues to increase at stimulation rates higher than necessary to elicit maximal tetanized force (5) (Fig. 6.6A). Similar findings have been observed in whole-muscle preparations and during contraction of human skeletal muscle *in vivo*. Very high MU firing rates, 100 to 400 Hz, may transiently occur at the onset of maximal contraction (6), which likely serves to increase initial RFD rather than increasing maximal contraction force per se. Further support

of a close linkage between maximal MU firing frequency and contractile RFD comes from the finding that resistance training can induce concurrent increases in RFD and maximal MU firing frequency (6).

A large muscle mass (high CSA) will result in a high numerical RFD simply because of a greater capacity for force development. Considering the influence of muscle fiber type, a high proportion of type II MHC isoforms also is associated with a high RFD (7,8) (Fig. 6.6B). This influence of MHC isoform composition on RFD is mainly explained by a markedly faster crossbridge cycling rate in the type II muscle fibers than in type I fibers. In consequence, the maximal muscle force that can be reached during rapid movements, hence short contraction times (<250 ms), is closely related to the relative content of fast type II MHC isoforms in the muscle (9) (Fig. 6.3).

Parallelism between the rate of EMG and rate of force development has previously been proposed to exist. In support of this notion, concurrent increases in RFD and integrated EMG (including rate of EMG rise) have been observed following resistance training (4,6,10). In functional terms, the training-induced increase in RFD (Fig. 6.5B) is accompanied by an increased contractile impulse ($\int$ force dt) in the initial phase of muscle contraction (0–200 ms), which not only increases the muscle force and power generated during rapid limb movements but also contributes to increase maximal unloaded limb movement speed (4). Notably, a high level of contractile RFD is as vital to the trained athlete as to

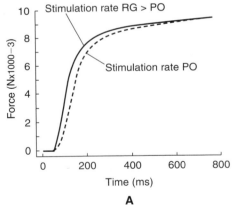

A

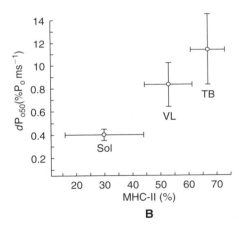

B

FIGURE 6.6 Influence of neural activation and muscle fiber type composition on contractile rate of force development (RFD). **A.** Force-time curves recorded for isolated motor units in the rat soleus muscle when activated at the minimum stimulation frequency needed to elicit maximal tetanic fusion (P_O) and when activated at a supramaximal rate (RG). RFD is greater at supramaximal rate of stimulation. *(Modified from Nelson AG. Supramaximal activation increases motor unit velocity of unloaded shortening. J Appl Biomech 1996;12:285–291.)* **B.** Relationship between RFD and fiber type (MHC isoform) composition. Peak RFD (dP_{o50}) was recorded in human skeletal muscles *in vivo* (soleus, Sol; lateral vastus, VL; triceps brachii, TB) using electrically evoked muscle activation at 50 Hz pulse stimulation rate. A high proportion of fast type II MHC isoforms is associated with a high RFD. *(Modified from Harridge SDR. The muscle contractile system and its adaptation to training. In Marconnet P, Saltin B, Komi PV, Poortmans J, eds. Human Muscular Function During Dynamic Exercise. Basel: Karger, 1996;82–94.)*

the aging individual who needs to control and counteract unexpected perturbations in postural balance.

Contractile Force and Power Generation in Relation to MHC Isoform Composition

In human skeletal muscle fibers, the myosin molecule is composed of the MHC (molecular weight approximately 200 kDa) and two distinct types of myosin light chains (MLC) (alkali and regulatory, each approximately 20 kDa). Various types of myosin analogues (isoforms) have been identified in adult human skeletal muscle fibers. Classifying these myosins with respect to molecular density yields a separation into three distinct isoforms: MHC I, MHC IIA, and MHC IIX. Furthermore, the embryonic MHC isoform may in rare circumstances be transiently expressed in response to certain types of muscle injury associated with severe eccentric overloading. Muscle fiber type distribution, as determined by myosin ATPase histochemistry, is closely related to the specific composition of MHC isoforms (9,11). However, the analysis of MHC composition appears to provide a more consistent measure of fiber type, as it accounts more sensitively for the coexpression of various MHC isoforms within the single muscle cell (12).

Importantly, the various myosin isoforms show distinct mechanical properties with respect to maximal shortening speed and power generation, force–velocity characteristics, RFD, ATP consumption, and economy of contraction. As such, the specific expression of various MHC isoforms in the muscle fiber becomes a major determinant of its mechanical output. In human skeletal muscle, the enormous range in functional properties between the different fiber types is mainly explained by differences in MHC composition (13).

Maximal Unloaded Shortening Velocity: Influence of MHC Composition

In isolated human muscle fibers, maximal unloaded shortening velocity (V_o) is found to increase in the order MHC IIX greater than IIA greater than I (7,14–16) (Table 6.1). This fiber type difference in V_o does not seem to depend on differences in sarcomeric structure, as similar results have been produced when the maximal sliding velocity of actin propelled by myosin was measured using *in vitro* motility assays (13).

In nonhuman animal muscle (rat, rabbit), a large variability of V_o can be observed for muscle fibers with identical MHC content, which may be accounted for by differences in MLC isoform composition (MLC3f). However, for human muscle fibers at normal physiological conditions, alkali and regulatory MLCs do not explain the variability in V_o observed for a given MHC isoform composition (16,17). This suggests that MLCs have only a minor regulatory role, if any, for the maximal shortening velocity of human skeletal fibers (13). As discussed later, the reliance of V_o on MHC composition exerts a significant influence on the specific force–velocity and power–velocity relationships of the single muscle fibers, which have substantial functional consequence for the mechanical performance of the whole muscle. Furthermore, this effect of MHC isoform composition on contractile muscle properties appears to manifest itself both during contraction of a single muscle fiber *in vitro* (Fig. 6.7) and during contraction of the intact muscle *in vivo* (Fig. 6.3).

Force and Power Relationships: Influence of MHC Composition, Functional Implications

Combined with analysis of muscle MHC isoform composition, recent experiments on single skinned muscle fibers

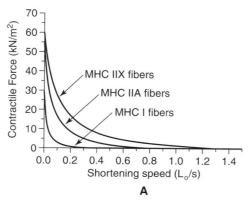
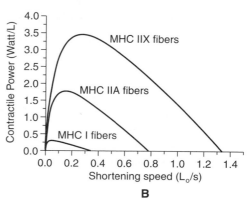

FIGURE 6.7 Force-velocity (**A**) and power-velocity (**B**) relationships obtained for single human muscle fibers. Graphs were generated by use of equations presented in Box 6.1 and Figure 6.2, using curve coefficients reported in Table 6.1. Notice the marked difference in maximal power generation between type I, IIA, and IIX fibers. Also, at the speed of peak power of the type IIX muscle fibers, type I fibers contribute almost no contractile power.

have expanded our understanding of the molecular, structural, and functional heterogeneity of skeletal muscle fibers. In the skinned fiber preparation, single fibers are dissected and the sarcolemma removed by chemical agents to leave the contractile myofibrillar system intact. With the skinned fiber technique it is possible to examine V_o and the contractile force–velocity and power–velocity properties in human muscle fibers of varying MHC isoform composition. However, the experimental conditions of the skinned fiber preparation do not readily resemble those of intact muscle fibers *in vivo*. A low temperature (12–15°C) is needed to keep the skinned fibers stable, whereas increasing the temperature from 12 to 22°C results in a fivefold and twofold increase in V_o and maximal isometric tension (F_o), respectively. Furthermore, some expansion (swelling) of the contractile filament space occurs, and that in turn influences the measurements of specific tension (F_o/CSA) and V_o. Nevertheless, the skinned fiber preparation provides a valuable method to evaluate the relative influence of fiber type composition (i.e., MHC isoform composition) on central aspects of contractile muscle performance (V_o, F_o, force–velocity properties).

The force–velocity properties of single muscle fibers can be described by the classical hyperbolic relationship for shortening contractions that was initially described by Hill (1). Further, contractile power can be derived as the product between muscle force and shortening speed (Fig. 6.2) (Milestone of Discovery). While the convexity constant a determines the specific shape of the force–velocity and power–velocity curves (Fig. 6.2), values for this parameter as well as for V_o and F_o have been obtained for single fibers with different MHC composition (Table 6.1) to yield the specific force–velocity and power–velocity relationship for human muscle fibers with different MHC isoform content (Fig. 6.7).

During concentric muscle contraction, muscle fiber contraction force is highly dependent on MHC isoform composition. Thus, at a given shortening speed muscle fibers dominated by the fast MHC II isoforms are capable of generating substantially higher forces than fibers dominated by the slow MHC I isoform, with MHC IIX fibers producing even greater forces than MHC IIA fibers (Fig. 6.7A). This difference in concentric force production between muscle fibers with different MHC composition is closely related to the difference in maximal shortening speed, which varies also in the order MHC I less than IIA less than IIX (Fig. 6.8A). In addition, expressed relative to the CSA of the muscle fiber, maximal isometric contraction force appears to differ in the order MHC I less than MHC II (Fig. 6.7A). The influence of MHC isoform composition on contractile muscle fiber performance relies for the most part on fiber type–related differences in maximal crossbridge cycling rate and actomyosin kinetics (attachment–detachment rate constants), while fiber type–related differences in intracellular Ca^{++} handling could possibly have an additional contribution. Notably, these molecular and cellular factors may manifest themselves also at the integrated macroscopic level, as concentric muscle force measured *in vivo* also appears to be influenced by MHC isoform composition (Fig. 6.3).

The power output normalized to fiber CSA is substantially higher in type II than in type I fibers, as a ninefold difference in contractile peak power can be observed between type I and IIX fibers (Figs. 6.7B and 6.8B) (15). Seen in a functional perspective, the recruitment of type II fibers at increasing contraction intensity will increase the magnitude of contractile power production even more, since the type II units contain a higher number of muscle fibers than the type I units. Furthermore, the speed of optimal power production

TABLE 6.1	Maximal Unloaded Shortening Velocity (V_o expressed in fiber lengths per second) and Convexity Constant a (a/F_o) Reported in the Literature for Single Human Muscle Fibers			
	Larsson & Moss (16)	Harridge et al. (7)	Bottinelli et al. (14)	Bottinelli et al. (15)
MHC I	V_o **0.3**[n = 32]	V_o **0.29**[n = 24]	V_o **0.26**[n = 24]	V_o **0.29**[n = 21] a/F_o 0.032
MHC I–IIA	—	V_o **0.96**[n = 3]	V_o **0.52**[n = 7]	—
MHC IIA	V_o **1.0**[n = 22]	V_o **1.09**[n = 10]	V_o **1.12**[n = 20]	V_o **1.26**[n = 14] a/F_o 0.063
MHC IIA–IIX	—	V_o **1.93**[n = 7]	V_o **2.14**[n = 12]	—
MHC IIX	V_o **3.1**[n = 7]	—	V_o **2.42**[n = 4]	V_o **3.07**[n = 9] a/F_o 0.072
	skinned fibers, Human muscle: VL, soleus	*skinned fibers, Human muscle: VL*	*skinned fibers, Human muscle: VL*	*skinned fibers, Human muscle: VL*

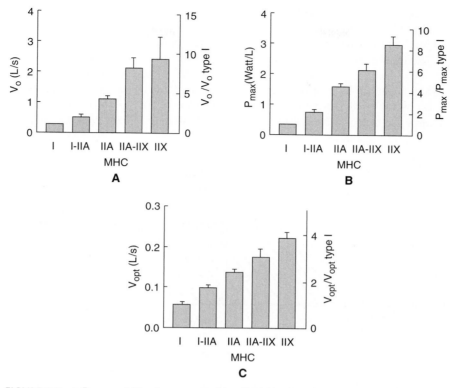

FIGURE 6.8 Influence of fiber type composition (MHC isoforms) on the contractile properties of human skeletal muscle. **A.** Maximal unloaded shortening velocity (V_o) of single human muscle fibers in relation to MHC isoform composition. V_o was measured by the slack-test method. Compared to the type I fiber, V_o is fourfold and ninefold greater in the type IIA and IIX fibers, respectively. (Reprinted with permission from Bottinelli R. Functional heterogeneity of mammalian single muscle fibers: do myosin isoforms tell the whole story? Pflüger's Arch 2001; 443:6–17.) **B** and **C.** Maximal contractile power generation, P_{max} (**B**) and muscle fiber shortening speed V_{opt} at P_{max} (**C**). A ninefold difference in peak power generation exists between type I and type IIA or IIX fibers, respectively. Likewise, optimum shortening speed at peak power (V_{opt}) differs between type I, IIA, and IIX fibers by a factor of two to four. *(Modified from Bottinelli R, Pellegrino MA, Canepari R, et al. Specific contributions of various muscle fiber types to human muscle performance: an in vitro study. J Electromyogr Kinesiol 1999;9:87–95.)*

is greatly increased with the gradual recruitment of type II units, as fiber shortening velocity at P_{max} is fivefold to sixfold higher in type IIX than type I fibers (Fig. 6.8C) (15). Since the highest energetic efficiency of contraction is achieved at a shortening velocity close to V_{opt}, the most economical speed of contraction also will increase with the gradual recruitment of type II units. Consequently, because of their individual reliance on MHC isoform composition, all of these intrinsic parameters seem to contribute in a synergistic manner to the contractile properties of the whole muscle, which in turn allows it to meet the functional demands at a wide range of movement speeds.

Notably, V_o appears to be reduced in the aging muscle. Thus, single muscle fibers dominated by MHC I and MHC IIA isoforms showed slower V_o in old (about 75 years) than in young (about 30 years) individuals (17), suggesting that

qualitative differences in contractile properties may exist between young and aging muscle fibers.

Muscle Architecture: Implications for Performance, Adaptive Changes Induced by Training

Most human skeletal muscles are pennate; that is, muscle fibers are spatially oriented with an angle relative to the aponeurosis or tendon at which they insert (Fig. 6.9). As a result, the total physiological CSA of the muscle greatly exceeds its anatomical CSA, which enables the muscle to exert much higher contractile forces than a nonpennate muscle with similar anatomical CSA. Importantly, an increased muscle fiber pennation angle, for example induced by resistance training, allows for an increased physiological muscle CSA per volume unit of muscle, which per se will result in a rise in maximal contractile muscle force (Fig. 6.9).

Muscle fiber pennation angle can be measured during muscle contraction *in vivo* by use of high-resolution ultrasonography (Fig. 6.9), either at rest or at varied levels of muscle tension, and at various muscle lengths (joint angles). Furthermore, ultrasound imaging has allowed examination of the strain characteristics of human tendon and aponeurosis structures *in vivo*. Also recently, ultrasonography has been used to investigate the adaptive change in muscle fiber pennation angle in response to long-term training. It was found that in the triceps brachii and vastus lateralis muscles, hypertrophy was accompanied by substantial increases in fiber

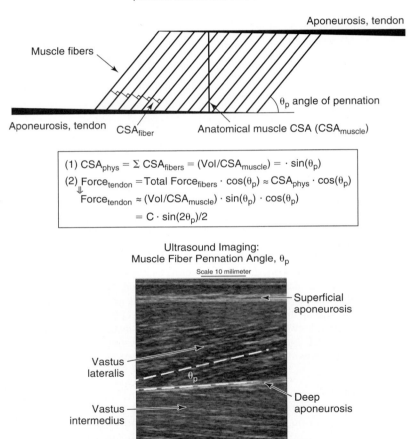

Human Skeletal Muscle
pennate muscle architecture

Aponeurosis, tendon

Muscle fibers

θ_p angle of pennation

Aponeurosis, tendon CSA_{fiber} Anatomical muscle CSA (CSA_{muscle})

(1) $CSA_{phys} = \Sigma\, CSA_{fibers} = (Vol/CSA_{muscle}) = \cdot \sin(\theta_p)$

(2) $Force_{tendon} = Total\, Force_{fibers} \cdot \cos(\theta_p) \approx CSA_{phys} \cdot \cos(\theta_p)$

$\quad\quad Force_{tendon} \approx (Vol/CSA_{muscle}) \cdot \sin(\theta_p) \cdot \cos(\theta_p)$

$\quad\quad\quad = C \cdot \sin(2\theta_p)/2$

Ultrasound Imaging:
Muscle Fiber Pennation Angle, θ_p

Scale 10 milimeter

Superficial aponeurosis

Vastus lateralis

θ_p

Vastus intermedius

Deep aponeurosis

FIGURE 6.9 Simplified diagram of pennate skeletal muscle in which fibers are oriented with an angle (pennation angle θ_p) relative to the longitudinal axis of the muscle (*top*). The total muscle contraction force varies in proportion to the summed area of all of the muscle fibers (nonreduced physiological CSA, CSAphys), which for a muscle with a given volume (Vol) and anatomical CSA (CSAmuscle) increases in proportion to $\sin(\theta_p)$ (Equation 1). However, the effective muscle fiber force to the tendon or aponeurosis is reduced at increased θ_p (Equation 2). As a result, force in the tendon will increase in proportion to $\sin(2\theta_p)$. *Bottom.* Sagittal plane ultrasonography (US) image obtained at 50% femur length in the resting vastus lateralis muscle of the left leg. (*US image modified from Aagaard P, Andersen JL, Leffers AM, et al. A mechanism for increased contractile strength of human pennate muscle in response to strength training: Changes in muscle architecture. J Physiol [Lond] 2001;534.2:613–623.*)

pennation angle after a period of resistance training (18,19), which contributed to the training-induced increase in maximal muscle force.

The increase in muscle fiber pennation angle observed with resistance training explains why the increase in single-muscle-fiber CSA measured in muscle biopsies (reflecting the change in physiological CSA) may well exceed the concurrent increase in muscle CSA observed by magnetic resonance imaging (reflecting the change in anatomical CSA) (18). Consequently, measurements of muscle CSA or volume obtained by magnetic resonance imaging or computed tomography may not readily replace the information obtained by measurements of single-muscle fiber area using muscle biopsy sampling.

At first glance, muscles with a large fiber pennation angle would be expected to have a low maximal origin-to-insertion shortening speed because of the less effective projection of muscle fiber shortening relative to the longitudinal axis of the muscle (Fig. 6.9). However, the continuous change (increase) in fiber pennation angle during the shortening movement appears to induce a rotational wiperlike motion of the muscle fibers relative to the aponeurosis or tendon. This angular sweep motion contributes effectively to the origin–insertion speed of the muscle, in fact to the extent that the overall shortening speed of the muscle may well exceed the maximal shortening speed of the single muscle fibers (20). As a result of their architectural design, therefore, pennate muscles are not compromised with respect to origin–insertion contraction speed. Rather, pennate muscles show a lower origin–insertion length change than do nonpennate muscles of similar fiber length.

Endurance in Relation to Muscle Metabolic Characteristics and MHC Isoform Composition

In discussion of endurance performance it is useful to include information from sport. One sport discipline that is easy to analyze is running. Running distance and time to perform are recorded, and average running speed can be calculated. Figure 6.10A shows data for the world records for various distances, and it is clear that there is a hyperbolic relationship between running speed and endurance performance. A central component in such a relationship is the capacity of the muscles.

Indirect evidence of the importance of the characteristics of the muscles for performance can be obtained from the observation that for elite runners there is a relationship between running distance and fiber type composition, that is, the relative content of type I, IIA, and IIX muscle fibers. Figure 6.11 shows that successful short-distance runners have many type II fibers, whereas for the longest distances (lower mean speed) it is better to have many type I fibers. However, for each running distance there is a large variation among elite athletes (Fig. 6.11), showing that the fiber type distribution is not the only factor that determines running performance. One explanation is that the separation into three fiber types on the basis of ATPase histochemical staining is too arbitrary. Another more important reason is that distinct adaptations for each muscle fiber occur with training.

A similar relationship between exercise intensity and performance, as observed during whole-body exercise (Fig. 6.10A), appears to be present on examination of the isolated

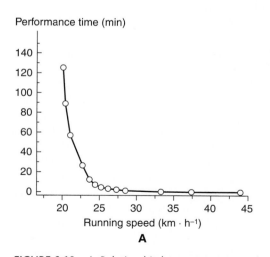

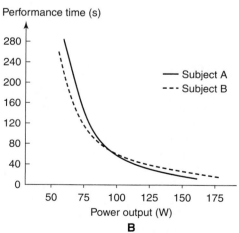

FIGURE 6.10 **A.** Relationship between mean running speed and world record times for different running distances. **B.** Relationship between work and intensity and time to exhaustion during one-legged knee exterior exercise for two subjects. Subect A (full line) performs better than subject B (dotted line) at low work loads and vice versa at high work intensities. Thus, human skeletal muscle displays different resistance to fatigue whether the exercise is performed at a low or high work load intensity.

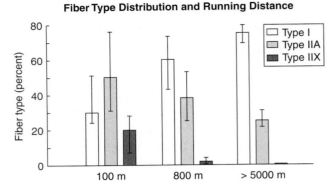

FIGURE 6.11 Relationship between running distance and fiber type distribution in elite runners. Means and range for different studies are listed. For the 100-m runners, the proportion of type I, IIA, and IIX, muscle fibers was 30, 50, and 20%, respectively (range 24–51%, 31–76%, and 43–73%). For the 800-m runners, the proportion of type I, IIA, and IIX was 60, 38, and 2%, respectively (range 43–74%, 25–53%, and 0–4%). For those who ran 5000 meters or more, the proportion of type I, IIA, and IIX was 75, 25, and 0%, respectively (range 69–79%, 21–31%, and 0%).

muscle. This relationship is illustrated in Figure 6.10B, which shows the performance at different exercise intensities for two subjects. Both demonstrated a hyperbolic relationship between power output and muscular endurance. Interestingly, one subject performed better than the other at low exercise intensities, while it was vice versa at high exercise intensities. This illustrates that a muscle has different resistance to fatigue with a low than with a high power output. How short-term and long-term exercise performance may be limited and how fatigue is related to the characteristics of the muscle are discussed later. Exercise can also be classified as being submaximal or supramaximal, which represents intensities lower and higher, respectively, than levels that elicit maximal aerobic power responses (maximum oxygen uptake).

Performance With Short-Term Activities

To understand what limits performance during short-term heavy exercise it is important to consider what causes fatigue during intense exercise. During maximal exercise, muscle power output peaks within a few seconds and then declines. Thus fatigue, defined as a loss of force output, occurs even within 5 seconds of maximal exercise. It is difficult to identify a single factor responsible for the reduction in performance during heavy exercise. Fatigue may be caused by reduced neural activation of the muscle. It may be cortical, but it appears that in well-motivated subjects, a substantial component of fatigue can be localized in the muscle. The area of central fatigue, including the significance of afferent activity, will not be covered here. This chapter discusses only a few possible causes of fatigue in relation to muscle characteristics and the adaptations that occur with chronic exercise

(training) and inactivity (detraining). For a detailed discussion of muscle fatigue, see Chapter 8.

Accumulation of Potassium in Muscle Interstitium and Performance

In recent years much focus has been on the importance of potassium in the development of muscle fatigue during exercise. During muscle activity, potassium is released from the intracellular to the extracellular space (interstitium) via voltage-dependent K^+ channels activated during propagation of action potentials. Potassium may also be released through K^+-ATP channels during exercise. A continuous efflux of potassium from the exercising muscle, together with a limited reuptake and release to the venous blood, leads to a progressive accumulation of potassium in the interstitium, which may be implicated in the fatigue process. Thus, extracellular accumulation of potassium impairs membrane excitability (21). Recently it has been demonstrated that interstitial potassium concentrations (K^+_{int}) in human skeletal muscle can reach values over 12 mmol · L^{-1} during heavy exercise (22), which is considerably higher than extracellular concentrations that have been shown to reduce contractility in isolated muscles. It is probably not the accumulation of extracellular potassium alone that causes fatigue in human muscle but also a decrease in intracellular potassium (K^+_{cyt}) and the simultaneous intracellular accumulation of Na^+ and lowering of extracellular Na^+ as a result of the translocation of Na^+. Together these changes lead to a significant increase (less negative) in the electrical membrane potential (Em), which can be calculated to be beyond −60 mV *in vivo*. At such high Em a large reduction in tetanic force has been reported *in vitro*. The K^+-depressed force is due to reduced Ca^{++} release within the muscle cells caused by an altered action potential profile (phase 1) and the presence of inexcitable muscle fibers as a result of an increased action potential threshold (phase 2).

It is well known that exercise training increases performance. If accumulation of potassium is a key factor in the development of fatigue, theoretically a reduced release of potassium from the muscle cells and/or an increased removal of potassium from the muscle interstitium should delay muscle fatigue after a period of training. Actually, it has recently been demonstrated in humans that high-intensity dynamic intermittent training (about 130% of $\dot{V}O_{2max}$) reduced the accumulation of potassium in skeletal muscle interstitium during both light and heavy exercise, which was associated with an enhanced work capacity (23). This finding supports the hypothesis that interstitial potassium accumulation is closely involved in the development of fatigue. Furthermore, training resulted in higher muscular levels of both the Na^+-K^+-ATPase α_1- and α_2-subunits, whereas the release of potassium to the blood was not changed. Thus, the reduced accumulation of potassium was likely due to a greater reuptake of potassium by the contracting muscles as a result of a greater Na^+-K^+-pump activity. A number of other studies have also shown that various types of exercise training lead to an increased amount of Na^+-K^+-ATPase α_1- and α_2-subunits in human skeletal muscle (24).

During exercise potassium may also be released from the muscle cell through the K^+-ATP channels, which are presented in human skeletal muscle (25). The K^+-ATP channels are inhibited by ATP, and this effect is reversed by lowering pH. Thus, the K^+-ATP channels may be activated in metabolically exhausted muscle fibers, and the activity of the channels contributes to the decline in force during fatigue in frog muscle. Although the number of K^+-ATP channels does not appear to change with heavy intermittent training (25), they may play a role in improving performance after training (discussed later in the chapter).

Muscle Lactate, pH, and Contractile Performance

High-intensity exercise is associated with a large production of lactate and concomitant elevation in acidity within the contracting muscles. Decreases in muscle pH from about 7.1 down to about 6.5 have been observed, which may affect muscle performance, as low pH has an inhibitory effect on various functions within the muscle cell (see Chapter 8). Thus, it is generally believed that lactic acid accumulation and low pH cause fatigue. However, a number of *in vivo* studies have demonstrated that lactate and pH are not the exclusive determinants of fatigue (26). On the other hand, this does not mean that pH is unimportant in the development of fatigue. In fact, major changes in muscle lactate and H^+ turnover occur after a period of heavy dynamic intermittent training, which may be important for the improvement in performance after training (discussed later).

The muscle buffer capacity *in vivo* is expressed as the ratio between the accumulation of lactate in the muscle and the observed change in muscle H^+. Thus, the buffer capacity is also influenced by transmembrane fluxes of ions. Trained subjects demonstrate a higher muscle buffer capacity than untrained subjects. Similarly, it has been observed that after a period of heavy, intense dynamic training, the subjects had a greater accumulation of lactate for the same change in muscle pH during a 30-second sprint, indicating an elevated buffer capacity (27). This is in part due to an elevated amount of muscle carnosine and histidine, which increase the buffering of H^+. Nevertheless, it appears that the major effect of heavy intermittent training is a higher transport of lactate and H^+ out of the muscle cell as a result of an elevated level of the monocarboxylate transporters MCT1 and MCT4 (28). These transporters release H^+ and lactate in a 1:1 manner and account for a considerable part of the efflux of lactate and H^+ during exercise. A higher muscle buffer capacity with training will delay the fall in muscle pH during heavy exercise, which probably diminishes the release of potas-

sium through the K^+ channels, delaying the point when K^+_{int} and K^+_{cyt} are reaching critical values. Hence, although a lowered muscle pH per se may not cause muscle fatigue, it may contribute to a decrease in muscle performance by increasing the release of potassium from the muscle cells.

Other Factors and Muscle Performance

Muscle fatigue during intense exercise does not appear to be related to lack of energy, since muscle ATP remains high at exhaustion during heavy voluntary exercise (26) and no single muscle fiber seems to be depleted for ATP even during electrical stimulation that results in a large decline in force. On the other hand, at the point of exhaustion many individual fibers are creatine phosphate (CP) depleted, which cannot exclude a role of lowered muscle CP in the development of fatigue. This is supported by the observation that oral intake of creatine over some days, which leads to elevated muscle CP and creatine levels, is associated with increased performance during heavy intermittent exercise. However, at the initial part of exercise muscle CP decreases rapidly, and exercise can be continued even with low levels of CP. Thus, low CP seems not to be a limiting factor during a single high-intensity exercise bout, but it may contribute to a reduced performance during repeated intense exercise. Little or no change in the concentration of CP and ATP is observed with high-intensity training (29). In contrast, such training elevates the level of enzymes related to the anaerobic production of energy, such as the activity of creatine kinase (CK) and phosphofructokinase (PFK). An increase in these enzymes implies that a certain change in an activator results in a higher rate of CP breakdown and glycolysis, respectively. However, the activity of these anaerobic enzymes is high even for untrained subjects, and the adaptations do not seem to be important to an increase in performance after a period of training. Actually, a 16% increase in the activity of PFK has been observed after a period of heavy intermittent training without a change in sprint performance.

Training at a high intensity increases the stores of muscle glycogen within the trained muscles, which appears to occur in all fiber types. However, it is not likely to affect performance during an acute exercise bout, since it has been demonstrated that development of fatigue during intense exercise depends on the initial muscle glycogen concentration only when it is low, that is, below 50 mmol $\cdot$ kg^{-1} dw (26).

Endurance Performance With Long-Term Activities

Muscle fatigue in an exercise event lasting more than 30 minutes seems to be related to depleted or partly depleted muscle glycogen storage or, if the exercise is performed for hours, lowered blood glucose levels. Thus, it has been demonstrated in a number of studies that the time to exhaustion with continuous and intermittent long-term exercise is prolonged when the subjects have ingested a high-carbohydrate diet in the preceding days (30). However, other factors with long-term exercise are also associated with muscular fatigue. For example, it is well recognized that during high thermal stress, elevated brain temperatures will cause termination of the exercise.

The primary factors setting an athlete's pace in a long-term exercise event are maximum oxygen uptake and movement economy (energy cost for a specific work requirement). The duration a pace can be maintained is a function of the magnitude of the glycogen storage within the muscles and the effectiveness of the way it is spared. These two factors establish the relative work rate, and the duration it can be maintained. Therefore, performance in long-term exercise is related to the initial muscle level of glycogen stores, substrate utilization, and the economy of the contracting muscles. These aspects are emphasized next, in the discussion of muscle characteristics and adaptation with training.

Substrate Utilization and Muscle Adaptations With Endurance Training

The degree of carbohydrate metabolism depends on the exercise intensity. The higher the intensity, the greater the carbohydrate oxidation, both in absolute and relative terms, and lactate production (see Chapters 17 and 19). With endurance training, carbohydrate metabolism is markedly altered, fat oxidation is significantly elevated, and lactate production in the muscle is lowered. A number of cellular changes are associated with this shift in metabolism, including proliferation of capillaries, an increase in the number of mitochondria, and an elevation in their content and enzymes.

MUSCLE CAPILLARIES   For an untrained muscle the number of capillaries around type I fibers is higher than for type II fibers. However, the distribution of type I and type II fibers throughout the muscle is heterogeneous. Thus, one capillary often supplies both type I and type II fibers. With aerobic training the number of capillaries around both type I and type II fibers increases, and the difference between the fiber types becomes less marked and may disappear.

The higher number of capillaries after a period of endurance training leads to a greater capillary volume, which in turn results in a longer capillary mean transit time (MTT = capillary blood volume/muscle blood flow) at a given muscle blood flow. Also, the capillary surface area is enlarged, and if the increase in capillaries exceeds the increase in muscle fiber size, the diffusion distance from capillary to mitochondria becomes smaller. All of these factors contribute to improve the conditions of exchange between blood and muscle and benefit the extraction of oxygen. However, the most important effect is probably making it possible to elevate the uptake of substrates, especially free fatty acids (FFA), from the bloodstream. In this way the higher number

of capillaries contributes to greater fat oxidation and lowered glycogen utilization at a given submaximal exercise intensity after a period of training.

MITOCHONDRIAL ACTIVITY AND ENZYMES   The mitochondrial content for untrained individuals is different in the various muscle fiber types. Thus, type I fibers have higher levels of oxidative enzymes, such as citrate synthase (CS) and succinate dehydrogenase (SDH), as well as higher levels of β-hydroxy acyl coenzyme A dehydrogenase (HAD). On the other hand, the level of glycolytic enzymes, such as phosphorylase and PFK, is higher in type II fibers. These factors reflect that the type I fibers have a higher oxidative capacity than the type II fibers, which conversely have a greater ability to perform anaerobic exercise . However, by training it is possible to change this balance.

Regular dynamic exercise can induce an increase in limb skeletal muscle mitochondria and tissue oxidative capacity (see Chapter 21). In highly endurance-trained individuals there is little difference in oxidative enzyme levels between the three fiber types. Furthermore, trained subjects demonstrate SDH levels in the type II fibers that are considerably higher than the SDH levels observed in type I fibers of untrained subjects, showing that muscle fibers have a wide adaptation to training. This is also illustrated by the finding that a group of top-class Tour de France cyclists in the preparation period from February to July increased the activity of enzymes (CS and HAD) that are markers for muscle mitochondrial content by approximately 60%, with only a concurrent 5% increase in maximum oxygen uptake (31). Furthermore, the level of mitochondrial enzymes at the period of competition was more than fourfold higher than for sedentary men. A high level of oxidative enzymes is important in endurance activities because they can lead to elevated fat oxidation, hence reduce the utilization of muscle glycogen and elevate long-term exercise performance. There is indirect evidence that this is the case. In a study runners were forced to be inactive for 2 weeks, and it was observed that endurance performance measured as time to exhaustion during running on a treadmill was reduced from 18 to 13.5 minutes (25%). This finding was associated with a 24% reduction in the activity of oxidative enzyme, whereas the runners had only a 3% drop in maximum oxygen uptake (32).

Reduced lactate production at a given submaximal exercise intensity after endurance training is accomplished by lowering the rate of glycolysis and by reduced activity of lactate dehydrogenase LDH_{4-5} isozyme and elevated activity of LDH_{1-2}. An increase in the capacity in one of the shuttle systems for reduced nicotinic acid dehydrogenase (NADH) and an enlarged muscle mitochondrial volume reduce the accumulation of NADH in the cytosol, and thereby also diminish the production of lactate during exercise.

MUSCLE EFFICIENCY   For exercise lasting more than 1 minute most energy is provided by aerobic metabolism. Pulmonary oxygen uptake per power output is higher at heavy than light submaximal exercise, which may be related to additional fiber type II recruitment with increasing power outputs. Thus, it is well established from *in vitro* studies that the energy cost of contraction differs between muscle fiber types, with type II fibers showing a larger oxygen uptake and heat production per work unit at low contraction speeds. Supporting evidence exists for a similar relationship in human muscle (33). Thus, it was demonstrated that the oxygen cost of dynamic exercise was elevated when more type II fibers were recruited because of prior type I glycogen depletion, suggesting that the type II fibers *in vivo* have a greater oxygen uptake at a given power output.

When exercise continues at a given relative high submaximal exercise intensity, pulmonary oxygen uptake progressively increases. The extra oxygen used is called the slow component of oxygen uptake. It has been demonstrated that most of the slow component of oxygen uptake can be attributed to the active muscles (34). Based on the observation that the magnitude of the slow component of oxygen uptake is a function of the relative exercise intensity and that the fraction of type II fibers are positively correlated to the amplitude of slow component, it has been suggested that progressive type II fiber recruitment explains the slow component of oxygen uptake. In support of this hypothesis, the slow component was observed only during moderate-intensity exercise that activated type II fibers because the type I fibers had been depleted the day before by long-term moderate-intensity exercise (33). It is not clear whether the number of active type II fibers increases during exercise or whether the oxygen requirement of each of the already active fibers rises over time. There exists, however, some indirect evidence of a change in recruitment pattern during various phases of submaximal exercise that causes a slow-component oxygen uptake. Determinations of surface electromyography and contrast shifts in magnetic resonance imaging suggest a gradually increased muscle activation during intense submaximal exercise. Measurements of metabolites in individual fibers confirmed these findings. Thus, it was demonstrated that more fibers, particularly type II fibers, were recruited in 3 to 6 minutes of intense submaximal exercise in association with a pronounced slow component of oxygen uptake (35). The need to recruit additional fibers may be due to (*a*) some fibers not working at their optimal shortening velocity as exercise progress and/or (*b*) some fibers no longer contributing to the force development (not contracting). The previously contracted fibers still have an elevated oxygen uptake because of their energy demand related to resynthesis of energy-rich phosphates and to reestablishment of ion homeostasis. For example, it well known that noncrossbridge ATP activity, mainly Ca^{++} and Na^+-K^+ pump ATPase, can account for a substantial fraction of the total energy turnover (20–40%).

It is also possible that the oxygen requirement of the contracting fibers increases over time. *In vitro* studies have shown that the fraction of noncrossbridge ATPase activity increases markedly during a series of intense contractions. Furthermore, the mitochondrial efficiency, defined as a decrease in ATP resynthesized per unit of oxygen used, may decrease during intense submaximal exercise and thereby contribute to the slow component of oxygen uptake. *In vitro* studies have revealed that a number of substances, including Ca^{++}, P_i, H^+, and reactive oxygen species, which are elevated during intense exercise, can attenuate mitochondrial enzyme activities and uncouple skeletal muscle mitochondrial respiration, contributing to a reduction in mitochondrial efficiency. Several mechanisms may be involved, including opening of the permeability transition pore (PTP), which has been shown to function as a fast-release Ca^{++} channel in the inner mitochondrial membrane. Maximal opening of PTP to its 1500-Da conductance state may cause uncoupling of mitochondrial respiration and loss of coenzymes from the mitochondrial matrix. However, it is unknown to what extent mitochondrial enzyme activities are affected and whether mitochondrial phosphate to oxygen ratio (P/O) is lowered during continuous intense submaximal exercise.

Several *in vitro* studies have shown differences between mitochondria derived from type I and type II fibers. For example, mitochondria from type II fibers contain a larger amount of uncoupling protein 3 (UCP-3) and a higher activity of α-glycerophosphate dehydrogenase (α-GPD) both in rats and humans. Additionally, the ratio of mitochondrial α-GPD relative to pyruvate dehydrogenase was shown to be elevated after intense submaximal exercise, which suggests that uncoupling of mitochondria may occur during exercise, leading to an elevate drift in oxygen uptake.

A period of dynamic exercise training appears to have no effect on oxygen uptake during submaximal exercise at low intensities. However, the oxygen uptake increases more rapidly in the initial phase of exercise, and the slow component of oxygen uptake occurs at higher work intensities. This may be due to adaptations in type II fibers with training, but little is known about such an effect.

SUMMARY

In single human muscle fibers the specific composition of MHC isoforms determines the contractile force–velocity and power–velocity properties. At the whole-muscle level these properties are dynamically modulated by the specific pattern of neural muscle fiber innervation. Resistance training induces adaptive changes in maximal eccentric muscle strength, which mainly rely on changes in neural function. Likewise, explosive muscle strength (maximal RFD) is found to increase following resistance training. Changes in muscle architecture (fiber pennation angle) may also occur with resistance training and contribute to the training-induced increase in maximal muscle force, power, and RFD. The increase in muscle fiber pennation angle allows single-muscle fiber area and hence maximal contractile force to increase disproportionally more than anatomical muscle CSA.

The distinct metabolic and enzymatic characteristics of the various fiber types play a decisive role in the endurance performance observed during both short-term and long-term exercise. Accumulation of potassium in the interstitial space is implemented in the development of fatigue during heavy exercise. Potassium pumps in the human sarcolemma are elevated with heavy training. This can explain the adaptive reduction in interstitial potassium accumulation and elevated performance. Likewise, intense intermittent training elevates transport of lactate and hydrogen ions out of the muscle cell as a result of an increased number of transporters. The concurrent rise in muscle buffer capacity delays the fall in muscle pH during intense exercise, hence delaying the onset of fatigue. The activity of anaerobic key enzymes, such as CK and PFK, increases after anaerobic exercise regimens. During prolonged exercise, maximum rate of oxygen uptake, movement economy, and substrate utilization are the main factors that determine endurance performance. Endurance training increases maximum oxygen uptake and increases muscle capillaries and mitochondrial content. In turn, these changes lead to elevated muscle fat oxidation and better endurance performance. Mechanical efficiency of muscle contraction is affected by the pattern of type I versus type II fiber recruitment, since mechanical efficiency seems to differ between fiber types.

A MILESTONE OF DISCOVERY

During their life span all living animals, including the human being, learn that light loads can be moved at greater speeds than heavy ones. As the load gradually increases, movement speed slows down until no movement can occur. As described for the first time in detail by Hill in 1938, there is a reciprocal relationship between contractile muscle force and shortening speed, and it relies on inherent mechanical muscle properties. In his previous work in the early 1920s Hill, and others with him, suggested that maximal muscle activation always elicited maximal muscle force but that during shortening some of this force was used to overcome viscoelastic resistance within the muscle itself. Further, it was thought that the magnitude of viscous resistance progressively increased with increase in muscle shortening speed, causing muscle force to decrease. Based on the viscosity hypothesis, the relationship between contraction force and speed of shortening was expected to be linear. However, early experiments performed on isolated frog and cat muscles clearly showed a nonlinear concave relationship. In his later experiments, Hill developed a rapid technique for precise thermodynamic muscle measurements, which made it possible to record the heat produced by the frog sartorius muscle during slow and fast shortening contractions *in vitro* (1). Using this technique, Hill was able to measure the rate of heat release and contractile work performed by the muscle at different speeds of shortening, which led to the classical hyperbolic relationship between contractile muscle force (F) and shortening speed ($\dot{V}$) during isotonic contraction:

$$(F+a)(V+b) = \text{constant} = (F_o + a)b$$

where F = contraction force; $\dot{V}$ = velocity of shortening; F_o = force exerted at zero speed, or maximal isometric tension; a = the convexity constant, which determines the convexity of the force–velocity curve; constant b = V_o a / F_o, with V_o denoting the shortening velocity at zero muscle force, or maximal unloaded short-

ening speed (1). Rearranging this equation to express muscle force F as a function of shortening speed $\dot{V}$ yields (graph shown in Fig. 6.2):

$$F = c/(V+b) - a \text{ in which } c = \text{constant} = (F_o + a)b$$

These equations, which later became known as the force–velocity relationship of skeletal muscle, are important for a number of reasons. First, the close association to the shortening heat released by the muscle suggested that the relationship reflected molecular crossbridge dynamics, which was later verified. Second, the relationship precisely describes the mechanical behavior of the muscle when contracting against different loads. Thus, once the force–velocity relationship is established for a given muscle, concentric muscle force at given contraction speed can be predicted. Third, the force–velocity relationship reveals precise information about the magnitude of contractile power that can be generated by the muscle when it is contracting at a given shortening speed, as the power–velocity relationship is derived from the force–velocity relation by calculating the product between muscle force and shortening speed at a given speed (Fig. 6.2):

$$\text{Power} = FV = cV/[((V+b)-a)] \text{ in which } c = (F_o + a)b$$

The importance and relevance of the work published by Hill in 1938 extends into the present. Thus, for more than 60 years the force–velocity and power–velocity relationships have been intensively used to examine and characterize the contractile behavior of skeletal muscle, also addressing the influence of fiber type composition (Fig. 6.7).

Hill AV. The heat of shortening and the dynamic constants of muscle. Proc Royal Soc Lond Series B 1938;126:136–195.

REFERENCES

1. Hill AV. The heat of shortening and the dynamic constants of muscle. Proc R Soc Lond Ser B 1938;126: 136–195.

2. Katz B. The relation between force and speed in muscular contraction. J Physiol (Lond) 1939;96:45–64.

3. Westing SH, Seger JY, Thorstensson A. Effects of electrical stimulation on eccentric and concentric torque-velocity relationships during knee extension in man. Acta Physiol Scand 1990;140:17–22.

4. Aagaard P, Simonsen EB, Magnusson SP, et al. Increased rate of force development and neural drive of human skeletal muscle following resistance training. J Appl Physiol 2002;93:1318–1326.

5. Nelson AG. Supramaximal activation increases motor unit velocity of unloaded shortening. J Appl Biomech 1996;12:285–291.

6. Van Cutsem M, Duchateau J, Hainaut K. Changes in single motor unit behavior contribute to the increase in contraction speed after dynamic training in humans. J Physiol (Lond) 1998;513.1:295–305.

7. Harridge SDR, Bottinelli R, Canepari M, et al. Whole-muscle and single-fibre contractile properties and myosin heavy chain isoforms in humans. Pflüger's Arch 1996;432: 913–920.

8. Harridge SDR. The muscle contractile system and its adaptation to training. In Marconnet P, Saltin B, Komi PV, Poortmans J, eds. Human muscular function during dynamic exercise. Basel: Karger, 1996;82–94.

9. Aagaard P, Andersen JL. Correlation between contractile strength and myosin heavy chain isoform composition in human skeletal muscle. Med Sci Sports Exerc 1998;30:1217–1222.

10. Häkkinen K, Komi PV. Training induced changes in neuromuscular performance under voluntary and reflex conditions. Eur J Appl Physiol 1986;55:147–155.

11. Staron RS, Leonardi MJ, Karapondo DL, et al. Strength and skeletal muscle adaptations in heavy-resistance trained women after detraining and retraining. J Appl Physiol 1991;70:631–640.

12. Klitgaard H, Bergman O, Betto R, et al. Co-existence of myosin heavy chain I and IIa isoforms in human skeletal muscle fibres with endurance training. Pflüger's Arch 1990;416:470–472.

13. Bottinelli R. Functional heterogeneity of mammalian single muscle fibers: do myosin isoforms tell the whole story? Pflüger's Arch 2001;443:6–17.

14. Bottinelli R, Canepari R, Pellegrino MA, et al. Force-velocity properties of human skeletal muscle fibres: myosin heavy chain isoform and temperature dependence. J Physiol (Lond) 1996;495:573–586.

15. Bottinelli R, Pellegrino MA, Canepari R, et al. Specific contributions of various muscle fibre types to human muscle performance: an in vitro study. J Electromyogr Kinesiol 1999;9:87–95.

16. Larsson L, Moss RL. Maximum velocity of shortening in relation to myosin isoform composition in single fibres from human skeletal muscles. J Physiol (Lond) 1993;472: 595–614.

17. Larsson L, Xiaopeng L, Frontera WR. Effects of aging on shortening velocity and myosin isoform composition in single human skeletal muscle cells. Am J Physiol 1997;272:C638–C649.

18. Aagaard P, Andersen JL, Leffers AM, et al. A mechanism for increased contractile strength of human pennate muscle in response to strength training: changes in muscle architecture. J Physiol (Lond) 2001;534.2: 613–623.

19. Kawakami Y, Abe T, Kuno S, et al. Training induced changes in muscle architecture and specific tension. Eur J Appl Physiol 1995;72:37–43.

20. Gans C. Fiber architecture and muscle function. Physiol Rev 1982;10:160–207.

21. Fitts RH. Cellular mechanisms of muscle fatigue. Physiol Rev 1994;74: 49–94.

22. Nordsborg N, Mohr M, Pedersen LD, et al. Muscle interstitial potassium kinetics during intense exhaustive exercise: effect of previous arm exercise. Am J Physiol 2003;285: R143–R148.

23. Nielsen JJ, Mohr M, Klarskov C, et al. Effects of high-intensity intermittent training on potassium kinetics and performance in human skeletal muscle. J Physiol (Lond) 2004;554.3:857–870.

24. McKenna MJ, Harmer AR, Fraser SF, et al. Effects of training on potassium, calcium and hydrogen ion regulation in skeletal muscle and blood during exercise. Acta Physiol Scand 1996;156:335–346.

25. Nielsen JJ, Kristensen M, Hellsten Y, et al. Localization and function of ATP-sensitive potassium channels in human skeletal muscle. Am J Physiol 2003;284: R558–R563.

26. Bangsbo J, Graham TE, Kiens B, et al. Elevated muscle glycogen and anaerobic energy production during exhaustive exercise in man. J Physiol (Lond) 1992;451: 205–227.

27. Nevill ME, Boobis LH, Brooks S, et al. Effect of training on muscle metabolism during treadmill sprinting. J Appl Physiol 1989;67:2376–2382.

28. Pilegaard H, Domino K, Noland T, et al. Effect of high intensity exercise training on lactate/H^+ transport capacity in human skeletal muscle. Am J Physiol 1999;276: E255–E261.

29. Reilly T, Bangsbo J. Anaerobic and aerobic training. In Elliott B, ed. Applied Sport Science: Training in Sport. West Sussex, England: John Wiley & Sons, 1998;351–409.

30. Graham TE, Adamo KB. Dietary carbohydrate and its effects on metabolism and substrate stores in sedentary and active individuals. Can J Appl Physiol 1999;24: 393–415.

31. Sjøgaard G. Muscle morphology and metabolic potential in elite road cyclists during a season. Int J Sports Med 1984;5:250–254.

32. Houston ME, Bentzen H, Larsen H. Interrelationship between skeletal muscle adaptations and performance as studied by detraining and retraining. Acta Physiol Scand 1979;105:163–170.

33. Krustrup P, Söderlund K, Mohr M, et al. Slow-twitch fiber glycogen depletion elevates moderate-exercise fast-twitch fiber activity and O_2 uptake. Med Sci Sports Exerc 2004;36:973–982.

34. Poole DC. Role of exercising muscle in slow component of $\dot{V}O_2$. Med Sci Sports Exerc 1994;26:1335–1340.

35. Krustrup P, Söderlund K, Mohr M, et al. The slow component of oxygen uptake during intense, sub-maximal exercise in man is associated with additional fibre recruitment. Pflüger's Arch 2004;448:452–456.

CHAPTER 7

The Muscular System: The Control of Muscle Mass

Richard Tsika

Introduction

An extraordinary characteristic of adult skeletal muscle is its intrinsic ability to adapt to a broad range of physiological stimuli, such as those produced by various exercise paradigms. For example, increased skeletal muscle work load (force times distance) as imposed by various weight training regimens has a profound effect on both mass (hypertrophy) and strength (force production) (1,2). This type of adaptation to weight training is so well known it is legendary. Milo of Crotona, a sixth century B.C. Greek athlete, reportedly acquired the strength to carry a bull around a stadium by lifting the bull daily from the time it was a newborn calf, thereby gradually accommodating to the increased load as the calf increased in weight (3). Conversely, decreased muscle loading associated with inactivity resulting from normal aging processes, immobilization due to injury, various systemic diseases, and the less frequently encountered exposure to zero gravity (space travel) leads to the undesirable decline in muscle mass (atrophy) and function (1). Because of obvious ethical considerations, rigorous biochemical and molecular studies concerning altered muscle loading conditions have used animal models as opposed to human subjects. Nevertheless, the relentless advancements in biotechnology over the past decade, including the powerful genetic methodology of transgenesis, allowed scientists to unravel complex molecular mechanisms underlying the biochemical

and physiological adaptations that occur in muscle following alterations in load-bearing activity. This chapter focuses on some of the most recent and remarkable discoveries that form just the beginning of our insight into the control of muscle mass.

Hypertrophy

Hypertrophy of adult skeletal muscle is a complex biological response wherein the cross-sectional area of each fiber in a given muscle increases (Fig. 7.1, A–D). This enlargement in adult rodent (rat and mouse) muscle size does not involve an increase in muscle fiber (individual cell) number, a process referred to as hyperplasia. Because adult skeletal muscle fibers are terminally differentiated, they have lost the ability to proliferate, and thus any increase in size due to increased work load must occur without increased numbers of cells.

General Physiological and Biochemical Properties of Skeletal Muscle

Skeletal muscle can be categorized into two broad types, slow twitch and fast twitch. The combined use of histochemical (myofibrillar ATPase), immunohistochemical (anti-MHC) (Table 7.1) and electrophoretic techniques has demonstrated that adult rat and mouse hindlimb muscle ex-

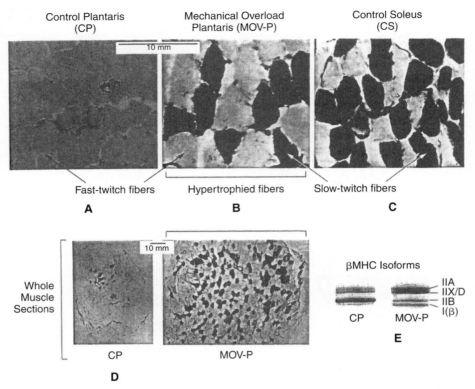

FIGURE 7.1 Cross-section of control and hypertrophied hindlimb muscle with corresponding isomyosin profile. **A** to **C.** Muscle sections subjected to acid-stable myosin ATPase histochemistry, which results in dark staining of only slow-twitch fibers. A 10-mm bar shows the approximate magnification for all three panels. **A.** Control plantaris. **B.** Hypertrophied plantaris that resulted from mechanical overload (MOV). **C.** Control soleus. (Reprinted with permission from Wiedenman JL, Tiska GL, Gao L, et al. Muscle specific and inducible expression of 293-base pair beta-myosin heavy chain promoter in transgenic mice. Am J Physiol 1996;271:R688–R685.) **D.** Cross-sections of both control and hypertrophied whole plantaris muscle. **A** to **D.** Approximate doubling of fiber size in the hypertrophied plantaris compared to control sections. In addition to increased fiber size the MOV-induced hypertrophied sections show that some fibers undergo a fast-to-slow phenotypic transition. **E.** Further evidence of this fiber type switch: induction of the βMHC (type I isoprotein), an increase in type IIA and IIX/D isoproteins, and a decrease in the fast type IIB isoproteins in the MOV-P muscle extract.

presses four major MHC isoforms designated as fast type IIB, IIX/D, IIA, and slow type I (β) (Fig. 7.1E). The heterogeneous spectrum of vertebrate sarcomeric MHC isoforms and their differential expression pattern underlie the broad classification scheme that distinguishes four primary adult skeletal muscle fiber types, also termed fast-twitch IIB, IIX/D, IIA, and slow-twitch type I. Each of these fiber types displays unique properties with respect to size, metabolism, fatigability, and intrinsic contractile properties, the last of which is in part determined by their MHC content (1,4,5). In addition, hybrid fibers that coexpress multiple MHC isoforms have been identified, and the relative population of these fibers increases in response to perturbations such as increased and decreased muscle loading states (1,4). The notion that each MHC serves a physiological role is underscored by the classic finding that actin-activated myosin

ATPase and unloaded shortening velocity (V_{max}) are highly correlated to the amount and type of isomyosin or MHC in a given muscle or muscle fiber (6). Evidence gathered from other studies on both animal and *in vitro* models have provided ample evidence that the amount and type of MHC in a muscle's contractile apparatus has functional significance as well as producing the physiological consequences of alterations in MHC composition, whether induced by physiological stimuli, disease, or mutation (natural or by gene targeting) (1,5–7).

Experimental Models

Over the years several animal models have been developed for the purpose of elucidating the cellular, biochemical, and molecular mechanisms involved in skeletal muscle remod-

TABLE 7.1	Frequently Used Terms and Abbreviations
Term	**Definition**
DNA regulatory element	Site of protein binding; also called cis-acting element
Frameshift mutation	A mutation that occurs due to insertion or deletion of nucleotides resulting in a changed codon
Kinase	Enzyme that adds a phosphate to a substrate
Phosphatase	Enzyme that removes a phosphate from a substrate
Ras	A monomeric GTP-binding protein
Work	Force times distance

Abbreviation	**Definition**
Akt	Protein kinase B
ATP	Adenosine triphosphate
βA/T	Beta A/T—rich element
CaMK	Calcium–calmodulin protein kinase
CNBP	cellular nucleic acid binding protein
CsA	Cyclosporin A
dMCAT	Distal MCAT
eIF-2B	Eukaryotic translation initiation factor 2B
eIF-4E	Eukaryotic translation initiation factor 4E
EMG	Electromyography
ERK	Extracellular signal-regulated kinase
GATA	Denotes a GATA nucleotide
GDF-8	Growth differentiation factor-8; also termed myostatin
GPDH	α-Glycerophosphate dehydrogenase
G3PDH	Glyceraldehyde-3-phosphate dehydrogenase
GSK-3β	Glycogen-synthase kinase-3β
HDAC	Histone deacetylase
HS	Hindlimb suspension
IGF-1	Insulinlike growth factor-1
MAFbx	Muscle atrophy F-box; also called atrogin-1
MAPK	Mitogen-activated protein kinase
MCAT	Muscle-CAT
MCIP-1	Modulatory calcineurin-interacting protein-1
MCK	Muscle creatine kinase
MEF2	Myocyte enhancer factor-2
MGF	Mechano growth factor
MHC	Myosin heavy chain
MOV	Mechanical overload
mTOR	Mammalian target of rapamycin
MuRF1	Muscle ring finger 1
NFAT	Nuclear factor of activated T-cell
NWB	Non–weight bearing
pal-Mt	palindromic myotube element
PGAM-M	phosphoglycerate mutase
PHAS-1	Phosphorylated heat- and acid-stable protein-1; also known as 4E-BP1
PI(3)K	Phosphatidylinositol-3-OH-kinase
PKB	A cytosolic protein kinase recruited to the membrane when PI3K is activated (also known as AKT)
p70S6K	Kinase that phosphorylates the S6 subunit of ribosomes
SCF	Skp1, Cullin I, F-box (type E3 ligase complex)
Sp-1	Specific protein-1
SRF	Serum response factor
TEF-1	Transcriptional enhancer factor-1
TGF-β	Transforming growth factor-β
V_{max}	Maximum unloaded shortening velocity
YB-1	Y box protein

eling in response to increased muscle loading. These models include stretch, resistance exercise, and compensatory overload (2). Evidence gathered from these studies has revealed that although the contractile activity and magnitude of work overload imposed differs between these diverse models, all skeletal muscles adapt with varying degrees of hypertrophic growth, increased strength, and a fast-to-slow phenotype transition (2). The compensatory overload model produces the most profound changes in skeletal muscle hypertrophy and phenotype, and because of this feature, this model has been frequently used to characterize physiological and biochemical adaptations to increased muscle loading (Fig. 7.2). More recently this model has been combined with transgenesis to elucidate *in vivo* complex integrated biological responses such as cell signaling and transcriptional regulation (8,9). Thus, compensatory overload is the focus of this section, where sustained adaptation induced by chronic work load is concerned. In some cases, acute adaptations are discussed. For a detailed description of the stretch or resistance exercise models of muscle hypertrophy and the adaptations associated with each of these models, consult the outstanding reviews of Booth and Baldwin (1), Timson (2), and Baldwin and Haddad (4).

The Compensatory Overload Model and Skeletal Muscle Adaptations

In the rodent (mouse, rat) model of compensatory overload, a chronic increase in muscle loading is induced by the sur-

gical removal of a given muscle's synergists (Fig. 7.2). For example, compensatory overload of the rodent fast-twitch plantaris muscle involves the surgical removal of its synergists, the soleus and gastrocnemius (2). In this case, the imposition of chronic loading demands that the remaining fast-twitch plantaris muscle (used in high-force locomotor activity) take over the functional duties normally performed by the slow-twitch soleus (used for chronic postural maintenance) and mixed–fiber type gastrocnemius (locomotor movements) muscles. Because this model requires the plantaris muscle to perform the duties of the soleus and gastrocnemius muscles and to develop a sustained increase in force, it has also been referred to as functional overload or MOV. In this chapter, this model is called MOV. The MOV model can be used to induce hypertrophy and fiber phenotype switches in both slow-twitch muscle (e.g., soleus) and fast-twitch muscle (e.g., plantaris). Even though the soleus muscle is already primarily composed of type I fibers (85% type I in rat; 50–70% type I in mouse), the direction of the fiber type shift remains fast to slow twitch. However, because the adult rodent fast-twitch plantaris muscle is composed primarily of fast type II fibers (95%), it is the preferred muscle with which to study load-induced enlargement and fast-to-slow phenotype switches.

MOV is a physiological stimulus associated with a rapid increase in muscle mass. Notably, the rapid enlargement that occurs within the first week post MOV is accompanied by inflammatory edema, and therefore assessments of true muscle hypertrophy (protein accretion) during this early time should be viewed with caution (2). Nevertheless, a steady-state hypertrophy of the adult MOV plantaris muscle appears to occur 6 to 9 weeks post overload (1,10). This enlargement is achieved by an increase in the rate of protein synthesis, primarily resulting in an increase in the cross-sectional area (sarcomeres in parallel) of all existing fibers, whereas models of stretch hypertrophy largely result in increased muscle length (primarily sarcomeres in series) (2). The MOV-induced protein accretion is coincident with increases in essential contractile proteins that when assembled into sarcomeres (smallest force-generating units of striated muscle), enhance the force-generating capacity of the hypertrophied plantaris muscle. The adaptation in contractile properties within the MOV plantaris muscle includes increases in absolute peak tension and maximal tetanic isometric force, while the unloaded shortening velocity (V_{max}) is decreased (6). Consistent with a decrease in V_{max}, the actin-activated myosin ATPase activity is also decreased (1,2). The latter adaptations are consistent with a fast-to-slow fiber type transition, which has been confirmed by histochemical staining for myofibrillar ATPase, MHC immunohistochemistry, and electrophoretic separation of native myosin and MHC isoforms (Fig. 7.1) (1). Concurrent with a fast-to-slow phenotype remodeling, a change in innervation pattern or total electrical activity of the MOV muscle has been observed (11).

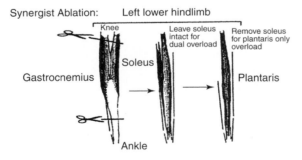

Mechanical Overload Model (MOV)

Synergist Ablation: Left lower hindlimb

Removes 85%: Gastrocnemius (mixed), Soleus (Type I)
Retains   15%: Plantaris (Type II)

Imposes:
   Chronic mechanical overload

Induces:
   Hypertrophy of all muscle fibers
   Fiber type transitions:

Fast-glycolytic   Slow-oxidative

Type IIB → IIX/D → IIA → Type I

FIGURE 7.2 Significant features of the mechanical overload model used to induce both skeletal muscle hypertrophy and fiber phenotype fast-to-slow changes.

MOV as a Complex Externally Imposed Stimulus Which Activates Numerous Signals

Because MOV is a complex external stimulus associated with the activation of numerous signals, it is not possible to accurately replicate all of its effects using cell culture systems. This is illustrated by the fact that adult-stage muscle phenotypes, fiber type transitions, and equivalent loading conditions cannot be duplicated with myogenic cells in culture. Further limitations are that many control mechanisms associated with hormonal (endocrine), circulatory, and neural input and important communication between different cell types are not represented in permanent cell lines or primary cells in culture. Thus, the elucidation of the regulatory mechanisms that control skeletal muscle adaptations in response to MOV requires the use of rat or mouse models. Also, with intact animals, any adaptation that occurs in response to MOV is the result of an integrated physiological response that includes input (independent and convergent signals) from but not limited to the following:

1. Increased levels of load bearing
2. Increased electrical activation (as measured by EMG signal)
3. Autocrine (e.g., IGF-1, prostaglandins) signals
4. An acute immune response associated with cytokine secretion (interlukin-6, leukemia inhibitory factor)

5. Growth factors
6. Rapid and transient induction (1–48 hours) of immediate early response genes (c-fos, c-myc, Erg1) thought to be involved in the growth response
7. Decreased expression (within first 2 days) of enzymes representative of a glycolytic profile (GPDH, G3PDH, MCK) that may represent a metabolic signal for a switch to a more oxidative (slow) phenotype
8. Activation of integrin signaling cascades within the first week
9. Regulation of myostatin
10. Activation of satellite cells and putative endogenous muscle stem cells (2,8,11–15)
11. Likely other as yet unidentified stimuli (Fig. 7.3)

It is clear from this list that identification of precise regulatory mechanisms controlling load-induced skeletal muscle remodeling (hypertrophy and phenotype) will be a challenging task, since this process involves the differential expression of hundreds of genes representing numerous subcellular systems. Regardless of inherent complications with intact animal model usage, the importance of these models lies in the fact that they are not discrete and thus are relatively likely to mimic human activity that requires sustained increases in force development (load). Despite difficulties, significant advances have been made in defining cell signaling pathways activated by MOV (see section "Intracellular Signal Transduction

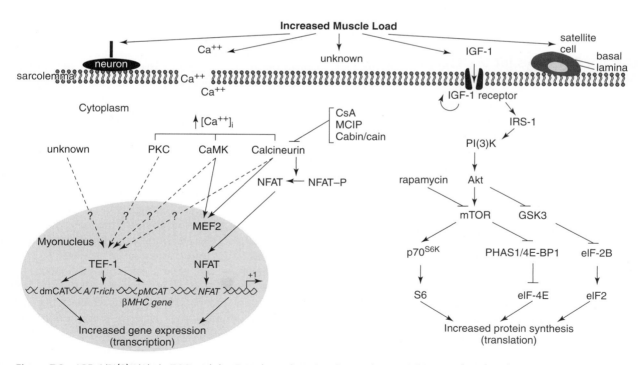

Figure 7.3 IGF-1/PI(3)K/Akt/mTOR and the Ca^{++}-dependent signaling pathways Calcineurin (CaN) and CaMK. These signaling pathways may be involved in growth (IGF-1/PI[3]K/Akt/mTOR), phenotype changes (Calcineurin [CaN] and CaMK) or possibly both. Intracellular signaling pathways recently shown to be associated with load-induced hypertrophic growth and fiber type transitions are shown (muscle remodeling).

Pathways"), and the involvement of satellite cells in the development of skeletal muscle hypertrophy.

Regarding the latter, satellite cells represent a population of mononucleated cells that are distinct from multinucleated adult skeletal muscle fibers. Satellite cells are normally quiescent and reside between the muscle cell sarcolemma and basal lamina (14). When activated in response to MOV, these cells proliferate, and eventually their progeny fuse to existing muscle fibers and provide additional nuclei that are necessary to maintain the ratio of nuclei to cytoplasm. Because adult skeletal muscle cells cannot divide, they require the activation and incorporation of satellite cells to undergo hypertrophic growth in response to increased load-bearing stimuli such as MOV (14). Experiments have shown that irradiation of skeletal muscle to destroy the satellite cell population eliminates MOV-induced hypertrophy and increased numbers of myonuclei (14). On the other hand, while irradiation blocked MOV-induced skeletal muscle hypertrophy, it did not alter the fast-to-slow transition in MHC expression. This raises the question to what extent satellite cells participate in the fast-to-slow phenotype transitions (12). While numerous signals have been implicated in satellite cell activation, those directly involved in the MOV response are not well defined. Some evidence supports a role for IGF-1 and a macrophage response involving secretion of cytokines (14). Additional work will be required to precisely delineate MOV-induced signals involved in satellite cell activation and to resolve issues regarding cross-talk between signaling pathways involved in directing hypertrophic growth versus phenotype transitions.

Molecular Pathways for Skeletal Muscle Hypertrophy

All eukaryotic cells have the innate ability to respond to a broad range of extracellular stimuli, ultimately resulting in a suitable physiological response. This action occurs via the integration of multiple intracellular signaling pathways and gene networks to modulate the activity of transcription factors and cellular proteins involved in protein synthesis and degradation (Fig. 7.3).

Intracellular Signal Transduction Pathways

A well-known response to external signals is the activation of intracellular protein kinases and phosphatases, which modulate the phosphorylation status of a multitude of intracellular and nuclear molecules. Ultimately, these modifications alter the function of the target protein. For example, phosphorylation or dephosphorylation can alter the DNA binding activity of a transcription factor, its subcellular location, its stability, or whether it forms dimers. In addition to phosphorylation and dephosphorylation, other post-translational modifications such as glycosylation, lipidation, acetylation, or sumolation have been shown to alter a given

protein's activity. This section addresses some of the most intensely studied intracellular signaling pathways thought to control skeletal muscle hypertrophy and phenotype.

CALCINEURIN: A Ca++-DEPENDENT SIGNALING PATHWAY

Calcineurin is a cytoplasmic calcium- and calmodulin-dependent serine–threonine protein phosphatase. The functional role of calcineurin was first delineated in T cells, where increased levels of intracellular calcium were found to mediate the interaction between calmodulin and calcineurin, leading to calcineurin activation. Mechanistically, cytoplasmic NFAT proteins are dephosphorylated by activated calcineurin, allowing their translocation into the nucleus, where they combine with other transcription factors to activate target gene transcription (16,17). Since calcium is known to regulate many cellular processes in striated muscle, the question arose whether the calcineurin signaling pathway also functioned in striated muscle. The work of Molkentin and colleagues (18) provided the first evidence that calcineurin was involved in the development of cardiac hypertrophy. This was followed by the observation of Chin and associates (19), whose work implicated a role for this enzyme in determining skeletal muscle fiber type. The latter conclusion was based on the finding that treatment of rats with CsA, an inhibitor of calcineurin activity, led to a decrease in the proportion of slow fibers populating the soleus muscle while the proportion of fast fibers increased. Additionally, cell culture experiments implicated the calcineurin–NFAT pathway in modulating both skeletal muscle phenotype and the development of IGF-1–induced hypertrophy (16,17).

Since these initial observations, numerous research teams have investigated the role of calcineurin in determining skeletal muscle fiber type gene expression and the induction of hypertrophy. This work has led to a proposed model postulating that calcium-mobilizing signals evoked by stimuli such as chronic low-frequency motor nerve stimulation, MOV, or voluntary wheel running induce a sustained low-amplitude elevation in intracellular calcium levels and that this in turn stimulates both the calcineurin and CaMK signaling pathways. Activation of these two signaling pathways leads to induction of hypertrophic growth and the transcriptional activation of slow fiber genes mediated by downstream modulators comprising various members of the NFAT and MEF2 transcription factor families (16,17). The transcriptional activity of nuclear MEF2 is enhanced by calcineurin in two ways: (a) by its dephosphorylation and (b) by direct interaction with nuclear DNA–bound NFAT. CaMK is also thought to activate the transcriptional activity of DNA-bound MEF2 by disrupting MEF2's association with HDACs, which act to suppress the transcriptional activation function of MEF2. Recently, a previously unidentified HDAC kinase has been proposed to play a role similar to that of CaMK (17). However, this overall model is not without controversy.

Although initial evidence implicated a primary role for calcineurin in mediating skeletal muscle hypertrophy and phenotype, a number of recent studies have shown that while this pathway may play a central role in the development of many forms of cardiac hypertrophy, it is not necessarily required for the development of skeletal muscle hypertrophy or fiber type shifts. On the other hand, an equal number of studies support a role for calcineurin as a mediator of skeletal muscle hypertrophy and/or phenotype transitions (17). While it is difficult to attribute a definitive role to calcineurin at this time, it seems reasonable that this calcium-activated pathway may be activated by MOV, a perturbation known to be associated with stimuli (IGF-1, increase motor nerve activity) that reportedly increase sustained low-amplitude levels of intracellular calcium. A definitive statement as to whether calcineurin plays a role in skeletal muscle hypertrophy and/or phenotypic transitions will require the use of nonlethal tissue-specific and inducible gene targeting in mice that are devoid or nearly devoid of calcineurin. These mice could be subjected to MOV and other forms of exercise known to induce hypertrophy and fiber type transitions. In addition, more knowledge of the downstream gene targets of NFAT and MEF2 will be necessary for a better understanding of its role in modulating fast and slow phenotype switches in response to various physiological perturbations. Continued investigations will also be required to elucidate additional downstream effectors (transcription factors) of calcineurin signaling and for a clearer picture of how calcineurin signaling integrates with other signaling pathways shown to be involved in both hypertrophic growth and phenotype transitions.

CALCIUM–CALMODULIN PROTEIN KINASE: A CA^{++}-DEPENDENT SIGNALING PATHWAY

The activity of CaMK, like calcineurin, is regulated by intracellular calcium, although the amount and type of calcium signal differs. Whereas calcineurin is activated by sustained low-amplitude calcium signals, CaMK is presumably activated by short-duration, high-amplitude calcium signals (16,17). As previously described, CaMK is thought to enhance MEF2 transcriptional activity by disrupting its interaction with HDACs, which function as transcriptional repressors. New evidence suggests that this role may also be played by a recently reported unidentified HDAC-kinase. The activation of MEF2 has been tied to skeletal muscle fiber type gene expression based on a number of observations:

1. MOV, chronic low-frequency nerve stimulation, voluntary wheel running, and overexpression of an activated calcineurin protein resulted in decreased nuclear MEF2 phosphorylation (16,20) (supports role for calcineurin).
2. Electrophoretic mobility shift assays, which are designed to examine DNA–protein interaction, have shown that the degree of MEF2 protein binding at

MEF2 elements does not change in response to these perturbations (16) (indicates a release of HDAC transcriptional repression supporting a role for CaMK).
3. These same perturbations activated a MEF2-dependent reporter transgene in transgenic mice (termed *MEF2-sensor* mice) (20), and this effect was blocked by treatment with CsA and by transgenic expression of MCIP-1 (16) (supports a role for calcineurin and CaMK).

However, conclusions concerning MEF2 involvement in regulating slow fiber gene expression based on the results obtained with the MEF2-sensor transgenic mice must be viewed with caution, since it was recently shown that all four TEF-1 family members avidly bind the desmin MEF2 element used in the MEF2 sensor transgene (see section "Transcriptional regulation of the βMHC gene in response to MOV") (20). Here again, there is more work to be done to sort out roles for this pathway in the transduction of exercise-induced signals into growth or phenotypic transitions.

RAS–MITOGEN-ACTIVATED PROTEIN KINASE PATHWAY

The important influence of neural input on modulating muscle phenotype has been recognized since the early studies of Buller and associates (21), which demonstrated that fast muscles take on slow-twitch contractile properties following cross-innervation with a slow motor neuron and vice versa. To determine the signaling pathways involved in this process, Murgia and colleagues (22) investigated the role of the Ras-MAPK pathway, previously shown to be activated by electrostimulation of muscle. Use of several Ras mutants allowed these researchers to show that the Ras-MAPK pathway mimics the effects of slow nerve innervation, thereby implicating its role in regulating nerve-dependent slow-muscle gene expression (22). A constitutively activated Ras mutant was found to activate the ERK pathway (a MAPK pathway), which reproduced the effect of slow motor nerve input by activating slow myosin expression and decreasing fast myosin expression in denervated regeneration muscle. In contrast, slow myosin expression was blocked in innervated muscle that overexpressed a dominant negative mutant of Ras (interferes with Ras signaling). This observation is relevant to many exercise models and specifically to the overload model, since MOV is associated with an increase in motor nerve activity as measured by EMG signal.

INSULIN-LIKE GROWTH FACTOR-1, PHOSPHATIDYLINOSITOL-3-OH-KINASE, PROTEIN KINASE B, MAMMALIAN TARGET OF RAPAMYCIN PATHWAY

IGF-1 has been shown to serve important functional roles during myogenesis and in adult muscle in response to muscle injury and growth-inducing stimuli such as MOV. In particular, one isoform of IGF-1 is up-regulated in skeletal muscle only in response to mechanical stimuli and thus has been termed *mechano growth factor* (23). Studies on transgenic mice have shown that IGF-1 overexpression results in skeletal muscle hypertrophy, and IGF-1 has also been shown to stimulate satellite cell proliferation, which may contribute to its hypertrophic effect on muscle (Fig. 7.3).

Observations that IGF-1 has the potential to improve skeletal muscle regenerative capacity in injured, diseased (mdx [muscular dystrophy]) and aged mice have prompted considerable interest in deciphering the downstream signaling pathway or pathways activated by IGF-1 leading to skeletal muscle hypertrophy. Briefly, the signaling pathway downstream from IGF-1 binding to its membrane receptor (a receptor tyrosine kinase) involves the serial activation of several downstream kinases (PI[3]K, Akt, mTOR, and p70^{S6K}) leading to increased protein synthesis, a necessary step in the development of skeletal muscle hypertrophy (Fig. 7.3). Studies on myogenic cells in culture have reported that IGF-1 signaling involves the calcium-activated calcineurin pathway (24); however, the findings of others dispute this observation by showing that treatment of cells with CsA did not block IGF-1–mediated hypertrophy of myotubes (24). Instead, the latter studies provided strong evidence for a PI(3)K–Akt–mTOR pathway by showing increased phosphorylation of these downstream IGF-1 effectors following treatment of cells with IGF-1 and by demonstrating that CsA treatment did not block this response nor could a calcium ionophore induce this response (24). The involvement of this pathway in inducing skeletal muscle hypertrophy was further supported by animal studies wherein the levels of Akt phosphorylation were found to be increased in response to MOV, and treatment with the mTOR inhibitor rapamycin nearly eliminated hypertrophy of the MOV plantaris muscle (24). The overexpression of a constitutively active form of Akt in adult mouse skeletal muscle was also found to induce hypertrophy and to prevent atrophy (24). In addition, constitutively active PI(3)K, the upstream activator of Akt, was also shown to prevent muscle atrophy (24). Collectively, activation of the Akt pathway led to activation of mTOR, which in turn activates its target, p70^{S6K}, and inhibits PHAS-1/4E-BPI, which are necessary steps for increased protein synthesis and thus hypertrophy. Further support for the involvement of the Akt pathway in muscle growth comes from experiments in which double Akt knockout mice (Akt1$^{-/-}$ × Akt2$^{-/-}$) showed striking muscle atrophy (25).

MYOSTATIN: GROWTH DIFFERENTIATION FACTOR-8   Myostatin, or GDF-8, is a member of the TGF-β family, and like other members of this family, it is secreted. The expression of myostatin is primarily restricted to muscle from early embryonic development to adult life. The targeted deletion of myostatin resulted in a highly muscled mouse phenotype that resembled a phenotype observed in two breeds of cattle (Belgian Blue and Piedmontese) as early as 1807 (15). This naturally occurring phenotype in cattle was described as an inheritable condition of hyperplasia (increase in cell number) as opposed to hypertrophy (increase in cell size, as seen

with MOV) in 1982 and hence termed *double muscling*. Collectively, the finding that the absence of biologically active myostatin, whether due to a natural gene mutation (frameshift mutation due to 11-nucleotide deletion in cattle) or via gene targeting, led to increased muscle mass indicated that myostatin is a negative regulator of muscle growth. Thus, because of myostatin's obvious potential therapeutic value as a countermeasure of muscle wasting diseases, much effort has focused on elucidating signaling components of the myostatin pathway to be used as targets to block myostatin's negative influence on muscle growth.

Transcriptional Control of Skeletal Muscle Hypertrophy

An important aspect of understanding how skeletal muscle hypertrophy and phenotype are controlled undoubtedly involves the transcriptional regulation of muscle genes representing contractile proteins that constitute, in part, the protein accretion necessary for enlargement and for increased force development. Although the protein products of these muscle genes must be assembled in precise stoichiometric amounts to produce sarcomeres, no common genetic regulatory program for controlling muscle gene transcription has been identified. An explanation may be derived from the following observations: (*a*) Most muscle genes are in different parts of the genome that may not be transcriptionally activated by the same signals. (*b*) While some promoter and enhancer regions of muscle genes share conserved DNA regulatory elements (sites of protein binding, also called cis-acting element), not all muscle genes contain these regulatory elements within their control regions. (*c*) The existence of a conserved element within a gene's control region does not necessarily imply a functional role for this element under all physiological conditions (Fig. 7.4).

GENERAL SKELETAL MUSCLE TRANSCRIPTIONAL REGULATION
Although no genetic regulatory program composed of a common set of cis-acting elements and trans-acting factors that regulates all muscle genes has been elucidated, recent efforts have revealed some common aspects of transcriptional control that appear to be shared by all muscle genes. It is now clear that the initiation and maintenance of skeletal muscle cell differentiation, growth, and adult specification (fiber type) involves the activation of subsets of genes by the combined action of sequence-specific DNA-binding transcription factors and chromatin remodeling enzymes. The DNA sequences that regulate gene expression are generally located 5′ to its start site of transcription (also termed CAP site, +1), and are composed of a mosaic pattern of regulatory elements that can be distributed distally or appear clustered in the proximal promoter. However, these regulatory modules can also be located 3′ to the structural gene or within introns (Fig. 7.4A).

General Gene Structure

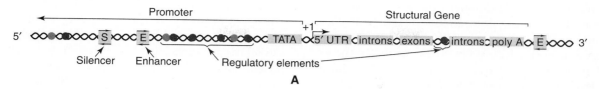

Silencer   Enhancer   Regulatory elements

A

βMyosin Heavy Chain Proximal Promotor

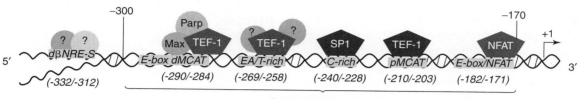

βMHC Control Region

B

FIGURE 7.4 The modular nature of gene control regions. **A.** The general structure of a gene and the hypothetical location of regulatory regions that can influence its expression in a manner specific to tissue, developmental stage, and perturbation. The modular arrangement of regulatory regions and elements allows for the integration of combinatorial signals in a gene-specific manner. **B.** A minimal human βMHC promoter previously shown to direct the expression of a reporter gene in a pattern that mimics the expression pattern of the endogenous βMHC promoter throughout development and in response to MOV. Numerous studies on the βMHC promoter have identified the presence of a strong positive muscle-specific control region (−300/−170) that is highly conserved in sequence and location across species. The regulatory elements comprising this control region and their cognate binding factors are shown. This region contains highly conserved distal muscle-CAT (dMCAT; −290/−284), A/T-rich (βA/T-rich −269/−258; also called GATA), C-rich (−244/−233), proximal MCAT (pMCAT; −210/−203) and E-box/NFAT elements (−182/−171). In addition, a negative element resides immediately upstream from the dMCAT element and is termed dβNRE-S (−332/−312).

Ample evidence supports the notion that the modular arrangement of clustered or discrete cis-acting elements provides an elegant mechanism by which the location, time, and magnitude of gene expression can be precisely regulated during development and in response to various physiological and pathophysiological stimuli (26). For example, activation of tissue-specific gene transcription involves the assembly of unique combinations of transcription factors at distinct sets of cis-acting DNA elements within promoter and enhancer regions. These DNA–protein interactions become a dynamic foundation for transcription. Cis-acting elements within these regulatory regions appear to be arranged such that either independent and/or simultaneous signals can be accommodated through the recruitment of transcriptional cofactors. Such an arrangement of elements also facilitates protein–protein interactions between bound factors. The multiprotein complexes that assemble at these various regulatory modules involve the collaborative interaction of transcription factors that are expressed ubiquitously (e.g., Sp1, MEF2, NFAT, SRF), in a tissue-specific manner (e.g., MyoD, GATA4), or activated by intrinsic or extrinsic signals. Other features that add specificity to complex gene regulation:

1. The existence of overlapping cis-acting elements (composite elements)

2. The relatedness in nucleotide composition between various cis-acting DNA regulatory elements
3. Cis-element sequence similarity does not always predicting which transcription factor will bind
4. Sequences flanking a regulatory element having profound effects on transcription factor binding
5. The possible combination of interactions that can occur between different classes of transcription factors
6. The involvement of coactivator and corepressor protein factors that can function via protein–protein interactions to bring about altered transcriptional specificity and efficiency

As can be seen in (Fig. 7.4B), all of the aforementioned regulatory features exist in the 5′-flanking region of the βMHC5′ activating gene. In addition, the βMHC is a quintessential marker of the slow muscle phenotype and is very responsive to load; thus it represents an excellent model gene system to illustrate transcriptional regulation in response to MOV.

TRANSCRIPTIONAL REGULATION OF THE βMHC GENE IN RESPONSE TO MOV   One of the most physiologically significant changes that occur in the rodent MOV plantaris muscle is a striking induction of βMHC gene expression, a MHC that is virtually nonexistent in this muscle. This adaptation has been documented by measured increases in endogenous βMHC mRNA, protein, and βMHC transgene expression (1,4,27,28). A transgenic analysis of both mouse and human βMHC promoters has delineated a minimal 293-bp human βMHC promoter that mimicked the expression pattern of the endogenous βMHC gene during early development (fetal heart and hindlimb), in adult type I fibers, and in response to MOV (27,29). Transgenic mutagenesis studies revealed that the dMCAT and NFAT elements were not required for MOV responsiveness or basal slow fiber expression; however, the βA/T-rich element was found to be required for constitutive (basal) slow muscle expression and possibly MOV responsiveness of the minimal 293 bp βMHC transgene (20,28,29). Subsequently, *in vitro* DNA–protein interaction studies provided support for the notion that the βA/T-rich element contributes to MOV induction by showing enriched binding of two distinct nuclear proteins only when using MOV plantaris nuclear extract (30). Surprisingly, the transcription factors MEF2 and GATA predicted to bind the βA/T-rich element (a composite GATA/MEF2-like element) did not bind this element when using control or MOV nuclear extracts. A yeast 1-hybrid screen of an MOV plantaris cDNA library identified TEF-1, also termed TEAD-1, a factor previously thought to bind only MCAT elements, as one of the βA/T-rich binding factors (20). The functional significance of TEF-1 binding to the βA/T-rich element was demonstrated in transient expression assays wherein overexpression of TEF-1 isoforms was shown to trans-activate βMHC reporter genes as well as TEF-1 dependent heterologous promoters.

An observation from these studies that is relevant to the complexity and control of skeletal muscle plasticity was that TEF-1 proteins were shown to bind a broad subset of A/T-rich and MEF2 sites as well as the pal-Mt element in the control region of other genes representative of the slow phenotype. Several of these elements displayed enriched TEF-1 binding only when using MOV plantaris nuclear extract. Of particular interest was the finding that the desmin pal-Mt element, which overlaps the desmin MEF2 element used to construct the MEF2-sensor transgene, bound TEF-1 protein as opposed to MEF2 during use of a variety of muscle nuclear extracts, including MOV plantaris (20). Importantly, up-regulation of the desmin MEF2-dependent transgene (MEF2-sensor mice) has been used in numerous studies as a marker of enhanced MEF2 transcriptional activation (recall that MEF2 is a downstream target of the calcineurin/CaMK pathways) in response to several exercise paradigms including electrical stimulation, voluntary wheel running, and MOV (16,17,20). It is intriguing to imagine that in adult skeletal muscle MEF2 and TEF proteins may compete for MEF2 site occupancy, depending on the activity state of a given skeletal muscle. For example, MOV may induce TEF-1 protein binding at the desmin MEF2–Mt element, whereas voluntary wheel running or motor nerve pacing may induce MEF2 activity. Clearly, additional work will is necessary to clarify whether

TEF-1 or MEF2 occupies these MEF2 binding sites in fast versus slow muscle and under various conditions of muscle activity. In any event, the specific binding of TEF-1 to a variety of MEF2, A/T-rich, and MCAT elements under control and MOV conditions (20,29), strongly suggests that TEF-1 proteins may serve a broader role than previously thought in striated and smooth muscle gene regulation under basal and hypertrophic conditions.

Atrophy

Atrophy is defined as a decrease in the cross-sectional area of all existing muscle fibers without the loss of number of muscle fibers (Fig. 7.5).

Experimental Models

The response of adult skeletal muscle to NWB activity has been extensively studied using several models that include ground-based HS, limb immobilization with muscle in a shortened position, bed rest, spinal cord isolation or transection, and space flight. Several excellent reviews provide a more comprehensive description of the experimental models used to impose muscle disuse and the physiological consequences of muscle inactivity (1,4,31). This section provides current information on the mechanistic basis underlying muscle atrophy and phenotype switches in response to NWB activity induced by HS.

The Non–Weight-Bearing Model and Skeletal Muscle Adaptations

While both fast- and slow-twitch muscle fibers are sensitive to NWB activity, muscles (soleus) or muscle regions composed mainly of slow-twitch type I fibers, which function primarily during postural and low-intensity locomotor activity, have been shown to be more susceptible. In general, this is evidenced by a rapid loss in muscle mass (cross-sectional area), a decrease in bone density, and an altered protein phenotype that correlates with a slow-to-fast change in proteins representing various subcellular systems, such as sarcomeres, glycolytic and oxidative enzymes, sarcoplasmic reticulum, and t-tubules. This shift toward a fast-twitch phenotype is characterized in part by an increase in maximum unloaded shortening velocity (V_{max}), faster contraction and relaxation times, and a greater susceptibility to fatigue (1,4). Furthermore, recent quantitative EMG measurements provided evidence that the total amount and pattern of electrical activity is significantly decreased in the NWB rat soleus and plantaris muscles throughout the period of hindlimb unweighting (32). Thus, it is not surprising that chronically innervated postural muscles such as the soleus are most susceptible to the effects of NWB activity (Fig. 7.6)

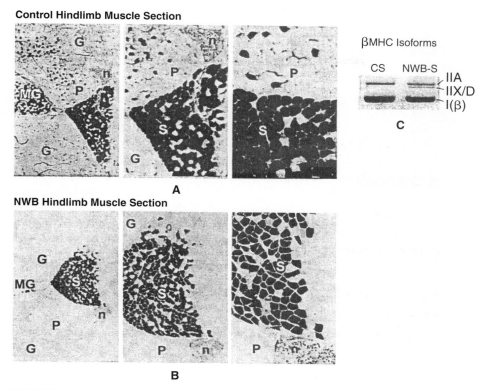

FIGURE 7.5   Cross-section of control and non–weight-bearing (NWB) hindlimb muscle with corresponding isomyosin profile. *Right to left.* Sections at increasing magnification of hindlimb skeletal muscles subjected to acid-stable ATPase histochemistry. **A.** Control muscles including the gastrocnemius (G), medial portion of the gastrocnemius (MG), plantaris (P), and soleus (S). The major nerve that runs parallel and directly adjacent to the bone is labeled *n.* **B.** The same skeletal muscles, G, MG, P, and S, subjected to 2 weeks of hindlimb suspended (HS) induced NWB. Fiber size has been significantly reduced in the NWB muscles compared to control tissues, and some fibers have undergone a slow-to-fast fiber type transition distinguished by a decrease in the number of dark stained fibers. **C.** A reduced amount of βMHC (type I fibers) and type IIA isoproteins and an induction of the type IIX/D isoprotein in the NWB-S muscle, which is consistent with slow-to-fast fiber type transition.

Prevention of Skeletal Muscle Atrophy: Countermeasures

Over the past decade, in an attempt to identify and test potential countermeasures for NWB atrophy and phenotype changes, numerous studies have shown the direct relationship between various types and combinations of postural loading and the preservation of muscle mass. The underlying common result in all of these studies is that successful countermeasures contain some form of mechanical loading, such as surgically induced mechanical overload, intermittent weight-bearing activity, centrifugation to reload muscles, or some combination of either hindlimb unweighting with mechanical overload or administration of anabolic adjuvants.

Simultaneous Imposition of Overload and Non–Weight Bearing

In this countermeasure model, the rat fast-twitch plantaris muscle was mechanically overloaded and simultaneously subjected to HS so that for 6 weeks the animals were never allowed to bear weight. Whereas MOV alone results in plantaris hypertrophy of 80 to 100% and NWB alone results in approximately 20% atrophy, the combined models resulted in a modest 18% increase in normalized plantaris weight. In addition, native slow myosin content (5%), which is normally completely repressed under NWB conditions, was restored to levels that were slightly above those observed for controls. In a similar study, only 2 weeks of the simultaneous imposition of MOV and HS countered the loss in absolute and normalized mouse soleus weight but did not prevent decreased βMHC transgene expression (33). The latter finding emphasizes that the hypertrophic stimulus of MOV was not an efficient countermeasure against the NWB-induced phenotype switch, which assuredly contributes to the NWB soleus muscle's diminished functional capacity. Furthermore, these results suggest that there is a mechanistic divergence

Non–Weight Bearing (NWB)

Hindlimb
suspension:

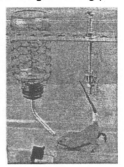

Imposes:
Chronic non–weight-bearing (NWB) activity

Induces:
Atrophy of all hindlimb muscles: (predominantly Type I)

Fiber type transitions:

Slow oxidative   Fast glycolytic

Type I $\longrightarrow$ Type IIA $\longrightarrow$ IIX/D $\longrightarrow$ IIB

FIGURE 7.6 Significant features of the non–weight-bearing (NWB) hindlimb suspension (HS) model used to induce both skeletal muscle atrophy and fiber phenotype slow-to-fast changes. The HS model is a noninvasive model that induces near maximum NWB changes in muscle mass and phenotype within 2 weeks in either rats or mice. If it is done correctly, the animal has ability to feed and drink ad libitum and can rotate 360°. Here this is accomplished with a simple sewing bobbin and a paper clip attached to a bolt and a series of locking nuts (33). Because the tail is an important component of thermoregulation, as much as possible should remain exposed. Here athletic tape is applied over thick soft cotton gauze that does not exceed an inch in width placed at the base of the tail. Not shown: with mice, four suspension stations easily fit into a double-size breeding cage, which allows mice to socialize without climbing, so their hindlimbs do not bear weight. Animals' hindlimb suspended in this manner remain healthy and active throughout the experimental period.

in the control of gene transcription leading to phenotypic transitions versus hypertrophic growth.

SEQUENTIAL OVERLOAD, NON–WEIGHT BEARING When two diverse models of muscle usage (MOV for 12 weeks immediately followed by 7 weeks of NWB) were combined sequentially, a significant increase (27%) in normalized rat plantaris weight and a slight increase in slow myosin content were observed, which indicated that the effects of loading could not be completely regressed by NWB (10).

By linking two diverse models of muscle usage (MOV induced by synergist ablation and NWB induced by HS) either simultaneously or sequentially, both slow myosin content and normalized muscle weights were not only pre-

served but increased. These results are presumably due to two factors:

1. The imposition of a chronic stretch induced a mechanical load imposed by the antagonistic muscles (tibialis anterior). Support for this notion comes from the observation of a 29% decrease in the weight of the tibialis anterior muscle (muscles in shortened position show accelerated degradation).
2. Although these rats (MOV plus NWB) were not allowed to bear weight, these animals continued to use their hindlimbs in kicking movements during which the hindlimbs were fully extended. This type of activity may have contributed to the low-level chronic mechanical stress, thereby preserving muscle mass and slow myosin content.

Other paradigms involving intermittent periods of mechanical loading, such as artificially-induced gravity by centrifugation, intermittent periods of ground support (4 times a day for 10 minutes for 7 days) and treadmill running have resulted in partial attenuation of soleus muscle atrophy.

ANABOLIC STEROIDS OR GROWTH HORMONE AND NON–WEIGHT BEARING Combining anabolic steroid, a well known adjuvant used to induce muscle growth, with NWB, revealed that anabolic steroid enhanced both body and plantaris muscle weights in both control and HS rats (34). Further increases were observed when anabolic steroid administration was combined with the simultaneous perturbation of MOV and NWB induced by HS. In contrast, results using the soleus revealed that anabolic steroid treatment in combination with HS provided no apparent influence on muscle weight or protein accumulation, nor did they appear to preferentially affect the percentages of myosin isoform content (34). Studies using intermittent loading (ladder-climbing resistance exercise) have shown that the independent effects of either intermittent resistance exercise or growth hormone provided at best minimal countermeasure effects for sparing muscle mass. However, the combination of these two perturbations appeared to have strong interactive effects in preserving muscle mass and protein content (4).

In the absence of muscle loading, growth hormone treatment alone did not prevent soleus muscle atrophy during a 4-day space flight. Furthermore, it was shown that mice harboring a transgene that specifically targeted IGF-I overexpression to skeletal muscle had normal body weights, while skeletal myofibers were hypertrophied (15–20%). Interestingly, when these same transgenic mice were subjected to 14 days of HS, targeted overexpression of IGF-I to skeletal muscle was not sufficient to attenuate NWB-induced muscle atrophy (4). Importantly, these studies illustrate that a hypertrophic stimulus may not necessarily serve as an efficient countermeasure against NWB atrophy.

Review of the literature makes it clear that considerable effort has been spent trying to identify suitable countermeasures to prevent or attenuate muscle atrophy as a result of NWB activity. Although mechanical load appears to be important for maintaining muscle mass, the use of countermeasures employing muscle loading to prevent muscle atrophy may not always be possible, or in the case of astronauts, may be too time consuming. Nevertheless, the continued quest to find a countermeasure coupled with the advancements in biotechnology has led to some progress in deciphering the mechanistic basis (signaling molecules and transcription factors) underlying muscle atrophy, thereby identifying potential protein targets for pharmacological intervention.

Molecular Pathways for Skeletal Muscle Atrophy

It is well known that various forms of muscle inactivity or disuse, as with disease, injury, aging, space travel, and sedentary life style, results in loss of both muscle mass and functional capacity. This entails a dramatic molecular remodeling, regardless of how muscle disuse commenced. The combination of mechanisms required to precisely orchestrate increased synthesis of newly required proteins, decreased synthesis of proteins no longer needed, and up-regulation of degradation pathways requires the integrated input from numerous signaling pathways that ultimately influence transcriptional regulation.

Intracellular Signal Transduction

The obvious value of elucidating the mechanistic basis controlling the amount and type of protein regulated in response to stimuli that result in skeletal muscle atrophy and

changes in phenotype has focused the attention of many researchers on a variety of signaling pathways. As a result, a plethora of data have emerged (1,4) and accumulated research generally supports the notion that while the rate of protein synthesis is decreased in response to disuse, it appears that most of the observed loss in skeletal muscle mass is the result of increased protein degradation (1).

EVIDENCE FOR DECREASED PROTEIN SYNTHESIS: AKT–MTOR–P70^{S6K} PATHWAY Since the Akt signaling pathway and its downstream targets, GSK-3β and mTOR, as well as the mTOR effectors p70^{S6K} and PHAS-1/4E-BPI, were found to be instrumental in regulating muscle hypertrophy via increased protein synthesis, this signaling pathway represented a logical place to begin investigation into the mechanistic basis underlying decreased skeletal muscle mass following inactivity (Fig. 7.3). In response to HS, Akt protein and Akt and p70^{S6K} protein phosphorylation levels in the rat gastrocnemius muscle were observed to be decreased, while levels of eIF4E-bound PHAS-1/4E-BPI were increased (24). Importantly, these modifications in response to HS were reverted in the gastrocnemius muscles of rats recovering from HS. Collectively, these data reveal an important mechanism associated with HS that selects for decreased protein translation and thus decreased protein synthesis.

EVIDENCE FOR INCREASED PROTEIN DEGRADATION: UBIQUITIN–PROTEOSOME PATHWAY Although there are several degradation pathways (lysosomal, cytosolic calcium dependent) operating in skeletal muscle, the ATP-dependent ubiquitin–proteosome pathway is thought to be the primary degradation pathway used in response to NWB induced by HS (Fig. 7.7) (35).

Ubiquitin Proteolytic Mechanism

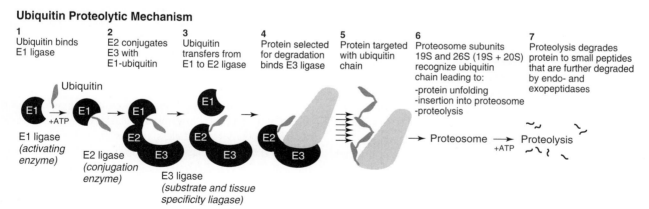

1
Ubiquitin binds E1 ligase

2
E2 conjugates E3 with E1-ubiquitin

3
Ubiquitin transfers from E1 to E2 ligase

4
Protein selected for degradation binds E3 ligase

5
Protein targeted with ubiquitin chain

6
Proteosome subunits 19S and 26S (19S + 20S) recognize ubiquitin chain leading to:
-protein unfolding
-insertion into proteosome
-proteolysis

7
Proteolysis degrades protein to small peptides that are further degraded by endo- and exopeptidases

FIGURE 7.7 Ubiquitin-proteosome mechanism. Ubiquitination-proteasome–mediated protein degradation is an ATP-dependent highly selective process with multiple components. Ubiquitin acts as a target signal for the proteosome when it is in a polyubiquitin chain bound to the protein selected for degradation. Three types of ubiquitin ligases are involved: (a) E1 ligase is the activating ligase which binds ubiquitin. (b) E2 ligase is a conjugating enzyme that combines the E2/E3 ligase complex to the E1-ubiquitin complex. (c) The E3 tissue and substrate specific ligase. Proteosome subunits 19S recognize polyubiquitin chains and initiate a process of protein unfolding, insertion into the core (20S) proteosome, and proteolysis. This results in degradation of targeted protein into small peptides. Peptides undergo further degradation via endopeptidases and exopeptidases.

Ubiquitin is a small protein that is recognized by the proteosome when it is bound in a multiple-ubiquitin complex with the protein selected for degradation. The proteosome is a large structure composed of 19S ubiquitin recognition subunits and a 20S core protein degradation subunit, which degrades targeted substrates into smaller peptides (24,35). Ubiquitination and subsequent degradation of substrates are both ATP-dependent processes. The exact mechanism that activates the ATP-dependent ubiquitin–proteosome pathway in NWB muscle has not been delineated; however, numerous studies have shown that various catabolic stimuli (sepsis, cancer, dexamethasone) are associated with increased levels of proteins in this pathway and up-regulation of ubiquitin mRNA and E3 ubiquitin–protein ligases. Available evidence will support the notion that increases in mRNAs encoding pathway components in response to catabolic inducing signals are regulated at the level of gene transcription. For example, glucocorticoid treatment of cultured L6 rat myotubes has been shown to transcriptionally induce the UbC gene, which encodes ubiquitin C. Expression of the UbC gene was shown to involve activation of the MAP kinase signaling pathway and enriched binding of the ubiquitously expressed (Sp-1) transcription factor at several Sp-1 elements (Fig. 7.8) (35). Whether or not the MAP kinase–Sp-1 pathway is activated in NWB muscle remains to be determined.

Recent research has led to the identification of two distinct ubiquitin proteins ligases, termed MuRF1 and atrogin-1, also called MAFbx. Both are E3 ligases; however, MuRF1 has been shown to act as a monomeric E3 ligase, while MAFbx contains an F-box and is a component of an SCF (Skp1, Cullin I, F-box) type E3 ligase complex. Interestingly, their expression is restricted to striated muscle and is rapidly up-regulated in response to several models of inactivity, including HS (24). In a test of the function of MAFbx, its overexpression in cultures of differentiated myogenic cells resulted in smaller myotubes. A further test of the role of these two ubiquitin ligases *in vivo* was undertaken by generating genetically altered mice that carried null mutations of these gene loci. Mice carrying null mutations of either MuRF1 or MAFbx were found to partially prevent losses in muscle mass (36–56%, respectively) in response to muscle inactivity (24). These *in vivo* functional studies provide evidence that these two ubiquitin ligases play a significant role in targeting protein substrates for degradation via the ATP-dependent ubiquitin–proteosome pathway during skeletal muscle atrophy.

Transcriptional Control of Skeletal Muscle Atrophy

It is clear that the regulation of protein synthesis and degradation are key processes controlling muscle growth, hypertrophy, and atrophy. The recent identification of two ubiquitin protein ligases (MuRF1 and MAFbx) whose expression levels are significantly up-regulated in response to NWB prompts

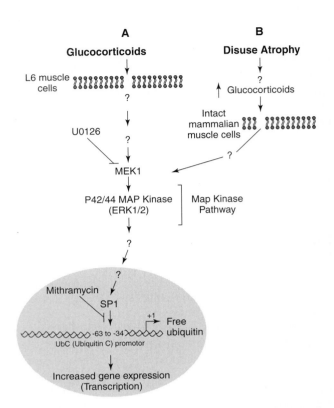

FIGURE 7.8 Map kinase/SP1 pathway regulation of ubiquitin C showing components shown to be involved in the production of increased levels of free ubiquitin. In response to treatment of glucocorticoids using L6 cells in culture, U0126 was shown to block MEK1 activation of ERK1, which indicates that members of the Map kinase signaling pathway are involved in glucocorticoid-stimulated regulation of ubiquitin. Mithramycin was shown to block SP1 binding to the UbC (ubiquitin C gene) promoter region (−63 to −34), showing specificity of SP1 involvement in up-regulating ubiquitin gene transcription. Although these experiments have been done only in cell culture to date, it is possible that this pathway is activated in intact mammalian muscle to produce the increased levels of ubiquitin necessary for greater protein degradation requirements leading to reduced muscle mass.

important questions as to whether their up-regulation is controlled at the level of transcription; such studies as yet have not been conducted. Nevertheless, transcriptional regulation was initially thought to play only a minor role, if any, in the remodeling of NWB skeletal muscle. However, recent evidence suggests that transcription is an important control point at which myofibrillar protein phenotype transitions are regulated, along with the expression of various components of the ubiquitin–proteosome pathway. This section discusses transcriptional regulation of the βMHC gene, since this gene has been the most extensively studied under NWB conditions.

TRANSCRIPTIONAL REGULATION OF THE βMHC GENE NWB imposed by HS is associated with a striking shift in MHC isoform expression that favors an increased proportion of fast MHC and a decrease in slow type I MHC (βMHC) (1,4,33). The decrease in βMHC expression observed in the NWB rodent soleus muscle has been measured at the protein and mRNA levels, suggesting that transcription in part serves a regulatory role in modulating βMHC expression. This notion was first confirmed *in vivo* when the analysis of transgenic mice harboring two different transgenes composed of either 5600 or 600 base pairs of βMHC promoter region demonstrated a significant decrease in expression following 14 days of HS (33). Since that initial observation, other reports using direct DNA injection into NWB rat soleus muscle have shown decreased expression of βMHC reporter genes (4) and increased expression of proteins representative of the fast phenotype (MHC IIB, PGAM-M). Additional transgenic and DNA–protein interaction studies showed that while the 600 bp of βMHC promoter region was sufficient to direct decreased βMHC transgene transcription in response to NWB, mutation of three highly conserved cis-acting elements (dMCAT, C-rich, and pMCAT, or βe3) (Fig. 7.4*B*) within the βMHC control region did not interfere with this process (33). A further search for the cis-element or elements responsible for NWB decreased expression led to the identification of a negative element that displayed binding only on the sense strand and was thus termed distal β-negative regulatory element sense strand (dβNRE-S,–332 to–311) (Fig. 7.4*B*) (27). In DNA–protein interaction studies, this element demonstrated highly enriched binding of two distinct nuclear proteins only when NWB soleus nuclear extract was used. Further, these two proteins were found to be antigenically distinct from CNBP and YB-1, two single-stranded DNA-binding proteins previously shown to bind this element when using heart nuclear extract. Further work will be necessary to identify these unknown proteins. Subsequent transgenic analysis revealed that regulatory element or elements downstream from the dβNRE-S element were also involved in NWB-induced decreased βMHC transgene expression (Fig. 7.4*B*). This latter study also revealed that while the pMCAT element appeared to play an important role in regulating decreased expression of rat βMHC reporter genes, it was not involved in NWB-induced human βMHC transgene expression. Collectively, this series of studies has provided important insight into the mechanisms controlling βMHC transcription in response to NWB activity: (*a*) Decreased expression of the βMHC gene involves transcriptional regulation. (*b*) βMHC DNA regulatory elements responsive to NWB were distinct and segregated from those identified to be MOV responsive, showing that the molecular mechanisms controlling gene expression during atrophy versus hypertrophy are different. (*c*) The presence of a regulatory element does not necessarily imply a function for all genes or for the same gene in different species.

Unfortunately, only a paucity of transcriptional regulation data is available regarding muscle atrophy; however, recently several laboratories, sparked by the discovery of the muscle ligases MuRF1 or MAFbx, have begun to investigate this important topic. A great deal of effort will have to be devoted to identifying transcriptional control mechanisms involved during the regulation of atrophy in response to various modes of muscle inactivity.

SUMMARY

This chapter provides a perspective of current ideas about cellular and molecular mechanisms that are involved in the control of skeletal muscle mass and phenotype. Research in this area is in its infancy, having only begun a decade ago. Nevertheless, several important concepts can be gleaned from this research:

1. No single signaling pathway, transcription factor, or DNA regulatory element (silver bullet) will universally account for the unique adaptations that occur in both muscle size and phenotype in response to altered states of muscle loading.
2. It is inappropriate to declare that the molecular responses to one perturbation are universal for all exercise modes or species.
3. Since hundreds of proteins and genes are involved in the physiological adaptations occurring during exercise, it is difficult to precisely assign any single mechanism exclusively to growth or phenotype changes.
4. While it is clear that skeletal muscle hypertrophy and atrophy involve signaling pathways that coordinately regulate protein synthesis and degradation, transcriptional regulation also plays an important role in the regulation of muscle mass.
5. Despite massive effort, controversy still exists over the precise role that the calcium-dependent CaMK and calcineurin pathways play in the control of skeletal muscle phenotype and mass.
6. The modular arrangement of DNA regulatory elements (promoter or enhancer/silencer regions) optimizes combined interactions between DNA-bound transcription factors and allows responsiveness to independent or multiple stimuli (single and converging signaling pathways) in the control of skeletal muscle gene transcription.
7. Exercise adaptations involve one or more complex mechanisms (see discussion on MEF2 sensor mice), and thus conclusions should remain conservative.

The future challenge for researchers will be to extend existing correlative observations to causative mechanisms that control skeletal muscle mass and phenotype. As future work emerges, these delineations will undoubtedly become less tangled and more comprehensive, an understanding worth obtaining since our collective health is at stake.

A MILESTONE OF DISCOVERY

Although in 1961 regeneration of skeletal muscle following injury was recognized, the mechanistic basis underlying this process remained largely unknown. The first mechanistic insight into skeletal muscle regeneration came from Alexander Mauro's electron microscopy studies of frog muscle, which discovered a new muscle cell type primarily consisting of a nucleus (with little cytoplasmic volume) external to the mature skeletal muscle fiber. This cell would have appeared to be a peripheral nucleus in the muscle fiber except for its position between the skeletal muscle fiber plasma membrane and the basal lamina; this unique location likely underlies the name *satellite cells* given by Mauro. Although experimental evidence concerning the function of satellite cells was completely absent at this time, Mauro advanced several insightful hypotheses concerning their role in skeletal muscle regeneration. To fully appreciate the accuracy of his insight, the following excerpts are provided:

> [M]ore in keeping with conventional notions of cytology, is that the satellite cells are remnants from the embryonic development of the multinucleate muscle cell which results from the process of fusion of individual myoblasts. Thus the satellite cells are merely dormant myoblast that failed to fuse with other myoblasts and are ready to recapitulate the embryonic development of skeletal muscle fiber when the main multinucleate cell is damaged. . . .
>
> [S]atellite cells are "wandering" cells that have penetrated the basement membrane and are lying underneath it ready to be mobilized into activity under the proper conditions. . . .
>
> [C]ardiac muscle has not revealed . . . satellite cells. It is exciting to speculate whether the apparent inability of cardiac muscle cells to regenerate is related to the absence of satellite cells.

We now know that satellite cells first appear at about day 17 during mouse embryonic development and reside between the basal lamina and the mature muscle fiber as inactive myoblasts. When satellite cells are activated, they

1. Recapitulate the developmental program that resembles a program initiated in muscle progenitor cells during myogenesis.
2. Proliferate and replenish the satellite cell pool, fuse to generate myotubes that mature into myofibers, and migrate to sites of muscle damage, where they fuse and participate in the regenerative process.

As yet, a cardiac cell equivalent to the skeletal muscle satellite cell has not been identified, and damaged heart muscle is incapable of regenerating.

Mauro's discovery of satellite cells has stimulated decades of research. This research has directly extended our fundamental knowledge of the role satellite cells play in the repair of mature skeletal muscle and their involvement in adult muscle hypertrophy. Because of their unique features, these cells have been used in transplantation studies with the goal to repair damaged cardiac muscle or to ameliorate skeletal muscle disease states such as muscular dystrophy. Furthermore, this research has led to the exciting identification of putative stem cells in several adult tissues, including skeletal muscle, and in some cases, these stem cells have been postulated to find their way to areas of damaged muscle via the circulation. Collectively, this ongoing work holds tremendous promise for future remedies expected to rectify an assortment of debilitating myopathies.

Mauro A. Satellite cell of skeletal muscle fibers. J Biophys Biochem Cytol 1961;9:493–495.

ACKNOWLEDGMENTS

My laboratory is supported by the University of Missouri-Columbia and by the National Institutes of Health for investigating molecular mechanisms involved in skeletal muscle hypertrophy (R01-AR41464-012) and atrophy (R01-AR45217.04). I apologize to many colleagues whose work because of space limitations has not been referenced.

REFERENCES

1. Booth FW, Baldwin KM. Exercise: regulation and integration of multiple systems. In Rowell LB, Shephard JT, eds. Muscle Plasticity: Energy Demand and Supply Processes. Handbook of Physiology. New York: Oxford University, 1996;1075–1123.
2. Timson BF. Evaluation of animal models for the study of exercise-induced muscle enlargement. J Appl Physiol 1990;69:1935–1945.
3. Crowther NB. Weightlifting in antiquity: achievement and training. In McAuslen I, Walcot P, eds. Greece and Rome, vol XXIV. Oxford, UK: Oxford University, 1977;111–120.
4. Baldwin KM, Haddad F. Plasticity in skeletal, cardiac, and smooth muscle. Invited review: effects of different activity and inactivity paradigms on myosin heavy chain gene expression in striated muscle. J Appl Physiol 2001;90:345–357.
5. Schiaffino S, Reggiani C. Molecular diversity of myofibrillar proteins: gene regulation and functional significance. Physiol Rev 1996;76:371–432.
6. Barany M. 1967. ATPase activity of myosin correlated with speed of muscle shortening. J Gen Physiol 1967;5:197–218.
7. Sartorius CA, Lu BD, Acakpo-Satchivi L, et al. Myosin heavy chains IIa and IId are functionally distinct in the mouse. J Cell Biol 1998;141:943–953.
8. Tsika RW, Gao L. Metabolic and contractile protein adaptations in response to increased mechanical loading. In Maughan RJ, Shirreffs SM, eds. Biochemistry of Exercise. Champaign, IL: Human Kinetics, 1996;205–215.

9. Tsika RW, Hauschka SD, Gao L. M-creatine kinase gene expression in mechanically overloaded skeletal muscle of transgenic mice. Am J Physiol 1995;269:C665–C674.

10. Tsika RW, Herrick RE, Baldwin KM. Time course adaptation in rat skeletal muscle isomyosins during compensatory growth and regression. J Appl Physiol 1987;63:2111–2121.

11. Gardiner PF, Michel RN, Browman F, et al. Increased EMG of rat plantaris during locomotion following surgical removal of its synergists. Brain Res 1986;380:114–121.

12. Adams GR, Caiozzo VJ, Haddad F, et al. Cellular and molecular responses to increased skeletal muscle loading after irradiation. Am J Physiol 2002;283:C1182–C1195.

13. Carson JA, Wei L. Invited review: Integrin signaling's potential for mediating gene expression in hypertrophying skeletal muscle. J Appl Physiol 2000;88:337–343.

14. Hawke TJ, Garry DJ. Invited review: Myogenic satellite cells: physiology to molecular biology. J Appl Physiol 2001;91:534–551.

15. McPherron AC, Lawler AM, Lee SJ. Regulation of skeletal muscle mass in mice by a new TGF-β superfamily member. Nature 1997;387:83–90.

16. Crabtree GR, Olson EN. Review: NFAT signaling: choreographing the social lives of cells. Cell 2002;109:S67–S79.

17. Olson EN, Williams RS. Calcineurin signaling and muscle remodeling. Cell 2000;101:689–692.

18. Molkentin JD, Lu JR, Antos CL, et al. A calcineurin-dependent transcriptional pathway for cardiac hypertrophy. Cell 1998;93:215–228.

19. Chin ER, Olson EN, Richardson JA, et al. A calcineurin-dependent transcriptional pathway controls skeletal muscle fiber type. Genes Dev 1998;12:2499–2509.

20. Karasseva N, Tsika G, Ji J, et al. Transcription enhancer factor 1 binds multiple muscle MEF2 and A/T-rich elements during fast-to-slow skeletal muscle fiber type transitions. Molec Cell Biol 2003;23:5143–5164.

21. Buller AJ, Eccles JC, Eccles RM. Interactions between motoneurones and muscles in respect of the characteristic speeds of their responses. J Physiol (Lond) 1960;150:417–439.

22. Murgia M, Serrano AL, Calabria E, et al. Ras is involved in nerve-activity-dependent regulation of muscle genes. Nature Cell Biol 2000;2:142–147.

23. Goldspink G. Gene expression in muscle in response to exercise. J Muscle Res Cell Motil 2003;24:121–126.

24. Glass DJ. Review: Molecular mechanisms modulating muscle mass. Trends Molec Med 2003;9:344–350.

25. Peng XD, Xu PZ, Chen ML, et al. Dwarfism, impaired skin development, skeletal muscle atrophy, delayed bone development, and impeded adipogenesis in mice lacking Akt1 and Akt2. Genes Devel 2003;17:1352–1365.

26. Firulli AB, Olson EN. Modular regulation of muscle gene transcription: a mechanism for muscle cell diversity. Trends Genet 1997;13:364–369.

27. McCarthy JJ, Vyas DR, Tsika GL, et al. Segregated regulatory elements direct β-myosin heavy chain expression in response to altered muscle activity. J Biol Chem 1999;274:14270–14279.

28. Tsika GL, Wiedenman JL, Gao L, et al. Induction of β-MHC transgene in overloaded skeletal muscle is not eliminated by mutation of conserved elements. Am J Physiol 1996;271:C690–C699.

29. Vyas DR, McCarthy JJ, Tsika GL, et al. Multiprotein complex formation at the β myosin heavy chain distal muscle CAT element correlates with slow muscle expression but not mechanical overload responsiveness. J Biol Chem 2001;276:1173–1184.

30. Vyas DR, McCarthy JJ, Tsika RW. Nuclear protein binding at the β-myosin heavy chain A/T-rich element is enriched following increased skeletal muscle activity. J Biol Chem 1999;274:30832–30842.

31. Morey-Holton ER, Globus RK. Invited review: Hindlimb unloading rodent model: technical aspects. J Appl Physiol 2002;92:1367–1377.

32. Riley DA, Slocum GR, Bain JLW, et al. Rat hindlimb unloading: soleus histochemistry, ultrastructure, and electromyography. J Appl Physiol 1990;69:58–66.

33. McCarthy JJ, Fox AM, Tsika GL, et al. βMyHC transgene expression in suspended and mechanically overloaded/suspended soleus muscle of transgenic mice. Am J Physiol 1997;41:R1552–R1561.

34. Tsika RW, Herrick RE, Baldwin KM. Effect of anabolic steroids on skeletal muscle mass during hindlimb suspension. J Appl Physiol 1987;63:2122–2127.

35. Price SR. Increased transcription of ubiquitin-proteosome system components: molecular responses associated with muscle atrophy. Int J Biochem Cell Biol 2003;35:617–628.

CHAPTER 8

The Muscular System: Fatigue Processes

ROBERT H. FITTS

Introduction

In 1983, Edwards (1) defined muscle fatigue as the inability to maintain the required power output, and thus the degree of fatigue depends on the extent of decline in both force and velocity. The 1990 NHLBI (Table 8.1) workshop on respiratory muscle (2) defined fatigue as "a condition in which there is a loss in the capacity for developing force and/or velocity of a muscle, resulting from muscle activity under load which is reversible by rest." The last phrase distinguishes fatigue from muscle weakness or damage, in which the capacity for rested muscle to generate force is impaired. This definition implies that fatigue can exist before performance declines or task failure occurs. In this chapter, fatigue is defined as described by Edwards (1) with the clarifier that the process is reversible. Clearly, the etiology of muscle fatigue is an important question, as the decline in force, velocity, and power that define fatigue often lead to serious limitations in muscle and whole-body performance (3,4). Despite the obvious importance of this field and considerable research, the cellular causes of muscle fatigue remain controversial. The etiology of muscle fatigue depends on the individual's state of fitness, the fiber type composition of the involved muscles, dietary status, and the intensity and duration of the exercise. For example, the factors causing fatigue during prolonged exercise differ from those precipitating fatigue in high-intensity contractile activity. The problem is complex because muscle fatigue may result from deleterious alterations in the muscle itself (peripheral fatigue) and/or from changes in the nervous system (central fatigue). Additionally, because fatigue often results from the effects of multiple factors acting at various sites and in some cases interacting synergistically, it has been difficult to unequivocally identify the causative factors (3,5). In 1984, Bigland-Ritchie (6) identified the major potential sites of fatigue as (a) excitatory input to higher motor centers, (b) excitatory drive to lower motor neurons, (c) motor neuron excitability, (d) neuromuscular transmission, (e) sarcolemma excitability, (f) E-C coupling, (g) contractile mechanisms, and (h) metabolic energy supply and metabolite accumulation. As shown in Figure 8.1A, these sites represent all of the steps involved in voluntary force production. While data support a role for each of these sites in the fatigue process, in highly motivated athletes, sites 5 to 8 appear most important (3,7,8). Although the cellular etiologies of fatigue with high-intensity compared to prolonged exercise are clearly different, both result in losses in force, velocity, and power. This chapter first describes the functional changes that characterize fatigue and follows with a consideration of the cellular mechanisms thought to be responsible for fatigue. Some examples of how fatigue is altered by programs of exercise training are discussed.

TABLE 8.1	List of Abbreviations
ADP	Adenosine diphosphate
AM	Actomyosin
AMP	Adenosine monophosphate
ATP	Adenosine triphosphate
AP	Action potential
a/P_0	Describes the degree of curvature of the Hill force–velocity curve, where "a" is a force constant
ΔC	Concentration gradient
Ca^{++}_i	Intracellular Ca^{++} transient
CaPi	Calcium phosphate
CICR	Calcium-induced calcium release
CK^{-1}	Creatine kinase deficient
CNS	Central nervous system
CT	Time in milliseconds from initiation of isometric twitch to peak twitch tension
DHP	Dihydropyridine
$+dP/dt$	Peak rate of tension development
$-dP/dt$	Peak rate of tension decline
E-C	Excitation–contraction
FFA	Free fatty acid
Hz	Stimulation frequency per second
$([K^+]I)$	Interstitial potassium
k_{tr}	Rate constant of tension redevelopment following rapid release and then extension of a muscle fiber
LFF	Low-frequency fatigue
mM	millimolar
α-MN	α-Motor neuron
ML/s	Muscle lengths per second
MPD	myophosphorylase deficient
MVC	Maximal voluntary contraction
NADH	nicotinic acid dehydrogenase
NHLBI	National Heart, Lung and Blood Institute
N-M	Neuromuscular
PC	Phosphocreatine
pCa	Negative log of the calcium concentration
pH	Negative log of the hydrogen ion concentration
P_i	Inorganic phosphate
P_0	Peak isometric tetanic tension
P_t	Peak isometric twitch tension
ROS	Reactive oxygen species
$\frac{1}{2}$ RT	Time in milliseconds for relaxation from peak twitch tension to one-half of peak tension
SR	Sarcoplasmic reticulum
V_m	Membrane potential
V_{max}	Maximal velocity of muscle or fiber shortening determined by the Hill plot
$\dot{V}_0$	Maximal velocity of muscle or fiber shortening determined by the slack test

The Effect of Fatigue on Muscle Mechanics

Animal and human studies have shown that force, velocity, and power decline with fatigue, with the degree of change dependent on the fiber composition of the muscle. The studies on muscle fatigue in animals have used isolated single fibers (both living and skinned fiber preparations), whole muscles *in vitro,* and anesthetized *in situ* preparations (3,5,9–11). Human studies, on the other hand, have for the most part been per-

formed using *in vivo* exercise paradigms and muscle tests and/ or organelle isolated from muscle biopsies (3,8,12–15). Two general types of contraction (isometric and isotonic) have been evaluated, and for the most part the alterations in contractile function with fatigue have been observed to be similar regardless of the species studied (3). When both peak force and velocity were compared, it has been generally observed that force declined sooner and to a greater extent than velocity (16). Since peak power depends on both, it was compromised to a greater extent than either force or velocity. When different muscles are compared, slow oxidative muscles, such as the

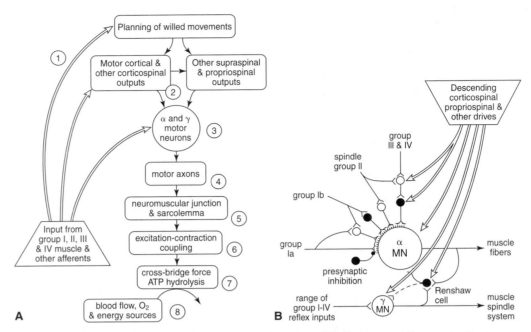

FIGURE 8.1 **A.** Potential sites of central (events 1–4) and peripheral (events 5–8) fatigue. Feedback from skeletal muscle (event 1) is shown acting at three levels in the central nervous system. **B.** Summary of inputs to α- and γ-motor neurons for an agonist muscle. Cells with solid circles are inhibitory. Presynaptic inhibition is shown acting selectively on the afferent paths to motor neurons. (*Modified from Gandevia SC. Spinal and supraspinal factors in human muscle fatigue. Physiol Rev 2001;81:1735.*)

soleus, are more resistant to fatigue than fast muscles, such as the tibialis anterior. Consistent with this, slow motor units, containing oxidative type I fibers, are more resistant to fatigue than motor units composed of fast type II fibers. Among fast motor units, the type IIX units showed resistance to fatigue that was intermediate between the highly fatigable type IIB and the relatively fatigue-resistant type IIA motor units (3).

Each contractile property (e.g., maximal shortening velocity, peak force, twitch duration) depends on specific cellular and molecular events associated with the crossbridge cycle. Although the molecular details of the crossbridge cycle are not yet fully understood, a kinetic model of actin and myosin interaction in skeletal muscle has been developed (17) (Fig. 8.2). When myosin initially binds to actin, the actomyosin (AM · ADP · P_i) is in a weakly bound low-force state, and with the subsequent release of P_i (step 5, Figure 8.2), the crossbridge transforms into a strongly bound high-force state (AM' · ADP). The latter is thought to be the dominant form during a maximal isometric contraction. The rate of transition (difference between the forward and backward rate constants of step 5 in Fig. 8.2) is thought to limit the peak rate of force development (+dP/dt). In contrast, the maximal unloaded shortening velocity (V_0) is highly correlated with and likely limited by the actomyosin–ATP hydrolysis rate, which in turn appears limited by the ADP dissociation step (Fig. 8.2, step 7). This kinetic scheme has

proved useful in assessing the cellular mechanisms of muscle fatigue for factors acting at the crossbridge (3).

Isometric Twitch and Tetanic Contractile Properties

During exercise limb skeletal muscles go through a shortening and lengthening cycle and for a portion of the cycle may

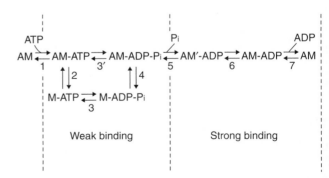

FIGURE 8.2 Actomyosin ATP hydrolysis reaction during contraction in skeletal muscle, where A is actin and M is the myosin head (myosin S1). Scheme is adapted from current models of ATP hydrolysis. (*Modified from Metzger JM, Moss RL. pH modulation of the kinetics of a Ca⁺⁺-sensitive crossbridge state transition in mammalian single skeletal muscle fibres. J Physiol (Lond) 1990;428:761.*)

contract isometrically. The α-MN activation frequency varies from 10 to 50 Hz for slow and from 30 to more than 100 Hz for fast motor units, with force output dependent on the activation frequency and the number of recruited units. It is clear that muscles are never activated with single action potential or twitch contractions. However the evaluation of isometric twitch properties before and after fatigue has proved useful in identifying the cellular sites of fatigue. Figure 8.3A shows representative isometric twitches recorded before and immediately following fatigue produced by in situ stimulation (2) (100-ms fused contractions per second for 5 minutes) of rat slow-twitch soleus muscles. As shown, P_t is generally depressed following fatiguing contractile activity. However, since Pt is influenced by muscle temperature (which increases during contractile activity), dP/dt, and the duration of the intracellular Ca^{++} transient, it does not always reflect the degree of fatigue-induced decline in either the number of crossbridges that can be activated or the force per bridge. Other features of a twitch post fatigue are prolonged contraction (CT) and ½ RT and reductions in the peak rate of tension development (+dP/dt) and decline (−dP/dt). In addition, when fatigue is produced in vitro one generally observes a prolonged twitch (total time for contraction and relaxation). With in situ stimulation, the CT and 1/2 RT are usually prolonged, but the total twitch duration may remain unaltered (Fig. 8.3A). Relaxation appears to slow in direct proportion to the degree of fatigue and is exacerbated when intracellular acidosis develops (pH < 6.9). The changes in the twitch with fatigue reflect the intracellular Ca^{++} transient (Ca^{++}_i), which has a reduced amplitude, a slower onset and rate of decline, and a prolonged duration in fatigued muscle fibers (9,18). The reduced P_t is a direct result of the decline in the amplitude of the Ca^{++}_i. The amount of Ca^{++} released in response to a single stimulus (twitch response) or even low-frequency activation (10–20 Hz) places the muscle fiber on the steep region of the pCa–force relationship (Fig. 8.4) such that a small decline in the amplitude of the Ca^{++}_i elicits a large drop in force.

P_0 before and immediately following fatigue for the slow type I soleus muscle is shown in Figure 8.3B. The decline in P_0 (34% in this example) is a universal observation for fatigued muscles and muscle fibers: by definition a fatigued muscle must have a reduced P_0. The decline in P_0 with fatigue can be explained only by a decline in the force per crossbridge and/or the number of crossbridges in the high-force states (AM′ − ADP and AM − ADP states shown in Fig. 8.2). Figure 8.4 summarizes the mechanisms involved in the reduction of isometric force with fatigue. The initial decline in force (mechanism 1, Fig. 8.4) occurs as a result of a reduction in maximal isometric force (inhibition of step 5, Fig. 8.2). Simultaneously, the Ca^{++}–force relationship shifts right (mechanism 2, Fig. 8.4), but this has no immediate consequence, as the amplitude of the Ca^{++}_i is still high. However, late in fatigue, the amplitude of the Ca^{++}_i declines (mechanism 3, Fig. 8.4) and force is depressed by the combined effect of mechanisms 2 and 3. A combination of mechanisms

1 to 3 causes peak tension to decline along the broken line shown in Figure 8.4.

In nonfatigued muscles, the peak rate of tension development (+dP/dt) is limited by the rate of crossbridge transition from the low- to the high-force state, which depends on the difference between the forward and reverse rate constants of step 5, Figure 8.2. With contraction, the forward rate constant is accelerated by both cytoplasmic Ca^{++} and the number of strongly bound crossbridges, both of which decrease with fatigue. In high-intensity exercise, the decline in +dP/dt with fatigue could also be mediated by an increase in H^+ and P_i. The observation that +dP/dt divided by P_0 [(+dP/dt)/P_0] was not altered by fatigue suggests that the reduced +dP/dt resulted primarily from the decline in P_0, which in turn was caused by the fatigue-induced reduction in the number of strongly bound high-force crossbridges. Of course the latter depends on the concentration of cytoplasmic Ca^{++}, pH, and P_i (see "Crossbridge Mechanism of Fatigue"). In contrast, −dP/dt declines considerably more than force, and in the example shown in Figure 8.3B the values were 28 and 66% of those before fatigue for −dP/dt and P_0, respectively. The depression in −dP/dt with fatigue is even greater in fast muscles. This suggests a slower dissociation of actin from myosin in fatigued muscle cells, which could reflect a direct effect on the crossbridge detachment rate and/or a reduced rate of Ca^{++} reuptake by the SR pumps. The rate of Ca^{++} dissociation from troponin is thought to be too fast to be rate limiting (5). Relaxation from a tetanus generally occurs in 3 phases:

Phase 1, no change in force following the final action potential
Phase 2, a slow, linear drop
Phase 3, a final rapid exponential decline

With fatigue each of these phases slows, and the distinction between them is less clear (5). During phase 2 the sarcomere length remains constant and the force decline is thought to reflect the rate of crossbridge detachment. The time course of the decline in force is delayed compared to the predicted force, which is determined from the known relationship between the intracellular Ca^{++} content and force in the steady state (pCa–force relationship). It has been hypothesized that the delay between the predicted force and measured force reflects the crossbridge detachment time. The observation that this delay increases in fatigued muscle fibers suggests that the slowed relaxation is caused in part by a reduced crossbridge dissociation rate (5).

Force–Velocity and Force–Power Relationship

Since the work of Hill (19) it has been known that the force–velocity relationship is hyperbolic, with the maximal velocity of shortening (V_{max}) obtained at zero load. The curvature of the relationship is described by the a/P_0 ratio, where "a" is a force constant of the Hill equation, and a higher ratio reflects less curvature (19). Fast-twitch muscles are characterized by a high V_{max} and a/P_0 ratio in which the former is

SOLEUS

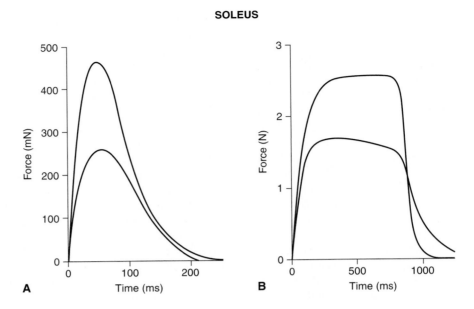

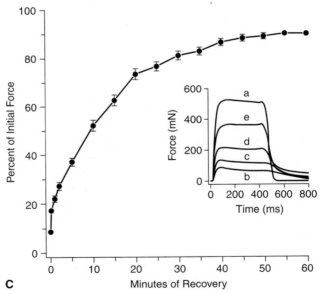

FIGURE 8.3 Isometric twitch (**A**) and tetanic (**B**) contraction of the rat soleus before and immediately following 5 minutes of *in situ* stimulation (2/s, 100 ms trains at 150 Hz for 5 minutes). Control and fatigued values were, respectively, twitch tension (P_t), 462 and 260 mN; contraction time (CT), 43 and 54 ms; One-half relaxation time ($\frac{1}{2}$RT), 60 and 74 ms; tetanic tension (P_0), 2.57 and 1.71 N; peak rate of tetanic tension development (+dP/dt), 25.0 and 22.1 N/s; peak rate of tetanic tension decline (−dP/dt), 27.5 and 7.6 N/s. **C.** Recovery of force production of frog semitendinosus (percent of initial force) after stimulation. Values are means ± SE. Inset: tetanus records at prefatigued (a) and at 10 seconds (b), 60 seconds (c), 5 minutes (d), and 20 minutes (e) of recovery. Peak tetanic tension returned to prefatigued value by 45 minutes. *(Fig. 8.3C is modified from Thompson LV, Balog EM, Riley DA, et al. Muscle fatigue in frog semitendinosus: alterations in contractile function. Am J Physiol 1992;262:C1504.)*

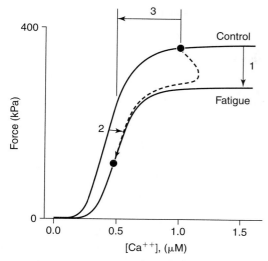

FIGURE 8.4 A plot of tetanic force versus intracellular calcium (Ca^{++}_i) summarizing the mechanisms involved in the reduction of isometric force in fatigue: (1) reduced maximal force, (2) reduced myofibrillar Ca^{++} sensitivity, and (3) reduced tetanic (Ca^{++}_i). *Broken line*, the normal pattern during fatigue. *Arrow*, the direction of time. (*Modified from Allen DG, Lännergren J, Westerblad H. Muscle cell function during prolonged activity: cellular mechanisms of fatigue. Exp Physiol 1995;80:507.*)

limited by the myofibrillar ATPase activity. Hence, V_{max} reflects the crossbridge cycle speed, which is considerably higher in fast- than in slow-twitch muscle. Figure 8.5, *A* and *B* shows representative force–velocity curves for the rat slow-twitch soleus and fast-twitch plantaris.

To compare the two muscles, V_{max} is expressed in muscle lengths per second. In this example, the fast plantaris showed a 2.7 higher V_{max} than the soleus. V_{max} is known to underestimate the true unloaded maximal shortening velocity (V_0) obtained by the slack test method, in which slow type I fibers have been shown to be one-third and one-sixth as fast as the fast type IIA and IIX fiber types, respectively.

With the development of muscle fatigue, force usually declines sooner and to a greater extent than shortening velocity. In the example shown, the soleus P_0 fell by 34% (Fig. 8.3B), compared to an 8% drop in V_{max} (Fig. 8.5A). While force always declines first, V_{max} may ultimately drop by an amount equal to that observed for force (5). However, muscles contracting *in vivo* never have zero loads; thus, it is important to assess whether the curvature as reflected by the a/P_0 ratio changes with fatigue. In fast muscles, the a/P_0 ratio is threefold to fourfold higher than in slow muscle (compare solid lines Fig, 8.5, *A* and *B*, where the ratio was 0.129 and 0.521 for the soleus and plantaris, respectively). Consequently, individuals with a high percentage of fast-twitch fibers can generate higher velocity and power at a given relative load than those with predominantly slow-twitch fibers. There are

few data assessing the affect of fatigue on the a/P_0 ratio. Since the extremes of the force–velocity relationship (V_{max} and P_0) in response to a given contractile paradigm are more resistant to change in slow than in fast muscles, one might expect a similar difference in the stability of the a/P_0 ratio. This appears to be the case. In the data shown in Figure 8.5, the a/P_0 ratio was relatively unaltered by fatigue in the soleus (0.129 vs. 0.117) but declined to 0.147 in the plantaris. These data suggest that with fatigue the fast plantaris lost its ability to maintain relatively high velocities at moderate loads. The importance of this is that peak power is obtained at moderate loads and velocities (generally between 25 and 40% of V_{max} and P_0).

To prevent muscle fatigue and a deterioration of performance, one must maintain peak power. Although peak power can be determined from the force–velocity relationship, few studies have actually assessed peak power or its change with fatigue. In human muscle, peak power varies with fiber type, with a ratio of 10:5:1 for the type IIX, IIA, and I fibers, respectively. Recovery from fatigue generally shows a fast (complete in < 2 minutes) and a slow component (1–2 hours) with the former particularly apparent in fast muscles (Fig. 8.3C). Because of the rapid recovery phase, it is difficult to acquire power curves post fatigue. Nonetheless, it can be accomplished, and representative data are shown in Figure 8.5, C and D for the soleus and plantaris muscles, respectively. With fatigue, the reduced peak power results from a decline in both the tension and velocity. The latter is particularly important in fast muscles because of the decline in the a/P_0 ratio. As fatigue develops, peak power declines and is obtained at progressively lower shortening velocities, making only slower movements effective.

Central Fatigue

Since the early twentieth century, it has been recognized that changes in the afferent input to the CNS or events within the CNS itself can contribute to fatigue. This component of fatigue has been referred to as *central fatigue*. The relative importance of central versus peripheral fatigue is still unsettled and clearly depends on the work situation (competitive sport versus every day activities) and the motivation of the individual. Most agree that central fatigue likely plays a minor role in limiting the performance of the highly trained athlete but is likely more important in repetitive tasks performed in the workplace (3,7,8). The cellular sites responsible for central fatigue have not been elucidated but could involve alterations in (*a*) afferent inputs from group I to IV muscle afferents, (*b*) suprasegmental centers involved in planning of willed movements, (*c*) motor cortical and other corticospinal outputs, (*d*) other supraspinal and propriospinal outputs, and (*e*) α- and γ-motor neurons or their axons (Fig. 8.1A). Merton (20) and others (8) used electrical stimulation of motor nerves to demonstrate that voluntary activation could

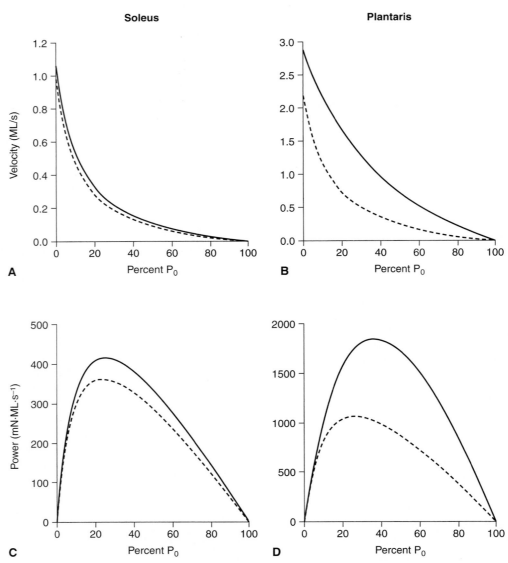

FIGURE 8.5 Force–velocity (traces **A** and **B**) and force-power (traces **C** and **D**) relationships for rat soleus (**A** and **C**) and plantaris (**B** and **D**) muscles before (*solid lines*) and immediately following fatigue (*broken lines*) produced by *in situ* stimulation (2/s, 100 ms trains at 150 Hz [soleus] or 200 Hz [plantaris] for 5 minutes). Control and fatigued values were, respectively, soleus (**A**) maximal shortening velocity (V_{max}), 1.06 and 0.98 muscle lengths (ML) per second; a/P_0, 0.129 and 0.117; plantaris (**B**) V_{max}, 2.91 and 2.22 ML/s; a/P_0, 0.521 and 0.147; soleus (**C**) peak power, 415 and 361 mN · ML · s^{-1}; plantaris (**D**) peak power, 1848 and 1072 mN · ML · s^{-1}.

maximally activate a muscle and that central fatigue did not exist during a MVC. The latter conclusion was based on the observation that a twitch produced by nerve stimulation during a MVC did not elicit additional force (twitch interpolation technique) even when significant peripheral fatigue had developed. Since the initial studies of Merton (20), the resolution of the recording systems has improved, and the twitch interpolation technique has been applied to numerous muscles. It is now generally accepted that the extent to which voluntary activation can produce peak force varies be-

tween muscles (8). For example, it has been demonstrated that it is more difficult to elicit maximal force by voluntary activation in the ankle plantar flexors than the ankle dorsiflexors. With improved recording techniques, twitch interpolation has established the occurrence of central fatigue in several muscle groups, including elbow flexors, ankle plantar flexors and dorsiflexors, and quadriceps muscles (8).

The identification of specific sites involved in central fatigue is problematic, as it is difficult to separate factors mediated by changes in afferent inputs from suprasegmental alterations. The problem is exacerbated by the fact that the intrinsic properties of α-motor neurons can contribute to motor output. Figure 8.1B shows a summary of inputs to the α- and γ-motor neurons and demonstrates the complexity of the circuits affecting α-motor neuron excitability. It is well established that during a sustained maximal voluntary effort the firing rate of α-motor neurons declines. This response was termed muscular wisdom, as it was thought not to cause but rather protect against fatigue by matching the motor nerve firing rate to the slowed force transient of the fatiguing muscle. Bigland-Ritchie and associates (21) hypothesized that the reduced firing rate resulted from an increased activation of group III and IV muscle afferents that were activated by metabolic factors, such as an increase in extracellular K+. This hypothesis was supported by their observation that the firing rate did not recover during 3 minutes of rest while muscle blood flow was occluded but did upon resumption of blood flow.

Proponents of a significant role for central fatigue suggest that the decline in α-motor neuron firing rate is excessive and results in reduced force caused by too low a firing rate and/or a reduction in the number of active motor neurons (8). The supporting evidence is that a significant twitch interpolation can be observed and that motor cortical stimulus can increase the force output of the fatigued muscle. It seems likely (although not proved) that there is a net decline in α-motor neuron facilitation due to the combined effects of reduced IA (muscle spindle) afferent input and increased activation of group III and IV muscle afferents activating inhibitory interneurons (Fig. 8.1B). Additionally, maintained activation of an α-motor neuron results in a decreased firing rate due to intrinsic property of the cell. Collectively, these changes would reduce the likelihood of a MVC producing optimal activation of the α-motor neuron pool. The observation that an extrinsic motor cortical stimulus can increase the force output of a muscle suggests that pathways proximal to the corticospinal outputs (Fig. 8.1A) contribute to central fatigue.

Given the current state of knowledge, it is not possible to determine the importance of central fatigue in limiting human performance. The increase in force in response to peripheral motor nerve or CNS motor cortical paths suggests at most a 10% contribution to the fatigue-induced decline in force. Research is needed to establish that the observed changes in CNS function are causative and not simply correlative with fatigue and to identify the exact cellular sites involved in central fatigue.

Substrates and Fatigue With Heavy-Intensity Exercise

Fatigue caused by peripheral cellular events may have a site of origin at the crossbridge, E-C processes, and/or cell metabolic pathways. With heavy exercise the muscle high-energy phosphates, ATP, and PC decrease, while P_i, ADP, lactate, and H+

all increase as fatigue develops. All of these changes have been suggested as possible fatigue-inducing factors (3,5).

To avoid fatigue, adequate tissue ATP levels must be maintained, as this substrate supplies the immediate source of energy for force generation by the myosin crossbridges. ATP is also needed in the functioning of the sodium–potassium pump (Fig. 8.6, 5), which is essential in the maintenance of a normal sarcolemma and t-tubular AP. Additionally, ATP stabilizes the SR Ca++ release channel and is a substrate of the SR ATPase and thus is required in the process of Ca++ release and reuptake by the SR (Fig. 8.6, points 4 and 6). A disturbance in any of these processes could lead to muscle fatigue. It is well established that whole-cell ATP content declines during heavy contractile activity and that it can drop from about 5 to 1.5 mM. However, even the latter would be more than 100-fold higher than that required for full crossbridge activation, sufficient for normal Na+-K+ pump, SR pump, and Ca++ release channel function. Consequently, for low ATP to be a factor in fatigue, its distribution would have to show considerable compartmentalization so that the ATP content around ion pumps and SR Ca++ channels was below the cell average. As will be discussed in the section on E-C coupling, there is some evidence that compartmentalization of ATP does exist and that low ATP may inhibit SR Ca++ release. Nonetheless, a cause-and-effect relationship between low cell ATP and muscle fatigue has not been demonstrated. In fact, the classic experiments of Karlsson and Saltin (15) illustrate the absence of a correlation between changes in ATP and performance. In this research, the needle biopsy technique was used to evaluate substrate changes after dynamic exercise to exhaustion at three exercise intensities. After 2 minutes of exercise, ATP and PC were depleted to the same extent at all loads; however, fatigue occurred only with the highest workload. These results are equivocal, since the biopsy was acquired some seconds after exercise ceased, and the sample represented an average tissue ATP that might not reflect the concentration existing at the crossbridges, sarcolemma, or the SR. However, in vitro studies in which the muscles were quick-frozen while contracting also failed to show a correlation between ATP and force (3).

Although PC is known to decline with heavy exercise, the time course of decline differs from that observed for tension, making a casual relationship unlikely (3). PC facilitates the movement of high-energy phosphates from the mitochondria to the sites of utilization, a process called the PC-ATP shuttle. A critically low PC level may disrupt this shuttle system and slow the rate of ADP rephosphorylation to ATP. This could lead to critically low ATP at various subcellular sites. The interpretation of whole-muscle determinations of ATP and PC are further complicated, as compartmentalization may exist between as well as within fibers. Consequently, a high mean value post fatigue may not be representative of the most fatigued cells. Although low ATP may inhibit ion pumps and SR Ca++ release, it seems unlikely that ATP content surrounding the crossbridges would be low enough to

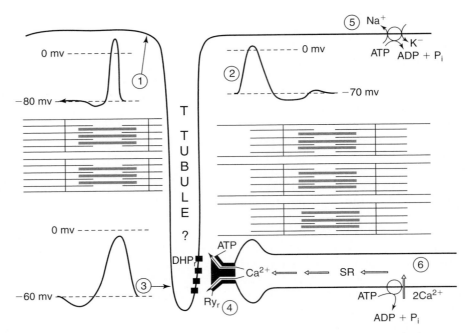

FIGURE 8.6   E-C coupling showing a representative sarcolemma action potential (AP) at rest (1) and following fatigue (2). It is unknown how fatigue affects the AP in the depths of the t-tubule (3); hence, the displayed record is theoretical and not an actual measured AP. The SR Ca⁺⁺ release channel (ryanodine receptor) is shown as 4; 5 and 6 represent the sarcolemma Na⁺-K⁺ pump and the SR ATPase pump, respectively. The question mark indicates that the composition of the extracellular fluid in the depths of the t-tubule in a fatigued muscle is unknown. The broken lines across each AP represent the resting and zero overshoot potentials. *(Modified from Fitts RH. Cellular, molecular, and metabolic basis of muscle fatigue. In Rowell LB, Shepherd JT, eds. Handbook of Physiology, Section 12. Exercise: Regulation and Integration of Multiple Systems. New York: Oxford University, 1995;1157.)*

directly inhibit force production (22). The prevailing evidence suggests that fatigue produced by other factors reduces the ATP utilization rate before ATP becomes limiting at the crossbridge (3).

The role of increased ADP levels in the development of muscle fatigue is not well understood. It has been calculated that with PC depletion and the relatively low activity of myokinase, ADP could rise from about 10 μM to 2 to 3 mM during heavy contractile activity (23). Although high ADP has been shown to increase force and depress velocity (5), the primary effect of mM ADP may be on the SR pump (see "SR ATPase Pump").

Intense stimulation of skeletal muscle activates glycolysis, hence a high rate of lactic acid production. The acid immediately dissociates into lactate and free H⁺, and cell pH declines from 7.0 to values as low as 6.2 (3). In the early twentieth century, lactic acid was linked to fatigue, and following the work of A. V. Hill in the late 1920s the lactic acid theory of muscle fatigue was highly popular. It is now generally thought that the component of fatigue correlated with lactate results from the effects of an increased free H⁺ (low pH) rather than lactate or the undissociated lactic acid.

The H⁺ ion could elicit fatigue by inhibiting

1. Crossbridges
2. Ca⁺⁺ binding to troponin
3. Na⁺-K⁺ pumps
4. SR pumps
5. Glycolysis

Crossbridges and Ca⁺⁺ binding to troponin are considered in the section "Crossbridge Mechanism of Fatigue," and Na⁺-K⁺ and SR pumps in the section "Excitation–Contraction Coupling." Regarding glycolysis, two observations support the hypothesis that an elevated H⁺ ion concentration inhibits glycolysis. First, lactate formation during muscle stimulation stopped when the intracellular pH dropped to 6.3 (22). Second, during a 60-second measurement period, Hermansen and Osnes (14) found no change in the pH of the most acidic homogenates of fatigued muscle, while the pH values of the homogenates from resting muscle showed a marked fall due to significant glycolysis. However, the observations that the changes in ATP were not correlated with either work capacity or force during recovery argues against an important role for H⁺ inhibition of glycolysis in the fatigue process. If the inhibition of glycolysis were causative in fatigue, the decline in tissue ATP would likely reach limiting levels. Consequently, a significant correlation between force and ATP would exist during the development and recovery from fatigue.

Excitation–Contraction Coupling

The major components of a muscle cell involved in E-C coupling include the neuromuscular (N-M) junction, the surface membrane, the t-tubules, and the SR membranes, including the Ca++ release channels (ryanodine receptor) and the Ca++ pump proteins. Except for the N-M junction all have been suggested to play a role in muscle fatigue, particularly fatigue induced by high-intensity contractile activity. Although the amount of transmitter released from the motor nerve endings may decline with high frequencies of activation, transmission block at the N-M junction has not been observed (3,20). The primary observations supporting a role for E-C coupling failure in muscle fatigue are as follows: (*a*) The drop in force with electrical stimulation in single fibers is associated with a decline in the amplitude of the Ca++ transient. (*b*) Direct release of Ca++ from the SR by caffeine increases intracellular Ca++ and to a large extent reverses the decline in force (Fig. 8.7).

Sarcolemma and t-Tubular Membrane Action Potential

In nonfatigued muscle, the surface (sarcolemma) membrane AP propagates down into the t-tubules, where the depolarization triggers a voltage-driven conformational change in an intramembranous t-tubular protein (DHP receptor). This t-tubular charge movement in turn triggers Ca++ release from adjacent SR Ca++ release channels, producing a uniform activation of the entire fiber (3). It is well documented that with heavy exercise, the resting potential of skeletal muscle fibers depolarizes by 10 to 20 mV and that the amplitude and duration of the AP are depressed and prolonged, respectively. A schematic representation of this change is shown in Figure 8.6, where points 1 and 2 show AP before and after fatigue, respectively. In this example, fatigue has resulted in a 10-mV depolarization of the resting membrane potential (V_m), and the overshoot of the AP has been reduced from +30 mV to a few millivolts above zero. It has been suggested but not proved that these changes in the sarcolemma and t-tubular V_m and AP induce fatigue either by preventing propagation of the AP into the depths of the fiber or by inhibiting the t-tubular charge sensor, which in turn reduces SR Ca++ release

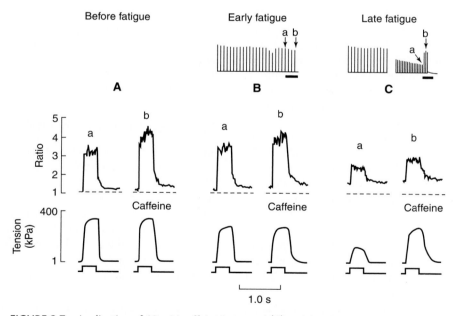

FIGURE 8.7 Application of 10 mM caffeine in control (**A**) and during two successive fatigue runs (**B** and **C**). Bars below tension records (*top*) indicate caffeine exposure during fatiguing stimulation; caffeine was applied after 22 fatiguing tetani (**B**) and when tetanic tension was depressed to 0.36 P_0 by 187 tetani (**C**). Fluorescence ratio and tension records from tetani elicited before application of caffeine (a) and in presence of caffeine (b) (*middle* and *bottom*). Broken lines represent resting ratio in control prefatigued fiber; stimulation periods are displayed below tension records. Tetanic ratio increase induced by caffeine in late fatigue was accompanied by a substantially enhanced tension production, whereas tension was not markedly affected by increased ratios in the other two states. (*Modified from Westerblad H, Allen DG. Changes of myoplasmic calcium concentration during fatigue in single mouse muscle fibers. J Gen Physiol 1991;98:625.*)

(Fig. 8.6, no. 4). The problem is likely to be exacerbated in centrally located myofibrils (22). This hypothesis, termed the membrane mechanism of muscle fatigue (24), would allow contractions at reduced rates and forces while preventing catastrophic changes in cellular homeostasis that might lead to cell damage. The primary support for this theory comes from the observations that high frequency stimulation can (*a*) produce a spatial gradient of Ca^{++} with higher concentrations near the fiber surface and (*b*) induce central core wavy myofibrils as a result of activation of peripheral but not central fibrils (3,5). The extent of wavy myofibril formation has been shown to increase in parallel with the development of muscle fatigue and to be prevented by direct release of Ca^{++} from the SR by caffeine.

The fatigue-induced depolarization of the sarcolemma and t-tubule resting potential and the reduced AP spike height are caused by an increase in extracellular K^+ and intracellular Na^+, respectively. The loss of intracellular K^+ with contractile activity is considerably greater than can be attributed to the K^+ efflux during the APs, which suggests that an increased K^+ conductance contributes to the buildup in extracellular K^+ and thus V_m depolarization as fatigue develops. Additionally, a decline in Na^+ conductance contributes to the reduced AP spike height and conduction velocity. It is clear from these data that the sarcolemma and t-tubular Na^+-K^+ pumps (Fig. 8.6, point 5) fail to keep pace with the K^+ efflux and Na^+ influx during high-frequency activation. The insufficient pump activity might result from a reduced ATP/ADP + P_i ratio and/or elevated H^+ in the intracellular fluid surrounding the membrane pumps. This problem would be exacerbated in the depths of the fiber, where the t-tubular Na^+-K^+ pump density is low and diffusion limitation likely increases extracellular K^+. The extent of V_m depolarization and decline in the action potential overshoot in the depths of the t-tubules has not been established, but it is plausible the V_m would be more depolarized and the AP amplitude less than in the sarcolemma (Fig. 8.6, no. 3). As depicted by the question mark in Figure 8.6, the ionic conditions in the t-tubular lumen following intense contractile activity are unknown. It is particularly important to know what happens to lumen K^+ and Ca^{++}. If either lumen K^+ or Ca^{++} builds up, the AP propagation could be blocked from reaching the depths of the fiber (3). Additionally, depolarization to values more positive than −60 mV would cause inactivation of the DHP receptor (4).

Heavy exercise is known to cause a considerable increase in ([K^+]I) in human skeletal muscle, and Nielsen and associates (25) recently demonstrated that heavy one-legged exercise-training for 7 weeks reduced the rate of ([K^+]I) increase the trained compared to the control leg. These authors also found an increased Na^+–K^+–ATPase pump protein, and hypothesized that the slower increase in ([K^+]I) in the trained leg was caused by a greater reuptake of K^+ due to a higher activity of the muscle Na^+–K^+–ATPase pumps. Consistent with the membrane mechanism of muscle fatigue, the trained leg showed a 28% longer time to fatigue during an incremental exercise test, and at the point of fatigue the ([K^+]I) levels were similar in the two legs.

The t-Tubular Charge Sensor

The t-tubular DHP receptor (charge sensor) is stabilized by the negative resting potential and mM extracellular Ca^{++} found in nonfatigued fibers and inactivated by depolarization or zero extracellular Ca^{++} (3). It is unknown how t-tubular lumen Ca^{++} changes with fatigue. An increase in intracellular Ca^{++} would be expected to activate the t-tubular Ca^{++}–ATPase pump and increase lumen Ca^{++}. However, t-tubular Ca^{++} channels are opened by the AP depolarization, and the electrochemical gradient favors Ca^{++} influx. Small increases in t-tubular Ca^{++} (about 5 mM) would shift the activation potential about 15 mV more positive and help prevent depolarization-induced inactivation by stabilizing the charge sensor. The former would not contribute to fatigue, as threshold would still be reached by −20 mV and even the most fatigued muscle fibers show AP spikes near zero. Fatigued fibers do exhibit a positive shift in the activation threshold (26), which supports the hypothesis that extracellular Ca^{++} increases. The available evidence suggests that the t-tubular charge sensor is robust and unlikely to be inactivated even in highly fatigued muscle fibers. A significant decline in the amplitude of the Ca^{++}_i was observed in the absence of any change in t-tubular charge movement (27). The result did not rule out a partial inactivation of the charge sensor by cell depolarization in fatigued cells, as charge movement and Ca^{++} release were measured at a −80 mV holding potential. The result does indicate that problems in SR Ca^{++} release persisted in the fatigued cells with a normal t-tubular charge.

The SR Ca^{++} Release Channel

In the past 20 years, considerable progress has been made in understanding the molecular mechanism by which t-tubules charge induces SR Ca^{++} release. The important proteins at the T-SR junction have been identified, and it is now clear that the t-tubular charge sensor lies directly opposite and may contact the junctional foot protein (ryanodine receptor), which makes up the Ca^{++} release channel of the SR (Fig. 8.6, point 4). The exact mechanism of transduction across the T-SR junction and the stoichiometric relationship between DHP receptor and the SR Ca^{++} release channel (the ryanodine receptor) in mammalian muscle have not been established. In the toadfish swim bladder the ratio is 1:2, indicating that only one-half of the Ca^{++} release channels are regulated by the t-tubular charge sensor (3). It seems likely that the channels not facing DHP receptors are activated by Ca^{++} released from the neighboring voltage-regulated SR channels, a process termed CICR. While the relative importance of the voltage- versus CICR-regulated processes has not been established in human muscle fibers, the latter process exists in fibers isolated from human muscle and likely makes an important contribution to SR Ca^{++} channel opening in these fibers (28).

A consistent observation is that the amplitude of the Ca^{++} transient decreases as fatigue develops. While the problem may be caused in part by a blockage of the t-tubular AP or reduced t-tubular charge movement, considerable support exists for the hypothesis that the primary problem involves a direct inhibition of Ca^{++} release from the SR Ca^{++} release channel (ryanodine receptor). The intracellular Ca^{++} content depends upon the relative activity of Ca^{++} release from the SR, and Ca^{++} removal processes. The latter consists of the activity of the SR Ca^{++} pump and Ca^{++}-binding proteins, particularly parvalbumin in fast muscles. Calcium release (or flux) from the SR depends on channel permeability and the ΔC between SR lumen and intracellular fluid. The permeability is regulated by interplay between opening of the SR calcium release channels and channel inactivation.

A fatigue-induced decline in the amplitude of the Ca^{++} transient could be caused by a reduction in ΔC or by factors that decrease channel activation (either directly or by inhibiting t-tubular charge) or increase channel inactivation. Additionally, considering that force is related to intracellular Ca^{++}, which in turn depends on the Ca^{++} release and removal fluxes, any influences that decrease removal of Ca^{++} will tend to prolong the Ca^{++} transient and slow relaxation.

Concentration Gradient Across the SR

The ΔC depends on the SR Ca^{++} content; a reduction in SR Ca^{++} decreases ΔC and thus release. Eberstein and Sandow (29) showed in the early 1960s that fatigue did not completely deplete the SR of Ca^{++}, as caffeine, a compound that acts directly on the SR to induce Ca^{++} release, reversed the tension loss in fatigued fibers. Later this was directly confirmed by the simultaneous measurement of force and intracellular Ca^{++} following caffeine administration to a single fiber (Fig. 8.7C). The reduction of SR Ca^{++} during continuous contractile activity is likely due in part to an increased binding of Ca^{++} to the intracellular Ca^{++}-binding proteins parvalbumin (fast fibers only) and the SR pump. Consequently, during activation free Ca^{++} would be removed more slowly. Additionally, the SR Ca^{++} pump rate may be slowed in fatigued muscle fibers, further reducing SR Ca^{++} stores and decreasing ΔC and Ca^{++} release. These mechanisms would increase the resting intracellular Ca^{++} (3,9). The net effect is that Ca^{++} would be displaced from the release pool (SR store) to the removal pool, where it is unavailable for release. These events would explain the observed prolongation in the Ca^{++} transient (9,18), twitch duration (3,5), and the relaxation time following a tetanic contraction in fatigued muscle (Fig. 8.3).

Besides the redistribution of Ca^{++} from the SR to intracellular buffers, recent evidence suggests that the ΔC for SR Ca^{++} can be further reduced during heavy exercise by P_i precipitation of SR Ca^{++} (11,30). It is well documented that intense contractile activity leads to increases in intracellular P_i that can approach 30 mM (3). The hypothesis is that P_i enters the SR and at concentrations above 6 mM begins to form an insoluble precipitate of calcium phosphate (CaP_i). This reduces the amount of releasable Ca^{++} (lowers ΔC) and depresses the amplitude of the Ca^{++} transient, which contributes to the development of muscle fatigue. Figure 8.8 provides a concise summary of the role of P_i in reducing SR Ca^{++} release. The traces shown in Figure 8.8A were taken from the experiment of Fryer and associates (30) and demonstrate the depressive effect of 50 mM P_i exposure on a subsequent caffeine contracture. Figure 8.8B shows how P_i reduced the releasable pool of SR Ca^{++} by lowering free Ca^{++} as well as the fraction bound to calsequestrin. According to Duke and Steele (31) the Ca-P_i precipitation may be reduced and less likely to contribute to fatigue in PC-depleted cells. Their data suggest that the dominant influence of P_i in PC-depleted cells is the activation of SR Ca^{++} efflux via pump reversal. This P_i-induced pump reversal required high ADP, which only occurred in PC-depleted cells. Rather than inhibiting Ca^{++} release, this effect would contribute to the progressive increase in resting Ca^{++} and prolongation of muscle relaxation observed during the development of fatigue. The relative importance of these competing mechanisms to the development of muscle fatigue will depend on the degree of increase in P_i and ADP as well as the extent of PC depletion.

Inhibition of SR Ca^{++} Opening by Ions and Substrates

The observation that fatigued muscles exposed to caffeine (Fig. 8.7) show recovery of Ca^{++} release and force demonstrates that SR Ca^{++} stores were not depleted and that a reduced ΔC can not totally explain the inhibition of SR Ca^{++} release. Studies of SR vesicles and isolated SR Ca^{++} release channels have demonstrated channel activity to be modulated by intracellular ions and substrates to include glycogen, ATP, Mg^{++}, H^+, and Ca^{++}. A reduced pH has been shown to inhibit channel open probability with near zero activation at pH 6.2. However, when intact fibers were made acidotic, the amplitude of the Ca^{++}_i was increased, and low pH had no effect on SR Ca^{++} release in skinned fibers. These data suggest that the low pH is unlikely to affect the SR Ca^{++} release channel or the amplitude of the Ca^{++}_i during in vivo contractile activity. The hypothesis with the most experimental support is that the SR Ca^{++} release channel is inhibited during fatigue by the combined affect of an increased Mg^{++} and a reduced ATP (5,9). The most convincing evidence comes from studies of skinned muscle fiber, in which potential fatigue factors can be individual or collectively altered. Using this technique, Blazev and Lamb (32) observed that a decline in cell ATP to 0.5 mM had no effect, but when it was combined with an increased Mg^{++} (3 mM), significant inhibition of Ca^{++} release was observed (32). Since much of the intracellular Mg^{++} is bound to ATP, the drop in cell ATP with intense exercise is mirrored by an increase in free Mg^{++}. Allen and associates (5) used changes in Mg^{++} to model cell ATP in single mouse fibers and found a linear relationship between the fall in ATP and the amplitude of

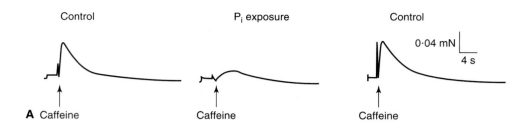

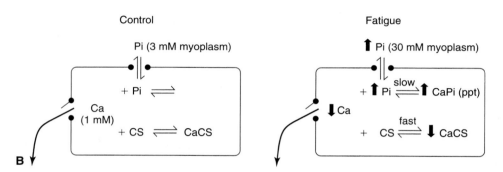

FIGURE 8.8 **A.** Force records from skinned fibers with intact SR. Caffeine was used to release SR Ca^{++}, producing the contractures shown; thus the size of the contracture is an indication of the Ca^{++} available for release in the SR. In the middle record, the muscle was exposed to 50 mM P_i for 20 seconds; the P_i was then washed off and caffeine applied. **B.** Ca^{++} and P_i movements across the SR membrane and binding sites within the SR. Under control conditions $[P_i]myo = [P_i]SR = 3$ mM and $[Ca^{++}]SR = 1$ mM. Thus, $[Ca^{++}]SR \times [P_i]SR = 3$ mM^2. Because this is below the solubility product of CaPi (which is 6 mM^2), none of this product is present. Ca^{++} in the SR, however, binds rapidly and reversibly to calsequestrin (CS), so that there is a large pool of CaCS that buffers $[Ca^{++}]SR$. When the SR Ca^{++} release channel opens, a large flux of Ca^{++} into the myoplasm occurs because $[Ca^{++}]SR$ is high and is maintained high by the buffering of CaCS. In fatigue $[P_i]myo$ is 30 mM, and P_i enters the SR via anion channels. Once $[P_i]SR$ exceeds 6 mM, the product of $[Ca^{++}]SR \times [P_i]SR$ exceeds the solubility product of CaPi, and precipitation of CaPi starts to occur slowly in the SR. As a consequence $[Ca^{++}]SR$ and CaCS fall, and when the SR Ca^{++} release channels are open, the flux is smaller, because $[Ca^{++}]SR$ is lower and the buffering of $[Ca^{++}]SR$ by CaCS is reduced. Dissociation of CaPi is assumed to be too slow to contribute to Ca^{++} release. *Heavy arrows,* changes of key concentrations during fatigue. *(Modified from Allen DG, Westerblad H. Role of phosphate and calcium stores in muscle fatigue. J Physiol (Lond) 2001;536:657–665. Data in part A adapted with permission from Fryer MW, Owen VJ, Lamb GD, et al. Effects of creatine phosphate and P_i on Ca^{++} movements and tension development in rat skinned skeletal muscle fibres. J Physiol (Lond) 1995;482:659.)*

the Ca^{++}_i. A decline in the amplitude of the Ca^{++}_i could be caused by a reduced SR Ca^{++} release flux and/or by an increase in the intracellular Ca^{++} buffer capacity. However, the latter seems unlikely in that intracellular acidosis and the reduction in strongly bound crossbridges associated with heavy activity would reduce Ca^{++} buffering by reducing Ca^{++} affinity for troponin-C (5). With the exception of conditions that elicit low-frequency fatigue, activity-induced depression in SR Ca^{++} release recovers rapidly by a process that can be blocked by metabolic inhibitors, observations consistent with the low ATP, high Mg^{++} hypothesis. Since even in the most fatigued cells ATP content remained above 1.5 mM, the hypothesis requires that ATP be compartmentalized, with lower levels surrounding the SR release channels. The data of Han and

associates (33) provide support for this hypothesis. They demonstrated that skeletal muscle triads contain a compartmentalized glycolytic reaction sequence and that the ATP formed in the triadic gap appears restricted and unavailable for reactions elsewhere in the cell. The likelihood of compartmentalization would increase in fatigue as PC content and the effectiveness of the PC shuttle declined.

Studies employing CK-deficient mice have provided evidence that the fatigue-induced decline in SR Ca^{++} release can be explained by the combined effect of CaP_i precipitation within the SR and low ATP, high Mg^{++} inhibition of the SR release channel (9). This conclusion is based on the observation that CK-deficient mice but not control mice showed a rapid decline in Ca^{++}_i and force in response to heavy contractile activity, while with less intense stimulation the CK-deficient mice were less fatigable than control mice. The CK-deficient mice would be unable to buffer the decline in ATP, which would increase the direct inhibition of low ATP on the SR release channel. However, intracellular P_i would remain low, preventing the C_a-P_i–mediated reduction in SR Ca^{++} release.

With intense stimulation, fibers show a rapid decline in SR Ca^{++} release and in the fraction of Ca^{++} that can be directly released by caffeine or other drugs. However, in glycogen-depleted fibers the Ca^{++}_i falls rapidly, but the SR Ca^{++} store is not depleted. Furthermore, recovery of both peak force and Ca^{++}_i is slowed in fibers bathed in glucose-free solutions (34). The reduced Ca^{++} release in the low glycogen fibers was observed in the presence of high ATP. These observations suggest that cell glycogen or some intermediate of glycogen metabolism is required for optimal regulation of the SR Ca^{++} release channel. Glycogen is known to be associated with the T-SR junctional complex, and some critical level maybe necessary for maintenance of the structural integrity of the complex.

It is not known whether the inhibition of SR Ca^{++} release with fatigue can be delayed or reduced by programs of dynamic exercise training. However, based on the known metabolic adaptations, exercise training should prove beneficial. The exercise training–induced increase in muscle mitochondria would allow a given tissue respiratory rate to be established with less of a rise in cell ADP, P_i, and Mg^{++} while maintaining a higher ATP (35). With heavy exercise, this should reduce the likelihood of a C_a-P_i mediated reduction in SR Ca^{++} release or a direct inhibition of release by the combined affects of high Mg^{++} and low ATP. During prolonged dynamic exercise, any mechanism inhibiting SR Ca^{++} release that is coupled to glycogen depletion would be delayed by dynamic exercise training by the slower rate of muscle glycogen depletion in the muscle of the trained individual (12, 35).

SR ATPase Pump

Fatigue is known to be associated with a prolonged relaxation time resulting from a reduced rate of SR Ca^{++} reuptake. With heavy exercise, the inhibited SR pump function has been linked to the combined affects of the increase in H^+, P_i, and ADP. Low pH is known to inhibit the SR ATPase and Ca^{++} pump rate, with the latter declining by twofold between pH 7.1 and 6.6 and by an additional twofold between 6.6 and 6.1 (5). Further support for a role for low pH in prolonging muscle relaxation time comes from the observation that with stimulation iodoacetic acid–poisoned muscles underwent a 50% fall in tension but no change in pH or relaxation time (3). However, clearly other factors are involved, as MPD subjects showed a slowed relaxation with no change in pH.

High P_i appears to inhibit the SR pump and increase Ca^{++} leak through the SR Ca^{++} release channel to the intracellular fluid. The latter is thought to be responsible for the increase and slowing in Ca^{++}_i observed early in fatigue in control (Fig. 8.7B), but not CK-deficient muscle fibers (9).

Recently, Macdonald and Stephenson (23) showed 1 mM ADP to decrease by fourfold the ability of the SR to load Ca^{++}. Only 10 to 30% of this effect was caused by a reduced SR pump rate, while the rest was attributed to a marked increase in the leak of Ca^{++} from the SR. High ADP apparently increased the Ca^{++}-Ca^{++} exchange function of the SR, which moved Ca^{++} from the SR lumen (high concentration) to the myoplasm (low concentration). This Ca^{++} movement was caused not by a reversal of the SR pump, as ATP was not synthesized, but by pump slippage allowing Ca^{++} leak into the cytosol. The reduced SR pump rate could be in part due to the reduced free energy of ATP hydrolysis as the ATP/ADP + P_i ratio declines with fatigue (3).

Low-Frequency Fatigue

Following certain contractile paradigms (elicited both *in vivo* in humans and *in vitro* in animals) muscle force required several hours to days to recover, and the delayed recovery was especially apparent at low activation frequencies (36,37). The etiology of this condition, termed low-frequency fatigue, is still not understood. Since the amplitude of the Ca^{++} transient is depressed and recovery slow, the mechanism is thought to involve a structural alteration of either the SR Ca^{++} release channel and/or associated proteins (36,37). This structural change reduces the amplitude of the Ca^{++} transient for all stimulation frequencies, but due to the shape of the pCa-force relationship a major depression of force is only observed at low frequencies. Bruton and associates (36) reviewed the literature in this field and concluded that short-term increases in intracellular Ca^{++} in the vicinity of the triads might initiate low-frequency fatigue. The primary evidence for this was the observation that mM Ca^{++} abolished E-C coupling in isolated peeled single fibers, while caffeine contractures were maintained. Although the mechanism likely requires an elevated intracellular Ca^{++}, the exact process involved is unclear. The most likely candidates are Ca^{++}-mediated events involving calmodulin, calcium-activated lipases, or reactive oxygen species (36).

It is well established that calmodulin plays a dual role in the regulation of the SR Ca^{++} release channel (36). Calmodulin binding activates or inhibits channel opening at low and high cytoplasmic Ca^{++}, respectively. In a nonfatigued fiber, this process likely contributes to the cyclic activation and inactivation of the release channel. There is no evidence linking Ca^{++}-calmodulin to an altered ryanodine receptor function during low-frequency fatigue (36). However, the possibility exists that elevated cytoplasmic Ca^{++} associated with fatigue leads to an altered calmodulin binding such that the channel is harder to activate. Reactive oxygen species (ROS) such as hydrogen peroxide (H_2O_2) are produced during oxidative metabolism and their rate of production increases with the work intensity in skeletal muscle. Studies in the mid-1990s suggested that ROS inhibited SR Ca^{++} release in skinned fibers, thus contributing to fatigue (36).

More recently, Andrade and associates (38) found that brief exposures to H_2O_2 had no effect on the amplitude of the Ca^{++} transient but significantly increased force. This response was biphasic, as longer exposures to H_2O_2 caused a small increase in myoplasmic Ca^{++} with large declines in force. The latter effect was completely reversible by the reductant dithiothreitol (DTT). The authors concluded that the main effect of ROS was to alter the myofibrillar Ca^{++} sensitivity and that the effect on SR Ca^{++} release was minor. Since low-frequency fatigue is thought to be caused by inhibition of the SR Ca^{++} release channel, these data do not support a primary role for ROS in the etiology of low-frequency fatigue.

Crossbridge Mechanism of Fatigue

Muscle contraction involves the hydrolysis of ATP to produce energy for crossbridge cycling with a resulting increase in ADP, P_i, and H^+. All three increase in proportion to the intensity of the work performed, and because of the CK reaction, they show an inverse relation to PC. The initial decline in force with intense stimulation of individual muscle fibers (Fig. 8.7B) occurs with no change in the amplitude of the Ca^{++}_i, and it is thought to be mediated by the combined effects of an increase in P_i and H^+ (5). Both ions have been shown to directly reduce the peak force of single skinned fibers (Fig. 8.9), presumably by inhibiting or reversing the crossbridge transition from the low- to the high-force state (Fig. 8.2, step 5) and/or by reducing the force per cross-

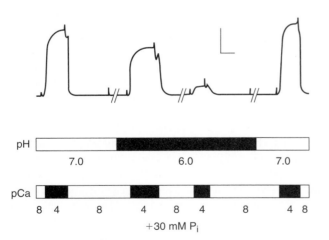

FIGURE 8.9 Effect of P_i and pH on maximal Ca^{++}-activated force, pCa 4.0, of skinned muscle fiber. The recording shows the typical effects of pH 6.0 alone and in combination with 30 mM P_i on maximal force of a fast-twitch skeletal muscle fiber. Calibration bars show 50 mg and 10 seconds, and spikes on record are solution exchange artifacts. For concision, record shown is not continuous but has been truncated at interrupted lines. (*Modified from Nosek TM, Fender KY, Godt RE. It is diprotonated inorganic phosphate that depresses force in skinned skeletal muscle fibers. Science 1987;236:191.*)

bridge. There is no conclusive evidence as to which mechanism is most important, and it may differ between ions and muscle temperature. Most single-fiber studies have been performed at 15°C. At that temperature, a drop in fiber pH has been shown to reduce the force per crossbridge in both fast- and slow-twitch fibers, while the number of strong (high force) crossbridges was reduced only in fast fibers (17). Metzger and Moss (17) observed that for the fast fiber type, the k_{tr} following a rapid slack and reextension of fiber length was depressed at pH 6.2 compared to 7.0 at suboptimal (pCa > 5.0) but not maximal levels of Ca^{++} activation. From this they concluded that protons have a direct depressant effect upon the forward rate constant for the transition between the weak and strong binding states of the crossbridge (Fig. 8.2, step 5). In contrast, P_i is thought to reduce P_0 and increase k_{tr} by accelerating the reversal of step 5 (Fig. 8.2). In addition to reducing the number of strong binding (high force) crossbridges, P_i may also reduce the force per bridge (3).

An increased H^+ not only depresses force but also inhibits myofibrillar ATPase activity, which contributes to the fatigue-induced drop in V_0. Thus H^+ affects at least two steps in the crossbridge cycle (Fig. 8.2, steps 5 and 7), while an increase in P_i depresses force (step 5) but has no effect on V_0 (step 7). As can be seen in Figure 8.9, the effects of pH and P_i on fiber force are additive, with considerably greater depression in force observed with both ions than with either one alone (39).

The fatigue-induced decline in peak power (Fig. 8.5) can at least in part be attributed to the direct effects of H^+ and P_i on crossbridge kinetics (Fig. 8.2, steps 5 and 7) and the resulting depression of force and velocity. Although this has not yet been determined, it is also possible that the reduced a/P_0 ratio observed in fatigued fast-twitch muscle (Fig. 8.5B) is caused by the increase in H^+ and P_i.

In addition to a direct affect on peak force, both H^+ and P_i shift the pCa–force relationship to the right, such that higher free Ca^{++} is required to reach a given tension. For low pH, this effect is mediated in part by competitive inhibition of Ca^{++} binding to troponin-C. The observations that high Ca^{++} (pCa 4.5) cannot eliminate the effect and that rigor tension is reduced by 33% at pH 6.2 compared to 7.0 suggest that factors in addition to competitive inhibition of Ca^{++} binding to troponin-C are involved. The decline in the number of high-force crossbridges (caused by both H^+ and P_i) reduces the thick filament–mediated cooperativity between regulatory thin filament sites, and this is thought to contribute directly to the right shift in the pCa–force relationship. This effect is shown as point 2 in Figure 8.4. Since the amplitude of the Ca^{++}_i transient is known to decline with fatigue (Fig. 8.4, point 3, and Fig. 8.7), the right shift in the pCa–force relationship exacerbates the fatigue-inducing affects of H^+ and P_i. Additionally, at less than maximal Ca^{++} concentrations, the pH- and P_i-induced right shift in the pCa–force relationship would contribute to the decline in ktr (and presumably +dP/dt), as the forward rate constant of step 5 (Fig. 8.2) would be slowed by the reduction in the number of strong binding high-force crossbridges (17). In the fast fiber types, a drop in cell pH could also directly depress k_{tr} by inhibiting the forward rate constant of step 5 (Fig. 8.2).

In contrast, a rise in ADP would increase force by reducing the rate of step 7 (Fig. 8.2), thus increasing the number of crossbridges in the high force states (AM′ · ADP and AM · ADP). Since step 7 is thought to be rate limiting to the overall crossbridge cycle speed, an increase in ADP contributes to the decline in fiber V_0.

In recent years, the importance of low pH in the etiology of muscle fatigue has been questioned (34). The challenge to the hypothesis that low pH contributes to fatigue has come from the observations that the inhibitory effects of low pH on P_0 and V_0 are reduced as the temperature increases from 10 to 30°C. However, these studies have not considered the effects of low pH on peak power or the combined effects of a reduced Ca^{++} release, low pH, and an elevated P_i. Recent evidence suggests that the H^+- and P_i-induced right shift in the pCa–force relationship may be greater at temperatures closer to physiological (30°C). As a consequence, the reduced amplitude of the Ca^{++}_i with fatigue would depress force to a greater extent at physiological temperatures (combined effects of points 2 and 3, Figure 8.4). Thus it is premature to dismiss the direct effects of H^+ on the crossbridge as an important player in muscle fatigue.

There is no evidence on whether programs of regular exercise training cause any direct effects on the interaction between putative fatigue factors and either steps of the crossbridge cycle or the pCa–force relationship. However, dynamic exercise training is known to increase mitochondrial content in all fiber types, and consequently during exercise, trained individuals show less of an increase in muscle ADP, AMP, and P_i and a reduced glycolysis (35). The latter would also reduce the increase in cell lactate and H^+ at the same absolute or even relative workload. One would also expect to see higher cell ATP and less of an increase in Mg^{++}. All of these changes would reduce muscle fatigue by limiting the known deleterious affects of low ATP and high Mg^{++}, H^+, P_i, and ADP.

Prolonged Exercise and Fatigue

Despite more than a century of research, the etiology of fatigue with prolonged dynamic exercise is not fully understood. Hypoglycemia and/or high core temperature can limit endurance-type exercises, but with adequate carbohydrate and water intake during dynamic exercise, fatigue from these factors can generally be prevented (12). At submaximal workloads the inability to continue exercise is frequently correlated with and perhaps caused by muscle glycogen depletion. With exercise intensities below 50 or above 90% of one's maximal oxygen consumption, ample muscle glycogen remains at exhaustion (12). In addition to glycogen depletion, SR function has frequently been found to be compromised following prolonged dynamic exercise.

Glycogen Depletion

Since the development of the needle biopsy technique, multiple studies have found a correlation between muscle glycogen depletion and fatigue with dynamic exercise. Despite this a cause-and-effect relationship has not been demonstrated. However, the observation that regular exercise training reduces the rate of glycogen utilization, delays glycogen depletion, and increases exercise time to exhaustion supports the hypothesis that muscle glycogen depletion is an important factor in fatigue. Although muscle glycogen is an important fuel source, it is not clear why cell metabolism could not proceed with free fatty acids (blood and cellular) and blood glucose as substrates for energy. Carbohydrate feedings throughout exercise prevents hypoglycemia and delays fatigue by 30 to 60 minutes but does not alter the rate of muscle glycogen depletion or prevent fatigue (12). During prolonged dynamic exercise, after the first 2 hours, the primary carbohydrate fuel source switches from muscle glycogen to blood glucose. With blood glucose as the primary carbohydrate fuel source, Coyle (12) found that even trained cyclists could not maintain exercise intensities above 74% of maximal oxygen consumption. This suggests that the metabolism of blood-borne substrates (both glucose and free fatty acids) is simply too slow to maintain heavy exercise intensities. An increased reliance on fat oxidation would further reduce an individual's work capacity as less ATP is generated per liter of oxygen consumed.

It seems unlikely that glycogen depletion is the sole cause of fatigue with prolonged dynamic exercise but rather that it triggers additional events leading to fatigue. One hypothesis is that a certain level of muscle glycogen metabolism is required to maintain Krebs cycle intermediates at a level adequate for the optimal production of NADH and electron transport rate. Consistent with this is the observation that the concentration of Krebs cycle intermediates declined with prolonged dynamic exercise (40). Besides reducing carbon chain precursors for the production of Krebs cycle intermediates, glycogen depletion has been shown to be associated with an increased production of branch chain amino acids from Krebs cycle intermediates (41). The increase in branch chain amino acid aminotransferase reactions induced by glycogen depletion would contribute to the reduction in Krebs cycle intermediates.

With prolonged exercise and the resulting glycogen depletion there is an increased reliance on free fatty acid metabolism. Maintenance of high oxidation rates may be limited by the muscle cell's ability to translocate free fatty acids into the mitochondria. The enzyme catalyzing this step, carnitine acyltransferase I, is thought to be rate limiting for free fatty acid oxidation. In the latter stages of dynamic exercise this step may be unable to keep up with the increased demand for fat oxidation. Support for this possibility comes from the observation that carnitine administration delayed fatigue in the isolated soleus muscle (42).

It is well documented that regular exercise training delays fatigue during dynamic exercise and that the rate of muscle and liver glycogen depletion with exercise is slowed as a result of reduced carbohydrate and increased fat metabolism in trained individuals (35). It is generally thought that this glycogen-sparing effect is important in delaying muscle fatigue, but as discussed here, the exact mechanism or mechanisms linking glycogen depletion with the inability to continue exercise has not been established.

SR Function

Of all of the intracellular organelles, the SR appears particularly vulnerable to deleterious changes with prolonged dynamic exercise. Except for conditions that elicit low-frequency fatigue there is little or no information on whether prolonged exercise inhibits SR Ca^{++} release. In contrast, considerable data in animals and humans show a reduced SR pump function. SR vesicles isolated from muscles fatigued by prolonged exercise show a reduced Ca^{++} uptake rate, which is generally but not always related to reduced SR ATPase activity (3,13,43). A reduced SR Ca^{++} uptake with no change in ATPase activity suggests either an uncoupling of the transport or a leaky vesicle whereby Ca^{++} fluxes back into the intracellular fluid. This plus the observation of a reduced SR yield (44) suggests that the SR may be structurally damaged, perhaps by the activation of proteases. The disruption in SR function appears more related to the degree of activity and not necessarily glycogen depletion. In rats swum to exhaustion, glycogen depletion was observed in muscles representative of all fiber types, but SR Ca^{++} uptake was depressed in vesicles isolated from the slow type I soleus and fast type IIA deep region of the vastus lateralis, but not the fast type IIB/IIX superficial region of the vastus lateralis (44). Presumably the latter muscle was recruited less during the exhaustive swim. It is still possible that glycogen somehow stabilized the SR membranes and that following glycogen depletion other factors led to its disruption.

Other Factors

Glycogen depletion and a compromised SR function may not be exclusive factors mediating fatigue during prolonged dynamic exercise. A controversial area is whether or not prolonged exercise leads to mitochondrial swelling and a reduced oxidative capacity. Structural and functional data both support and refute this hypothesis (3). Studies on skinned fibers isolated from human muscle following exhaustive bicycle exercise showed increased respiration in the absence of ADP but no change in maximal ADP-stimulated respiration (45). This observation suggests that fatigue-induced changes in mitochondria are unlikely to limit ATP production or performance.

The myofibrils appear relatively resistant to fatigue induced by prolonged exercise (3,44). Myofibrils isolated from fast and slow muscles of rats swum to exhaustion showed no change in ATPase activity, and despite a 26% drop in peak force, the maximal shortening velocity of the soleus was un-

altered (44). However, force and power loss resulting from eccentrically induced muscle fiber damage can be easily mistaken for fatigue. The former can occur during either intensive heavy or prolonged dynamic exercise and does involve disruption of myofibrils (3). From a performance standpoint it is irrelevant whether the loss of power was caused by fiber damage or fatigue except that the former requires a considerably longer recovery period (days as opposed to hours).

SUMMARY

The mechanisms of muscle fatigue are complex and depend on the type of exercise (heavy-intensity versus prolonged dynamic), one's state of fitness, and the fiber type composition of the muscle. As shown in Figure 8.1, it is clear that fatigue is not caused by a single entity but rather by various factors acting at multiple sites of both central and peripheral origin. This chapter reviews both central and peripheral factors and provides evidence that at least in well-motivated athletes, peripheral events within the muscle are most important in eliciting fatigue. In short-duration, heavy-contractile activity the initial phase of fatigue appears to be mediated by the combined effects of an elevated H^+, P_i, and ADP acting at the crossbridge to reduce force, velocity, and power. Late in fatigue, the process is dominated by a precipitous fall in SR Ca^{++} release, which when combined with the right shift in the pCa–force relation causes a large drop in force. A reduced SR Ca^{++} release is also of prime importance in the etiology of low-frequency fatigue, a special condition in which force is reduced in response to low but not high activation frequencies. Fatigue from prolonged dynamic exercise is highly correlated with and likely at least in part caused by muscle glycogen depletion. With reduced glycogen, muscles depend more on bloodborne substrates (glucose and free fatty acids), and this necessitates a reduced work rate. Carbohydrate supplementation can delay but not prevent fatigue, and thus other factors must contribute to fatigue. It may be that glycogen depletion limits the production of Krebs cycle intermediates, which leads to a reduced NADH production and electron transport rate. Prolonged dynamic exercise may disrupt organelles, with the SR appearing particularly susceptible, as depression in both SR ATPase activity and Ca^{++} uptake are known to occur. It will be important to understand the nature of the decline in SR Ca^{++} release with heavy exercise and low-frequency fatigue and the relationship of muscle glycogen depletion to the onset of other important factors (such as an altered SR pump function) in mediating fatigue during prolonged exercise. Programs of regular exercise training are known to delay the onset and reduce the extent of fatigue that occurs with both short-duration heavy and moderate-intensity prolonged exercise. However, additional research is needed to determine whether or not exercise training can reduce either the fatigue-inducing effects of H^+ and P_i at the crossbridge or the factors involved in the inhibition of SR function.

A MILESTONE OF DISCOVERY

For more than 100 years muscle fatigue had been characterized by a loss of peak force and a prolonged relaxation transient, and for the first 70 years of the twentieth century the leading hypothesis was that fatigue resulting from high-intensity contractile activity was caused by lactic acid. The first indication that Ca^{++} release from the SR and the resulting intracellular calcium transient might be involved in the fatigue process came in 1963. At that time, Eberstein and Sandow (29) observed that caffeine, a compound stimulating direct release of Ca^{++} from the SR, could reverse the tension loss of fatigued fibers. This result, along with the observation of Grabowski and colleagues (26) that fatigued fibers exposed to high K^+ responded with high-force contractures, demonstrated that muscle fatigue was not caused by depletion of releasable Ca^{++} from the SR. Two years prior to the milestone work of Westerblad and Allen (18), Allen and associates (10) dissected single fibers from *Xenopus* lumbrical muscles and microinjected the fibers with the photoprotein aequorin to measure the myoplasmic Ca^{++}_i in rested and fatigued cells. The important observations were that the characteristic reduction in force and slowing of relaxation in the fatigued fibers was associated with a decline in the amplitude and a slowing of the rate of decline in the aequorin light signal. This was the first indication that fatigue may be mediated by a decline in SR Ca^{++} release. About the same time, Lännergren and Westerblad (46) developed the single-fiber technique in mammals with a mouse foot muscle. They observed that fatigue occurred in three phases:

Phase 1, an early 10% drop in tension
Phase 2, a plateau period
Phase 3, a rapid decline in force

Westerblad and Allen (18) studied the same preparation to test the hypotheses that phase 1 was independent of SR Ca^{++} release and that phase 3 was a direct result of a decline in the amplitude of the Ca^{++}_i. They were the first to use the fluorescent indicator Fura-2 to measure the amplitude of the Ca^{++}_i. Figure 8.7 demonstrates the important results: (*a*) Early fatigue occurred while the amplitude of the Ca^{++}_i increased (Fig. 8.7*B*). (*b*) The precipitous drop in tension late in fatigue was caused by a reduced Ca^{++}_i (Fig. 8.7*C*). This point was proved by the application of caffeine, which increased the amplitude of the Ca^{++}_i and restored force (Fig. 8.7*C*). Another important finding was that the sensitivity of the myofilaments to Ca^{++} was reduced such that in fatigued fibers less force was obtained at a given Ca^{++} concentration. This group and others have since shown that the early fatigue is associated with increases in H^+, P_i, and ADP acting directly on the crossbridge (Fig. 8.2). Perhaps the most important consequence of this work was that it focused the attention of this field on the role of E-C coupling (and in particular SR Ca^{++} release) in mediating fatigue. Subsequent studies have looked for the factor or factors inhibiting SR Ca^{++} release, and an extensive list has been studied (low ATP, high Mg^{++}, ROS). A disappointment is that to date no factor has been unequivocally linked to the inhibition of the SR Ca^{++} release.

Westerblad H, Allen DG. Changes of myoplasmic calcium concentration during fatigue in single mouse muscle fibers. J Gen Physiol 1991;98:615–635.

ACKNOWLEDGMENTS

I thank Janell Romatowski, who helped in the preparation of the figures, and my former graduate students who participated in the laboratory's muscle fatigue research. My research has been sponsored by NASA and NIH.

REFERENCES

1. Edwards RHT. Biochemical basis of fatigue in exercise performance: catastrophe theory of muscular fatigue. In Knuttgen HG, ed. Biochemistry of Exercise. Champaign, IL: Human Kinetics, 1983;3–28.
2. National Heart, Lung and Blood Institute Workshop Summary. Am Rev Respir Dis 1990;142:474–480.
3. Fitts RH. Cellular Mechanisms of muscle fatigue. Physiol Rev 1994;74:49–94.
4. Fitts RH, Balog EM. Effect of intracellular and extracellular ion changes on E-C coupling and skeletal muscle fatigue. Acta Physiol Scand 1996;156:169–181.
5. Allen DG, Lännergren J, Westerblad H. Muscle cell function during prolonged activity: cellular mechanisms of fatigue. Exp Physiol 1995;80:497–527.
6. Bigland-Ritchie B. Muscle fatigue and the influence of changing neural drive. Clin Chest Med 1984;5:21–34.
7. Enoka RM, Stuart DG. Neurobiology of muscle fatigue. J Appl Physiol 1992;72:1631–1648.
8. Gandevia SC. Spinal and supraspinal factors in human muscle fatigue. Physiol Rev 2001;81:1725–1789.
9. Allen DG, Kabbara AA, Westerblad H. Muscle fatigue: the role of intracellular calcium stores. Can J Appl Physiol 2002;27:83–96.
10. Allen DG, Lee JA, Westerblad H. Intracellular calcium and tension during fatigue in isolated single muscle fibres from *Xenopus laevis*. J Physiol (Lond) 1989;415:433–458.
11. Allen DG, Westerblad H. Role of phosphate and calcium stores in muscle fatigue. J Physiol (Lond) 2001;536:657–665.
12. Coyle EF. Carbohydrate metabolism and fatigue. In Atlan G, Beliveau L, Bouissou P, eds. Muscle Fatigue: Biochemical and Physiological Aspects. Paris: Masson, 1991;153–164.
13. Gollnick PD, Körge P, Karpakka J, et al. Elongation of skeletal muscle relaxation during exercise is linked to reduced

calcium uptake by the sarcoplasmic reticulum in man. Acta Physiol Scand 1991;142:135–136.

14. Hermansen L, Osnes J. Blood and muscle pH after maximal exercise in man. J Appl Physiol 1972;32:302–308.

15. Karlsson J, Saltin B. Lactate, ATP, and CP in working muscles during exhaustive exercise in man. J Appl Physiol 1970;29:598–602.

16. Edman KAP, Mattiazzi AR. Effects of fatigue and altered pH on isometric force and velocity of shortening at zero load in frog muscle fibers. J Mus Res Cell Mot 1981;2:321–334.

17. Metzger JM, Moss RL. pH modulation of the kinetics of a Ca^{++}-sensitive crossbridge state transition in mammalian single skeletal muscle fibres. J Physiol (Lond) 1990;428:751–764.

18. Westerblad H, Allen DG. Changes of myoplasmic calcium concentration during fatigue in single mouse muscle fibers. J Gen Physiol 1991;98:615–635.

19. Hill AV. The heat of shortening and the dynamic constants of muscle. Proc R Soc B 1938;126:136–195.

20. Merton PA. Voluntary strength and fatigue. J Physiol (Lond) 1954;123:553–564.

21. Bigland-Ritchie B, Dawson NJ, Johannson RS, et al. Reflex origin for the slowing of motoneurone firing rates in fatigue of human voluntary contractions. J Physiol (Lond) 1986;379:451–459.

22. Fitts RH. Mechanisms of muscular fatigue. In Poortmans JR, ed. Principles of Exercise Biochemistry. Basel: Karger: Med Sport Sci 2004;46:279–300.

23. Macdonald WA, Stephenson DG. Effects of ADP on sarcoplasmic reticulum function in mechanically skinned skeletal muscle fibres of the rat. J Physiol (Lond) 2001;532:499–508.

24. Lindinger MI, Sjøgaard G. Potassium regulation during exercise recovery. Sports Med 1991;11:382–401.

25. Nielsen JJ, Mohr M, Klarskov C, et al. Effects of high-intensity intermittent training on potassium kinetics and performance in human skeletal muscle. J Physiol (Lond) 2003;554:857–870.

26. Grabowski W, Lobsiger EA, Lüttgau HC. The effect of repetitive stimulation at low frequencies upon the electrical and mechanical activity of single muscle fibers. Pflügers Arch 1972;334:222–239.

27. Gyorke S. Effects of repeated tetanic stimulation on excitation-contraction coupling in cut muscle fibers of the frog. J Physiol (Lond) 1993;464:699–710.

28. Melzer W, Herrmann-Frank A, Lüttgau H Ch. The role of Ca^{++} ions in excitation-contraction coupling of skeletal muscle fibres. Biochim Biophys Acta 1995;1241:59–116.

29. Eberstein A, Sandow A. Fatigue mechanisms in muscle fibers. In Gutmann E, Hnik P, eds. The Effect of Use and Disuse on Neuromuscular Function. Prague: Czech Academy of Science, 1963;515–526.

30. Fryer MW, Owen VJ, Lamb GD, et al. Effects of creatine phosphate and P_i on Ca^{++} movements and tension develop-

ment in rat skinned skeletal muscle fibres. J Physiol (Lond) 1995;482:123–140.

31. Duke AM, Steele DS. Interdependent effects of inorganic phosphate and creatine phosphate on sarcoplasmic reticulum Ca^{++} regulation in mechanically skinned rat skeletal muscle. J Physiol (Lond) 2001;531:729–742.

32. Blazev R, Lamb GD. Low [ATP] and elevated [Mg^{++}] reduce depolarization-induced Ca^{++} release in rat skinned skeletal muscle fibres. J Physiol (Lond) 1999;520:203–215.

33. Han JW, Thieleczek R, Varsányi RM, et al. Compartmentalized ATP synthesis in skeletal muscle triads. Biochemistry 1992;31:377–384.

34. Westerblad H, Allen DG, Bruton JD, et al. Mechanisms underlying the reduction of isometric force in skeletal muscle fatigue. Acta Physiol Scand 1998;162:253–260.

35. Holloszy JO, Coyle EF. Adaptations of skeletal muscle to endurance exercise and their metabolic consequences. J Appl Physiol 1984;56:831–838.

36. Bruton JD, Lännergren L, Westerblad H. Mechanisms underlying the slow recovery of force after fatigue: importance of intracellular calcium. Acta Physiol Scand 1998;162:285–293.

37. Westerblad H, Bruton JD, Allen DG, et al. Functional significance of Ca^{++} in long-lasting fatigue of skeletal muscle. Eur J Appl Physiol 2000;83:166–174.

38. Andrade FH, Reid MB, Allen DG, et al. Effect of hydrogen peroxide and dithiothreitol on contractile function of single skeletal muscle fibres from the mouse. J Physiol (Lond) 1998;509:565–575.

39. Nosek TM, Fender KY, Godt RE. It is diprotonated inorganic phosphate that depresses force in skinned skeletal muscle fibers. Science 1987;236:191–193.

40. Sahlin K, Katz A, Broberg S. Tricarboxylic acid cycle intermediates in human muscle during prolonged exercise. Am J Physiol 1990;259:C834–C841.

41. Wagenmakers AJM, Beckers EJ, Brouns F, et al. Carbohydrate supplementation, glycogen depletion, and amino acid metabolism during exercise. Am J Physiol 1991;260:E883–E890.

42. Brass EP, Scarrow AM, Ruff LJ, et al. Carnitine delays rat skeletal muscle fatigue in vivo. J Appl Physiol 1993;75:1595–1600.

43. Tupling R, Green H, Grant S, et al. Postcontractile force depression in humans is associated with an impairment in SR Ca^{++} pump function. Am J Physiol 2000;278:R87–R94.

44. Fitts RH, Courtright JB, Kim DH, et al. Muscle fatigue with prolonged exercise: contractile and biochemical alterations. Am J Physiol 1982;242:C65–C73.

45. Tonkonogi M, Harris B, Sahlin K. Mitochondrial oxidative function in human saponin-skinned muscle fibres: effects of prolonged exercise. J Physiol (Lond) 1998;510:279–286.

46. Lännergren J, Westerblad H. Force decline due to fatigue and intracellular acidification in isolated fibers of mouse skeletal muscle. J Physiol (Lond) 1991;434:307–322.

The Autonomic Nervous System

DOUGLAS R. SEALS

Introduction

Through its efferent parasympathetic and sympathetic nervous system (SNS) arms, the autonomic nervous system (ANS) is an important tool that the central nervous system (CNS) uses to maintain organismic homeostasis at rest and during challenges imposed by acute changes in physiological state, such as physical exercise. This homeostatic regulatory control is achieved primarily through cardiovascular, metabolic, and thermoregulatory adjustments produced by specific changes in the activity of the vagus nerves to the heart, and the sympathetic nerves to the heart, other internal organs, and arterial blood vessels. The physiological effects of the ANS depend on both (a) the change in the activities of the autonomic nerves and their release of neurotransmitters and (b) the responsiveness of the peripheral tissues to this neurochemical stimulus (1). The importance of the ANS in mediating the physiological adjustments to exercise has been established by experiments in which the ANS has been eliminated by pharmacological blockade of peripheral adrenergic receptors or by surgical ablation of ANS structures (2–4).

Cardiovascular Effects

The influence of the ANS on cardiovascular and thermoregulatory control during exercise is reviewed in detail elsewhere (1,5,6). Decreases in cardiac vagal nerve activity to the sinoatrial node and ventricular muscle of the heart during exercise reduce the tonic suppressive influence of the vagus nerve on heart rate and ventricular contractility, respectively. Complementary activation of sympathetic nerves to these cardiac tissues, along with SNS stimulation of epinephrine release from the adrenal medulla, further increase heart rate and ventricular contractility during exercise, primarily via stimulation of the β-adrenergic receptor signaling pathway. (There is a modest α-adrenergic contribution to left ventricular contractility.) Together, these changes in ANS activity serve to increase heart rate, left ventricular stroke volume, and cardiac output. The latter, in turn, plays a critical role in supporting systemic arterial blood pressure (and therefore vital organ perfusion), augmenting blood flow to the heart, respiratory muscles, and active locomotor muscles to help meet their increased metabolic (oxygen and energy substrate) demands, and increasing blood flow to the cutaneous circulation for heat dissipation. Activation of sympathetic nerves to arterial resistance vessels (arterioles) in response to exercise produces region-specific vasoconstriction via stimulation of α-adrenergic receptor signaling, thus mediating the redistribution of the increased cardiac output away from tissues in which metabolic rate is not elevated (e.g., gut, liver, and kidneys) while contributing to the augmentation of active muscle blood flow. This vasoconstriction also serves to maintain both cardiac output (by supporting, along with the active muscle pump, cardiac filling pressure) and systemic vascular resistance (conductance) and therefore systemic arterial perfusion pressure in the face of marked vasodilation in active muscle.

Metabolic Effects

As reviewed in detail previously, activation of the sympathoadrenal system has physiologically significant effects on metabolism during exercise (1,5,7). These effects are mediated both by the direct influences of SNS activity and circulating epinephrine on target tissues in the periphery and by the indirect effects of the SNS (e.g., inhibition of insulin release, stimulation of glucagon release) on those tissues. The influence of the sympathoadrenal system on metabolism during exercise includes the following:

- Stimulation of β-adrenergic mediated lipolysis in adipose tissue with a consequent increase in circulating free fatty acid concentrations
- Stimulation of hepatic glycogenolysis via activation of glycogen phosphorylase and hepatic gluconeogenesis via activation of phosphoenolpyruvate carboxykinase (in combination with glucagon release from the pancreas)
- Modulation of substrate metabolism in active skeletal muscle (β-adrenergic–stimulated glucose uptake and utilization and glycogenolysis; fat and protein utilization) and as a consequence lactate release from muscle
- Potential role for α-adrenergic modulation of lipolysis and hepatic gluconeogenesis

Maximal Aerobic Capacity and Exercise Performance

The importance of the ANS in determining maximal aerobic exercise capacity and the ability to perform submaximal exercise has been studied in both experimental animals and human subjects. Surgical ablation of ANS structures and pharmacological blockade have been used to study these issues in experimental animals, whereas pharmacological blockade has been used in investigations of human subjects (discussed later). The key findings on this topic have been reviewed in detail recently by Tipton (8). In dogs, both vagotomy and sympathectomy are associated with reductions in work performance (8). Similarly, Robinson (9) reported in 1953 that pharmacological blockade of the effects of the cardiac vagus reduces maximal oxygen consumption (by about 10% on average) and exercise performance in humans, although a subsequent systematic investigation reported no effects of vagal blockade on oxygen consumption or exercise work time (10). Pharmacological blockade of the sympathetic β-adrenergic system in untrained young adults causes about 5 to 15% reductions in maximal oxygen consumption (2,11). Submaximal and maximal dynamic exercise performance appear to be reduced 10 to 50% during

β-adrenergic receptor blockade, that is, in most cases much more than the associated reduction in maximal aerobic capacity (8). In endurance exercise–trained runners, the reductions in maximal oxygen consumption during exercise with nonspecific β-adrenergic receptor blockade are greater than those observed in untrained subjects under the same conditions (12). These impaired exercise responses upon removal of the sympathetic β-adrenergic system are associated with reductions in cardiac output and leg blood flow, although metabolic changes resulting in enhanced muscle fatigue also may be involved (8). Thus, a substantial body of experimental evidence supports a critical role for the sympathetic β-adrenergic system and to a lesser extent the cardiac vagus in determining maximal aerobic capacity and the ability to perform both submaximal and maximal dynamic exercise.

Exercise Training

These collective ANS adjustments to acute physical activity can be modified after a period of regular performance of exercise. Such adaptations are most clearly expressed during performance of the same absolute submaximal workload of large-muscle dynamic exercise after aerobic endurance training. Tonic (resting) ANS activity and/or the physiological response to a given level of ANS activity during exercise also may be influenced by habitually performed exercise.

Chapter Objectives and Outline

The primary goal of this chapter is to describe the changes in ANS activity that produce the physiological adjustments necessary to maintain homeostasis in response to conventional forms of acute large-muscle dynamic exercise and the peripheral and CNS mechanisms that mediate those changes in ANS activity. A secondary aim is to describe the influence of chronically performed exercise on the changes in ANS activity evoked during acute submaximal exercise and the CNS mechanisms involved. The possible effects of habitual exercise on ANS activity and ANS-mediated physiological function under resting conditions also will be considered. To achieve these objectives the chapter is divided into four sections:

- A description of the methods needed to understand the data on exercise and the ANS
- A discussion of the ANS adjustments to acute exercise
- A discussion of the ANS adaptations to chronic exercise
- An overall summary

Measurement of ANS Activity

To properly interpret the experimental evidence upon which our understanding of ANS physiology during exercise is based, we begin with a brief discussion of the methods for assessing ANS activity, particularly in human subjects. These measurements of cardiac vagal and SNS–adrenal medullary activity have been performed during both actual exercise and simulated exercise (e.g., electrical stimulation of motor areas in the brain or peripheral muscle contraction and intent to perform exercise during muscle paralysis).

Assessment of Cardiac Vagal Activity

Cardiac vagal influences on the heart at rest and during exercise have been studied using two main experimental approaches.

Muscarinic Receptor Antagonists

The most direct approach involves administration of the muscarinic receptor antagonist atropine sulfate (4,9,13). Atropine competes with acetylcholine, the neurotransmitter released from cardiac vagal nerves, for binding to postjunctional muscarinic receptors in the heart, including the sinoatrial node and ventricular muscle. When atropine is administered prior to the beginning of exercise, baseline heart rate is increased as a result of removal of the tonic suppressive effect imposed by the cardiac vagal nerves. Any direct or indirect (e.g., heart rate–related) anti-inotropic effect of vagal activity on the left ventricle also is removed, but this is difficult to demonstrate under normal (intact) in vivo conditions, likely because the consequent reduced filling period decreases preload (decreased Frank Starling effect) and negates any augmentation of intrinsic contractility. The increase in baseline heart rate with administration of atropine therefore represents the tonic influence of the cardiac vagus on cardiac chronotropic function. Thus, any increases in heart rate observed during subsequent exercise can be reasonably interpreted as being mediated by nonvagal ANS (i.e., sympathoadrenal) mechanisms. A seldom-used variation of this approach involves giving atropine during rather than before exercise (14,15). Under these conditions, the increase in heart rate upon acute administration of atropine would be interpreted as reflecting the influence of the cardiac vagus at that specific intensity and/or duration of exercise. The strength of this overall experimental approach involving the use of atropine is the ability to directly block the actions of the vagus nerves in mediating cardiac function, especially the control of heart rate. Limitations include

- The side effects of atropine that particularly in humans necessitate doses that produce incomplete blockade of muscarinic receptors
- Changes in baseline heart rate produced by administration of atropine in attempts to interpret heart rate responses to exercise
- The risks to human subjects of inducing cardiac events as a result of the changes in sympathovagal balance, especially in patients with existing disease or other high-risk groups (e.g., elderly subjects)

- Potential problems with interpretation based on the fact that at low doses atropine possesses vagomimetic properties, whereas at higher doses its actions are vagolytic

Heart Rate Variability

A second approach for assessing the influence of the cardiac vagus on the modulation of heart rate is to measure heart rate variability (HRV), that is, the beat-to-beat variation in the length of cardiac cycles (14,16,17). This can be done using either time (usually expressed as the absolute length and standard deviation of the R-R intervals) or frequency (power spectral analysis of R-R interval frequency content) domain analyses. In general, the interpretation is that the greater the HRV, the greater the modulatory influence of the cardiac vagus on heart rate. Greater HRV would be reflected either by an increased standard deviation of R-R intervals or an increased power at the respiratory frequency (high-frequency power of the R-R intervals, 0.15–0.50 Hz). The primary advantage of this approach is its noninvasive nature, making it attractive to use in high-risk subject groups and/or under laboratory conditions in which the clinical support required to safely oversee the administration of cardiovascular drugs such as atropine is not available. The primary disadvantage of these measures is their indirect nature, that is, that nonvagal influences could affect the values obtained, especially during exercise, with its concomitant changes in hemodynamic function and breathing (18). Measurement errors, superimposed motion, and/or physiological artifacts and the dependence of some methods on steady-state exercise conditions represent additional limitations of this approach.

Assessment of Sympathoadrenal Activity

Initially, indirect approaches based on changes in cardiovascular function from resting conditions in response to exercise were used. These included increases in heart rate, arterial blood pressure, and regional vascular resistance (inactive limbs and internal organs). Although the latter continues to be a useful marker of exercise-evoked increases in SNS vasoconstrictor activity to resistance vessels, a general limitation of all such methods is the fact that these and other cardiovascular functions are or can be under certain conditions influenced by mechanisms independent of the SNS.

Plasma Norepinephrine Concentrations

With the development of sensitive radioenzymatic assays in the 1970s and later high-performance liquid chromatography (HPLC) it became possible to estimate SNS activation during exercise from measurements of plasma concentrations of norepinephrine (PNE) (1,5). Norepinephrine is the primary neurotransmitter released from postganglionic SNS neurons in response sympathetic nerve discharge. Thus, increases in PNE from baseline resting conditions have been used to assess the activation of the SNS in response to various types, intensities, and durations of acute exercise (1,5). In general, this approach appears to yield accurate estimates of SNS activity, particularly during moderate to maximal intensities of large-muscle dynamic exercise that produce marked increases in PNE. However, PNE is the product of a complex process that involves norepinephrine (NE) release from postganglionic sympathetic nerve terminals in response to sympathetic nerve discharge (including prejunctional modulation of that release), NE uptake back into those nerve terminals (80–90% of release), extraneuronal metabolism of NE, diffusion of the remaining NE into the plasma compartment, and clearance of NE from the systemic circulation (19,20). As such, inaccuracies can occur in comparisons of individuals or groups that differ in any step in this process. Moreover, about 50% of the PNE obtained from antecubital venous blood samples (the most common sampling site) is derived from the NE released by the sympathetic nerves in the arm and therefore may not accurately reflect average systemic (whole-body) SNS activity (19). Nevertheless, most of the available experimental data providing insight into the activation of the SNS during exercise is based on PNE.

Plasma Norepinephrine Spillover

A more accurate method of assessing SNS activity using circulating concentrations of NE involves determination of rates of NE spillover (appearance) into the plasma compartment (19,20). These values are obtained from measurements of arterial and venous PNE, extraction of NE by the tissues (using tritiated NE), and plasma flow, and they are independent of any effects on NE clearance. NE spillover can be determined from measurements obtained from the systemic circulation (i.e., whole-body or total NE spillover) or from specific regional circulations (heart, kidneys, liver, gut, limbs). The limitations of this approach include the following:

- Invasiveness of the blood sampling required, typically requiring both arterial and venous catheters (although blood from arterialized hand veins also has been used); also, for regional NE spillover measurements, the venous catheter must be in a vein draining the organ or tissue of interest
- Costs of tritiated NE
- Need to measure regional or systemic plasma flow

In some regional circulations, simple arteriovenous differences in PNE have been used to estimate SNS activity (19,20); however, such measures do not take into account the influence of NE uptake into tissues, which could theoretically confound the results obtained. In experimental animals, regional SNS activity also has been assessed with measurements of NE turnover using isotope labeling and extraction and analysis of specific tissues or organs (21).

Neuropeptide Y

Neuropeptide Y (NPY) is a cotransmitter stored in sympathetic nerve endings that is released only during high frequencies of sympathetic nerve discharge. It has a much longer half-life and is believed to produce stronger and more sustained vasoconstriction than NE (22). Thus, increases in plasma concentrations and/or spillover of NPY would be interpreted as reflecting high levels of SNS activation during exercise (23,24).

Neural Recording of SNS Activity

The only direct method of assessing peripheral SNS activity during exercise is through recordings of the discharge rates of postganglionic sympathetic nerves. In humans, the technique of positioning the tip of a microelectrode in a peripheral nerve has been used to record SNS activity to skeletal muscle arterioles or the skin in primarily inactive limbs during exercise (25), whereas recordings of SNS activity have been obtained from internal organs in experimental animals. The key advantage of this overall approach is that it yields intraneural recordings of actual SNS activity rather than estimating SNS activity from neurochemical plasma markers or cardiovascular functions that are influenced by SNS activity. These recordings of peripheral SNS activity are believed to reflect SNS outflow from the CNS. Disadvantages of human subject microneurography include the following:

- Inability to assess SNS activity to internal organs
- Difficulty in maintaining neural recordings, even from inactive limbs, during conventional forms of large-muscle dynamic exercise because of excessive body movement, which tends to dislodge the electrode from its recording site
- Expense associated with the hardware and software necessary for data acquisition and analysis
- Substantial investigator training, experience, and skill required to obtain interpretable recordings on a consistent basis
- Invasiveness of the procedure, which causes temporary local side effects in a small percentage of subjects

Whole-nerve recordings of SNS activity from internal organs in experimental animals require highly invasive surgery to isolate and position the recording electrode on the internal organ nerve in question, postsurgical care and recovery of the animal, and considerable investment in equipment and investigator skill.

Low-frequency Power of HRV

Measurements of the low-frequency power of HRV also have been used to assess cardiac sympathetic modulation of heart rate (as well as overall cardiac SNS tone) (20). However, although noninvasive and convenient, there is considerable controversy as to the validity of these measurements as reflecting cardiac sympathetic modulation of heart rate (20). As such, the use of low-frequency power of HRV for this purpose has not received widespread support from knowledgeable investigators in the field.

Plasma Concentrations and Secretion of Epinephrine

Release of epinephrine from the adrenal medulla has most commonly been assessed by measurement of plasma epinephrine (PE) concentrations via radioenzymatic assay or HPLC (19,26). The strength of this approach is that PE accurately reflects the circulating concentrations of this hormone available to bind to β-adrenergic receptors in the systemic circulation both under resting baseline conditions and during exercise. Thus, if the circulating concentrations of epinephrine are most important for providing insight into the research question being addressed, measurement of PE is appropriate. However, the same limitation associated with interpretation of PNE applies to these measurements. That is, PE reflects the balance between the respective rates at which epinephrine is released from the adrenal medulla and the clearance of epinephrine from the plasma compartment (19,26). Therefore, accurate determinations of actual epinephrine release from the adrenal medulla during exercise cannot be made from PE. This is the case particularly when individuals or groups in a study sample differ in PE clearance. Rather, precise assessment of epinephrine secretion from the adrenal medulla at rest and during exercise requires measurement of total PE kinetics using tritiated epinephrine (26).

Adrenergic Receptor Antagonists

As is the case with the use of atropine to block cardiac vagal influences, various drugs can be used to block the peripheral effects of sympathoadrenal system activation during exercise, most commonly β- and α-adrenergic receptor antagonists (e.g., propranolol, phentolamine) (8,20). As with atropine, these drugs can be administered either before (most common) or during exercise to assess the involvement of the sympathoadrenal system in mediating the physiological responses observed. That is, any differences in the cardiovascular or other physiological adjustments to exercise in the presence compared with the absence of these antagonists are interpreted as indicating the specific contribution of the sympathoadrenal stimulus (neuronally released NE, circulating NE and epinephrine) and peripheral adrenergic (β- and/or α-adrenergic receptor) signaling pathway in question. Again, the ability to block sympathoadrenal system activation of specific peripheral adrenergic signaling pathways is the primary advantage of this approach. The primary disadvantages include the following:

- Changes in baseline cardiovascular function produced by administration of these cardiac and/or vasoactive agents, which can make interpretation of resting-to-exercise changes in cardiovascular function challenging (also a problem with atropine)
- Side effects of the drugs
- Acute circulatory risks of these agents
- Clinical support requirements for administering the drugs to human subjects

Assessment of Overall ANS Effects: Surgical Ablation of Parasympathetic (Vagal) and SNS Structures

This experimental approach has been recently reviewed in detail by Tipton (8). A classic approach to determining the importance of specific anatomical structures, including the ANS, in producing specific physiological functions involves surgical ablation (lesioning) of those structures. Using this approach, the physiological adjustments to exercise are established in the intact (control) state and after removal of ANS structures of interest. Any difference in a physiological response in the presence compared with the absence of the structure in question is interpreted as evidence that the structure is required for the normal expression of the response during exercise. The strength of this approach is the ability to remove the effect of a specific structure and directly determine the effect of its absence on a particular physiological response to exercise. Two obvious limitations of this model are the facts that it only can be used in experimental animals (although specific human genetic- and disease-based research models of ANS lesions exist) and the inability to study the same animal under control (intact) and experimental (lesioned) conditions in a randomized order. Another limitation is the possibility that other structures compensate for the absence of the ablated structure (redundancy of control). In this scenario, the physiological response to exercise in the experimental (ablation) condition is normal, and the conclusion might be made that the structure in question is not normally involved in the neural regulation of the response. However, the structure may indeed normally be involved in the control of the exercise response, but this contribution cannot be shown because of redundant control mechanisms. Therefore, the appropriate interpretation for this type of outcome of an experiment using this approach is that the structure in question "is not necessary" to produce the response during exercise, that is, that the response does not depend on that structure. In other words, if the response is abolished after elimination of the structure, the interpretation of the experiment is definitive. If the response remains intact in the absence of the structure, the interpretation is not definitive. This same limitation also applies to the use of adrenergic receptor antagonists described earlier.

Transgenic Animals

Finally, use of transgenic animals represents a relatively new experimental approach to altering elements of the ANS, such as adrenergic receptors (27), that play a role in physiological function. ANS structures and/or elements of their signaling pathways can be eliminated (knock-out models) or alternatively, overexpressed. In these models genetically modified animals are compared with intact control (wild type) animals. Any differences in the responses to exercise would be attributed to the absence or overexpression of the ANS structure or pathway in question. The strength of such approaches is the ability to directionally modify a specific ANS influence. The primary limitation is the possibility that other systems may adapt to help compensate for the genetic modification, thus altering their normal contributions to physiological control and masking the usual effect of the genetically altered influence.

ANS Changes During Acute Exercise

Conventional Whole-Body Dynamic Exercise

Cardiac Vagal Modulation of Heart Rate

ONSET OF EXERCISE   At the onset of dynamic exercise cardiac vagal modulation of heart rate is reduced, presumably reflecting a decrease in efferent cardiac vagal nerve activity. This concept is consistent with at least two lines of experimental evidence:

1. Cardiac vagal–related expressions of HRV decrease from rest with the initiation of exercise (14,17,28) (Fig. 9.1).
2. Administration of atropine prior to exercise eliminates the abrupt increase in heart rate observed with the initiation of exercise (4,29) (Fig. 9.2).

Together, this evidence indicates that reduced cardiac vagal modulation of heart rate (reduced efferent cardiac vagal nerve activity) is the key mechanism involved in mediating the tachycardia associated with the onset of exercise.

EXERCISE INTENSITY   Increasing exercise intensity is associated with a progressive, even exponential reduction in cardiac vagal modulation of heart rate, presumably reflecting a progressive reduction in cardiac vagal nerve activity. The experimental evidence supporting this conclusion includes the following:

1. Progressively greater reductions in cardiac vagal–related expressions of HRV increase with increasing intensities of exercise (14,28,30) (Figs. 9.1 and 9.3).
2. When compared with normal intact (control) conditions, after pretreatment with atropine, the increase in heart rate from rest in response to incremental exercise is either abolished or reduced during mild to moderate-intensity workloads but is progressively less affected with further increases in workload to maximum (4,9,29) (Figs. 9.4 and 9.5).

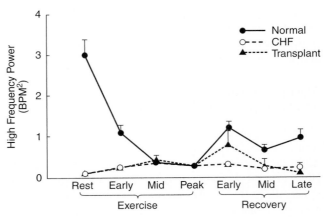

FIGURE 9.1   High-frequency power of the heart rate variability in groups of normal adult humans and patients with congestive heart failure (CHF) (*left*) or heart transplantation (*right*) at rest prior to continuous incremental exercise, during the second to third minutes of the initial and lightest intensity of continuous incremental leg cycling exercise (early), during a workload about halfway from the lightest to the peak workload (mid), during the peak workload attained, and during early (minutes 1 to 2), middle (minutes 4 to 5), and late (minutes 8 to 9) post exercise recovery. Note in particular (*a*) the marked reduction in high-frequency power from rest to the initial few minutes of light exercise, reflecting a striking reduction in cardiac vagal modulation of heart rate evoked by the initiation of exercise, and (*b*) the further stepwise reductions in cardiac vagal modulation of heart rate with increasing exercise intensity and duration in the normal subjects. The patients lacked significant cardiac vagal modulation of heart rate at rest, during exercise, and during post-exercise recovery. (*Modified with permission from Arai Y, Saul JP, Albrecht P, et al. Modulation of cardiac autonomic activity during and immediately after exercise. Am J Physiol 1989;256:H135.*)

Reductions in cardiac vagal–related expressions of HRV from baseline (resting) levels have been observed experimentally at exercise intensities as low as about 20% of maximal oxygen consumption ($\dot{V}_{O_{2max}}$) (4,14,28). It is likely, however, that reductions in cardiac vagal modulation of heart rate occur at any exercise intensity that evokes an increase in heart rate above resting levels. Much of the reduction in cardiac vagal modulation of heart rate from resting levels appears to occur by intensities of exercise associated with increases in heart rate up to about 100 beats per minute (4,22,28). However, based on the following facts, it appears that at least some cardiac vagal modulation of heart rate is retained even during heavy submaximal intensities of dynamic exercise:

- Heart rate increases significantly during strenuous exercise after administration of atropine (9,14,15)
- Significant HRV remains during higher-intensity exercise in dogs (14) (Fig. 9.3)

As emphasized by O'Leary and colleagues (15), the retention of at least some cardiac vagal modulation of heart rate dur-

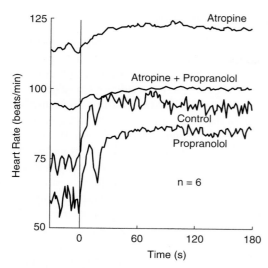

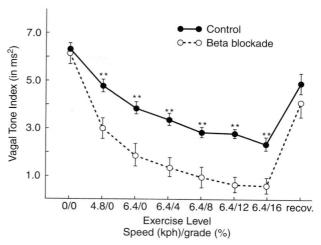

FIGURE 9.2 Heart rate responses from rest (left of the 0 time point) during the initial 3 minutes of light dynamic leg cycling exercise (50 W) in healthy young men under control (no drug) conditions and after pretreatment with atropine alone (removes cardiac vagal influence), propranolol alone (removes β-adrenergic receptor signaling pathway), or combined atropine and propranolol. Blockade of the vagal influence with atropine caused a marked increase in heart rate at rest but significantly blunted the normal increase in heart rate at the onset of exercise, suggesting that vagal withdrawal mediates the tachycardia normally observed with the initiation of exercise. In contrast, propranolol lowered resting heart rate but did not influence the heart rate response to exercise, suggesting that increases in cardiac sympathetic nerve activity and β-adrenergic receptor signaling do not contribute to the tachycardia produced upon initiation of exercise. *(Modified from Fagraeus L, Linnarsson D. Autonomic origin of heart rate fluctuations at the onset of muscular exercise. J Appl Physiol 1976;40:680.)*

FIGURE 9.3 Changes in the vagal tone index based on analysis of heart rate variability from rest during incremental treadmill running in healthy mongrel dogs under control conditions and after pretreatment with propranolol, a nonspecific β-adrenergic receptor antagonist. Note in particular in the normal (control) condition (*a*) the progressive reduction in cardiac vagal tone index from rest during exercise of increasing intensity, suggesting an important role for cardiac vagal withdrawal in mediating the progressive tachycardia observed with increasing exercise intensity, and (*b*) that significant vagal tone remains during heavy submaximal exercise. *(Modified from Billman GE, Dujardin JP. Dynamic changes in cardiac vagal tone as measured by time-series analysis. Am J Physiol 1990;258:H898.)*

ing heavy submaximal exercise may be advantageous in that it would provide the ability to evoke a rapid arterial baroreflex–mediated increase in heart rate and cardiac output in the case of hypotension (the arterial baroreflex requires cardiac vagal withdrawal to produce rapid tachycardia). At maximal exercise intensities in humans there is no obvious remaining cardiac vagal modulation of heart rate based on these observations:

- Atropine administration has no effect on maximal heart rate (9) (Fig. 9.5).
- Relatively little HRV exists during peak cycling exercise in healthy humans (28) (Fig. 9.1).

PROLONGED SUBMAXIMAL EXERCISE   There is little or no direct information on cardiac vagal modulation of heart rate

during prolonged (>30 minutes) dynamic exercise performed at a fixed submaximal intensity. This is unfortunate, given the fact that this type of exercise is most often performed for purposes of maintaining optimal health and fitness. Based on the facts that (*a*) some reserve for cardiac vagal modulation of heart rate remains up to heavy submaximal intensities of exercise (9,14,15) and (*b*) heart rate continues to rise above early steady-state levels during prolonged submaximal exercise (6), one might reasonably speculate that at least part of this progressive tachycardia with sustained exercise is mediated by further reductions in cardiac vagal modulation of heart rate. Preliminary observations showing progressively greater reductions in HRV during prolonged fixed-intensity submaximal running exercise in dogs support this postulate (personal communication from Professor George E. Billman of The Ohio State University, 9/2003) (Fig. 9.6). The contribution of cardiac vagal withdrawal to the increase in heart rate during prolonged submaximal exercise would depend, at least in part, on the intensity of exercise and therefore on the early steady-state exercise heart rate. The greater the latter, the smaller the cardiac vagal modulation early in exercise, the smaller the possible contribution of additional vagal withdrawal to any further tachycardia with continuing exercise, and vice versa.

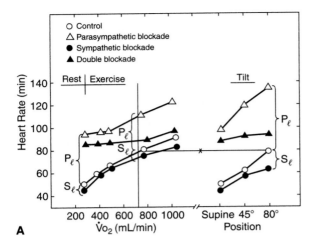

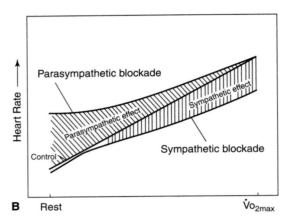

FIGURE 9.4 **A.** Heart rate during dynamic leg cycling exercise of increasing intensity in primarily healthy young men under control (no drug) conditions and after pretreatment with atropine alone (parasympathetic blockade—removes cardiac vagal influence), propranolol alone (sympathetic blockade—removes β-adrenergic receptor signaling pathway), or combined atropine and propranolol (double blockade) (*left side, top*). Blockade of the vagal influence with atropine caused a marked increase in heart rate at rest but significantly blunted the normal increase in heart rate with increasing exercise intensities, suggesting that vagal withdrawal mediates the tachycardia normally observed with light to moderate intensity exercise. In contrast, propranolol lowered resting heart rate slightly, did not influence the heart rate response to mild to moderate submaximal exercise (suggesting that increases in cardiac sympathetic nerve activity and/or circulating epinephrine and β-adrenergic receptor signaling do not contribute to the tachycardia occurring at these exercise intensities), but reduced heart rate at heavier submaximal exercise intensities, suggesting an important role for this mechanism in mediating the tachycardia under these conditions. **B.** The relative influences of cardiac vagal withdrawal (parasympathetic effect) and sympathetic β-adrenergic stimulation (sympathetic effect) in mediating the increases in heart rate observed during exercise of increasing intensity. (*Modified with permission from Robinson BF, Epstein SE, Beiser GD, et al. Control of heart rate by the autonomic nervous system. Studies in man on the interrelation between baroreceptor mechanisms and exercise. Circ Res 1966;19:400–411.*)

Sympathoadrenal Response

ONSET OF EXERCISE The integrative response of the efferent SNS at the onset of conventional large-muscle dynamic exercise is unclear based on the available experimental evidence. Specifically, there is evidence for selective regional (tissue or organ specific) but not diffuse (systemic) SNS activation with the initiation of exercise. In experimental animals, renal SNS activity increases with the initiation of exercise (31,32), and recent findings demonstrate that cardiac SNS activity increases at the onset of light to moderate treadmill exercise (33). In human subjects, skin SNS activity, at least SNS sudomotor (sweat gland) activity, increases with the onset of isometric handgrip exercise in humans (34), but there are no direct (microneurographic) recordings of skin SNA at the onset of conventional large-muscle dynamic exercise. In contrast, results of experiments employing direct recordings of SNS activity to inactive skeletal muscle demonstrate a reduction in SNS activity from baseline resting levels early during dynamic exercise (35,36). Indeed, SNS activity to inactive muscle in the arms decreases consistently from resting control levels during preparation for exercise and remains below resting control levels during the first minute of upright leg cycling exercise at intensities up to 80% of maximum (35) (Fig. 9.7).

Moreover, in human subjects SNS β-adrenergic blockade does not affect the increase in heart rate at the onset of upright leg cycling exercise (29), indicating no physiologically relevant increase in cardiac SNA (at least to the sinoatrial node) with the initiation of conventional dynamic exercise (Fig. 9.2). Due to technical limitations, it is unknown whether a SNS-mediated increase in epinephrine secretion from the adrenal medulla occurs at the onset of exercise. If so, this likely occurs only in response to heavy submaximal or maximal intensities of exercise and/or during sudden movement associated with a fight-or-flight response.

The lack of a consistent or uniform SNS response at the onset of exercise could be physiological; that is, tissue- or organ-selective SNS activation may be evoked in order to meet specific needs aimed at preserving homeostasis. For example, increases in SNS outflow to the heart would stimulate heart rate and increase cardiac output, and renal SNS activation would produce vasoconstriction in the kidney, which would allow the increased cardiac output to be preferentially distributed to active muscle. Inhibition of SNS activity to muscle would acutely decrease vasoconstrictor tone, thus reducing opposition to locally mediated vasodilation in active muscle. On the other hand, the increase in cardiac SNS activity observed at the onset of treadmill exercise in conscious cats (33) is at odds with the fact that β-adrenergic blockade does not affect the heart rate response to the onset of large-muscle dynamic exercise in humans (29). The information needed to clarify these issues is not likely to be acquired in the foreseeable future because technical limitations restrict our ability to directly assess internal organ sympathetic

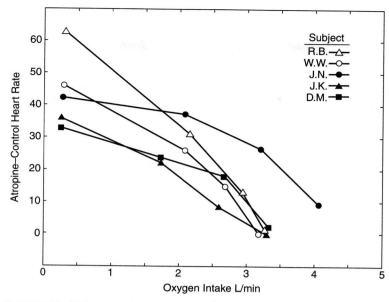

FIGURE 9.5 Differences in heart rate during treadmill running in five healthy men during cardiac vagal blockade (pretreatment with atropine) compared with control (intact cardiac vagal tone). Note (*a*) the differences in heart rate between vagal blockade and control become less with increasing exercise intensities, demonstrating progressive cardiac vagal withdrawal; and (*b*) in four of the five men there was no observable vagal influence remaining at maximal exercise (far right data points on individual lines). (*Modified from Robinson S, M Pearcy, F Brueckman, et al. Effects of atropine on heart rate and oxygen intake in working man. J Appl Physiol 1953;5:510.*)

(heart, kidney, gut) and adrenal medullary (epinephrine secretion) adjustments at the onset of large-muscle dynamic exercise in humans.

EXERCISE INTENSITY In general, in humans SNS activation occurs at exercise intensities ranging from about 25 to 50% of maximum work capacity (1,6,25), that is, at exercise intensities associated with heart rates above 100 beats per minute (6,22). The increase in SNS activity during these intensities of exercise appears to be widespread, including active and inactive skeletal muscle, the kidneys, the splanchnic region, the heart, the spleen, and the skin (6,19,37). Epinephrine secretion from the adrenal medulla also is increased during moderate to heavy exercise (typically 50% of $\dot{V}O_{2max}$ or above) (21,26,38). Sympathoadrenal activation becomes progressively greater as exercise intensity increases from threshold levels up to maximum. The overall evidence supporting sympathoadrenal system activation in response to moderate to heavy submaximal intensities of dynamic exercise includes the following:

- Progressively greater increases in PNE (e.g., from 1.4 nmol/L at rest to 20 nmol/L at maximum) and PE (e.g., from 0.25 nmol/L at rest to 2 nmol/L at maximum) with increasing exercise intensities up to maximum in humans (39–41) (Figs. 9.8 and 9.9)

- Increases in total (whole-body) PNE (24,37,42) and PE (26) spillover rates from rest to exercise in humans that become greater with increasing exercise intensity (Fig. 9.10)

- Increases in directly recorded SNS activity to inactive skeletal muscle (muscle sympathetic nerve activity [MSNA]) from rest with increasing intensities of exercise in humans (35,43,44) (Fig. 9.11)

- Intensity-dependent increases in PNE arteriovenous difference and/or spillover to active and inactive skeletal muscle (45,46) (Fig. 9.12), the kidneys (24,37,45) (Fig. 9.9), the hepatomesenteric region (liver and gut) (47), and/or the heart (37,45) from rest to exercise in humans

- Intensity-dependent increases in renal SNS activity (31,32) and increases in liver NE spillover (48) with treadmill running in experimental animals, and progressive inactive limb, renal, and splanchnic vasoconstriction and increases in plasma renin activity and angiotensin II concentrations from rest with increasing exercise intensities in humans and experimental animals (22,24) (Figs. 9.9 and 9.13)

- Increases in plasma concentrations of NPY from rest in response to heavy submaximal and maximal intensities of exercise in humans (23,24) (Fig. 9.9).

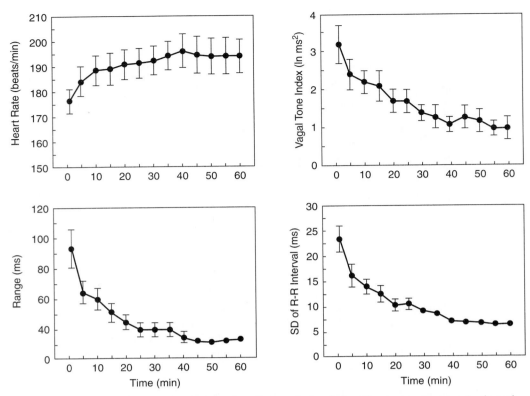

FIGURE 9.6 Heart rate and three measures of cardiac vagal tone during 60 minutes of submaximal treadmill running (6.4 kpm at a 10% grade) in 13 dogs. The upward drift in heart rate is associated with reductions in cardiac vagal tone during the initial 40 minutes of exercise, and both responses plateau over the last 20 minutes. These observations support the idea that cardiac vagal withdrawal plays an important role in mediating the heart rate drift during prolonged submaximal exercise. (*Unpublished data and figure courtesy of Professor George Billman of The Ohio State University.*)

It is important to appreciate that the active limbs are a major target of the increase in SNS vasoconstrictor activity and a major source of the increase in PNE spillover during moderate and higher-intensity dynamic exercise in humans (19,46,49) (Fig. 9.12). Indeed, Esler and associates (19) have estimated, based on measurements of total and regional PNE kinetics, that the skeletal muscle circulation accounts for about 60% of NE released from sympathetic nerve endings during submaximal large-muscle dynamic exercise. It is believed that this is an essential ANS adjustment to exercise because it counteracts locally mediated active muscle vasodilation (22,49). If unchecked by SNS-evoked vasoconstriction, the increases in active muscle and total vascular conductance would reduce arterial blood pressure (i.e., vital organ perfusion pressure for the brain and heart), threatening overall homeostasis.

PROLONGED SUBMAXIMAL EXERCISE Insight regarding the sympathoadrenal system adjustments to prolonged large-muscle dynamic exercise is largely limited to investigations assessing the changes in PNE and PE from rest during fixed moderate submaximal exercise (40,50,51). Galbo (5) and

Galbo and colleagues (40) observed that PNE increases progressively during 180 minutes of submaximal dynamic exercise (Fig. 9.14), supporting the idea of increasing SNS activation during prolonged exercise. Results of other studies (50,51) involving submaximal exercise sustained for more than 45 minutes generally are in agreement with this finding. In healthy young adults, the rise in PNE above baseline control levels has been observed as early as 10 minutes after the onset of exercise, and there is a clearly significant increase in PNE by 20 minutes (50). Continuous increases in PE also are observed during prolonged submaximal exercise (40,51), indicating time-dependent increases in epinephrine secretion from the adrenal medulla under these conditions. (Epinephrine release also can be triggered by hypoglycemia during prolonged exercise.) Plasma concentrations of NPY appear to increase with exercise duration during moderate to heavy exercise intensities (23).

A limited amount of data from measurements of PNE kinetics and/or inactive MSNA during submaximal exercise supports the observations on PNE. During 30 minutes of mild-intensity leg cycling (25% of peak power output) PNE increases significantly above baseline by 15 minutes and

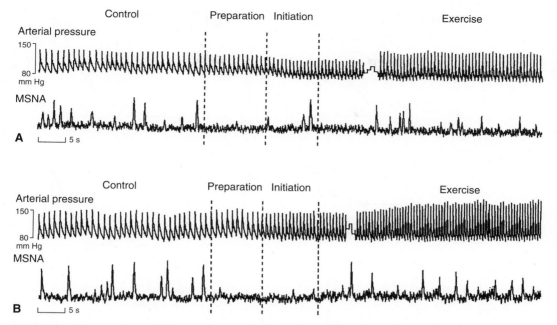

FIGURE 9.7 Microneurographic (intraneural) recordings of inactive MSNA from the radial nerve in the arm during resting control, preparation for, and initiation of light (**A**) and moderate (**B**) intensity leg cycling exercise in a healthy young subject. Note the marked inhibition of MSNA during preparation for and initiation of exercise compared with resting control. During the early (first minute) exercise period MSNA remained suppressed during light intensity exercise, but it returned toward resting control levels at the higher exercise intensity. *(Modified from Callister R, Ng AV, Seals DR. Arm sympathetic nerve activity during preparation for and initiation of leg-cycling exercise in humans. J Appl Physiol 1994;77:1406.)*

remains close to that elevated level thereafter (42) (Fig. 9.10). During moderate-intensity cycling (65% of peak power output), however, the initial increase in PNE is greater and the subsequent rise over time is much steeper than that observed during mild exercise (Fig. 9.10). At both intensities the increase in PNE is either solely or primarily medi-

ated by increases in total PNE spillover, because total PNE clearance is either unchanged (mild intensity) or only slight reduced (moderate intensity) from baseline levels during exercise (Fig. 9.10). These observations indicate that changes in PNE during prolonged exercise generally appear to reflect increases in SNS activity as estimated by

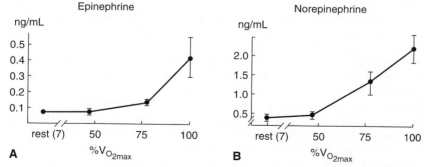

FIGURE 9.8 Plasma epinephrine and norepinephrine concentrations obtained from antecubital venous blood samples on healthy young adults at rest and during incremental treadmill running. Note the progressive increases in the concentrations of these catecholamines with increasing exercise intensity. *(Modified from Galbo H. Hormonal and metabolic adaptation to exercise. Stuttgart, New York: Thieme-Stratton, 1983;7. Based on data from Galbo H, Holst JJ, Christensen NJ. Glucagon and plasma catecholamine responses to graded and prolonged exercise in man. J Appl Physiol 1975;38:70–76.)*

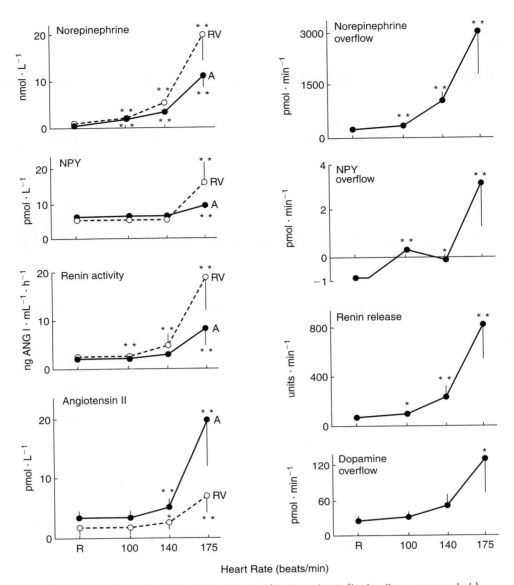

FIGURE 9.9 *Left. Arterial (solid lines, closed symbols)* and renal vein *(broken lines, open symbols)* plasma concentrations of norepinephrine, neuropeptide Y (NPY), renin activity, and angiotensin II. *Right.* Renal overflows of norepinephrine, NPY, renin, and dopamine, at rest (R) and during leg cycling exercise at increasing levels of heart rate equivalent to 30, 60, and 80 to 90% of maximum workload in healthy young men. With increasing exercise intensity there are progressive increases in (a) total norepinephrine overflow, reflecting increasing net whole-body sympathetic activation; (b) renal norepinephrine and dopamine overflow and renin release, reflecting increasing renal sympathetic nerve activation; and (c) increasing systemic and renal NPY overflow at the highest exercise intensity reflecting very high net whole-body and renal sympathetic activation, respectively, during heavy submaximal to nearly maximal exercise intensities. *(Reprinted with permission from Rowell LB, O'Leary DS, Kellogg DL. Integration of cardiovascular control systems in dynamic exercise. In Rowell LB, Shepherd JT, eds. Handbook of Physiology, section 12: Exercise: Regulation and Integration of Multiple Systems. New York: Oxford University, 1996;783. Based on data from Tidgren B, Hjemdahl P, Theodorsson E, et al. Renal neurohormonal and vascular responses to dynamic exercise in humans. J Appl Physiol 1991;70:2279–2286.)*

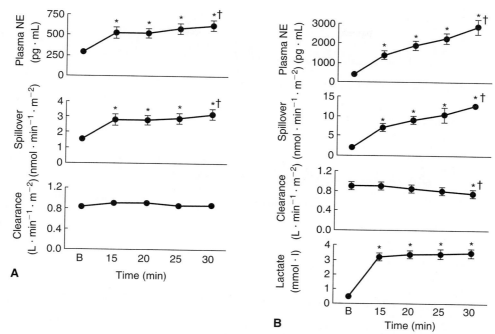

FIGURE 9.10   Plasma norepinephrine concentrations, total (whole-body) spillover, and clearance in healthy young adults at rest and during 30 minutes of leg cycling performed at (**A**) a light (25% of maximum workload) and (**B**) a moderate (65% of maximum workload) exercise intensity. During light exercise, plasma norepinephrine concentrations are increased modestly (about 100% above rest) by 15 minutes of exercise mediated by an increase in norepinephrine spillover, reflecting an increase in net systemic sympathetic nervous system activation, which plateaus during the remainder of the exercise period. In contrast, moderate exercise results in a much more marked (about 10-fold above rest) and progressive increase in sympathetic activation throughout the 30-minute exercise period. This progressive sympathetic activation is dissociated from the corresponding increase in plasma lactate concentration, a byproduct and marker of glycolytic metabolism. *(Modified with permission from Leuenberger U, Sinoway L, Gubin S, et al. Effects of exercise intensity and duration on norepinephrine spillover and clearance in humans. J Appl Physiol 1993;75:670, 671.)*

changes in total PNE spillover. One target of the increase in overall SNS outflow during prolonged submaximal exercise appears to be inactive skeletal muscle, as indicated by significant increases in inactive arm MSNA during 30 minutes of light to moderate leg cycling exercise (52). Taken together, these findings support the idea of progressive time-dependent sympathoadrenal system activation during prolonged submaximal exercise. The results also indicate that the greater the submaximal intensity, the greater the additional sympathoadrenal activation that occurs from early on to the end of the exercise period.

RELATION TO PLASMA LACTATE RESPONSE   There is a body of experimental evidence supporting the view that the increases in PNE and PE during incremental submaximal exercise are strongly related to the corresponding increases in plasma lactate concentrations (40,53). These findings suggest a physiological connection between sympathoadrenal system activation and glycolytic metabolism during exercise. One explanation for this association is that sympathoadrenal

activation, particularly increases in PE, stimulates β-adrenergic activation of phosphorylase, which in turn stimulates glycogenolysis in skeletal muscle and perhaps the kidneys, resulting in enhanced glycolytic flux and consequent formation of lactate (53). In contrast, it has been noted that SNS activation occurs at exercise intensities associated with heart rates of about 100 beats per minute (i.e., as low as 25–40% of peak or maximum $\dot{V}O_{2max}$), whereas significant increases in plasma lactate concentrations typically are not observed until significantly higher exercise intensities (e.g., heart rates of about 140–150 beats per minute) (6,22,42) (Figs. 9.10 and 9.13). Moreover, during 30 minutes of moderate-intensity leg cycling, both PNE and total PNE spillover increases progressively, whereas plasma lactate concentrations are increased above baseline early in exercise and remain at that level throughout exercise (42). These seemingly disparate observations may be explained by the fact that muscle lactate turnover increases even at mild exercise intensities, which is not immediately reflected by changes in plasma concentrations.

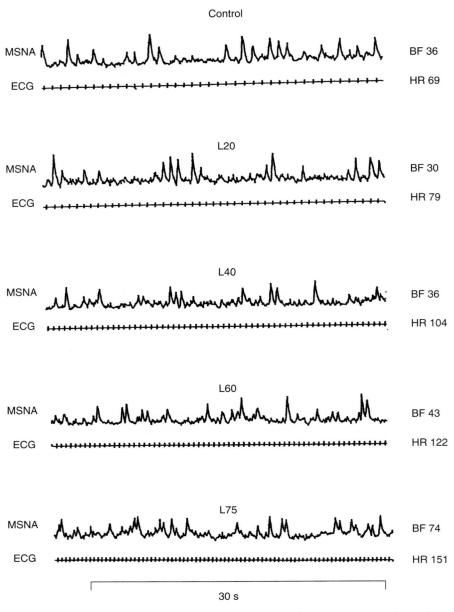

FIGURE 9.11 Tracings from microneurographic recordings of inactive MSNA in the median nerve of the arm (*top to bottom*) during resting control conditions and increasing intensities of leg cycling exercise (20–75% of maximum workload) in one subject. Compared with rest, MSNA is slightly reduced during light exercise, increasing progressively thereafter with increases in exercise intensity. *(Modified from Saito M, Tsukanaka A, Yanagihara D, et al. Muscle sympathetic nerve responses to graded leg cycling. J Appl Physiol 1993;75:664.)*

SYMPATHOLYSIS The term *sympatholysis*, or *functional sympatholysis*, refers to the idea that vasodilation of arterioles induced by locally released metabolic factors (e.g., potassium and hydrogen ions, adenosine, and hyperosmolarity) can prevent SNS-mediated vasoconstriction, either by inhibiting NE release from sympathetic nerve endings or by blocking the effects of NE release on postjunctional α-adrenergic receptors (22,49,54). The physiological context in which this issue has received most interest is that of metabolic vasodilation interfering with the SNS vasoconstriction in active skeletal muscle arterioles. As emphasized by Joyner and Thomas (54), this idea is attractive because it provides an additional regulatory mechanism by which the increase in cardiac output generated during exercise can be preferentially distributed to the active skeletal muscles and away from regions not requiring augmented flow in the face of wide-

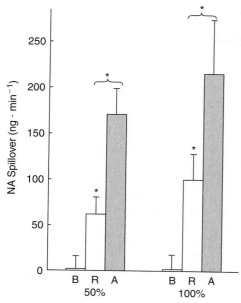

FIGURE 9.12 Noradrenaline (NA), or norepinephrine, spillover rates during one-legged knee extension exercise performed for 10 minutes at each of two intensities (50% and 100% of maximum workload) in healthy young men. Measurements were made under basal control conditions before exercise in the pooled (average of both) legs (B), in the resting leg during contralateral leg exercise (R), and in the active leg during exercise (A). NA spillover was progressively greater from rest to light to maximal intensities, reflecting incremental sympathetic activation to the legs across these conditions. Importantly, at both intensities sympathetic activation to the active (exercising) leg was much greater than that to the resting leg. *(Modified from Savard G, Strange S, Kiens B, et al. Noradrenaline spillover during exercise in active versus resting skeletal muscle in man. Acta Physiol Scand 1987;131:512.)*

the interpretation of data in this area (e.g., the use of vascular conductance vs. vascular resistance) (22), it is well established that high local concentrations of vasodilatory metabolites, as produced during strenuous exercise, can reduce SNS-adrenergic vasoconstriction in active muscle (22). However, it also is clear that vasodilatory metabolites cannot completely abolish SNS-mediated vasoconstriction (22). It now has been shown (22,49,54) that sympatholysis most likely occurs in terminal arterioles via interactions with α_2-adrenergic receptors, which are more responsive to vasodilatory metabolites than are α_1-adrenergic receptors (which predominate in the larger more proximal arterioles). Differences in α-adrenergic receptor subtype density also may explain why sympatholysis has been observed in white glycolytic fibers (in which α_2-adrenergic receptors predominate), but not red oxidative fibers (primarily α_1-adrenergic receptors) in experimental animals (22). This proposed selective effect of sympatholysis on terminal arterioles via interactions with α_2-adrenergic receptors—but not in more proximal arterial vessels predominated by α_1-adrenergic receptors—may explain how functional sympatholysis can provide a mechanism for precise local control of active muscle blood flow while not interfering with the ability to limit total vascular conductance during large-muscle dynamic exercise (54). Specifically, recent evidence (54) indicates that sympatholysis occurs only in the smallest arterioles in

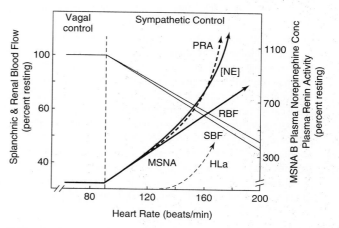

FIGURE 9.13 Summary of sympathetic responses to large-muscle dynamic exercise of increasing intensity. Diffuse sympathetic activation begins at moderate exercise intensities associated with heart rates above 100 beats per minute and increases exponentially up to maximal exercise intensities, as indicated by reductions in splanchnic (SBF) and renal (RBF) blood flow and corresponding increases in plasma renin activity (PRA), norepinephrine (NE), and MSNA. The increase in lactic acid (HLa) occurs at a higher intensity (associated with heart rates of 130–140 beats per minute) than sympathetic activation. *(Modified from Rowell LB, O'Leary DS, Kellogg DL. Integration of cardiovascular control systems in dynamic exercise. In Rowell LB, Shepherd JT, eds. Handbook of physiology section 12: Exercise: Regulation and Integration of Multiple Systems. New York: Oxford University, 1996, 782.)*

spread SNS activation. That is, functional sympatholysis would provide active muscle a powerful local mechanism for more precisely regulating blood flow to meet its metabolic demands. The potential disadvantage of such a mechanism would be the inability to produce SNS-mediated vasoconstriction in active muscle to limit the increase in systemic vascular conductance that can threaten arterial blood pressure and therefore vital organ perfusion (54). Under these conditions, the CNS must be able to produce effective SNS vasoconstriction in active muscle.

The concept of sympatholysis, which is discussed in depth elsewhere (22,49,54), remains controversial, with evidence that has been interpreted as both supporting and refuting the hypothesis. Although methodology issues affect

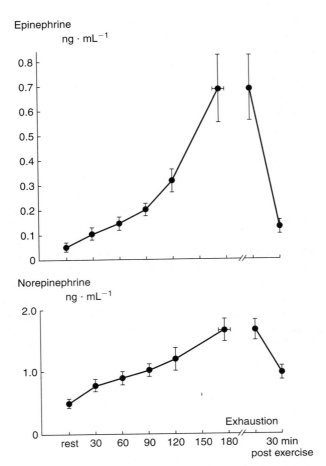

FIGURE 9.14 Plasma epinephrine (*top*) and norepinephrine (*bottom*) concentrations at rest and during 3 hours of continuous treadmill running at an intensity associated with 60% of maximal oxygen consumption in healthy young adults. Note the progressive increases in the plasma concentrations of these catecholamines, reflecting progressively increasing sympathoadrenal system activation during prolonged moderate submaximal exercise. (*Modified from Galbo H. Hormonal and Metabolic Adaptation to Exercise. Stuttgart, New York: Thieme-Stratton, 1983;7. Based on data from Galbo H, Holst JJ, Christensen NJ. Glucagon and plasma catecholamine responses to graded and prolonged exercise in man. J Appl Physiol 1975;38:70–76.*)

contracting muscle, whereas SNS vasoconstriction in the more proximal arterioles and feed arteries is largely preserved. This scheme, therefore, provides an overall regulatory model by which functional sympatholysis can operate to ensure proper control of active muscle blood flow without threatening systemic cardiovascular homeostasis during large-muscle dynamic exercise (54).

Modulatory Factors

Several factors or conditions can modify the ANS adjustments to acute exercise.

ABSOLUTE VERSUS RELATIVE EXERCISE INTENSITIES Comparing individual subjects at the same absolute submaximal exercise intensity or level of $\dot{V}O_2$ results in marked variability among individuals in the ANS responses to exercise. This has been most thoroughly documented with regard to the plasma catecholamine responses to incremental exercise. In general, expressing these responses as a function of the percent of $\dot{V}O_{2max}$ of the subject markedly reduces this variability (1,26,41). Such observations provide support for the widely held concept that the magnitude of the ANS adjustments to submaximal exercise is primarily determined by the relative (percent of maximum) rather than the absolute intensity (5,26,41). The absolute work rate or level of $\dot{V}O_2$, however, does appear to contribute to the ANS response to exercise. One line of evidence supporting this idea is that during different types of dynamic exercise performed at the same percent of maximum, the increase in PNE is greater when the absolute workload or $\dot{V}O_2$ is greater (55). As such, it is likely that both the relative and the absolute workload determine the ANS response to submaximal dynamic exercise, with the former having the stronger influence.

SUBJECT GENDER The available data indicate that the plasma catecholamine responses to dynamic exercise may differ in men and women. PNE and PE have been found to be higher in men than in women at various intensities of large-muscle dynamic exercise (56), including at the same relative workloads (56), although in another study no gender-related differences were reported (1). When observed, the greater PNE and PE in men may be explained by the higher maximal aerobic exercise capacity in men. That is, the same relative workload in men and women represents a much greater absolute exercise stimulus in the men because of their higher maximal aerobic exercise capacity. Thus, women may undergo less sympathoadrenal system activation than men during large-muscle dynamic exercise performed at the same percent of maximal aerobic capacity.

SIZE OF THE ACTIVE MUSCLE MASS The sympathoadrenal response to dynamic exercise is influenced by the size of the active muscle mass. Specifically, the increases in PNE and PE are greater when the same absolute workload is performed by a smaller compared with a larger muscle mass (1,49,55). Thus, the greater amount of work performed and energy demand per unit of active muscle mass, the greater the activation of the sympathoadrenal system. Alternatively, when dynamic exercise is performed with different sized muscle masses (e.g., 1-arm vs. 1-leg vs. 2-leg cycling) at the same relative intensity (i.e., the same percent of maximum for each respective mode of exercise), the magnitude of the increases in plasma catecholamine concentrations from rest to exercise are progressively greater with increasing size of the active muscle mass (55). Under these conditions the larger muscle mass exercise is associated with a greater absolute workload and level of $\dot{V}O_2$. The augmented SNS activation with the larger muscle mass exercise likely is necessary to produce vasoconstriction to counteract the greater active muscle vasodilation and therefore challenge to arterial blood pressure maintenance.

AMBIENT TEMPERATURE AND INTERNAL BODY TEMPERATURE

ANS adjustments to dynamic exercise are influenced by both ambient and internal body temperature. With regard to the parasympathetic nervous system, HRV is lower during exercise performed in the heat than in thermoneutral control conditions (16). Indeed, there is an inverse relation between the high-frequency power of the HRV and rectal temperature during exercise (16). Thus, cardiac vagal modulation of heart rate is lower during exercise performed in warm ambient temperatures, which results in a higher internal body temperature than exercise under cool conditions. Both temperature extremes appear to influence the sympathoadrenal response to dynamic exercise in that the plasma catecholamine responses to exercise are augmented in temperature extremes compared to thermoneutral control conditions (5,16,57). The increased sympathoadrenal activation during exercise in warm conditions may be driven by the need to maintain arterial blood pressure in the face of marked cutaneous vasodilation produced for thermoregulatory needs. In particular, this requires a strong SNS-mediated vasoconstriction in the splanchnic and renal circulations (6,22). Increases in body temperature and the consequent cutaneous vasodilation and effects on arterial blood pressure may also act to stimulate SNS vasoconstrictor nerve activity during prolonged submaximal dynamic exercise performed in thermoneutral ambient conditions (50,52). The augmented sympathoadrenal activation during exercise performed in the cold likely is the result of an increase in baseline activity associated with the independent effects of cold. The increase in SNS activity during exercise in the cold is directed in part to the peripheral arterial blood vessels to maintain a high level of peripheral vasoconstriction to preserve internal body temperature by limiting access of the warm core blood to the cool body surface.

BODY POSITION AND STATE OF HYDRATION

The increase in PNE is greater during dynamic exercise performed upright than supine (1,57,58). This augmented SNS response to exercise in the upright position likely is mediated in part by a greater baseline SNS activity as the result of reduced baroreflex inhibition of SNS outflow (baroreflex unloading). Greater SNS-mediated peripheral vasoconstriction is required to maintain arterial blood pressure in the upright body position (6). Body posture also modifies the SNS response to mild dynamic leg exercise (36), possibly via interactions with cardiopulmonary baroreceptors (discussed later). Exercise performed in the dehydrated state also is associated with an augmented PNE response over that of a hydrated state (1,5). This greater level of SNS activity is required to produce the elevated vasoconstrictor state necessary to maintain arterial blood pressure in the face of a reduced intravascular volume.

DIET, PLASMA GLUCOSE, AND CAFFEINE INGESTION

The ANS response to exercise also appears to be influenced by the composition of energy intake and circulating plasma glucose concentrations. For example, the increase in PE is greater when exercise is performed in a state of reduced circulating glucose (1,5). This augmented sympathoadrenal response to exercise with reduced availability of carbohydrate is likely mediated in part by the independent effects of hypoglycemia (1,5). Finally, caffeine ingestion appears to augment the PNE and/or PE responses to large-muscle dynamic exercise (59).

HYPOXIA AND HYPEROXIA

The ANS responses to exercise are modified by the level of inspired oxygen. Specifically, cardiac vagal modulation of heart rate is reduced and the increase in plasma catecholamine concentrations is augmented during exercise in low inspired oxygen (hypoxia or hypoxemia) conditions, and the reverse is true in hyperoxic states (6,60). This topic is covered in more detail in Chapter 27.

Small-Muscle Dynamic and Isometric Exercise

Dynamic exercise performed with a small muscle mass (e.g., rhythmic handgrip exercise) or isometric exercise has been used frequently to study the regulation of ANS-mediated physiological function during exercise (25,49,55). However, these types of exercise are not performed commonly in daily life. Therefore, only a brief description of the ANS adjustments is warranted here.

Many of the adjustments that occur during more conventional forms of dynamic exercise apply to small-muscle dynamic and isometric exercise. Cardiac vagal modulation of heart rate is reduced at the onset of these types of exercise and is responsible for the associated tachycardia (3,13,49). When these forms of exercise are sustained, eventually SNS activity and possibly PE will increase and stimulate heart rate via the β-adrenergic signaling pathway (3). Thus, as with more conventional forms of dynamic exercise, both withdrawal of cardiac vagal modulation and an increase in sympathoadrenal–β-adrenergic activation are responsible for the tachycardia associated with small-muscle dynamic and isometric exercise.

With regard to the sympathoadrenal system, in general little or no activation is observed during mild (nonfatiguing) intensities and durations of small-muscle dynamic and isometric exercise and early on during contractions that eventually result in active muscle fatigue (1,25,26). However, total PNE spillover, cardiac NE spillover, inactive MSNA (Fig. 9.15), skin sudomotor SNS activity, and epinephrine secretion from the adrenal medulla all are stimulated at intensities and durations associated with muscle fatigue (25,34,61),

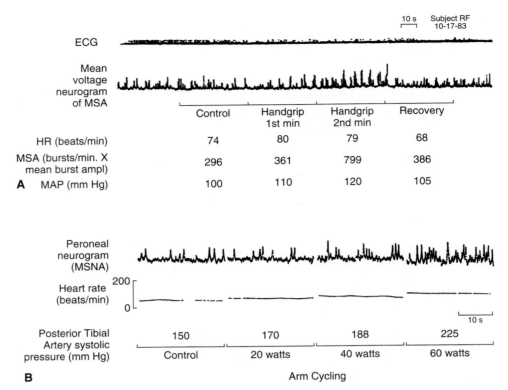

FIGURE 9.15 A. Peroneal neurogram of inactive leg muscle sympathetic nerve activity (MSA) in a healthy young subject at rest (control), during 2 minutes of an isometric handgrip muscle contraction sustained at 30% of maximal voluntary contraction and during 2 minutes of relaxation (recovery) with corresponding mean values for heart rate (HR), MSA, and mean arterial pressure (MAP). MSA does not increase during the initial portion of the contraction period but becomes progressively stimulated during the second minute of the contraction. *(Reprinted with permission from Mark AL, Victor RG, Nerhed C, et al. Neurographic studies of the mechanisms of sympathetic nerve responses to static exercise in humans. Circ Res 1985;57:463. Subsequently published by Seals DR, Victor RG. Regulation of muscle sympathetic nerve activity during exercise in humans. Exerc Sport Sci Rev 1991;19: 313–349.)* **B.** Peroneal neurogram of inactive leg MSNA in a healthy young subject at rest (control) and during the final 30s of two-arm cycling performed for 2 minutes each at 20, 40, and 60 watts (about 20, 35, and 50% of maximum workload). MSNA does not increase above control levels during light intensity submaximal arm cycling but increases progressively during the two higher submaximal workloads. *(From Victor RG, Seals DR, Mark AL. Differential control of heart rate and sympathetic nerve activity during dynamic exercise: Insight from direct intraneural recordings in humans. J Clin Invest 1987;79:508–516. Modified with permission from Seals DR, Victor RG, Regulation of muscle sympathetic nerve activity during exercise in humans. Exerc Sport Sci Rev 1991;19:319.)*

consistent with widespread sympathoadrenal system activation. During such sustained submaximal contractions the increase in MSNA to the inactive limb parallels increases in active muscle electromyographic activity (62) (Fig. 9.16) and perceived sensations of fatigue (63), indicating a physiological coupling between SNS activation and muscle fatigue. Renal SNS activity appears to increase immediately before or at the onset of brief voluntary isometric contractions in conscious cats (64). The increases in PNE, PE, and the spillover rates of the major catecholamines are relatively small compared with those produced by conventional whole-body dynamic exercise (1,49,55), likely due to the absence of extensive active muscle vasodilation in exercises that involve a small muscle mass (22,49). Generally, the greater the active muscle mass involved in isometric contractions, the greater the magnitude of the increase in SNS activity produced (25).

These ANS adjustments to small-muscle dynamic and isometric exercise are critical for mediating the well-established cardiovascular responses to these types of exercise, including increases in heart rate, cardiac output, and a marked elevation in arterial blood pressure. Indeed, these cardiovascular responses are eliminated when the sympathoadrenal–adrenergic signaling pathways are blocked by adrenergic receptor antagonists, such as the combination of phentolamine and propranolol (3,13).

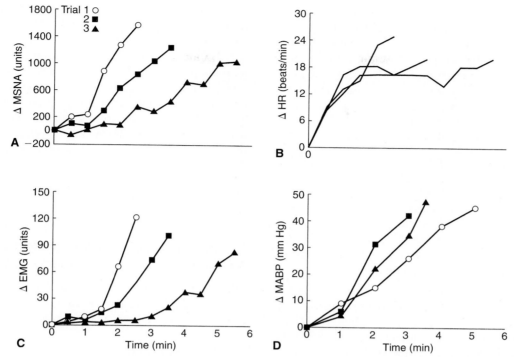

FIGURE 9.16   Changes from resting control levels in (**A**) inactive leg MSNA, (**B**) heart rate (HR), (**C**) contracting forearm muscle electromyographic (EMG) activity, and (**D**) mean arterial blood pressure (MABP) during three successive trials of isometric handgrip sustained at 30% of maximal voluntary contraction, each performed to exhaustion in one young healthy adult. Note the tight temporal coupling between MSNA and EMG within and among the trials, suggesting a physiological link between the onset and development of local muscle fatigue and activation of the sympathetic nervous system during small-muscle mass exercise. In contrast, changes in EMG were not consistently associated with increases in HR or MABP. (*Modified with permission from Seals DR, Enoka RM. Sympathetic activation associated with increases in EMG during fatiguing exercise. J Appl Physiol 1989;66:90.*)

Mechanisms Controlling the ANS Adjustments to Acute Exercise

Brain Regions and Neuromodulators Involved in ANS Control During Exercise

The anatomical areas of the brain involved in mediating the ANS adjustments to acute exercise have been discussed in detail elsewhere (65–67). This issue has been studied in both anesthetized animals during electrical stimulation of muscle contractions and in conscious animals during exercise (e.g., treadmill running). Identification of brain sites activated by exercise has been performed using several experimental approaches, including the following (65–67):

- Comparing ANS responses to exercise (e.g., actual exercise, electrically stimulated muscle contractions, local arterial injections of reflex-activating metabolites into the skeletal muscle circulation) with and without anatomical or pharmacological lesioning of selected areas of the brain, including the use of electrolytic and chemical lesions, synaptic blocking agents, and various agonists or antagonists (in some cases specific receptor antagonists were used to produce exercise responses)

- Recordings of single neuronal activity in various sites in the brain during electrically induced muscle contractions

- Global metabolic labeling of brain sites (e.g., with 2-deoxyglucose or using c-fos immunocytochemistry) during exercise or electrically stimulated contractions compared with resting conditions

- Microdialysis of catecholamines from specific areas of the brain

There are limitations in interpreting these data, including (*a*) the ability to generalize results obtained from electrically induced muscle contractions to actual exercise and the nonspecific stress responses associated with forced treadmill running in experimental animals to the responses to voluntary exercise in humans and (*b*) the inability to determine whether the activated neurons are inhibitory or excitatory for ANS responses when using brain labeling techniques during actual exercise. Nevertheless, these technically challenging studies have provided substantial insight into the nature of the CNS nuclei that determine ANS outflow to the periphery during exercise, either by generating excitatory or inhibitory action potentials or by processing sensory feedback from receptors in the peripheral nervous system. Based on evidence obtained from these experimental models, specific areas of the brain activated during exercise that appear to be linked to the stimulation of exercise-associated ANS-cardiorespiratory responses include the following (Fig. 9.17):

Diencephalon: Areas of the ventromedial caudal hypothalamus involved in classic defense reactions as well as hypothalamic locomotor regions (posterior and lateral hypothalamus), possibly activated via inhibition of GABAergic cells (65). Neurons in the caudal hypothalamus are stimulated by feedback from contracting hindlimb muscles (discussed later) and therefore appear to be activated by those neural inputs (65,67).

Midbrain and pons: The periaqueductal gray matter appears to be among the most activated areas in the midbrain region during exercise (65). Both the medial and lateral aspects of the cuneiform nucleus, that is, the so called mesencephalic locomotor region that evokes locomotion upon stimulation (65,67), demonstrates significant activation during exercise (65). The lateral parabrachial neurons in this area also appear to be stimulated by exercise (65).

Medulla: Several areas of the medulla appear to be activated during exercise:

- The dorsal column nuclei, particularly in the nucleus gracilis (65).
- The medial aspect of the nucleus of the tractus solitarius (65), possibly linked to stimulation of baroreceptor and/or chemoreceptor feedback (discussed later).
- The rostral and caudal ventrolateral medulla. These areas have direct projections to the spinal cord intermediolateral cell column and have been implicated as a major region involved in the stimulation of preganglionic sympathetic neurons and the regulation of SNS outflow to the periphery under a number of conditions. Activation of cells in the caudal ventrolateral medulla as well as the sympathoexcitatory parapyramidal region also appears to occur with exercise (65).
- The raphe nuclei and ventromedial medulla are activated during exercise, possibly via the stimulation of reflexes produced by muscle contraction during exercise (65).

Thus, as summarized by Iwamoto and colleagues (65), ANS-mediated cardiorespiratory adjustments to exercise appear to be controlled by selected nuclei in several areas of the brain, including the hypothalamic locomotor region, periaqueductal gray matter, rostral ventrolateral medulla, ventral midline medulla, and parapyramidal region (Fig. 9.17).

However, the separate and interactive roles of these specific regions of the brain in producing the ANS responses to exercise remain to be ascertained.

There is relatively little information available as to the receptor–neurochemical signaling pathways involved in the transduction of neural information generated or received by these regions of the brain into ANS outflow during exercise. Evidence obtained from studies in experimental animals during real or simulated (e.g., electrically induced muscle contractions) exercise supports a role for several of the prominent CNS neurotransmitter systems, including noradrenergic (68–70), dopaminergic (68), serotonergic (68), and GABAergic (71,72) in the regulation of the ANS responses to exercise.

Central and Peripheral Neural Mechanisms Mediating the ANS Adjustments to Exercise

The central and peripheral neural mechanisms involved in the control of the ANS adjustments to exercise are summarized next. This topic has been reviewed extensively (49,66,67).

Central Command

Central command, as initially envisioned by Krogh and Lindhard (6) and discussed by Rowell, refers to a CNS-generated signal that is believed to be a primary stimulus mediating the ANS adjustments to exercise (25,49,67). Central command is thought to originate in the nuclei in the brain (e.g., primary motor cortex) involved in producing the neural excitation leading to activation of motor nerves and muscle contraction. These areas include nuclei in the cerebral cortex (primary motor cortex), diencephalon (hypothalamic and subthalamic locomotor regions), mesencephalon (mesencephalic locomotor region), and selected portions of the pons, medulla (pontomedullary locomotor strip), and possibly the amygdala (67). The basic concept is that this descending central motor command signal is generated in response to the intent to exercise and not only results in appropriate activation of spinal motor units and muscle but also causes stimulation of areas of the brain involved in the regulation of ANS outflow to the periphery (Fig. 9.18). As such, the central command signal is believed to produce the initial motor and ANS effector responses to the initiation of exercise. This signal could then be adjusted as exercise is sustained and also could be complemented by various sources of sensory feedback to achieve the appropriate overall set of physiological responses in a particular exercise state. This is an attractive regulatory control hypothesis for at least three reasons:

- It provides a means by which the CNS can play an active role in the maintenance of overall physiological homeostasis during the stress of exercise.
- It provides a feed-forward neural mechanism by which the necessary ANS adjustments can be produced at the initiation of exercise.

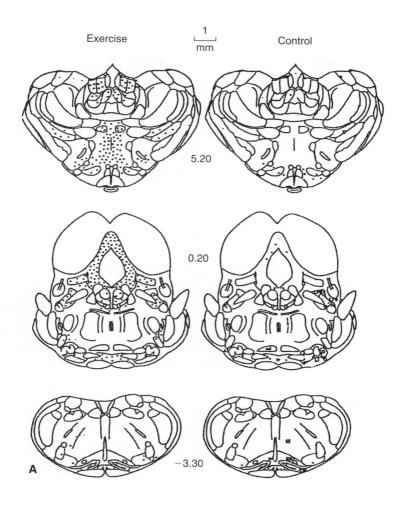

Brain area:	Experimental evidence for involvement:		
	Fos labeling	Single unit recordings	Blocking agents or lesions
Rostral ventrolateral medulla	X	X	X
Lateral tegmental field	X	X	X
Raphe nuclei	X	X	
Caudal hypothalamus and locomotor region	X	X	X
	X		
Mesencephalic locomotor region	X	X	X
Periaqueductal gray matter	X	X	X
Nucleus of the solitary tract	X		

B

FIGURE 9.17 (A) Representative Fos data of selected standard rat brain stereotactic planes in separate animals either in response to a single bout of treadmill running or during resting control: 5.20 is the level of the caudal hypothalamus, 0.28 is midbrain, and −3.30 is rostral medulla. Each dot signifies two cells. The control animal showed little or no Fos immunoreactivity labeling compared to the exercised animal in the following areas: rostral ventrolateral medulla; lateral tegmental field area just lateral to Gi); raphe nuclei; caudal hypothalamus, including locomotor region (ventromedial part of 5.2 level); mesencephalic locomotor region (cuneiform); periaqueductal gray matter (dorsomedial part of 0.28 level surrounding cerebral aqueduct). At these levels the lateral tegmental field, raphe nuclei, and medial nucleus of the solitary tract (a sensory relay) were not labeled but were at other levels and in other animals. (Stereotactic figures and other abbreviations are adapted from Paxinos G, Watson C. The rat brain in stereotaxic coordinates, 2nd ed. Orlando: Academic Press, 1986. *Modified with permission from Iwamoto GA, Wappel SM, Fox GM, et al. Identification of diencephalic and brainstem cardiorespiratory areas activated during exercise. Brain Res 1996;726:113, 115, 116.* **B.** *Summary of evidence supporting the activation of selective brain sites during acute exercise. (Unpublished table courtesy of Professor Gary Iwamoto of the University of Illinois.)*

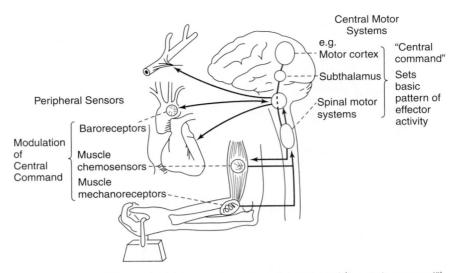

FIGURE 9.18   Possible interactions among central motor command ("central command"), arterial baroreflexes, and active muscle chemoreflexes and mechanoreflexes in controlling ANS efferent activity during exercise. In this scheme, central command would be responsible for the feed-forward stimulation of ANS changes at initiation of and during exercise. In contrast, the arterial baroreflexes and active muscle reflexes would provide fine-tuning feedback from the periphery that would modify the effects of central command to produce the most appropriate combination of ANS responses for maintaining overall physiological homeostasis. *(Modified with permission from Rowell LB. Human cardiovascular control. New York: Oxford University, 1993;442.)*

- It provides a control system in which the magnitude of the ANS adjustments can be graded to the exercise stimulus and, therefore better meet the specific physiological demands imposed by the nature of the exercise being performed.

There is considerable experimental evidence that central command can influence the ANS responses to voluntary exercise and/or muscle contraction. The prevailing view is that central command is a key or the key mechanism responsible for the reduction in cardiac vagal modulation of heart rate with exercise, which contributes importantly to increases in cardiac output, particularly in the early period of exercise and at mild to moderate intensities (22,25,49). In contrast, central command is believed to contribute little to the stimulation of sympathoadrenal system activity during exercise (22,25,49).

The experimental findings supporting a significant modulatory effect of central command on the ANS during exercise include the following:

- Exercise-like responses to intended muscle activity; that is, muscle contraction is prevented by administration of neuromuscular blocking agents, so that no feedback from active muscle is possible, which isolates the effects of central command. Under these conditions, a normal increase in heart rate is observed during attempted handgrip exercise (13,73) (Fig. 9.19). The increase in heart rate is abolished by

pretreatment with atropine but unaffected by β-adrenergic receptor antagonists (13,73), indicating that withdrawal of cardiac vagal modulation of heart rate is the key mechanism by which central command produces tachycardia during exercise.

- Augmented ANS responses with increases in voluntary effort (central command) during performance of a constant muscle force contraction (i.e., manipulation of central command with fixed muscle afferent feedback) using partial neuromuscular blockade. Partial neuromuscular blockade, which requires increased voluntary effort to achieve and maintain a particular submaximal force, is associated with an augmented arterial blood pressure response to isometric exercise in humans (6,49); this blood pressure response is mediated primarily by a reduction in cardiac vagal modulation of heart rate and increase in cardiac output.

- Normal ANS and cardiovascular responses to exercise performed by limbs without intact sensory feedback, which demonstrates the ability of central command to evoke the necessary adjustments to exercise without feedback from active muscle (74) (Fig. 9.20).

- Both imagined exercise (central command in the absence of muscle activity) (75) and perceived increases in effort during constant submaximal-intensity leg cycling exercise while under hypnosis (increased central command with fixed active muscle feedback)

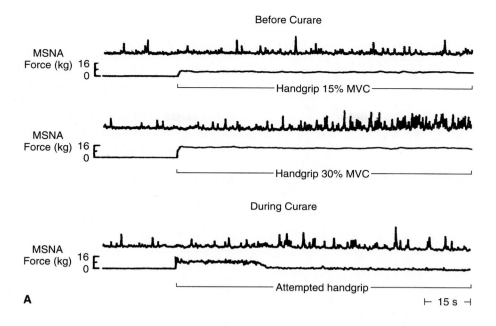

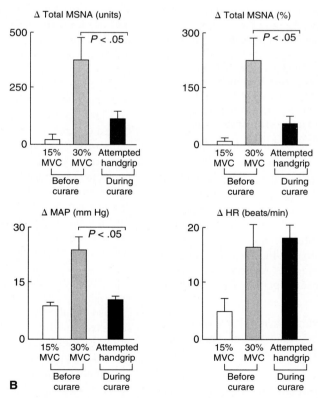

FIGURE 9.19   **A.** Tracings of peroneal (inactive leg) MSNA and force before and during isometric handgrip contractions performed at 15% (*top*) and 30% (*middle*) of maximal voluntary contraction (MVC) prior to curare infusion (partial neuromuscular blockade), and attempted handgrip during curare infusion (*bottom*) in 1 subject. MSNA increased during handgrip at 30% MVC but not at 15% MVC. During partial neuromuscular blockade, which eliminated the ability to produce even the normal 15% of MVC handgrip force (removing active muscle reflex feedback and isolating the influence of central command), MSNA increased only slightly despite maximal effort (intent to perform the contraction), suggesting that even maximal levels of central command have little effect on MSNA. **B.** Mean changes in MSNA, mean arterial blood pressure (MAP), and heart rate (HR) in response to the same conditions. Although attempted handgrip contraction had little effect on MSNA, it produced normal increases in HR (abolished with atropine), indicating a primary influence of central command in producing cardiac vagal withdrawal-mediated tachycardia during exercise. *(Modified with permission from Victor RG, SL Pryor, NH Secher, et al. Effects of partial neuromuscular blockade on sympathetic nerve responses to static exercise in humans. Circ Res 1989;65:471–472)*

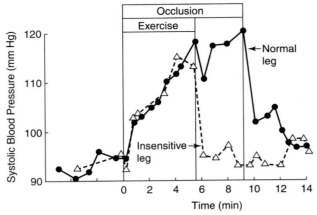

FIGURE 9.20 Systolic blood pressure responses to leg exercise and postexercise leg ischemia performed with a normal leg (intact central command and active muscle reflex feedback) and a leg without functional sensory afferent feedback (intact central command without active muscle reflex feedback). Note the normal blood pressure response to exercise of the leg with sensory loss, suggesting that central command alone can produce this autonomically mediated cardiovascular response to exercise. Also note the importance of sensory afferent feedback in maintaining blood pressure elevations during postexercise ischemia via the muscle chemoreflex. *(Modified from Rowell LB. Human circulation regulation during physical stress. New York: Oxford University, 1986;213–416. Adapted from Alam M, Smirk FH. Unilateral loss of a blood pressure raising, pulse accelerating, reflex from voluntary muscle due to a lesion of the spinal cord. Clin Sci 1938;3:297.)*

(76) increase heart rate, blood pressure, and blood flow to cortical regions of the brain thought to be involved in mediating the effects of central command.

- In experimental animals, electrical stimulation of the CNS sites (e.g., subthalamus) thought to be involved in central command–induced ANS physiological adjustments produce exercise-like motor, cardiorespiratory, neuroendocrine, and metabolic responses (65,67).

Experimental evidence supporting the view that central command has little if any role in the stimulation of sympathoadrenal system activity during exercise includes these points:

- Even maximal levels of central command (i.e., maximal voluntary effort to perform handgrip exercise with total neuromuscular blockade) has a relatively small effect on MSNA (73) (Fig. 9.19).
- No increase in MSNA takes place during the initiation of exercise or during mild intensities of exercise despite physiologically significant central command–evoked cardiac vagal withdrawal–mediated increases in heart rate (73) (Figs. 9.11, 9.15, and 9.19).

As described earlier, renal SNS activity may increase soon after the initiation of exercise, at least in experimental ani-

mals (31,32). It could be argued that this is mediated by central command, although muscle mechanoreflexes and/or baroreflexes (discussed later) also could produce this response. There also is evidence that central command can stimulate SNS activity to skin during voluntary and electrically stimulated isometric muscle contractions and "intended" exercise models (34,77).

Active Muscle Reflexes

As reviewed in detail previously (25,49,66), there is extensive experimental evidence that feedback from active skeletal muscles can influence the ANS-physiological adjustments to exercise and therefore serve as the other primary CNS exercise signal along with central command. The peripheral neural substrate providing this feedback is group III and IV sensory nerves, which are stimulated by chemical, mechanical, and/or thermal stimuli produced by active muscle (25,49,66). The feedback is reflex in origin: Excitatory action potentials from muscle sensory afferents project to the brain via synaptic transmissions in the dorsal root of the spinal cord. This exerts effects on specific nuclei in the brain (primarily caudal and rostral aspects of the ventrolateral medulla) (66), which in turn inhibit vagal and/or stimulate sympathetic preganglionic neurons, thus producing selective efferent ANS responses to target tissues in the periphery (e.g., heart and arterial vasculature).

This type of exercise-evoked CNS signal is attractive from a control system perspective because it would theoretically provide information from active muscle as to the appropriateness of the central command (feed-forward controller) produced ANS-physiological adjustments to exercise. In this way, the initial, grosser ANS-physiological activation generated by central command could be fine-tuned by information from the active muscle fibers (Fig. 9.18). Feedback indicating, for example, a mismatch between active muscle oxygen demand and delivery could produce the necessary ANS-cardiovascular adjustments to augment active muscle perfusion. Thus, active muscle feedback would complement the central command signal, providing more precise regulatory control for maintaining active muscle homeostasis during the changing metabolic demands imposed by the exercise state.

Two primary classifications of these reflexes have been identified: (*a*) those activated by chemical stimuli produced as a consequence of active muscle metabolism and (*b*) mechanical stimuli generated by the contracting muscle fibers (Fig. 9.18). The possible involvement of these reflexes, as well as active muscle thermoreflexes, in ANS control during exercise has been discussed in detail elsewhere (25,49,66).

Muscle Chemoreflexes, or Muscle Metaboreflexes

Muscle chemoreflexes appear to be activated when the metabolic state of the active muscle fibers changes during exercise in a manner that reflects an adverse (unwanted) internal metabolic environment posing a potential challenge to the maintenance of homeostasis. Under these conditions, the metabolism of the active muscle fibers will shift from oxidative to more glycolysis-driven ATP production, and the metabolic milieu both within the muscle cell and in the interstitial fluid surrounding those muscle fibers will change accordingly. The altered chemical composition of the interstitium stimulates the endings of group III and IV sensory neurons in the extracellular space surrounding these muscle fibers, increasing their discharge rates and initiating a reflex modulation of efferent ANS activity. The basic idea is that this reflex provides a local sensor to monitor the biochemical state of the active muscle fibers and transduce to the CNS information concerning the functional status of those cells. Thus, if inadequate oxygen delivery results in shifts in intracellular metabolism and corresponding changes in the interstitial fluid reflecting a mismatch with oxygen demand, the reflex would attempt to correct this error by stimulating ANS-cardiovascular adjustments resulting in increased perfusion of the active muscle fibers.

The specific biochemical changes that occur in the interstitium to activate chemically sensitive group III and IV nerve endings and engage this reflex have been discussed (22,25,66). These putative changes include increases in interstitial concentrations of carbon dioxide, hydrogen ion, lactic acid, arachidonic acid, potassium, phosphate, cyclooxygenase products, bradykinin, and prostaglandins (22,66), whereas changes in adenosine do not appear to be involved (78). Increases in potassium concentrations likely have only transient, if any, effects in stimulating these sensory afferents (22). Although a reduction in pH appears to be a key step in activating this reflex (discussed in the Milestone of Discovery), hydrogen ion itself may actually stimulate not chemically sensitive afferents during exercise but rather the conversion of monoprotonated phosphate to its diprotonated form (H_2PO_4) (22,66,79). At this time, the individual chemical triggers and/or interactions that result in muscle chemoreflex activation *in vivo* during exercise are only partially understood.

The specific ANS effects of muscle chemoreflex activation appear to involve primarily increases in SNS activity, with no obvious effect on cardiac vagal modulation of heart rate (25,49,66). Initially, the muscle chemoreflex was believed to have no effect on SNS modulation of heart rate, but more recent investigations demonstrated an influence on SNS β-adrenergic modulation of heart rate with exercise (22). Experimental evidence supporting the ability of muscle chemoreflexes to influence the SNS adjustments to exercise include the following:

- During small-muscle dynamic and isometric exercise (44,62,63) (Figs. 9.15, 9.16, and 9.19A), (a) the absence of any increase in MSNA during the initial period of exercise that precedes accumulation of muscle chemoreflex activating metabolites and (b) a progressive and marked increase in MSNA thereafter as exercise is sustained, coinciding with the development of muscle fatigue and perceptions of muscle discomfort consistent with buildup of glycolytic metabolites. This temporal pattern of the MSNA response is consistent with the correspondingly delayed pattern of activation of chemically sensitive muscle afferents when stimulated by isometric contractions in anesthetized cats (49,66).

- Augmentation of the MSNA (inactive limb vasoconstrictor) and/or arterial blood pressure responses during exercise performed with compared to without partial or complete occlusion of blood flow to the active limbs (25,49,80); the occlusion of blood flow both increases the production and traps the buildup of muscle chemoreflex–activating metabolites in the active muscles.

- Maintenance of the exercise-induced elevation in MSNA, inactive limb vasoconstriction, and arterial blood pressure during a period of post-exercise occlusion of blood flow to the previously active limb (i.e., as compared with a non–blood flow occluded recovery period post-exercise) (25,74,80) (Fig. 9.20). During post-exercise occlusion, the muscle chemoreflex remains activated in the absence of central command or other exercise-dependent CNS stimuli (i.e., muscle mechanoreflex input, discussed later).

- During isometric and dynamic handgrip exercise, increases in MSNA and inactive limb vascular resistance are consistently related to the intracellular hydrogen ion accumulation and pH (i.e., chemoreflex activating stimuli) of the active forearm muscles (81,82) (see figures in Milestone of Discovery). In contrast, in patients with muscle phosphorylase deficiency (McArdle's disease), who cannot break down glycogen, produce lactic acid, or therefore increase hydrogen ion (reduce pH) during exercise (i.e., cannot activate the muscle chemoreflex), there is no increase in MSNA during the same handgrip exercise stimulus that results in a doubling of MSNA in normal subjects (83).

- In dogs, activation of muscle chemoreflexes (via occlusion of the terminal aorta) during treadmill running produces cardiac SNS–mediated coronary artery vasoconstriction (84) as well as increases in arterial blood pressure and systematic vascular resistance (22).

The concept that acidotic active skeletal muscle could trigger a reflex that would stimulate SNS vasoconstriction and augment arterial perfusion pressure is attractive from a control theory perspective when considered together with functional sympatholysis. That is, the SNS activation evoked by the reflex would produce widespread vasoconstriction except in tissues under increased metabolic demand, such as active skeletal muscle. In the latter, functional sympatholysis would secure increased blood flow for the most metabolically active tissues.

Despite a substantial body of experimental evidence demonstrating that activation of muscle chemoreflexes affects the ANS-cardiovascular responses to exercise, we still lack a clear understanding of the role, if any, these reflexes play in cardiovascular control during conventional large-muscle dynamic exercise. It is well established that these reflexes stimulate SNS activity in experimental animals and/or humans during these events:

- Fatiguing levels of isometric exercise, that is, exercise in which the sustained contractions mechanically compress arteries, resulting in a natural restriction in blood flow (Figs. 9.15A, 9.16, and 9.19)
- Fatiguing levels of dynamic exercise performed with small muscle groups (e.g., handgrip and arm cycling), that is, exercise in which the demand for energy production per active muscle fiber is great and therefore glycolytic flux and intracellular acid production and accumulation are high within the active muscles (Fig. 9.15B)
- Large-muscle dynamic exercise performed under conditions of mild to severe occlusion of active muscle blood flow (22,49)

However, although muscle chemoreflexes can influence the ANS responses to exercise, that does not necessarily mean that they actually contribute to ANS-cardiovascular regulation during conventional forms of dynamic exercise performed without artificial occlusion of active muscle blood flow. At present, we have no direct or convincing evidence that the muscle chemoreflex is normally engaged during the submaximal levels of large-muscle dynamic exercise typically performed by humans for health and fitness purposes. These forms of exercise are not obviously associated with restricted active muscle perfusion or with excessive accumulation of glycolytic metabolites or reductions in pH. If the muscle chemoreflex were activated during normal (free flow) large-muscle dynamic exercise, this likely would be limited to heavy submaximal and/or maximal intensities of work.

Muscle Mechanoreflexes

The possible involvement of active muscle mechanoreflexes in ANS-cardiovascular control during exercise has been discussed previously (22,49,66). These reflexes are stimulated by mechanical stimuli (stretch and/or compression) in the active muscle fibers that activate mechanically sensitive group III and IV afferents. Evidence that these reflexes can modulate ANS adjustments to exercise includes:

- Stimulation of mechanically sensitive group III and IV sensory afferents produces a reflex increase in systolic arterial blood pressure (presumably mediated by the ANS) in experimental animals (22,49,66); compression or increases in the intravascular volume of the active forearm muscles during exercise augments MSNA in humans (22,85).
- The onset of electrically induced muscle contraction in humans (i.e., in the absence of central command and before the possible activation of muscle chemoreflexes) is associated with an increase in heart rate (22,25,49), a response shown to be mediated by cardiac vagal withdrawal (13) and an increase in skin (sudomotor) SNS activity (34).
- Brief muscle contractions are associated with corresponding bursts of cardiac SNS activity in cats; the magnitude of the increase in cardiac sympathetic nerve discharge is positively related to the muscle tension produced (22,49,66).

As with muscle chemoreflexes, the actual involvement of muscle mechanoreflexes in ANS-cardiovascular control during conventional forms of dynamic exercise is unknown. Mechanically sensitive muscle afferents appear to be active only at the onset of exercise, with their discharge rates returning rapidly to resting control levels (22,49,66). Therefore, any involvement of these potential signals would likely be confined to the initiation of exercise, severely limiting the possible scope of this mechanism in contributing to ANS control during sustained exercise.

Muscle Thermoreflexes

In addition to responding to chemical and/or mechanical stimuli, many group III and IV sensory afferents are thermosensitive (22,66). Because active muscle temperatures can increase significantly during sustained moderate to heavy submaximal exercise, it is possible that these afferents could be stimulated and provide feedback to the CNS regarding the thermal status of the active muscle fibers (22). While this remains a possibility, experimental findings are insufficient to determine the role of this mechanism in ANS-cardiovascular control during exercise.

Arterial Baroreflexes

Arterial baroreflexes evoke beat-to-beat changes in cardiac vagal modulation of heart rate as well as SNS activity to the heart and vasculature in response to changes in arterial blood pressure (6,22,49). Specifically, increases in arterial blood pressure would deform the walls of the aortic arch and carotid sinus, in which these mechanically sensitive receptors are located, stimulating their afferent nerve endings and signaling the CNS to increase cardiac vagal modulation of heart rate and decrease SNS activity to the heart and vasculature. These reflex ANS adjustments would act to reduce cardiac output (by decreasing heart rate and left ventricular contractility) and systemic vascular resistance (by dilating arterial resistance vessels), thus lowering arterial blood pressure. The opposite ANS-cardiovascular adjustments are induced in response to reductions in arterial blood pressure, which deactivates the arterial baroreflex.

The role of the arterial baroreflex in ANS-cardiovascular control during exercise (Fig. 9.18) has been reviewed in great detail by Rowell (6,49) and Rowell and colleagues (22). Because systolic and arterial pulse pressures increase during conventional forms of large-muscle dynamic exercise and because both systolic and diastolic blood pressure increase during small-muscle dynamic and isometric contractions, originally it was believed that the arterial baroreflex was inhibited during exercise. However, it now is understood that the arterial baroreflex is simply reset to regulate arterial blood pressure at a higher operating point during exercise (6,22,49) (Fig. 9.21). Indeed, it has been established that not only does the arterial baroreflex operate normally during exercise but also an intact arterial baroreflex is essential for producing the ANS-cardiovascular adjustments necessary to exercise. The primary experimental evidence for this conclusion comes from studies on animals in which arterial blood pressure falls markedly with the onset of large-muscle dynamic exercise following denervation of the sinoaortic and cardiopulmonary baroreceptors (22,49,86) (Fig. 9.22). Although blood pressure returns toward normal levels during moderate to heavy submaximal exercise in these animals, during light exercise blood pressure remains below control levels and demonstrates unusual instability (22,49,86). The key concept advanced from this research is that the arterial baroreflex is essential for maintaining arterial blood pressure at the onset of large-muscle dynamic exercise and throughout at least lower-intensity dynamic exercise. This is because the

arterial baroreflex counteracts the extensive active muscle vasodilation and increase in total vascular conductance produced during exercise by evoking reflex decreases in cardiac vagal modulation of heart rate and increases in SNS vasoconstriction (6,22,49). With the onset of exercise the arterial baroreflex is reset, likely by central command (discussed later), to a higher operating pressure, resulting in the prevailing blood pressure being perceived as hypotension and evoking ANS-cardiovascular responses aimed at raising arterial pressure. Therefore, the contemporary view is that the arterial baroreflex does not oppose the ANS-cardiovascular adjustments by which arterial blood pressure is increased during exercise but rather actually supports ANS-cardiovascular evoked increases in arterial pressure with exercise.

Cardiopulmonary Baroreflexes

Cardiopulmonary baroreflexes monitor cardiopulmonary blood volume by sensing changes in the filling pressure (distension) of the chambers of the heart and pulmonary arteries and veins, as well as cardiac contractility and afterload (6,22,86). Increases in these stimuli activate mechanically sensitive receptors in these structures, stimulating vagal afferent fibers that signal the CNS to inhibit SNS activity. The latter results in systemic vasodilation and a reduction in systemic vascular resistance. This in turn increases the compliance of the arterial circulation and reduces the normal displacement of blood to the venous circulation and its return to the heart and pulmonary circulation, thus reducing cardiopulmonary blood volume. The release of extracellular fluid–regulating hormones also is modulated by this reflex in a manner that would act to facilitate water and sodium excretion under these conditions of hypervolemia. The opposite set of responses would be evoked in response to reductions in cardiopulmonary blood volume. These reflexes operate in an integrative fashion with arterial baroreflexes, generally one reflex opposing the effects of the other.

The possible involvement of these homeostatic reflexes in ANS-cardiovascular control during exercise has been reviewed in detail by Rowell (6,49), Rowell and colleagues (22), and Tipton (8). Because of active skeletal muscle pump–evoked increases in cardiac filling (preload) and contractility during conventional forms of upright dynamic exercise in humans, it might reasonably be assumed that these reflexes actively inhibit SNS outflow under these conditions. The possible modulatory effects of cardiopulmonary baroreflexes on the ANS-cardiovascular adjustments to exercise have been studied in both humans and experimental animals. The results of these studies are equivocal, with evidence both supporting and refuting a physiologically significant effect of cardiopulmonary baroreflexes in ANS control during exercise (6,22,49). The most compelling evidence for the involvement of this reflex in modulating ANS function during exercise in humans comes from observations of inhibition of inactive MSNA during the onset and early phase of upright

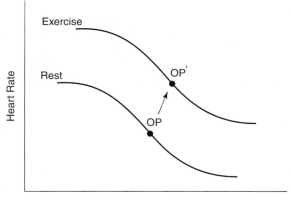

FIGURE 9.21 Resetting of the arterial baroreflex operating point (OP) for control of heart rate upward and to the right with acute exercise. *(Modified with permission from O'Leary D. Heart rate control during exercise by baroreceptors and skeletal muscle afferents. Med Sci Sports Exerc 1996;28:212.)*

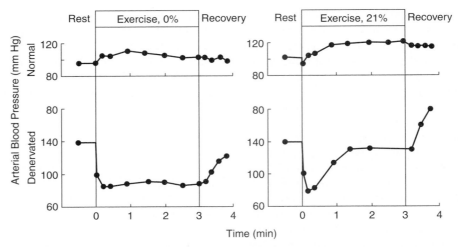

FIGURE 9.22 Arterial blood pressure at rest (left of 0 time points) and in response to light (0% grade, *left*) and heavier (21% grade, *right*) submaximal treadmill exercise (5.5 km · hr⁻¹) in healthy dogs with either intact (*top*) or denervated (*bottom*) baroreflexes. Note the immediate fall in blood pressure at the onset of both intensities of exercise in the barodenervated state. Blood pressure remains below resting control levels throughout light exercise but returns toward resting levels after the initial minute of heavier exercise, probably as a result of increased central command and/or muscle chemoreflex activation arising from the effect of low arterial blood pressure on active muscle blood flow. *(Modified with permission from Rowell LB. Human circulation regulation during physical stress. New York: Oxford University, 1986;320. Adapted from Melcher A, Donald DE. Maintained ability of carotid baroreflex to regulate arterial pressure during exercise. Am J Physiol 1981;241:H838–H849.)*

dynamic exercise (22,35,36). The theory advanced is that the activation of the muscle pump with the initiation of dynamic exercise would augment cardiac filling and central blood volume, stimulating these mechanoreceptors and producing reflex SNS inhibition. However, this muscle pump–produced increase in blood volume in the central circulation at the onset of dynamic exercise also increases cardiac output and systolic blood pressure and therefore likely causes distension of the aortic arch and carotid sinus regions, possibly activating the arterial baroreflex and producing sympathoinhibition via that mechanism (22). Thus, it is unclear whether cardiopulmonary baroreflexes play an important role in ANS-cardiovascular regulation during exercise, independent of arterial baroreflexes.

Central Thermoreflexes

The role of central thermoreflexes in ANS-cardiovascular control during exercise has been reviewed in detail by Rowell (6) and Rowell and colleagues (22). These reflexes modulate neural vasoconstrictor and vasodilator outflow to the cutaneous circulation to ensure optimal circulatory conditions for heat dissipation during exercise, particularly that performed in warm ambient conditions. In performing these regulatory functions, central thermoreflexes interact with arterial and cardiopulmonary baroreflexes and other neural inputs to the CNS during exercise to maintain internal

homeostasis. During sustained submaximal exercise in warm ambient conditions, cutaneous vasomotor outflow is adjusted to allow increased blood flow and volume to the skin circulation (6,22). If sufficiently great, this redistribution of the cardiac output to the skin can restrict active muscle blood flow, producing competition between exercise signals (central command and active muscle reflexes) aimed at ensuring perfusion of the contracting muscle fibers and thermal inputs charged with maintaining core temperature within the appropriate range. Moreover, the increased cutaneous vascular conductance during exercise in the heat acts to lower systemic vascular resistance, threatening arterial blood pressure, particularly in the face of marked active muscle vasodilation. Thus, under these conditions, a robust interaction occurs among exercise-specific and exercise-nonspecific neural inputs to the CNS, each attempting to produce ANS-cardiovascular responses to meet their particular homeostatic needs. The CNS must interpret these competing signals and generate efferent ANS outflow that attempts to support these diverse demands on the systemic circulation. In general, it appears that the top regulatory priority of the CNS is the maintenance of arterial blood pressure to ensure perfusion of vital organs followed in order by maintenance of internal body temperature and support of active locomotor muscle blood flow. Thus, the ability to sustain exercise is sacrificed first, for example, via SNS vasoconstriction of active muscle blood flow in order to maintain systemic vascular resistance and arterial blood pressure and to provide flow to the cutaneous circulation for thermoregulation. If necessary, the skin will undergo vasoconstriction to protect systemic arterial pressure, but vital organ perfusion will be protected at all costs.

Arterial Chemoreflexes

Arterial chemoreflexes monitor and help maintain arterial oxygen and carbon dioxide levels and pH within their respective homeostatic ranges via effects on pulmonary ventilation and arterial blood acid-base balance (6,66). Stimulation of arterial chemoreflexes also has pronounced effects on the ANS, a key feature of which appears to be SNS activation by hypoxia, hypercapnia, and/or acidosis (6,66). Because exercise normally is associated with maintenance of PaO_2, normal or reduced arterial carbon dioxide, and maintenance of blood pH within acceptable ranges, the arterial chemoreflexes are not normally activated and therefore likely do not play an important role in ANS control during conventional submaximal exercise at sea level or mild elevations in altitude. However, arterial chemoreflexes may be activated during exercise performed upon acute exposure to higher altitudes in normal subjects (i.e., before compensatory adaptations), during exercise in patients with lung disease demonstrating arterial hypoxemia and/or hypercapnia, and/or during heavy submaximal and maximal exercise in endurance-trained athletes who demonstrate hypoxemia under these conditions. Moreover, experimentally induced acidosis augments the PNE response (87), and experimentally produced alkalosis can attenuate the PNE and PE responses (88) to leg cycling exercise in humans, consistent with the concept that arterial chemoreflexes can influence sympathoadrenal responses to exercise under conditions of altered systemic acid-base balance.

Lung Inflation Reflexes and Respiratory Metaboreflexes

In anesthetized animals, lung inflation stimulates vagal afferent nerves projecting to the CNS, producing a reflex inhibition of efferent SNS activity (6,66). Similarly, in humans MSNA is inhibited during inspiration and stimulated during expiration under resting conditions (89). Breathing (6) also influences cardiac vagal modulation of heart rate. Because breathing frequency, tidal volume, and minute ventilation all increase during exercise, it is possible that reflexes activated by lung inflation participate in ANS control during exercise. There is little information providing insight into this possibility. In healthy humans, simulated exercise hyperpnea (i.e., isocapnic high-frequency elevated tidal volume breathing) has no obvious influence on mean levels of MSNA at rest or during muscle metaboreflex activation produced by either isometric handgrip exercise or ischemia of the previously active forearm post handgrip (89). Thus, at present there is no

compelling evidence that stimulation of lung inflation reflexes modulates SNS activity during exercise. However, studying cardiopulmonary interactions during exercise is extremely challenging, and data obtained with present experimental models often are difficult to interpret. In contrast, the work of Dempsey and colleagues (90) is consistent with the existence of a "respiratory muscle chemoreflex" (respiratory metaboreflex). The concept, as recently summarized (91) (Fig. 9.23), is that such a reflex can be activated during heavy submaximal and/or maximal exercise that is associated with a sustained elevation in work of breathing and development of respiratory muscle fatigue. Under these conditions, glycolytic metabolites may stimulate group III and IV phrenic afferents, increasing their discharge to the

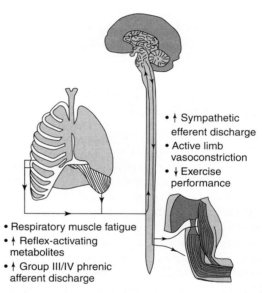

- ↑ Sympathetic efferent discharge
- Active limb vasoconstriction
- ↓ Exercise performance

- Respiratory muscle fatigue
- ↑ Reflex-activating metabolites
- ↑ Group III/IV phrenic afferent discharge

FIGURE 9.23 Key elements of a potential respiratory muscle metaboreflex. The concept is that sustained high-volume ventilation during exercise, particularly during high resistance to flow, could produce respiratory muscle fatigue with an associated increase in glycolytic metabolism, increased production, release and accumulation of reflex-activating (glycolytic) metabolites, and consequent activation of chemically sensitive group III/IV respiratory muscle sensory afferents. The latter would project to the CNS, producing a reflex increase in efferent sympathetic activity evoking peripheral vasoconstriction, including in arterioles perfusing the active locomotor muscles. This vasoconstriction would reduce active locomotor muscle blood flow, potentially providing increased flow and oxygen delivery to the respiratory muscles to maintain ventilation and therefore arterial blood gases and acid-base balance within ranges consistent with homeostasis. *(Modified from Seals DR. Robin Hood for the lungs? A respiratory metaboreflex that "steals" blood flow from locomotor muscles. J Physiol [Lond] 2001;537:2.)*

CNS and evoking a reflex excitation of efferent SNS activity to peripheral tissues, including the active locomotor muscles. The latter would produce active muscle vasoconstriction and a reduction in blood flow with a consequent reduction in exercise performance. This vasoconstriction would act to redistribute cardiac output to the respiratory muscles, increasing their blood flow in an attempt to address the flow error via a classic muscle chemoreflex response. Teleologically, this respiratory muscle metaboreflex could have as its primary regulatory aim the preservation of respiratory muscle perfusion during physiological states in which there is competition for cardiac output with locomotor muscles. Because the respiratory muscles are essential for producing pulmonary ventilation at the necessary levels to maintain arterial blood gases and pH, the proper perfusion of the respiratory muscles should be a high priority for maintaining organismic homeostasis. Under these conditions, it could be argued that blood flow to the locomotor muscles and support of locomotion would constitute a far less important regulatory goal.

Integrative Control of the ANS Adjustments to Exercise

How do these CNS inputs control ANS function during exercise? Which of these signals actually contribute to integrative ANS-cardiovascular regulation during conventional forms of large-muscle dynamic exercise? Which are not actively involved, perhaps participating only under specific or unusual exercise conditions? We do not know. However, Rowell (49) has advanced an overall model as to how the ANS adjustments to large-muscle dynamic exercise may be mediated. This hypothesis represents the most compelling integrative scheme attempting to explain the primary signals involved and how those signals may interact to produce these ANS adjustments to exercise.

In this theory, the central command (feed-forward) signal generated with the onset of exercise would cause the arterial baroreflex to be reset to a higher operating pressure (Fig. 9.24). Under these conditions, the prevailing arterial blood pressure would be interpreted by the CNS as hy-

potension, and reflex ANS adjustments would be evoked to increase blood pressure to the new operating point to correct the presumed blood pressure error (Fig. 9.25). Because cardiac vagal modulation of heart rate is the fastest ANS adjustment available to the arterial baroreflex for correcting blood pressure errors, the hypothesis is that cardiac vagal withdrawal–mediated increases in heart rate and cardiac output are produced initially to raise arterial blood pressure to the new exercise operating point (there also is evidence that central command can directly stimulate cardiac vagal withdrawal with the initiation of exercise independent of arterial baroreflex resetting) (22). Based on data from studies in experimental animals (31–33), an increase in cardiac and/or renal SNS activity may also be part of this initial ANS response to resetting of the arterial baroreflex operating pressure with the initiation of exercise (22). In any case, the key concept is that vagally mediated tachycardia and an increase in cardiac output would be the primary mechanism by which blood pressure would increase at the onset of exercise via central command–evoked arterial baroreflex resetting. The augmentation of cardiac output also would increase blood flow to active muscle, thus initiating a necessary increase in oxygen delivery to meet the increased metabolic demands of muscle activity.

Rowell's model (Fig. 9.25) also predicts that if the exercise intensity is within the range in which the increases in heart rate required to raise cardiac output and arterial blood pressure could be met solely by cardiac vagal withdrawal (i.e., up to about 100 beats per minute), little or no sympathoadrenal system activation would be required. Additional increases in exercise intensity would require further increases in the central motor command signal, producing further resetting of the arterial baroreflex to progressively higher operating pressures. At these greater intensities of exercise the required increases in arterial blood pressure cannot be met by cardiac vagal withdrawal–mediated tachycardia-induced increases in cardiac output. Rather, increases in SNS activity to the heart would be required to further augment cardiac output via β-adrenergic stimulation of heart rate and left ventricular contractility. At heavy submaximal to maximal exercise intensities, SNS stimulation of epinephrine se-

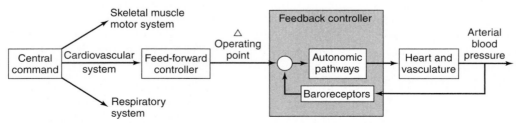

FIGURE 9.24 Hypothesized effect of central command in stimulating ANS adjustments to exercise via both direct effects on ANS controllers in the CNS and indirectly by eliciting a resetting of the arterial baroreflex operating point, which in turn influences ANS adjustments during exercise. *(Modified with permission from Rowell LB. Human Cardiovascular Control. New York: Oxford University, 1993;463.)*

The ANS adaptations to exercise training and information concerning the underlying mechanisms are discussed in the following sections. Unless otherwise stated, *exercise training* will refer to the chronic performance of sustained large-muscle dynamic exercise, that is, aerobic or endurance exercise. The term *exercise-trained state* refers either to the physiological state after a period of regular exercise within a particular individual or group (i.e., after vs. before an exercise intervention) or to the physiological state of exercise-trained adults compared with sedentary age- and gender-matched peers (i.e., cross-sectional comparison of exercise-trained and sedentary subjects). Findings supporting the conclusions are based on research involving both experimental animals and human subjects, generally healthy young and middle-aged adults. The reader is referred to selective previous reviews of this topic for additional information (1,6,17).

Cardiac Vagal Modulation of Heart Rate

At Rest

Cardiac vagal modulation of heart rate appears to be increased under tonic (resting) conditions after a period of exercise training in some experimental animals and human subjects. The experimental evidence supporting such an adaptation includes the following:

- Greater increases in heart rate in response to acute intravenous administration of atropine at rest in the exercise-trained than in the sedentary state (17,92,93)
- Greater heart rate variability at rest (17,94,95) and over the entire day (96) in the exercise-trained than in the sedentary state
- Higher cardiac acetylcholine concentrations in the exercise-trained than in the sedentary state (97).

However, there is a significant body of evidence that does not support enhanced cardiac vagal tone in the endurance-trained state, including observations of similar heart rate increases in response to atropine in the trained and untrained states (17,98). The reasons for the lack of consistent findings likely include at least two factors (17):

- Between-study differences in the strength of the exercise training stimulus (i.e., differences in the duration, intensity, frequency, and/or length of exercise training); a milder exercise stress may produce no adaptation or possibly only a small adaptation that could be missed because of normal measurement error and variability among subjects.
- Law of initial baseline; that is, subjects with low cardiac vagal modulatory tone at baseline (before the initiation of exercise training) would have the most potential for adaptation (increase in vagal tone with training), and vice versa.

Accordingly, the greatest possibility of an increase in cardiac vagal modulation of heart rate would be under these conditions:

- Subjects with very low baseline levels (e.g., older adults or patients with cardiovascular diseases) undergoing strenuous and prolonged exercise training
- Comparing highly endurance exercise-trained with very sedentary adults

Thus, the role of increased cardiac vagal modulation of heart rate in the so-called training bradycardia (lower resting heart rate in the exercise-trained state) is not uniformly clear. The available evidence supports the view that this mechanism could contribute to the resting bradycardia in some endurance-trained subjects, but not necessarily in all. In the absence of such an effect, current evidence supports an important role for a reduction in the intrinsic heart rate (i.e., heart rate in the absence of extrinsic [autonomic-adrenergic] influences) in mediating the training bradycardia (92,98,99).

Also, recent findings (100) provide compelling support for the likelihood that intense and sustained endurance training, so-called overtraining, in athletes results in reduced HRV and therefore reduced cardiac vagal modulation of heart rate, decreased cardiovagal baroreflex sensitivity, and an associated increase in resting heart rate. Thus, excessive exercise training may produce at least a temporary physiological stress state characterized by reduced cardiac vagal tone and a shift in cardiac ANS balance toward an increased cardiac SNS predominance.

During Acute Exercise

Surprisingly, there are no data directly addressing the effects of endurance training on cardiac vagal modulation of heart rate during performance of acute submaximal exercise. With this critical limitation noted, it seems reasonable to speculate that there would be greater cardiac vagal modulation of heart rate (greater vagal tone) during the same absolute submaximal workload in the exercise-trained compared with the sedentary state. At the same relative submaximal workload (same percent of maximal exercise capacity), one would predict that cardiac vagal modulation of heart rate would be similar in the exercise-trained and untrained states. This speculation is consistent with the following facts:

- Heart rate is lower and unchanged, respectively, during submaximal dynamic exercise performed at the same absolute and relative work rates in the endurance-trained than in the sedentary state (6,22).
- HRV at the offset of acute submaximal exercise is higher after than before exercise training (17,95).

If true, this means that the range of heart rate, oxygen consumption, and absolute submaximal workloads over which cardiac vagal modulation of heart rate occurs would be increased after exercise training as a result of this adaptation (22).

Sympathoadrenal System Activity at Rest and Throughout a Day

Although there appears to be widespread belief that sympathoadrenal system and/or SNS activity is lower in the exercise-trained than in the sedentary state under resting conditions, the actual data related to this issue are remarkably inconsistent. With regard to the SNS, PNE has been reported to be either unchanged (101,102) (Fig. 9.26) or lower (39,103) in the exercise-trained than in the sedentary state. There are few data on total PNE spillover rate, a more precise measure of average whole-body SNS activity than PNE, comparing the exercise-trained and sedentary states. In young adults, a reduction in total PNE spillover rate at rest has been reported after a period of daily exercise training (103), but findings are inconsistent as to the effects of less frequent (3 days a week) training (99,103) (Fig. 9.27). In contrast, in older adults total PNE spillover rate at rest has been found to be either elevated (104) or

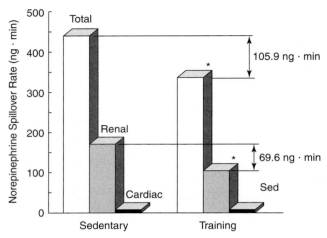

FIGURE 9.27   Total, renal, and cardiac norepinephrine spillover rates determined during resting conditions before and after endurance exercise training in healthy young and middle-aged men. Total norepinephrine spillover rate was lower after training, mediated largely by a corresponding reduction in renal norepinephrine spillover rate, indicating training-associated reductions in average whole-body and kidney sympathetic activity at rest. In contrast, cardiac norepinephrine spillover rate, which was already low in the sedentary state, was not further reduced after exercise training, suggesting no effect of regular endurance exercise on cardiac sympathetic activity in healthy men of this age. *(Modified with permission from Meredith TT, Friberg P, Jennings GL, et al. Exercise training lowers resting renal but not cardiac sympathetic activity in humans. Hypertension 1991;18:579.)*

not different (105) in the exercise-trained compared with the untrained state.

With reference to possible changes in regional SNS activity under resting conditions, a reduction in renal PNE spillover rate has been reported in young adult males after endurance exercise training compared with a period of sedentary living (99); the decrease in renal PNE spillover accounted for about two-thirds of the reduction in total PNE spillover rate after training (Fig. 9.27). MSNA generally has been found not to be different in the exercise-trained and sedentary states in young adult human subjects (106,107). MSNA has been reported to be higher in endurance-trained than in sedentary older adults, primarily as a result of greater levels of MSNA in endurance-trained women than in their untrained peers (101). In contrast, MSNA does not appear to be different in middle-aged and older endurance-trained men compared with sedentary men (101,108). In experimental animals, NE content and/or turnover has been found to be elevated in the brain (109), not different in the liver (21,110), but lower in the spleen (109) in the endurance-trained state.

Findings concerning the effects of exercise training on SNS activity to the heart also are inconsistent. Observations of (a) a smaller reduction in heart rate in response to acute β-adrenergic receptor blockade in the exercise-trained than in sedentary states (92) and (b) reduced NE content (111)

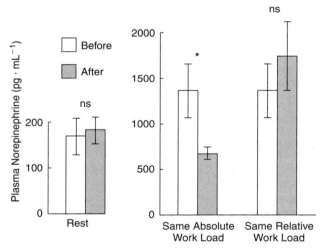

FIGURE 9.26   Plasma norepinephrine concentrations determined under resting conditions (*left*) and during submaximal leg cycling exercise (*right*) performed at the same absolute and relative (percent of maximum) intensities before and after endurance exercise training in 10 healthy young and middle-aged men. Plasma norepinephrine concentrations were not different under resting conditions or during exercise performed at the same relative workload before and after exercise training, indicating unchanged sympathetic activity with endurance training under these conditions. In contrast, plasma norepinephrine concentrations were lower at the same absolute submaximal workload after compared with before exercise training, indicating a markedly lower sympathetic activity after training under this condition. *(Modified with permission from Peronnet F, Cleroux J, Perrault H, et al. Plasma norepinephrine response to exercise before and after training in humans. J Appl Physiol 1981;51:813.)*

and turnover (109) in whole-heart preparations and in right atrium (but not whole heart) β-adrenergic receptor density and affinity (112) in exercise-trained than in untrained experimental animals indicate a reduction in cardiac SNS tone with endurance training.

However, findings of (*a*) no difference in heart rate in response to β-adrenergic receptor blockade (98), (*b*) no change in cardiac PNE spillover rate (99), and (*c*) no difference (21,110) or increased (109) NE content of the heart in the exercise-trained compared with sedentary states do not support an exercise training–associated reduction in cardiac SNS tone. Thus, the role of reduced sympathoadrenal β-adrenergic modulation of heart rate in contributing to the training bradycardia observed in the exercise-trained state is not clear. This mechanism could play some role, but the available experimental evidence is more consistent for enhanced cardiac vagal modulation and, particularly, a reduction in intrinsic heart rate in mediating the training bradycardia observed at rest.

Under resting conditions epinephrine secretion from the adrenal medulla appears to be either unchanged or augmented in the endurance exercise–trained compared with the sedentary state. PE generally has been found to be not different in the trained and untrained states (41,99,103), nor is tissue epinephrine content in the adrenal medulla different in exercise-trained compared with sedentary rats under resting conditions (21). In contrast, there is evidence supporting enhanced epinephrine secretion rate from the adrenal medulla in the endurance-trained state (26), including elevated PE and increased epinephrine secretion, with unchanged epinephrine clearance.

PNE and PE over an entire 24-hour period in endurance exercise-trained and untrained young males have been established using serial blood sampling (113). Normal daily exercise training sessions were included in the analysis. Peak plasma concentrations of the catecholamines were much greater in the trained males as a result of their exercise training session. Mean 24-hour PNE and PE were twice as great in the trained as in the untrained men (Fig. 9.28), despite similar mean levels of heart rate. These higher mean 24-hour plasma catecholamine concentrations in the exercise-trained men were only slightly influenced by the increases occurring during their training session. The markedly higher PNE concentrations in the trained men were not likely explained by correspondingly reduced PNE clearance rates, because the latter has been reported to be unchanged in the endurance-trained state. These unique data therefore support the possibility that average daily sympathoadrenal system activity actually is greater in the endurance exercise-trained than in the sedentary state.

During Acute Exercise

The most consistently observed sympathoadrenal system adaptation to aerobic endurance exercise training is lower

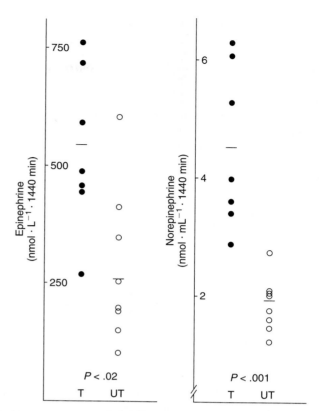

FIGURE 9.28 Mean 24-hour plasma epinephrine (*left*) and norepinephrine (*right*) concentrations in groups of endurance exercise–trained (T) and untrained (UT) healthy young men. The average 24-hour concentrations of these catecholamines were much higher in the endurance-trained than in the untrained men, suggesting that trained men have greater daily sympathoadrenal system activity and consequent circulating plasma epinephrine and norepinephrine levels than untrained men. *(Modified from Dela F, Mikines KJ, Von Linstow M, Galbo H. Heart rate and plasma catecholamines during 24 h of everyday life in trained and untrained men. J Appl Physiol 1992;73:2392.)*

PNE and PE during performance of the same absolute submaximal exercise condition in the trained than in the untrained state (39,102,114) (Fig. 9.26). This adaptation is observed at moderate to heavy submaximal exercise intensities that evoke significant sympathoadrenal system activation (i.e., increases in PNE and PE above resting levels) in the untrained state. The magnitude of the adaptations depends at least in part on the size of the increase in maximal aerobic capacity with exercise training: the greater this increase, the greater the reduction in submaximal exercise PNE and PE in response to training. This is because the greater the increase in maximal aerobic capacity, the smaller the stress that the same absolute submaximal exercise load imposes in the exercise-trained compared with the untrained state. The temporal pattern of this adaptation has not been extensively studied, but reductions in PNE and PE have been observed to be complete by the third week of a 7-week intensive endurance training program (114); heart rate continued to decrease and $\dot{V}O_{2max}$ continued to increase after the third week, thus dissociating these adaptations in the sympathoadrenal system, control of heart rate, and maximal aerobic capacity (Fig. 9.29). These training-induced reductions in PNE and PE during submaximal exercise are abolished after a period of no exercise training (115). PE has been reported to be augmented in endurance-trained compared with untrained subjects during prolonged submaximal ex-

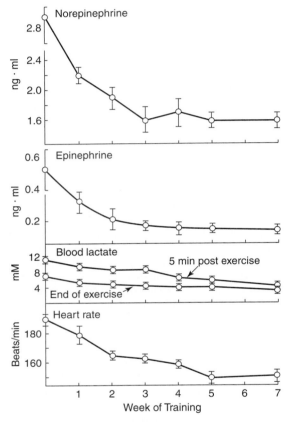

FIGURE 9.29 Changes in plasma norepinephrine and epinephrine, blood lactate, and heart rate during leg cycling exercise performed at the same absolute submaximal workload before (far left vertical axis points) and weekly throughout an intense 7-week exercise training program in healthy young men. Plasma norepinephrine and epinephrine concentrations during exercise decreased significantly throughout the initial 3 weeks of training and remained unchanged thereafter, indicating that this sympathoadrenal system adaptation was complete by the third week of exercise training. In contrast, exercise heart rate continued to decrease until the fifth week of training, suggesting that nonsympathetic mechanisms contribute to reductions in heart rate after the third week of training. (*Modified from Winder WW, Hagberg JM, Hickson RC, et al. Time course of sympathoadrenal adaptation to endurance exercise training in man. J Appl Physiol 1978;45:372.*)

ercise performed to exhaustion (26), consistent with the concept of an increased capacity for adrenal medullary secretion of epinephrine in the exercise-trained state.

PNE and PE usually are not different during exercise performed at the same relative submaximal workload (percent of maximal exercise capacity) (Fig. 9.26) or at maximum in the exercise-trained and sedentary states (39,41,102), although greater levels of PNE and/or PE also have been observed under these conditions (26,116). Greater PNE at the same relative submaximal exercise intensity and/or at maximum following endurance training may be linked to the greater absolute work rates and $\dot{V}O_2$, and a consequent greater active muscle mass compared with the untrained state (116). This would in turn require greater active muscle blood flow and vascular conductance, producing a greater threat to the maintenance of arterial blood pressure in the trained state. To maintain total vascular conductance and arterial blood pressure in the face of greater active muscle vasodilation, the arterial baroreflex would allow a correspondingly greater increase in SNS vasoconstrictor activity, which accounts for the higher PNE values in the trained state under these conditions.

The effects of these sympathoadrenal system adaptations to exercise training on cardiovascular function during acute exercise include the following (6,8):

- Less inactive muscle and internal organ (renal, splanchnic) vasoconstriction during the same absolute submaximal workload in the trained state as a consequence of the reduced SNS activity
- Similar (or slightly greater) inactive muscle and internal organ (renal, splanchnic) vasoconstriction during the same relative workload in the trained state as a consequence of the similar (or slightly greater) SNS activity
- The slope of the line relating renal and splanchnic blood flow to percent of $\dot{V}O_{2max}$ is unchanged with exercise training; thus, a greater absolute workload can be performed with the same increase in SNS activity and associated renal and splanchnic vasoconstriction (6,22)
- Sympathoadrenal system activation occurs at a higher absolute submaximal workload after endurance training, although the heart rate–SNS activity relation is not altered in the exercise-trained state (6,22)

Role of the Sympathoadrenal System in Mediating Physiological Adaptations to Exercise Training

The role of an intact sympathoadrenal system in mediating the physiological adaptations to aerobic endurance exercise training is controversial (8). As limited evidence supports the need for an intact SNS in producing the bradycardia and other cardiovascular adaptations associated with endurance training (117,118). This information is obtained by comparing the physiological responses to exercise training in experimental animals or humans with either an intact sympathoadrenal system or the absence of a functional sympathoadrenal system produced by SNS denervation, adrenalectomy, or adrenergic receptor blockade. The observation that chronic infusion of dobutamine, a β-adrenergic receptor agonist, can produce exercise training–like cardiovascular adaptations also is consistent with the idea that sympathoadrenal system stimulation of the β-adrenergic signaling pathways in the heart and other key peripheral tissues is an important mechanism in mediating the cardiovascular adaptations to exercise training (119). However, there is alternative experimental support for the position that the physiological adaptations to exercise training, including increases in maximal aerobic capacity, can be produced without an intact sympathoadrenal system, including in the absence of β-adrenergic system signaling (8,11). Thus, at present this issue remains controversial.

Influence of Resistance Exercise Training on Sympathoadrenal System Function

There is a limited amount of information on the effects of resistance exercise training on sympathoadrenal activity. With regard to whole-body measures of sympathoadrenal activity, PNE and PE concentrations at rest are not different in the resistance exercise–trained compared with the untrained state (120,121). PNE and PE during the same absolute submaximal workloads of large muscle dynamic exercise also are the same before and after resistance exercise training (121). Concerning regional SNS activity, recently MSNA determined under resting conditions was found to be unchanged after resistance exercise training in young adults (122). Thus, based on the available experimental evidence, resistance exercise training does not appear to influence sympathoadrenal system activity under resting conditions or during conventional submaximal dynamic exercise. Sympathoadrenal system activation could be reduced during acute submaximal resistance exercise in the resistance exercise–trained state, that is, when the trained muscles are performing the same absolute submaximal level of resistance exercise as in the untrained state. However, this remains to be established experimentally.

Central and Peripheral Neural Mechanisms Mediating the ANS Adaptations to Large-Muscle Dynamic Exercise Training

Any changes in efferent ANS activity in the exercise-trained compared with the untrained state must be mediated by corresponding changes in the peripheral nervous system and/or CNS mechanisms that control that activity under the specific set of physiological conditions in which the ANS adaptation is observed. As such, exercise training–related changes in ANS activity observed under resting conditions would be mediated by changes in CNS nuclei involved in automatic

rhythm generation of ANS activity (i.e., vagal and SNS preganglionic nerve activity) and/or sensory afferent feedback from tonic homeostatic reflexes (e.g., baroreflexes, arterial chemoreflexes). Of course, indirect cardiovascular measures of ANS activity, such as HRV, also are subject to nonneural peripheral adaptations (e.g., changes in muscarinic receptor density or sensitivity). Exercise training–associated changes in ANS activity during acute exercise could be mediated by changes in these tonic control mechanisms but also are affected by changes in neural signals specific to physical exercise (i.e., central command and feedback from active muscle reflexes). Therefore, insight into the mechanisms responsible for training-evoked changes in ANS activity comes from these putative influences.

ANS Adaptations Observed Under Resting Conditions

For at least two reasons it is difficult to speculate about the mechanisms that may mediate ANS adaptations to exercise training observed under resting conditions. First, as noted earlier, these adaptations have not been observed consistently, particularly in human subjects. Second, unlike adaptations observed under conditions of submaximal exercise, there are not one or two specific signals that are believed to dominant ANS control under resting conditions but rather an integration of basic CNS outflow tonically modulated by feedback input from a number of homeostatic reflexes. When observed, increased HRV and reduced PNE may be mediated in part by increased vagal and reduced SNS activity from hypothalamic, medullary, and possibly other regions of the subcortical brain known to control tonic ANS outflow (123). However, increased cardiac vagal modulation of heart rate also could be mediated in part by peripheral adaptations in acetylcholine release from the vagus nerve and/or muscarinic receptor density and affinity for and sensitivity to acetylcholine. Similarly, reduced PNE could be mediated in part by training-associated changes in presynaptic modulation of NE release from sympathetic nerve endings (i.e., reduced NE release per unit sympathetic nerve discharge).

Possible changes in baroreflex control of heart rate and SNS activity at rest in the exercise-trained and untrained states have been studied extensively in both human subjects and experimental animals. As discussed in detail recently (124), the results of studies in humans indicate that baroreflex control of ANS-cardiovascular function (i.e., heart rate, MSNA, and/or arterial blood pressure) is increased (125), unchanged (108,124), or reduced (126) in the exercise-trained versus sedentary state. Findings from investigations in experimental animals are much more consistent, indicating impaired baroreflex control of the circulation in the endurance exercise–trained condition (127). However, the potential mechanistic role of changes in baroreflex function (when observed) in mediating the ANS-cardiovascular adaptations to endurance exercise training under resting conditions (when observed) has not been established.

Finally, inconsistency in ANS activity, particularly SNS activity, under resting conditions in the exercise-trained and untrained conditions could be mediated in part by changes in the state of energy flux. Energy flux refers to the absolute levels of energy intake and energy expenditure during a period of energy balance. A state of high-energy flux would be associated with high daily energy expenditure (e.g., as a result of daily endurance exercise training) and correspondingly high-energy intake required to maintain energy balance, and vice versa. High-energy flux states involving regular large-muscle dynamic exercise are associated with correspondingly greater levels of SNS activity (based on PNE values) and resting metabolic rate compared with a low-energy flux state involving sedentary energy-balanced conditions (128). Accordingly, this poorly appreciated influence on the ANS should be considered in attempts to interpret findings related especially to the effects of endurance training on resting SNS activity.

ANS Adaptations Observed During Submaximal Exercise

As emphasized earlier, the most consistently evident ANS adaptations to exercise training are the (presumed) higher levels of cardiac vagal modulation of heart rate and the well-established lower overall sympathoadrenal system activity at the same absolute submaximal workload in the exercise-trained compared with the untrained state. Because central motor command, feedback from active muscle reflexes, and feedback from arterial baroreflexes are believed to be the three major neural signals mediating the ANS adjustments to acute exercise (49,66,67), most of the related experimental results to date concern the possible involvement of these mechanisms.

CENTRAL COMMAND During exercise central command is believed to (22,49):

- Directly or indirectly (via baroreflex resetting) stimulate a reduction in cardiac vagal activity, with a resulting increase in heart rate
- Indirectly (via baroreflex resetting) stimulate increases sympathoadrenal activity, with resulting increases in heart rate and region-specific vasoconstriction

Therefore, one might reasonably hypothesize that a reduced level of central command is a key mechanism underlying the lower heart rate, PNE, renal and splanchnic vasoconstriction, and PE observed during the same absolute submaximal exercise load in the endurance-trained compared with the sedentary state. Three primary lines of experimental evidence support such an idea:

1. Reduced heart rate and blood pressure responses to the same absolute submaximal bout of dynamic cy-

cling exercise performed with the untrained leg after compared with before one-leg exercise training (129). The interpretation of such results is that because the untrained leg has not undergone metabolic or other adaptations that occur in the trained leg, the feedback from the active muscles of the untrained leg during acute exercise should be the same before and after the period of exercise training. As such, the mechanism mediating the lower ANS-evoked cardiovascular adjustments to acute exercise with the untrained leg after contralateral leg training must involve a CNS-based adaptation, presumably a lower central motor command mediated by some type of crossover effect on the untrained limb.

2. Reduced heart rate and diastolic blood pressure responses to voluntary but not electrically stimulated (involuntary) submaximal isometric exercise in the untrained limb after compared with before exercise training of the contralateral trained limb (130). The fact that the attenuated heart rate and diastolic blood pressure responses in the untrained limb after contralateral limb training was not observed during involuntary exercise (i.e., when only feedback from active muscle reflexes were stimulating ANS responses) implicates a lower level of central command in mediating the adaptations observed during voluntary exercise of the untrained limb post training.

3. Lower active muscle electromyographic (EMG) activity during performance of the same submaximal muscle activity in the endurance-trained compared with the untrained state (131). Active muscle EMG activity has been used as an indirect measure of central command; thus, a lower level of EMG during exercise is interpreted as representing a lower level of central command in the exercise-trained state.

FEEDBACK FROM ACTIVE MUSCLE REFLEXES Feedback from active muscle reflexes, particularly from muscle chemoreflex activation, can stimulate SNS outflow to the heart (raising heart rate) and to the arterial blood vessels (producing vasoconstriction in inactive muscle, the kidney, and the splanchnic circulations), although the contributions of these mechanisms during conventional large-muscle dynamic exercise are not clear (discussed earlier). Thus, it is possible that reduced SNS-mediated responses to acute exercise in the endurance-trained compared with the untrained state could be the result of reduced feedback from active muscle reflexes. Experimental evidence supporting this possibility includes these findings:

1. Greater reductions in heart rate and arterial blood pressure during the same absolute level of submaximal leg cycling exercise performed with the trained limb versus the untrained limb after compared with before one-leg endurance training (132). The idea is that because of CNS crossover effects produced by

training, central command should be similarly reduced during performance of acute exercise with the trained and untrained limbs following exercise training. Therefore, any differences observed in ANS-mediated responses can be attributed to less feedback from active muscle reflexes.

2. Reductions in muscle lactate concentrations during acute submaximal large-muscle dynamic exercise as well as less hyperemia post exercise in the active muscles following exercise training (132,133). Because muscle chemoreflex activation during exercise is related to the extent of glycolytic metabolism and the production and accumulation of glycolytic metabolites, as well as to mismatches between oxygen demand and delivery, these observations suggest a metabolic state in the active muscles following training consistent with less muscle chemoreflex activation.

3. Reduced MSNA response to small-muscle dynamic exercise after training (134) associated with evidence for reduced active muscle chemoreflex (e.g., reduced accumulation of reflex-activating metabolites) (135) and possibly mechanoreflex (134) activation.

Based on the discussion of the involvement in these reflexes in ANS control during acute exercise presented earlier in this chapter, changes in these mechanisms likely play a more important role in mediating ANS adaptations to small-muscle and perhaps very high-intensity large-muscle exercise training than the adaptations observed in response to conventional intensities and durations of large-muscle endurance training.

BAROREFLEXES   As discussed previously, the resetting of the arterial baroreflex to a higher operating pressure from rest may be a key mechanism by which the ANS adjustments, particularly increases in SNS activity, to acute large-muscle dynamic exercise are mediated. Thus, changes in baroreflex function could contribute to or even explain the ANS adaptations observed during the same absolute intensity of submaximal exercise in the endurance-trained compared with the sedentary state. Unfortunately, direct experimental evidence is not available either to support or to refute this possibility, because studies to date have investigated baroreflex function in the trained and untrained states only under resting conditions (discussed earlier).

INTEGRATIVE MODEL EXPLAINING TRAINING-ASSOCIATED ANS ADAPTATIONS DURING SUBMAXIMAL DYNAMIC EXERCISE   A key question, therefore, remains unanswered: how are the smaller withdrawal of cardiac vagal nerve activity and sympathoadrenal system activation observed during the same absolute submaximal level of large-muscle dynamic exercise in the endurance-trained state mediated? Again, we don't know. However, using the previous discussion in this

chapter as the basic substrate, we can construct a working model that attempts to explain how these adaptations may be produced.

In the regulatory scheme advanced by Rowell (49) (Fig. 9.25), the increase in heart rate during exercise requiring levels below 100 beats per minute is mediated by central command–stimulated cardiac vagal withdrawal. Exercise requiring greater increases in heart rate also necessitates activation of the SNS, which produces further increases in heart rate and cardiac output along with vasoconstriction in the inactive skeletal muscle, renal, and splanchnic circulations. At least the SNS activation appears to involve a resetting of the arterial baroreflex to a higher operating pressure. Given this scenario, it seems reasonable to hypothesize that the ANS adaptations to endurance training that are expressed during the performance of submaximal exercise are mediated by changes to these two key control mechanisms, central command and arterial baroreflex resetting. For example, a lower central motor command in the trained state would presumably cause less CNS-mediated cardiac vagal withdrawal and therefore result in the lower heart rate observed during submaximal exercise. In addition, the lower central command would cause less resetting of the arterial baroreflex, and therefore, the operating point for arterial blood pressure would be lower during submaximal exercise in the endurance-trained than in the sedentary state. During submaximal exercise performed at heart rates below 100 beats per minute (in the untrained state), less withdrawal of cardiac vagal activity and a smaller increase in heart rate would be required in the endurance-trained state to achieve the lower exercise-associated operating pressure. This would explain the lower heart rate and arterial blood pressure in the endurance-trained versus untrained state during mild to moderate submaximal exercise. During higher intensities of exercise requiring SNS activation, the smaller central command–mediated arterial baroreflex resetting would explain not only greater cardiac vagal tone in the endurance-trained state but also the accompanying smaller increases in SNS activity to the heart and peripheral arterial vessels. That is, compared with the untrained state, less SNS activation (less NE release from sympathetic nerve endings and less epinephrine secretion from the adrenal medulla) would be needed because less of an increase in heart rate and regional vasoconstriction would be required to attain the lower operating pressure in the exercise-trained state. This would explain the smaller sympathoadrenal–β-adrenergic stimulation of heart rate, SNS-mediated α-adrenergic reductions in regional blood flow and vascular conductance (i.e., increases in vascular resistance), and increases in PNE and PE during moderate to heavy submaximal exercise observed in the endurance-trained state. Thus, in this regulatory scheme, the key mechanism involved in producing the ANS adaptations observed during submaximal large-muscle dynamic exercise in the trained state is a smaller central motor command.

ROLE OF REDUCED CNS NEURONAL ACTIVATION IN ANS ADAPTATIONS OBSERVED DURING SUBMAXIMAL EXERCISE

Regardless of the exact mechanisms that contribute to the ANS adaptations to training observed during submaximal exercise, one would hypothesize that neuronal activity in selective regions of the brain involved in ANS-cardiorespiratory control during exercise would be different in the endurance-trained compared with the sedentary state. In particular, it might be postulated that areas of the brain implicated in stimulating SNS outflow to the heart and arterial blood vessels during exercise would demonstrate less activation during submaximal exercise in the trained state. Recent work from the laboratory of Iwamoto and colleagues (123) provide experimental evidence for this concept. Fos-like (c-Fos) immunocytochemistry was used to establish putative neuronal activation in specific regions of the brain thought to be involved in ANS-cardiorespiratory control during exercise. Rats who underwent spontaneous (voluntary) wheel running training were compared with sedentary controls during wheel running at the same submaximal running velocity. Submaximal exercise resulted in what can be presumed to be less neuronal activation in the posterior (caudal) hypothalamus, periaqueductal gray, nucleus of the tractus solitarius, and the rostral ventrolateral medulla in the exercise-trained compared with the sedentary rats (Fig. 9.30). Thus, based on these results, neuronal activation in selective sites at all levels of the CNS appears to be lower during submaximal dynamic exercise in the endurance-trained than in the sedentary state. This altered state of CNS activation likely is mediated by some combination of reduced central command, less arterial baroreflex resetting, and possibly reduced excitatory feedback from the active muscles.

Endurance Training and Tissue Responsiveness to Adrenergic Stimulation

There is extensive experimental literature concerning the effects of endurance exercise training on tissue responsiveness to adrenergic receptor stimulation. Unfortunately, overall the results of this research are highly inconsistent.

Endurance Training and Vascular Responsiveness to α-Adrenergic Stimulation

The influence of the endurance exercise–trained state on vascular responsiveness to α-adrenergic stimulation has been studied by examining the vasoconstrictor response of isolated arterial blood vessels, specific regional circulations, or the overall (systemic) circulation to specific α-adrenergic agonists (typically phenylephrine) or to NE, a nonspecific adrenergic agonist. The advantage of agonists such as phenylephrine is greater specificity for the α-adrenergic receptor (i.e., the associated vasoconstrictor response is presumed to be largely or solely mediated by this receptor signaling system); the disadvantage is some potential nonspecific

β-adrenergic agonist effects and the fact that phenylephrine is not a natural endogenous (physiological) agonist but rather a pharmacological stimulus. The advantage of NE is that it is the primary neurotransmitter released from postganglionic sympathetic nerve endings that binds to α-adrenergic receptors and evokes physiological vasoconstriction, although the actions of exogenously administered NE are thought to be somewhat different from those of neuronally released NE. (This can be avoided by administering drugs that stimulate endogenous NE release from sympathetic nerve endings such as hexamethonium.) The major disadvantage of NE as an α-adrenergic receptor agonist is that it also is an agonist for β-adrenergic receptors. Because of this, the vasoconstrictor effects of NE mediated by stimulation of α-adrenergic receptors cannot be isolated because of the potential for concomitant stimulation of vasodilation via β_2-adrenergic receptors.

Vasoconstrictor responsiveness to phenylephrine has been found to be reduced (136), not different (124,127,137), or enhanced (26,138) in the endurance-trained compared with the untrained state. Similarly, vasoconstrictor responsiveness to NE has been reported to be impaired (139), not different (127), or increased (140) in the exercise-trained state. When exercise training–associated reductions in vasoconstrictor responsiveness to α-adrenergic receptor stimulation are observed, there is evidence that the reductions are mediated by increased nitric oxide–dependent endothelial vasodilatory tone (136). However, the overall results concerning the relation between endurance exercise training and vascular responsiveness to α-adrenergic receptor stimulation are equivocal.

Endurance Training and Tissue Responsiveness to β-Adrenergic Stimulation

The effects of endurance exercise training on tissue responsiveness to β-adrenergic receptor stimulation has been studied by measuring cardiac (heart rate, ventricular contractility) and/or vascular (vasodilation in arterial blood vessels or the overall arterial circulation) responses to infusion of β-adrenergic receptor agonists, such as isoproterenol or dobutamine. Cardiac responses are mediated by both β_1- (primarily) and β_2-adrenergic receptors, whereas peripheral vasodilation is mediated by β_2-adrenergic receptors. Most often the nonselective β-adrenergic receptor agonist isoproterenol has been used to determine both cardiac and peripheral vascular responsiveness.

Using these methods, cardiac and vascular responsiveness to β-adrenergic receptor stimulation has been found to be reduced (112,138,141), not different (142, 143), or augmented (144,145) in the exercise-trained versus sedentary state. Similarly, β-adrenergic receptor density and affinity have been reported to be decreased (141), not different (138,143), or increased (146). Thus, as with vasoconstrictor responsiveness to α-adrenergic receptor

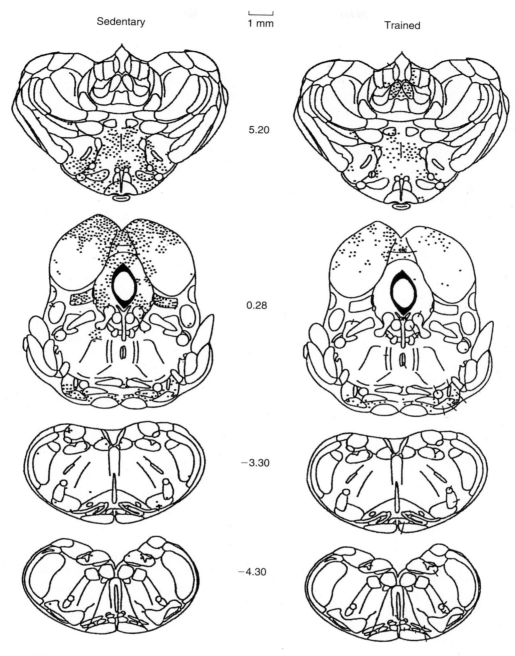

Sedentary   1 mm   Trained

5.20

0.28

−3.30

−4.30

FIGURE 9.30 Representative Fos data contrasting a single bout of exercise wheel activity at a fixed submaximal speed in an endurance exercise–trained and an untrained rat in selected standard rat brain stereotactic planes: 5.20 is the level of the caudal hypothalamus, 0.28 is midbrain, −3.30 is the rostral medulla, and −4.30 is the caudal medulla. Each dot signifies three cells. Each of the following areas showed a statistically significant reduction in Fos immunoreactivity in the trained versus the sedentary animals in response to the exercise bout: rostral ventrolateral medulla; caudal hypothalamus and locomotor region (ventromedial part of 5.2 level); mesencephalic locomotor region (cuneiform); periaqueductal gray matter (dorsal medial part of 0.28 level surrounding cerebral aqueduct) and medial nucleus of the tractus solitarius. While most are ANS-associated sites, the tractus solitarius is a sensory relay. Areas showing large reductions in activity that did not quite reach levels of statistical significance included the lateral hypothalamus and cuneiform nucleus (mesencephalic locomotor region). *(Stereotactic figures adapted from Paxinos G, Watson C. The rat brain in stereotaxic coordinates, 2nd ed. Orlando: Academic Press, 1986. Modified with permission from Ichiyama RM, Gilbert AB, Waldrop TG, et al. Changes in the exercise activation of diencephalic and brainstem cardiorespiratory areas after training. Brain Res 2002;947:230.)*

stimulation, the results of investigations concerning the effects of the endurance-trained state on cardiac and vascular responsiveness to β-adrenergic receptor stimulation, as well as on β-adrenergic receptor properties, are equivocal.

Sources of Variability in Data Concerning Endurance Training and Tissue Responsiveness to Adrenergic Stimulation

Because tissue responsiveness to SNS adrenergic stimulation plays such a key role in the ANS-mediated physiological adaptations to exercise training, it is important to understand the potential sources of the variability in the experimental results just described. These sources include the following:

- Use of various experimental animal models and human subjects (species differences).
- Local versus systemic arterial administration of adrenergic receptor agonists.
- Systemic infusion of adrenergic agonists with intact versus absent baroreflexes; intact baroreflexes will actively counterregulate agonist-induced changes in arterial blood pressure by evoking ANS adjustments, which in turn confound interpretation of the results (124,137,147).
- Use of selective (e.g., specific β₁-adrenergic) versus nonselective (e.g., nonspecific β₁- and β₂-adrenergic) agonists causes stimulation of different receptor populations.
- Use of cross-sectional compared with intervention study designs.
- Comparisons of responses between different cardiovascular tissues (e.g., heart versus peripheral arterial blood vessels) or different functions within the same organ (e.g., heart rate versus left ventricular contractile response).
- Differences in baseline adrenergic responsiveness in the untrained subject groups among studies as a result of differences in age, degree of sedentary lifestyle (deconditioning), and so on.
- Differences in fiber type of the muscles in which blood flow measurements are made in animal studies (148).

SUMMARY

The ANS plays an important role in mediating the cardiovascular, thermoregulatory, and metabolic adjustments required to maintain internal homeostasis during acute physical exercise. These ANS-mediated physiological adjustments are necessary to achieve one's true maximal aerobic capacity and submaximal endurance exercise performance. A variety of experimental approaches, each with its own strengths and limitations, have been used to study the ANS at rest and during acute exercise. Using these methods, experimental evidence has established that cardiac vagal activity is reduced at the onset of even mild exercise, which produces an immediate increase in heart rate and cardiac output, providing blood flow to active muscle while supporting arterial blood pressure in the face of active muscle vasodilation–associated increases in total vascular conductance. Activation of the sympathoadrenal system occurs at moderate to heavy submaximal exercise intensities, further increasing cardiac output via stimulation of heart rate and left ventricular contractility. This sympathoadrenal activation also produces vasoconstriction of arterioles that (a) redistributes the increased cardiac output away from certain regional circulations (kidney, gut, inactive muscle) to active muscle and (b) restricts active muscle vasodilation to maintain systemic vascular resistance and most important, arterial blood pressure at levels required for proper perfusion of vital organs. The temporal pattern and magnitude of these ANS adjustments during acute exercise are determined by a number of modulatory influences, including the intensity and duration of the exercise, gender, type of exercise, size of the active muscle mass, ambient temperature, and body position, among others. The ANS adjustments to acute exercise are stimulated by central command signals generated as part of neuromuscular activation; these central command signals are modulated by several sources of sensory afferent feedback from the periphery to the CNS, including active muscle reflexes and arterial baroreflexes. The key interaction may involve central command–induced resetting of the arterial baroreflex operating pressure. These collective CNS inputs modify the neuronal activity of various regions of the brain involved in ANS-cardiorespiratory control to produce the appropriate ANS adjustments during acute exercise. Repeated performance of large-muscle dynamic exercise results in specific ANS adaptations that are intended to accommodate the demands of the exercise and allow the exercise to be sustained while reducing tissue stress, thus increasing the resistance of the body to loss of homeostasis. Such ANS adaptations are most consistently evident during submaximal exercise performed at the same absolute intensity and duration in the exercise-trained and the sedentary state. Under these exercise conditions there is less of a reduction in cardiac vagal modulation of heart rate and a smaller sympathoadrenal activation in the endurance-trained state. These reduced ANS adjustments to submaximal exercise in the trained state are associated with correspondingly reduced neuronal activation in regions of the brain involved in the control of ANS outflow to the periphery. This reduced neuronal activation in the trained state is most likely mediated by a smaller level of central command and arterial baroreflex resetting during the same submaximal exercise condition. The role of changes in tissue responsiveness to adrenergic receptor stimulation in mediating the ANS adaptations to endurance exercise training has not been established.

The Milestone of Discovery experiment on the ANS and exercise actually is two novel complementary experiments, both conducted by Professor Ron Victor and colleagues at Southwestern Medical School in Dallas. Victor has performed some of the most compelling science from the mid-1980s to date on the topic of CNS control of ANS adjustments to exercise. The two studies highlighted in this section address a critical but unanswered question at the time: the nature of the intracellular biochemical events that are responsible for activation of active muscle chemoreflexes during exercise in humans. These investigations were chosen for their use of novel experimental approaches, how well they complement each other (i.e., when considered together their findings provide much more definitive insight into the question than either alone), and the influence of the results on our understanding of the physiology of these events and on future research in this area.

Both investigations focus on the association between isometric exercise—induced increases in glycolysis, consequent generation of hydrogen ion and reductions in pH, and the increases in efferent SNS activity (inactive MSNA). In the first study, published in 1988, Victor and his colleagues performed simultaneous measurements of phosphorous nuclear magnetic resonance spectroscopy (31P-NMR) in the active forearm muscle and MSNA in the peroneal nerve of an inactive leg during sustained submaximal isometric and rhythmic handgrip exercise in healthy young adult humans. During both types of exercise, increases in MSNA coincided with intracellular accumulation of hydrogen ion and reductions in pH in the active forearm muscles. During sustained exercise MSNA correlated strongly with reductions in intracellular pH (Fig. 9.31). Their primary conclusion was that stimulation of SNS outflow during exercise-evoked muscle chemoreflex activation is coupled to intracellular accumulation of hydrogen ions.

In the second study, published in 1990, Victor and his colleagues used an "experiment of nature" to independently confirm these initial observations. Specifically, they studied the physiological responses to isometric handgrip exercise in groups of normal subjects and in patients with muscle phosphorylase deficiency. This disorder, McArdle's disease, is an inborn enzymatic defect of skeletal muscle that prevents glycolysis and therefore hydrogen ion

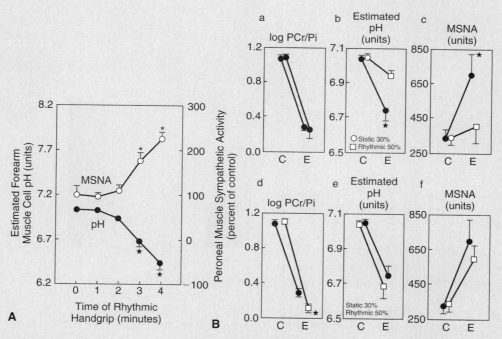

FIGURE 9.31 (Milestone). **A.** Active forearm muscle pH and peroneal (inactive leg) MSNA during 4 minutes of rhythmic handgrip exercise (2 minutes at 30% MVC followed by 2 minutes at 50% MVC) performed by healthy young subjects. Note the tight association between the exercise-induced reductions in pH and increases in MSNA. **B.** MSNA changes from resting control levels in response to handgrip exercise with (*a–c*) comparable reductions in [PCr]/[Pi] or with (*d–f*) comparable reductions in pH. The MSNA responses were consistently associated with changes in pH but not with changes in [PCr]/[Pi]. *(Modified from Victor RG, Bertocci LA, Pryor SL, et al. Sympathetic nerve discharge is coupled to muscle cell pH during exercise in humans. J Clin Invest 1988;82:1301–1305, as published by Seals DR, Victor RG. Regulation of sympathetic nerve activity during exercise in humans. Exerc Sport Sci Rev 1991;19:336.)*

(continued)

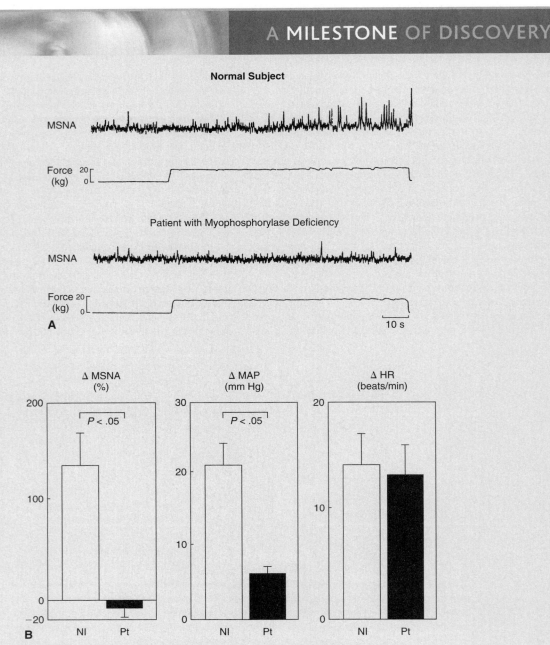

FIGURE 9.32 (Milestone). **A.** Peroneal MSNA and handgrip force before and during 90 seconds of isometric handgrip exercise at 30% of MVC in a normal subject (*top*) and a patient with myophosphorylase deficiency (*below*). The MSNA increased during handgrip exercise in the normal subject but not in the patient. **B.** Increases above resting control levels of MSNA, mean arterial blood pressure (MAP), and heart rate (HR) during isometric handgrip exercise in groups of normal subjects (NI) and patients (Pt). In contrast to the normal subjects, the patients failed to evoke any increase in MSNA, produced an attenuated MAP response, but demonstrated normal tachycardia during handgrip exercise. (*Modified from Pryor SL, Lewis SF, Haller, et al RG. Impairment of sympathetic activation during static exercise in patients with muscle phosphorylase deficiency (McArdle's disease). J Clin Invest 1990;85:1444–1449 as published by Seals DR, Victor RG. Regulation of muscle sympathetic nerve activity during exercise in humans. Exerc Sport Sci Rev 1991;19:339.*)

A MILESTONE OF DISCOVERY

accumulation and reductions in pH during exercise. Normal subjects demonstrated exercise-induced reductions in active forearm muscle pH and corresponding increases in inactive peroneal MSNA. In contrast, during exercise the patients with McArdle's disease did not produce a reduction in active forearm muscle pH, nor did they demonstrate increases in peroneal MSNA (Fig. 9.32). These findings confirmed that muscle chemoreflex–evoked stimulation of inactive MSNA depends on augmentation of intracellular glycolysis and reduction in pH in the active muscles.

The key conclusion from these studies, which were confirmed and subsequently extended and refined by the elegant work of MacLean and colleagues (78) and Sinoway and associates (79,81), was that intracellular biochemical events linked to the stimulation of active muscle glycolysis are important mechanisms underlying activation of muscle chemoreflexes and the increase in MSNA during small-muscle exercise in humans.

Victor RG, Bertocci LA, Pryor SL, Nunnally RL. Sympathetic nerve discharge is coupled to muscle cell pH during exercise in humans. J Clin Invest 1988;82:1301–1305.

Pryor SL, Lewis SF, Haller RG, et al. Impairment of sympathetic activation during static exercise in patients with muscle phosphorylase deficiency (McArdle's disease). J Clin Invest 1990;85:1444–1449.

ACKNOWLEDGMENTS

I thank John Carson for obtaining and summarizing the existing experimental literature related to the ANS and exercise upon which much of the content of this chapter is based. I also thank Ashley Depaulis for her assistance with the bibliography, Professor Gary Iwamoto from the University of Illinois for his important contributions related to the sections on CNS control of the ANS with acute and chronic exercise, and Professor George Billman from Ohio State University for his preliminary data concerning cardiac vagal modulation of heart rate during prolonged submaximal exercise. Finally, I thank Professor Charles Tipton for his personal insight into the content presented in this chapter and Professor Robert Mazzeo for his editing of selected sections.

REFERENCES

1. Christensen NJ, Galbo H. Sympathetic nervous activity during exercise. Annu Rev Physiol 1983;45:139–153.
2. Epstein S, Robinson BF, Kahler RL, et al. Effects of beta-adrenergic blockade on the cardiac response to maximal and submaximal exercise in man. J Clin Invest 1965;44:1745–1753.
3. Martin CE, Shaver JA, Leon DF, et al. Autonomic mechanisms in hemodynamic responses to isometric exercise. J Clin Invest 1974;54:104–115.
4. Robinson BF, Epstein SE, Beiser GD, et al. Control of heart rate by the autonomic nervous system: Studies in man on the interrelation between baroreceptor mechanisms and exercise. Circ Res 1966;19:400–411.
5. Galbo H. Hormonal and Metabolic Adaptation to Exercise. Stuttgart, New York: Thieme-Stratton, 1983;1–116.
6. Rowell LB. Human Circulation Regulation During Physical Stress. New York: Oxford University, 1986; 213–416.
7. Nonogaki K. New insights into sympathetic regulation of glucose and fat metabolism. Diabetologia 2000;43:533–549.
8. Tipton CM. The autonomic nervous system. In Tipton CM, ed. Exercise Physiology: People and Ideas. New York: Oxford University, 2003;188–254.
9. Robinson S, Pearcy M, Brueckman F, et al. Effects of atropine on heart rate and oxygen intake in working man. J Appl Physiol 1953;5:508–512.
10. Ekblom B, Goldbarg AN, Kilbom A, Astrand PO. Effects of atropine and propranolol on the oxygen transport system during exercise in man. Scand J Clin Lab Invest 1972;30:35–42.
11. Wilmore JH, Ewy GA, Freund BJ, et al. Cardiorespiratory alterations consequent to endurance exercise training during chronic beta-adrenergic blockade with atenolol and propranolol. Am J Cardiol 1985;55:142D–148D.
12. Joyner MJ, Freund BJ, Jilka SM, et al. Effects of beta-blockade on exercise capacity of trained and untrained men: a hemodynamic comparison. J Appl Physiol 1986;60:1429–1434.
13. Freyschuss U. Elicitation of heart rate and blood pressure increase on muscle contraction. J Appl Physiol 1970;28:758–761.
14. Billman GE, Dujardin JP. Dynamic changes in cardiac vagal tone as measured by time-series analysis. Am J Physiol 1990;258:H896–H902.
15. O'Leary D, Rossi N, Churchill P. Substantial cardiac parasympathetic activity exists during heavy dynamic exercise in dogs. Am J Physiol 1997;273: H2135–H2140.
16. Brenner IK, Thomas S, Shephard RJ. Autonomic regulation of the circulation during exercise and heat exposure: inferences from heart rate variability. Sports Med 1998;26:85–99.
17. Carter JB, Banister EW, Blaber AP. Effect of endurance exercise on autonomic control of heart rate. Sports Med 2003;33:33–46.
18. Casadei B, Cochrane S, Johnston J, et al. Pitfalls in the interpretation of spectral analysis of the heart rate variability

during exercise in humans. Acta Physiol Scand 1995;153: 125–131.

19. Esler M, Jennings G, Lambert G, et al. Overflow of catecholamine neurotransmitters to the circulation: source, fate, and functions. Physiol Rev 1990;70:963–985.

20. Grassi G, Esler M. How to assess sympathetic activity in humans. J Hypertens 1999;17:719–734.

21. Mazzeo RS. Catecholamine responses to acute and chronic exercise. Med Sci Sports Exerc 1991;23:839–845.

22. Rowell LB, O'Leary DS, Kellogg DL. Integration of cardiovascular control systems in dynamic exercise. In Rowell LB, Shepherd JT, eds. Handbook of Physiology, Section 12: Exercise: Regulation and Integration of Multiple Systems. New York: Oxford University, 1996;770–838.

23. Pernow J, Lundberg JM, Kaijser L, et al. Plasma neuropeptide Y-like immunoreactivity and catecholamines during various degrees of sympathetic activation in man. Clin Physiol 1986;6:561–578.

24. Tidgren B, Hjemdahl P, Theodorsson E, et al. Renal neurohormonal and vascular responses to dynamic exercise in humans. J Appl Physiol 1991;70:2279–2286.

25. Seals DR, Victor RG. Regulation of Muscle Sympathetic Nerve Activity During Exercise in Humans. Dubuque: Brown & Benchmark, 1991;319–349.

26. Kjaer M. Epinephrine and some other hormonal responses to exercise in man: with special reference to physical training. Int. J Sports Med 1989;10:2–15.

27. Bachman E, Zhang DHC, Cinti S, et al. Beta-AR signaling required for diet-induced thermogenesis and obesity resistance. Science 2002;297:843–845.

28. Arai Y, Saul JP, Albrecht P, et al. Modulation of cardiac autonomic activity during and immediately after exercise. Am J Physiol 1989;256:H132–H141.

29. Fagraeus L, Linnarsson D. Autonomic origin of heart rate fluctuations at the onset of muscular exercise. J Appl Physiol 1976;40:679–682.

30. Yamamoto Y, Hughson R, Peterson J. Autonomic control of heart rate during exercise studied by heart rate variability spectral analysis. J Appl Physiol 1991;71:1136–1142.

31. DiCarlo SE, Bishop VS. Onset of exercise shifts operating point of arterial baroreflex to higher pressures. Am J Physiol 1992;262:H303–H307.

32. O'Hagan KP, Bell LB, Mittelstadt SW, et al. Effect of dynamic exercise on renal sympathetic nerve activity in conscious rabbits. J Appl Physiol 1993;74:2099–2104.

33. Tsuchimochi H, Matsukawa K, Komine H, et al. Direct measurement of cardiac sympathetic efferent nerve activity during dynamic exercise. Am J Physiol 2002;283:H1896–H1906.

34. Saito M, Naito M, Mano T. Different responses in skin and muscle sympathetic nerve activity to static muscle contraction. J Appl Physiol 1990;69:2085–2090.

35. Callister R, Ng AV, Seals DR. Arm sympathetic nerve activity during preparation for and initiation of leg-cycling exercise in humans. J Appl Physiol 1994;77:1403–1410.

36. Ray CA, Rea RF, Clary MP, et al. Muscle sympathetic nerve responses to dynamic one-legged exercise: effect of body posture. Am J Physiol 1993;264:H1–H7.

37. Hasking G, Esler M, Jennings G, et al. Norepinephrine spillover to plasma during steady-state supine bicycle exercise. Comparison of patients with congestive heart failure and normal subjects. Circulation 1988;78:516–521.

38. Esler M, Kaye D, Thompson J, et al. Effects of aging on epinephrine secretion, and on regional release of epinephrine from the human heart. J Clin Endocr Metab 1995;80:435–442.

39. Bloom SR, Johnson RH, Park DM, et al. Differences in the metabolic and hormonal response to exercise between racing cyclists and untrained individuals. J Physiol (Lond) 1976;258:1–18.

40. Galbo H, Holst JJ, Christensen NJ. Glucagon and plasma catecholamine responses to graded and prolonged exercise in man. J Appl Physiol 1975;38:70–76.

41. Lehmann M, Keul J, Huber G, et al. Plasma catecholamines in trained and untrained volunteers during graduated exercise. Int J Sports Med 1981;2:143–147.

42. Leuenberger U, Sinoway L, Gubin S, et al. Effects of exercise intensity and duration on norepinephrine spillover and clearance in humans. J Appl Physiol 1993;75: 668–674.

43. Saito M, Tsukanaka A, Yanagihara D, et al. Muscle sympathetic nerve responses to graded leg cycling. J Appl Physiol 1993;75:663–667.

44. Victor RG, Seals DR, Mark AL. Differential control of heart rate and sympathetic nerve activity during dynamic exercise: insight from direct intraneural recordings in humans. J Clin Invest 1987;79:508–516.

45. Manhem P, Lecerof H, Hokfelt B. Plasma catecholamine levels in the coronary sinus, the left renal vein and peripheral vessels in healthy males at rest and during exercise. Acta Physiol Scand 1978;104:364–369.

46. Savard G, Strange S, Kiens B, et al. Noradrenaline spillover during exercise in active versus resting skeletal muscle in man. Acta Physiol Scand 1987;131:507–515.

47. Mazzeo RS, Rajkumar C, Jennings G, et al. Norepinephrine spillover at rest and during submaximal exercise in young and old subjects. J Appl Physiol 1997;82:1869–1874.

48. Coker RH, Krishna MG, Zinker BA, et al. Sympathetic drive to liver and nonhepatic splanchnic tissue during prolonged exercise is increased in diabetes. Metabolism 1997;46:1327–1332.

49. Rowell LB. Human Cardiovascular Control. New York: Oxford University, 1993;162–479.

50. Davy K, Johnson D, Seals D. Cardiovascular, plasma norepinephrine, and thermal adjustments to prolonged exercise in young and older healthy humans. Clin Physiol 1995;15:169–181.

51. Hagberg JM, Seals DR, Yerg JE, et al. Metabolic responses to exercise in young and older athletes and sedentary men. J Appl Physiol 1988;65:900–908.

52. Saito M, Sone R, Ikeda M, et al. Sympathetic outflow to the skeletal muscle in humans increases during prolonged light exercise. J Appl Physiol 1997;82: 1237–1243.

53. Mazzeo RS, Marshall P. Influence of plasma catecholamines on the lactate threshold during graded exercise. J Appl Physiol 1989;67:1319–1322.

54. Joyner MJ, Thomas GD. Having it both ways? Vasoconstriction in contracting muscles. J Physiol (Lond) 2003;550:333.

55. Blomqvist CG, Lewis SF, Taylor WF, et al. Similarity of the hemodynamic responses to static and dynamic exercise of small muscle groups. Circ Res 1981;48:187–92.

56. McMurray RG, Forsythe WA, Mar MH, et al. Exercise intensity-related responses of beta-endorphin and catecholamines. Med Sci Sports Exerc 1987;19:570–574.

57. Galbo H, Houston ME, Christensen NJ, et al. The effect of water temperature on the hormonal response to prolonged swimming. Acta Physiol Scand 1979;105:326–337.

58. Watson RD, Hamilton CA, Jones DH, et al. Sequential changes in plasma noradrenaline during bicycle exercise. Clin Sci 1980;58:37–43.

59. Anderson DE, Hickey MS. Effects of caffeine on the metabolic and catecholamine responses to exercise in 5 and 28 degrees C. Med Sci Sports Exerc 1994;26:453–458.

60. Escourrou P, Johnson D, Rowell L. Hypoxemia increases plasma catecholamine concentrations in exercising humans. J Appl Physiol 1984;57:1507–1511.

61. Esler MD, Thompson JM, Turner AG, et al. Effects of aging on the responsiveness of the human cardiac sympathetic nerves to stressors. Circulation 1995;91:351–358.

62. Seals DR, Enoka RM. Sympathetic activation associated with increases in EMG during fatiguing exercise. J Appl Physiol 1989;66:88–95.

63. Saito M, Mano T, Iwase S. Sympathetic nerve activity related to local fatigue sensation during static contraction. J Appl Physiol 1989;67:980–984.

64. Matsukawa K, Mitchell JH, Wall PT, et al. The effect of static exercise on renal sympathetic nerve activity in conscious cats. J Physiol (Lond) 1991;434:453–467.

65. Iwamoto GA, Wappel SM, Fox GM, et al. Identification of diencephalic and brainstem cardiorespiratory areas activated during exercise. Brain Res 1996;726:109–122.

66. Kaufman MP, Forster H. Reflexes controlling circulatory, ventilatory and airway responses to exercise. In Rowell LB, Shepherd JT, eds. Handbook of Physiology, Section 12: Exercise: Regulation and Integration of Multiple Systems. New York: Oxford University, 1996;381–447.

67. Waldrop T, Eldridge FL, Iwamoto GA, et al. Central neural control of respiration and circulation during exercise. In Rowell LB, Shepherd JT, eds. Handbook of Physiology, Section 12: Exercise: Regulation and Integration of Multiple Systems. New York: Oxford University, 1996;333–380.

68. Elam M, Svensson TH, Thoren P. Brain monoamine metabolism is altered in rats following spontaneous, long-distance running. Acta Physiol Scand 1987;30:313–316.

69. Pagliari R, Peyrin L. Norepinephrine release in the rat frontal cortex under treadmill exercise: a study with microdialysis. J Appl Physiol 1995;78:2121–2130.

70. Scheurink AJ, Steffens AB, Gaykema RP. Hypothalamic adrenoceptors mediate sympathoadrenal activity in exercising rats. Am J Physiol 1990;259:R470–R477.

71. Overton JM, Redding M, Yancey S, et al. Hypothalamic GABAergic influences on treadmill exercise responses in rats. Brain Res Bull 1994;33:517–522.

72. Potts JT. Exercise and sensory integration: role of the nucleus tractus solitarius. Ann NY Acad Sci 2001;940:221–236.

73. Victor RG, Pryor SL, Secher NH, et al. Effects of partial neuromuscular blockade on sympathetic nerve responses to static exercise in humans. Circ Res 1989;65:468–476.

74. Alam M, Smirk FH. Unilateral loss of a blood pressure raising, pulse accelerating, reflex from voluntary muscle due to a lesion of the spinal cord. Clin Sci 1938;3:247–252.

75. Williamson J, McColl R, Mathews D, et al. Brain activation by central command during actual and imagined handgrip under hypnosis. J Appl Physiol 2002;92:1317–1324.

76. Williamson J, McColl R, Mathews D, et al. Hypnotic manipulation of effort sense during dynamic exercise: cardiovascular responses and brain activation. J Appl Physiol 2001;90:1392–1399.

77. Vissing SF, Hjortso EM. Central motor command activates sympathetic outflow to the cutaneous circulation in humans. J Physiol (Lond) 1996;492:931–939.

78. MacLean DA, Vickery LM, Sinoway LI. Elevated interstitial adenosine concentrations do not activate the muscle reflex. Am J Physiol 2001;280:H546–H553.

79. Sinoway LI, Smith MB, Enders B, et al. Role of diprotonated phosphate in evoking muscle reflex responses in cats and humans. Am J Physiol 1994;267:H770–778.

80. Alam M, Smirk FH. Observations in man upon a blood pressure raising reflex arising from the voluntary muscles. J Physiol (Lond) 1937;89:372–383.

81. Sinoway LI, Prophet S, Gorman I, et al. Muscle acidosis during static exercise is associated with calf vasoconstriction. J Appl Physiol 1989;66:429–436.

82. Victor RG, Bertocci LA, Pryor SL, et al. Sympathetic nerve discharge is coupled to muscle cell pH during exercise in humans. J Clin Invest 1988;82:1301–1305.

83. Pryor SL, Lewis SF, Haller, et al RG. Impairment of sympathetic activation during static exercise in patients with muscle phosphorylase deficiency (McArdle's disease). J Clin Invest 1990;85:1444–1449.

84. Ansorge E, Shah S, Augustyniak R, et al. Muscle metaboreflex control of coronary blood flow. Am J Physiol 2002;283:H526–H532.

85. Herr MD, Imadojemu V, Kunselman AR, et al. Characteristics of the muscle mechanoreflex during quadriceps contractions in humans. J Appl Physiol 1999;86:767–772.

86. Melcher A, Donald DE. Maintained ability of carotid baroreflex to regulate arterial pressure during exercise. Am J Physiol 1981;241:H838–H849.

87. Goldsmith SR, Iber C, McArthur CD, et al. Influence of acid-base status on plasma catecholamines during exercise in normal humans. Am J Physiol 1990;258:R1411–R1416.

88. Bouissou P, Defer G, Guezennec CY, et al. Metabolic and blood catecholamine responses to exercise during alkalosis. Med Sci Sports Exerc 1988;20:228–232.

89. Seals DR, Suwarno NO, Dempsey JA. Influence of lung volume on sympathetic nerve discharge in normal humans. Cardiovasc Res 1990;67:130–141.

90. Rodman J, Henderson K, Smith C, et al. Cardiovascular effects of the respiratory muscle metaboreflexes in dogs: rest and exercise. J Appl Physiol 2003;95:1159–1169.

91. Seals DR. Robin Hood for the lungs? A respiratory metaboreflex that "steals" blood flow from locomotor muscles. J Physiol (Lond) 2001;537:2.

92. Ekblom B, Kilbom A, Soltysiak J. Physical training, brady-cardia, and autonomic nervous system. Scand J Clin Lab Invest 1973;32:251–256.

93. Frick MH, Elovainio RO, Somer T. The mechanism of bradycardia evoked by physical training. Cardiology 1967;51:46–54.

94. Kenney WL. Parasympathetic control of resting heart rate: relationship to aerobic power. Med Sci Sports Exerc 1985;17:451–455.

95. Yamamoto K, Miyachi M, Saitoh T, et al. Effects of endurance training on resting and post-exercise cardiac autonomic control. Med Sci Sports Exerc 2001;33:1496–1502.

96. Goldsmith R, Bigger J, Steinman R, et al. Comparison of 24–hour parasympathetic activity in endurance-trained and untrained young men. J Am Coll Cardiol 1992;20:552–558.

97. Herrlich HC, Raab W, Gigee W. Influence of muscular training and of catecholamines on cardiac acetylcholine and cholinesterase. Arch Intern Pharmacodyn 1960;129:201–215.

98. Katona PG, McLean M, Dighton DH, et al. Sympathetic and parasympathetic cardiac control in athletes and nonathletes at rest. J Appl Physiol 1982;52:1652–1657.

99. Meredith TT, Friberg P, Jennings GL, et al. Exercise training lowers resting renal but not cardiac sympathetic activity in humans. Hypertension 1991;18:575–582.

100. Iellamo F, Legramante JM, Pigozzi F, et al. Conversion from vagal to sympathetic predominance with strenuous training in high-performance world class athletes. Circulation 2002;105:2719–2724.

101. Ng AV, Callister R, Johnson DG, et al. Endurance exercise training is associated with elevated basal sympathetic nerve activity in healthy older humans. J Appl Physiol 1994;77:1366–1374.

102. Peronnet F, Cleroux J, Perrault H, et al. Plasma norepinephrine response to exercise before and after training in humans. J Appl Physiol 1981;51:812–815.

103. Jennings G, Nelson L, Nestel P, et al. The effects of changes in physical activity on major cardiovascular risk factors, hemodynamics, sympathetic function, and glucose utilization in man: a controlled study of four levels of activity. Circulation 1986;73:30–40.

104. Poehlman E, Danforth E. Endurance training increases metabolic rate and norepinephrine appearance rate in older individuals. Am J Physiol 1991;261:E233–E239.

105. Marker J, Cryer P, Clutter W. Simplified measurement of norepinephrine kinetics: application to studies of aging and exercise training. Am J Physiol 1994;267:E380–E387.

106. Seals DR. Sympathetic neural adjustments to stress in physically trained and untrained humans. Hypertension 1991;17:36–43.

107. Svedenhag J, Wallin BG, Sundlof G, et al. Skeletal muscle sympathetic activity at rest in trained and untrained subjects. Acta Physiol Scand 1984;120:499–504.

108. Sheldahl LM, Ebert TJ, Cox B, et al. Effect of aerobic training on baroreflex regulation of cardiac and sympathetic function. J Appl Physiol 1994;76:158–165.

109. Ostman-Smith I. Adaptive changes in the sympathetic nervous system and some effector organs of the rat following long term exercise or cold acclimation and the role of cardiac sympathetic nerves in the genesis of compensatory cardiac hypertrophy. Acta Physiol Scand Suppl 1979;477:1–118.

110. Mazzeo RS, Grantham PA. Norepinephrine turnover in various tissues at rest and during exercise: evidence for a training effect. Metabolism 1989;38:479–483.

111. DeSchryver C, DeHerdt P, Lammerant J. Effect of physical training on cardiac catecholamine concentrations. Nature 1967;214:907–908.

112. Hammond HK, White FC, Brunton LL, et al. Association of decreased myocardial beta-receptors and chronotropic response to isoproterenol and exercise in pigs following chronic dynamic exercise. Circ Res 1987;60:720–726.

113. Dela F, Mikines KJ, Von Linstow M, et al. Heart rate and plasma catecholamines during 24 h of everyday life in trained and untrained men. J Appl Physiol 1992;73:2389–2395.

114. Winder WW, Hagberg JM, Hickson RC, et al. Time course of sympathoadrenal adaptation to endurance exercise training in man. J Appl Physiol 1978;45:370–374.

115. Hagberg JM, Hickson RC, McLane JA, et al. Disappearance of norepinephrine from the circulation following strenuous exercise. J Appl Physiol 1979;47:1311–1314.

116. Greiwe JS, Hickner RC, Shah SD, et al. Norepinephrine response to exercise at the same relative intensity before and after endurance exercise training. J Appl Physiol 1999;86:531–535.

117. Ordway GA, Charles JB, Randall DC, et al. Heart rate adaptation to exercise training in cardiac-denervated dogs. J Appl Physiol 1982;52:1586–1590.

118. Wolfel EE, Hiatt WR, Brammell HL, et al. Effects of selective and nonselective beta-adrenergic blockade on mechanisms of exercise conditioning. Circulation 1986;74:664–674.

119. Liang C, Tuttle RR, Hood WB Jr, et al. Conditioning effects of chronic infusions of dobutamine. Comparison with exercise training. J Clin Invest 1979;64:613–619.

120. Fry AC, Kraemer WJ, Van Borselen F, et al. Catecholamine responses to short-term high-intensity resistance exercise overtraining. J Appl Physiol 1994;77:941–946.

121. Peronnet F, Thibault G, Perrault H, et al. Sympathetic response to maximal bicycle exercise before and after leg strength training. Eur J Appl Physiol 1986;55:1–4.

122. Carter JR, Ray CA, Downs EM, et al. Strength training reduces arterial blood pressure but not sympathetic neural activity in young normotensive subjects. J Appl Physiol 2002;94:2212–2216.

123. Ichiyama RM, Gilbert AB, Waldrop TG, et al. Changes in the exercise activation of diencephalic and brainstem cardiorespiratory areas after training. Brain Res 2002;947:225–233.

124. Christou DD, Jones PP, Seals DR. Baroreflex buffering in sedentary and endurance exercise-trained healthy men. Hypertension 2003;41:1219–1222.

125. Grassi G, Seravalle G, Calhoun D, et al. Physical training and baroreceptor control of sympathetic nerve activity in humans. Hypertension 1994;23:294–301.

126. Smith SA, Querry RG, Fadel PJ, et al. Differential baroreflex control of heart rate in sedentary and aerobically fit individuals. Med Sci Sports Exerc 2000;32:1419–1430.

127. Bedford TG, Tipton CM. Exercise training and the arterial baroreflex. J Appl Physiol 1987;63:1926–1932.

128. Bullough RC, Gillette CA, Harris MA, et al. Interaction of acute changes in exercise energy expenditure and energy intake on resting metabolic rate. Am J Clin Nutr 1995;61:473–481.

129. Clausen JP, Klausen K, Rasmussen B, et al. Central and peripheral circulatory changes after training of the arms or the legs. Am J Physiol 1973;225:675–682.

130. Fisher WJ, White MJ. Training-induced adaptations in the central command and peripheral reflex components of the pressor response to isometric exercise of the human triceps surae. J Physiol (Lond) 1999;520:621–628.

131. Hakkinen K, Komi PV. Electromyographic changes during strength training and detraining. Med Sci Sports Exerc 1983;15:455–460.

132. Saltin B, Nazar K, Costill DL, et al. The nature of the training response, peripheral and central adaptation to one-legged exercise. Acta Physiol Scand 1976;96:289–305.

133. Elsner R, Carlson L. Post exercise hyperemia in trained and untrained subjects. J Appl Physiol 1962;17:436–440.

134. Sinoway L, Shenberger J, Leaman G, et al. Forearm training attenuates sympathetic responses to prolonged rhythmic forearm exercise. J Appl Physiol 1996;81:1778–1784.

135. Mostoufi-Moab S, Widmaier EJ, Cornett JA, et al. Forearm training reduces the exercise pressor reflex during ischemic rhythmic handgrip. J Appl Physiol 1998;84:277–283.

136. Delp MD, McAllister RM, Laughlin H. Exercise training alters endothelium-dependent vasoreactivity of rat abdominal aorta. J Appl Physiol 1993;75:1354–1363.

137. Jones PP, Shapiro LF, Keisling GA, et al. Is autonomic support of arterial blood pressure related to habitual exercise status in healthy men? J Physiol (Lond) 2002;540:701–706.

138. Svedenhag J, Martinsson A, Ekblom B, et al. Altered cardiovascular responsiveness to adrenoceptor agonists in endurance-trained men. J Appl Physiol 1991;70:531–538.

139. Wiegman DL, Harris PD, Joshua IG, et al. Decreased vascular sensitivity to norepinephrine following exercise training. J Appl Physiol 1981;51:282–287.

140. LeBlanc J, Boulay M, Dulac S, et al. Metabolic and cardiovascular responses to norepinephrine in trained and non-trained human subjects. J Appl Physiol 1977;42:166–173.

141. Sylvestre-Gervais L, Nadeau A, Nguyen MH, et al. Effects of physical training on beta-adrenergic receptors in rat myocardial tissue. Cardiovasc Res 1982;16:530–534.

142. Stratton JR, Cerqueira MD, Schwartz RS, et al. Differences in cardiovascular responses to isoproterenol in relation to age and exercise training in healthy men. Circulation 1992;86:504–512.

143. Williams RS, Schaible TF, Bishop T, et al. Effects of endurance training on cholinergic and adrenergic receptors of rat heart. J Mol Cell Cardiol 1984;16:395–403.

144. Hopkins MG, Spina RJ, Ehsani AA. Enhanced beta-adrenergic-mediated cardiovascular responses in endurance athletes. J Appl Physiol 1996;80:516–521.

145. Lash JM. Exercise training enhances adrenergic constriction and dilation in the rat spinotrapezius muscle. J Appl Physiol 1998;85:168–174.

146. Lehmann M, Dickhuth HH, Schmid P, et al. Plasma catecholamines, beta-adrenergic receptors, and isoproterenol sensitivity in endurance trained and non-endurance trained volunteers. Eur J Appl Physiol 1984;52:362–369.

147. Evans J, Funk J, Charles J, et al. Endurance training in dogs increases vascular responsiveness to an alpha-1 agonist. J Appl Physiol 1988;65:625–632.

148. Plourde G, Rousseau-Migneron S, Nadeau A. Effect of endurance training on beta-adrenergic system in three different skeletal muscles. J Appl Physiol 1993;74:1641–1646.

CHAPTER 10

The Respiratory System

JEROME A. DEMPSEY, JORDAN D. MILLER, AND LEE M. ROMER

Introduction

Exercise Demands on the Respiratory System

The structure and function of the lung parenchyma, airways, and respiratory muscles and the regulation of respiratory muscle activity by the autonomic nervous system are solely responsible for the first two major steps in oxygen transport from the inspired air to muscle mitochondria. These steps include (a) the difference in oxygen pressure (PO_2) from inspired air to alveolar gas, which is determined solely by the precision with which alveolar ventilation matches tissue metabolic requirements, and (b) the transfer of oxygen from alveolar gas to pulmonary capillary to systemic arterial blood, as determined primarily by the distribution of ventilation to perfusion throughout the lungs' myriad branchings of blood vessels and airways and its 300 million alveolar-capillary gas exchange interfaces. These same respiratory structures are also solely responsible for the precise regulation of carbon dioxide levels in the body (and for much of the regulation of pH). They perform this function by controlling the elimination of carbon dioxide from mixed venous blood, again by providing adequate and precise amounts of ventilation of the alveolar spaces. It is not enough that these structures and controllers simply maintain arterial blood gas homeostasis on a second-by-second basis; this must also be accomplished at a minimum energy expense to the organism. That is, respiratory muscle work must be minimized and breathing remain a truly automatic, involuntary act. Additionally, pulmonary vascular resistance and pressure must remain low so as to avoid excessive loads on the right heart or trauma to the delicate alveolar–capillary interface. At rest, these goals are readily met with use of a minuscule fraction of the structural and functional capabilities of the respiratory system. It is for the extreme challenge presented by the increased metabolic requirements of dynamic muscular exercise that the structure and neural regulation of the respiratory system are ideally designed.

Consider some of the major challenges to the respiratory system presented by heavy intensity exercise:

- Increased muscle metabolism causes mixed venous oxygen content to fall to less than one-fifth of its resting value and mixed venous PCO_2 to double.
- Cardiac output increases to 5 to 6 times resting values, and since all of the cardiac output must go through the lungs all of the time, this poses substantial threats, not only to the time available in the pulmonary capillaries for gas exchange but also to the regulation of pulmonary vascular resistance and capillary pressure and therefore to the containment of plasma water within the pulmonary vasculature.
- Ventilatory requirements of 20 to 30 times rest must be met while the increase in mechanical work required for each breath is minimized. To these ends the medullary respiratory network must integrate a host of sensory feedback and feed-forward stimuli (a) to

ensure that ventilation is driven precisely in proportion to metabolic requirements and (b) to preserve precise synchronization of respiratory motor output to the upper airway and to the primary and accessory pump muscles of the chest and abdominal walls.

- The work produced by both the locomotor muscles and the respiratory muscles increases several fold, and the blood flow requirements of both sets of these essential muscles must be met.

This chapter examines how the healthy human respiratory system is structured and how it is regulated by the nervous system to meet these exercise requirements. Emphasis is on the respiratory physiology of the normal untrained young adult exercising near sea level. However, we will also consider the special needs and adaptations of the respiratory system that accompany healthy aging and physical training and the special circumstances that determine the balance (or imbalance) achieved between metabolic demand and respiratory system capacity in the highly trained endurance athlete.

Control of Breathing

In healthy humans, breathing in all physiological states (including wakefulness, sleep, and exercise) is a remarkably well-controlled phenomenon. Consider that although the partial pressure of oxygen (PO_2) and carbon dioxide (PCO_2) within the alveoli are regulated precisely within a few millimeters of mercury, we are rarely consciously aware of taking a breath, and we effortlessly speak, cough, chew, swallow, and breathe, all through the same airway and using many of the same muscles. The control system that allows this multitasking with such precision and efficiency consists of three highly integrative, overlapping levels of control:

- The central controller (or driver) of respiratory rhythm and pattern
- Sensory inputs
- Distribution and synchronization of respiratory motor output to the appropriate respiratory muscles

A schematic of most known components of the control system coupled with a sketch of the motor pathways from the brain to the respiratory muscles is shown in Figure 10.1. We briefly describe each of these components and the nature of their interactions before attempting to put them together to consider the complex mechanisms of exercise hyperpnea.

The Central Controller of Respiratory Rhythm and Pattern

Nearly a century of research using neural lesioning and intracellular and extracellular neural recordings in mammalian preparations *in vivo* and more recently *in vitro* and *in situ* has begun to unmask at least a significant portion of the complex mystery surrounding the morphology and physiology

of the central respiratory pattern generator. Eupneic breathing rhythm appears to reflect the output of a pontomedullary neuronal circuit. Within the ventral lateral medulla a tiny area labeled the pre-Bötzinger complex and an even smaller adjacent area contain a combination of pacemaker-like neurons linked to a neural network. Together, this hybrid pacemaker and network system is capable of generating an oscillatory, respiratory-like rhythm (1). The rostral area of the pons is also capable of generating a respiratory rhythm (2). Ablation of either of these areas greatly disrupts the normal eupneic rhythm and it seems likely—although very controversial—that the entire pontomedullary network is required for central generation of the respiratory rhythm.

The underlying rhythm from this network is relayed to larger adjacent networks of respiratory premotor medullary neurons (called the ventral respiratory group and the ventral lateral nucleus of the solitary tract). Within these neuronal networks the respiratory pattern is further sculpted in response to several types of sensory inputs, which are added to the basic rhythm (discussed later). This rhythmic pattern is passed on via the spinal cord to the phrenic, intercostal, and abdominal motor nerves, which in turn drive the respiratory pump muscles to generate the appropriate level of negative intrathoracic pressure for a breath. In addition, this same pattern of respiratory output is directed in parallel to cranial motor neurons, which lie primarily in the nucleus ambiguus and project out cranial nerves IX to XII to innervate skeletal muscles of the upper airway, tongue, and smooth involuntary muscles of the trachea and bronchi.

Central Control of the Pattern of Distribution of Efferent Respiratory Motor Output

Although the breathing rhythm is conceptually simple (good air in, bad air out) the pattern of respiratory motor output from premotor neurons in the medulla must be much more than a simple sine wave. Indeed, a carefully sculpted, patterned output containing essential features such as precise timing and amplitude of pump muscle contractions and carefully controlled coordination of activation of the rib cage and the diaphragm musculature is necessary. Equally important, the motor control of the skeletal muscles regulating the extrathoracic (upper) airway, which run from the tip of the nares (alae nasae) to the larynx (posterior cricoarytenoid) must be synchronized precisely with the chest wall pump muscles. This coordination ensures that the upper airway is prepared (via dilation and stiffening) for the subatmospheric intrathoracic pressure generated by the pump muscles with each inspiration.

This precise coordination of motor output requires not only several different types of premotor neurons in the medullary pattern generator but also a means for these neurons to know precisely what each other is doing throughout every millisecond of the breath. Six types of neurons within the central pattern generator have been identified with some (but not complete) certainty: three for inspiration and three for

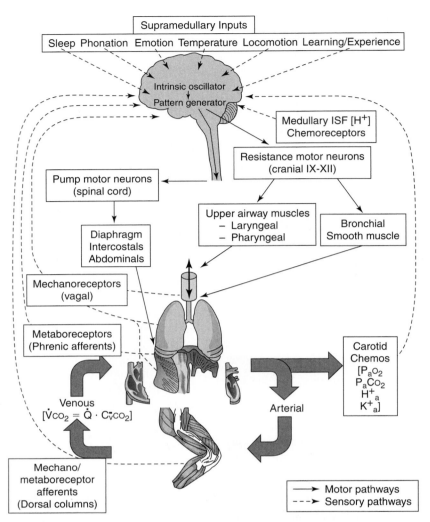

FIGURE 10.1 The three major components of the control system for breathing.
1. *Central controller.* These neurons are in the ventral lateral medulla, consisting of intrinsic oscillator pacemaker neurons and a neuronal network for pattern generation. (Fig. 10.2, *A*). 2. *Sensory inputs* from the periphery, including carotid chemoreceptors, mechanoreceptors from the lung and respiratory and locomotor muscles, metaboreceptors from the respiratory and locomotor muscles, and an additional set of chemoreceptors bathed by the brain's interstitial fluid and located primarily throughout the medulla. Additional inputs to the respiratory pattern generator include those from supramedullary areas of the higher central nervous system, including those from locomotor areas. 3. *Efferent motor outputs* carried in cranial and spinal nerves from the medullary pattern generator are shown to innervate the skeletal muscles of the upper airway and the bronchial smooth muscle as well as the respiratory pump muscles of the chest wall and abdomen.

expiration (Fig. 10.2*A*). Inspiratory and expiratory premotor neurons do not discharge simultaneously, but rather one set of neurons is silent while the other is active (Fig. 10.2*B*). Furthermore, note in Figure 10.2*C* that the onset of inspiratory activity in cranial nerves (innervating the muscles of the upper airway) precedes that of the phrenic nerves. Such coordination among neuronal activities ensures a smooth, mechanically efficient, and effective breath, and it is critically dependent upon the principle of reciprocal inhibition among neurons. For example, the discharge of the inspiratory augmenting neuronal activity inhibits all expiratory neuronal activity and vice versa.

In summary, the past decade has brought significant advances in our understanding of the cellular neuroanatomical basis for respiratory rhythm generation. Nevertheless, considerable controversy exists in this field and huge gaps

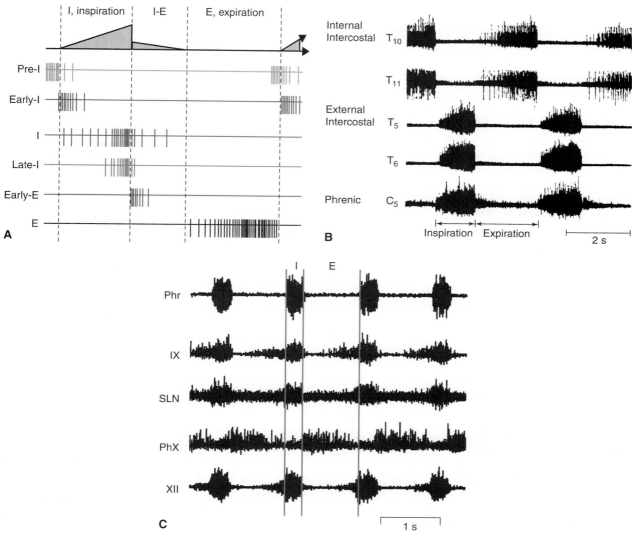

FIGURE 10.2   A. Patterns of discharge of the phrenic nerve (gray area at top) and of brainstem respiratory neurons (traces at bottom) are shown to distinguish three stages in the respiratory cycle, namely inspiration, inspiration-expiration transitions, and expiration, along with six types of respiratory neurons, three during inspiration and three during different phases of expiration. *(Reprinted with permission from Hilaire G, Pasaro R. Genesis and control of the respiratory rhythm in adult mammals. News Physiol Sci 2003;18:24.)* **B.** Spinal respiratory motor nerve activities to the expiratory intercostals (T10 and T11), the inspiratory intercostals (T5 and T6), and the phrenic nerve to the diaphragm. Note the apparent reciprocal inhibition of expiratory nerve activity by inspiratory nerve activity and vice versa. Also, in the phrenic nerve activity the continued activity into early expiration, commonly called post-inspiratory activity of the diaphragm. This activity is abruptly inhibited when ventilation is increased during exercise. *(Reprinted with permission from Hlastala MP, Berger AJ. Physiology of respiration. New York: Oxford University, 1996; 173.)* **C.** Coordination among respiratory motor activities: raw nerve recordings in cranial nerves and the phrenic nerve. The vertical red lines indicate phase transitions between inspiration (I) and expiration (E). The onset of inspiratory activity in cranial nerves to the muscles of the upper airway precedes the onset of activity in the phrenic nerve to the diaphragm. IX, glossopharyngeal nerve innervating muscles of the pharynx and tongue; PhX, pharyngeal branch of the vagus nerve; SLN, superior laryngeal nerve innervating muscles of the larynx and constrictor muscles of the pharynx; XII, hypoglossal nerve innervating intrinsic muscles of the tongue and neighboring pharyngeal muscles. *(Reprinted with permission from Hayashi F, McCrimmon DR. Respiratory motor responses to cranial nerve afferent stimulation in rats. Am J Physiol 1996;271:R1056.)*

in our knowledge persist, even on such fundamental questions as the minimal pontomedullary structures required for the eupneic rhythm. We also have no information on the principles governing exactly how these neuronal networks integrate the underlying rhythm with the multitude of demands imposed by the many and varied sensory inputs to produce the desired breath. A major problem is that while *in vitro* and *in situ* preparations offer great advantages in terms of increased feasibility of intracellular recordings and expanded possibilities for precise ablation and experimental manipulation, these reduced preparations are also unphysiological, and to a highly variable and often indeterminate degree. For example, *in vitro* brainstem spinal cord preparations have no blood supply and are therefore anoxic at their inner core. Furthermore, these preparations are extremely limited in the extent to which they can mimic the ever-changing respiratory behaviors of the *in vivo* state, such as those that occur with hyperpnea. Perhaps even the specific types of neurons (Fig. 10.2A) may take on different roles as total respiratory drive is changed, and each neuronal type may contribute to more than one phase of activity during the respiratory cycle. Almost all *in vivo* preparations used to study rhythm generation require anesthesia or decerebration, procedures which greatly obtund the sensitivity and stability of the neuronal networks under study. A very few chronically instrumented unanesthetized preparations are available and have provided valuable although limited data thus far on the nature of respiratory rhythm genesis in both waking and sleeping states (3).

Sensory Inputs to the Central Pattern Generator

Sensory inputs to the medulla originating in the periphery, the higher central nervous system (CNS), and the medulla itself are essential for the organism to breathe and for respiratory pattern and rhythm to respond appropriately to all physiological states. It is claimed by scientists working with *in vitro* preparations that sensory afferents are not required for formation of the basic respiratory pattern because the respiratory-like rhythm from the phrenic nerve was shown to persist when the preparation was fully deafferented (4). However, the rhythm of the *in vitro* preparation is absolutely dependent upon the addition of a significant concentration of carbon dioxide in the bathing medium; hence, at least one type of sensory input is required for rhythmic respiratory motor output.

We now briefly describe two types of sensory inputs—chemical and mechanical—and leave consideration of sensory inputs related to locomotion to our later discussion of exercise hyperpnea.

Chemoreceptors

Mammals have two types of chemoreceptors. One set is in the periphery and is exposed to arterial blood, and the other is central in the medulla and bathed by brain interstitial fluid.

The carotid bodies lie bilaterally at the bifurcations of the common carotid arteries and sense changes in P_{O_2}, P_{CO_2}, and pH of the arterial blood on the way to the brain (Fig. 10.2). In turn, sensory activity is carried via cranial nerve IX to stimulate the brainstem medullary respiratory neurons and influence motor nerve activity to the respiratory muscles. These small (1-mm diameter) organs receive the highest blood flow per gram of tissue of any organ. These receptors are especially important because they are the only ones responsible for rapidly stimulating ventilation in the presence of oxygen lack. There are neurons in the ventral medulla that can sense oxygen lack, but it is not yet established what role they play in regulating breathing in the intact awake animal when both the central chemoreceptors and the brain are hypoxic.

Figure 10.3B shows the curvilinear response of ventilation to reductions in arterial oxygen pressure (Pa_{O_2}). Normally, arterial carbon dioxide pressure (Pa_{CO_2}) would be reduced when alveolar ventilation ($\dot{V}_A$) was stimulated, but in this case, Pa_{CO_2} was held constant by adding carbon dioxide to the inspired air (so as to demonstrate the full strength of the hypoxic stimulus). The ventilatory response to hypoxia is curvilinear; under isocapnic conditions the response becomes quite brisk at 60 mm Hg Pa_{O_2}. This Pa_{O_2} corresponds to the shoulder of the oxyhemoglobin dissociation curve, below which oxyhemoglobin saturation drops severely and tissue hypoxia probably occurs. Also, reduced P_{O_2} and increased P_{CO_2} both stimulate ventilation via the carotid body, and when applied together, that is, during "asphyxia," they have powerful synergistic effects on ventilatory output (5). The carotid chemoreceptors also respond briskly to ionic changes in the arterial blood, especially metabolically induced changes in pH, that is, metabolic acidosis or alkalosis. Furthermore, with short-term acute changes in metabolic acid-base status, the carotid chemoreceptors are solely responsible for the ventilatory response. Carotid chemoreceptors respond to a reduced P_{O_2} in their environment but do not respond to a reduction in arterial oxygen content *per se* when it is caused by decreased hemoglobin concentration.

How chemoreception occurs within the carotid bodies remains somewhat of a mystery. The microscopic anatomy of this remarkable sensor reveals two types of cells, with the peripheral nerve endings terminating in the type I cells. The sensory nerve fibers emerging from the carotid chemoreceptors join those of the carotid baroreceptors to form the carotid sinus nerve. The cell bodies of this nerve are located in the petrosal sensory ganglion of cranial nerve IX. Oxygen-sensitive potassium channels have recently been discovered within the carotid body cells. Somehow, a low P_{O_2} reduces potassium currents, thereby causing these type I cells to depolarize. As firing frequency increases with hypoxia, calcium enters the cell and causes the release of neurotransmitters that are important in transduction of the signal from the carotid body cells to the sensory nerve fiber.

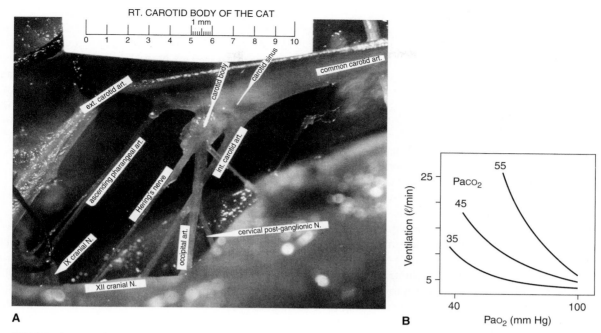

FIGURE 10.3   A. The intact carotid chemoreceptor in the cat. Head is to the left and heart to the right. Note the highly vascularized carotid body at the bifurcation of the common carotid artery. The sensory carotid sinus nerve, labeled here as its older designation, Hering's nerve, projects to the ninth nerve (glossopharyngeal), which in turn projects to the petrosal ganglion and then to the nucleus of the solitary tract. *(Courtesy of Dr. E. H. Vidruk of the University of Wisconsin at Madison.)* **B.** Effects of hypoxia and carbon dioxide on minute ventilation in the normal healthy human. As Pa_{O_2} is reduced (by gradually reducing inspired P_{O_2}), ventilation increases in a hyperbolic fashion. This effect of hypoxia on ventilation is enhanced by increasing arterial P_{CO_2}. Thus in the lowest response curve, arterial P_{CO_2} is maintained at 35 mm Hg and at the highest response curve at 55 mm Hg. These differences in carbon dioxide are achieved by adding carbon dioxide to the inspired gas as the P_{O_2} is reduced. Note the strong interactive (greater than additive) effect of carbon dioxide on the hypoxic ventilatory response.

Some of the **medullary chemoreceptors** have yet to be isolated anatomically, although several locations near the ventrolateral surface of the medulla are very sensitive to changes in interstitial brain fluid pH, especially when pH is changed by an excess or decrease in P_{CO_2} (6) (Fig. 10.3B). The cerebral fluid environment of these medullary chemoreceptors has a closely regulated ionic composition because of the selective permeability of the capillary endothelium of cerebral blood vessels, that is, the so-called blood-brain barrier. Thus, metabolic acids and bases in the plasma enter the brain interstitial fluid very slowly, whereas carbon dioxide crosses readily and changes the pH of the medullary interstitial fluid very quickly and substantially, as the low protein content of cerebrospinal fluid makes it a very poorly buffered fluid.

Collectively, the ventilatory response to increased carbon dioxide in the arterial blood and the brain is a result of both peripheral carotid chemoreceptor and the central medullary chemoreceptor stimulation. In the steady state, after several minutes of a raised Pa_{CO_2}, the medullary chemoreceptors are the major contributors to the increased ventilation. However, the carotid chemoreceptors still respond very strongly to small increases and decreases in Pa_{CO_2}. Furthermore, when

Pa_{CO_2} is changing dynamically, the carotid chemoreceptors are the sole initiators of the ventilatory response.

The ventilatory response to inhaled carbon dioxide is much more linear than to hypoxia. This likely reflects the fact that even very small changes in carbon dioxide will change plasma and tissue pH and the sensitive ventilatory response to acute changes in carbon dioxide is designed to defend pH. On the other hand, when Pa_{O_2} is reduced, the high affinity of hemoglobin for oxygen at Pa_{O_2} levels greater than 70 mm Hg prevents appreciable reductions in oxyhemoglobin saturation and systemic oxygen transport until Pa_{O_2} is greatly reduced. Thus, the ventilatory response to "pure" hypoxemia is more linearly related to the percentage of oxyhemoglobin saturation.

Chemoreceptors perform classical negative feedback control of breathing, so that they are intimately involved as error detectors every time breathing is changed. For example, if for any reason alveolar ventilation is increased or reduced out of proportion to tissue carbon dioxide production or oxygen consumption, alveolar and arterial P_{CO_2} and P_{O_2} will rise or fall, respectively. Within the circulation time from the alveoli to the carotid chemoreceptor (<10 seconds) the carotid chemoreceptors will react and change phrenic nerve output and ventilation in a direction to restore the

PCO_2 to its normal range. Roughly 15 to 20 seconds later, the medullary chemoreceptors will follow suit and respond to the lingering changes in PCO_2. Accordingly, these chemoreceptors are the vigilant guardians of their own chemical environment and—as we shall see—are important to the regulation of exercise ventilation.

Mechanical Feedback

To maintain precise and mechanically efficient control of breathing, it is crucial that the pattern generating neurons in the medulla be constantly made aware of the mechanical state of the lung and the mechanical and metabolic state of the respiratory muscles. Accordingly, the lung and airways are richly innervated by vagal afferents serving several types of receptors and afferent fibers. The slowly adapting fibers in the lung perform a unique role in the control of breathing efficiency, because they respond to lung stretch and volume by providing feedback to the medulla via the vagus nerves to inhibit inspiration. This inhibitory effect limits end-inspiratory lung volume, usually to the linear portion of the lung's compliance curve, thereby avoiding the increased stiffness of the lung at high lung volumes. Input from the pontine respiratory neurons to the medullary pattern generator provides an additional source of inhibition to inspiration. Lung stretch receptors also provide an excitatory input to the medullary respiratory neurons in response to lung deflation; thus they may be responsible for activating augmented inspirations (or sighs), which occur periodically to prevent excessive airway narrowing at low lung volumes. Additional vagally mediated receptors in the lung parenchyma include unmyelinated C-fiber endings, which respond to changes in lung interstitial fluid pressure and have marked effects on ventilatory drive and frequency. Finally, many other receptors in the intrathoracic airways are sensitive to pressure deformation of the mucosal wall, particulate matter, temperature, and so on, most of which cause coughing or changes in bronchial smooth muscle tone to protect the lung from injury and foreign matter.

Respiratory muscles, including the diaphragm and abdominal muscles, have receptors that are sensitive to both mechanical changes (type III afferents) and to metabolic changes (type IV afferents) in the contracting muscle and send feedback to the medulla via afferent fibers within the major motor nerves, such as the phrenic, which innervates the diaphragm. Feedback from these receptors exerts significant effects on the control of both ventilation and the circulation (discussed in the section "Cardiorespiratory Interactions," later in the chapter). Afferent feedback from upper airway skeletal muscles, responding to pressure and airway wall deformation, is also very important for the activation of cranial nerve motor activity directed at stiffening and abducting the pharyngeal and laryngeal musculature for purposes of protecting upper airway patency.

Significant influences from these types of mechanoreceptor feedback on the control of breathing are well established for laboratory mammals, including rats, cats, dogs, and others. Vagal feedback from lung stretch has also been shown to be very powerful in the newborn human. However, the role of these mechanoreceptor feedback mechanisms in adult humans is less well established. Recent work using mechanical ventilators to alter tidal volumes in sleeping humans (to avoid behavioral responses to lung inflation) and in patients with denervated transplanted lungs has suggested that the pulmonary stretch reflex does play a role in inhibiting inspiratory ventilatory drive in adult humans, although the sensitivity to changes in lung volume appears to be significantly less than in most laboratory mammals (7).

Memory Effects of Ventilatory Stimuli: Short-Term Potentiation

The full effects of any given stimulus to breathe (e.g., chemoreceptor stimulation) or inhibition to breathe (e.g., vagal feedback) on respiratory motor output last beyond the time of application of the stimulus. Examples of this memory response are shown during and following electrical stimulation of the carotid sinus nerve in the anesthetized animal (i.e., mimicking carotid body stimulation) and also following brief hypoxic ventilatory stimulation in the sleeping human (8) (Fig. 10.4, A and B). These aftereffects on respiratory motor output also occur in response to a wide variety of sensory stimuli, including those from central chemoreceptors or skeletal muscle (excitatory) or from vagal or superior laryngeal nerves (inhibitory). So just as activation of a synapse and the firing of any neuron leaves behind an altered state of the neuron, or a memory of the preceding excitatory events, the network of neurons in the respiratory pattern generator also displays an intrinsic after-discharge, or short-term potentiation (STP), in response to its own neuronal activity. These lingering aftereffects are attributed to changes in the presynaptic membrane, as repetitive neuronal firing causes gradual accumulation of Ca^{++} and increased neurotransmitter release, and the slow exponential decline in neural discharge is attributable to a slow removal of Ca^{++} from nerve terminals.

The implications of STP for understanding the control of breathing are many, including the realization that the full ventilatory response to a given stimulus does not occur immediately and that STP acts as a self-amplifying effect to boost the ventilatory output. STP also acts as a smoothing or stabilizing effect on the ventilatory response, preventing overshoots and undershoots in ventilation during periods of transition between increases and decreases in ventilatory stimuli.

Exercise Hyperpnea

Requirements for Hyperpnea

The extra ventilation generated during exercise must accomplish two aims. First, increased alveolar ventilation must be proportional to the increase in VCO_2 and VO_2 demanded by the muscular work according to the strict rules of the

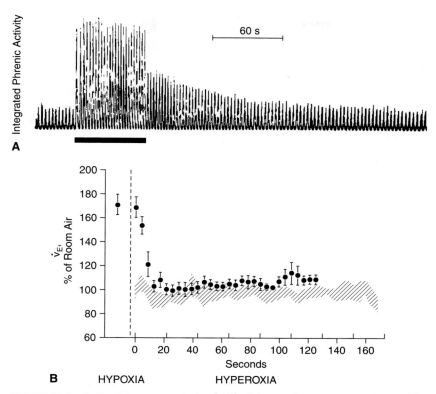

FIGURE 10.4 **A.** Short-term potentiation (STP) of the ventilatory response to carotid chemoreceptor stimulation. Electrical stimulation of the carotid sinus nerve was used to suddenly increase carotid sinus nerve activity and to suddenly withdraw that activity in the anesthetized cat. Phrenic nerve activity increased during carotid sinus nerve stimulation and then slowly dissipated to return to control several seconds following the sudden cessation of carotid sinus nerve stimulation. *(Reprinted with permission from Eldridge FL, Gill-Kumar P. Lack of effect of vagal afferent input on central neural respiratory after discharge. J Appl Physiol 1978;45:342.)* **B.** Similar STP-like effects have been shown in sleeping humans using brief periods of isocapneic hypoxia to stimulate ventilation and then inspiration of hyperoxic gas to achieve sudden cessation of carotid chemoreceptor stimulation. Note that 45 seconds of isocapneic hypoxia increased ventilation ($\dot{V}_E$) to 170% of baseline $\dot{V}_E$. Then, after the third breath of hyperoxia, $\dot{V}_E$ remained more than 20% greater than control and did not return completely to control (hatched area) until the ninth hyperoxic recovery breath following hypoxia. *(Reprinted with permission from Badr MS, Skatrud JB, Dempsey JA. Determinants of poststimulus potentiation in humans during NREM sleep. J Appl Physiol 1992;73:1963.)*

alveolar gas equations. These relationships are also shown graphically in Figure 10.5.

$$\text{Alveolar } P_{O_2}/P_{CO_2} \approx \text{metabolic requirement}$$
$$\div \text{ventilatory supply}$$
$$P_{CO_2} = \left[\dot{V}_{CO_2} \div \dot{V}_A\right] K$$
$$P_{aO_2} = P_{IO_2} - \left[\dot{V}_{O_2} \div \dot{V}_A\right] K$$
$$[\text{Equation 10.1}]$$

where $\dot{V}_{CO_2}$ = volume of carbon dioxide expired per minute, $\dot{V}_A$ = alveolar ventilation, K = constant = 0.863, $\dot{V}_{O_2}$ = volume of oxygen consumed per minute.

Calculation of alveolar gases may be made from these equations if $\dot{V}_{O_2}$ and $\dot{V}_{CO_2}$ are expressed in milliliters per meter and $\dot{V}_A$ is expressed in liters per minute. The constant K then becomes 0.863. For example, if the inspired P_{O_2} is 150 mm Hg, $\dot{V}_{O_2}$ is 240 mL · min⁻¹ STPD, and $\dot{V}_A$ is 4.0 L · min⁻¹ BTPS, alveolar P_{O_2} is 98 mm Hg. The same applies to the calculation of alveolar P_{O_2}, only this is simplified because carbon dioxide is virtually absent in the inspired air.

Problem: Use Equation 10.1 and inspired P_{O_2} to calculate what would happen to alveolar P_{CO_2} and P_{O_2} if, for example, you exercise at a very mild intensity requiring a fourfold increase from rest in $\dot{V}_{O_2}$ and $\dot{V}_{CO_2}$ (e.g., $\dot{V}_{O_2}$ and $\dot{V}_{CO_2}$ = 0.25 L · min⁻¹ at rest and 1.0 L · min⁻¹ during exercise) but failed to increase your $\dot{V}_A$ above a resting level of 4.0 L · min⁻¹. Further, determine how much you would have to increase $\dot{V}_A$ during

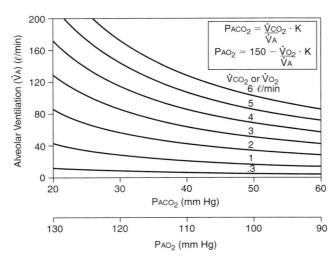

FIGURE 10.5 Graphical representation of the relationships between alveolar ventilation and $P_{A_{CO_2}}$ at varying $\dot{V}_{O_2}$ and between alveolar ventilation and $P_{A_{CO_2}}$ at varying $\dot{V}_{CO_2}$. All $P_{A_{CO_2}}$ values are for breathing room air near sea level. To estimate total ventilation during exercise from the alveolar ventilation, multiply the $\dot{V}_A$ by 1.15. This assumes an average dead space to tidal volume ratio (V_D/V_T) of 0.15 throughout exercise. Because of the hyperbolic nature of $\dot{V}_A$ to Pa_{CO_2}, note the following circumstances. In a normally fit subject at a $\dot{V}_{CO_2}$ of 3.5 L · min⁻¹ at maximum exercise, this requires an alveolar ventilation of about 80 L · min⁻¹ to maintain Pa_{CO_2} constant at resting value, that is, 40 mm Hg. To achieve an average degree of hyperventilation at maximum exercise, which would drive Pa_{CO_2} down to about 30 mm Hg, an alveolar ventilation of about 95 to 100 L · min⁻¹ is required (and a total minute ventilation of 100 to 115 L · min⁻¹). Contrast this ventilatory requirement to that in a highly trained individual of similar body mass to the untrained but with a $\dot{V}_{CO_2}$ of 6 L · min⁻¹. To achieve the same amount of alveolar hyperventilation (Pa_{CO_2} = 30 mm Hg and Pa_{O_2} = 120 mm Hg) the highly trained subject would require an alveolar ventilation of 180 L · min⁻¹, or slightly over 200 L · min⁻¹ total ventilation.

this same level of exercise to maintain alveolar P_{CO_2} and P_{O_2} precisely at their resting levels.

Clearly then, to protect the alveolar gases, that is, the first line of defense in the oxygen transport system, you must increase your $\dot{V}_A$ quickly and precisely in tune with the metabolic requirement. Picture the alveolar gas as a compartment of gas that resides between the conducting airways (source of fresh inspired air and of dead space air) and the pulmonary capillaries (source of metabolic carbon dioxide brought to the lung in the venous blood and oxygen taken up from the lung). If the alveolar gases are not protected, Pa_{O_2} and Pa_{CO_2} will quickly deteriorate, and oxygen transport to tissue and elimination of carbon dioxide and tissue acid-base status will be severely compromised. Also, recall that all of the total ventilation ($\dot{V}_E = f_R \times V_T$, where $\dot{V}_E$ is minute ventilation, f_R is respiratory frequency, and V_T is tidal volume) does not completely aerate the alveoli; rather, about

one-third of each breath in the resting subject is dead space air, defined as gas low in oxygen and high in carbon dioxide that remains in the lungs' conducting airways at end of expiration and must be inhaled into the alveoli on each subsequent inspiration. Each breath has a dead space volume (V_D) that does not fully aerate the alveoli; thus the higher the breathing frequency the greater the contribution of dead space ventilation to total ventilation.

$$\begin{bmatrix} \text{Alveolar ventilation } (\dot{V}_A)(L \cdot min^{-1}) = f_R \times \dot{V}_E \\ \times (1 - V_D/V_T) \end{bmatrix}$$
[Equation 10.2]

Fortunately, this dead space gas, as a fraction of the increasing tidal volume, is reduced during exercise at a time when the demand for $\dot{V}_A$ is high.

The second requisite of the exercise hyperpnea is that the work and metabolic cost of the augmented ventilation be minimized. We simply cannot expend a great deal of energy and devote an excessive portion of our cardiac output to our respiratory muscles during exercise, when the blood flow and $\dot{V}_{O_2}$ of locomotor muscles must be a top priority. Furthermore, we cannot afford to be made aware of our breathing effort to the point of even mild distraction from the locomotor tasks at hand.

The Optimal Response Strategy

So given these multiple requisites, the ideal hyperpneic response to increasing exercise intensities would contain the following features. First, $\dot{V}_A$ must increase in proportion to metabolic requirements so that alveolar gases are maintained or improved. The increase in $\dot{V}_A$ must not be too much (energetically wasteful, creating hypocapnia and alkalosis) or too little (causing hypercapnia, acidosis, and hypoxemia), and the speed of the response must be neither too slow nor too fast.

Second, during exercise of heavy or prolonged intensities or varying durations, the control system must be sensitive to and capable of responding to any special needs for extra alveolar ventilation beyond the basic metabolic requirements of a rising tissue carbon dioxide production.

Third, a carefully selected combination of increased frequency and tidal volume must be achieved, taking into account the need for minimizing dead space ventilation (i.e., the increase in breathing frequency (f_b) should not be excessive). At the same time, this combination protects against an excessive increase in V_T, which would require excessive generation of subatmospheric intrathoracic pressures and therefore large amounts of work by the inspiratory muscles (discussed later).

Fourth, the work of breathing must be shared and carefully coordinated among all inspiratory, expiratory, and airway muscles. Further, respiratory muscle length must be carefully guarded and optimized so that force production is maximized for a given motor command.

Finally, underlying a precise neural control system for regulating ventilation and breathing pattern must be adequate structural capacities of the respiratory muscles. They must be capable of producing and sustaining the large forces necessary for changing intrathoracic pressure as required across the continuum of demands for ventilation with increasing exercise intensity. Similarly, lung and airway structural capacities must be capable of responding to the pressure changes and producing the appropriate volumes and flow rates.

This combination of a highly sensitive multifaceted control system with an adequately structured lung and chest wall exists in healthy subjects across most of the lifespan. The result is—with few exceptions—a nearly perfect and highly efficient ventilatory response to exercise. We now describe this response and examine in detail some of the proposed underlying mechanisms.

The Primary Stimulus for Exercise Hyperpnea

In Figure 10.6, *A* and *B* and in Table 10.1 are shown the well-established hallmarks of the ventilatory response to mild and moderate dynamic exercise requiring less than 60% $\dot{V}O_{2max}$. First, ventilation increases abruptly from resting levels at the onset of exercise and then increases more gradually over time until a steady state is achieved. Second, the steady-state ventilatory response is almost directly in proportion to the increase in $\dot{V}CO_2$. Accordingly, throughout the range of mild to moderate exercise, alveolar PO_2 is controlled within 5 to 10% of resting levels, and the control of $PaCO_2$, PaO_2 and pH is also tightly regulated. This tight relationship between $\dot{V}A$ and $\dot{V}CO_2$ holds for all types of large-muscle exercise, such as cycling, walking, and running. However, a tendency for a mild hyperventilatory response to exercise is fairly common during running (rather than walking) and during exercise with smaller muscle groups, such as with the arms in humans. Most fur-bearing quadrupeds also show a moderate degree of hyperventilation and respiratory alkalosis during mild exercise. The time course of the ventilatory response to exercise onset (from a baseline of rest) is very fast, usually faster than the concomitant rate of rise of cardiac output and $\dot{V}CO_2$, resulting in transient levels of mild hypocapnia. However, if an increase in exercise intensity is initiated from milder exercise (rather than rest) the increase in $\dot{V}A$ is in closer proportion to the increase in $\dot{V}CO_2$, and $PaCO_2$ changes very little. This difference between ventilatory changes from the resting to the exercise baseline suggests that some extra behavioral response may be causing the transient hyperventilation often noted in the transition from rest to exercise.

For more than 130 years physiologists have been fascinated with the power and precision of this hyperpneic response to exercise, and many have asked the same question, namely: What mechanism will stimulate ventilation in direct proportion to the increasing production of carbon dioxide by the working muscles?

Several candidate stimuli and heated controversies have emerged; they are based on ingenious experiments performed using humans and animal models. The primary candidates include the following:

- Carbon dioxide flow ($\dot{Q} \cdot C\bar{v}CO_2$) (where $\dot{Q}$ = pulmonary blood flow in liters/minute and $C\bar{v}CO_2$ = CO_2 content in the mixed venous blood in mL CO_2/100 mL blood). Ventilation may be influenced by the sensing of this signal (or either of its components) by afferents located within the lung or in circulation on either the right or left side of the lung.
- Locomotor muscle mechanoreceptors and metaboreceptors sensitive to the muscle's work rate, muscle metabolite accumulation, and/or blood vessel distension
- Central locomotor command proportional to the work rate required by the locomotor muscles

Of course, all of these potential mechanisms occur simultaneously during exercise. So the experimental approach to teasing out a role for each of these stimuli has been to isolate the specific stimulus and determine whether it alone will produce a physiological, hyperpneic, exerciselike response.

Carbon Dioxide Flow to the Lung

This humoral mechanism is extremely attractive because of the nearly perfect correlation of increases in $\dot{V}A$ to $\dot{V}CO_2$ with steady-state exercise and because the proposed primary driver to increasing $\dot{V}A$ (i.e., carbon dioxide) is also the controlled variable. Now, how can one isolate this humoral stimulus and yet be sure that any change in carbon dioxide is not seen on the arterial (as well as the venous) side of the circulation by the carotid chemoreceptors? Remember, $PaCO_2$ remains very constant during exercise, and therefore any significant changes in $PaCO_2$ (or PaO_2 or arterial pH) would not mimic the exercise response and would bring additional chemoreceptors into play that would not ordinarily be a factor. The approach has been to use an extracorporeal gas exchanger in resting experimental animals (dogs or sheep) attached to the inferior vena cava so that mixed venous carbon dioxide and/or blood flow could be raised or lowered over a limited range. When carbon dioxide flow to the lung $C\bar{v}CO_2 \cdot \dot{Q}$) was changed in either the resting awake or anesthetized animal, $\dot{V}A$ changed in proportion to the change in $\dot{V}CO_2$. Amazingly, in one study using docile, awake sheep, as CO_2 was scrubbed from the venous return, $\dot{V}A$ fell until prolonged apneas ensued (9). Other investigators argued that very small changes in $PaCO_2$ occurred during venous loading and unloading and that these changes were sufficient to explain much or all of the observed ventilatory response. One answer to this controversy was to use two extracorporeal gas exchangers in the anesthetized animal—one to change $C\bar{v}CO_2 \cdot \dot{Q}$ and the other to control carotid arterial blood gases (to be absolutely sure that the $PaCO_2$ was maintained constant at baseline values). Even

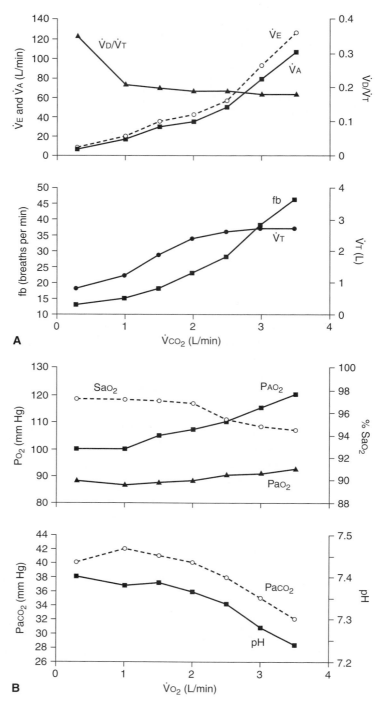

FIGURE 10.6 **A.** Ventilatory responses to progressive increases in work rate in a normal trained healthy young man ($\dot{V}_{O_{2max}} = 45$ mL $\cdot$ kg^{-1} $\cdot$ min^{-1}). $\dot{V}_E$, total minute ventilation; $\dot{V}_A$, alveolar ventilation; V_D/V_T, dead space to tidal volume ratio; fb, breathing frequency; V_T = tidal volume; $\dot{V}_{CO_2}$, CO_2 production. **B.** Arterial blood gases and acid-base status during progressive steady-state increases in work rate. Sa_{O_2}, percent oxyhemoglobin saturation; $P_{A_{O_2}}$, alveolar oxygen; Pa_{O_2}, arterial P_{O_2}; Pa_{CO_2}, arterial P_{CO_2}; pH, arterial pH. The fall in pH at the two heaviest work rates is caused by a rise in the concentration of lactic acid and a reduction in plasma [HCO^3] in arterial blood. Pa_{CO_2} is fairly constant over the first four work rates but falls commensurately with the metabolic acidosis at the two heaviest work rates. Thus the arterial blood acid-base status at the final two workloads is primary metabolic acidosis partially compensated by hyperventilation (and hypocapnia).

| TABLE 10.1 | Representative Mean Values for Ventilation, Pulmonary Gas Exchange, Arterial and Mixed Venous Blood Characteristics, and the Pulmonary Circulation at Rest and During Submaximal and Maximal Exercise at Sea Level |

						Highly Trained Athletes*	
% $\dot{V}O_{2max}$	Rest	Mild	Moderate	Heavy	Maximum	Sa O_2 = 95%	Sa O_2 = 88%
Breathing pattern							
$\dot{V}O_2$ (L · min^{-1})	0.30	0.90	1.80	2.70	3.00	5.25	5.25
$\dot{V}CO_2$ (L · min^{-1})	0.24	0.77	1.71	2.85	3.30	6.04	6.04
$\dot{V}E$ (L · min^{-1})	8.0	22.00	51.00	90.00	113.00	183	168
$\dot{V}A$ (L · min^{-1})	5.3	18.00	41.00	74.00	93.00	150	138
V_T (L)	0.65	1.20	2.20	2.70	2.70	3.1	2.9
fb	12.0	18.00	23.00	33.00	42.00	59	58
V_D/V_T	0.35	0.21	0.19	0.18	0.18	.18	.18
EELV (% TLC)	0.50	0.46	0.44	0.42	0.42	.48	.48
Gas exchange and arterial blood characteristics							
PaO_2 (mm Hg)	91	93	92	92	92	85	70
PAO_2 (mm Hg)	96	101	107	114	117	115	112
$PaCO_2$ (mm Hg)	39	38	36	33	31	35	38
A-aDO_2 (mm Hg)	5	8	15	22	25	30	42
pH	7.4	7.38	7.34	7.29	7.28	7.27	7.27
SaO_2 (%)	97	97	96.5	95.5	95	95	88
$\dot{V}A/\dot{Q}$	1.1	2	3	3.7	4.4	4.4	4.1
Arterial O_2, mL O_2 · 100 mL^{-1}	20.5	20.5	20.4	20.2	20.1	20.1	18.6
Mixed venous O_2 (mL O_2 · 100 mL^{-1}	16	9.5	7.4	5.1	4.1	3.1	1.6
Pulmonary circulation							
CO (L · min^{-1})	5	9	14	20	21	34	34
PCBV (mL)	83	107	137	173	180	220 to 260	220–260
Mean red cell transit time (s)	1.0	0.71	0.59	0.52	0.51	.39 to .45	.39 to .45
Ppa (mm Hg)	12	16	21	27	28	41	41
PVR (mm Hg · L · min^{-1})	2.4	1.76	1.49	1.35	1.33	1.21	1.21

Subjects were healthy untrained young adults aged 30 years, body mass 70 kg, $\dot{V}O_{2max}$ 40–45 mL · kg^{-1} · min^{-1}). Also shown are representative mean values during maximal exercise in highly trained athletes aged 30 years, body mass 70 kg, $\dot{V}O_{2max}$ 75 mL · kg^{-1} · min^{-1}. One group had an arterial oxyhemoglobin saturation of 95% and another of 88%. Endurance-trained subjects with high $\dot{V}O_{2max}$ show a diverse pulmonary gas exchange response at maximum exercise, as evidenced by the significant arterial hypoxemia in some but not in others.
$\dot{V}E$, minute ventilation; $\dot{V}A$, alveolar ventilation; V_T, tidal volume; fb, breathing frequency; V_D/V_T, fraction of dead space to tidal volume; EELV, end-expiratory lung volume; PaO_2, partial pressure of arterial oxygen; PAO_2, partial pressure of alveolar oxygen; $PaCO_2$, partial pressure of arterial carbon dioxide; A-aDO_2, alveolar to arterial PO_2 difference; SaO_2, saturation of hemoglobin with oxygen; $\dot{V}A:\dot{Q}$, relation of alveolar ventilation to perfusion; CO, cardiac output; PCBV, pulmonary capillary blood volume; Ppa, pulmonary artery pressure; PVR, pulmonary vascular resistance.
Pulmonary capillary blood volume calculated from Hsia CC, McBrayer DG, Ramanathan M. Reference values of pulmonary diffusing capacity during exercise by a rebreathing technique. Am J Respir Crit Care Med 1995;152:658–665.
Mean pressure in the pulmonary artery and pulmonary vascular resistance calculated from Reeves JT, Dempsey JA, Grover RF. Pulmonary circulation during exercise. In Weir EK, Reeves JT, eds. Pulmonary Vascular Physiology and Pathophysiology. New York: Marcel Dekker, 1989;107–133.
Cardiac output calculated from Rowell L. Human Cardiovascular Control. New York: Oxford University, 1993;162–203.
All other data compiled from authors' laboratory.

with these stringent controls, significant ventilatory responses to changes in pulmonary $C\bar{v}CO_2 \cdot \dot{Q}$, *per se*, were still obtained (10).

Other approaches examining the carbon dioxide flow hypothesis in resting humans have documented a proportional sensitivity of ventilation to small changes in carbon dioxide flow, including the following:

- The increased isocapnic ventilatory response to increases in $\dot{V}CO_2$ and respiratory quotient induced by augmenting the proportion of carbohydrate in the diet.
- The reduction in ventilation (and unstable breathing) produced in renal dialysis patients produced by lowering the carbon dioxide in the dialysate (and therefore in the venous return).

- The increase in ventilation occurring in proportion to the coincident increase in $\dot{V}CO_2$ caused by electrically stimulating the lower limb muscles to contract in patients with complete spinal cord lesions. Carbon dioxide flow would be the main mechanism for the hyperpnea in the absence of functional afferent neural pathways from contracting limbs to medulla and with no apparent central command (also discussed later).

There is little doubt, then, that carbon dioxide flow *per se* (i.e., without accompanying locomotion) does influence ventilation, but how? Several possible mechanisms have been investigated. For example, vagally mediated feedback receptors do exist on both the right and left sides of the pulmonary circulation; they mediate increases in ventilation in response to infused acid solutions and to changes in vascular pressures. Furthermore, the phasic ventilation of the lung causes intrabreath fluctuations in alveolar and also in systemic $PaCO_2$ and PaO_2, and these fluctuations are sensed by and can influence the sensory output from the carotid chemoreceptors. These PCO_2 fluctuations are augmented around a constant mean value as carbon dioxide returning to the lungs increases during exercise.

To summarize, both correlational data linking $\dot{V}CO_2$ to $\dot{V}A$ during whole-body dynamic exercise and the logical appeal of self-regulation of carbon dioxide as the dependent variable are excellent points in support of carbon dioxide flow–linked mechanisms. Furthermore, as outlined previously, isolated studies in the resting (and usually anesthetized) animal show that feedback receptors on both the right and left side of the circulations do exist and are ideally situated to influence ventilation quickly in response to each of the components of carbon dioxide flow. This broaches the next question: is the sensitivity of these receptors sufficient to produce the 10- to 12-fold increases in steady-state ventilation above resting levels that accompany light to moderate dynamic exercise?

The bulk of evidence speaks against such a major role in exercise hyperpnea for these carbon dioxide flow feedback receptors (10). For example, artificially controlling stroke volume, cardiac output, and therefore carbon dioxide flow in exercising animals did not produce concomitant or proportional changes in $\dot{V}A$. (11). Also, the extracorporeal gas exchange studies in awake animals (as cited earlier) were conducted over quite narrow ranges of increasing $\dot{V}CO_2$, in which even small changes in $PaCO_2$, (i.e., within the measurement error) could have explained the entire observed ventilatory response. Furthermore, enhanced fluctuations in $PaCO_2$ and arterial pH were shown *to modulate but not to stimulate* ventilation to a significant extent. Finally, these chemoreceptors (or flow measurement receptors) are not required for the normal hyperpnea, as shown by the normal isocapnic ventilatory responses to steady-state exercise obtained in human heart and/or heart-lung transplant recipients, in humans with denervated carotid bodies studied following surgery, or an animal model studied both before and after vagal or carotid body denervations.

Conclusion

Collectively, we think the findings in both animal models and humans point to an essential role for carbon dioxide flow ($\dot{V}CO_2$), possibly mediated via right-sided feedback receptors, in the very sensitive regulation of breathing near resting eupneic levels. This metabolic rate effect on normal eupnea may be viewed as forming the essential underpinning to the control of breathing. In fact, this metabolic rate effect also remains a very important determinant of ventilatory output, even in the presence of other strong stimuli, such as hypoxia, which has the dual effect of simultaneously increasing chemoreceptor stimulation and reducing whole-body metabolic rate (14). However, the control of exercise hyperpnea clearly requires additional more powerful stimuli to ventilation, which are engaged by the act of locomotion. At first glance it may appear as though these mostly nonmetabolic locomotor-linked stimuli do not fit with the logical arterial blood gas homeostatic role for hyperpnea (as was clearly the case for carbon dioxide flow). Indeed, it is logical that the controlled variable (PCO_2) should also have a major say in its means of control (i.e., alveolar ventilation). On the other hand, with dynamic exercise there is also a highly predictable and linear relationship between increasing work rate and metabolic rate. Accordingly, the tight relationship of increasing $\dot{V}A$ to $\dot{V}CO_2$ may be attributed more to strictly locomotor-related rather than to metabolic or cardiovascular linked ventilatory control mechanisms. We now examine these locomotor-linked mechanisms.

Feedback From Working Locomotor Muscles

It is well established from studies in anesthetized animals and in isolated muscle that various types of receptors in limb skeletal muscle and tendons are sensitive to mechanical events (stretch, pressure, tension), to metabolic changes produced by contracting limb skeletal muscle (lactic acid and bradykinin), and also to the venous vascular distention caused by increasing muscle blood flow (15). The most important nerve fibers sensing these perturbations in muscle are those that are very thinly myelinated or unmyelinated, classified as type III (primarily mechanical) and type IV (primarily metabolic), respectively. These skeletal muscle afferents synapse in the laminae of the dorsal horn of the spinal cord and project to the medulla, including the nucleus of the solitary tract relay area, which also receives other cardiopulmonary afferents carried in the vagus and glossopharyngeal nerves. When these afferent fibers are adequately stimulated, electrically, pharmacologically, or via perfusion of acid or other metabolites into their arterial blood supply, phrenic nerve activity and breathing frequency increase, as do sympathetic nerve activity, systemic vascular resistance, and blood pressure. These cardiorespiratory responses are prevented by ganglionic blockade or by lesioning of the sensory nervous pathways. Furthermore, when muscle contraction was caused by direct electrical stimulation and the venous efflu-ent blood from the working muscle was directed to another animal via cross circulation anastomosis—thereby eliminat-ing the carbon dioxide flow stimulus—hyperpnea was read-ily achieved. There is also limited evidence in humans supporting a significant role for peripheral muscle feedback in exercise hyperpnea, including the hyperpneic responses to electrical stimulation of muscle and to muscle ischemia.

This evidence shows that ventilatory and especially cir-culatory responses to stimuli originating in the locomotor muscle do occur; but what are these stimuli and how effective are they during physiological exercise? First, it seems as though a sensitive and potent stimulus for activating the type III and IV sensory afferents is simply rhythmic muscle contraction. This was demonstrated by stimulating motor areas of the higher CNS in the decorticate cat and observing activation of type III and IV afferents in the biceps femoris muscle during evoked rhythmic contractions, even of mild intensity (16). Increasing the force of limb muscle contraction *per se* has lit-tle effect on ventilatory output, whereas frequency of limb movement and changes in the distention of veins within the muscle and/or intramuscular pressure appear to have marked effects on stimulating the sensory afferent input to the medulla and increasing ventilation. The proposed relationship of mus-cle venous distention and muscle blood flow to sensory out-put and ventilatory drive is attractive in a teleological sense because it links muscle blood flow to the hyperpnea and blood flow is a critical variable in determining carbon dioxide flow to the lung. Furthermore, many of the type III and IV fibers terminate within the adventitia of the venous vascula-ture of the muscle and respond to the mechanical changes as-sociated with venous distention (17).

In summary, when rhythmic muscle contraction is viewed as an isolated stimulus, it appears as though it pro-vides sufficient sensory feedback stimulation to increase ven-tilation. This feedback mechanism also has appeal simply because there are extremely vast numbers of these afferent re-ceptors throughout the large mass of skeletal muscle tissue, and they are therefore available for substantial sensory input during muscle contraction. The relatively recent evidence linking local muscle blood flow and muscle receptors to ex-ercise hyperpnea is especially worth further investigation be-cause it incorporates a powerful feedback effect—relative to previously proposed carbon dioxide flow mechanisms operat-ing in the central circulation or at the carotid chemoreceptors (see previous section)—to explain the $\dot{V}A$–$\dot{V}CO_2$ relationship. As to the relative role of this mechanism in the total scheme of exercise hyperpnea, we speculate that it contributes a sig-nificant portion of both the immediate increase in ventilation at exercise onset and the sustained hyperpnea in the steady state. This proposed feedback role for hyperpnea, while a sig-nificant one, contrasts with the more critical dependence of sympathetic vasoconstrictor outflow responses on these feed-back influences from metabolite accumulation in the con-tracting muscles.

Central Command and Exercise Hyperpnea

The third proposal for a major locomotor-induced primary stimulus to exercise hyperpnea is the *feed-forward* pathway, as opposed to the feedback pathways provided by the car-bon dioxide flow and muscle mechanoreceptors and me-taboreceptors. This stimulus is called *central command,* denoting the cardiorespiratory responses caused by direct action of the supramedullary locomotor center neurons on respiratory pattern–generating medullary neurons, whose output in turn regulates respiratory motor output to the air-way and chest wall muscles (and parasympathetic and sym-pathetic efferent output to the heart and blood vessels). Thus, central command involves a parallel simultaneous excitation of the neuronal circuits containing locomotion and cardiorespiratory neurons. Anatomically, several motor areas involved in this response have been identified in mul-tilabel nerve tracing studies. These motor areas are located principally in discrete regions of the hypothalamus, in the diencephalon of the midbrain, and in the premotor cortex; they project to the medullary cardiorespiratory neurons and also directly to cervical and lumbar spinal motor neurons.

Just as in the two hypotheses discussed earlier, to de-termine a role for central command in exercise hyperpnea requires isolation of the specific stimulus. The concept of a central command over cardiorespiratory function was first suggested prior to the last century (18) and named cortical ir-radiation. It was not until the past 2 decades that researchers devised methods using first electrical and then pharmaco-logical stimulation of these specific CNS locomotor regions in unanesthetized, decorticate cats to cause rhythmic loco-motion of the limbs similar to that produced voluntarily (19). When locomotion was initiated via this type of hypo-thalamic stimulation, phrenic nerve activity and cardiac out-put increased, and blood flow was redistributed from inactive to active tissues. Most important, these exercise-like cardio-respiratory changes occurred even when limb muscles were paralyzed (i.e., so-called fictive locomotion), thereby pro-viding strong evidence that central command was capable—by itself—of producing normal exercise hyperpnea (see Milestone of Discovery). These impressive findings were confirmed in several laboratories using the decorticate ani-mal central command model. However, skepticism contin-ues, especially concerning how precisely this model mimics actual physiological dynamic exercise.

In humans there is circumstantial evidence favoring a significant role for central command in exercise hyperpnea. Most often cited are the very fast ventilatory responses at ex-ercise onset and cessation, which appear to be almost antic-ipatory of these exercise transitions and apparently occur faster than any feedback mechanism could operate (18). Furthermore, exercise following partial muscle paralysis caused a fast-onset hyperventilatory response, which was at-tributed to the additional central command required to re-cruit more muscle motor units in an attempt to produce a given amount of force in the compromised muscle. Also, studies using hypnotic suggestion of exercise have been used in resting humans to uncouple feedback from central command. Merely the suggestion of exercise in a resting subject or of heavier exercise in the mildly exercising subject caused exerciselike tachycardia and increased ventilation (i.e., hyperventilation) in the absence of any (or further) muscular contraction or increase in $\dot{V}CO_2$. Also, neuroimaging techniques measuring brain blood flow distribution showed that several motor cortical areas were activated by this imagined exercise (20). These cortical areas were also activated with purely volitional hyperventilation. Whether these are the same higher CNS areas and pathways activated by the true central command during normal physiological exercise is a question that must be answered before these types of findings can be applied with confidence to the exercise hyperpnea question.

The Hyperventilation of Heavy Exercise and Prolonged Exercise: When $\dot{V}A$ Increases More Than $\dot{V}CO_2$

As exercise intensity increases beyond 50 to 60% of $\dot{V}O_{2max}$, ventilation first increases out of proportion with respect to $\dot{V}O_2$ (causing alveolar PO_2 to rise) and then, at a slightly higher workload, disproportionately more with respect to $\dot{V}CO_2$ (causing alveolar PCO_2 to fall). The degree of hyperventilation can be substantial, sufficient to drive $PaCO_2$ 8 to 15 mm Hg below resting normocapnic values at maximal exercise. What causes this extra drive to breathe? The popular choice for the past 60 years or so has been metabolic acidosis, because arterial plasma lactic acid and H^+ begin to rise with the onset of the hyperventilatory response. Reasonably, the hyperventilation is viewed as a ventilatory compensation (i.e., reduced $PaCO_2$) for a primary metabolic acidosis. Furthermore, since carotid chemoreceptors are exposed to the metabolic acidosis, they are the logical choice as the main transducer of the hyperventilatory response. On the other hand, the brain interstitial fluid that bathes the medullary chemoreceptors is protected from fast, acute increases in circulating lactic acid by the blood-brain barrier. Two types of clinical models also support this hypothesis, as neither the mildly asthmatic patient with denervated carotid bodies (21) nor the rare patient with normal lungs but a demonstrated absence of ventilatory response to chemoreceptor stimuli (carbon dioxide or hypoxia) show a hyperventilatory response to heavy exercise—even though they both have a normal isocapnic hyperpnea in mild exercise. Accordingly, unlike the dilemma of hyperpnea of moderate-intensity exercise, the hyperventilation of heavy dynamic exercise would at first glance appear to have a clearly defined stimulus and reflex receptor site.

Unfortunately, several lines of evidence preclude such a clearcut conclusion. First, neither metabolic acidosis nor the carotid bodies were shown to be **required** for the hyperventilatory response to heavy exercise. When dietary-induced

glycogen depletion was used to prevent almost all of the exercise-induced increase in lactic acid, a normal hyperventilatory response persisted (22). Furthermore, when exercising animals were studied before and after carotid body denervation, the animals' ventilatory response to heavy exercise was, if anything, slightly *greater* following carotid body denervation, despite similar levels of metabolic acidosis. (23). These data conflict with the cross-sectional evidence in the carotid body–denervated humans cited earlier. Inspiring hyperoxic gases, which greatly reduce the tonic activity and responsiveness of the carotid chemoreceptors, caused transient reductions in ventilation in heavy exercise; however, similar thresholds of exercise intensity were shown to exist for the onset of hyperventilation in hyperoxic as well as normoxic exercise.

What can we conclude from these conflicting data? Given the well-described ventilatory response of the carotid chemoreceptors to circulating hydrogen ions, it is safe to say that the carotid chemoreceptors are involved to a significant extent in the ventilatory response to heavy exercise. However, the metabolic acidosis alone is unlikely to be a sufficiently strong stimulus to explain the 20 to 30% extra increase in ventilation (20–40 L · min^{-1} $\dot{V}E$ in healthy young subjects) observed during high-intensity exercise. Additional carotid body stimuli, such as increasing concentrations of norepinephrine and potassium, occur in heavy dynamic exercise. Also, other powerful locomotor-linked nonchemoreceptor stimuli might come into play to cause hyperventilation. For example, as limb locomotor muscle fatigue occurs in heavy intensity exercise, more central command must be generated to maintain locomotor muscle force, and this would be expected to have a coincident augmenting effect on respiratory motor output. There is no direct evidence to support this suggestion, but in exercising humans, electromyography of the limb locomotor muscles (vastus lateralis muscle) showed a marked increase in activity versus work rate—suggesting an increase in central command—coincident with the onset of high-intensity exercise and the onset of hyperventilation (24). Similarly, heavy exercise causes substantial metabolite accumulation in working skeletal muscle, which would certainly stimulate muscle metaboreceptors and perhaps contribute to the extra ventilatory response, as they do to the increase in sympathetic afferent activity accompanying heavy exercise.

In summary, the hyperventilation of heavy dynamic exercise presents as many as or perhaps even more opportunities for known feed-forward and feedback sensory inputs to influence ventilation than the isocapnic hyperpnea of moderate exercise. The major obvious difference is that in heavy exercise we have large changes in additional known chemoreceptor stimuli in arterial blood, which surely contribute to some extent to the hyperventilatory response. However, the available evidence also points to the additional (and perhaps interactive) strong ascending influences of augmented feedback from fatiguing locomotor muscles and descending influences from central command. Logically, this central command influence may also rely critically on stored information from past memorable experiences of heavy exercise intensities (discussed later).

Finally, sustaining constant work-rate exercise at heavy intensities (>75% $\dot{V}_{O_{2max}}$) beyond about 5 to 10 minutes causes a time-dependent tachypneic (i.e., increased breathing frequency) hyperventilatory response. An important difference between short- and long-term high intensity exercise is that arterial [H⁺] may actually be falling in the long term as opposed to rising in short-term heavy exercise. This is because the net release of lactic acid from the working muscle may actually fall over time at constant workloads, and the level of hypocapnia resulting from hyperventilation becomes the dominant determinant of arterial [H⁺] (25). Nevertheless, carotid chemoreceptor stimuli in the form of time-dependent increases in circulating norepinephrine and potassium continue to be present in long-term exercise, in addition to the potentially augmented central command influences associated with locomotor limb fatigue. An additional consideration here is the time-dependent rise in core and blood temperature, which has a unique effect among ventilatory stimuli in humans in that it produces a predominant tachypnea rather than a tidal volume response. Furthermore, preventing most of this temperature increase via skin cooling was shown to prevent some of the time-dependent tachypneic hyperventilation in long-term exercise (26). Exactly where the increase in temperature might be acting to cause hyperventilation is uncertain. Perhaps this tachypneic response is stimulated by increased hypothalamic temperature and serves as a thermoregulatory response for selective brain cooling (27), analogous to that commonly experienced in the fur-bearing, panting animal.

Summary: Interim Proposal and Future Considerations

After more than a century of investigation, is the mechanism of exercise hyperpnea still a true dilemma and an ultra secret—as expressed 2 decades ago by the late Frederick Grodins (1915–1989), one of the pioneering modelers of the ventilatory control system? Not completely! On the positive side we clearly have two candidates in the locomotor-linked stimuli, namely central command (feed-forward) and muscle receptors (feedback). When studied in isolation, each is capable of producing fast and significant increases in respiratory motor output and ventilation. The findings that hypothalamic locomotor centers received sensory input from skeletal muscle receptors also shows the presence of the neural circuitry for providing interaction between these two main drives to breathe (28). Thus, we propose that these two major stimuli act together to provide the primary stimulus to exercise hyperpnea, perhaps with backup error detection by carotid chemoreceptors to provide fine tuning of the ventilatory response to ensure sufficient and precise normocapnic hyperpnea. This combination of stimuli provides an explanation for the first (fast) phase of increased ventilation at exercise onset and the final normocapnic steady-state ventilation achieved at a given exercise intensity. The memory or self-amplifying effect of short-term potentiation (discussed previously) would account for the gradual time-dependent increase in ventilation between exercise onset and steady state and also explain the lack of large transient overshoots and undershoots in ventilation in transitional phases at exercise onset, upon achievement of the steady-state, and during recovery from dynamic exercise.

Summary

We propose this control scheme for hyperpnea as an interim working hypothesis. Future research should also consider the following findings.

When either of these two primary mechanisms is removed, via lesioning of the spinal cord (in the case of feedback) or destruction of hypothalamic locomotor center neurons (in the case of central command), the ventilatory response to exercise remains near normal (29). Apparently, then, *neither input is required* for normal exercise hyperpnea. Perhaps we can explain this finding by the concept of redundant biological mechanisms or the multifaceted effects of lesioning (see comment in Box 10.1 about denervation effects). Both of these concerns are reasonable and important. At the same time, it is difficult to accept any given mechanism as the *primary* driver of such a substantial physiological response when it is not also an *obligatory* mechanism!

Attempts have been made to test how these two powerful locomotor-linked ventilatory stimuli might interact as we propose they do during normal exercise. This was accomplished by activation of each of the mechanisms separately and then together in anesthetized animals (30). Surprisingly, the sum of the response of each of the mechanisms acting alone was always greater than the two acting simultaneously. Strong interactive effects of combined ventilatory stimuli do commonly occur, for example, with all carotid chemoreceptor stimuli. However, there is as yet no direct evidence that this synergistic effect on ventilation occurs between the two locomotor-linked ventilatory stimuli.

An emerging concept is based on the capability of the organism to make accurate ventilatory responses to locomotion without guidance from identifiable error signals (see lesioning studies earlier in the chapter). This concept proposes that it is unlikely that the brain—in our case the medullary respiratory controller—solves complex differential equations in response to the many sensory inputs it receives from the higher CNS motor areas, muscular contraction, chemoreceptors, and short-term potentiation during dynamic exercise. Rather, the brain learns to make accurate ventilatory responses by trial and error, correcting them time after time during maturation. That is, the CNS anticipates present and future needs based on experience (31).

Box 10.1 — THE UNFORTUNATE DRAWBACK TO DENERVATION EXPERIMENTS

Denervation experiments such as these obviously provide very important understanding to the relative importance of certain sensory pathways. However, negative results allow only the conclusion that these receptors are not required and do not rule out a significant role for these receptors in the intact subject. The key problem with such preparations is that removal of these sensory inputs is most certainly not the only significant change in the neural control system as a result of the denervations. To the contrary, sensory pathways such as those contained in vagal or carotid sinus nerves contain important tonic inputs to the medulla under normal intact conditions; accordingly, when they are denervated and this input is removed, adaptive changes are likely to occur either at the level of the neurons that generate central integrative respiratory patterns or by up-regulation of other sensory receptors. For example, carotid body denervation was shown by histological studies to have marked detrimental effects on the metabolic integrity (and therefore the neuronal function) of the medullary rhythm-generating neurons in the pre-Bötzinger complex (12) and over time also caused sensitization of the other sites of peripheral chemoreception in aortic chemoreceptors (13).

The identified sensory inputs for hyperpnea, as detailed in the foregoing sections, would certainly be important, especially during the learning-maturation phase, for the CNS to have knowledge of its "errors." However, it is also proposed that the brain must rely on stored information to achieve error-free regulation (31,32). This idea of learning the appropriate exercise hyperpneic response has been named *adaptive feed-forward control*. As implied from the cardiorespiratory responses and neuroimaging findings obtained during exercise suggested under hypnosis (discussed previously), the prefrontal cortex may be a critical area for encoding a respiratory motor program that evolves as motor tasks are learned in development (20). Further tests of these intriguing but still highly theoretical hypotheses will occur as our knowledge of the neurophysiology of learning and memory evolves.

Mechanics of Breathing in Dynamic Exercise

The lungs are inflated by negative pressure respiration, whereby intrapleural and then alveolar pressures are reduced below atmospheric pressure by the expanding action of the inspiratory muscles on the chest wall. When the inspiratory muscles contract, they must provide sufficient force to overcome two mechanical impedances in the lung, namely, (*a*) resistance to flow through the airways and (*b*) the lung's elastic recoil forces, which—when unopposed by the outward recoil of the chest wall—will cause the lung to collapse to its smallest volume. A balance between lung inward recoil and chest wall outward recoil occurs at the lung's functional residual capacity (FRC), that is, the lung volume averaging 45 to 50% of total lung capacity and from which under quiet resting conditions each inspiration is initiated. This elastic characteristic for any given lung volume is defined by the lung compliance, which is calculated as the change in volume divided by a given change in pleural pressure (Δ volume/Δ pressure).

The compliance of the lung decreases exponentially with increasing lung volume, which makes the lung stiff at high lung volumes. The resistance to flow through the airways is expressed in centimeters of water per liter per second and is determined primarily by the radius of the airway, according to Poiseuille's law, which governs flow through rigid tubes. Airway caliber increases linearly (and resistance to flow decreases) as lung volume increases.

Given the huge demands of exercise for increases in both tidal volume and flow rate, it is extremely important that these elastic and resistive characteristics are regulated so as to minimize the magnitude of intrapleural pressure changes, hence prevent excessive amounts of work by the respiratory muscles. For the most part, these goals are met during exercise, because the lungs, airways, and parenchymal tissue are anatomically suited to the increased ventilatory demands and also because the nervous control of breathing pattern and airway caliber is nearly optimal. We now address each of these anatomical and physiological characteristics in detail.

Control of Airway Caliber

Even though the rate of airflow increases as much as fivefold to sixfold during moderate and up to tenfold during high-intensity dynamic exercise and airflow turbulence increases, the total resistance to airflow remains fairly constant. Thus, when airway resistance is compared at identical flow rates between rest and exercise, airway resistance is remarkably lower during exercise. This reduced resistance to airflow reflects a major effect of exercise on both the stiffening (i.e., the airway is less collapsible) and dilating of the upper and lower airways.

Extrathoracic Airway Caliber

The upper airways consist of the nose, mouth, pharynx, and larynx, and their diameters are regulated by more than 20 pairs of skeletal muscles innervated by the cranial nerves (discussed previously). This complex upper airway structure is responsible for phonation, swallowing, coughing, and mastication, in addition to being a critical conduit for airflow. It also offers a tortuous and potentially high-resistance breathing route, especially in the human. However, several key mechanisms activated during exercise ensure a low-resistance upper airway. First, the major route of airflow switches from predominantly nasal at rest to predominantly oral during even light exercise requiring about 25 to 50 L · min⁻¹ V̇E. This switch largely bypasses the nasal cavity, which possesses the smallest cross-sectional area in the upper airway. Cessation of nasal airflow is accomplished by activation of pharyngeal muscles, which bring the soft pallet into contact with the posterior pharyngeal wall. The diameter of the oral pharynx is enlarged and stiffened largely via activation of the genioglossus muscle, which controls tongue position, and other palatal and pharyngeal muscles. The fact that the activation of the pharyngeal muscles slightly precedes that of the respiratory pump muscles (Fig. 10.2*C*) is extremely important, because this allows the airway to be stiffened and prevents airway narrowing and/or collapse in the face of the highly subatmospheric intrathoracic pressures generated by the inspiratory muscles during dynamic exercise.

Finally, the cartilaginous larynx connects the pharynx with the trachea. The valvelike regulation of the laryngeal vocal folds, principally by the posterior cricoarytenoid and the thyroarytenoid muscles, is a key determinant of upper airway resistance. At rest, the glottal laryngeal opening widens on inspiration and narrows on expiration, providing a slight brake on expiratory airflow—presumably to prevent end-expiratory lung volume from dropping below FRC. During exercise, with increased frequency and shortened inspiratory and expiratory times, the glottal opening is widened and there is little or no narrowing on expiration (Fig. 10.7).

There are multiple levels of control of the diameter and compliance of the upper airway during dynamic exercise. First, activation of the nasal, pharyngeal, and laryngeal skeletal muscles is under very similar feed-forward and feedback control (via the cranial nerves) as explained in detail earlier for the respiratory pump muscles during exercise. Output from the medullary respiratory pattern generator is the primary determinant of the timing and magnitude of the contractions of all the respiratory muscles, including those of the upper airway and of the chest wall (Fig. 10.1). Sympathetic activation during dynamic exercise also causes vasoconstriction of the nasal mucosa, thereby increasing nasal airway diameter and reducing nasal resistance. Finally, purely mechanical forces associated with increased chest wall inspiratory pump muscle contractions are also important to increasing laryngeal diameter by means of caudal traction on the trachea (i.e., the so-called tracheal tug).

Bronchial Caliber

Intrathoracic airway caliber is under the control of involuntary smooth muscle. A powerful dilation of the bronchi occurs during exercise at all intensities, and this has been observed

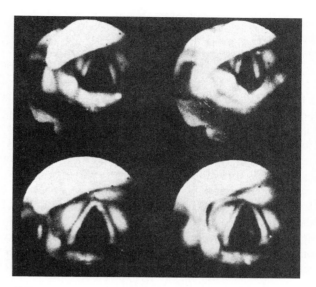

FIGURE 10.7   Position of the human vocal chords as viewed through a laryngoscope during mid inspiration (left side) and mid expiration (right side) from typical breaths at rest (eupneic breathing) (top panel) and during moderate exercise (hyperpnea) (bottom panel). The vocal chords are much more abducted during hyperpneic ventilation in exercise than at rest. The major effect of hyperpnea on the position of the vocal chords occurred during expiration: they narrowed markedly at rest during expiration but underwent only minor amounts of narrowing during exercise. *(Reprinted with permission from England SJ, Bartlett D Jr. Changes in respiratory movements of the human vocal cords during hyperpnea. J Appl Physiol 1982;52:782.)*

by measurements of airway mechanics either during or immediately following exercise in healthy nonasthmatic subjects. Both the maximal amount of air forced out of the lungs during 1 second (FEV₁) and the maximum flow–volume loop (FVC), both of which are indices of bronchial caliber, increase during and following exercise. Several mechanisms contribute to this exercise-induced bronchodilation. The most important is the immediate and sustained withdrawal of vagal parasympathetic tone to the airways. This vagal withdrawal occurs primarily reflexively via neural feedback from limb locomotor muscle mechanoreceptor activation at exercise onset (23). This mechanism is also responsible in part for the reduced vagal efferent output to the heart during exercise, which increases heart rate. The passive stretching of the lung which occurs with increasing VT will also contribute to bronchiolar smooth muscle relaxation and airway dilation (discussed later).

Pure mechanical effects on the bronchi also occur with increased VT. Due to the strong interdependence between the airway and the lung parenchyma, an increased VT will tether open the bronchi. In addition, recent findings using airway smooth muscle strip preparations *in vitro* have shown that even small amounts of airway stretch result in reductions in bronchial smooth muscle crossbridge formation (by disturbing the bronchiolar smooth muscle latch state), and these reductions decrease smooth muscle stiffness and promote bronchial smooth muscle relaxation (33).

Although major changes in airway caliber and resistance do occur during dynamic exercise, the elastic characteristics of the lung and chest wall remain essentially unaltered. Thus the respiratory system compliance and therefore total lung capacity remain unchanged during and following exercise. However, the elastic work performed by the respiratory muscles on the lungs and chest wall is also critically dependent upon the operating lung volume. If hyperinflation occurs secondary to expiratory flow limitation, lung compliance will be reduced during tidal breathing and the elastic work of breathing markedly increased. Additionally, reductions in vital capacity following maximum short-term and heavy long-term exercise may occur, as maximum expiratory flow rates are reduced at low lung volumes as a result of small-airway narrowing (also discussed later).

Breathing Patterns and Lung Volumes

In addition to the total amount of ventilation required and the mechanical characteristics of the lung and airways, precisely how the timing and amplitude of *each* breath is sculpted during exercise is a critical determinant of the amount of mechanical work required by the respiratory muscles. The important variables requiring control under these conditions include tidal, end-inspiratory, and end-

expiratory lung volumes, inspiratory and expiratory flow rates, and breath timing and duty cycle.

As shown in Figure 10.8, in light to moderate exercise the increase in $\dot{V}_E$ is achieved by increases in both frequency and V_T ($\dot{V}_E = fb \cdot V_T$), whereas at higher intensities V_T tends to level off, and an increase in frequency accounts for all of the further increase in $\dot{V}_E$. This pattern of breathing also occurs over time during high-intensity endurance exercise. Increases in breathing frequency are brought about by reductions in both inspiratory and expiratory times. The breathing duty cycle, which is defined as the inspiratory time divided by the total breath time (T_I/T_{TOT}), is increased slightly, but most of the total breath time remains in expiration and the T_I is maintained at less than 50% of the total breath time. Finally, as noted in Figure 10.8, the increase in V_T is reached by both reductions in end-expiratory lung volume below FRC (achieved by activation of the expiratory muscles beginning at light exercise intensities) and by increases in end-inspiratory lung volume.

Are these changes in breath timing and lung volume important to ensuring optimal mechanics of breathing during exercise? First, the choice of increased V_T rather than just increased frequency to achieve increased $\dot{V}_E$ means that the increase in dead space ventilation is minimized and effective alveolar ventilation is maximized ($\dot{V}_A = fb \cdot [V_T - V_D]$). This choice of breathing pattern clearly optimizes the gas exchange function of the lung and also minimizes flow rate and the flow-resistive work of breathing. Moreover, the facts that

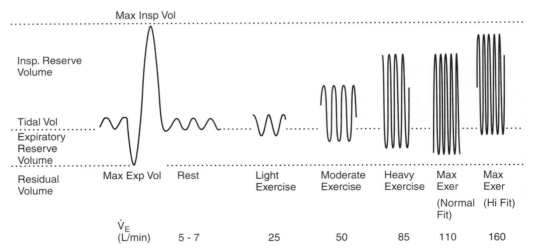

FIGURE 10.8 Changes in breathing pattern during exercise. The spirogram on the left is from a resting subject showing normal tidal volume, maximum expiration to residual lung volume, then maximal inspiration to total lung capacity. With light to heavy exercise (in both normal and highly fit subjects) the increase in ventilation is achieved by both an increase in breathing frequency and an increase in tidal volume. Tidal volume increases because of progressive encroachment on both the expiratory and inspiratory reserve volume as end-expiratory lung volume is reduced. This reduced end-expiratory lung volume is also maintained at maximum exercise in the normally fit subject ($\dot{V}_{O_{2max}} = 45$ mL $\cdot$ kg^{-1} $\cdot$ min^{-1}). In the highly fit subject ($\dot{V}_{O_{2max}} = 75$ mL $\cdot$ kg^{-1} $\cdot$ min^{-1}) the ventilation, frequency, and V_T are all higher than in the normally fit subject. Also, in the highly fit subject at maximum exercise end-expiratory lung volume was increased to near resting values because of expiratory flow limitation. (Also see Fig. 10.9.)

the increase in V_T is limited to 70% of vital capacity during heavier exercise and that end-expiratory lung volume is reduced below resting levels throughout exercise (Fig. 10.8) are very important in minimizing the elastic component of the work of breathing (Box 10.2).

Why are these changes in tidal and lung volumes during heavy exercise such important determinants of both the work and the perception of your breathing? First, it is important that you are accomplishing an increased tidal volume on the linear (and therefore most compliant) portion of the respiratory system pressure–volume relationship (or compliance curve); that is, the least amount of negative intrathoracic pressure has to be generated by the inspiratory muscles for a given increase in volume. Second, the reduced end-expiratory lung volume, achieved via activation of the abdominal expiratory muscles, means that intra-abdominal pressure is elevated and the diaphragm and other inspiratory muscles are lengthened at end expiration. As with any skeletal muscle, the greater the length, the greater the capability for force generation at any given motor input. Third, the act of expiration and the reduced end-expiratory lung volume below relaxation FRC allow for the storage of elastic energy in the chest wall during expiration, and this energy can be used to produce a significant portion of the work required during the ensuing inspiration, therefore potentially sparing the inspiratory muscles. Fourth, the fact that inspiratory time remains less than one-half the total time for a breath is important to preserving blood flow to the diaphragm, because forceful diaphragmatic contractions will increase intra-abdominal pressure, compress the vessels supplying the diaphragm, and reduce its blood flow. Thus the shorter the inspiration, the lesser the reduction in diaphragmatic blood flow, and the longer the expiration, the more time for recovery of blood flow to the diaphragm.

Flow–Volume Relationships

The maximum volitional flow–volume envelope is commonly used to quantify the maximum limits of the lung and respiratory muscles for these variables (Fig. 10.9). Inspiratory flow rate is limited primarily by the ability of the inspiratory muscles to generate negative intrathoracic pressure, which is the key determinant of the pressure gradient for airflow between the atmosphere and the alveoli. Thus, as inspiratory effort and the magnitude of the subatmospheric intrathoracic pressures increase, flow rate increases at any given lung volume. In contrast, expiratory flow rate is dependent upon the force of expiratory muscle effort *only* very early in expiration (i.e., near the peak flow rate at a high lung volume). Over most of the ensuing forced expiration, flow rate at any given lung volume is determined by the pressure difference across the airway. This so-called transmural pressure is the difference between the intra-airway pressure (being determined by the lungs' elastic recoil) and the collapsing positive intrathoracic pressure outside the airway (being determined by the compressive forces produced by expiratory muscles of the chest wall). Thus, in contrast to inspiration, maximum expiratory flow rate at any given lung volume is reached when expiratory muscle pressure and effort are only a small portion of the maximum achievable pressure. The lowest expiratory muscle pressure that generates maximum expiratory flow is termed maximum effective pressure, because any extra expiratory muscle effort beyond this point will cause airway narrowing or collapse and will not increase flow rate any further.

In Figure 10.9 inspiratory and expiratory flow rates increase progressively during incremental exercise, gradually reducing end-expiratory lung volume and increasing end-inspiratory lung volume (34). The maximum pressures at any given flow rate and lung volume are also shown for inspiration and expiration (detailed explanation in the legend to Fig. 10.9). For young adult untrained healthy subjects with normal $\dot{V}_{O_{2max}}$ and maximum $\dot{V}_E$ of about 110 to 120 L · min^{-1}, the maximum mechanical limits of the flow–volume envelope are not reached even during maximal exercise. End-expiratory lung volume stays below resting levels and end-inspiratory lung volume is 70 to 80% of total lung capacity. Further, inspiratory muscle force is only 50 to 60% of the maximum capacity for force generation by these muscles. Clearly then, the maximum mechanical capability of the inspiratory muscles to produce maximum flow rate substantially exceeds the ventilatory requirements normally observed

Box 10.2

To appreciate the importance of these changes in lung volume to the work required for breathing, try this experiment on yourself. Voluntarily increase your V_T about three times above your resting level for just five or six breaths. Do this starting at three different beginning end-expiratory lung volumes (a) from your normal relaxed end-expiratory lung volume (or FRC), (b) from your residual lung volume, and (c) from an end-expiratory lung volume that is well above your relaxation FRC and about halfway between FRC and TLC. Accomplish this latter end-expiratory lung volume by first breathing in to well above FRC and then hold your breath for a second or two before you start your high–tidal volume breaths. Now you should be able to appreciate how much more effort it takes to accomplish the same V_T starting in a hyperinflated state versus starting in a normal or a deflated lung volume.

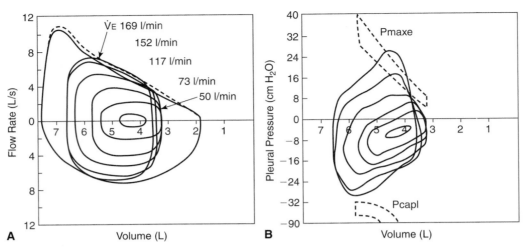

FIGURE 10.9   Flow-to-volume and pressure-to-volume relationships in the young healthy adult at rest and exercise. For the flow-to-volume relationship the maximum outer envelope is obtained by a maximal volitional inspiratory and expiratory effort both before exercise (*solid line*) and immediately following exercise (*broken line*). For the pressure-to-volume relationships only tidal breaths at rest through maximum exercise are shown. In addition is shown the maximum inspiratory pleural (esophageal) pressures (Pcapi) at the specific peak volume and flow rate achieved during tidal breathing in heavy exercise. Up to a $\dot{V}E$ of 117 L · min⁻¹, which would approximate that in a normally fit young adult, the inspiratory and expiratory flow volume limits have not been reached, and the pressures reached by the inspiratory muscles are only 40 to 50% of capacity. The more highly trained subject is shown achieving ventilations in excess of 150 L · min⁻¹ at higher metabolic rates. Under these conditions the tidal flow-to-volume loop encroaches on the maximum flow-to-volume envelope, end-expiratory lung volume rises, and the inspiratory muscles at maximum exercise are approaching 90% of their dynamic capacity for force output and velocity of shortening. The broken area on the expiratory side indicates an expiratory pressure (for any given lung volume) beyond which extra expiratory muscle effort will not produce a higher flow rate. In almost all instances up to 150 L · min⁻¹ $\dot{V}E$ this critical expiratory pressure is not exceeded, but it is exceeded slightly in the highly trained athlete at maximum exercise.

during exercise—at least in the normally fit, healthy subject. However, in more highly trained subjects, $\dot{V}O_{2max}$ and $\dot{V}E$ increase further, while the maximum flow–volume envelope is unchanged from that of the untrained normal subject. Accordingly, the expiratory flow during tidal breathing now commonly intersects with the maximum flow–volume envelope. End-expiratory lung volume is now forced upward so that there will be room within the maximum flow–volume envelope to increase flow rate further. However, this extra flow rate and ventilation are accomplished at the expense of lung hyperinflation (Box 10.2). Indeed, breathing at a higher lung volume means the lung is stiffer during tidal inspiration and inspiratory muscles are shorter, with less force-generating capability (Fig. 10.9). We further address this point of mechanical ventilatory limitation in the section "Limiting Factors," later in the chapter.

Respiratory Pump Muscles in Exercise

Ventilatory requirements are directly served by several groups of skeletal muscles, namely upper airway dilators and stiffeners (as described earlier) and four main groups of respiratory pump muscles, namely the diaphragm, rib cage in-

spiratory muscles, and rib cage and abdominal expiratory muscles. The diaphragm is a remarkable skeletal muscle, designed to work rhythmically throughout life and to handle the high ventilatory demands of dynamic exercise. The fatigue-resistant nature of the diaphragm derives from its relatively high oxidative capacity (as compared to most limb locomotor muscles of similar mixed fiber type) and also to the short capillary-to-mitochondrial diffusion distances for oxygen achieved by the very low muscle fiber cross-sectional area–capillary ratios. Furthermore, the recruitment order of motor units for the diaphragm follows the size principle based on increasing axonal conduction velocity. Accordingly, for most ventilatory behaviors, the fatigue-resistant type I slow twitch and intermediate type IIA fibers are recruited first, followed by more fatigable type IIB/X fibers with increasing levels of force production.

Respiratory Pump Muscle Recruitment Patterns

To provide mechanically efficient increases in VT and fb during exercise requires the following:

- Both the force output and the velocity of shortening of the pump muscles must increase.

- The volumes of both the rib cage and the abdominal compartments must change progressively.
- The fiber lengths of the respiratory muscles must be regulated at nearly optimal lengths.
- The respiratory system compliance (Δ volume/ Δ pressure) must remain high so that minimal amounts of pressure are needed for changes in tidal volume.

The combined and highly coordinated actions of the diaphragm, rib cage, and abdominal muscles accomplish all of these required responses to exercise. It is not possible to measure length changes or the actual force production of the respiratory muscles in humans, but appropriate placements of balloon catheters provide estimates of the pressure production resulting from the contraction of inspiratory muscles. This is achieved by measurements of pleural pressure (Ppl; esophageal balloon) and abdominal pressure (P_{ABD}; gastric balloon), with the subsequent calculation of transdiaphragmatic pressure (P_{DIA}; the difference between the abdominal and pleural pressure). Accurate measures of rib cage and abdominal volume changes are extremely difficult, especially during exercise. The most accurate estimates to date have been made through the use of three-dimensional video tracking of reflective markers placed at many locations over the upper and lower rib cage and abdomen (35).

We know that at rest motor command from the medulla activates the phrenic motor neurons and in turn shortens the diaphragm, whose descent expands the thoracic cavity and causes a more negative pleural pressure. P_{ABD} increases as the diaphragm shortens and descends toward the abdominal cavity, and P_{DIA} increases throughout inspiration. Thus, at rest the diaphragm is the major force generator, the rib cage muscles are a minor force generator, and expiratory muscles are inactive, as expiration is passive. With mild dynamic exercise and throughout further increases in exercise intensity, increased motor command is distributed to all three sets of respiratory pump muscles, but now the diaphragm is no longer the only major force developer. Although the work performed by the diaphragm increases more than tenfold during exercise, it now acts as the major flow producer by increasing its velocity of shortening (discussed later), whereas the rib cage muscles (i.e., intercostals) now become the major force producer to expand rib cage volume and reduce Ppl during inspiration. Furthermore, the abdominal expiratory muscles (primarily the internal and external obliques and transversus abdominus) now become major force producers to reduce abdominal and rib cage volumes and to increase P_{ABD} during active expiration. We now address how the active expiration achieved by the abdominal expiratory muscles influences the function of the diaphragm during dynamic exercise.

The expiratory abdominal muscles (primarily the transversus abdominus and external and internal oblique muscles) in many ways are important to diaphragmatic function during exercise. Active expiration begins even with light exercise, causing P_{ABD} to move in an increasingly positive direction and abdominal compartment volume to be reduced during expiration. At the end of the active expiration, the expiratory muscles relax rapidly and the abdominal wall recoils outward. Thus, during inspiration P_{ABD} initially falls as abdominal volume increases, and this occurs coincidentally with the falling Ppl. Thus, the contracting, descending diaphragm is not faced with an increasing P_{ABD} and is therefore unloaded during inspiration and capable of generating a high velocity of shortening. In addition, as mentioned earlier, the phasic activation of the abdominal muscles during expiration reduces end-expiratory lung volume and also aids the diaphragm in two other important ways during exercise: (*a*) With increasing P_{ABD} and stretching the diaphragm on expiration, at the onset of the ensuing inspiration diaphragmatic descent will occur purely passively, that is, prior to the initiation of active diaphragmatic contraction, which occurs over most of the inspiratory period. (*b*) The diaphragm and other inspiratory muscles are lengthened to nearly optimal length in preparation for their own active force generation during the ensuing inspiration.

In weight-supported locomotion, such as in jogging or running, in both humans and quadrupeds the abdominal muscles are tonically activated, and mean levels of intra-abdominal pressure also increase. The resultant stiffening of the abdominal wall and increased mean P_{ABD} mean that the abdominal cavity acts as a shock absorber during exercise, by absorbing and therefore substantially lessening the concussive forces transmitted to the vertebral column and cranium from the impact of each foot plant.

Respiratory Muscle Energetics

The inspiratory and expiratory muscles of the rib cage, diaphragm, and abdomen perform both elastic work to produce lung expansion during inspiration and resistive work to produce increases in inspiratory and expiratory flow rates, the latter increasing nonlinearly at very high exercise intensities as flow rates become fully turbulent and especially when expiratory flow limitation is present. Accordingly, total respiratory muscle work increases several fold from resting levels to heavy intensity dynamic exercise.

Estimates of the oxygen cost of this increase in ventilatory work (Fig. 10.10) averaged 1.8 mL $\dot{V}O_2 \cdot L^{-1} \dot{V}E \cdot min^{-1}$ during light and moderate exercise. Thereafter, the oxygen cost of breathing rose out of proportion to the increasing $\dot{V}E$ and averaged 2.9 mL $\dot{V}O_2 \cdot L^{-1} \dot{V}E \cdot min^{-1}$ at maximal exercise. Much of this extra work is required for increased flow-resistive work as flow rates rise and fully turbulent flow occurs in the airways. As a fraction of total body $\dot{V}O_2$, the oxygen cost of exercise hyperpnea averaged 3 to 5% in moderate exercise and 8 to 10% at a normal $\dot{V}O_{2max}$ in untrained young adults (at $\dot{V}O_{2max}$ 40–50 mL $\cdot$ kg$^{-1} \cdot$ min^{-1}). The values for respiratory muscle $\dot{V}O_2$ during maximal exercise were highly variable among subjects, with some highly fit subjects ($\dot{V}O_{2max} > 60$ mL $\cdot$ kg$^{-1} \cdot$ min^{-1}) requiring 13 to 16% of the total $\dot{V}O_{2max}$ (36).

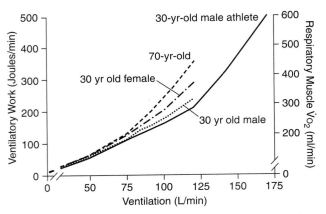

FIGURE 10.10 The work of breathing and the oxygen cost of breathing at different levels of steady-state ventilation during exercise in four different types of subjects. In the 30-year-old untrained male at $\dot{V}O_{2max}$ the oxygen cost of breathing approximates 10% of the $\dot{V}O_{2max}$, whereas in the 70-year-old and 30-year-old highly fit women (at comparable $\dot{V}O_{2max}$ as the young adult normally fit male) the work of breathing and the oxygen cost of breathing is significantly higher. In the highly trained young endurance athlete working at much higher $\dot{V}O_{2max}$ (75 mL $\cdot$ kg^{-1} $\cdot$ min^{-1}) and at much higher minute ventilation the oxygen cost of breathing approaches 15 to 16% of the $\dot{V}O_{2max}$.

Exercise effects on the metabolism of respiratory muscles as compared to locomotor muscles of similar fiber type have received some attention in studies using rats in which diaphragm tissue was assayed at rest and after exhausting exercise. Other studies have used ponies and sheep whose arterial to venous differences in metabolites were examined across the diaphragm. Heavy prolonged exercise causes significant glycogen depletion in all fiber types of the diaphragm, implying that all fiber types were recruited during exercise. However, in almost all studies, glycogen depletion in the diaphragm was substantially less than in locomotor muscles, and at end of exercise a substantial amount of glycogen was still present in the diaphragm. Interestingly, high levels of lactic acid accumulated in the diaphragm during heavy sustained exercise, demonstrating that as with cardiac muscle, the diaphragm appears to take up and utilize lactate effectively as a metabolic substrate (37). Recent evidence from homogenates of costal diaphragm obtained following brief maximal dynamic exercise in rodents showed a significant reduction in Ca^{++} uptake and release paralleled by decreased activity of the sarcoplasmic reticulum (SR) Ca^{++}-adenosine triphosphatase (ATPase) (38). These attenuations of the SR function also occur in maximally exercising limb muscle and are believed to play a critical role in reduction of force development and muscle fatigue (39) (also discussed later).

Respiratory Muscle Blood Flow

Blood flow to all skeletal muscles during exercise increases with increasing metabolic requirements. The magnitude of this increase is dependent upon the net influences of the specific muscle's arteriolar smooth muscle response to local vasodilators (such as nitric oxide and muscle metabolites) and to sympathetic vasoconstrictor activity. These opposing influences both increase along with exercise intensity (40). The network of blood vessels supplying blood flow to the diaphragm is extensive, including tributaries from the phrenic, lobar, and mammary arteries.

Data on respiratory muscle blood flow and $\dot{V}O_2$ during exercise are derived from experimental animals (Table 10.1) using radiolabeled microspheres to determine local blood flow and cannulation of the phrenic vein to obtain arterial-to-venous oxygen differences across the diaphragm. In this way, diaphragm $\dot{V}O_2$ may be obtained ($\dot{V}O_2$ = blood flow $\cdot$ a – v – O_2 difference). Although exercise effects varied greatly *among* species and *within* species, it is clear that vascular conductances and blood flow (per 100 g of tissue) to the inspiratory and expiratory muscles increase substantially, probably to a similar extent as to limb locomotor muscles. Diaphragm $\dot{V}O_2$ also increased to many times rest values as a result of both increased blood flow and increased oxygen extraction, also similar to the locomotor muscles. In total, during maximum dynamic exercise, blood flow to the inspiratory and expiratory muscles approximated 15 to 16% of the total cardiac output.

This fraction of cardiac output devoted to respiratory muscles in running equines as measured with microspheres (41) is similar to that estimated indirectly in humans from measuring the reduction in cardiac output and $\dot{V}O_2$ after a mechanical ventilator was used to unload the respiratory muscles during maximum exercise (Fig. 10.11) (42). Furthermore, these fractions of the total $\dot{V}O_2$ devoted to breathing agree closely with those obtained by measuring the increase in $\dot{V}O_2$ when the work of breathing during exercise was mimicked voluntarily by resting subjects (Fig. 10.10). Certainly none of these methods is without some error in estimating the total blood flow devoted to breathing during exercise. For example, the blood flow measured in the designated respiratory muscles of the abdomen and rib cage in the exercising quadrupeds is likely devoted to a significant extent to trunk stabilization and locomotion (see discussion of abdominal muscles, earlier in the chapter); furthermore, a portion of the reductions in stroke volume and cardiac output achieved via mechanical unloading of the respiratory muscles in the humans was likely due to reductions in the negativity of intrathoracic pressure (see section "Cardiorespiratory Interactions"). So for now we can only conclude that a highly significant portion of the total cardiac output and total $\dot{V}O_2$, probably in the range of 10 to 16% (depending on the maximum metabolic and ventilatory requirements of the individual), is devoted to inspiratory and expiratory muscle work during maximum exercise. How these requirements for blood flow by the respiratory muscles may actually compete with the limb locomotor muscles for a share of the cardiac output is considered later in the chapter.

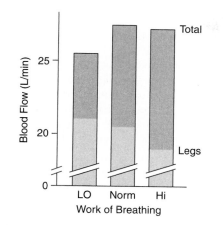

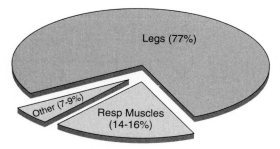

FIGURE 10.11 Effects of respiratory muscle work during exercise on cardiac output and its distribution in highly fit adult male subjects cycling at $\dot{V}_{O_{2max}}$ ($\dot{V}_{O_2}$ = 65 mL · kg^{-1} · min^{-1}; cardiac output = 28 L · min^{-1}). The estimated distribution of blood flow to the limb locomotor and to the respiratory muscles is shown in the pie chart. These estimates come from three sources: (a) the oxygen cost of breathing at maximum exercise (36), (b) measurements based on microsphere distribution to the respiratory muscles during maximum exercise in the equine (41), and (c) the change in cardiac output and in limb muscle blood flow determined in response to unloading of the respiratory muscles during maximum exercise (42,79). These effects of respiratory muscle unloading at maximum exercise on limb blood flow and on total cardiac output are shown in the insert. With reduced respiratory muscle work, that is, unloading, the total cardiac output falls and the limb muscle blood flow rises, whereas with respiratory muscle loading and increased work of breathing at maximum exercise, the maximum cardiac output remains unchanged but the limb blood flow is reduced.

Respiratory Muscle Fatigue

Muscle fatigue is universally defined as a reduction in force output and/or the velocity of shortening in response to a given (usually supra-maximal) stimulus that recovers with rest. Maximum force output is determined objectively by applying supra-maximal stimulation to the motor nerves to the muscle in question.

Compared to the limb muscles, it is difficult to objectively assess fatigue of the diaphragm because both the muscle and the motor nerves are relatively inaccessible. Thus, force development across the muscle is estimated by measuring the pressure difference between the esophageal and gastric pressures, and supra-maximal stimulation is achieved by bilateral electrical or magnetic stimulation of the phrenic nerves (BPNS) at one or more stimulation frequencies (43). Controlling muscle length by close monitoring of lung volume prior to BPNS is an important part of this test.

These BPNS techniques have been applied before and after exercise in humans over the past decade, with the following findings (44, 45). Following short-term, progressive exercise up to high intensities in untrained or trained subjects, maximally stimulated diaphragmatic force output was not reduced consistently in all or even most subjects. Similarly, at the end of constant-load exhaustive exercise at intensities less than 80% of $\dot{V}_{O_{2max}}$, supramaximally stimulated Pdi was also not affected. However, following sustained exercise intensities greater than 80 to 85% of $\dot{V}_{O_{2max}}$ continued to exhaustion, reductions of 15 to 50% in stimulated Pdi were consistently obtained in the immediate period post exercise. Stimulated Pdi did not return to control values before exercise until 1 to 2 hours following exercise. When hypoxic gas mixtures were breathed during exercise, diaphragmatic fatigue occurred with shorter work times, and recovery of the stimulated Pdi took longer.

What factors contribute to exercise-induced diaphragmatic fatigue? The ventilatory parameters that lead to diaphragmatic fatigue have been determined for subjects at rest who voluntarily control their breath timing and respiratory muscle force production. The key parameters include the breathing frequency, the ratio of force (Pdi) developed with tidal breathing to maximum force available (as determined by the maximum Pdi developed via maximum inspiratory effort against a closed airway) and the duty cycle of the breath (T_I/T_{TOT}). The product of these latter two variables is the so-called tension–time index of the diaphragm (46). Combinations of these factors produced voluntarily in healthy subjects at rest breathing against resistance can certainly cause diaphragmatic fatigue. However, at rest diaphragmatic fatigue does not occur until the forces developed by the diaphragm are substantially greater than those present with tidal breathing during whole-body exercise at intensities that caused exercise-induced diaphragmatic fatigue.

Why is the fatigue threshold of force production for the diaphragm so much lower during whole-body exercise than at rest? The probable explanation of this quite substantial effect of whole-body exercise on diaphragm fatigability is that at rest, the volitional increases in diaphragmatic work mean large shares of the total cardiac output are devoted to the diaphragm, whereas during exercise the diaphragm must compete with locomotor muscles for their share of the available cardiac output. The less the blood flow to the diaphragm, the less the oxygen transport and carbon dioxide removal, the greater the likelihood of fatigue.

The physiological consequences of exercise-induced diaphragm fatigue are not entirely clear. First, diaphragm fatigue is defined as a significant reduction in maximum force output in response to BPNS or in maximum velocity of shortening which is reversible by rest. Fatigue is not synonymous with task failure of the muscle. That is, the diaphragm is certainly compromised but is still able to continue much of its function. In fact, objective evidence of diaphragm fatigue commonly occurs long before the subject is unable to maintain a given force output (i.e., task failure). Two consequences of diaphragmatic fatigue that occur during prolonged heavy exercise are (*a*) a decrease in relative contribution of the diaphragm to total ventilation over time as accessory inspiratory and expiratory muscles are recruited to deliver a progressive hyperventilatory response and (*b*) an increase in breathing frequency. Both of these effects would be expected to reduce the mechanical efficiency of breathing in heavy prolonged exercise (see "Limiting Factors" section).

Exercise-induced transient abdominal pain, or the so-called abdominal stitch, is commonly felt during sustained heavy exercise. It may be associated with some aspect of diaphragmatic contraction and/or fatigue during exercise. This sharp, stabbing pain occurs in the lumbar region of the abdomen and may also involve shoulder tip pain, occurs commonly in exercise involving repetitive torso movements, is exacerbated by fluid ingestion and distention of the stomach, and is relieved by physical measures that reduce abdominal volume (such as abdominal strapping). Ischemia of the diaphragm has been cited as a possible cause, but this seems unlikely. More likely causes include irritation of the ligaments extending from the diaphragm to the abdominal viscera, which may be provoked by repeated diaphragm shortening. Alternatively, irritation of the abdominal portion of the parietal peritoneum may be caused by increased abdominal pressure and stomach distention (47).

Neural Regulation of Breathing Pattern and Respiratory Muscle Recruitment

What mechanisms within the ventilatory control system are responsible for the timing of the respiratory pattern and the actions of the inspiratory and expiratory muscles? Vagally mediated feedback from lung stretch and airway receptors (Fig. 10.1) have been studied in exercising animals whose vagus nerves may be isolated, placed in a skin flap in the neck, and blocked quickly and reversibly by external cooling. In humans, patients with transplanted denervated lungs have been studied, and topical airway anesthesia has also been used to block feedback from the lung in normal intact humans. These data show that blockade of the vagal feedback causes frequency to slow and tidal volume to increase via increases in end-inspiratory lung volume, thereby demonstrating that vagal feedback was critical to limiting the in-

crease in tidal volume, at least during moderate exercise. Furthermore, phasic expiratory abdominal muscle activity was stimulated and rib cage expiratory muscle activity inhibited by vagal feedback during exercise. Since active expiration begins even in very light exercise, these findings suggest that vagal feedback control of active expiration via the abdominal expiratory muscles is highly sensitive to even small changes in lung stretch in both humans and dogs. Feed-forward activation of abdominal expiratory muscles, originating from locomotor areas of the higher CNS commensurate with the onset of locomotion, may also account for some of this early activation of expiratory abdominal muscle activity.

The control of breathing pattern appears to be more complex at higher exercise intensities, especially when expiratory flow limitation first appears, as evidenced by the intersection of the tidal flow–volume loop with the maximum volitional loop (Fig. 10.9). Key questions here include the following: What constrains the expiratory muscles from developing excessive pressures beyond those effective in increasing expiratory flow rate? Is there neural feedback control over the hyperinflation that occurs as airways narrow during expiration (i.e., *avoiding* impending flow limitation), or does this hyperinflation occur simply because of mechanical constraint on expiratory flow rate imposed by the narrowed airways (i.e., forcing lung volume upward)? With high exercise intensities the powerful combination of chemoreceptors and locomotor-linked drives to breathe become intense, producing hyperventilation. However, the responsiveness of tidal volume and frequency to these stimuli is mechanically constrained in many subjects with a greater than average $\dot{V}O_{2max}$. This constraint has been demonstrated by showing that the slope of the tidal volume and ventilatory responses to added inspired carbon dioxide is reduced during heavy exercise versus that in mild or moderate exercise; and that this ventilatory response to carbon dioxide during heavy exercise is enhanced if the maximum flow–volume envelope is enlarged and flow limitation is relieved by breathing He-O$_2$, a low-density gas mixture (48).

What about feedback from the inspiratory and expiratory muscles themselves to control breathing pattern and/or respiratory muscle recruitment? As with any negative feedback system, it makes sense that the best source of feedback should be from the structures that are the most affected by the efferent motor output, in this case, the respiratory muscles. Just as with limb skeletal muscles, there are high densities of sensory nerve endings in the diaphragm, intercostals, and abdominal expiratory muscles, including type III and IV afferents and Golgi tendon organs. Furthermore, recent evidence in anesthetized preparations shows that the type IV receptors in the diaphragm are activated by fatiguing the diaphragm (49), and accumulation of lactic acid in the diaphragm muscle may actually inhibit phrenic nerve activity (50). Perhaps this inhibitory feedback from a fatiguing diaphragm may be an attempt to spare this crucial inspiratory muscle from further fatigue (or even damage). So the potential for significant feedback reflex effects from the respiratory muscles themselves on cardiorespiratory control is clearly present. These feedback influences from the diaphragm appear to be similar but probably less effective—at least over the control of ventilation—than the feedback from similar receptors in working limb skeletal muscle.

Locomotor–Respiratory Coupling

Just as there is a dual role for respiratory abdominal and rib cage muscles in assisting locomotion, it has also been claimed that locomotion affects breathing pattern and ventilation. There are certainly examples of clear entrainment of respiratory frequency with stride frequency. For example, in bipedal humans, such entrainment occurs on occasion—but is not observed consistently. This entrainment seems to occur most often in running (vs. cycling) and at high intensities in experienced versus novice athletes. In quadrupeds, 1:1 respiratory locomotor coupling is observed consistently only in galloping animals, such as horses. In the canine such strict entrainment is rare, as very high breathing frequencies, in the 2- to 5-Hz range (which occur with panting), are common for purposes of thermal regulation.

Contributions of locomotor forces during running to the generation of airflow is commonly claimed in both humans and quadrupeds, based on the concept that the to-and-fro movements of the liver act as a "visceral piston" against the diaphragm. However, extensive electromyographic evidence in exercising dogs shows that each inspiration, regardless of breathing frequency, is accompanied by diaphragmatic electrical activity and active shortening of the diaphragm (51). Furthermore, in running humans, airflow associated only with the foot plant was shown to contribute less than 1 to 2% of the total tidal volume generated during active inspiration. So while there are certainly important mechanical links between locomotion and respiratory muscle function, exercise hyperpnea and breathing pattern during exercise are not commonly determined by the mechanical consequences of locomotor activity. Thus, neural control mechanisms are clearly required for this coupling between the two motor systems, respiration and locomotion. Again, the usual suspects invoked to explain this coupling are central locomotor "command" and peripheral feedback. A recent study used an *in vitro* brainstem–spinal cord preparation and electrical stimulation of sensory afferent pathways to simulate the effects of muscle contraction (52). They showed that an intact rhythmic sensory feedback input from hindlimb muscles was essential to respiratory–locomotor coupling.

This neuroanatomical linkage originating in proprioceptor afferents from the lumbar spinal cord, with sensory input to the medullary respiratory network and motor output to phrenic motor neurons and diaphragm, may provide the basis for respiratory–locomotor coupling in many mammals. Certainly these types of findings represent an impor-

tant advance in understanding because of the unique capability of these preparations to isolate and separate specific mechanisms. However, whether the demonstrated dominance of peripheral over central locomotor input on respiratory rhythm will hold during actual dynamic exercise in the intact animal remains untested.

Conscious Perception of the Drive and Effort to Breathe

In our discussions of the control of breathing and exercise hyperpnea we have exclusively emphasized the brainstem as the sole depository of afferent inputs from reflex receptors in the periphery and from higher locomotor centers. However, common experience tells us that the cerebral cortex must also receive information related to the effort to breathe. For example, we commonly do express an awareness of an increased effort to breathe at moderate exercise intensities (i.e., usually above work rates where $\dot{V}E$ increases slightly more than $\dot{V}O_2$). Also, with further increases in exercise intensity, most healthy persons will eventually express an unpleasant sensation commonly called shortness of breath, breathlessness, or dyspnea. This dyspneic sensation assumes great significance to daily living in many patients with pulmonary or cardiac disease, who often have debilitating and truly painful levels of dyspnea during exercise of even mild intensity. Such symptoms become the major limitation to exercise performance and likely play a role in the conscious decisions on the part of these patients whether to engage in exercise in their daily living. It is also likely that these cortical perceptions of breathing effort play some significant role in determining breathing frequency and V_T in an attempt to minimize breathing discomfort. It is now common in routine exercise testing protocols to assess subjective perceptions of dyspnea (in addition to those of limb effort and discomfort) using various types of rating scales.

There is a sound anatomical and neurophysiological basis for the higher CNS to be made aware of excessive sensory input associated with breathing efforts and ventilatory stimuli. This evidence shows that sensory input received by the medullary pattern generator, in addition to providing motor output to stimulate the respiratory muscles, also gives rise to neural information that is relayed to and perceived by higher (supramedullary) nervous system structures as an unpleasant sensation emanating from increased respiratory drive and/or effort. That these neural pathways from the medulla to higher centers do exist is shown by the activation of rhythmic neuronal activity in mesencephalic and thalamic neurons in response to peripheral chemostimulation (53).

The mechanisms underlying the perception of breathlessness remain a mystery. Is dyspnea due only to the magnitude of sensory input? What types of input are important? What is the role of efferent motor output to the respiratory pump muscles in the perception of respiratory effort, and how does one distinguish the effects of a high motor output from that due to the summation of massive sensory inputs alone to the higher CNS? Since only humans can provide feedback concerning their perception of effort, remarkable experiments have been conducted in such models as patients with spinal cord lesions as high as C1-C2, experimental respiratory muscle paralysis in normal subjects, and patients with heart-lung transplants. Most evidence supports an important role for mechanoreceptor afferent feedback from respiratory muscles, rib cage, and lung volume accompanying the hyperpnea of exercise. Furthermore, a long-held concept is that sensations of dyspnea are most likely to occur when there is a marked discrepancy between the magnitude of the central neural drive and/or the neuromuscular effort exerted by the respiratory muscles on the one hand and the ventilation (volume and flow rate) achieved on the other. This discrepancy and the ensuing unpleasant and often even painful perception of breathing has been aptly attributed to "unsatisfied inspiratory efforts" (54).

This combination of factors is most commonly encountered in patients with lung, chest wall, or cardiac diseases because of mechanical impedances to lung expansion (decreased compliance) or to airflow (higher resistance), especially when the drives to breathe and the ventilatory requirements are augmented during exercise. However, this discrepancy between neural input and ventilatory output also occurs in healthy subjects at high ventilatory demands in heavy exercise, especially when lung volume hyperinflation occurs in the face of expiratory flow limitation. Heavy exercise in the hypoxia of high altitudes often elicits extreme dyspneic sensations, probably owing to the extremely high sensory inputs emanating from hypoxemic and acidotic carotid chemoreceptors in combination with the markedly increased levels of respiratory muscle work.

Pulmonary Gas Exchange

The Demands Imposed on the Lung by Exercise

Exercise places huge demands on the lung. First, the lung is faced with a large progressive decline in oxygenation ($P\bar{v}O_2$ reduced to < 20 mm Hg) and rise in carbon dioxide ($P\bar{v}CO_2$ rising to > 75 mm Hg), as the locomotor muscles utilize oxygen and produce carbon dioxide in large amounts (Table 10.1). Second, because of the rising pulmonary blood flow the lung has a greatly reduced time in which to equilibrate the deoxygenated mixed venous blood with the alveolar gas in order to maintain PaO_2 (and $PaCO_2$) near resting levels. Third, because the lung is in series with the left heart, *it is the only organ that must accommodate all of the cardiac output all of the time;* so as cardiac output increases more than fourfold to fivefold over resting levels during heavy exercise, so must the flow of blood through the pulmonary vasculature increase to an identical extent. This huge increase in flow has the potential to increase pulmonary vascular pressures substantially, thereby increasing the load placed on the right ventricle and also presenting a large hydrostatic pressure gradient that could force plasma water out of the vasculature and into the alveoli. The exudation of even small amounts of fluid into the alveoli would substantially reduce the diffusion of oxygen into the pulmonary capillaries, resulting in severe arterial hypoxemia.

We know that these dire events do not occur in the normal healthy lung even in heavy exercise, as PaO_2 is (with some exceptions) maintained near resting levels and the increase in pulmonary capillary pressures is usually limited to less than double its resting value. Pulmonary vascular resistance falls dramatically as cardiac output rises. The alveoli remain dry. An understanding of the unique microstructure of the healthy gas–blood interface in the lung is important to appreciate this remarkable homeostatic response. Key features of these structures are summarized next.

Lung Structure Suits Function

The structure of the pulmonary circulation is unique and aimed at preserving a low vascular resistance and providing maximum alveolar–capillary surface area for diffusion (Fig. 10.12). To this end vessels are thin-walled and highly compliant in the lung, and they contain relatively little smooth muscle. At rest, the average resistance to blood flow in the pulmonary vasculature is only about one-tenth that in the systemic circulation (Box 10.3).

The pulmonary arterioles at the entrance to the lung's gas exchange area do contain smooth muscle and will respond vigorously to local alveolar hypoxia or carbon dioxide accumulation. While this smooth muscle is innervated by motor nerves from the sympathetic branch of the autonomic nervous system, pulmonary arterioles do not constrict vigorously with reflex sympathetic activation, unlike arterioles in the systemic circulation. This lack of sympathetic vasoconstrictor influence is very important to maintaining a low resistance in the pulmonary vasculature during exercise, because this circulation does not share in the exercise-induced increase in efferent sympathetic vasoconstrictor activity imposed on the systemic vasculature.

The pulmonary circulation includes an extensive interdigitating capillary network within the alveolar walls (Fig. 10.12B). This capillary network has been likened more to sheets of blood than to individual channels, with its huge surface area of many square meters containing only 70 to 90 mL of blood (or only 2% of the total circulating blood volume) under resting conditions. This blood volume in the pulmonary capillaries can expand more than threefold with only very small changes in perfusion pressure, as pulmonary blood flow rises linearly with increasing work rate.

It is important to gas exchange that the alveoli be kept dry, and to this end capillary perfusion pressures are maintained relatively low during exercise. At rest there is a small outward flow of plasma fluid (about 10–20 mL/hour) from the capillaries into the interstitial space of the alveolar wall,

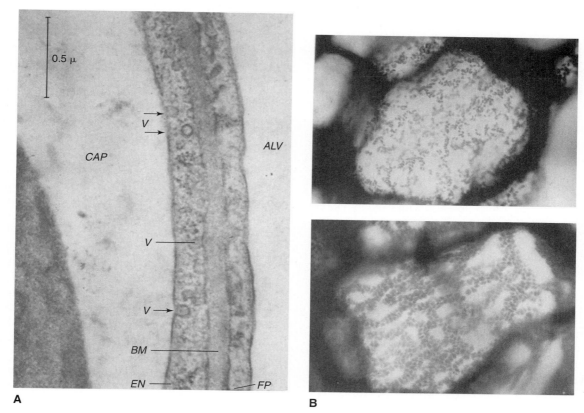

FIGURE 10.12 **A.** The alveolar–capillary blood gas barrier and the alveolar-to-capillary diffusion pathway. Alv, alveolar gas; EP, alveolar epithelium; BM, basement membrane; EN, capillary endothelium; CAP, capillary. In the capillary, the clear area is plasma and the darker area is the corner of a red blood cell in the left bottom corner. Between the alveolar epithelium and the capillary endothelium lies the interstitial fluid space, which is important to lymphatic drainage of extravascular lung water. **B.** Single alveolar walls face on to show the extent of filling of the capillary network. *Top.* Capillaries are less well filled with erythrocytes than they might be in a midgravitational zone of the lung in the resting human. *Bottom.* Alveoli under higher flow conditions (such as with exercise), in which the capillary network is fully recruited and distended. The capillary network around each alveolus forms a nearly continuous sheet of blood when all capillaries are recruited, as in the high flow condition.

which passes into the perivascular and peribronchiolar spaces of the lung (Fig. 10.12A). In turn, the lymphatic system transports fluid from the interstitial spaces out of the lung to the hilar lymph nodes. The flow of lymph will increase substantially with increasing cardiac output as hydrostatic pressure rises in the capillaries and the alveolar capillary surface expands. This lymphatic "storm sewer" is vitally important to *preventing exudation of fluid into the alveoli* during exercise (55).

The alveolar–capillary barrier must be both *extremely thin,* so that diffusion distance is kept to a minimum, and *very strong,* so that it does not break down when capillary pressures are raised with increases in blood flow through the lung. This barrier is indeed extremely thin, less than a fraction of the

Box 10.3

SYSTEMIC VERSUS PULMONARY VASCULAR RESISTANCE

Systemic vascular resistance = (aortic pressure – right atrial pressure) ÷ blood flow = (90 mm Hg – 3 mm Hg) ÷ 5 L/min = 17 mm Hg · L · min^{-1}

Pulmonary vascular resistance = (pulmonary artery pressure – left atrial pressure) ÷ blood flow = (14 mm Hg – 8 mm Hg) ÷ 5 L · min^{-1} = 1.2 mm Hg · L · min^{-1}

thickness of a human hair; however, strength to this barrier is supplied by an extremely thin layer of collagen tissue (56).

Pulmonary Vascular Response to Exercise and the Blood–Gas Barrier

The net driving force for blood flow through the lung is the pressure difference between the pulmonary artery (Ppa) and the pulmonary capillary (Pcap). The Ppa is measured directly via right heart catheterization, and the Pcap is estimated from the so-called wedge pressure, obtained when a balloon-tipped catheter is advanced into a lobar branch of the Ppa. Changes in wedge pressure with exercise closely approximate those in left ventricular end-diastolic pressure.

The changes in pulmonary vascular pressures during steady-state upright exercise are shown in Figure 10.13. With the onset of mild exercise there is a parallel rise in both pulmonary arterial and wedge pressure with no change in the driving pressure (Ppa − Pcap) across the lung. Nevertheless, pulmonary blood flow increases, indicating an abrupt fall in pulmonary vascular resistance (PVR). This reduced resistance reflects an increase in cross-sectional area of the pulmonary vasculature as more capillaries are recruited, especially in the lung apices, and with distention of already recruited capillaries (Fig. 10.12B). As exercise intensity increases further, the linear increase in blood flow through the lung is achieved with

only minor further reductions in PVR, principally by increasing the driving pressure within the pulmonary vasculature.

With progressive increases in exercise intensity, the purely mechanical effects of a rising left atrial filling pressure and pulmonary capillary pressure secondary to the increase in pulmonary blood flow exert the dominant effect on recruitment and distension of the delicate, thin-walled, highly compliant lung capillaries. The rise in left atrial pressure also accounts for almost all of the upstream increase in Ppa.

An increased shear stress on the pulmonary vasculature induces release of potent vasodilators such as nitric oxide from the vascular endothelium. However, these humoral vasodilators are of only minor importance in regulating pulmonary hemodynamics during progressive intensity exercise. During prolonged constant-load exercise, pulmonary vascular resistance falls over time, and this may involve active vasodilation secondary to the release of vasodilators from the endothelium.

The rate of fluid filtration from the pulmonary vasculature is governed by classical Starling forces, which include the hydrostatic pressure gradient from vessel lumen to interstitial fluid space, the oncotic pressures governing reabsorption into the capillary, and the permeability of the blood–gas barrier (Box 10.4).

Contrary to earlier concepts, it is now clear that heavy dynamic exercise places significant stress on the integrity of the blood-gas barrier. First, pulmonary capillary wedge pressures in maximum exercise often exceed 20 mm Hg in untrained subjects (at cardiac outputs about 25 L · min⁻¹) and 30 to 35 mm Hg in highly trained subjects (at cardiac outputs of 30–35 L · min⁻¹). These higher capillary wedge pressures are approaching those shown to cause fluid accumulation in isolated lung lobes. Second, lungs stretched to extreme volumes (as may occur with dynamic hyperinflation in high-intensity exercise) will narrow capillaries, may increase pulmonary vascular resistance, and may also increase the permeability of the pulmonary capillaries in the alveolar walls by increasing the longitudinal tension in the alveolar walls. In addition, the alveolar-capillary surface area increases substantially with capillary recruitment during exercise, thereby promoting increased fluid flux across the blood-gas barrier.

So what are the consequences of these changes in extravascular fluid flux and high capillary pressures in the lung? When extravascular fluid does accumulate, it appears first as interstitial fluid cuffs that surround larger vessels and airways outside the alveolar–capillary region. With further transvascular fluid flux, alveolar flooding may occur. Since it is not possible to precisely measure extravascular lung water *in vivo*, we do not know for sure whether heavy exercise causes accumulation of extravascular fluid. However, it seems unlikely that substantial fluid accumulation is reached during exercise, because fluid reabsorption from the interstitial space is enhanced by an increased capillary osmotic pressure gradient and the thoracic lymph flow also rises several orders of magnitude and in proportion to the increased pulmonary blood flow. The tremendous reserve capacity of

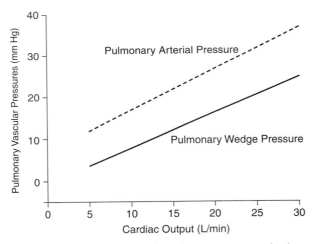

FIGURE 10.13 Pressures in the pulmonary artery and pulmonary capillaries (wedge pressures) and pulmonary vascular resistance in young male and female subjects during progressive steady-state exercise, plotted against increasing cardiac output. The relationships between the increasing pulmonary blood flow and the increasing vascular pressures were such that pulmonary vascular resistance fell from rest to moderate exercise and remained low through heavy exercise intensities. *(Data are reprinted with permission from Reeves JT, Dempsey JA, Grover RF. Pulmonary circulation during exercise. In Weir EK, Reeves JT, eds. Pulmonary Vascular Physiology and Pathophysiology. New York: Marcel Dekker, 1989, 107–133.)*

the thoracic lymphatic drainage is a key mechanism in keeping the lung dry even at very high exercise intensities (55).

However, there are examples of pulmonary capillary stress failure during extreme dynamic exercise when cardiac output and capillary hydrostatic pressures are extraordinarily high (Fig. 10.14, *A* and *B*). First, maximal exhaustive exercise in elite competitive cyclists forces red blood cells and protein across the blood-gas barrier; they appear in bronchial alveolar lavage fluid obtained following the exercise (57). In the Thoroughbred horse, even submaximal exercise routinely causes widespread alveolar hemorrhage. In this equine athlete, the enormous cardiac output achieved (>750 L · min^{-1} at a $\dot{V}_{O_{2max}}$ >160 ml · kg^{-1} · min^{-1}) relative to the morphometric dimensions of the pulmonary vasculature results in left atrial pressures above 70 mm Hg, Ppa above 120 mm

Hg, and pulmonary capillary pressures approximating 100 mm Hg (these exceed by several fold those in humans, as shown in Fig. 10.13 and Table 10.1). The capillary stress failure occurs because of intracellular disruptions in both endothelial and epithelial cells. Once the capillary pressures are reduced to normal following this extreme dynamic exercise, these intracellular disruptions rapidly close.

Regulation of the Alveolar to Arterial P$_{O_2}$ Difference and Arterial P$_{O_2}$ During Exercise, Diffusion, $\dot{V}/\dot{Q}$ Distribution, and Shunt

Determinants of the A-aD$_{O_2}$

The alveolar to arterial P$_{O_2}$ difference (A-aD$_{O_2}$) is a measurement of the efficiency of pulmonary gas exchange. Its magni-

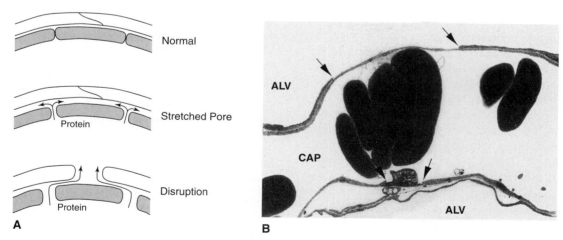

A   **B**

FIGURE 10.14   A. Three hypothetical stages of pulmonary edema caused by increasing capillary transmural pressure. *Top.* Normal morphology, which is associated with low protein hydrostatic edema when capillary pressure is raised. *Center.* Pore stretching with increased permeability of endothelium and leakage of protein into interstitium; epithelium remains intact. *Bottom.* Endothelial and epithelial disruption caused by stress failure and consequent movement of protein into alveolar spaces. *(Reprinted with permission from West JB, Tsukimoto K, Mathieu-Costello O, et al. Stress failure in pulmonary capillaries. J Appl Physiol 1991;70:1740.)* **B.** Stress failure in pulmonary capillaries in response to very high capillary transmural pressures caused by experimentally increasing perfusion pressure in an *in situ* perfused rabbit lung preparation. Both the alveolar epithelial layer (*right*) and capillary endothelial layer (*left*) are disrupted with a platelet shown close to the basement membrane. *(Reprinted with permission from West JB, Tsukimoto K, Mathieu-Costello O, et al. Stress failure in pulmonary capillaries. J Appl Physiol 1991;70:1733.)*

tude is determined primarily by the uniformity with which $\dot{V}_A$ is distributed with respect to $\dot{Q}$ throughout the lungs' 300 million alveolar capillary gas exchange units. In intact humans, given the complexity and enormity of the gas exchange area, the $\dot{V}/\dot{Q}$ distribution cannot be quantified with great precision, but it can be estimated in two ways. First, lung imaging of inhaled and infused radioactive tracers yields useful information on topographical gravity-dependent distribution of $\dot{V}/\dot{Q}$; however, this approach lacks resolution because of the large tissue volumes that must be averaged. A second approach uses infused inert gases (i.e., those that do not combine with hemoglobin) of varying solubility to provide a near-continuous measurement of the distribution of $\dot{V}/\dot{Q}$ throughout the lung. This multiple inert gas technique is based on the principle that the excretion and retention of each of the inert gases by the lung depends upon the magnitude of the $\dot{V}/\dot{Q}$ ratio and the solubility of the gas (58).

Second, the A-aDO$_2$ can be widened by the extrapulmonary shunting of deoxygenated mixed venous blood, which bypasses the pulmonary capillaries. To date, the only such significant shunt of deoxygenated venous blood known for sure to be present in healthy humans is that of the Thebesian venous drainage, originating in the coronary vasculature and emptying into the left ventricle. This is estimated to constitute 1 to 2% of the resting cardiac output. Estimating the exact amount of shunt (intrapulmonary and extrapulmonary) is usually done by determining the effects of breathing high concentrations of oxygen on PaO$_2$ and on the A-aDO$_2$ and is based on the premise that increases in alveolar PO$_2$ to more than 600 mm Hg will readily correct any contributions to the A-aDO$_2$ of simply low (but > 0) $\dot{V}/\dot{Q}$ regions or deficient diffusion capacity (discussed later). Primarily because of the great difficulty encountered in measuring very high levels of PO$_2$ in blood and several of the assumptions that must be made, this technique is of questionable value in quantifying shunts less than 10% of cardiac output.

Finally, the third determinant of the A-aDO$_2$ is the diffusion equilibrium of alveolar gas with end-pulmonary capillary blood, as determined by the alveolar capillary surface area, the diffusion gradient (from alveolar to capillary PO$_2$) and the time available for equilibration in the pulmonary capillary (Fig. 10.15). The available diffusion surface area in the lung may be estimated by inspiring small concentrations of carbon monoxide and measuring its rate of disappearance from the lung, because carbon monoxide uptake is dependent upon the rate of diffusion from alveolar gas to capillary blood.

The contribution of $\dot{V}/\dot{Q}$ nonuniformity and shunt to the A-aDO$_2$ may be calculated by knowing the mixed venous oxygen content, the $\dot{V}/\dot{Q}$ distribution, and the shunt fraction. Any remaining A-aDO$_2$ not attributable to $\dot{V}/\dot{Q}$ or shunt is commonly attributed to diffusion disequilibrium.

At rest, the A-aDO$_2$ averages 5 to 15 mm Hg in normal, healthy nonsmoking young adults and rises another 5 to 10 mm Hg or so by age 70. That the A-aDO$_2$ is this narrow is truly amazing, given the marked topographical heterogeneity

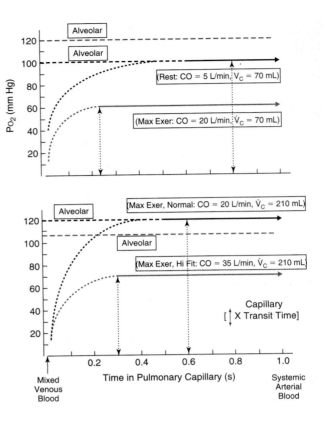

FIGURE 10.15 Time course of equilibration of mixed venous blood with alveolar gas in the pulmonary capillary at varying cardiac outputs, pulmonary capillary blood volumes (VC), and degrees of alveolar hyperventilation (and alveolar PO$_2$.) *Top.* A normally fit subject at rest and at maximum exercise, with normal increases in cardiac output, alveolar ventilation, and alveolar PO$_2$ but assuming a pulmonary capillary blood volume fixed at resting levels. The capillary transit time is greatly reduced from rest to exercise because cardiac output increased without a corresponding increase in pulmonary capillary blood volume. This theoretical example emphasizes the importance of the normal pulmonary capillary expansion to gas exchange during exercise. *Bottom.* Contrast between a normally fit subject and a highly fit subject at $\dot{V}O_{2max}$. Pulmonary capillary blood volumes are assumed to be similar in the two subjects, but $\dot{V}O_{2max}$ and therefore maximum cardiac output is substantially greater in the highly fit subject. In addition, the highly fit subject has not hyperventilated to the same extent as the normally fit subject. Note the slower rate of equilibration of mixed venous blood with alveolar oxygen in the pulmonary capillary and the markedly shortened transit time in the pulmonary capillary; this is due to a cardiac output that increased out of proportion to the pulmonary capillary blood volume. Arterial hypoxemia occurs because pulmonary capillary blood reached the end of the pulmonary capillary before it reached equilibration with alveolar gas. This scenario represents one theoretical explanation for arterial hypoxemia in heavy exercise in highly trained subjects.

from lung apex to base in the distribution of $\dot{V}_A$ (fourfold to fivefold difference), $\dot{Q}$ (ninefold difference), and $\dot{V}/\dot{Q}$ (3–4 at the apex vs. 0.8 at the lung bases). Furthermore, even in the healthy lung there is also structural heterogeneity in vessels and airways, which gives rise to nongravitational maldistribution of $\dot{V}_A$ and $\dot{Q}$ distribution within any lung region (59). Nonetheless, the inert gas measurements show us that functional $\dot{V}/\dot{Q}$ distribution is really rather narrow in the healthy lung at rest, with an average $\dot{V}/\dot{Q}$ ratio of about 0.8 to 0.9 and a variation about this mean from about 0.4 to

1.3 $\dot{V}/\dot{Q}$. This $\dot{V}/\dot{Q}$ distribution could account for about half of the resting A-aDo$_2$; the remainder is likely due to the small anatomical shunt, with no portion of the A-aDo$_2$ attributable to diffusion disequilibrium at rest (Fig. 10.16).

Why the Increased A-aDo$_2$ During Dynamic Exercise?

A-aDo$_2$ begins to rise with mild exercise and continues to widen to average 20 to 30 mm Hg at maximal exercise in the

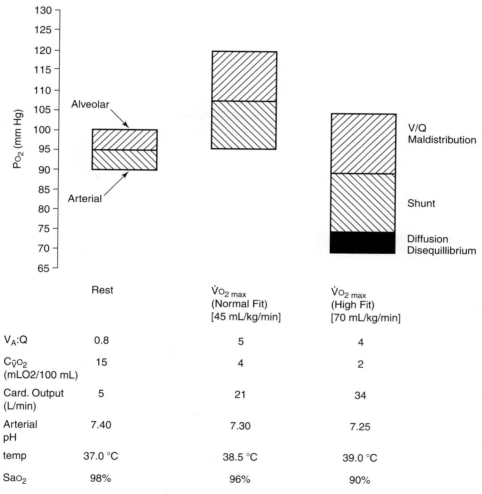

	Rest	$\dot{V}o_{2\ max}$ (Normal Fit) [45 mL/kg/min]	$\dot{V}o_{2\ max}$ (High Fit) [70 mL/kg/min]
$V_A{:}Q$	0.8	5	4
$C\bar{v}o_2$ (mLO2/100 mL)	15	4	2
Card. Output (L/min)	5	21	34
Arterial pH	7.40	7.30	7.25
temp	37.0 °C	38.5 °C	39.0 °C
Sao$_2$	98%	96%	90%

FIGURE 10.16 Causes of the increase in the alveolar to arterial Po$_2$ difference and the reduction in percent Oxyhemoglobin saturation during maximum exercise in a normally fit and a highly fit subject with exercise-induced arterial hypoxemia (EIAH). In the normally fit subject the increase in the A-aDo$_2$ at maximum exercise was due to approximately equal contributions from V/Q lack of uniformity and a small anatomical shunt of mixed venous blood. Both contributions to the A-aDo$_2$ from these sources are magnified because of the exercise-induced reductions in mixed venous oxygen content ($C\bar{v}o_2$). In the highly fit subject most of the A-aDo$_2$ is also caused by shunt and V/Q maldistribution, but in addition it has been proposed that an alveolar capillary diffusion disequilibrium is present, perhaps because of the shortened red cell transit time (Fig. 10.15). The reduced Pao$_2$ in the highly fit is also due to less hyperventilation, as noted by the lower alveolar Po$_2$. The reduced Sao$_2$ is due almost equally to the reduced Pao$_2$ and to the rightward shift in the hemoglobin-oxygen dissociation curve in arterial blood because of the combination of metabolic acidosis and increased temperature.

normally fit subject and to as much as 35 to 50 mm Hg at higher $\dot{V}O_{2max}$ in a significant number (but not all) of highly fit subjects. In most subjects the increased A-aDO_2 consists only of a rise in PAO_2, because $\dot{V}A$ increases out of proportion to $\dot{V}O_2$, and arterial PO_2 is maintained near resting levels. In the extreme cases of A-aDO_2 widening, arterial hypoxemia does occur (PAO_2 20–30 mm Hg less than resting levels and percent oxyhemoglobin saturation $SaO_2 < 94\%$) and is often exacerbated by a minimal hyperventilatory response (and therefore minimal rise in alveolar PO_2).

So we can now examine the three major determinants of A-aDO_2 (as discussed earlier) to determine why pulmonary gas exchange becomes more inefficient as exercise intensity increases (Fig. 10.16). First, a small but significant increase, about 20 to 30%, occurs in the overall nonuniformity of $\dot{V}/\dot{Q}$ distribution throughout the lung with moderate to heavy exercise (as determined via the inert gas method). Interestingly, topographical (or gravity dependent) $\dot{V}/\dot{Q}$ distribution becomes much more uniform during exercise, as perfusion to lung apices is greatly improved by an increased pulmonary arterial pressure coincident with the increase in cardiac output (Fig. 10.13). Accordingly, we presume that the increased heterogeneity in overall $\dot{V}/\dot{Q}$ distribution must derive from greater nonuniformity within *isogravitational* lung regions. The reasons for this small increase in $\dot{V}/\dot{Q}$ nonuniformity are unknown, but the possibilities range from release of inflammatory mediators in the airways and/or vasculature, which would increase local resistances to airflow or blood flow, to fluid accumulation (or cuffing of plasma water around small vessels and airways). The most likely explanation is simply the normal anatomical heterogeneity of vessel and airway diameters and compliances within specific isogravitational lung regions in all healthy subjects. The effect of even these small increases in $\dot{V}/\dot{Q}$ lack of uniformity on the A-aDO_2 is magnified during exercise by the progressively reduced mixed venous oxygen content resulting from the increased extraction of oxygen by the working muscles (Table 10.1).

Although these combined effects of $\dot{V}/\dot{Q}$ heterogeneity and reduced $C\bar{v}O_2$ alone would tend to widen A-aDO_2 and reduce PaO_2 during exercise, these effects are opposed by the disproportionate increase in total $\dot{V}A$ relative to cardiac output (and to $\dot{V}O_2$). This means that mean $\dot{V}/\dot{Q}$ increases from less than 1.0 at rest to 4 to 5 in heavy exercise. Accordingly, even the lowest $\dot{V}/\dot{Q}$ regions of the lung during exercise are greater in magnitude (and therefore well ventilated with high alveolar PO_2) than the highest $\dot{V}/\dot{Q}$ regions at rest. Thus the ventilatory response to exercise is a key protector of pulmonary gas exchange and arterial PO_2 during exercise.

While $\dot{V}/\dot{Q}$ nonuniformity accounts for about half of the increase in A-aDO_2 with exercise, what accounts for the remainder of the increase? Two popular postulates are diffusion disequilibrium and intrapulmonary or extrapulmonary shunts. To date there has been no definitive way to precisely partition these potential contributions to the A-aDO_2.

Extrapulmonary shunting must be a significant contributor to the increased A-aDO_2, because we know that venous drainage from the coronary sinuses to the left ventricle via the Thebesian veins does exist in the human. Furthermore, as myocardial $\dot{V}O_2$ increases during exercise, the oxygen content of coronary sinus effluent blood must fall and the absolute flow of shunted blood increases. Other potential conduits for shunting mixed venous blood via intrapulmonary or extrapulmonary routes may actually open up during exercise as cardiac output and pulmonary arterial pressure increase (60). However, this latter possibility has not been tested directly.

Can alveolar–capillary diffusion disequilibrium occur during exercise and explain a portion of the widened A-aDO_2? This will depend upon the rate of equilibration of mixed venous blood with alveolar PO_2 (i.e., diffusion capacity) and the time available in the pulmonary capillary allowed for this equilibrium to occur (Fig. 10.15). The transit time of the red blood cell in the pulmonary capillary depends critically upon how closely changes in pulmonary capillary blood volume match those in cardiac output during exercise.

$$\text{Mean transit time of the pulmonary capillaries (s)}$$
$$= \text{pulmonary capillary blood volume (mL)}$$
$$\div \text{pulmonary blood flow (mL s}^{-1}\text{)}$$

So for example, at rest:

$$\text{Transit time} = 70 \text{ mL} \div 5000 \text{ mL min}^{-1}$$

Thus

$$\text{transit time} = 70 \text{ mL} \div 83 \text{ mL s}^{-1} = 0.8 \text{ s}$$

If one exercises at high intensities, so that cardiac output increases to 20 L · min^{-1} and pulmonary capillary blood volume does not change from resting levels, the mean transit time would fall to about 0.2 seconds, and there is an excellent chance that diffusion equilibrium of capillary blood with alveolar gas would occur (Fig. 10.15). However, four important adaptations during exercise counteract this potential diffusion disequilibrium in the pulmonary capillary. First, alveolar–capillary surface area increases, which greatly increases the *diffusion capacity* of the lung (i.e., oxygen diffused and taken up by the capillary blood per millimeter of mercury of diffusion gradient). Second, the extremely short alveolar–capillary diffusion distance is preserved by preventing plasma fluid from entering the alveoli via reductions in pulmonary vascular resistance combined with high lymphatic drainage of the lung interstitium (discussed previously). Third, the alveolar PO_2 increases (via hyperventilation) as the venous PO_2 falls (via muscle oxygen extraction), increasing the diffusion gradient of alveolar to capillary PO_2. Finally, pulmonary capillary blood volume gradually expands as capillaries are recruited with increased cardiac output and reaches values of 200 to 250 mL in normal-sized adults (or about 3 times resting values). This expanded pulmonary capillary volume (Vc) probably approaches the maximum morphological capacity of the entire pulmonary capillary vasculature during maximal exercise. That is, all capillaries are recruited and maximally distended (Fig. 10.12*B*). Thus at 20 L · min^{-1} cardiac output, mean transit time is 0.5 to 0.6 seconds and diffusion equilibrium is readily achieved in the pulmonary capillaries. Estimates of the influence of these changes on the rate of and time for equilibration of oxygen in the pulmonary capillaries are shown schematically in Figure 10.15.

To summarize, the A-aDO$_2$ of 20 to 25 mm Hg achieved in most healthy, untrained subjects at $\dot{V}O_{2max}$ is attributable primarily to the combination of a nonuniform $\dot{V}/\dot{Q}$ and a reduced $C\bar{v}O_2$ plus some significant (but still unquantified) contribution from anatomical shunts (Fig. 10.16). Diffusion limitation is unlikely to be a significant factor in these subjects. However in some trained subjects who widen their A-aDO$_2$ to more than 30 mm Hg at their higher $\dot{V}O_{2max}$, there is a greater probability that diffusion equilibrium is not complete, at least in part because of the extremely short capillary transit times. This may occur in these subjects because their maximum cardiac output is higher than in the untrained, while their maximum pulmonary capillary blood volume may only approximate that in the untrained subject (see "Exercise Training Effects"). In addition, many of these trained subjects also have little or no hyperventilatory response to heavy exercise, so alveolar PO$_2$ is less than normal, as is the alveolar to capillary diffusion gradient.

Finally, the ratio of Vc to blood flow (Vc:$\dot{Q}$), is likely to be distributed heterogeneously throughout the lung. Accordingly, the distribution of red cell transit times will also be heterogenous. In turn, during heavy exercise (and especially in the highly fit subject who has exercise-induced arterial hypoxemia, or EIAH) when calculated mean transit time is barely sufficient to ensure diffusion equilibrium, it is likely that at least a small (but significant) portion of capillary blood flow will perfuse gas exchange areas with a low Vc and therefore markedly shorten transit time. In these areas of the lung, diffusion equilibrium may not occur. In the face of a falling $C\bar{v}O_2$, these small areas of the lung with very short transit times would be expected to contribute significantly to the widened overall A-aDO$_2$.

Respiratory–Cardiovascular Interactions During Dynamic Exercise

It makes sense that the functions of the respiratory and cardiovascular systems should be tightly linked and that their neural control systems communicate, simply because both organ systems acting together are the major determinants of oxygen and carbon dioxide transport (oxygen transport equals arterial oxygen content times blood flow). It would serve no useful purpose to activate one system at the onset of exercise, for example an increase in $\dot{V}O_2$ and cardiac out-

put, without increasing ventilation to maintain arterial oxygen content. Accordingly, there is ample evidence to show that the two primary mechanisms proposed for exercise hyperpnea also have major cardiovascular influences during exercise: (*a*) Central locomotor command has parallel neural pathways to medullary neural networks, which in turn affect increases in both ventilation and cardiac output. (*b*) Activation of type III and IV afferents in contracting limb skeletal muscle reflexively increase both ventilation and sympathetic efferent vasoconstrictor activities. Further, one important trigger for these afferents is the venous distention in muscle that is secondary to increased muscle blood flow (15). There are many other such examples of respiratory–cardiovascular interactions operating during dynamic exercise. We briefly address two fundamental interactions. One is an important determinant of venous return and cardiac output via mechanical heart-lung interdependencies, and the other may influence sympathetic vasoconstrictor outflow and blood flow distribution during exercise via mechanoreflexes and metaboreflexes from the respiratory muscles.

Mechanical Interactions Between the Respiratory and Circulatory Systems (Fig. 10.17)

The performance of the right and left ventricles is in large part determined by the influence of two factors: end-diastolic volume (i.e., preload), and systolic wall stress (i.e., afterload). Perhaps the greatest challenge to understanding cardiopulmonary interactions is forcing yourself to think in terms of *transmural* pressures (inside pressure minus outside pressure). The heart, situated within the intrathoracic space, is unavoidably exposed to excursions in intrathoracic pressure, and its juxtaposition to the lungs in the cardiac fossa provides an additional mechanical interface. At any given point in the respiratory cycle, cardiac preload and afterload will be a function of not only *intracardiac* pressure but also intrathoracic pressure (P$_{ITP}$) and lung surface–cardiac fossa pressure (P$_{lung}$). Similar relationships hold true for the transmural wall stress across the blood vessels within the abdominal compartment or rib cage, which can also be influenced by P$_{ITP}$, P$_{lung}$, or abdominal pressure (P$_{ABD}$). To facilitate the understanding of the basic mechanical interactions between the pulmonary and circulatory systems, the effects of inspiratory and expiratory pressure production are first discussed in the resting human.

Mechanical Effects of P$_{ITP}$ and P$_{lung}$ on Cardiac Preload and Afterload at Rest

During inspiration, the negative pressure generated in the intrathoracic space widens the pressure gradient across the walls of the heart. Such a widened transmural pressure is thought to improve ventricular filling by lowering the pressures within the heart's chambers and augmenting cardiac

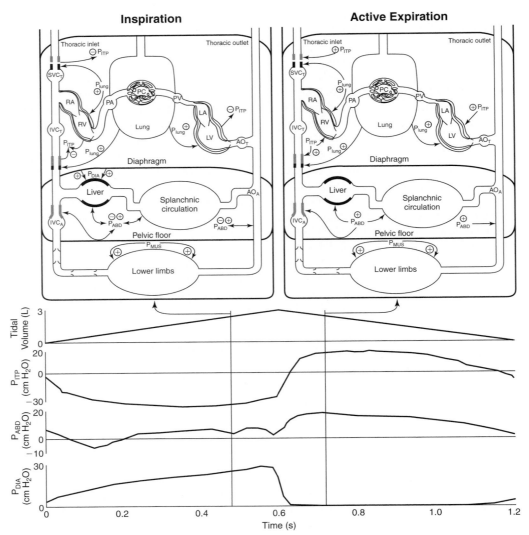

FIGURE 10.17 The cardiovascular effects of respiratory muscle pressure production during high intensity exercise (>90% $\dot{V}O_{2max}$, $f_b = 50$ br · min^{-1}) at the same lung volume during inspiration and expiration. During inspiration, intrathoracic pressure (P_{ITP}) can decrease to less than −30 cm H_2O, resulting in a substantial widening of the pressure gradient across the walls of the heart (denoted by a negative sign). During expiration, P_{ITP} becomes positive, decreasing the transmural pressure across the walls of the heart (denoted by a positive sign). These shifts in P_{ITP} also result in significant changes in the transmural pressure across the thoracic inferior and superior vena cavae (IVC_T and SVC_T, respectively), which can markedly alter the resistance to venous return via changing vessel cross-sectional area. P_{lung} increases exponentially with increases in lung volume and will have a compressive effect on the heart and great vessels. However, its magnitude is likely to be far less than that of P_{ITP} except in cases of severe dynamic hyperinflation. The contraction of the abdominal muscles shifts intraabdominal pressure (P_{ABD}) positive during expiration, resulting in compression of the vasculature within the abdominal compartment and driving of end-expiratory lung volume below functional residual capacity. This contributes to the biphasic P_{ABD} pattern observed during inspiration, as the relaxation of the abdominal muscles during early inspiration results in a rapid outward recoiling of the abdominal wall and a reduction in P_{ABD}. This occurs in spite of contraction of the diaphragm (increasing P_{DIA}), as its descent lags behind the outward movement of the abdominal wall until later during inspiration, when further increases in P_{DIA} elicit roughly proportional increases in P_{ABD}. While increases in P_{DIA} consistently reduce blood flow through the liver via compression of the hepatic sinusoids, the dynamics of P_{ABD} result in distention of the abdominal inferior vena cava (IVC_A) during early inspiration (when P_{ABD} is decreased), followed by moderate compression of the IVC_A during the last half of inspiration (when P_{ABD} is increasing). P_{ABD} is smaller at all time points during inspiration than at expiration, resulting in a *relative* distention of the IVC_A throughout inspiration. The modulatory effects of P_{ITP} and P_{ABD} on venous return from the lower limbs are lower than during rest because of the powerful rhythmic contraction of the locomotor muscles, which compresses the veins within them and forces blood toward the heart.

preload. Of particular importance are the reductions in right atrial pressure during inspiration, which widen the pressure gradient for venous return from the limbs and splanchnic vasculature and increase the return of blood to the heart. However, the increases in ventricular preload during inspiration due to a reduced P_{ITP} can be limited by increases in lung surface pressures as the cardiac fossa becomes less compliant with increasing lung volumes (61). These increases in lung surface pressure usually become significant only at higher lung volumes (e.g., >75% total lung capacity), and the transmural pressure across the walls of the heart is predominantly influenced by changes in P_{ITP}. During the ensuing expiration, ventricular filling is impeded by a narrowing of the transmural pressure gradient due to a positive shift in P_{ITP}, which also reduces the pressure gradient for venous return.

During systole, the reductions in P_{ITP} during inspiration widen the transmural pressure gradient across the walls of the heart and actually *hinder* ventricular emptying. Conversely, during expiration, the positive shift in P_{ITP} can actually *aid* the emptying of the ventricle by the narrowing of the transmural pressure gradient (i.e., the positive P_{ITP} pushes inward on the ventricle as it contracts inward). Although increases in intrathoracic pressure during expiration may increase stroke volume very transiently (e.g., modulation over the course of a breath), the volume of blood ejected from the heart with each contraction is largely dependent upon ventricular preload, *and reductions in cardiac preload will usually predominate over reductions in transmural wall stress because of the dependence of stroke volume upon the Frank-Starling mechanism in normal, healthy humans (67).*

Mechanical Effects of Diaphragm Contraction and P_{ABD} on Venous Return at Rest

While the previous section implies that reductions in P_{ITP} always increase venous return to the heart, increases in inferior vena caval blood flow are not always observed during inspiration at rest. This is primarily because increases in P_{ABD} due to diaphragmatic descent can compress the abdominal inferior vena cava and impede venous return from the lower limb (62). Further complicating matters is the observation that diaphragmatic contraction decreases venous return from the splanchnic circulation via compression of the liver, with this phenomenon occurring independently of changes in P_{ABD} (63). A third and final consideration in the prediction of the effects of breathing on venous return is the blood volume status of the inferior vena cava. If abdominal vena caval blood volume is high (e.g., immediately preceding an inspiration at rest), increases in P_{ABD} will translocate a relatively large volume of blood up toward the heart during inspiration as a result of the compression of the abdominal vena cava (with the venous valves preventing retrograde flow), resulting in increases in venous return.

However, if blood volume is low (e.g., at end-inspiration at rest), a relatively small volume of blood will be translocated upward, and venous return will decrease during inspiration as a result of a decreased blood flow *through* the inferior vena cava (64).

So predicting the effect of inspiration or expiration on cardiac filling and emptying requires knowledge not only of the magnitude and directionality of P_{ITP} and lung surface pressure but also the of P_{ABD} and transdiaphragmatic pressure (P_{DIA}). Reductions in P_{ITP} cannot increase venous return from the lower limbs and splanchnic vasculature without permissive changes in P_{ABD} and P_{DIA}. The role of blood volume in the cardiovascular response to changes in P_{ITP}, P_{ABD}, and P_{DIA} is only beginning to be understood but is likely to play a significant role as well.

Most of these mechanisms have been derived or elucidated using anesthetized, paralyzed, and/or open-chested animals. While such reduced preparations have provided a strong foundation to build on and are fundamental to one's understanding of cardiopulmonary interactions, it is very difficult (and often inappropriate) to extrapolate from these findings and predict the effects of the pressures produced by the respiratory muscles on the heart and great vessels during dynamic exercise.

Mechanical Effects of Respiratory Muscle Pressure Production on Cardiovascular Function During Dynamic Exercise

To facilitate understanding of the principles of mechanical cardiopulmonary interactions, all of the preceding discussion has focused on the effects of respiratory muscle pressure on cardiovascular function at rest. When considering these interactions during exercise, one must account for the mechanical effects of the phasic contraction of the locomotor muscles, which push blood back to the heart (Fig. 10.17). This is frequently referred to as the skeletal muscle pump, and it is thought to be critical in the maintenance of venous return during upright exercise. In fact, the rhythmic contraction of the lower limb locomotor muscles alone can empty more than 25% of the blood volume contained in the lower limb vasculature. With such a powerful force pushing blood back to the heart, are the negative pressures produced during inspiration actually *required* for normal venous return and cardiac output during exercise? An idealistic approach to answering this question involves the analysis of both within-breath and steady-state cardiac function.

The examination of within-breath modulation of cardiovascular function by breathing is quite useful, as the marked modulation of venous return and cardiac output implies that the cardiovascular system is susceptible to manipulation by respiratory pressure. Unfortunately, technical limitations have resulted in few data examining the within-breath effects of respiration on cardiovascular function during whole body exercise. While early measures of inferior vena cava blood *velocity* implied a profound modulatory effect of respiration on venous return (65) during cycling exercise, it is difficult to translate these measures into blood flow, given the high compliance of the veins and relatively large changes in venous cross-sectional area that occur over the course of a breath. Nonetheless, this observation suggests that altering respiratory muscle pressure production experimentally could have significant effects on cardiac function in the steady state.

There are few experimental data on the effects of respiratory muscle pressure on steady-state cardiac output (i.e., blood *flow*). Perhaps the most insightful intervention has been the application of positive pressure mechanical ventilation during inspiration, which makes intrathoracic pressure less negative during inspiration by forcing air into the lungs. Under these conditions, significant *decreases in stroke volume and cardiac output* have been observed in the maximally exercising human, likely because a less negative intrathoracic pressure limits cardiac preload (i.e., reduces ventricular transmural pressure during diastole) (Fig. 10.17) (42). These data provide strong support to the hypothesis that the pressures produced by the respiratory muscles during inspiration can contribute significantly to the normal cardiac output and stroke volume responses to dynamic exercise.

You may wonder how the negative P_{ITP} during inspiration can facilitate venous return from the exercising limbs if P_{ABD} increases with diaphragmatic contraction. The answer lies in the mechanics used to minimize the work of breathing during exercise. Even at the onset of light exercise, expiration becomes active, P_{ABD} becomes positive, and the contraction of the abdominal muscles forces end-expiratory lung volume below functional residual capacity. Now, when the abdominal muscles relax, the abdominal wall quickly moves outward, and P_{ABD} actually *decreases* during inspiration (Fig. 10.17). This occurs despite the contraction of the diaphragm, as the outward movement of the abdominal wall is faster than the descent of the diaphragm. During very heavy exercise, P_{ABD} can actually become *negative* (Figure 10.17), which would widen the transmural pressure gradient across the inferior vena cava, preventing its collapse and allowing the reductions in P_{ITP} (which in turn reduce right atrial pressure) to facilitate the return of blood to the heart from the locomotor limbs.

While there are few data concerning the effects of respiratory pressure production during active expiration on cardiac function, it is likely that the excessively high positive expiratory pressures produced during maximal exercise in athletes with expiratory flow limitation and patients with chronic obstructive pulmonary disease (COPD) limit cardiac filling by increasing *mean* P_{ITP} (i.e., the average P_{ITP} over the course of the respiratory cycle). When expiratory flow limitation is severe and dynamic hyperinflation is present, increases in pressure on the lung surface and cardiac fossa may also contribute to compromised diastolic filling during exercise.

Ventricular Interdependence and the Matching of Right and Left Ventricular Stroke Volumes Over Time

While breathing can have a profound modulatory effect upon cardiac preload by changing the transmural pressure across the right and left ventricular free walls, the effects of inspiration and expiration on ventricular filling are limited by an intrinsic autoregulatory cardiac mechanism termed *ventricular interdependence;* that is, the preload of one ventricle affects the other. Simply put, the filling of one ventricle shifts their common wall—the interventricular septum—toward the opposite ventricle, which limits its filling. The magnitude of the septal shift depends in large part upon septal compliance, in addition to the individual elastances of the right and left ventricular free walls, and will also be markedly affected by the degree to which the pericardium constrains the heart (66). For example, with high levels of pericardial constraint (which may occur during maximal exercise), the only way the right ventricle can increase its filling is by shifting the septal wall leftward, which in turn impedes left ventricular filling. However, when pericardial constraint is low, it is more likely that the right ventricular free wall will move outward to accommodate the increased end-diastolic volume, and left ventricular filling is not likely to be substantially compromised. In any event, this reciprocal relationship between right and left ventricular filling serves to equalize stroke volumes over time, as reductions in the output of one ventricle will inevitably reduce the filling of the other, and vice versa.

While this section highlights some of the most common direct mechanical effects of respiratory pressure production on cardiovascular function, it is by no means comprehensive. A nearly endless number of permutations exist for each variable we have discussed, all yielding slightly different cardiovascular effects both over the course of a breath and over time. However, the fact remains that our understanding of most of these effects is poor, as data on whole-body exercise in humans are limited. For detailed discussions of many of these topics in reduced animal preparations, see Scharf and associates (67). In the next section, we discuss an equally important component of ventricular afterload that may be affected by respiratory influences on autonomic function—the resistance of the skeletal muscle vascular beds.

Respiration-Induced Autonomic Effects on Cardiovascular Function

Breathing has significant influences over sympathetic vasoconstrictor outflow and heart rate, which are manifested in two ways. First, a modulatory influence on sympathetic nerve activity and heart rate occurs within each respiratory cycle; second, overall levels of sympathetic nerve activity are increased and systemic vasoconstriction occurs when respiratory muscles undergo heavy sustained dynamic exercise.

Within-Breath Cardiovascular Modulation

In humans, muscle sympathetic nerve activity (MSNA) to a resting limb as measured via microneurography (40) is markedly depressed throughout the latter half of inspiration and early expiration and rises and peaks during mid to late expiration. The modulatory effect of respiration on MSNA is critically dependent on lung volume, with both tidal volume and the lung volume from which inspiration begins being important determinants of the extent of modulation (68). However, the magnitude of central respiratory motor output does not affect the modulation of MSNA over the course of a breath (68). These observations demonstrate that lung stretch is important to MSNA inhibition during inspiration and to its modulation over the course of a breath. The neural pathway controlling this feedback modulation originates in the pulmonary stretch receptors in the lung parenchyma, travels through the vagus nerves to the nucleus of the solitary tract (NTS), and eventually meets a common pool of cardiorespiratory interneurons in the medulla. These interneurons in turn affect output from the NTS and contribute to the control of the spinal preganglionic neurons that regulate systemic vascular sympathetic tone. The most important influence of lung stretch on sympathetic nerve activity is probably through its effectiveness in modulating the sympathetic responses to baroreceptor input to the NTS, which is markedly depressed during inspiration and augmented during expiration (69).

A second well-known respiratory influence is the parasympathetically mediated within-breath variation in heart rate, or so-called respiratory–sinus arrhythmia (RSA). RSA is markedly dependent on tidal volume and requires intact feedback from pulmonary stretch receptors in the human, as shown by the absence of RSA in lung-denervated transplant patients (70). However, unlike the respiratory modulation of sympathetic activity, central respiratory motor output (or respiratory drive) also has significant influences on RSA. Collectively, these examples of within-breath modulation clearly document a strong respiratory influence on both parasympathetic and sympathetically mediated cardiovascular function in the human.

Metabo-chemoreceptor Effects on Sympathetic Vasoconstrictor Outflow and Blood Flow Distribution

As detailed in the chapter on autonomic control (40), mechanoreceptors and metaboreceptors in the working skeletal muscle, together with central command from locomotor areas of the higher CNS, are important determinants of sympathetic vasoconstrictor outflow to the cardiac and systemic vasculature during exercise of all intensities, especially during high-intensity exercise (71). These are the same feed-forward and feedback mechanisms we previously discussed in detail as potential primary determinants of exer-

cise hyperpnea. It is believed that augmentation of sympathetic outflow during dynamic exercise occurs in part by the integration of feedback (from muscle) and feed-forward (from higher CNS locomotor centers) signals at the level of the NTS in the lateral medulla, which in turn results in the resetting of the baroreceptor set point (72). However, intact baroreceptors are not *required* for an exercise-induced increase of sympathetic nerve activity (73).

Evidence from animal models has accumulated to demonstrate, not surprisingly, that mechanoreceptors and metaboreceptors are also present in great quantities in the diaphragm and other inspiratory and expiratory muscles, just as they are in limb skeletal muscles (Fig. 10.18). Furthermore, diaphragm metaboreceptor afferent activity relayed via afferent fibers in the phrenic nerve to the NTS is increased when diaphragm fatigue is produced in the anesthetized animal (50). In turn, when these metaboreceptors in the diaphragm or expiratory muscles are stimulated pharmacologically or with local lactic acid injections, increases occur in mean arterial pressure and in vascular resistance in several systemic vascular beds, including those in the limb muscle, renal, and mesenteric vasculatures (74,75). Also, when humans (at rest) fatigue their inspiratory or expiratory muscles by voluntarily breathing against resistance at a high level of respiratory motor output, MSNA in the resting limb increases and vascular conductance and blood flow fall in a time-dependent fashion (76,77). These findings with heavy dynamic exercise specifically of the respiratory muscles are similar to the increased MSNA (to resting limbs) that occurs secondary to rhythmic fatiguing contractions of the forearm musculature (40).

Certainly, the mechanisms are present for respiratory muscle afferent stimulation to contribute to the general increase in efferent sympathetic vasoconstrictor activity that occurs with exercise, so long as the exercise is sufficiently intense to activate respiratory muscle metaboreceptors. This activation may begin to occur in moderate exercise (16) but is much more likely to occur in sustained heavy exercise, when diaphragmatic fatigue is known to be present.

Central respiratory motor output is also very high during dynamic exercise, but in contrast to the excitatory effects of high central *locomotor* command on sympathetic efferent activity, there is no evidence that central *respiratory* motor output is excitatory in this regard. In fact, even at very high (voluntary) inspiratory efforts, MSNA is *reduced during inspiration,* apparently because of the dominant inhibitory effect of increased lung volume over augmented respiratory motor output on sympathetic efferent activity (68) (also discussed previously in the section "Within-Breath Modulation").

Another respiratory-related source of sympathetic activation in heavy dynamic exercise that is not often considered is the carotid chemoreceptors. These receptors are subjected to strong circulating humoral stimuli in heavy exercise (see "Exercise Hyperventilation"); and in addition to their role in ventilatory stimulation it is well documented that carotid

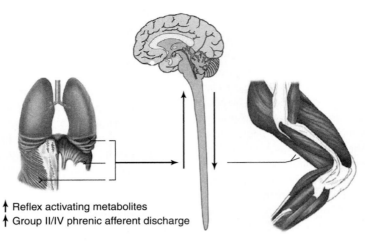

↑ Reflex activating metabolites
↑ Group II/IV phrenic afferent discharge

FIGURE 10.18 The diaphragm metaboreflex based on data in the resting human (77), the exercising dog (75), and the anesthetized dog (49,74). Collectively, these data show that either fatiguing contractions of the diaphragm or the local infusion of lactic acid into the phrenic artery increased the activity of type IV afferents in the diaphragm and triggered a supraspinal reflex that increased sympathetic nerve activity to the resting limb muscle vasculature and caused decreased vascular conductance and reduced blood flow to the limb both at rest and during mild exercise.

chemoreceptor stimulation has a strong sympathetic excitatory effect. The sympathoexcitation that occurs via carotid chemoreceptor and sinus nerve sensory stimulation is mediated via neural pathways that traverse the nucleus of the solitary tract and terminate upon the presympathetic neurons in the rostral ventral lateral medulla (78). This central pathway for sympathetic activation is quite separate from that for phrenic motor neuron activation (i.e., it is independent of the increases in respiratory muscle motor output). In fact, carotid chemoreceptor–mediated sympathetic excitation can occur even in the absence of medullary respiratory rhythm.

We now address what respiratory-related activations of sympathetic nerve activity may have to do with systemic blood flow distribution during dynamic exercise. Recall that the locomotor muscles receive more than 80% of the cardiac output during exercise. The magnitude of any increase in muscle blood flow depends upon the opposing effects of strong local vasodilators on the one hand versus the braking effects (and blood pressure–sparing effects) of sympathetic vasoconstrictor activity, both of which increase with increasing exercise intensity (40). This broaches the question whether the sympathetic excitation originating from respiratory muscle metaboreceptors (and/or carotid chemoreceptors) can overcome the regional vasodilator effects present in locomotor muscles and redistribute a portion of flow to the respiratory muscle vasculature.

Preceding sections have provided strong evidence that the respiratory muscles do the following:

1. Demand a significant amount of blood flow during dynamic exercise

2. Are richly innervated with afferent fibers that detect force and metabolite production and project to autonomic control centers in the medulla

3. Can elicit sympathetic activation in response to high, sustained levels of respiratory muscle work

4. Can reduce vascular conductance and blood flow to resting limb muscle

Collectively, these observations suggest that the respiratory muscles are well designed to compete for a significant fraction of cardiac output during maximal dynamic exercise, and there is a growing body of evidence that suggests that this may be the case. Certainly the 10 and 15% of total cardiac output devoted to the respiratory muscles must come from somewhere, and the locomotor muscles, with their high levels of blood flow (>80% of total cardiac output during maximal exercise), would appear to be the logical source.

The first observation that respiratory muscles could "steal" blood flow from the limbs came from studies using a mechanical ventilator to unload the respiratory muscles during exercise (79). When the work of breathing was reduced by about 50% during maximal exercise in fit humans, limb locomotor muscle blood flow and vascular conductance increased 7 to 10% and were proportional to decreases in norepinephrine spillover, an index of local sympathetic activity (Fig. 10.11). Further, limited data in dogs exercising at mild intensity (75) showed that activation of the respiratory muscle metaboreflex from the diaphragm or from the abdominal expiratory muscles (invoked via local lactic acidosis) caused vasoconstriction in the exercising hindlimb muscle and reduced blood flow a small but significant amount despite increases in systemic blood pressure.

However, the fact that phrenic afferent stimulation has been shown to increase sympathetic activity to *several* vascular beds (74) suggests that sympathetic activity is increasing globally. So how can blood flow be redistributed to the respiratory muscles via global sympathetic activation? This redistribution may be facilitated by regional differences in adrenergic receptor sensitivity. *In vitro* studies of isolated vessels have shown that α-adrenergic receptors in the diaphragm vasculature are less responsive to changes in catecholamines than in limb locomotor vasculature (80). Thus, at least theoretically, a global increase in sympathetic activity would result in greater vasoconstriction in the locomotor than respiratory muscle vasculature and in turn redirect blood flow to the respiratory muscles. However, technical limitations have precluded rigorous testing of these hypotheses *in vivo* during high-intensity dynamic exercise, a requisite for these concepts to progress beyond speculation from *in vitro* preparations.

Healthy Aging Effects on the Respiratory System at Rest and Exercise

Healthy aging causes substantial progressive deterioration in the structure and function of the lung parenchyma, airways, vasculature, and chest wall. Most of these changes begin in the mid-20s, with disproportionate changes in the fifth to sixth decades of life. In the lung, the two major structural changes with healthy aging (even in never-smokers) include the following:

1. Lung elastic recoil, likely due to a gradual loosening in the spatial arrangement and cross linking of the lungs' elastin collagen fiber network, is lost
2. Alveoli become less differentiated and increase in size

The number of alveoli and the total alveolar–capillary diffusion surface area falls with age, and this is reflected in a progressive reduction in the lung's diffusion capacity (81). Functionally, the loss of elastic recoil combined with reduced number of elastic attachments of supporting alveoli airways means that airways narrow excessively during forced expiration; thus older airways tend to close at higher lung volumes than in the young (Fig. 10.19A). Accordingly, distribution of inspired air and $\dot{V}/\dot{Q}$ becomes significantly more heterogeneous with aging. As the lung compliance increases with age, chest wall compliance is reduced secondary to costal cartilage calcification, a narrowing of intervertebral distances, and an increase in the anteroposterior diameter of the chest. Similarly, the compliance of pulmonary arterioles is reduced and pulmonary vascular resistance is increased; especially so as cardiac output increases during exercise.

Furthermore, the inspiratory muscles' capability to generate force is also markedly reduced with age.

These changes in the healthy lung and chest wall have significant implications for both the magnitude and the efficiency of the respiratory system's response to dynamic exercise. In contrast to the fairly uniform respiratory responses in young adults (discussed previously), the marked variability among individuals in the effects of aging on organ system function means that the response to exercise also varies widely among individuals. Nonetheless, some generalizations regarding healthy aging effects on the acute response to dynamic exercise can be drawn.

The overall ventilatory response to any given exercise work rate is increased in the aged because dead space ventilation ($\dot{V}D$) is increased both at rest and during exercise. $\dot{V}D/\dot{V}T$ averages .30 to .35 in the young adult at rest and .15 to .20 during exercise, whereas in the healthy, nonsmoking 70-year-old $\dot{V}D/\dot{V}T$ averages .40 to .50 at rest and .25 to .30 during exercise. This high $\dot{V}D/\dot{V}T$ likely reflects heterogeneous airway narrowing leading to a maldistribution of ventilation in the elderly, which persists during dynamic exercise. The limited vital capacity in the aged individual (because of increase in residual lung volume via loss of lung elastic recoil) limits the tidal volume response to exercise so that at any given $\dot{V}E$, breathing frequency is higher and tidal volume lower, thereby increasing anatomical dead space ventilation in the elderly. The end result is that alveolar ventilation is adequate to maintain arterial P_{CO_2} over all exercise intensities in most elderly subjects, but the total ventilatory response (alveolar plus dead space ventilation) in the aged is excessive and therefore inefficient.

Figure 10.19B shows average values for the flow–volume relationship at rest and during exercise for healthy 70-year-olds. The most striking contrast with younger subjects (Fig. 10.9) is that the elderly begin to experience significant expiratory flow limitation during submaximal exercise at relatively low ventilations (60–70 L $\cdot$ min^{-1}) and this flow limitation worsens as exercise intensity and $\dot{V}E$ increase further in fit elderly subjects (82). These responses are in sharp contrast to the typical 30-year-old, who does not begin to show any flow limitation until $\dot{V}E$ exceeds about 130 L $\cdot$ min^{-1} (Fig. 10.9). In summary, the exercise-induced flow limitation at low $\dot{V}E$ in the elderly results from a coincidence of two factors, namely:

1. A reduced lung elastic recoil and therefore reduced maximum flow–volume envelope
2. An augmented dead space ventilation and therefore hyperpneic response to exercise at any given work rate

The work of breathing is also increased at any given ventilation in the older exercising subject. Expiratory flow limitation accounts for much of this increase because it not only increases expiratory resistance but more importantly causes hyperinflation and therefore increases elastic work during inspiration. The consequence to the older flow-limited fit

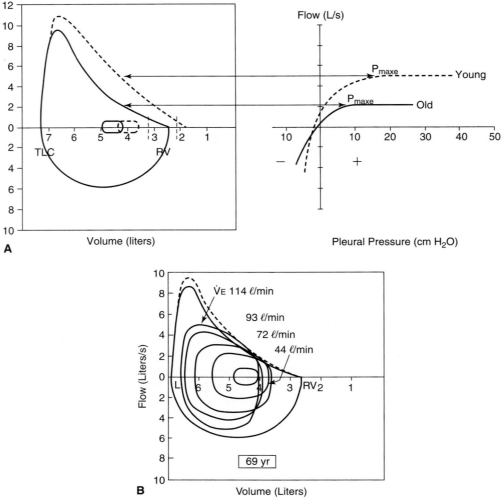

FIGURE 10.19   A. Maximum flow-to-volume loops and the isovolume, pressure-to-flow relationships in the 30-year-old and 70-year-old nonsmoking man. In the older subject the scooping in the expiratory limb of the maximum flow-to-volume loop indicates that airways are narrowing, reducing flow rate at any given lung volume during most of a forced expiration. *Right.* Expiratory flow increases with increasing expiratory effort up to the point of the critical closing pressure (P_{MAXE}), at which point, despite additional expiratory effort, airways narrow and close and no increase in flow rate is achieved. Note the much lower P_{MAXE} in the older subjects. *Left.* The end-expiratory lung volume is higher in the aged, as is the airway closing volume (broken line). These changes in the flow-to-volume loop, airway closing volume, and critical closing airway pressure occur with aging because of reduced lung elastic recoil. **B.** Flow-to-volume relationships at increasing levels of ventilation during steady-state exercise in the highly fit 69-year-old. Contrast these with Figure 10.9 in the younger subject. In the older subjects significant expiratory flow limitation begins at exercise ventilations (70 L · min⁻¹ or less) that are much lower than in the younger subject (> 100 L · min⁻¹.) Also, in the older subject, with the onset of the intersection of the tidal with the maximum expiratory flow volume loop, end-expiratory lung volume increases to and even in excess of resting levels. RV, residual lung volume; TLC, total lung capacity. *(Data are reprinted with permission from Johnson BD, Reddan WG, Seow KC, et al. Mechanical constraints on exercise hyperpnea in a fit aging population. Am Rev Respir Dis 1991;143:968–977.)*

subjects is that they must breathe along the upper, stiffer portion of the pressure–volume relationship of the lung (Box 10.2). Thus, what is originally initiated during exercise as a flow resistance problem on expiration in the heavy exercising healthy elderly subject leads to hyperinflation and an increase in the elastic load on inspiration. The lower compliance of the older subjects' chest wall also contributes to increased ventilatory work in exercise. It is presumed that this elevated respiratory muscle work will require greater oxygen consumption and blood flow by the respiratory muscles in the elderly during dynamic exercise. Furthermore, this elevated respiratory muscle work would contribute to perceptions of dyspnea.

Respiratory muscle efficiency is also affected because the relative lung hyperinflation means that the diaphragm and inspiratory muscles will be shortened and maximum force-generating capacity is reduced. Accordingly, during heavy dynamic exercise the inspiratory muscles are often working in excess of 80% of their dynamic capacity, in contrast with younger subjects at comparable $\dot{V}O_{2max}$ and $\dot{V}E_{max}$ who operate at 40 to 60% of maximum dynamic capacity for pressure generation (Fig. 10.9).

A limited number of measurements of arterial blood gases during exercise show that the A-aDO$_2$ is on average 8 to 12 mm Hg wider at any given $\dot{V}O_2$ (including $\dot{V}O_{2max}$) in 70-year-olds than in 30-year-olds. Normal, fit, healthy elderly do not experience EIAH, as is also the case with their younger healthy counterparts. In about 20 to 30% of highly active and fit elderly with a $\dot{V}O_{2max}$ 1.5 to 2 times that of age-matched controls (and about equal to normally fit 30-year-olds), A-aDO$_2$ exceeded 35 mm Hg (35–55 mm Hg), the exercise hyperventilation was limited (PaCO$_2$ 35–41 mm Hg), and arterial hypoxemia occurred (PaO$_2$ < 75 mm Hg, SaO$_2$ 85–93%). So just as with a significant fraction of highly trained younger subjects, elderly counterparts will experience EIAH for the same reasons: a widened A-aDO$_2$ and limited hyperventilation because of mechanical constraints. A major difference with the highly fit elderly is that the EIAH occurs in subjects with a much lower $\dot{V}O_{2max}$ (in the range of 40–55 mL · min^{-1} · kg^{-1}), whereas in young adults much higher levels of $\dot{V}O_{2max}$ are required before EIAH is observed.

Given the marked age-dependent effects on airway closure, ventilation distribution, and alveolar capillary diffusion surface (discussed previously), it is surprising that a much higher prevalence of excessive A-aDO$_2$ and inadequate hyperventilation are not observed in the healthy fit elderly. The simple explanation for these findings is that even though the lung and airways do indeed age, reductions in the maximal metabolic demands ($\dot{V}O_{2max}$) also occur with age at a rate equal to or greater than that of respiratory system deterioration. Accordingly, in most cases the maximal *demands* (for ventilation and alveolar to arterial oxygen transport) *relative to the capacity* for maximum air flow and alveolar capillary diffusion are no greater in the young than in the healthy elderly. There remain, however, exceptional highly active, highly fit elderly persons whose $\dot{V}O_{2max}$ (demand) declines substantially less than normal with age but whose age-dependent decline in structural capacities of the lung and airways is normal and unaffected by their lifelong physical training regimen, *per se* (82). EIAH and mechanical ventilatory constraint during maximal exercise are most likely to occur in these subjects and thus become a significant factor in exercise limitation.

The Effects of Dynamic Exercise Training on the Respiratory System

Lung and Airways

There is clear evidence that the cardiovascular and skeletal muscular systems adapt quickly and substantially to whole-body endurance exercise training (40,83). On the other hand, most evidence suggests that endurance training has little or no positive effects on the structure and function of the lung and airways. A striking example of the disparity between organ systems in their relative adaptabilities to increased metabolic demand was demonstrated in a series of studies comparing habitually active with relatively sedentary mammals of similar body size but with up to threefold differences in $\dot{V}O_{2max}$ (e.g., horse vs. cow; dog vs. goat). The higher $\dot{V}O_{2max}$ was accompanied by comparable increases in heart and limb muscle mitochondrial volume and capillary density in the athletic versus the sedentary animal but only 20 to 30% differences in the size of the lung's alveolar–capillary diffusion surface area (84). Further evidence that lung structure is mostly independent of habitual physical activity stems from studies that report nonsignificant changes in lung diffusion surface, airways, and pulmonary vasculature after chronic heavy exercise training in the maturing lung of rodents.

In humans, lung diffusion capacity and pulmonary capillary blood volume are not substantially different between endurance trained and healthy untrained subjects either at rest or during exercise. Furthermore, static lung volumes or maximum flow–volume loops of endurance trained human subjects are not different from those of normally fit individuals. There is recent evidence from *in vitro* studies in pigs to suggest that short-term training enhances vasorelaxation of the pulmonary artery via an increase in endothelial nitric oxide protein in the smooth muscle (85). These studies in pigs are the first to investigate training effects on the pulmonary vasculature. *In vivo* studies are required to determine the implications of these findings in isolated vessels to changes in pulmonary vascular resistance during exercise.

Swimmers may be an exception to the assertion that physical activity has minimal influence upon pulmonary structure and function. Swimmers tend to have larger lungs than the normal population (86). A limitation of these cross-sectional studies is that swimmers may have a strong genetic predisposition for large lungs. Whether static lung volumes can be improved by training during the period of lung growth remains to be determined. Longitudinal data from already fit adult subjects suggest that competitive swim training promotes slight but significant increases in static lung volumes (86). The mechanism responsible for these improvements in lung function is unclear, but during training swimmers inspire repeatedly to total lung capacity, which may result in an increased ability for swimmers to contract their inspiratory muscles to shorter lengths. Daily bouts of either voluntary hyperpnea or inspiratory flow resistive loading directed specifically at the inspiratory muscles have been shown to promote small but significant increases in both static and dynamic pulmonary function over several weeks (87).

Several studies have attempted to determine whether exercise training protects against the normal age-dependent deterioration in lung function (see section "Aging Effects," earlier). Cross-sectional comparisons of subjects with normal versus high $\dot{V}O_{2max}$ suggest that highly active elderly subjects have higher maximum expiratory flow rates and higher diffusion capacities than do less fit or sedentary subjects (88). At first glance, these findings suggest that age-dependent rates of decline in the lung elastic recoil and diffusion surface area are curtailed with habitual physical activity. In contrast, a longitudinal study of competitive distance runners in their sixth and seventh decades showed that chronic dynamic exercise training ensured high aerobic fitness but did not modify either the normal deterioration in resting lung function or the increased levels of ventilatory work during exercise that occur with healthy aging (48). Thus, the enhanced lung function of habitually active elderly subjects noted in cross-sectional studies was most likely *brought to,* rather than *resulted from,* their active lifestyle. The absence of a true training effect on the aging lung contrasts sharply with the beneficial effects of habitual exercise on aging influences on cardiac function, the systemic vasculature, limb skeletal muscle oxidative capacity and strength, and $\dot{V}O_{2max}$ (89).

Since the lung and airways do not change appreciably with dynamic exercise training, it is reasonable to question whether these structures adapt to other types of external stimuli. For example, humans native to high altitude, and to lesser extent lowlanders who reside for many years at high altitude, have higher lung diffusion capacities and pulmonary capillary blood volumes than their sea-level contemporaries (90). This enhanced diffusion capacity translated into a reduced A-aDo$_2$ and a more efficient gas exchange during exercise in hypoxia. Another stimulus to which the lungs adapt is calorie restriction (81). Studies on rodents show that calorie restriction increases the distance between alveolar walls and decreases alveolar surface area. Furthermore, these negative affects of calorie restriction are reversed with refeeding. Adaptation also occurs when a portion of lung is removed surgically (pneumonectomy). Compensatory growth of the

remaining lung occurs in response to this procedure in the form of an increased alveolar–capillary surface area. Finally, there are striking examples of genetic adaptation of the lung in some mammalian species with extremely high aerobic capacity. For example, in the prong-horned antelope (with a $\dot{V}O_{2max}$ >300 mL · kg^{-1} · min^{-1}), the alveolar–capillary surface area, like cardiovascular and muscle adaptations, is enlarged in proportion to the elevated $\dot{V}O_{2max}$.

So if the lung is indeed malleable to specific chronic stimuli, why does exercise training not elicit these kinds of adaptations in the lung and airways? An obvious explanation is that heavy dynamic exercise is not sufficiently stressful to warrant an adaptive morphological response. However, there is ample evidence that the limits of lung function and structure are being challenged, at least during heavy exercise in the highly trained human, as shown by the development of arterial hypoxemia, expiratory flow limitation, stress failure of the blood-gas barrier, and significant release of inflammatory mediators in the airways and pulmonary vasculature. In "superhuman" athletes, like the Thoroughbred horse, the lung parenchyma actually hemorrhages at multiple sites during exercise. One can imagine a significant scarring and stiffening of the lung parenchyma because of the repeated insults in these animals.

Limited evidence in human athletes suggests that instead of a positive adaptation to this repeated stress, a negative adaptation may actually occur in some susceptible athletes, especially when the endurance training is carried out in the presence of cold, dry air or urban pollutants. Recent lung biopsy studies in cross-country skiers show increased collagen deposition and remodeling in the bronchiolar airway walls (91). Perhaps repeated release of inflammatory mediators may be in part responsible for these structural changes. One wonders whether the high prevalence of asthmalike symptoms reported among populations of endurance athletes may be attributed in part to these training-induced structural changes. Furthermore, the finding that the widened A-aDo$_2$ and EIAH in many habitually active athletes occurs not only at their extraordinarily high peak work rates but also during moderate submaximal dynamic exercise implies an abnormal gas exchange function in these individuals. It is certainly within reason to suspect that the structural elements of the blood-gas barrier may undergo remodeling in response to the repeated stress accompanying heavy dynamic exercise.

In combination, these observations suggest that with exercise training not only does the lung lag behind the adaptations made by the cardiovascular system and the locomotor muscles but also the key elements of lung structure may be compromised or remodeled to the point where this interferes significantly with airway reactivity, ventilation and perfusion distribution, and gas exchange, even at submaximal requirements for oxygen transport. Confirmation of this postulate requires much more detailed longitudinal study of the lung and airways throughout training.

Respiratory Muscles

It is now clear that respiratory muscles are both metabolically and structurally plastic and respond to the regular contractile activity associated with whole body physical training (92). Evidence in rodents shows that heavy dynamic exercise training promotes 20 to 30% increases in mitochondrial enzyme activity within the costal diaphragm and also in specific accessory inspiratory (parasternal and external intercostals) and expiratory muscles (rectus abdominis and external oblique). The magnitude of these training-induced changes in oxidative capacity in the respiratory muscles are substantially less than those reported for limb locomotor muscles with fiber type composition similar to that of the diaphragm (e.g., plantaris). The differences in adaptation are likely attributable to differences in the work performed by diaphragm versus limbs during whole-body dynamic exercise training. In contrast to the changes in oxidative capacity, endurance training has little effect on most respiratory muscle glycolytic enzymes. However, training does elicit increases in the activities of key antioxidant enzymes within the diaphragm of rodents (93). This increased antioxidant capacity will improve the diaphragm's ability to scavenge reactive oxygen species and protect against the effects of exercise-induced oxidative stress, such as reductions in maximal tension and rate of force development, and early onset of fatigue. Endurance exercise training also promotes phenotypic adaptations in the diaphragm, as shown in a shift of type IIB to IIA in the fast myosin heavy chain isoforms. Furthermore, decreases occur in the cross-sectional area of costal diaphragm fibers, which results in a reduced distance from capillary to mitochondria for diffusion of gases, metabolites, and/or substrates in the diaphragm. Studies in rodents also show that the respiratory dilator muscles of the upper airway adapt to chronic dynamic exercise as shown by a fast-to-slow shift in the myosin heavy chain isoform phenotype,

together with an increase in oxidative and antioxidant capacities in the digastric and sternohyoid muscles (94).

Biopsy studies in humans attest to the plasticity of the diaphragm in response to chronic overload. Patients with COPD who underwent specific inspiratory muscle training via loaded breathing showed significant increases in the proportion of type I fibers and the size of type II fibers in the external intercostals (95). Furthermore, cross-sectional comparisons of diaphragm muscle biopsies in either chronic heart failure or severe COPD patients showed substantial increases in the proportion of type I fibers and the concentration of mitochondrial oxidative enzymes in the costal diaphragm, apparently resulting from the progressive increase in load placed on the respiratory muscles over several years or decades (96). Indirect evidence also shows that the respiratory muscles undergo a training effect following a whole-body dynamic exercise training regimen in healthy humans. The endurance-trained athlete will, like his or her sedentary counterparts, show significant diaphragm fatigue in response to heavy-intensity whole-body exercise continued to exhaustion. However, the endurance-trained athlete has diaphragm fatigue only at levels of total ventilation and respiratory muscle work that are far greater than in sedentary contemporaries (97) (also see Box 10.5 for further types of chronic respiratory muscle adaptations).

Although much attention has been paid to the diaphragmatic adaptations to chronic overload, little is known about the effects of detraining on diaphragmatic structure and function. Hemidiaphragmatic inactivity (induced by unilateral chemical blockade of phrenic nerve conduction or sectioning of the phrenic nerve) results in significant reductions in peak diaphragmatic force production and type II muscle fiber cross-sectional area in the inactive hemidiaphragm within 2 weeks (98). However, pure diaphragmatic quiescence (i.e., complete bilateral absence of diaphragmatic elec-

Box 10.5

EXAMPLES OF REMARKABLE PLASTICITY OF STRUCTURES AND FUNCTION IN THE DIAPHRAGM

Perhaps one of the most impressive diaphragmatic adaptations in an animal model of COPD is the loss of sarcomeres in series with elastase-induced emphysema. As lung elastic recoil decreases and more air is trapped in the lungs (i.e., FRC increases), the diaphragm is forced to operate at shorter lengths and in a flatter geometric configuration. In an attempt to optimize sarcomere length and force production under these conditions, sarcomeres are progressively lost from the diaphragmatic myofibrils in series (113). This allows the remaining sarcomeres to operate closer to their optimal length and shifts the length–tension relationship of the diaphragm to the left, with the magnitude of sarcomere loss being inversely proportional to the increase in FRC (114). Similar structural adaptations also seem to occur in the expiratory musculature with experimental COPD, as evidenced by the loss of sarcomeres in series in the transverse abdominis (115). Amazingly, following lung volume reduction surgery in these animals and the resulting reduction in FRC and lengthening of the diaphragm, diaphragmatic sarcomeres are added back in series, and the length–tension relationship of the diaphragm is shifted rightward (116).

trical activity) induced by mechanical ventilation for as little as 3 days results in significant myofibril damage and decreases in diaphragmatic force production by as much as 51% (99). Thus, removal of the normal phasic activation of the diaphragm has a substantial effect on its function in a relatively short time, with the period required for recovery from this damage remaining unclear.

Control of Breathing

Dynamic exercise training may influence the control of breathing. First, a consistent finding in the highly trained versus untrained subject is that ventilation is reduced during heavy exercise at any given absolute $\dot{V}O_2$ or power output. This is likely due to a reduction in one or more of the mechanisms purported to cause a hyperventilatory response to heavy exercise. These proposed mechanisms, which may be influenced by exercise training, include a reduction in circulating humoral stimuli, such as hydrogen ions, lactic acid, norepinephrine, or potassium, or reduced central motor command (at any given absolute power output) because limb fatigue is delayed to higher work rates in the highly fit. Second, the ventilatory response to hypoxia and inhaled carbon dioxide is known to be markedly heterogeneous in the normal healthy human population. Many endurance-trained athletes have been observed to have lower than average ventilatory responsiveness to these chemoreceptor stimuli, although this is certainly not a universal finding among highly fit endurance athletes. However in athletes who do show reduced ventilatory chemoresponsiveness, this characteristic may have practical limitations for gas exchange during exercise and perhaps even exercise performance. Specifically, a reduced hyperventilatory response in the presence of an excessive A-aDO$_2$ is responsible for exercise-induced arterial hypoxemia in some highly trained subjects. A portion of this inadequate hyperventilatory response is due to a mechanical constraint on exercise ventilation, primarily due to expiratory flow limitation (Fig. 10.9). However, purely mechanical constraint of ventilation does not account for all of the blunted hyperventilation during heavy exercise in these subjects with EIAH. In some subjects, failure to achieve sufficient hyperventilation occurs even when they are ventilating well within the maximal capacities defined by the envelope of their maximum flow–volume loop and when the pressures generated by their inspiratory muscles are substantially less than their capacity. Therefore, their failure to increase ventilation further may be due in part to their relative insensitivity to prevailing ventilatory stimuli, especially humoral stimuli, which are known to influence the carotid chemoreceptors.

The Respiratory System as a Limiting Factor to Dynamic Exercise in Health

It is generally agreed that $\dot{V}O_{2max}$ is in large part determined by systemic oxygen transport, that is, the product of maxi-

mal cardiac output ($\dot{Q}$) and arterial oxygen content (CaO$_2$), at least in normal adults with $\dot{V}O_{2max}$ in the range of 35 to 85 mL $\cdot$ kg^{-1} $\cdot$ min^{-1} (100,101). Support for this premise comes from findings showing a strong positive correlation across subjects of widely varying fitness levels between CaO$_2$ $\cdot$ $\dot{Q}_{max}$ and $\dot{V}O_{2max}$ (100). Experimental evidence in animals and humans also shows that as CaO$_2$ varies (via changes in the fractional oxygen concentration of inspired air or hemoglobin concentration) or $\dot{Q}_{max}$ is raised (via changing circulating blood volume or pericardectomy), $\dot{V}O_{2max}$ is also altered in accordance with the change in CaO$_2$ $\cdot$ $\dot{Q}$.

Of the two components of systemic oxygen transport, it is widely believed that maximum stroke volume, and therefore cardiac output, is the key limiting factor to maximum oxygen delivery in most healthy untrained young adults with a $\dot{V}O_{2max}$ in the normal range. As detailed throughout this chapter, the maintenance of CaO$_2$ is usually not a problem in health because the lung, airways, and respiratory muscles are in general structurally overbuilt with respect to maximum metabolic requirements for gas transport. Thus, a large diffusion surface area and a short alveolar–capillary diffusion distance, coupled with a substantial capacity for flow rate, volume, and ventilation because of a similarly overbuilt respiratory musculature and airway caliber, ensures that at $\dot{V}O_{2max}$: (*a*) The alveolar to arterial oxygen difference widens only two to three times resting levels. (*b*) Alveolar hyperventilation raises alveolar PO$_2$ sufficiently to compensate for the widened A-aDO$_2$, and arterial PO$_2$ and oxyhemoglobin saturation are maintained near resting levels.

On the other hand, evidence has accumulated to show that as aerobic capacity increases because of training or in already highly fit individuals, the healthy pulmonary system in some humans and some other mammals may not be so overbuilt with respect to metabolic requirements. As detailed in the section "Exercise Training" earlier in the chapter, the lung diffusion surface and airways and to a lesser extent even the respiratory muscles do not adapt to the training stimulus nearly to the same extent as do other links in the oxygen transport system. The result is that the respiratory system in many highly fit subjects is relatively underbuilt with respect to the extraordinarily high metabolic requirements and may contribute significantly to the limitations of exercise performance. Two specific types of respiratory system limitation to exercise have been identified to date, namely, (*a*) EIAH and (*b*) high levels of respiratory muscle work.

Dynamic EIAH in Trained Populations

Instances of arterial oxygen desaturation ranging from 3 to 15% below resting levels has been observed to occur at or near maximum exercise intensities in many—but certainly not all—habitually active highly trained subjects. EIAH has been reported most frequently in trained young males. However, recent studies of smaller numbers of trained females (102) and older trained adults (103) also reported a significant prevalence of EIAH, and the $\dot{V}O_{2max}$ in these subjects was substantially lower than in the young trained men with EIAH. Clearly, the true prevalence of EIAH and the susceptibility of various subpopulations to EIAH will require appropriate epidemiological studies. The Thoroughbred horse with a $\dot{V}O_{2max}$ twice that of even the most highly trained humans has a substantially underbuilt lung relative to its extraordinary metabolic requirements, Accordingly, all such horses studied to date demonstrate severe EIAH as well as marked carbon dioxide retention at moderately heavy to maximum exercise intensities (104).

In addition to the reduction in PaO_2 in subjects with EIAH, arterial oxyhemoglobin desaturation is further exaggerated by rightward shifts of the oxyhemoglobin dissociation curve as a result of the metabolic acidosis (pHa < 7.25) and increased temperature (+1.5 to 3°C > rest) that occur during heavy exercise. An excessively widened A-aDo$_2$ in heavy exercise is the most consistent contribution to EIAH. In addition, those with EIAH usually show a compromised hyperventilatory response to heavy exercise that is insufficient to raise alveolar PO_2 enough to prevent PaO_2 from falling in the face of a widened A-aDo$_2$. In turn, the mechanical limitations to inspiratory and expiratory flow rates are a major cause of the constrained hyperventilatory response.

The effect of EIAH on $\dot{V}O_{2max}$ was determined by preventing EIAH. This can be readily accomplished by modestly supplementing inspired oxygen to 3 to 5% above room air levels (105). Figure 10.20 shows the effect of preventing EIAH on $\dot{V}O_2$, which becomes significant near maximum exercise intensity. Studies in 40 to 50 subjects of varying fitness levels to date have shown that arterial oxyhemoglobin desaturation begins to have an effect on $\dot{V}O_{2max}$ when the desaturation level exceeds 3% below resting levels and that for every 1% reduction in SaO_2 below resting levels this results in a 1.5 to 2% decrement in the $\dot{V}O_{2max}$. The most commonly encountered levels of arterial oxyhemoglobin desaturation among fit males, females, and older subjects are usually modest, causing less than a 10% reduction in $\dot{V}O_{2max}$. A small but still significant number of endurance athletes have greater levels of oxyhemoglobin desaturation during maximal exercise, and the resulting decrement in $\dot{V}O_{2max}$ ranges from 8 to 15%. In the Thoroughbred horse, whose arterial oxyhemoglobin desaturates to almost 20% below resting levels at maximum exercise, $\dot{V}O_{2max}$ is reduced by 30% below levels achieved when EIAH is prevented. In athletes with high $\dot{V}O_{2max}$, exercising at even modest elevations in altitude (3000 to 5000 feet) exacerbates the severity of oxyhemoglobin desaturation substantially and further limits $\dot{V}O_{2max}$ (106–108). The reason EIAH causes a reduction in $\dot{V}O_{2max}$ is likely found in the Fick equation. That is, a reduced CaO_2 decreases oxygen transport to the working locomotor muscles, therefore reducing the maximal attainable a-vO$_2$ content difference across the working muscle, and in turn, $\dot{V}O_{2max}$ will fall (Fig. 10.19).

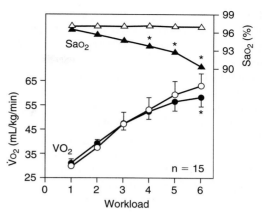

FIGURE 10.20 Effects of preventing exercise-induced arterial hypoxemia (EIAH) on $\dot{V}O_{2max}$ in 15 highly fit female subjects ($SaO_2 \leq 92\%$ at $\dot{V}O_{2max}$). Note the gradual reduction in SaO_2 with progressive increases in exercise above moderate intensity ($FIO_2 = 0.21$) (*solid triangles*). EIAH was prevented by breathing 0.26 FIO_2 (*open triangles*). At submaximal intensity, work rates preventing oxygen desaturation had no effect on $\dot{V}O_2$, whereas at peak work rates $\dot{V}O_2$ was significantly increased. Treadmill speed remained constant (6, 8, or 10 mph) throughout the test; the grade of the treadmill increased 2% each 2.5 minutes; asterisks denote a significant difference between $FIO_2 = 0.21$ and $FIO_2 = 0.26$ at the same workload (P < .05). *(Data are reprinted with permission from Dempsey JA, Wagner PD. Exercise-induced arterial hypoxemia. J Appl Physiol 1999;87:1999; and Harms CA, McClaran SR, Nickele GA, et al. Exercise-induced arterial hypoxaemia in healthy young women. J Physiol [Lond] 1998;507(Pt 2):622.)*

Exercise Limitation via High Levels of Respiratory Muscle Work

We have previously documented that heavy dynamic exercise causes substantial increases in the work of the inspiratory and expiratory muscles, both in normally fit human subjects and especially in the highly fit. These high levels of work require 10 to 16% of the maximum $\dot{V}O_2$ and of the maximum cardiac output. During sufficiently heavy prolonged dynamic exercise, the primary inspiratory muscle, the diaphragm, will fatigue. Further, experimentally relieving the work of the respiratory muscles (via mechanical ventilation) reduces cardiac output and $\dot{V}O_2$ and increases vascular conductance and blood flow to the limb locomotor muscles in heavy sustained exercise. Finally, maintaining the required levels of ventilation and the associated respiratory muscle work causes the subject to have intense perception of breathing effort, that is, exertional dyspnea. (For details see preceding section, "Respiratory Mechanics.")

The effects of these high levels of respiratory muscle work and/or fatigue and dyspneic perceptions on dynamic exercise performance have been assessed by use of a mechanical ventilator to unload the respiratory muscles and then determine the effects on time to exhaustion at a fixed high-intensity workload. As shown in Figure 10.21, unloading the respiratory muscles increased endurance time in most trials by a mean of 14%. The rate of rise of $\dot{V}O_2$ during exercise was reduced, as was the rate of rise of the subjects' perceptions of both respiratory and limb discomfort. When the work of breathing was increased with inspiratory resistors, performance time was reduced by 15%, and the rate of rise of $\dot{V}O_2$ versus time was increased, as were perceptions of respiratory and limb discomfort. These significant effects of respiratory muscle unloading on exercise performance are consistent with the deleterious effects on subsequent exercise performance of fatiguing the respiratory muscles (109). However, not all studies using unloading of the respiratory muscles showed improvement in performance, especially when the exercise intensities were substantially lower than those shown in Figure 10.21.

Of course, these studies do not tell us *why* high levels of respiratory work might affect endurance performance. Exercise-induced diaphragm fatigue is prevented by muscle unloading, but it is not clear why diaphragm fatigue *per se* should influence performance, because alveolar ventilation is not compromised (45). Perhaps a more likely link between respiratory muscle work and endurance exercise performance may be through its effects on limb vascular conductance and blood flow (see section "Cardiorespiratory Interactions," earlier in the chapter). Such reductions in limb flow would directly affect the susceptibility to fatigue in locomotor muscles and the perception of effort by these locomotor muscles. Another potential limiting factor is the extreme progressive dyspnea that occurs over time in heavy dynamic exercise, which was also substantially relieved by respiratory muscle unloading.

Can These Respiratory System Limitations to Exercise Be Avoided or Overcome?

We are not permitted to provide supplemental oxygen during competitive endurance exercise events, and we are unable to store previously inhaled hyperoxic gases within our body. Neither can one conceive of transporting a mechanical ventilator or breathing low-density gas mixtures to relieve the work of breathing during competition. Thus, while these ergogenic aids may be of substantial benefit to the supervised rehabilitation of patients with heart failure or COPD, the healthy athlete must seek other avenues of relief or avoidance of the proposed pulmonary limitations.

In the case of EIAH, the most practical advice to be gained by its measurement is its predictive capabilities. That is, endurance athletes who tend to desaturate even only marginally at sea level will in all likelihood desaturate substantially with even mild increases in altitude (106,108).

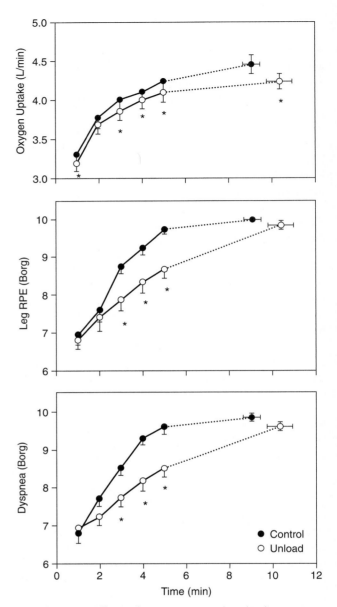

FIGURE 10.21 Effects of respiratory muscle unloading on endurance exercise performance. Exercise duration on the X-axis is plotted against $\dot{V}O_2$, ratings of perceived exertion of the limbs, and ratings of dyspnea under control conditions (*solid circles*) and during trials in which a mechanical ventilator was used to reduce the work of breathing by about 50% during exercise (*open circles*). The performance test consisted of pedaling a stationary bicycle beginning at 85% of $\dot{V}O_{2max}$ to volitional exhaustion. Unloading the work of breathing increased the exercise time to exhaustion by an average of 14% and reduced the rate of rise of perception of limb fatigue and the perception of dyspnea. $\dot{V}O_2$ was also reduced throughout most of the exercise by the respiratory muscle unloading. *(Data are reprinted with permission from Harms CA, Wetter TJ, St Croix CM, et al. Effects of respiratory muscle work on exercise performance. J Appl Physiol 2000;89:131–138.)*

Accordingly, when such athletes compete or train at even moderately high altitudes, they will be at a substantial disadvantage and should probably avoid such practices.

We know of no antidote to EIAH in susceptible subjects, although some attempts have been made by infusing alkalinizing agents, such as $NaHCO_2$. This will overcome a significant amount of the arterial oxyhemoglobin desaturation, that is, what is due to metabolic acidosis, but this might also interfere with offloading of oxygen at the muscle capillary or reduce respiratory drive and alveolar ventilation. Anti-inflammatory medications have been shown to reduce the A-aDo$_2$ and prevent EIAH in older master athletes (110) but have not been effective in younger subjects with EIAH (111). Of course, adding hemoglobin (and oxygen-carrying capacity) by intermittent hypoxic exposures or via the illegal practices of blood doping or exogenous erythropoietin would readily negate any reduction in arterial oxygen content secondary to EIAH.

Many have tested the hypothesis that specific respiratory muscle training (RMT) will enhance exercise performance, and the rationale for this belief may reside in the cardiovascular consequences of respiratory muscle work during heavy exercise, as described earlier. The logic is that RMT would increase the strength and/or endurance performance of the inspiratory and expiratory muscles; they would also be more fatigue resistant and perhaps even more mechanically efficient during whole-body heavy dynamic exercise. In turn, the more efficient, fatigue-resistant trained respiratory muscles would not require as large a fraction of cardiac output during exercise and/or accumulate metabolites as readily, thereby preventing any potential reflex vasoconstrictive effects on the locomotor muscle vasculature. Also, if locomotor and/or respiratory muscles are more fatigue resistant, this might also mean less sensory input from the contracting muscles to the CNS, resulting in a reduced intensity of perceptions of locomotor and respiratory effort at any given work rate or exercise duration.

Some or all of these potential effects of RMT also likely explain the positive effects on endurance exercise performance time of acutely unloading the respiratory muscles using positive pressure ventilation (see section "Limitations," earlier in the chapter). However, these experiments also showed that even with reductions in respiratory muscle work by as much as 40 to 60% and complete prevention of exercise-induced diaphragmatic fatigue, the increases in endurance time averaged slightly less than 15%, with no accompanying consistent effects on circulating lactate or ventilation. Furthermore, these positive effects of reducing respiratory muscle work on exercise performance or on diaphragmatic fatigue were not observed when whole-body exercise intensity to task failure was less than 80 to 85% of $\dot{V}O_{2max}$.

Some studies have found improvements in endurance performance together with reductions in circulating lactic acid concentrations and ventilation after several weeks of RMT. However this is not a consistent finding (112). A concern with most RMT studies is that endurance performance was evaluated using fixed–work rate tasks sustained to the limit of tolerance. Such tests do not accurately represent competitive endurance performance and are often unreliable. Unreliable performance tests, in combination with small sample sizes, may explain in part why some studies have reported improvements in exercise capacity but failed to achieve statistical significance. Also, the absence of placebo groups renders the findings of these studies difficult to interpret. Some more recent studies have used reliable and externally valid outcome measures (i.e., simulated time trial performance) in combination with a placebo-controlled experimental design, and most findings from these studies indicate that RMT has a small but likely significant effect on exercise performance. Future research on the effects of RMT must focus on objective, reliable outcomes for assessing both respiratory muscle and exercise performance. Future experimental designs should also explore possible underlying mechanisms—such as influences on respiratory muscle efficiency, on exercise-induced respiratory and/or limb muscle fatigue, and on blood flow distribution—which might explain any effects on exercise performance.

SUMMARY: NEED FOR FUTURE STUDY

It is important for the student of exercise physiology to appreciate that much of this field of study is relatively new. Accordingly, our understanding of even many fundamental problems concerning exercise and the respiratory system remain incompletely understood; furthermore, we are several steps away from applying much of our knowledge of basic physiology to improving or even understanding the performance of the competitive athlete. We conclude this chapter by addressing a few of the more pressing needs in this field.

- *Regulation of exercise hyperpnea.* Two major locomotor-linked mechanisms appear to account for much of the steady-state hyperpnea during exercise, but the key questions of how these inputs interact with one another and with other fine-tuning mechanisms remain unanswered. The influence of prior learning and the role of nervous system plasticity also are complex important questions concerning the mechanisms of hyperpnea. Innovative approaches employing unanesthetized, nervously intact preparations with control system sensitivities in the physiological range are needed.
- *Breathing mechanics and cardiorespiratory interactions.* Important reflex mechanisms originate in contracting inspiratory and expiratory muscles, which are capable of increasing sympathetic efferent vasoconstrictor activity. Under what conditions are these feedback receptors activated during whole body exercise, and what is their net influence on blood flow distribution to respiratory versus locomotor muscles? We also

know that large cyclical changes occur throughout the respiratory cycle in intrathoracic and intra-abdominal pressures during exercise, especially when expiratory flow limitation is present; however, the consequences of these changes in pressure on venous return from the contracting limbs and/or on left ventricular stroke volume have not been quantified.

- *Gas exchange.* It is surprising how little we understand of the structure of the pulmonary circulation in the face of an increase in cardiac output during dynamic exercise. If we could measure both the spatial distribution of pulmonary capillary blood volume and red cell transit time and could image arteriovenous anastomoses potentially capable of carrying deoxygenated mixed venous blood, perhaps we could explain the causes of gas exchange inefficiency and its marked individual variability during dynamic exercise.

- *Exercise training effects.* The structure of the airways and of the gas exchange surface area is usually viewed as unresponsive to the stimulus of exercise training. However, little attention has been paid to training effects on endothelial structure and reactivity in the pulmonary arterioles or in vessels regulating blood flow to the diaphragm and accessory respiratory muscles. Furthermore, recent evidence demonstrates that very heavy exercise training requirements may have deleterious effects on the airway epithelium and even on pulmonary gas exchange. The excellent animal models available to explore training effects on locomotor muscles and the systemic vasculature should be applied to these questions concerning training-induced structural changes in the lung airways and respiratory muscles.

- *Limiting factors.* Two types of limitations presented by the respiratory system have been identified in healthy humans exercising at or near sea level. EIAH will impose a significant but moderate limitation on $\dot{V}O_{2max}$, and this occurs only in habitually active, highly fit individuals. Also, high levels of fatiguing work by the respiratory muscles will limit performance time during high-intensity endurance exercise. What remains unknown is the cause of the marked variability in EIAH among trained subjects and the influence of EIAH on endurance exercise performance (as opposed to its effects on $\dot{V}O_{2max}$). It is also unknown whether exercise limitation via EIAH is a direct effect of limiting oxygen transport on the locomotor muscles *per se* or the hypoxemia acts indirectly via a hypoxic CNS, that is, so-called central fatigue. We also need to know whether the positive effects of reducing respiratory muscle work on exercise performance are attributable specifically to the relief of locomotor muscle fatigue (perhaps acting via changes in limb blood flow) or whether this is simply a perceptual benefit obtained via relieving the discomfort attending high levels of respiratory muscle work. Study of these same mechanisms also should be applied to the controversial problem of specific respiratory muscle training effects on exercise performance.

These are some of the key problems concerning the respiratory system biology of exercise that require attention in the healthy subject. Equally fascinating and even more challenging is the need to address similar questions in special populations (e.g., asthma, COPD, heart failure, healthy aging) and during exercise in extreme environments, such as at high altitudes, hyperbaria, heat, and cold.

A MILESTONE OF DISCOVERY

The question was whether central command of locomotion originating in the hypothalamic locomotor regions of the CNS also caused parallel activation of ventilation and circulation. By the end of the 1970s, neurochemical feedback from the periphery was the most popularly purported primary stimulus for exercise hyperpnea. However, Fred Eldridge, a Stanford-trained physician and professor of physiology at the University of North Carolina-Chapel Hill, believed strongly in the Krogh hypothesis of cortical irradiation as an explanation for exercise hyperpnea. Teaming with his research fellows, Tony Waldrop and David Millhorn, Eldridge expanded significantly on the original central command experiments conducted by Rushmer in anesthetized animals some 20 years earlier. The Eldridge model was the unanaesthetized decorticate cat (similar to a preparation described in the Russian literature), in which they used either electrical or pharmacological stimulation of the hypothalamic locomotor region to produce rhythmic limb contractions sufficient to cause revolutions of a treadmill belt. This caused immediate increases in $\dot{V}E$, cardiac output and blood pressure, analogous to the normal exercise response. Then, to completely isolate the central command stimulus, they paralyzed all skeletal muscles so that hypothalamic stimulation caused fictive locomotion. Amazingly, cardiorespiratory responses were identical to those obtained in the intact animal, that is, when both feed-forward and feedback stimulation were present (see Fig. 10.23)

These findings formally established central command as a significant player in exercise hyperpnea and served to stimulate

(continued)

the conduct of many subsequent studies throughout the 1980s and 1990s, which showed the following:

1. Other CNS areas, such as the mesencephalic locomotor areas and the amygdala, upon stimulation, also produced cardiorespiratory responses that were similar to those caused by stimulation of the hypothalamic areas.
2. Hypothalamic stimulation also engaged the parasympathetic and sympathetic nervous systems, leading to increases in cardiac output and a redistribution of systemic blood flow similar to that caused by normal exercise.
3. Descending projections were discovered linking the caudal hypothalamus to the cardiorespiratory medullary neurons.

4. Hypothalamic locomotor centers were shown to receive sensory input from skeletal muscle receptor afferents.

Nevertheless, lesioning of the hypothalamic locomotor areas did not prevent a normal cardiorespiratory response to exercise in the awake animal. It is likely, then, that these powerful central feed-forward and peripheral feedback mechanisms, which occur simultaneously during exercise, are somewhat redundant in terms of their functional influences on exercise hyperpnea (Figs. 10.22 and 10.23).

Eldridge FL, Millhorn DE, Waldrop TG. Exercise hyperpnea and locomotion: parallel activation from the hypothalamus. Science 1981;211:844–846.

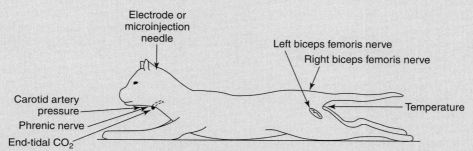

FIGURE 10.22 Decorticate, paralyzed, ventilated cat preparation used to study the cardiorespiratory effects of fictive locomotion. *(Reprinted with permission from Eldridge FL, Millhorn DE, Waldrop TG. Exercise hyperpnea and locomotion: parallel activation from the hypothalamus. Science 1981;211:845.)*

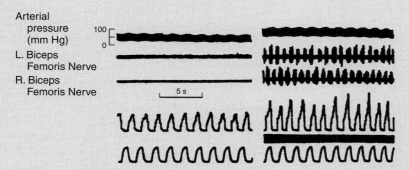

FIGURE 10.23 Respiratory, cardiovascular, and fictive locomotor responses dictated by stimulation of the hypothalamic locomotor region. *(Reprinted with permission from Eldridge FL, Millhorn DE, Waldrop TG. Exercise hyperpnea and locomotion: parallel activation from the hypothalamus. Science 1981;211:846.)*

ACKNOWLEDGMENTS

We acknowledge the expert assistance of Hans Haverkamp, David Pegelow, Tony Jacques, and Benjamin Dempsey in the preparation of this manuscript. Original work from our laboratory was financially supported by NHLBI and the American Heart Association.

REFERENCES

1. Smith JC, Ellenberger HH, Ballanyi K, et al. Pre-Bötzinger complex: a brainstem region that may generate respiratory rhythm in mammals. Science 1991;254:726–729.

2. St-John WM, Paton JF. Defining eupnea. Respir Physiol Neurobiol 2003;139:97–103.

3. Orem J, Netick A. Characteristics of midbrain respiratory neurons in sleep and wakefulness in the cat. Brain Res 1982;244:231–241.

4. Feldman JL, Mitchell GS, Nattie EE. Breathing: rhythmicity, plasticity, chemosensitivity. Annu Rev Neurosci 2003;26:239–266.

5. Lahiri S, DeLaney RG. Stimulus interaction in the responses of carotid body chemoreceptor single afferent fibers. Respir Physiol 1975;24:249–266.

6. Nattie E. Multiple sites for central chemoreception: their roles in response sensitivity and in sleep and wakefulness. Respir Physiol 2000;122:223–235.

7. Rice AJ, Nakayama HC, Haverkamp HC, et al. Controlled versus assisted mechanical ventilation effects on respiratory motor output in sleeping humans. Am J Respir Crit Care Med 2003;168:92–101.

8. Badr MS, Skatrud JB, Dempsey JA. Determinants of post-stimulus potentiation in humans during NREM sleep. J Appl Physiol 1992;73:1958–1971.

9. Phillipson EA, Duffin J, Cooper JD. Critical dependence of respiratory rhythmicity on metabolic CO_2 load. J Appl Physiol 1981;50:45–54.

10. Dempsey JA, Vidruk EH, Mitchell GS. Pulmonary control systems in exercise: update. Fed Proc 1985;44:2260–2270.

11. Huszczuk A, BJ Whipp, TD Adams, et al. Ventilatory control during exercise in calves with artificial hearts. J Appl Physiol 1990;68:2604–2611.

12. Liu Q, Kim J, Cinotte J, et al. Carotid body denervation effect on cytochrome oxidase activity in pre-Botzinger complex of developing rats. J Appl Physiol 2003;94:1115–1121.

13. Serra A, Brozoski D, Hodges M, et al. Effects of carotid and aortic chemoreceptor denervation in newborn piglets. J Appl Physiol 2002;92:893–900.

14. Olson Jr EB, Dempsey JA. Rat as a model for humanlike ventilatory adaptation to chronic hypoxia. J Appl Physiol 1978;44:763–769.

15. Haouzi P, Hill JM, Lewis BK, et al. Responses of group III and IV muscle afferents to distension of the peripheral vascular bed. J Appl Physiol 1999;87:545–553.

16. Pickar JG, Hill JM, Kaufman MP. Dynamic exercise stimulates group III muscle afferents. J Neurophysiol 1994;71:753–760.

17. Haouzi P, Chenuel B, Huszczuk A. Sensing vascular distension in skeletal muscle by slow conducting afferent fibers: neurophysiological basis and implication for respiratory control. J Appl Physiol 2004;96:407–418.

18. Krogh A, Lindhard J. The regulation of respiration and circulation during the initial stages of muscular work. J Physiol (Lond) 1913;47:112–136.

19. Eldridge FL, Millhorn DE, Waldrop TG. Exercise hyperpnea and locomotion: parallel activation from the hypothalamus. Science 1981;211:844–846.

20. Thornton JM, Guz A, Murphy K, et al. Identification of higher brain centres that may encode the cardiorespiratory response to exercise in humans. J Physiol (Lond) 2001;533:823–836.

21. Lugliani R, Whipp BJ, Seard C, et al. Effect of bilateral carotid-body resection on ventilatory control at rest and during exercise in man. N Engl J Med 1971;285:1105–1111.

22. Busse MW, Maassen N, Konrad H. Relation between plasma K^+ and ventilation during incremental exercise after glycogen depletion and repletion in man. J Physiol 1991;43:469–476.

23. Kaufman MP, Forster HV. Reflexes controlling circulatory, ventilatory and airway responses to exercise. In Rowell LB, Shepherd JT, eds. Handbook of Physiology. New York: Oxford University, 1996;381–447.

24. Mateika JH, Duffin J. Coincidental changes in ventilation and electromyographic activity during consecutive incremental exercise tests. Eur J Appl Physiol 1994;68:54–61.

25. Hanson P, Claremont A, Dempsey J, et al. Determinants and consequences of ventilatory responses to competitive endurance running. J Appl Physiol 1982;52:615–623.

26. MacDougall JD, Reddan WG, Layton CR, et al. Effects of metabolic hyperthermia on performance during heavy prolonged exercise. J Appl Physiol 1974;36:538–544.

27. White MD, Cabanac M. Exercise hyperpnea and hyperthermia in humans. J Appl Physiol 1996;81:1249–1254.

28. Waldrop TG, Mullins DC, Millhorn DE. Control of respiration by the hypothalamus and by feedback from contracting muscles in cats. Respir Physiol 1986;64:317–328.

29. Waldrop TG, Mullins DC, Henderson MC. Effects of hypothalamic lesions on the cardiorespiratory responses to muscular contraction. Respir Physiol 1986;66:215–224.

30. Waldrop TG, Eldridge F, Iwamoto G, et al. Central neural control of respiration and circulation during exercise. In Rowell LB, Shepherd JT, eds. Handbook of Physiology. New York: Oxford University, 1996;333–380.

31. Somjen GG. The missing error signal: regulation beyond negative feedback. News in Physiological Sciences 1992;7:15–19.

32. Houk JC. Control strategies in physiological systems. Faseb J 1988;2:97–107.

33. Fredberg JJ, Inouye D, Miller B, et al. Airway smooth muscle, tidal stretches, and dynamically determined contractile states. Am J Respir Crit Care Med 1997;156:1752–1759.

34. Johnson BD, Saupe KW, Dempsey JA. Mechanical constraints on exercise hyperpnea in endurance athletes. J Appl Physiol 1992;73:874–886.

35. Aliverti A, Cala SJ, Duranti R, et al. Human respiratory muscle actions and control during exercise. J Appl Physiol 1997;83:1256–1269.

36. Aaron EA. Seow KC, Johnson BD, et al. Oxygen cost of exercise hyperpnea: implications for performance. J Appl Physiol 1992;72:1818–1825.

37. Dempsey J, Adams L, Ainsworth D, et al. Airway, lung and respiratory muscle function during exercise. In Rowell LB, Shepherd JT, eds. Handbook of Physiology. New York: Oxford University, 1996;448–515.

38. Matsunaga S, Inashima S, Tsuchimochi H, et al. Altered sarcoplasmic reticulum function in rat diaphragm after high-intensity exercise. Acta Physiol Scand 2002;176: 227–232.

39. Hood DA, Irrcher I. The metabolic systems: training and mitochondrial biogenesis. In Tipton CM, ed. ASCM's Advanced Exercise Physiology. Baltimore: Lippincott Williams & Wilkins, 2006:437–452.

40. Seals DR. The autonomic nervous system. In Tipton CM, ed. ASCM's Advanced Exercise Physiology. Baltimore: Lippincott Williams & Wilkins, 2006:197–245.

41. Manohar M. Blood flow to the respiratory and limb muscles and to abdominal organs during maximal exertion in ponies. J Physiol (Lond) 1986;377:25–35.

42. Harms CA, Wetter TJ, McClaran SR, et al. Effects of respiratory muscle work on cardiac output and its distribution during maximal exercise. J Appl Physiol 1998;85:609–618.

43. Bellemare F, Bigland-Ritchie B. Central components of diaphragmatic fatigue assessed by phrenic nerve stimulation. J Appl Physiol 1987;62:1307–1316.

44. Babcock MA, Pegelow DF, McClaran SR, et al. Contribu-tion of diaphragmatic power output to exercise-induced diaphragm fatigue. J Appl Physiol 1995;78: 1710–1719.

45. Johnson BD, Babcock MA, Suman OE, et al. Exercise-induced diaphragmatic fatigue in healthy humans. J Physiol (Lond) 1993;460:385–405.

46. Bellemare F, Grassino A. Effect of pressure and timing of contraction on human diaphragm fatigue. J Appl Physiol 1982;53:1190–1195.

47. Morton DP, Callister R. Characteristics and etiology of exercise-related transient abdominal pain. Med Sci Sports Exerc 2000;32:432–438.

48. McClaran SR, Babcock MA, Pegelow DF, et al. Longitudinal effects of aging on lung function at rest and exercise in healthy active fit elderly adults. J Appl Physiol 1995;78:1957–1968.

49. Hill JM. Discharge of group IV phrenic afferent fibers increases during diaphragmatic fatigue. Brain Res 2000;856:240–244.

50. Jammes Y, Balzamo E. Changes in afferent and efferent phrenic activities with electrically induced diaphragmatic fatigue. J Appl Physiol 1992;73:894–902.

51. Ainsworth DM, Smith CA, Henderson KS, et al. Breathing during exercise in dogs: passive or active? J Appl Physiol 1996;81:586–595.

52. Morin D, Viala D. Coordinations of locomotor and respiratory rhythms in vitro are critically dependent on hindlimb sensory inputs. J Neurosci 2002;22:4756–4765.

53. Chen Z, Eldridge FL, Wagner PG. Respiratory-associated rhythmic firing of midbrain neurones in cats: relation to level of respiratory drive. J Physiol (Lond) 1991;437: 305–325.

54. O'Donnell DE, D'Arsigny C, Raj S, et al. Ventilatory assistance improves exercise endurance in stable congestive heart failure. Am J Respir Crit Care Med 1999;160:1804–1811.

55. Coates G, O'Brodovich H, Jefferies AL, et al. Effects of exercise on lung lymph flow in sheep and goats during normoxia and hypoxia. J Clin Invest 1984;4:133–141.

56. West JB. Invited review: Pulmonary capillary stress failure. J Appl Physiol 2000;89:2483–2489;discussion, 2497.

57. Hopkins SR, Schoene RB, Henderson WR, et al. Intense exercise impairs the integrity of the pulmonary blood-gas barrier in elite athletes. Am J Respir Crit Care Med 1997;155:1090–1094.

58. Wagner PD, Gale GE, Moon RE, et al. Pulmonary gas exchange in humans exercising at sea level and simulated altitude. J Appl Physiol 1986;61:260–270.

59. Sinclair SE, McKinney S, Glenny RW, et al. Exercise alters fractal dimension and spatial correlation of pulmonary blood flow in the horse. J Appl Physiol 2000;88: 2269–2278.

60. Tobin CE. Arteriovenous shunts in the peripheral pulmonary circulation in the human lung. Thorax 1966;21:197–204.

61. Lloyd TC. Respiratory system compliance as seen from the cardiac fossa. J Appl Physiol 1982;53:57–62.

62. Willeput R, Rondeux C, De Troyer A. Breathing affects venous return from legs in humans. J Appl Physiol 1984;57:971–976.

63. Moreno AH, Katz AI, Gold LD. An integrated approach to the study of the venous system with steps toward a detailed model of the dynamics of venous return to the right heart. IEEE Trans Biomed Eng 1969;16:308–324.

64. Takata M, Wise RA, Robotham JL. Effects of abdominal pressure on venous return: abdominal vascular zone conditions. J Appl Physiol 1990;69:1961–1972.

65. Wexler L, Bergel DH, Gabe IT, et al. Velocity of blood flow in normal human venae cavae. Circ Res 1968;23:349–359.

66. Belenkie I, Smith ER, Tyberg JV. Ventricular interaction: from bench to bedside. Ann Med 2001;33:236–241.

67. Scharf SM, Pinsky MR, Magder S, et al. Respiratory-Circulatory Interactions in Health and Disease. New York: Marcel Dekker, 2001.

68. St Croix CM, Satoh M, Morgan BJ, et al. Role of respiratory motor output in within-breath modulation of muscle sympathetic nerve activity in humans. Circ Res 1999;85:457–469.

69. Eckberg DL, Kifle YT, Roberts VL. Phase relationship between normal human respiration and baroreflex responsiveness. J Physiol (Lond) 1980;304:489–502.

70. Taha BH, Simon PM, Dempsey JA, et al. Respiratory sinus arrhythmia in humans: an obligatory role for vagal feedback from the lungs. J Appl Physiol 1995;78:638–645.

71. Tsuchimochi H, Matsukawa K, Komine H, et al. Direct measurement of cardiac sympathetic efferent nerve activity during dynamic exercise. Am J Physiol 2002;283: H1896–H1906.

72. Potts JT, Paton JF, Mitchell JH, et al. Contraction-sensitive skeletal muscle afferents inhibit arterial baroreceptor signalling in the nucleus of the solitary tract: role of intrinsic GABA interneurons. Neuroscience 2003;119:201–214.

73. Hajduczok G, Hade JS, Mark AL, et al. Central command increases sympathetic nerve activity during spontaneous locomotion in cats. Circ Res 1991;69:66–75.

74. Hussain SN, Chatillon A, Comtois A, et al. Chemical activation of thin-fiber phrenic afferents: 2. Cardiovascular responses. J Appl Physiol 1991;70:77–86.

75. Rodman JR, Henderson KS, Smith CA, et al. Cardiovascular effects of the respiratory muscle metaboreflexes in dogs: rest and exercise. J Appl Physiol 2003;95:1159–1169.

76. Sheel AW, Derchak PA, Morgan BJ, et al. Fatiguing inspiratory muscle work causes reflex reduction in resting leg blood flow in humans. J Physiol (Lond) 2001;537:277–289.

77. St Croix CM, BJ Morgan, TJ Wetter, et al. Fatiguing inspiratory muscle work causes reflex sympathetic activation in humans. J Physiol (Lond) 2000;529Pt 2:493–504.

78. Guyenet PG. Neural structures that mediate sympatho-excitation during hypoxia. Respir Physiol 2000;121: 147–162.

79. Harms CA, Babcock MA, McClaran SR, et al. Respiratory muscle work compromises leg blood flow during maximal exercise. J Appl Physiol 1997;82:1573–1583.

80. Aaker A, Laughlin MH. Diaphragm arterioles are less responsive to alpha1-adrenergic constriction than gastrocnemius arterioles. J Appl Physiol 2002;92: 1808–1816.

81. Massaro D, Massaro GD. Invited review: Pulmonary alveoli: formation, the "call for oxygen," and other regulators. Am J Physiol 2002;282:L345–358.

82. Johnson BD, Reddan WG, Seow KC, et al. Mechanical constraints on exercise hyperpnea in a fit aging population. Am Rev Respir Dis 1991;143:968–977.

83. Moore RL. The cardiovascular system: cardiac function. In Tipton CM, ed. ASCM's Advanced Exercise Physiology. Baltimore: Lippincott Williams & Wilkins, 2006:326–342.

84. Weibel ER, Taylor CR, Hoppeler H. Variations in function and design: testing symmorphosis in the respiratory system. Respir Physiol 1992;87:325–348.

85. Johnson LR, Rush JW, Turk JR, et al. Short-term exercise training increases ACh-induced relaxation and eNOS protein in porcine pulmonary arteries. J Appl Physiol 2001;90:1102–1110.

86. Clanton TL, Dixon GF, Drake J, et al. Effects of swim training on lung volumes and inspiratory muscle conditioning. J Appl Physiol 1987;62:39–46.

87. Leith DE, Bradley M. Ventilatory muscle strength and endurance training. J Appl Physiol 1976;41:508–516.

88. Hagberg JM, Yerg JE II, Seals DR. Pulmonary function in young and older athletes and untrained men. J Appl Physiol 1988;65:101–105.

89. DeSouza CA, Shapiro LF, Clevenger CM, et al. Regular aerobic exercise prevents and restores age-related declines in endothelium-dependent vasodilation in healthy men. Circulation 2000;102:1351–1357.

90. Dempsey JA, Reddan WG, Birnbaum ML, et al. Effects of acute through life-long hypoxic exposure on exercise pulmonary gas exchange. Respir Physiol 1971;13:62–89.

91. Karjalainen EM, Laitinen A, Sue-Chu M, et al. Evidence of airway inflammation and remodeling in ski athletes with and without bronchial hyperresponsiveness to methacholine. Am J Respir Crit Care Med 2000;161: 2086–2091.

92. Powers SK, Coombes J, Demirel H. Exercise training-induced changes in respiratory muscles. Sports Med 1997;24:120–131.

93. Powers SK, Shanely RA. Exercise-induced changes in diaphragmatic bioenergetic and antioxidant capacity. Exerc Sport Sci Rev 2002;30:69–74.

94. Vincent HK, Shanely RA, Stewart DJ, et al. Adaptation of upper airway muscles to chronic endurance exercise. Am J Respir Crit Care Med 2002;166:287–293.

95. Ramirez-Sarmiento A, Orozco-Levi M, Guell R, et al. Inspiratory muscle training in patients with chronic obstructive pulmonary disease: structural adaptation and physiologic outcomes. Am J Respir Crit Care Med 2002;166:1491–1497.

96. Levine S, Nguyen T, Shrager J, et al. Diaphragm adaptations elicited by severe chronic obstructive pulmonary disease: lessons for sports science. Exerc Sport Sci Rev 2001;29:71–75.

97. Babcock MA, Pegelow DF, Johnson BD, et al. Aerobic fitness effects on exercise-induced low-frequency diaphragm fatigue. J Appl Physiol 1996;81:2156–2164.

98. Zhan WZ, Sieck GC. Adaptations of diaphragm and medial gastrocnemius muscles to inactivity. J Appl Physiol 1992;72:1445–1453.

99. Sassoon CS, Caiozzo VJ, Manka A, et al. Altered diaphragm contractile properties with controlled mechanical ventilation. J Appl Physiol 2002;92:2585–2595.

100. Saltin B, Strange S. Maximal oxygen uptake: "old" and "new" arguments for a cardiovascular limitation. Med Sci Sports Exerc 1992;24:30–37.

101. Wagner PD. New ideas on limitations to $\dot{V}O_{2max}$. Exerc Sport Sci Rev 2000;28:10–14.

102. Harms CA, McClaran SR, Nickele GA, et al. Exercise-induced arterial hypoxaemia in healthy young women. J Physiol (Lond) 1998;507(Pt 2): 619–628.

103. Prefaut C, Anselme F, Caillaud C, et al. Exercise-induced hypoxemia in older athletes. J Appl Physiol 1994;76:120–126.

104. Bayly WM, Hodgson DR, Schulz DA, et al. Exercise-induced hypercapnia in the horse. J Appl Physiol 1989;67:1958–1966.

105. Dempsey JA, Wagner PD. Exercise-induced arterial hypoxemia. J Appl Physiol 1999;87:1997–2006.

106. Dempsey JA, Hanson PG, Henderson KS. Exercise-induced arterial hypoxaemia in healthy human subjects at sea level. J Physiol (Lond) 1984;355:161–175.

107. Gore CJ, Little SC, Hahn AG, et al. Reduced performance of male and female athletes at 580 m altitude. Eur J Appl Physiol 1997;75:136–143.

108. Lawler J, Powers SK, Thompson D. Linear relationship between $\dot{V}O_{2max}$ and $\dot{V}O_{2max}$ decrement during exposure to acute hypoxia. J Appl Physiol 1988;64: 1486–1492.

109. Sliwinski P, Yan S, Gauthier AP, et al. Influence of global inspiratory muscle fatigue on breathing during exercise. J Appl Physiol 1996;80:1270–1278.

110. Prefaut C, Anselme-Poujol F, Caillaud C. Inhibition of histamine release by nedocromil sodium reduces exercise-induced hypoxemia in master athletes. Med Sci Sports Exerc 1997;29:10–16.

111. Wetter TJ, Xiang Z, Sonetti DA, et al. Role of lung inflammatory mediators as a cause of exercise-induced arterial hypoxemia in young athletes. J Appl Physiol 2002;93:116–126.

112. McConnell AK, Romer LM. Respiratory muscle training in healthy humans: resolving the controversy. Int J Sports Med 2003;24:1–10.

113. Farkas GA, Roussos C. Adaptability of the hamster diaphragm to exercise and/or emphysema. J Appl Physiol 1982;53:1263–1272.

114. Farkas GA, Roussos C. Diaphragm in emphysematous hamsters: sarcomere adaptability. J Appl Physiol 1983;54:1635–1640.

115. Arnold JS, Thomas AJ, Kelsen SG. Length-tension relationship of abdominal expiratory muscles: effect of emphysema. J Appl Physiol 1987;62:739–745.

116. Shrager JB, Kim DK, Hashmi YJ, et al. Lung volume reduction surgery restores the normal diaphragmatic length-tension relationship in emphysematous rats. J Thorac Cardiovasc Surg 2001;121:217–224.

CHAPTER 11

The Oxygen Transport System: Integration of Functions

Peter D. Wagner

Introduction

This chapter focuses on the entire pathway for oxygen during exercise. The overall objective is to explain how oxygen transport is determined, with particular emphasis on maximal rates of transport. Implicit in this discussion will be how oxygen transport may become limited not only normally but also in pathological states. However, there will be no specific description of individual diseases, of which there are many, in which limited oxygen transport may at least in part govern maximal exercise capacity.

Maximal Versus Submaximal Exercise

Important to any discussion of oxygen transport is first distinguishing between *maximal* and *submaximal* exercise. Figure 11.1 indicates the common notion of how $\dot{V}O_2$ relates essentially linearly to power output as exercise intensity is increased (region between points A and B). This relationship reflects $\dot{V}O_2$ during a typical incremental test and ignores the upward drift in $\dot{V}O_2$ seen at high work loads that are maintained for several minutes. Above B, the relationship then levels off (region between points B and C). Point C indicates maximal exercise intensity, while the $\dot{V}O_2$ at the plateau is maximal, that is, $\dot{V}O_{2max}$.

Below B, the available capacity to move oxygen from the air to the mitochondria is not fully used. In this range, oxygen supply increases with exercise to match exactly the amount of oxygen required for any particular level of exercise (assuming steady state of oxygen use). Under such conditions, not all oxygen delivered to the muscles will be extracted, and any oxygen in muscle venous blood is simply not required by the mitochondria. Venous oxygen concentration is therefore a *dependent* variable, and oxygen demand by the muscles sets oxygen supply through the complex control systems that regulate ventilation, blood flow, and regional peripheral vascular resistance (1–4).

The region between B and C, however, must be considered differently. Two general scenarios are possible. One is that mitochondrial metabolic oxidative capacity to use oxygen has reached maximal values by point B (4 L · min⁻¹ in the example in Fig. 11.1). Implied here is that even if more oxygen were made available, it could not be used. Thus, in this case, availability of oxygen is not governing maximal exercise. As for submaximal conditions, the level of oxygen in the muscle venous blood is a *dependent* variable reflecting excess oxygen not usable by the mitochondria. In this scenario, if for example muscle blood flow rate could be increased, it would result only in a higher venous oxygen level. No change in $\dot{V}O_{2max}$ would occur.

The second possibility is that the plateau in $\dot{V}O_2$ reflects an inability to supply more oxygen to the mitochondria despite increasing demand created by higher work rates and

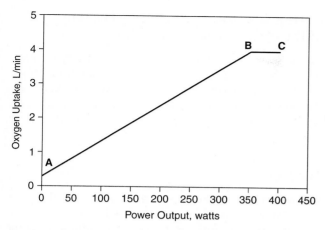

FIGURE 11.1 Expected relationship between exercise intensity (watts) and oxygen uptake (or consumption) from rest (A) to maximal exercise capacity (C). There is a linear increase over most of the range to satisfy the metabolic demands of the muscles, but at point B, oxygen uptake fails to rise further, indicating $\dot{V}O_{2max}$.

despite a higher metabolic capacity to use oxygen (than $4\,L\cdot min^{-1}$ in the case under discussion). This scenario defines oxygen supply limitation of $\dot{V}O_{2max}$. It implies that if more oxygen could be made available (by increasing oxygen delivery to the muscles), it would be used, and $\dot{V}O_2$ would rise.

One might think that if oxygen supply limitation were responsible for the plateau in $\dot{V}O_2$, muscle venous blood would have no oxygen left in it and that all oxygen reaching the muscles would be extracted for metabolic use. However, that is never the case (5–7). In fact, because the transfer of oxygen from blood to muscle cells is a diffusive process, high rates of oxygen transport demand a high average PO_2 in the muscle blood. This is because net oxygen flux depends on the PO_2 difference between the blood and the mitochondria. Thus, somewhat paradoxically, the higher the $\dot{V}O_{2max}$, the higher must be the average capillary PO_2 in a given muscle. Under such oxygen supply-limited conditions, the PO_2 of the venous blood (reflecting average microvascular values) is no longer a dependent variable passively reflecting a $\dot{V}O_2$ set by exercise demand but is a key determinant of ability to transport oxygen to the mitochondria by diffusion (8). In this way, muscle microvascular PO_2 becomes a factor determining $\dot{V}O_{2max}$ itself. This will be discussed in detail later.

When a subject exercises to exhaustion, one may never see a plateau of $\dot{V}O_2$. This means that symptoms have become severe enough to cause the subject to stop before (or possibly just at; one would not know) point B in Figure 11.1. In such a situation, the subject has reached peak $\dot{V}O_2$ and the term $\dot{V}O_{2max}$ should be avoided. If a plateau is seen, the subject has by definition reached $\dot{V}O_{2max}$. However, the mere presence of a plateau does not allow one to distinguish between metabolic capacity and oxygen supply limitation as the mechanism. This would take a second exercise test determining

whether $\dot{V}O_{2max}$ could be increased by augmenting oxygen availability (e.g., by exercising during pure oxygen breathing or after blood transfusion to increase hemoglobin levels). In metabolic limitation, $\dot{V}O_{2max}$ would not change, and muscle venous PO_2 would passively rise, reflecting constant $\dot{V}O_2$ in the face of a higher arterial oxygen concentration. In oxygen supply limitation, $\dot{V}O_{2max}$ would increase. So too would muscle venous PO_2 (reflecting the necessarily higher PO_2 gradient from blood to tissue). The laws of diffusion would predict that the increases in $\dot{V}O_{2max}$ and venous PO_2 would be roughly proportional, as shown later in this chapter. However, if one is to understand these concepts fully, the oxygen transport pathway itself must first be described.

The Oxygen Transport Pathway

A key concept underlying this chapter is that oxygen transport requires the integrated function of several tissues and organs working in an interdependent manner. Interdependent means that the function of any one such element of the pathway can affect the function of the others. The primary tissues and organs in question are the lungs, the heart and vasculature, the blood, and the muscles themselves (9). Secondary factors, such as the kidneys and skin, which over time play a role in fluid balance and thermoregulation, affect oxygen transport generally by affecting blood flow and/or hemoglobin concentration and are thus not separately considered in the following discussion.

The Oxygen Transport Pathway: In Series or in Parallel?

While it may be self-evident, it is important to point out that the primary tissues and organs involved in oxygen transport are arranged in *series* and not in *parallel* (Fig. 11.2). Thus, oxygen must first be inhaled into the alveoli (ventilation). Then it must pass into the blood (diffusion). Next it must bind to hemoglobin. After that cardiac activity moves it through the vasculature to the muscles (blood flow). Finally, oxygen must pass from the vasculature into the muscle cells and ultimately reach the mitochondria (diffusion). These separately identifiable processes occur in strict sequence, that is, in series. They do not form a parallel system of alternative pathways. The distinction is important because in a parallel system, in which any one step can be bypassed, a weakness in one parallel track might conceivably be made up by increased function of another, such that total system function remains intact. However, in a serial system, the function of the total system is strongly influenced by the function of the weakest step.

In a serial system, the overall throughput of the transported species cannot exceed that of the weakest step; in a parallel system, a weakness in an individual step might not reduce overall system function. For example, in the serial

Structures   **Functions**

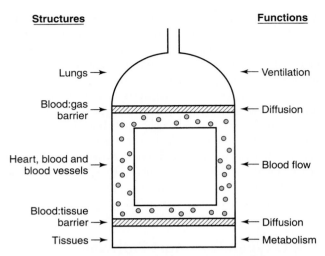

Lungs → ← Ventilation

Blood:gas barrier → ← Diffusion

Heart, blood and blood vessels → ← Blood flow

Blood:tissue barrier → ← Diffusion

Tissues → ← Metabolism

FIGURE 11.2   The oxygen transport pathway. Structures are shown on the left, transport functions on the right. The lungs, heart, blood vessels, blood, and muscles in series form an integrated transport system.

oxygen transport system, poor cardiac function and compromised muscle blood flow will constrain exercise capacity even if the lungs, blood, vasculature, and muscles are intact (10). Hypothetically, if the body had evolved with some kind of additional oxygen transport system that did not depend on the heart (e.g., absorption of oxygen through the skin), poor cardiac function might be compensated for by increased skin absorption of oxygen.

A different outcome occurs when the function of just one step is enhanced. For example, a substantial increase in cardiac function alone in a serial system may not translate into a corresponding gain in exercise capacity, because the remaining steps of the pathway have not increased to match the capacity of the heart. *Thus, impairment of any single component of the oxygen transport pathway can seriously reduce exercise capacity, but enhancement of a single component usually brings little benefit* (11). This is illustrated later in this chapter.

As mentioned, a critical feature of a serial transport system is that the function of any one step may be influenced by the function of any of the other steps in the chain. A good example again is cardiac function (but there are many others, described later). A change in blood flow may change red cell contact time in the microcirculation of both the lungs and the muscles. Since the oxygen exchange processes in the lungs and muscles are based on diffusion, length of red cell contact time may well affect the overall rate of oxygen transport across the lungs and/or into the muscles. Thus, while an increase in cardiac output may augment convective transport of oxygen around the body, it may at the same time impair diffusive equilibration of oxygen between lungs and blood or between blood and muscle, which will in part offset the gains in convective transport.

Critical Structure and Function Elements of the Oxygen Transport Pathway

In this section, the key functional (and underlying structural) aspects of each organ and tissue are briefly described. This is purely from the point of view of oxygen transport and should not be taken to supersede the far more detailed descriptions of these organs and tissues, especially their functional regulation, in other chapters in this volume.

The Lungs

As the first step in the oxygen transport chain, the lungs bring oxygen to the alveolar gas spaces by the highly regulated process of ventilation. Oxygen then diffuses from the alveolar gas into the pulmonary capillary blood and is transported to the left heart for distribution to the tissues and organs of the body. These processes are described in detail in Chapter 10.

Ventilation

The amount of fresh oxygen inhaled into the alveoli is not simply equal to the amount of oxygen that passes through the lips. This is because the airways between the lips and the closest alveoli have a combined volume of about 150 mL. Thus, no matter what the tidal volume, about 150 mL less than the tidal volume of fresh air actually reaches the alveoli with each breath. The total amount of ventilation passing the lips per minute is called *minute ventilation* ($\dot{V}E$), and it is the product of tidal volume and respiratory rate. The amount of fresh air entering the alveoli is the product of (tidal volume—conducting airway volume) and respiratory rate, and it is called *alveolar ventilation* ($\dot{V}A$). Only 21% of the molecules in air are oxygen, the rest being nitrogen with a few trace species of inert gases, pollutant gases, and carbon dioxide. The latter is negligible at 0.03%. Consequently, the amount of new oxygen reaching the alveoli per minute is given by the following formula:

$$\text{Alveolar } O_2 \text{ delivery} \cdot \text{min}^{-1} = \dot{V}A \times F_{IO_2}$$

[Equation 11.1]

where F_{IO_2} is the fractional concentration of oxygen in the air, that is, 0.21. It should be apparent that oxygen consumption by the body tissues cannot exceed the amount of fresh oxygen reaching the alveoli given in Equation 11.1.

However, because it is essential to the next step in the pathway (oxygen diffusion into the pulmonary capillary blood) to maintain a high alveolar P_{O_2}, maximal oxygen consumption must be far less than the limit given by Equation 11.1. A high alveolar P_{O_2} means that exhaled gas, which must come from the alveoli, has this high P_{O_2} as well. Thus, a large amount of inhaled oxygen is returned to the atmosphere in each and every breath. This is shown in Equation 11.2, which describes the net uptake of oxygen ($\dot{V}O_2$) as the difference between that inhaled (Equation 11.1) and that exhaled:

$$\dot{V}_{O_2} = \dot{V}_A \times F_{I_{O_2}} - \dot{V}_A \times F_{A_{O_2}}$$

[Equation 11.2]

where $F_{A_{O_2}}$ is the fractional concentration of oxygen in exhaled alveolar gas. $\dot{V}_A$ (alveolar ventilation) is taken to be the same for both inspiration and expiration. This is close to correct, the only discrepancy being any difference between rate of oxygen uptake and rate of carbon dioxide elimination.

Suppose at maximal exercise, alveolar ventilation is 150 L per minute. Equation 11.1 states that the amount of fresh oxygen reaching the alveoli will be 31.5 L per minute (0.21 × 150). $\dot{V}_{O_{2max}}$, however does not come close to such levels. Even Olympic champions do not have $\dot{V}_{O_2}$ levels beyond about 6 L per minute and hence each minute are returning to the air some 25 L of unused oxygen from alveolar gas. Equation 11.2 shows that when $\dot{V}_{O_{2max}}$ is 6 L per minute and $\dot{V}_A$ is 150 L per minute, the fractional alveolar oxygen concentration is 0.17. This corresponds to a high alveolar P_{O_2}, about 120 mm Hg, facilitating diffusion into the blood. Were an athlete able to absorb every molecule of inhaled oxygen, he or she could support a gold medal–winning 6 L per minute $\dot{V}_{O_2}$ breathing only about 29 L per minute of air! This would require exhaled gas to be devoid of oxygen, and thus alveolar P_{O_2} would be zero. Clearly, an energy-requiring oxygen transport pump would be needed to move oxygen into the blood if alveolar P_{O_2} were zero. The price for passive diffusion is high in terms of ventilatory requirements, 150/29, or about fivefold, in this example.

As exercise intensity rises, so too does ventilation. The relationship is tight, but how ventilation is regulated remains uncertain, with probably several redundant control systems in place (1). At light to moderate exercise levels that do not significantly elevate blood lactate concentrations, $\dot{V}_A$ rises roughly in proportion to exercise intensity such that alveolar and arterial P_{O_2} change little from values at rest (this would be expected from Equation 11.2 if $\dot{V}_{O_2}$ and $\dot{V}_A$ increase in proportion). Since a similar equation can be applied to carbon dioxide, a constant arterial P_{CO_2} would also be expected from this proportional increase in ventilation. However, at higher exercise intensities, when lactate is appearing in the blood, ventilation accelerates, causing alveolar P_{O_2} to rise and alveolar P_{CO_2} to fall. The benefit to gas exchange is a higher alveolar P_{O_2} for diffusion, but the cost is in higher ventilatory work.

Diffusion

Oxygen in the alveolar gas is constantly being moved across the blood-gas barrier into the pulmonary capillary blood. The transport process is passive diffusion (12). A net flux into the blood therefore *demands* a higher partial pressure of oxygen in the alveolar gas than the capillary blood. This is one disadvantage of diffusion (discussed earlier), the advantage of which is that it does not require energy (compare to energy-requiring renal ion pumps that regulate urine formation).

Alveolar P_{O_2} (normally about 100 torr) is indeed higher than the P_{O_2} of the mixed venous blood returning from the tissues and entering the pulmonary capillaries (normally about 40 torr). This is more than enough to assure adequate oxygen transfer into the blood, with diffusion equilibration occurring under most conditions. By this it is meant that the P_{O_2} in the end pulmonary capillary blood is essentially equal to that of the alveolar gas. In fact, in resting man, it takes only about 0.25 seconds for the P_{O_2} of a red cell to rise from mixed venous to alveolar levels. The time available at rest is much longer, about 0.75 seconds (13). We know that because the volume of blood in the pulmonary capillaries at any instant is about 75 mL, while the flow rate of blood through those capillaries (i.e., the cardiac output) totals about 6 L per minute. Mean transit time is their ratio: 75 mL/6 L per minute, or 0.75 seconds.

During exercise, pulmonary blood flow increases substantially, and the pulmonary capillary blood volume also expands (14) by a combination of capillary recruitment and distention. However, the relative increase in cardiac output outstrips that of capillary volume such that mean transit time falls to about 0.4 to 0.5 seconds (14). In addition, because mixed venous P_{O_2} falls during exercise, it takes longer than 0.25 seconds for capillary P_{O_2} to reach alveolar values. That means that at peak exercise, normal humans are on the brink of incomplete oxygen loading of red cells on the basis of limited contact time for red cells, and arterial P_{O_2} may fall as a result (15). This is a problem particularly for elite athletes because they tend to have quite high cardiac outputs yet not exceptionally large lungs. As a result, their red cell transit time is less than for a less fit person, and diffusion limitation may develop, commonly resulting in a fall in arterial P_{O_2}.

As ventilation increases with exercise intensity to maintain or even increase alveolar P_{O_2} above 100 torr and with muscle oxygen extraction also increasing (such that the mixed venous blood returns to the lungs at a P_{O_2} of often about 20 torr; discussed later), the diffusion gradient is enhanced over that at rest. The increase can be substantial. Thus at rest the initial alveolar-capillary P_{O_2} difference is as mentioned 100 − 40 = 60 torr. During heavy exercise, alveolar P_{O_2} is often 110 torr, while mixed venous P_{O_2} is 20 torr, and the initial gradient is thus 90 torr, fully 50% greater than at rest.

This increase in alveolar-venous P_{O_2} gradient in the lungs with exercise is a good example of the integrative nature of the oxygen transport system: ventilation and muscle oxygen extraction both increase, and these automatically enhance pulmonary oxygen uptake by diffusion when transport requirements increase.

Whether the diffusion process in the lungs is complete or not depends on several factors. These include not only the transit time and the alveolar and mixed venous oxygen levels as mentioned, but also the pulmonary diffusing capacity and the oxygen-hemoglobin binding characteristics in the red cell. The diffusing capacity is dictated by the alveolar structure, and indeed, the division of the lungs into a huge number of small, thin-walled alveoli is key. Fick's law of diffusion applied to the uptake of oxygen can be expressed as:

$$\dot{V}_{O_2} = k \times SA \times (P_{A O_2} - P_{c O_2})/d$$

[Equation 11.3]

where $\dot{V}_{O_2}$ = the rate at which oxygen crosses from alveolar gas ($P_{O_2} = P_{A O_2}$) into capillary blood ($P_{O_2} = P_{c O_2}$); SA = the total capillary surface area (essentially the total alveolar wall surface area because the capillary network is very dense); d = the thickness, about 0.3 μm, of the blood-gas barrier separating gas and blood; and k = a constant depicting the diffusive conductance of lung tissue per unit area and thickness. Given that the lung volume is about 4 L, if the lungs were constructed as a single large spherical alveolus, its radius would be about 10 cm and wall surface area just 1200 cm², or about 0.1 square meters. The lungs are, however, made up of 300 million alveoli, each of diameter 300 μm. Total volume of these alveoli is still only 4 L, but the total surface area comes to about 80 m², sufficient to enable a high $\dot{V}_{O_2}$ from Equation 11.3.

Equation 11.3 is easy in concept, but it is made complex by the fact that $P_{c O_2}$ is not constant, but rises continuously in a given red cell as that cell flows through the pulmonary capillary. When a red cell first enters the pulmonary capillary, its $P_{c O_2}$ is that of mixed venous blood (20–40 mm Hg). Since alveolar P_{O_2} is 100 to 120 mm Hg, diffusion of oxygen into the blood starts immediately. This raises $P_{c O_2}$, changing the numbers in Equation 11.3 to reduce the rate of oxygen transfer into the blood as the red cell continues through the capillary. This process can be described by a differential equation. If one is willing to approximate the oxyhemoglobin dissociation curve by a straight line of slope β, the capillary P_{O_2} at the end of the entire red cell transit through the network (here taken to be equal to systemic arterial P_{O_2}, $P_{a O_2}$) can be determined from an exponential equation (16):

$$P_{a O_2} = P_{A O_2} - (P_{A O_2} - P_{v O_2}) \times \exp[-D/(\beta \cdot \dot{Q})]$$

[Equation 11.4]

where $P_{A O_2}$ = alveolar and $P_{v O_2}$ mixed venous P_{O_2}; D = the diffusing capacity of the lungs (k × SA / d in Equation 11.3); $\dot{Q}$ = total cardiac output; and β = the average slope of the linearized oxyhemoglobin dissociation curve.

Equation 11.4 shows that the completeness of the diffusive process (i.e., how close $P_{a O_2}$ comes to $P_{A O_2}$) depends not only on the intrinsic diffusing capacity (D) of the lungs but also on both cardiac output ($\dot{Q}$) and on the average slope of the oxyhemoglobin dissociation curve (β). In particular, it is the *ratio* of D to (β$\dot{Q}$) that is the key determinant of diffusion limitation. In concept, therefore, diffusion limitation may occur when cardiac output and/or hemoglobin levels are high even if D is normal and may not occur when D is low if $\dot{Q}$ and/or β is also reduced. Once again, system component interdependence is evident: pulmonary oxygen uptake by diffusion depends on function of the lungs, blood, and heart, not on the lungs alone.

The Heart and Circulation

The control of cardiac output during exercise, like that of ventilation, is one of the most complex and least well understood elements of exercise physiology. The subject is well covered by Moore (17) and is not dealt with here except to state that there is a remarkably strong linear relationship between cardiac output and oxygen consumption across the domain from rest to maximal exercise. (See Chapter 12.) Cardiac output increases about 5 to 6 L per minute for every 1 L per minute of increase in $\dot{V}_{O_2}$ (3). Irrespective of the mechanisms controlling cardiac output, the Fick principle of mass conservation can be used to describe oxygen transport in the blood:

$$\dot{V}_{O_2} = \dot{Q} \times (C_{a O_2} - C_{v O_2})$$

[Equation 11.5]

where $C_{a O_2}$ and $C_{v O_2}$, respectively, = arterial and venous concentrations of oxygen. Neglecting oxygen physically dissolved in the blood (it is normally less than 2% of the total oxygen in the blood), these concentrations can be expressed in terms of hemoglobin concentration (Hb) and blood oxygen saturation of hemoglobin ($S_{a O_2}$ and $S_{v O_2}$, respectively) as follows:

$$C_{a O_2} = 1.39 \times Hb \times S_{a O_2}$$

[Equation 11.6]

$$C_{v O_2} = 1.39 \times Hb \times S_{v O_2}$$

[Equation 11.7]

In Equation 11.5, $\dot{V}_{O_2}$ represents the same rate of oxygen uptake as appears in Equation 11.2. Thus, Equations 11.2 and 11.5 are equivalent descriptions of oxygen uptake. Equation 11.5 represents the difference between the rate of delivery of oxygen to the tissues, $\dot{Q} \times C_{a O_2}$, and the rate of return of unused oxygen to the lungs from the tissues, $\dot{Q} \times C_{v O_2}$. It is useful to define systemic oxygen delivery ($\dot{Q}_{O_2}$) separately as follows:

$$\dot{Q}_{O_2} = \dot{Q} \times C_{a O_2} = 1.39 \times \dot{Q} \times Hb \times S_{a O_2}$$

[Equation 11.8]

$\dot{Q}_{O_2}$ in Equation 11.8 explicitly shows the rate of oxygen transport to the muscles as the product of transport variables pertinent to three different systems: cardiovascular, responsible for $\dot{Q}$; blood, responsible for hemoglobin; and lungs, determining $S_{a O_2}$ in concert with the heart and blood in accordance with Equation 11.4.

To this point, no distinction has been made between total cardiac output and pulmonary blood flow. In healthy normal subjects, these are indeed one and the same except for very small (about 1%) contributions to the systemic circulation from the bronchial and Thebesian veins consisting of deoxygenated blood that has not passed through the pulmonary capillary network. These so-called shunts can usually be neglected in the context of overall exercise physiology.

More important is the distinction between total cardiac output and muscle blood flow. At rest, when cardiac output is about 6 L per minute, muscle blood flow is less than 1 L per minute. Cardiac output and muscle blood flow are thus very different at rest. During maximal exercise in an average subject, cardiac output is some 20 to 25 L per minute. Only about 4 L per minute of that is not delivered to the exercising muscles, so that interchanging the terms *cardiac output* and *muscle blood flow* is not generally problematic. However, in patients with lung diseases such as COPD, with which the work of breathing is increased by airway obstruction, the respiratory muscles may require significantly more blood flow than in health. With cardiac function often also limited in such patients, it then becomes important not to equate exercising muscle blood flow with cardiac output. For research purposes involving blood flow studies, it is generally advisable to measure muscle blood flow directly and not equate it to some assumed fraction of cardiac output. Depending on conditions, that assumption may be seriously in error.

The Blood

Much of the role of the blood in transporting oxygen around the body has been laid out. Thus, hemoglobin levels play a role in the diffusion process in the lungs (and similarly in the muscles, shown later), as Equation 11.4 shows. How hemoglobin is important in systemic oxygen delivery was also mentioned (Equations 11.6–11.8). Additional important elements are the very shape of the oxyhemoglobin dissociation curve itself and the position of the dissociation curve as reflected in the P_{O_2} when oxygen saturation is 50% (P_{50}).

Shape of the Oxyhemoglobin Dissociation Curve

The shape of the curve is especially important in understanding both diffusive loading of oxygen in the lungs and diffusive unloading of oxygen in the muscles. The curve is nonlinear, as shown in Figure 11.3. On this figure are indicated typical exercise values for both venous and alveolar P_{O_2}. In the lungs, red cells take on oxygen so that their P_{O_2} rises from venous to alveolar along the dissociation curve; in the muscles, they give up their oxygen with P_{O_2} falling back to the venous level, again along the dissociation curve. One might therefore think that the diffusion processes are quantitatively similar in the lungs and muscles, just operating in opposite directions (so long as the diffusing capacities are similar). After all, at least at $\dot{V}_{O_{2max}}$, blood flow through the lungs and muscles is about the same, and the same dissociation curves must apply in both locations. Thus Equation 11.4, which also applies in principle to the muscles, as developed later, might suggest quantitative similarity in both directions, but this is not the case. Equation 11.4 remains useful in a conceptual sense, but accurate application to oxygen requires that the nonlinear nature of the oxyhemoglobin curve be allowed for.

When this is done, it becomes apparent that loading of oxygen in the lungs (for the same D, average β and Q̇) is

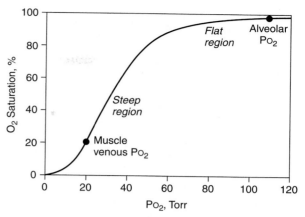

FIGURE 11.3   The oxyhemoglobin dissociation curve during exercise, showing blood oxygen saturation as a function of blood P_{O_2}. Solid circles indicate (*a*) alveolar P_{O_2} and the blood saturation that would correspond to it if end capillary P_{O_2} was equal to alveolar and (*b*) muscle venous P_{O_2} and saturation. Alveolar P_{O_2} is higher and venous P_{O_2} lower than at rest. Significance of the flat and steep regions of the curve is explained in the text.

faster than is unloading in the tissues. The explanation is as follows. In the lungs, as oxygen is loaded onto hemoglobin at the venous end of the capillary, oxygen concentration rises rapidly per unit rise in capillary P_{O_2} because the dissociation curve is steep. Thus, oxygen uptake is fast, yet the P_{O_2} difference between alveolar gas and the capillary blood is maintained until much of the oxygen has been loaded. Maintaining the P_{O_2} gradient facilitates diffusion (Equation 11.3). Now, when the oxygenated red cell reaches the muscle and starts offloading oxygen, it is happening on the flat part of the oxyhemoglobin curve. Thus, P_{O_2} is falling rapidly, while little oxygen is actually transferred from red cell to muscle cell. By the time significant amounts of oxygen are leaving the red cell, capillary P_{O_2} is quite low, and the diffusion gradient from blood to tissues is thus reduced. *The result is that the oxygen offloading process in the muscles is intrinsically slower than the oxygen loading process in the lungs because of the nonlinear shape of the oxyhemoglobin dissociation curve.* Figure 11.4 illustrates this for both the lungs and the tissues. The upper panel shows P_{O_2}, and the lower panel shows blood oxygen saturation. As a result, while diffusive loading of oxygen in the lungs is not often compromised (at least at sea level), incomplete diffusive unloading in the muscles is commonly observed and may limit overall oxygen availability to the muscle mitochondria during maximal exercise.

Of special interest is that at *altitude* (sufficient to cause alveolar P_{O_2} to fall to the steep part of the oxyhemoglobin curve), these differences no longer exist, because both pulmonary oxygen loading and muscle oxygen unloading are taking place completely on the linear, steep part of the dissociation curve. Under such conditions, diffusion limitation

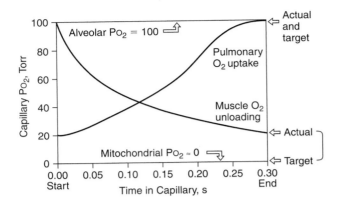

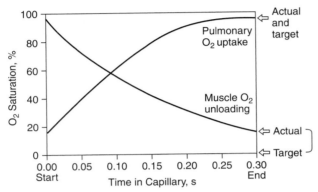

FIGURE 11.4 Calculated time course of P_{O_2} (*top*) and oxygen saturation (*bottom*) in a red cell passing through the lungs (rising curves) and muscles (falling curves) during exercise, assuming identical oxygen diffusional conductance in both locations. Transit time is estimated at 0.3 seconds in both. Full equilibration is reached in 0.3 seconds in the lungs (capillary and alveolar P_{O_2} the same) but not in the muscles (capillary P_{O_2} 20 torr, mitochondrial close to 0) despite the same assumed diffusing capacity. The explanation for the difference is in the shape of the oxyhemoglobin dissociation curve, discussed in the text.

becomes a problem for oxygen transport in *both* the lungs and the tissues (18).

While β and $\dot{Q}$ must be on average approximately the same for the lungs and the muscles, D may be different and might be imagined as compensating for the oxyhemoglobin curve if it were higher in muscle than lung. However, it turns out that lung and muscle diffusing capacities are fairly similar when measured during maximal whole-body exercise: some 80 to 100 mL oxygen per minute per millimeter of mercury in normal active human adults. Thus, such compensation is not apparent.

P_{50} of the Oxyhemoglobin Dissociation Curve

Quite separately from the events discussed in the previous section, the dissociation curve in each red cell undergoes substantial shifts as the red cells move between the muscles and the lungs every few seconds during exercise. In the mus-

cles, capillary P_{CO_2} rises and pH falls as a result of addition of metabolic carbon dioxide produced by the muscles as they consume oxygen. These conditions shift the oxyhemoglobin curve rightward. An additional rightward shift results from any associated increase in blood temperature and lactate level. A rightward shift means a lower oxygen saturation at a given P_{O_2}, which implies that more oxygen can be unloaded while still keeping the capillary P_{O_2} high to enable diffusive transport.

When the venous blood returns to the lungs, it gives up large amounts of carbon dioxide, which is exhaled. Thus, pulmonary capillary P_{CO_2} falls and pH rises, and there may be some cooling as well. These changes cause a leftward shift in the dissociation curve. This accentuates the curvature of the oxyhemoglobin dissociation relation and facilitates diffusive loading, as discussed in the preceding section.

Once again, the metabolic events in the muscles and respiratory events in the lungs each affect blood oxygen transport between the two organs, and in a mutually enhancing manner. This is yet another example of integration between the several components of the oxygen transport pathway.

The Muscles

The process of diffusive unloading of oxygen in the muscles is mentioned earlier. One can describe the diffusive process out of the blood in identical terms as used in Equations 11.3 and 11.4 for the lungs. The muscle equivalent of Equation 11.3 is

$$\dot{V}_{O_2} = k \times SA \times (P_{CO_2} - P_{mitO_2})/d$$
[Equation 11.9]

where $P_{CO_2} = P_{O_2}$ in the muscle capillary; $P_{mitO_2} =$ the mitochondrial P_{O_2}; k, SA, and d = the structural determinants of the muscle diffusing capacity, as for the lungs. We again assume that the oxyhemoglobin dissociation curve can be approximated by a straight line of slope β. By integrating this equation along the capillary, we end up with an equation similar to Equation 11.4 as follows (19):

$$P_{VO_2} = P_{mitO_2} + (P_{aO_2} - P_{mitO_2}) \times \exp\left[-D_M/\beta \cdot \dot{Q}\right]$$
[Equation 11.10]

where $P_{VO_2} =$ the effluent muscle venous P_{O_2}, $P_{aO_2} =$ the arterial P_{O_2}, $D_M =$ the muscle oxygen diffusing capacity, and $\dot{Q} =$ muscle blood flow. There is good evidence that even during moderate exercise, let alone at $\dot{V}_{O_2max}$, myoglobin-associated P_{O_2} is about 2 to 4 mm Hg or less (20,21), such that mitochondrial P_{O_2} is likely even lower. It can be neglected for simplicity, and Equation 11.10 becomes

$$P_{VO_2} = P_{aO_2} \times \exp\left[-D_M/(\beta \cdot \dot{Q})\right]$$
[Equation 11.11]

This expression, defining the diffusive behavior of the muscles, yet again points out that the muscle diffusive conductance, D_M, is just one of several factors that determine overall oxygen transport between the capillaries and mitochondria.

Some authors talk in terms of both central and peripheral factors in oxygen transport. In this construct, central factors include blood flow, hemoglobin level, and arterial P_{O_2} (i.e., Pa_{O_2}, β and $\dot{Q}$ in Equation 11.11), while D_M is the only peripheral factor involved. Thus, oxygen extraction, which determines Pv_{O_2}, is set by an *interaction* between central and peripheral factors, not by peripheral factors alone.

Other Factors Potentially Involved in Limiting Oxygen Transport

The discussion to this point has purposefully ignored two aspects of oxygen transport that may become important, if not in health then possibly in disease. These two aspects are heterogeneity of function in the lungs and in the muscles.

Pulmonary Heterogeneity

Diffusion limitation is not the only phenomenon that can cause arterial hypoxemia and reduced oxygen delivery to the tissues. Ventilation ($\dot{V}_A$) and blood flow ($\dot{Q}$) must be distributed relatively uniformly throughout the lungs to avoid hypoxemia. In fact, it is the distribution of $\dot{V}_A/\dot{Q}$ ratios that is key to the development of hypoxemia. In health, the amount of $\dot{V}_A/\dot{Q}$ heterogeneity is minor and plays essentially no role in limiting oxygen delivery to tissues (22). This may be very different in diseases of the lungs, with which $\dot{V}_A/\dot{Q}$ inequality can be extensive and hypoxemia severe (23). While quantifying how $\dot{V}_A/\dot{Q}$ ratios are distributed in the lung is complex, for present purposes it suffices to consider only the degree of hypoxemia $\dot{V}_A/\dot{Q}$ inequality causes. Thus, in all of the earlier equations, one can evaluate the effects of pulmonary dysfunction on oxygen transport by inserting the actual values of Pa_{O_2}.

Tissue Heterogeneity

While in the lungs the key is how ventilation is distributed in relation to blood flow, in the tissues the critical factor is how blood flow is distributed in relation to $\dot{V}_{O_2}$ (local metabolic rate). In the lungs, we can measure $\dot{V}_A/\dot{Q}$ inequality directly and allow for its effects on exercise through the reduction in arterial P_{O_2}. Unfortunately, $\dot{V}_{O_2}/\dot{Q}$ heterogeneity in the muscles is not yet easily measured. Preliminary findings from novel methods suggest measurable heterogeneity, but at a level that does not greatly affect oxygen transport (24,25).

A useful sense of the effects of such heterogeneity may be had by considering a simple two-compartment model (e.g., the two legs, to provide conceptually discrete compartments) in which blood flow distribution is progressively shifted from one leg to the other. In Figure 11.5, the outcome is shown in terms of effects on effluent muscle venous P_{O_2} (*top*) and muscle oxygen consumption (*bottom*). Arterial oxygen concentration is taken to be normal at 20 mL·dL^{-1}, and muscle venous oxygen concentration is assumed at 4 mL·dL^{-1}

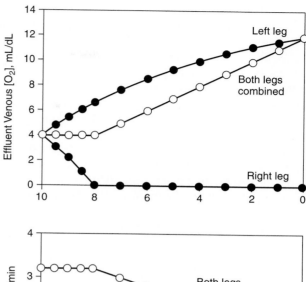

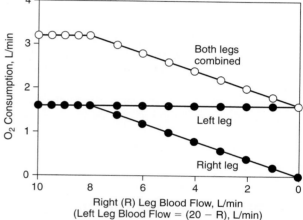

FIGURE 11.5   Calculation of the effects of a progressive shift in blood flow from the right to the left leg on the oxygen extraction and $\dot{V}_{O_2}$ of each leg and of both legs combined. Total flow (20 L per minute) and arterial oxygen levels (20 mL/dL) are held constant, as is metabolic potential to use oxygen in each leg (1.6 L per minute). For simplicity, the ability to unload oxygen by diffusion is assumed to be infinite. As much as 2 L per minute of flow can be shifted without consequence, and even if 4 L per minute were shifted (R at 6 L per minute and L at 14 L per minute), two-leg $\dot{V}_{O_2}$ would still be 2.8 L per minute, compared to 3.2 L per minute with equal flow.

in each leg when flow is evenly distributed. These are reasonable normal values, based on Equations 11.6 and 11.7, hemoglobin concentrations of 15 g/dL, and saturation levels in arterial blood of about 97% and in venous blood of about 20%. To the extent that [Hb] is generally lower in females, these estimates would be correspondingly reduced. Muscle metabolic potential to use oxygen is assumed equal in both legs at 1.6 L per minute. To keep it simple, no limit is imposed on the ability to offload oxygen by diffusion in either leg at any flow rate. Thus, for purposes of discussion, all oxygen could be extracted (even though this does not happen in reality). If blood flow (initially equally distributed) is shifted stepwise from the right to the left leg, keeping total blood flow constant at 20 L per minute, the outcome is as shown in the figure. Up to 2 L per minute (in this example) of blood flow can be redirected from right to left leg without consequence for $\dot{V}O_2$, because the flow reduction on the right is balanced by increased extraction until venous oxygen levels on the right side are zero. There is correspondingly less extraction at higher flows on the left, and combined venous oxygen levels and two-leg $\dot{V}O_2$ are unchanged. However, at greater levels of flow reduction on the right, since no further oxygen can be extracted, its $\dot{V}O_2$ must fall. The $\dot{V}O_2$ of both legs together thus also falls, and mixed venous oxygen levels rise. The interesting point is the ability of the system to maintain oxygen supply (in the absence of diffusion limitation as mentioned) in the presence of at least a moderate level of heterogeneity, 20% reduction in flow in the above example.

It is apparent that the effects of flow heterogeneity are dependent upon the inherent level of oxygen extraction and diffusion limitations to exchange. Thus, as oxygen extraction becomes more complete and/or there is a significant resistance to diffusive oxygen exchange, the ability of muscle to accommodate any flow heterogeneity without reduction in oxygen utilization is reduced. For the remainder of this chapter, we will assume that heterogeneity in both locations is insignificant, an assumption that in the future may have to be revisited.

Integrated Function of the Lungs, Heart, Vasculature, Blood, and Muscles

A Formal Mathematical Model of Maximal Oxygen Transport

The foregoing discussion has emphasized, mostly by examples, how the several tissues and organs involved in oxygen transport interact. If the transport system is considered to be a serial chain involving the lungs, heart, blood, and muscles, all operating as described under the conditions laid out in Equations 11.1 to 11.11, we can bring these equations together and see all of the interactions (18). Doing this also leads us to understand how the several elements of the system determine maximal oxygen availability. In this analysis we continue to make the approximations that the oxyhemoglobin dissociation curve is linear with slope β and that cardiac output and muscle blood flow are one and the same ($\dot{Q}$).

Equations 11.2, 11.4, 11.5, and 11.11 are reproduced:

$$\dot{V}O_2 = \dot{V}_A \times F_{IO_2} - \dot{V}_A \times F_{AO_2} = \dot{V}_A \times k \times \left(P_{IO_2} - P_{AO_2}\right)$$
[Equation 11.2]

$$\dot{V}O_2 = \dot{Q} \times \left(Ca_{O_2} - Cv_{O_2}\right) = \dot{Q} \times \beta \times \left(Pa_{O_2} - Pv_{O_2}\right)$$
[Equation 11.5]

$$Pa_{O_2} = P_{AO_2} - \left(P_{AO_2} - Pv_{O_2}\right) \times \exp\left[-D_L/(\beta \cdot \dot{Q})\right]$$
[Equation 11.4]

$$Pv_{O_2} = Pa_{O_2} \times \exp\left[-D_M/(\beta \cdot \dot{Q})\right]$$
[Equation 11.11]

Equations 11.2 and 11.5 define mass conservation of oxygen exchange between alveolar gas and capillary blood. In Equation 11.2, k relates fractional concentration, F, to partial pressure, P. Equation 11.4 defines arterial P_{O_2} as a function of the pulmonary diffusive process, where D_L is the lung diffusing capacity, written previously just as D. Equation 11.11 defines venous P_{O_2} as a function of the muscle diffusive process, where D_M is the muscle diffusing capacity, as written previously. Equations 11.2, 11.4, 11.5, and 11.11 form a set that all must be true simultaneously. Note that the same variables appear in more than one of the equations.

If we define values for inspired oxygen concentration (F_{IO_2}), alveolar ventilation ($\dot{V}_A$), muscle blood flow ($\dot{Q}$), β, and lung and muscle diffusing capacities (D_L and D_M, respectively), the four equations contain just four unknowns within them. They are oxygen uptake and consumption ($\dot{V}O_2$); and alveolar, arterial, and venous P_{O_2} values (P_{AO_2}, Pa_{O_2} and Pv_{O_2}, respectively). These four equations can thus be uniquely solved for these four unknowns. In other words, given the structural and functional parameters of the oxygen transport system (F_{IO_2}, $\dot{V}_A$, $\dot{Q}$, β, D_L and D_M), we can calculate maximal oxygen transport through the system by solving the equations. This will provide the only possible values for alveolar, arterial, and venous P_{O_2}, and the unique value of $\dot{V}O_{2max}$ associated with them.

The analytical solutions for the four variables are as follows:

$$P_{AO_2} = P_{IO_2} \times \dot{V}_A/\dot{Q} \times \left(1 - LM\right) / \\ \left[\left(\dot{V}_A/\dot{Q}\right)\left(1 - LM\right) + \lambda\left(1 - L\right)\left(1 - M\right)\right]$$
[Equation 11.12]

$$Pa_{O_2} = P_{IO_2} \times \dot{V}_A/\dot{Q} \times \left(1 - L\right) / \\ \left[\left(\dot{V}_A/\dot{Q}\right)\left(1 - LM\right) + \lambda\left(1 - L\right)\left(1 - M\right)\right]$$
[Equation 11.13]

$$Pv_{O_2} = P_{IO_2} \times \dot{V}_A/\dot{Q} \times M\left(1 - L\right) / \\ \left[\left(\dot{V}_A/\dot{Q}\right)\left(1 - LM\right) + \lambda\left(1 - L\right)\left(1 - M\right)\right]$$
[Equation 11.14]

$$\dot{V}O_2 = P_{IO_2} \times \dot{V}_A \times \beta\left(1 - L\right)\left(1 - M\right) / \\ \left[\dot{V}_A/\dot{Q} \times \left(1 - LM\right) + \lambda\left(1 - L\right)\left(1 - M\right)\right]$$
[Equation 11.15]

In these solutions, L is the abbreviation for the exponential term $\exp[-D_L/(\beta \cdot \dot{Q})]$, and M is the abbreviation for the exponential term $\exp[-D_M/(\beta \cdot \dot{Q})]$. P_{IO_2} is inspired partial pressure, proportional to F_{IO_2}, and λ is the slope of the oxyhemoglobin dissociation curve expressed in dimensionless units as a partition coefficient; λ is proportional to β, and at 37°C, $\lambda = 0.863 \beta$.

These solutions, while somewhat complex, clearly show how every conductance variable (F_{IO_2}, $\dot{V}_A$, $\dot{Q}$, β, D_L and D_M) has an explicit role in determining $\dot{V}_{O_{2max}}$.

This analysis points out that in such a serial system, it is inappropriate to ask the commonly expressed question, what is *the* limiting factor to $\dot{V}_{O_{2max}}$? Recognizing that $\dot{V}_{O_{2max}}$ is jointly and complexly set by all of these variables, the appropriate question is how each of the determining variables differently affects $\dot{V}_{O_{2max}}$.

Figure 11.6 illustrates, by plotting out values from Equation 11.15, how individual changes in each of the independent variables affect $\dot{V}_{O_{2max}}$. The figure shows, by the solid dot, the normal values of the transport variable in question plotted against the normal $\dot{V}_{O_{2max}}$. The relationships are similar for all five variables, and they indicate how $\dot{V}_{O_{2max}}$ will fall as the transport variable is reduced below normal (100%) and how it will rise as the variable is increased above normal. In general, a reduction in each has a substantial negative effect on $\dot{V}_{O_{2max}}$, while an increase has only a modest benefit. Such nonlinear behavior is typical of serial systems. The only variable that causes a linear response is F_{IO_2} itself, and in fact $\dot{V}_{O_{2max}}$ will be simply proportional to F_{IO_2} under the assumption of a linear oxyhemoglobin dissociation curve.

The value of this analysis is in pointing out, by means of algebraic equations, the principles underlying how maximal oxygen transport is determined. However, the unrealistic response to F_{IO_2} (whereby $\dot{V}_{O_{2max}}$ is calculated to increase in proportion to F_{IO_2} if the dissociation curve were indeed lin-

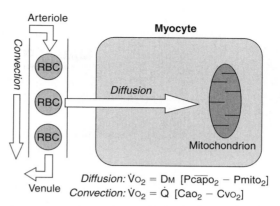

FIGURE 11.7 Oxygen transport by convection in the muscle microcirculation and diffusion between the microcirculation and mitochondria. The corresponding equations for oxygen flux ($\dot{V}_{O_2}$) are shown, providing the basis for the Fick diagram in Figure 11.8 and further explained in the text.

ear) points out the quantitative weakness in this analysis: that the oxyhemoglobin dissociation curve is nonlinear. Numerical modeling of the oxygen transport system allowing for the nonlinear nature of the oxyhemoglobin dissociation curve yields more meaningful outcomes (11). The general results are similar except for a much smaller calculated increase in $\dot{V}_{O_{2max}}$ as F_{IO_2} rises. This is explained by flattening of the oxyhemoglobin dissociation curve at high P_{O_2} (Fig. 11.3), such that arterial oxygen concentration is minimally raised as F_{IO_2} increases above that of room air.

Graphical Analysis of System Integration in Determining Maximal Oxygen Transport

Equations 11.12–11.15 provide direct, complete solutions for P_{O_2} in each compartment and for $\dot{V}_{O_{2max}}$, given the values of the conductance variables listed. However, algebraic analyses are not the easiest to assimilate, and the need for approximating the oxyhemoglobin curve by a straight line limits their utility. This has prompted development of a complementary graphical analysis of oxygen transport at the skeletal muscle capillary–fiber interface to provide the same general conclusions in a more accessible format (8). Moreover, this graphical analysis lends itself to the interpretation of actual experimental data and therefore is presented now, before the final section of this chapter, which deals with published studies.

Figure 11.7 shows the basis of this analysis, focusing on the muscle cell and its blood supply. There are two ways to describe the same flux rate of oxygen at this level. One is by means of the Fick principle, presented in Equation 11.5. This expresses *convective* transport of oxygen through the muscle circulation and simply defines mass conservation.

$$\dot{V}_{O_2} = \dot{Q} \times \left(C_{aO_2} - C_{vO_2} \right)$$

[Equation 11.5]

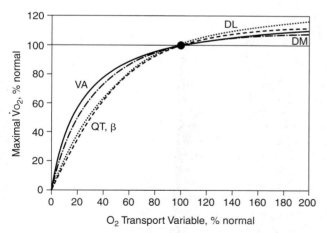

FIGURE 11.6 Theoretical calculations of dependence of maximal oxygen transport (and thus $\dot{V}_{O_{2max}}$) on changes in individual oxygen transport variables (VA, ventilation; QT, muscle blood flow; β, slope of the oxyhemoglobin dissociation curve; DL, lung diffusing capacity; DM, muscle diffusing capacity). For these calculations equation 15 was used, assuming a linear oxyhemoglobin dissociation curve. Solid circle indicates normal values. Each variable altered alone generally affects $\dot{V}_{O_{2max}}$ similarly, and even substantial increases in any single transport variable capacity offer little benefit to $\dot{V}_{O_{2max}}$. On the other hand, reduction in any one variable leads to a significant fall in $\dot{V}_{O_{2max}}$.

The second is by the Fick law of diffusion, presented in Equation 11.9. Given that capillary P_{O_2} falls as the red cell moves from the arterial to the venous end of the system, Equation 11.9 can be used to represent the entire process of *diffusive* efflux of oxygen along the length of the capillary by using the mean capillary P_{O_2} in the equation. This is indicated in Figure 11.7 by the bar above CAP and here as

$$\dot{V}_{O_2} = DM \times \left[\overline{P{CAP}}_{O_2} - PmitO_2 \right]$$

[Equation 11.16]

Mean capillary P_{O_2} is a conceptual variable, and it is useful to replace it with a measurable surrogate variable. We will assume that as conditions alter, mean capillary P_{O_2} and muscle venous P_{O_2} both change in proportion to one another, such that $\overline{P{CAP}}_{O_2} = k \times P_{vO_2}$. This is theoretically reasonable, and k can be calculated (normally it is approximately 2.0). Further, as was mentioned earlier, mitochondrial P_{O_2} is low enough that it may be neglected. Equation 11.9 can then be rewritten thus:

$$\dot{V}_{O_2} = DM \times k \times P_{vO_2}$$

[Equation 11.17]

Inspection of Equations 11.5 and 11.17 yields insight. If one considers a given situation in which muscle blood flow ($\dot{Q}$), arterial oxygen concentration (CaO_2), and muscle diffusing capacity (DM) are all defined, we have two equations in two unknowns. The unknowns are $\dot{V}_{O_2}$ and P_{vO_2}. Equation 11.5 is actually written in terms of venous oxygen concentration, CvO_2, and not partial pressure, P_{vO_2}. However, one can be calculated from the other from the known oxyhemoglobin dissociation curve.

To take this further is best done graphically, by plotting Equations 11.5 and 11.17 with P_{vO_2} on the abscissa and $\dot{V}_{O_2}$ on the ordinate. This is done in Figure 11.8. Equation 11.17 is simply a straight line passing through the origin and with slope equal to DM × k. It says that as mean capillary P_{O_2} is increased, so too is diffusive flux of oxygen from the capillaries to the mitochondria in a linearly proportional manner.

Equation 11.5 is more complicated. It shows the unique relationship between $\dot{V}_{O_2}$ and P_{vO_2} for given values of $\dot{Q}$ and CaO_2 (i.e., of oxygen delivery into the muscle microcirculation) as ordained by mass conservation. It has a negative slope because as P_{vO_2} (and thus CvO_2) is made higher, $\dot{V}_{O_2}$ determined from Equation 11.5 must be lower. It has the shape of an inverted oxyhemoglobin dissociation curve because the equation is written in terms of oxygen concentration, while the abscissa is P_{O_2}. Equation 11.5 says that as P_{vO_2} rises, $\dot{V}_{O_2}$ must fall, the *converse* of how P_{vO_2} and $\dot{V}_{O_2}$ relate in Equation 11.17. The highest point on this curve occurs at the lowest value of P_{vO_2}, namely zero. This would be the hypothetically greatest $\dot{V}_{O_2}$ that could occur, and would equal systemic oxygen delivery ($\dot{Q} \times CaO_2$). This would require that all oxygen be extracted from the muscle blood, which would in turn require an infinitely high diffusing capacity.

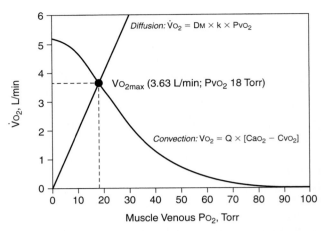

FIGURE 11.8   Fick diagram depicting the equations for diffusive and convective oxygen transport in the muscle. Maximal oxygen transport occurs where the two relationships intersect. This point, and thus $\dot{V}_{O_{2max}}$ and associated muscle venous P_{O_2}, depends on the values of muscle diffusional conductance (Dm), muscle blood flow ($\dot{Q}$) and arterial oxygen concentration (CaO_2). The particular example leads to a $\dot{V}_{O_{2max}}$ of 3.6 L per minute and a muscle venous P_{O_2} of 18 torr. See text for details.

The lowest point on this curve represents a $\dot{V}_{O_2}$ of zero, which would occur if no oxygen were taken out of the muscle blood. Thus, this point occurs at a P_{vO_2} equal to the arterial value. While both extremes are included in Figure 11.8, neither is attainable in reality.

Recall that Equations 11.5 and 11.17 must express the same rate of oxygen transport. That means that there is only one feasible condition in Figure 11.8 in which $\dot{V}_{O_2}$ is identical via the two equations—*at their point of intersection*. Thus this intersection point defines the maximal rate of oxygen transport through the system for the given values of $\dot{Q}$, CaO_2, and DM as the ordinate value of the point. The abscissa value of the same point is the *necessary* value of muscle effluent venous P_{O_2} that must exist to satisfy the equations.

This figure has been dubbed the Fick figure because it happens to be based on two equations that long have borne the name Fick, after the nineteenth-century German scientist Adolph Fick.

The intersection point, and thus maximal $\dot{V}_{O_2}$ (when $\dot{V}_{O_2}$ is limited by oxygen supply), is as stated, determined by three major variables: $\dot{Q}$, CaO_2, and DM. CaO_2 is itself determined by hemoglobin concentration and arterial oxygen saturation (Equation 11.6). Once again, the integration of the lungs, heart, blood, and muscles is apparent in how $\dot{V}_{O_{2max}}$ is determined by the values of the variables governing $\dot{Q}$, CaO_2 and DM.

In addition to showing the integrated nature of oxygen transport, what makes this figure so useful is its predictive value. Figure 11.9 shows how changes in the three primary determining variables would each affect $\dot{V}_{O_{2max}}$. Figure 11.9A shows how $\dot{V}_{O_{2max}}$ will fall as muscle oxygen diffusive conductance falls (by 50% in the example). The diffusive

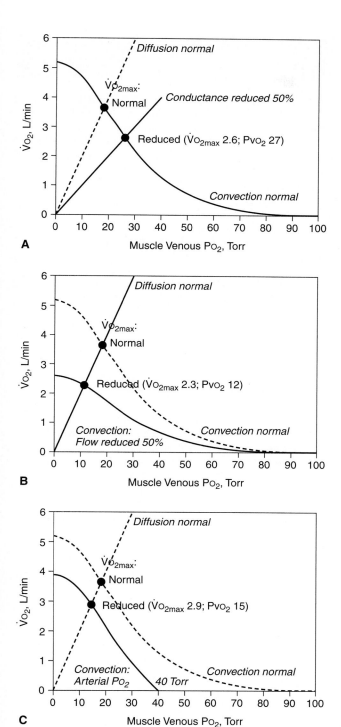

FIGURE 11.9 Fick diagrams exemplifying the effects of reduced diffusional conductance (**A**), muscle blood flow (**B**), and arterial P_{O_2} (**C**) on both $\dot{V}_{O_{2max}}$ and associated muscle venous P_{O_2}. Each panel shows significant reduction in $\dot{V}_{O_{2max}}$ when the corresponding oxygen transport variable is reduced. When blood flow or arterial P_{O_2} is reduced, $\dot{V}_{O_{2max}}$ and $P_{V_{O_2}}$ fall in proportion.

line has a lower slope, but the convective line is not affected, as neither $\dot{Q}$ nor Ca_{O_2} is altered. In this case, muscle venous P_{O_2} must rise. Figure 11.9B shows the effects of a 50% reduction in blood flow on $\dot{V}_{O_{2max}}$, in which case $\dot{V}_{O_{2max}}$ and muscle venous P_{O_2} must fall, and in a proportional manner, diffusive conductance and arterial P_{O_2} are unchanged. Figure 11.9C shows how a reduction in arterial P_{O_2}, as happens on ascent to altitude for example, will reduce $\dot{V}_{O_{2max}}$ and muscle venous P_{O_2}, again in proportion to one another. The predicted effects of such changes can be compared on this diagram to experimental interventions because both axes reflect measurable variables. Many other permutations of changes in $\dot{Q}$, Ca_{O_2}, and D_M can be imagined on such a diagram.

Experimental Evidence

The question answered here is the extent to which experimental evidence does or does not support the major premise of this chapter: that when $\dot{V}_{O_{2max}}$ is limited by oxygen supply, this happens in a predictable, quantifiable manner based on an integrated oxygen transport system.

The first and qualitative prediction is that $\dot{V}_{O_{2max}}$ can be altered by any of the identified components of the transport pathway. There is abundant evidence that this is true. In health, acute changes in F_{IO_2} in either direction alter $\dot{V}_{O_{2max}}$ in the same direction (26,27). An increase in cardiac output has been shown to increase $\dot{V}_{O_{2max}}$ in pericardiectomized dogs (28), and splenectomy reducing cardiac output (and hemoglobin concentration) in racehorses reduces $\dot{V}_{O_{2max}}$ (29). Increasing hemoglobin concentration by transfusion acutely increases $\dot{V}_{O_{2max}}$ (30), and muscle training, by increasing muscle oxygen diffusive conductance, shows that increases in this variable also increase $\dot{V}_{O_{2max}}$ (31). In lung disease, impaired ventilation is associated with reduced exercise capacity that can be somewhat augmented by increasing F_{IO_2} (32) (which demonstrates oxygen supply dependency in that setting). Also, reducing alveolar ventilation experimentally by imposing an external dead space in patients with lung disease reduces exercise capacity (33). Thus, it is quite clear that individually, any of the oxygen transport pathway variables discussed in this chapter has the potential to influence $\dot{V}_{O_{2max}}$.

A more quantitative approach poses the hypothesis that as arterial P_{O_2} is acutely lowered in normal subjects, $\dot{V}_{O_{2max}}$ will fall as predicted in Figure 11.9C. This has been shown on more than one occasion (7,26) when decreases in $\dot{V}_{O_{2max}}$ occur in close proportion to reductions in muscle venous P_{O_2}. The most accurate interpretation of these results is that the construct developed in this chapter is *not refuted* by data matching predictions. It would be overstepping what the data show to claim that the construct was *validated* by having data follow predictions. Thus, more critical is whether concordance with the behavior predicted from Figure 11.9C is truly the result of limited diffusion of oxygen out of the muscle microcirculation.

A MILESTONE OF DISCOVERY

It can be argued that the linear reduction in $\dot{V}O_{2max}$ with muscle venous PO_2, seen in Figure 11.9C as arterial PO_2, would also be expected if the problem with oxygen transport from capillary to mitochondria was heterogeneity of blood flow to metabolic rate and not diffusion limitation. This is difficult to resolve, but two reports in particular support the diffusion limitation hypothesis (34,35). In both cases, the P_{50} of the oxyhemoglobin dissociation curve was altered pharmacologically *while maintaining total systemic arterial oxygen delivery and arterial PO_2 unchanged.* Hogan and associates (34) reduced P_{50} using cyanate; Richardson and associates (35) raised P_{50} using methyl propionic acid. In such an experiment, the convection-based problem of $\dot{Q}/\dot{V}O_{2max}$ heterogeneity would *not* cause $\dot{V}O_{2max}$ to vary with P_{50}. On the other hand, if limited by diffusion, $\dot{V}O_{2max}$ would *increase with a right shift and decrease with a left shift* because such shifts would make for a higher (right shift) or lower (left shift) PO_2 gradient between the red cells and the muscle mitochondria. $\dot{V}O_{2max}$ was altered predictably by changes in P_{50} (34,35). To date, and without direct measurements of heterogeneity between perfusion and metabolism, this appears to be the best evidence supporting the idea that interaction between convection and diffusion in the movement of oxygen between the muscle microcirculation and the mitochondria is a critical determinant of maximal oxygen transport and thus of $\dot{V}O_{2max}$.

Hogan MC, Bebout DE, Wagner PD. Effect of increased Hb-O_2 affinity on $\dot{V}O_{2max}$ at constant O_2 delivery in dog muscle in situ. J Appl Physiol 1991;70:2656–2662.

Richardson RS, Tagore K, Haseler L, et al. Increased $\dot{V}O_{2max}$ with a right shifted Hb-O_2 dissociation curve at a constant oxygen delivery in dog muscle in situ. J Appl Physiol 1998;84:995–1002.

SUMMARY

This chapter examines the oxygen transport pathway in considerable detail. Using quantitative descriptions of the individual elements of the pathway, the complex interdependence of oxygen transport on each and every component of the pathway at every pathway step has been illustrated. This leads directly to a major conclusion: that $\dot{V}O_{2max}$, when limited by oxygen supply, is not governed by any single factor, such as cardiac output (or muscle blood flow), but depends on all transport variables in an integrated manner. The important tissues and organs determining oxygen transport are the lungs, the heart and circulation, the blood, and the muscles themselves. The principal determining variables are alveolar ventilation, cardiac output, pulmonary and muscle oxygen diffusive conductances, the shape and slope of the oxyhemoglobin dissociation curve, and obviously the inspired PO_2. Both analytical and graphical analyses have been presented for these complex interactions. Current experimental data support these models as a close approximation to the oxygen transport system.

The analytical approach shows that in an *in series* system, such as the oxygen transport pathway, reduced function of any single element has substantial negative influence on maximal oxygen transport. However, enhanced function of any single element provides relatively little increase in maximal oxygen transport. The graphical approach in particular, using the Fick diagram, is most helpful because it allows experimental data to be interpreted against theoretical expectations across a wide variety of physiological conditions.

REFERENCES

1. Dempsey JA, Miller JD, Romer LM. The respiratory system. In Tipton CM, ed. ASCM's Advanced Exercise Physiology. Baltimore: Lippincott Williams Wilkins, 2006:246–299.
2. Kaufman MP, Forster HV. Reflexes controlling circulatory, ventilatory and airway responses to exercise. In Rowell LB, Shepherd JT, eds. Handbook of Physiology. New York: Oxford University, 1996;381–447.
3. Rowell LB. Human Cardiovascular Control. New York: Oxford University, 1993.
4. Waldrop TG, Eldridge FL, Iwamoto GA, et al. Central neural control of respiration and circulation during exercise. In Rowell LB, Shepherd JT, eds. Handbook of Physiology. New York: Oxford University, 1996;333–380.
5. Knight DR, Poole DC, Schaffartzik W, et al. Relationship between body and leg $\dot{V}O_2$ during maximal cycle ergometry. J Appl Physiol 1992;73:1114–1121.
6. Richardson RS, Poole DC, Knight DR, et al. High muscle blood flow in man: is maximal O_2 extraction compromised? J Appl Physiol 1993;75:1911–1916.
7. Roca J, Hogan MC, Story D, et al. Evidence for tissue diffusion limitation of $\dot{V}O_{2max}$ in normal humans. J Appl Physiol 1989;67:291–299.
8. Wagner PD. Determinants of maximal oxygen transport and utilization. Annu Rev Physiol 1996;58:21–50.
9. Weibel ER. The Pathway for Oxygen: Structure and Function in the Mammalian Respiratory System. Cambridge, MA: Harvard University, 1984.
10. Barclay JK, Stainsby WN. The role of blood flow in limiting maximal metabolic rate in muscle. Med Sci Sports Exerc 1975;7:116–119.
11. Wagner PD. A theoretical analysis of factors determining $\dot{V}O_{2max}$ at sea level and altitude. Respir Physiol 1996;106:329–343.

12. Barcroft JA, Cooke A, Hartridge H, et al. The flow of oxygen through the pulmonary epithelium. J Physiol (Lond) 1920;53:450–472.

13. Roughton FJW, Forster RE. Relative importance of diffusion and chemical reaction rates determining rate of exchange of gases in the human lung with special reference to true diffusing capacity of pulmonary membrane and volume of blood in the lung capillaries. J Appl Physiol 1957;11:290–302.

14. Wu EY, Ramanathan M, Hsia CCW. Role of hematocrit in the recruitment of pulmonary diffusing capacity: comparison of human and dog. J Appl Physiol 1996;80:1014–1020.

15. Dempsey JA, Hanson PG, Henderson KS. Exercise-induced arterial hypoxemia in healthy human subjects at sea level. J Physiol (Lond) 1984;355:161–175.

16. Piiper J, Scheid P. Model for capillary-alveolar equilibration with special reference to O_2 uptake in hypoxia. Respir Physiol 1981;46:193–208.

17. Moore R. The cardiovascular system: cardiac function. In Tipton CM, ed. ACSM's Advanced Exercise Physiology. Baltimore: Lippincott Williams & Wilkins, 2006:326–342.

18. Wagner PD. Algebraic analysis of the determinants of $\dot{V}O_{2max}$. Respir Physiol 1993;93:221–237.

19. Piiper J, Meyer M, Scheid P. Dual role of diffusion in tissue gas exchange: blood-tissue equilibration and diffusion shunt. Respir Physiol 1984;56:131–144.

20. Honig CR, Gayeski TEJ, Federspiel WJ, et al. Muscle O_2 gradients from hemoglobin to cytochrome: new concepts, new complexities. Adv Exp Med Biol 1984;169:23–38.

21. Richardson RS, Noyszewski EA, Kendrick KF, et al. Myoglobin O_2 desaturation during exercise: evidence of limited O_2 transport. J Clin Invest 1995;96:1916–1926.

22. Gale GE, Torre-Bueno JR, Moon RE, et al. Ventilation/perfusion inequality in normal humans during exercise at sea level and simulated altitude. J Appl Physiol 1985;58:978–988.

23. Wagner PD, West JB. Ventilation-perfusion relationships. In West JB, ed. Ventilation, Blood Flow and Diffusion. New York: Academic Press, 1980;219–262.

24. Mizuno M, Kimura Y, Iwakawa T, et al. Regional differences in blood flow and oxygen consumption in resting muscle and their relationship during recovery from exhaustive exercise. J Appl Physiol 2003;95:2204–2210.

25. Richardson RS, Haseler LJ, Nygren AT, et al. Local perfusion and metabolic demand during exercise: a noninvasive MRI method of assessment. J Appl Physiol 2001;91:1845–1853.

26. Knight DR, Schaffartzik W, Poole DC, et al. Effects of hyperoxia on maximal leg O_2 supply and utilization in men. J Appl Physiol 1993;75:2586–2594.

27. Powers SK, Lawler J, Dempsey J, et al. Effects of incomplete pulmonary gas exchange on $\dot{V}O_{2max}$. J Appl Physiol 1989;66:2491–2495.

28. Stray-Gundersen J, Musch TI, Haidet GC, et al. The effect of pericardiectomy on maximal oxygen consumption and maximal cardiac output in untrained dogs. Circ Res 1986;58:523–530.

29. Wagner PD, Erickson BK, Kubo K, et al. Maximum O_2 transport and utilization before and after splenectomy. Equine Vet J 1995;18:82–89.

30. Buick FJ, Gledhill N, Froese AB, et al. Effect of induced erythrocythemia on aerobic work capacity. J Appl Physiol 1980;48:636–642.

31. Roca J, Agustí AGN, Alonso A, et al. Effects of training on muscle O_2 transport at $\dot{V}O_{2max}$. J Appl Physiol 1992;73:1067–1076.

32. Richardson RS, J Sheldon, DC Poole, et al. Evidence of skeletal muscle metabolic reserve during whole body exercise in patients with chronic obstructive pulmonary disease. Am J Respir Crit Care Med 1999;159:881–885.

33. Marciniuk DD, Watts RE, Gallagher CG. Dead space loading and exercise limitation in patients with interstitial lung disease. Chest 1994;105:183–189.

34. Hogan MC, Bebout DE, Wagner PD. Effect of increased Hb-O_2 affinity on $\dot{V}O_{2max}$ at constant O_2 delivery in dog muscle in situ. J Appl Physiol 1991;70:2656–2662.

35. Richardson RS, Tagore K, Haseler L, et al. Increased $\dot{V}O_{2max}$ with a right shifted Hb-O_2 dissociation curve at a constant O_2 delivery in dog muscle in situ. J Appl Physiol 1998;84:995–1002.

CHAPTER 12

The Cardiovascular System: Design and Control

DONAL S. O'LEARY AND JEFFREY T. POTTS

Introduction

Strenuous dynamic exercise presents one of the greatest challenges to cardiovascular control. In response to increasing work rates and oxygen consumption (e.g., treadmill running, bicycling), heart rate increases progressively towards maximal values. This tachycardia coupled with sustained or modestly increased stroke volume (amount of blood pumped by the heart with each heartbeat) causes large (fourfold to fivefold) increases in blood flow to the systemic circulation (cardiac output). Marked vasodilation occurs in the active skeletal muscles, such that virtually all of this increase in cardiac output is directed to the active muscles, although skin blood flow may also rise if internal temperature increases sufficiently. Blood flow to inactive areas (e.g., splanchnic, renal circulations) decreases as a result of substantial activation of the sympathetic nervous system, and this flow is redistributed to the active skeletal muscle as well. With the marked changes in autonomic nervous activity, increases in cardiac output, and vasoconstriction in inactive vascular beds, arterial pressure rises. With strenuous static muscle contraction, increases in heart rate and cardiac output also occur, as does vasoconstriction in inactive beds, but vasodilation within the active muscle becomes mechanically restricted, with strong static contractions due to the large increases in tissue pressure within the muscle, which compresses the blood vessels, and arterial systolic blood pressures may increase to extreme (about 400 mm Hg) levels.

The mechanisms mediating these substantial cardiovascular and autonomic responses to exercise are not completely understood, but they involve the action and likely interaction between three systems, central command, the arterial baroreflex, and activation of afferents within the active skeletal muscle (both mechanically sensitive and chemically sensitive receptors) (Fig. 12.1). This chapter focuses on what cardiovascular parameters are controlled during dynamic and resistance exercise and the mechanisms by which they are controlled. Given the limited space for this discussion, see other reviews for more detailed discussion (1,2).

Design: What Is Controlled?

The Pump: Control of Cardiac Output

Cardiac output is the amount of blood pumped by the heart into the systemic circulation per unit of time, most often expressed as liters per minute. Cardiac output can be calculated as the product of stroke volume (SV) and heart rate, that is, the amount of blood pumped per heartbeat times the number of times the heart contracts per unit of time (usually expressed as beats per minute [bpm])

$$CO = SV \times HR,$$

where CO = cardiac output and HR = heart rate. Thus, cardiac output can vary via changes in stroke volume, heart rate, or both.

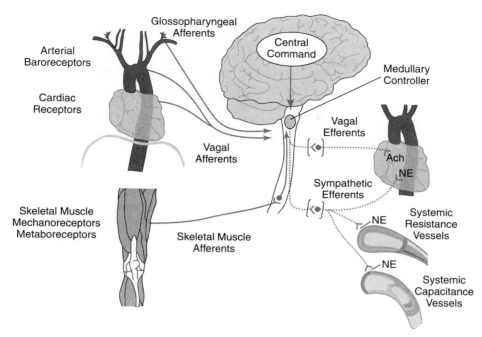

FIGURE 12.1 The mechanisms mediating the large cardiovascular responses to exercise. Activation of central command, skeletal muscle afferents, and resetting of the arterial and perhaps cardiopulmonary baroreflexes together affect central areas that control sympathetic and parasympathetic activity to the heart and peripheral blood vessels.

Control of Heart Rate

Heart rate is controlled primarily via changes in parasympathetic and sympathetic activity to the pacemaker area of the heart, the sinoatrial node. Increases in parasympathetic activity decrease heart rate, and increases in sympathetic activity increase heart rate. In resting humans, heart rate is well below the intrinsic heart rate because of significant tonic parasympathetic activity. Thus, in response to exercise, heart rate can increase via reductions in parasympathetic activity and via increases in sympathetic activity.

Control of Stroke Volume

As heart rate changes, SV can vary as a result of the changes in the time for filling of the ventricles. Figure 12.2 (solid line) shows the results of an experiment wherein heart rate was varied from about 40 to about 220 bpm in conscious dogs with atrioventricular block (3). As heart rate increased (via a pacemaker attached to the ventricles) from 40 to about 100 bpm, a fairly linear increase in CO occurred. However, from about 110 to about 180 bpm little further increase in CO occurred, because of the concomitant fall in SV as the filling time for the ventricles lessened. Above 180 bpm, further increases in heart rate actually caused decreases in CO because of the severe fall in SV as filling time decreased markedly. These are important considerations in understanding cardiac control mechanisms during exercise. Changes in heart rate

per se may be of little consequence in the steady-state control of CO unless other mechanisms are engaged to maintain or increase SV despite marked reductions in ventricular filling time. In contrast to the effects of heart rate *per se* on CO, the broken line in Figure 12.2 shows the changes in CO as a function of heart rate in conscious dogs during treadmill exercise. As heart rate increased from about 120 to the maximal level of about 280 bpm, substantial increases in CO occurred. In this setting, the increases in heart rate are accompanied by increases in ventricular performance, left ventricular filling pressure, and end diastolic volume, which together act to increase SV despite the markedly reduced ventricular filling time (from about 0.5 seconds at rest to < 0.1 seconds at maximal exercise). Similar results are observed during strong static muscle contractions (resistive exercise). Heart rate and CO increase while SV remains essentially constant.

Preload, Afterload, and Ventricular Contractility

Changes in ventricular filling can markedly affect stroke volume. Thus, as described earlier, as heart rate increases and ventricular filling time decreases, there can be less filling of the ventricles, less tension developed, and thus less ability to eject blood into the arterial circulation. This relationship between stroke volume and ventricular preload (ventricular volume immediately prior to contraction) can be modified via activation of the sympathetic nerves to the heart. With

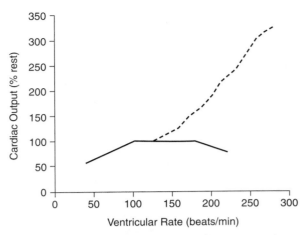

FIGURE 12.2 Relationship between cardiac output and ventricular rate when ventricular rate is altered via a pacemaker (*solid line*) versus during treadmill exercise to maximal exercise intensities in dogs. For the solid line, heart rate was varied via a pacemaker in conscious dogs with atrioventricular block (so that very low heart rates could be produced). As heart rate increases, initially increases in cardiac output occur, however above about 110 beats/min, little further increase in cardiac output occurs because of substantial decreases in stroke volume. Above 180 beats/min, further increases in heart rate actually decrease cardiac output because of severe reductions in stroke volume that result from limitations in ventricular filling time. *(Data from White S, Higgins CB, Vatner SF, et al. Effects of altering ventricular rate on blood flow distribution in conscious dogs. Am J Physiol 1971;221:H1402–H1407).* In contrast, during normal dynamic exercise (*broken line*), substantial increases in cardiac output occur with the normal tachycardia because of sustained or increased stroke volume with increases in heart rate. *(Data with permission from Musch TI, Friedman DB, Pitetti KH, et al. Regional distribution of blood flow of dogs during graded dynamic exercise. J Appl Physiol 1987;63:2269–2277.)*

the release of norepinephrine and stimulation of β-adrenergic receptors on the ventricular myocardium, the strength of each individual contraction increases and the relationship between SV and ventricular preload is improved, in that a larger SV will occur at a given preload. This represents an increase in ventricular contractility, also termed an increased inotropic state of the heart (see Chapter 13).

With each ventricular contraction, pressure inside the left ventricle must exceed pressure in the aorta before the aortic valve opens and blood can be expelled. Thus, changes in arterial pressure can also affect SV, termed afterload. At high arterial pressures, it takes longer to generate enough pressure to open the aortic valve, and the valve closes sooner. Therefore, the time during which ejection of blood can occur is lessened, and SV falls. This relationship between SV and afterload can also be modified by changes in ventricular contractility. With stimulation of sympathetic nerves to the heart and an increase in ventricular contractility, the heart becomes less sensitive to

changes in ventricular afterload, allowing the left ventricle to maintain SV over a wider range of arterial pressures.

The Peripheral Vasculature

Arterial Resistance

Control of the arterial resistance occurs primarily at the level of the arterioles. These are thick-walled vessels capable of marked changes in diameter. Inasmuch as the resistance to flow is inversely proportional to the radius of the blood vessel raised to the fourth power, even small changes in radius can yield large changes in resistance and therefore in blood flow. This relationship between flow and resistance is governed by a hydraulic analog of Ohm's law: perfusion pressure equals flow times resistance.

Changes in the level of activity of the vascular smooth muscle in the arterioles can vary as a result of changes in sympathetic activity to the arterioles (see Chapter 9). Sympathetic nerves innervate the peripheral blood vessels and release norepinephrine (NE) as the primary neurotransmitter. NE acts on α-receptors and elicits increased activity of the vascular smooth muscle, causing vasoconstriction, which decreases the radius of the arteriole. As described earlier, even small changes in radius can yield large changes in resistance and therefore blood flow (assuming a constant perfusion pressure, discussed in more depth later in the chapter).

Changes in the interstitial concentration of chemical substances release from cells can also modulate resistance. These metabolic vasodilators include bradykinin, prostaglandins, adenosine, K^+, carbon dioxide, and lactate, among others. Decreases in local P_{O_2} can also elicit release of adenosine triphosphate (ATP) from hemoglobin, which can activate purinergic receptors on the vascular smooth muscle, causing vasodilation. Furthermore, the endothelium lining the interior of the arterioles can also release a variety of substances that can affect vasomotor tone. Most notable is nitric oxide (NO). In response to increases in the shear stress, NO is released and causes vasodilation of the arterioles. Sheriff and associates (4) recently demonstrated that NO may contribute to the vasodilation in skeletal muscle accompanying mild to moderate treadmill exercise. The role of other endothelial factors, such as endothelin and endothelium-derived hyperpolarizing factor, in the regulation of skeletal muscle blood flow during exercise is unclear. Many if not all of the vasodilator substances described earlier likely contribute to the rapid vasodilation that occurs in skeletal muscle with the onset of dynamic exercise. With static muscle contractions, the production of metabolites also increases, but the vasodilation may be prevented mechanically by the increased muscle tissue pressure physically compressing the blood vessels.

Venous Capacitance

Approximately 70% of blood volume resides on the venous side of the circulation. Increased sympathetic activity to the veins results in mobilization of blood volume from the periphery to the central veins, which can aid in the increase of ventricular filling pressure and therefore SV. In addition, with locomotion, the repetitive dynamic contractions of the skeletal muscle act to squeeze the veins and pump the blood back toward the heart (this pumping of course occurs only once with static contractions). Thus, we have two pumps providing energy for movement of blood through the circulation during dynamic exercise: the heart and the skeletal muscle (5).

Reflex Control

The autonomic and neurohormonal responses to exercise are the result of the action and likely interaction among at least three systems: central command, the arterial baroreflex, and activation of skeletal muscle afferents (Fig. 12.1).

Central Command

Central command is the concept that the volition to exercise can elicit cardiovascular responses. This is a feed-forward system. The idea is that with activation of the motor cortex, there is a parallel activation of pathways that descend into the brainstem areas controlling sympathetic and parasympathetic activities.

Victor and colleagues (6) performed an insightful series of experiments that strongly support the concept that central command can cause substantial inhibition of parasympathetic activity; the role of central command in the control of sympathetic tone remains unclear. These investigators had subjects perform static forearm contractions before and after treatment with a neuromuscular blocker. In the control setting, the static contraction raised arterial pressure, heart rate, and sympathetic nerve activity to resting skeletal muscle. After neuromuscular blockade, the subjects attempted the contraction but were able to generate little if any force despite near maximal effort. In this setting of high levels of central command, the increase in arterial pressure and muscle sympathetic nerve activity were much smaller than in the control experiment; however, a similar increase in heart rate occurred. This rise in heart rate with attempted contractions could be blocked by an antagonist to the parasympathetic nerves and was unaffected by an antagonist to the cardiac sympathetic nerves. Thus, the increase in heart rate with strong activation of central command occurred via inhibition of tonic parasympathetic tone to the heart. Strong increases in central command can also elicit some increase in sympathetic tone (7). Thus, the initial rapid increase in heart rate at the initiation of exercise may stem from activation of central command causing rapid decreases in parasympathetic activity that will elicit very fast increases in heart rate.

Baroreflexes

Within the walls of the carotid sinus and aortic arch are receptors that sense the level of arterial pressure, termed the ar-

terial baroreceptors. In response to changes in arterial pressure (mean pressure as well as pulse pressure), the baroreceptors change their level of activity. For example, as pressure rises, the activity of the baroreceptors increases. This information is relayed to the brainstem via cranial nerves IX and X (for carotid and aortic arch baroreceptors, respectively) and a reflex increase in parasympathetic and decrease in sympathetic activity occurs. This causes heart rate and cardiac output to decrease and peripheral vasodilation of resistance and capacitance vessels, which decreases pressure. Opposite responses occur with decreases in blood pressure from the normal levels. Thus, the arterial baroreflex is the primary short-term controller of arterial pressure on a beat-to-beat basis. Removal of the arterial baroreceptors results in marked variability of arterial pressure at rest and during mild exercise.

For many years it was thought that since both heart rate and arterial pressure rise during exercise, the arterial baroreflex must be inhibited; otherwise the rise in arterial pressure would elicit a baroreflex reduction in heart rate. Much of the support for this concept came from a series of studies wherein the chronotropic responses to rapid increases in arterial pressure were observed in humans at rest and during dynamic exercise of various intensities (8). These studies concluded that the strength of the baroreflex was progressively lessened as exercise intensity increased. However, two factors can markedly affect the conclusions from these experiments: (*a*) Arterial pressure was raised rapidly via bolus intravenous infusion of a vasoconstrictor. (*b*) The chronotropic response was quantified as the change in interbeat interval (electrocardiographic R-R interval, the time between heartbeats). With the bolus method the changes in arterial pressure are so rapid that mainly only the parasympathetic component of the chronotropic response is observed because the speed of the sympathetic responses is much slower than the fast parasympathetic responses. Second, although R-R interval and heart rate are reciprocally related, they are often thought to be interchangeable. However, a reciprocal relationship is highly nonlinear. Figure 12.3 shows the relationship between R-R interval and heart rate. The problem in analysis comes when a large change in the baseline level occurs, as between rest and exercise. For example, assume that at rest heart rate is 60 bpm (R-R interval of 1000 ms) and that arterial pressure is raised by 10 mm Hg, causing a 10-bpm baroreflex bradycardia. Baroreflex sensitivity would be 1 bpm per millimeter of mercury, or 20.0 ms per millimeter of mercury. If in response to exercise, heart rate increases to 165 bpm (R-R interval = 363.6 ms) and the same 10-mm Hg increase in arterial pressure causes the same 10-bpm baroreflex bradycardia, then in terms of heart rate baroreflex strength is undiminished (again, 1 bpm per millimeter of mercury), whereas when analyzed in terms of R-R interval, baroreflex sensitivity is reduced nearly to one-tenth, to 2.3 ms per millimeter of mercury. Thus, the same data yield completely different conclusions when analyzed in terms of heart rate versus R-R interval. Which is correct? An important consideration is that heart rate is not the variable sensed and controlled by the arterial baroreflex; rather, that variable is arterial pressure.

In a classic study, Melcher and Donald (9) vascularly isolated the carotid sinus baroreceptors such that the pressure exposed to the carotid baroreceptors could be controlled in conscious animals at rest and during graded treadmill exercise. Thus, these investigators could change the pressure at the baroreceptors and observe the changes in systemic arterial pressure and heart rate. They found that the strength of the baroreflex was not reduced during exercise; rather, the reflex was reset to a higher pressure (see Milestone of Discovery). These conclusions have been confirmed by several other investigators in other species, including humans (10–13). Thus, rather than being turned off by exercise, the arterial baroreflex is reset to a higher pressure and now defends this higher pressure. Therefore, a portion of the rise in sympathetic activity and decrease in parasympathetic activity with exercise could be due to the resetting of the baroreflex; that is, rather than opposing the rise in pressure, the arterial baroreflex reinforces this increase.

There is controversy whether the strength or gain of the baroreflex decreases somewhat as exercise intensity approaches maximal levels. In a series of studies Raven and colleagues investigated carotid baroreflex control of heart rate and arterial pressure by manipulating the transmural pressure at the carotid sinuses by applying pressure or suction around the neck (11,13–16). They showed that as exercise intensity increased, the operating point (prevailing point on the stimulus–response relationship; point at which the reflex is operating) of the baroreflex moved away from the center of the carotid sinus pressure–heart rate relationship and toward the threshold for the baroreflex (Fig. 12.4). Thus, as exercise

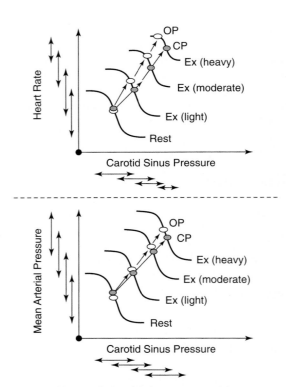

FIGURE 12.4 Relationship between carotid sinus pressure and heart rate (*top*) and carotid sinus pressure and mean arterial pressure (*bottom*) at rest and during graded exercise. At rest for both relationships, the operating point (OP) is at the high-gain portion of the curve near the center of the relationship (centering point, or CP). As exercise intensity rises, the OP for the heart rate responses moves away from the CP toward a lower-gain portion of the curve. Less movement of the OP for the mean arterial pressure responses occurs. For the heart rate responses, both the range of the responses (arrows on Y-axis) and the operating range (arrows on X-axis) decreases as exercise intensity rises, although no change in maximal gain was observed. Little change in either the response or operating ranges for the arterial pressure responses occurred. (*Figure 12.4 redrawn from unpublished figure courtesy of Dr. Peter B. Raven based on several recent studies from his laboratory, located at the University of North Texas Health Science Center in Fort Worth, Texas. Figure is based on investigation conducted in Raven's laboratory (13, 15, 16) or in colleague's laboratories where he was a co-investigator (11,14).*)

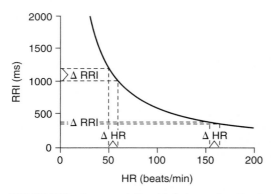

FIGURE 12.3 Inverse relationship between heartbeat interval (RRI) and heart rate (HR). *Solid line.* The line of identity between the two indices. *Broken lines.* When heart rate is low, a 10 bpm change in heart rate will yield a large change in RRI, whereas when the baseline level of heart rate is elevated, the same 10-bpm change in heart rate will be calculated as a very small change in RRI. (*Reprinted with permission from O'Leary DS. Med Sci Sports Exerc 1995;28:210–217.*)

intensity increased, the operating point moved from a high-gain portion of the curve (in the center) to a low-gain portion of the curve. Both the operating range (range of pressures over which the reflex is operating) and the response range (range of the heart rate response; maximal heart rate minus minimal heart rate) decreased at higher exercise intensities; however, the maximal gain (maximal slope of the curve; centering point) did not change, but the operating point became progressively displaced from the centering point as exercise intensity increased. Similar results were obtained by Iellamo and associates (17), who observed the chronotropic responses to small spontaneous changes in arterial pressure and found that the responses became smaller as exercise intensity increased. Theoretically, as heart rate approaches maximal levels, the operating point for the heart rate responses must move closer to the baroreflex threshold, inasmuch as further tachycardia becomes limited as the subject approaches maximal heart rate. Interestingly, the same large shift in the operating point with dynamic exercise was significantly less for the relationship between carotid sinus pressure and arterial pressure, and no changes in the operating or response ranges occurred (the arterial pressure response was shown to be virtually entirely due to changes in vasomotor tone, not cardiac output [11]). In this setting, effective baroreflex buffering of a hypotensive response could occur only via peripheral vasoconstriction (discussed later in the chapter).

Exercise Alters Baroreflex Mechanisms

With the large changes in cardiac output, heart rate, and regional blood flow accompanying exercise, the mechanisms mediating baroreflex responses can change between rest and exercise.

Heart Rate

In humans and other species such as dogs, resting heart rate is primarily under parasympathetic control. Thus baroreflex-mediated reductions in heart rate occur mainly if not solely via increases in the tonic parasympathetic activity, inasmuch as little if any sympathetic activity exists to be withdrawn, whereas baroreflex-mediated tachycardia can occur via both inhibition of the high tonic parasympathetic activity and increases in sympathetic tone. In contrast, during moderate to heavy exercise the baseline levels of autonomic activity to the heart have shifted. In this setting, parasympathetic activity is less (although not totally inhibited) and sympathetic activity is elevated. Thus both baroreflex-mediated tachycardia and bradycardia can occur via changes in both sympathetic and parasympathetic activity in response to both decreases and increases in arterial pressure, respectively (12).

Peripheral Vasculature

The most important component of the arterial baroreflex compensatory responses to a hypotensive challenge is peripheral vasoconstriction. In response to decreases in arterial pressure vasoconstriction occurs in virtually all vascular beds except the brain. The ability of vasoconstriction within a given vascular bed to affect arterial pressure depends on the extent of the vasoconstriction and on the fraction of the cardiac output directed to that vascular bed. This is an important consideration

because during dynamic exercise a greater and greater fraction of the cardiac output is directed to the active skeletal muscle as exercise intensity increases, such that at heavy exercise intensities active muscles receives more than 80% of cardiac output. Theoretically, in this setting, effective arterial pressure control can occur only via modulation of vascular tone within the active skeletal muscle. Yet this idea remains somewhat controversial because in 1962 Remensnyder and associates (18) concluded that the ability of skeletal muscle to vasoconstrict in response to sympathetic activation was depressed during exercise, termed functional sympatholysis. To some extent, however, this conclusion regarding the existence of sympatholysis may also depend on the method of data analysis (19). Blood flow can be affected by changes in both perfusion pressure and vasomotor tone, so an appropriate index quantifying vasoconstriction or dilation must reflect only changes in vasomotor tone. The two indices used are either vascular resistance (perfusion pressure divided by blood flow) or conductance (blood flow divided by perfusion pressure). As with the relationship between heart rate and R-R interval, discussed earlier, the reciprocal relationship between resistance and conductance is highly nonlinear. Thus, when marked changes in the baseline level of vasomotor tone occur (as within skeletal muscle between rest and exercise), opposite conclusions can be drawn regarding the magnitude of a vasomotor response when quantified according to the changes in resistance versus conductance. This apparent dichotomy is demonstrated in Figure 12.5. For simplicity we assume that arterial pressure remains constant. At both a low-flow (rest) and a high-flow (exercise) state, a 50% decrease in blood flow occurs in response to sympathetic activation. As can be seen, in terms of resistance a much larger change occurs during rest, whereas in terms of conductance a much greater change occurs during exercise. Which is correct? To make matters even more confusing, quantified as percent changes, the responses are exactly the same between the low- and high-flow states. Between rest and exercise, how can a vasomotor response be larger (Δ conductance), smaller (Δ resistance), and exactly the same (% Δ)? Clearly the conclusions depend on the definition of the term *vasoconstriction*. To resolve this apparent discrepancy, O'Leary (19) proposed that when large changes in blood flow occur between states, vascular conductance is the most appropriate index of vasomotor responses because at constant pressure, changes in conductance are linearly related to changes in flow. Furthermore, the effect of a given change in regional conductance on arterial pressure is much less dependent on the baseline level than that for resistance (19). Using a different approach, Collins and associates (20) directly quantified the contribution of vasoconstriction within skeletal muscle to the rise in arterial pressure with unloading of carotid baroreceptors at rest and during exercise. Since both total flow (cardiac output) and blood flow to the hindlimb skeletal muscles were measured, they could directly calculate what fraction of the carotid baroreflex pressor responses could be directly

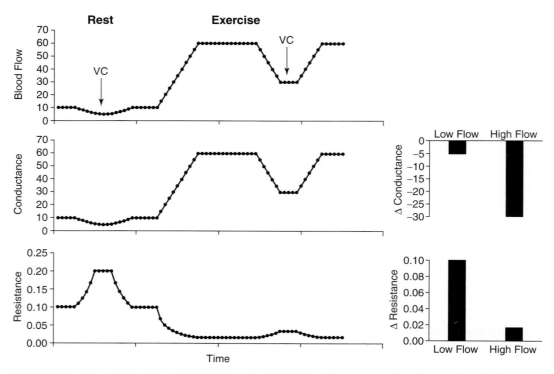

FIGURE 12.5 Theoretical effect of a 50% reduction in blood flow (VC at arrows) to skeletal muscle at rest and during exercise on the calculated changes in resistance and conductance. Opposite conclusions would be drawn using each index of the vasomotor response.

attributed to vasoconstriction in the hindlimb skeletal muscles. They concluded that as exercise intensity increased, vasoconstriction within the active skeletal muscle became progressively more important in mediating the rise in arterial pressure with unloading of the carotid baroreceptors. Importantly, these conclusions are independent of whether resistance or conductance are used for the calculations; that is, we are no longer trying to measure vasoconstriction but are evaluating changes in arterial pressure, which obeys Ohm's law whether you use resistance or conductance in the formulation. What is not known is whether this greater pressor effect of muscle vasoconstriction seen during exercise is produced by similar increases in sympathetic activity as seen at rest (e.g., little sympatholysis) or whether during dynamic exercise this greater pressor effect requires a much greater rise in sympathetic activity to overcome substantial sympatholysis.

Skeletal Muscle Afferents

Skeletal muscle is extensively supplied with afferents that sense both the mechanical and metabolic environment. These afferents are lightly myelinated (group III) and unmyelinated (group IV) fibers. In general the group III fibers tend to be more mechanosensitive and the group IV fibers more sensitive

to changes in the chemical environment (termed chemoreceptors or metaboreceptors). The larger group I and II fibers have no role in cardiovascular control (1).

Muscle Metaboreceptors

The cardiovascular effects of the skeletal muscle afferents were first discovered in 1937 by Alam and Smirk (21). They observed in humans that if blood flow to the active skeletal muscles was occluded at the cessation of exercise, arterial pressure remained elevated for as long as the occlusion was maintained. This technique of circulatory occlusion post exercise has been widely used to investigate the role of the muscle metaboreceptors, with the theory being that during the circulatory occlusion, metabolites responsible for activating the receptors (lactate, H$^+$, phosphate, bradykinin, and prostaglandins, among others) are entrapped within the formerly active muscle and maintain metaboreceptor activation. Activation of the muscle metaboreflex, especially with a large muscle mass, is capable of eliciting profound increases in sympathetic activity and arterial pressure. This rise in arterial pressure is buffered by arterial and cardiopulmonary reflexes. Left unbuffered by the arterial baroreflex, this reflex rivals that from cerebral ischemia in the ability to increase arterial pressure (20).

Metaboreflex activation increases cardiac output, heart rate, ventricular performance, peripheral vasoconstriction, and central blood volume mobilization, which raises arterial pressure, presumably in an attempt to increase blood flow to the ischemic muscles (22). The existence of circulatory occlusion responses to moderate to intense static muscle contractions post exercise provides compelling evidence that this reflex becomes activated in these settings. To what extent the muscle metaboreflex is normally activated during dynamic exercise is not well understood. Reductions in skeletal muscle blood flow during mild exercise do not cause metaboreflex responses until blood flow is reduced below a critical threshold level, which indicates that during mild exercise this reflex is not tonically active (2,21). However, as exercise intensity increases, the threshold level of skeletal muscle blood flow required to elicit reflex responses moves closer and closer to the normal level of flow, such that at moderate exercise intensities often no threshold is apparent; even small reductions in the normal level of flow elicit reflex cardiovascular responses. At even higher exercise intensities no threshold is detected (2,23). This indicates that either the reflex is indeed tonically active or that the reflex sits just at the blood flow threshold and any reduction in flow triggers metaboreflex responses. In pathophysiological states, such as peripheral claudication or heart failure, wherein the normal level of skeletal muscle blood flow is reduced, the muscle metaboreflex likely contributes to the exaggerated sympathetic activation observed in these settings.

One quandary in this area is that with sustained metaboreceptor activation during circulatory occlusion post exercise, whereas arterial pressure remains elevated, most often heart rate recovers toward resting values with a time course similar to that during the normal recovery from exercise (24). These results have led several investigators to conclude that this reflex (muscle metaboreflex) has little control over heart rate. In contrast, when blood flow to active muscle is reduced during sustained dynamic exercise, decreasing oxygen delivery and increasing metabolite production due to partial ischemia, substantial increases in heart rate and cardiac output are observed (2). This discrepancy has been resolved by studies wherein circulatory occlusion post exercise was performed after blockade of the parasympathetic nerves to the heart (2). In this setting, like arterial pressure, heart rate remains elevated for as long as the occlusion is maintained, indicating that sympathetic activity to the heart as well as to the peripheral vasculature remains elevated. The repeated observation of a fairly normal recovery of heart rate during circulatory occlusion post exercise likely stems from increases in parasympathetic activity, which can overwhelm the effects of sustained increases in sympathetic activity. The mechanisms mediating the rise in parasympathetic activity in this setting are not known but may stem from the loss of central command with the cessa-

tion of exercise. (As discussed earlier, activation of central command inhibits parasympathetic tone, so the reduction in central command would be expected to increase parasympathetic activity.) Or it may be due to the arterial baroreflex in an attempt to return arterial pressure to normal levels. This remains to be investigated.

Muscle Mechanoreceptors

Less is known about the normal role of mechanoreceptors in mediating the cardiovascular responses to dynamic and resistance exercise. Static muscle contraction likely activates both mechanoreceptors and metaboreceptors, although the time course of activation may be different, inasmuch as more time is required for generation of metabolites for metaboreflex activation (1). However, via tendon stretch, tension in the muscle can be increased without contraction, and this maneuver does elicit increases in sympathetic activity, heart rate, ventilation, and arterial pressure. To investigate differentiation between the roles of mechanoreceptors and metaboreceptors in mediating the responses to static muscle contraction, Hayes and Kaufman (25) observed the responses before and after infusion of gadolinium, which blocks mechanosensitive channels. Gadolinium significantly attenuated the rise in arterial pressure and heart rate in response to both static muscle contraction and tendon stretch, indicating that a portion of the cardiovascular response to static muscle contraction may be mediated via activation of the mechanoreceptors.

Interaction Between Central Command, Arterial Baroreflexes, and Skeletal Muscle Afferents

The reflex cardiovascular responses to exercise are likely the result of the action of and interaction between central command, the arterial baroreflex, and the activation of skeletal muscle afferents. With the transition from rest to mild dynamic exercise, the immediate rapid tachycardia is the result of rapid partial withdrawal of parasympathetic activity, which is likely due to activation of central command, rapid resetting of the arterial baroreflex, or activation of skeletal muscle mechanoreceptors. As exercise intensity progresses, marked sympathetic activation is not seen until moderate exercise intensities (although this can vary widely with species). This may be due to the ability to raise cardiac output via parasympathetic withdrawal in combination with the increased central blood volume mobilization arising from the skeletal muscle pump, which thereby maintains or increases ventricular filling pressure, allowing SV to be sustained despite the reduced filling time (2). If parasympathetic withdrawal increases cardiac output sufficiently to supply the active skeletal muscles with enough oxygen to prevent marked accumulation of ischemic metabolites, then the muscle metaboreflex is likely not strongly engaged. In addition, if the increase in cardiac output is large enough to raise arterial pressure toward the reset baroreflex set point, then the baroreflex is likely also not strongly engaged. Thus, little afferent signals would exist for substantial sympathetic activation via either the muscle metaboreflex or arterial baroreflex. (Whether muscle mechanoreflexes or central command could raise sympathetic activity in this setting is not well established.) With further increases in exercise intensity sympathetic activation is clearly evident. This increase in sympathetic tone could come about via further increases in central command, activation of skeletal muscle afferents, and/or resetting of the arterial baroreflex to a higher set point. With heavy or maximal exercise intensities parasympathetic activity is reduced to very low levels and sympathetic activity is greatly elevated. The relative roles for central command, skeletal muscle afferents, and the arterial baroreflex in this setting are not well understood, but it is likely that all are strongly activated and participate in the autonomic adjustments both to increase the delivery of oxygen to the active skeletal muscles and to maintain arterial pressure in the face of large peripheral vasodilation.

These reflexes also likely interact. Recent studies strongly support the concept that both activation of skeletal muscle afferents and central command can reset the arterial baroreflex (10). Furthermore, with strong stimulation of skeletal muscle afferents, the sympathetic activation is buffered by the arterial baroreflex: much larger pressor responses are observed after baroreceptor denervation (22,26). Thus, situations can exist when these reflexes are exerting changes in sympathetic activity in opposite directions. For example, during dynamic exercise in subjects with peripheral claudication or during intense static muscle contractions, the sympathetic activation due to strong metaboreflex activation may raise pressure above the baroreflex set point, and thus this increase in sympathetic activity would be partially suppressed by the baroreflex. It is likely that more often these reflexes are eliciting changes in autonomic outflow in the same direction as with the responses to graded exercise described earlier. In pathophysiological settings such as heart failure, enormous increases in sympathetic activity can occur during heavy exercise (27). In this setting, both arterial pressure (especially pulse pressure) and skeletal muscle blood flow are below normal levels. This likely results in strong activation of both the arterial baroreflex and the muscle metaboreflex to increase sympathetic activity, which can cause profound vasoconstriction in inactive vascular beds and even within the active skeletal muscle itself. This restraint of skeletal muscle vasodilation could exacerbate the situation, although it is possible that redistribution of flow within the muscles between motor units, which may be activated to different degrees, may occur to optimize the distribution of the restricted delivery of oxygen to areas most underperfused.

Dynamic Exercise Training and Reflex Cardiovascular Control

Dynamic exercise training increases the functional capacity of the cardiovascular system. The magnitude of such adaptations depends upon a number of factors, including the type of exercise (endurance vs. resistive), intensity, frequency, and duration of the stimulus, and genetic factors. Dynamic training provokes a host of structural and regulatory adaptations, including structural remodeling of the heart and blood vessels, which enhance delivery of oxygen and nutrients to skeletal muscle and improve work capacity (Fig. 12.6). In addition, dynamic training–induced adaptations in the autonomic nervous system alter the neural regulatory mechanisms controlling cardiac and vascular functions and improve morbidity and mortality in patients with cardiovascular disease. While these adaptations are generally thought to be beneficial, some dynamic training–induced effects may in fact be detrimental to reflex control of circulatory homeostasis. This section provides an overview of the changes in reflex control of the cardiovascular system that occur with dynamic exercise training, focusing predominantly on the arterial baroreceptor reflex.

Dynamic Exercise Training and Arterial Baroreflexes

Since the mid 1970s, a number of investigators have reported that dynamic exercise–trained subjects were less tolerant to an orthostatic challenge than were age-matched untrained subjects (28,29). While the cause of orthostatic intolerance, or the inability to maintain consciousness in the upright posture resulting from problems in blood pressure regulation, remains debated, there is no doubt that dynamic training–induced changes in the arterial baroreceptor reflex contribute to some degree to orthostatic hypotension. Evidence supporting this notion comes from longitudinal and cross-sectional training studies in animals and human subjects. Raven, Smith, and colleagues evaluated the effects of endurance exercise training on baroreflex control of blood pressure in human subjects using cross-sectional and longitudinal training studies. In cross-sectional studies, they reported that dynamic exercise-trained subjects exhibited attenuated tachycardic response to systemic hypotension (29, 30). However, when baroreflex function was evaluated in the same subjects during a longitudinal training study, dynamic exercise training failed to alter carotid baroreflex responsiveness (31). The discrepancy between these studies may be attributed to cross-sectional versus longitudinal study design. Alternatively, a more likely explanation may have been in the nature of the baroreceptor stimulus. In the former

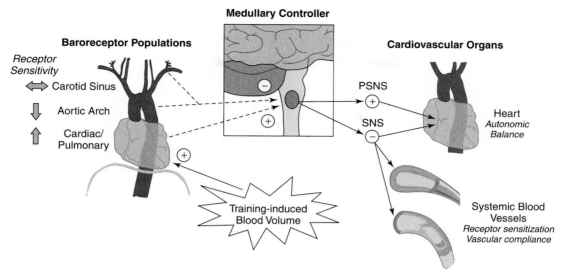

FIGURE 12.6 The important adaptive changes brought about by dynamic exercise training that alter baroreflex regulation of the cardiovascular system. Dynamic exercise training attenuates arterial (aortic) baroreflex responses and sensitizes cardiopulmonary afferents. This is accompanied by resting bradycardia, reduced sympathetic activity, and blunted cardiovascular responses to exercise. Mechanisms possibly contributing to training-induced changes in cardiovascular reflexes include altered baroreflex function, structural and/or autonomic changes to the heart and blood vessels, and altered hemodynamic responses during exercise.

study, lower-body negative pressure (LBNP) was used to provoke central and peripheral hypotension, which effectively deactivated both arterial (aortic, carotid sinus) and cardiopulmonary baroreceptors. In contrast, the latter study used the neck pressure suction technique to selectively manipulate carotid baroreceptors. Therefore, dynamic exercise training may have reduced baroreflex control of the circulation by preferentially altering a specific baroreceptor zone. To address this issue, Shi and colleagues (32) evaluated the effect of dynamic exercise training on the aortic baroreceptor reflex in a group of aerobically fit individuals. They reported blunted reflex bradycardia in response to activation of aortic baroreceptors. In contrast, carotid baroreflex responsiveness was unaltered in these subjects when compared to untrained sedentary individuals. These data suggest that the reported attenuation of reflex cardiovascular responses evoked by arterial baroreceptors in dynamic exercise–trained individuals may be attributed to selective adaptation of the aortic-cardiac baroreflex.

Dynamic Exercise Training and Cardiopulmonary Baroreflexes

Arterial baroreceptors are not the only baroreceptor population to sense changes in vascular pressure. Cardiopulmonary baroreceptors on the great veins, pulmonary artery, and heart respond to changes in central venous pressure. As such, they can signal changes in venous pressure to the central nervous system that occur in response to a distribution of circulating blood volume. Dynamic exercise training is associated with increased circulating blood volume, which may act as a stimulus for cardiopulmonary baroreceptors. Mack and colleagues (33) reported that cardiopulmonary baroreflex responses, measured from reflex changes in forearm blood flow during low-level LBNP (−10 to −20 torr), were reduced in response to dynamic exercise training. DiCarlo and colleagues examined the effect of dynamic exercise training on cardiac reflexes in chronically instrumented rabbits (34). They approached this problem by first training rabbits in dynamic exercise on a treadmill. They then altered central venous pressure during exercise while recording regional sympathetic nerve activities. They reported that baroreflex control of heart rate and sympathetic nerve activity were attenuated in dynamic exercise–trained rabbits and attributed this alteration to sensitization of cardiac vagal afferents. A similar inhibitory interaction has been reported in human subjects at rest and during dynamic exercise (15,16). Pawelczyk and Raven (16) also reported that the inhibitory interaction was absent in aerobically trained individuals. Together, these data indicate that dynamic exercise training altered reflex control of regional sympathetic outflow by sensitizing cardiac afferents and by interacting with the arterial baroreflex. Although the mechanism or mechanisms responsible for dynamic exercise training–induced alterations in the arterial baroreflex remain unknown, several possibilities have been proposed. First, dynamic exercise may sensitize cardiac afferents that will attenuate the arterial baroreflex by inhibiting baroreceptor neural circuits in the brain. Second, dynamic exercise training may upregulate the expression of inhibitory neurotransmitter systems (i.e., GABA, glycine) in the brain that suppress baroreflex function. Kramer, Waldrop, and colleagues recently provided evidence that dynamic exercise training in rats promoted inhibitory neurotransmission in the brain (35). While either of these mechanisms may explain the alterations in arterial baroreflex function, the definitive answer awaits future research.

Functional Implication of Dynamic Exercise Training, Baroreflexes, and Cardiovascular Homeostasis

Dynamic exercise training produces marked changes in the cardiovascular system and in neural reflexes responsible for its control. Structural changes in the heart and blood vessels promote improvements in cardiac function at rest and during exercise that lead to increased oxygen delivery and improved work capacity. The diminished sympathetic response during exercise in dynamic exercise–trained individuals may be attributed in part to elevated blood volume that supports a larger stroke volume and maintains greater activation of cardiopulmonary receptors. However, despite the apparent attributes of dynamic exercise training on many physiological systems, the fact remains that dynamic exercise–trained individuals have a reduced autonomic capacity to respond to an orthostatic challenge. Additionally, this is a significant problem for certain populations, especially for individuals who are exposed to high gravitational forces, such as high-performance pilots and astronauts. The cause or causes of orthostatic intolerance continue to be debated. However, it is likely that dynamic exercise–induced adaptations of the autonomic nervous system and other regulatory systems are involved.

Figure 12.6 summarizes the effects of dynamic exercise training on baroreflex control of the cardiovascular system. The major components include expansion of blood volume, structural adaptations to cardiovascular organs, and changes in neurally mediated reflex adjustments to the heart and peripheral vasculature. Likewise, the dynamic exercise training–induced increases in SV, along with altered sympathetic-parasympathetic balance, likely contribute to the reduction in exercise heart rate at a fixed submaximal intensity. The cellular mechanisms underlying dynamic exercise training–induced changes in baroreflex function remain to be elucidated. In addition, the contribution of the neurohumoral axis, which was not discussed here, must also be considered for complete understanding of the physiological adaptations that result from dynamic exercise training.

A MILESTONE OF DISCOVERY

As discussed in the section on baroreflexes, for many years it was thought that the arterial baroreflex was functionally inhibited (turned off) during exercise. This idea stemmed from two observations: (a) Both arterial pressure and heart rate increase during exercise; the baroreflex should inhibit any rise in heart rate with the increase in arterial pressure. (b) The increases in R-R interval (bradycardia) with rapid increases in arterial pressure became smaller and smaller as exercise intensity increased (8). The latter observation had been challenged, inasmuch as baroreflex-mediated heart rate responses were undiminished (Fig. 12.3). However, heart rate is neither sensed nor controlled by the arterial baroreflex; rather, arterial pressure is sensed and is controlled via changes in cardiac output and vasomotor tone.

In their study, Melcher and Donald used the innovative and technically demanding surgical approach of reversibly isolating the carotid sinuses to test the hypothesis that the carotid baroreflex remains functional during dynamic exercise. This technique allowed the vascular isolation of the carotid sinuses and thus pressure at the carotid baroreceptors to be controlled and the reflex changes in arterial pressure and heart rate observed. This was the first study to explore the entire range of baroreflex response at rest and during exercise. Importantly, this nearly heroic surgery allowed observations in a conscious animal running on a treadmill; thus, the detrimental effects of anesthesia and acute surgical trauma were avoided. Melcher and Donald found that baroreflex control of arterial pressure was reset upward to a higher pressure (later studies also showed a rightward shift in the curves, per Fig. 12.4). Importantly, they showed that the strength of the reflex (reflex gain) was undiminished from rest to heavy exercise. They also described how the baroreflex mediated changes in heart rate were time dependent, again reinforcing the problems of using heart rate for baroreflex analysis. Thus, these investigators conclusively demonstrated that the arterial baroreflex is not inhibited during exercise but rather the reflex is reset to a higher pressure in proportion to the exercise intensity. These observations, along with the innovative surgical techniques, have led many investigative teams to use similar approaches over the past 20 years or more to investigate the baroreflex, its action and interaction with other reflexes at rest, during exercise, and in pathophysiological conditions.

Melcher A, Donald DE. Maintained ability of carotid baroreflex to regulate arterial pressure during exercise. Am J Physiol 1981;241: H838–H849.

REFERENCES

1. Mitchell JH, Schmidt RF. Cardiovascular reflex control by afferent fibers from skeletal muscle receptors. In Shepherd JT, Abboud FM, eds. Handbook of Physiology, the Cardiovascular System, Peripheral Circulation and Organ Blood Flow. Bethesda, MD: American Physiological Society, 1983;623–658.

2. Rowell LB, O'Leary DS, Kellogg DL Jr. Integration of cardiovascular control systems in dynamic exercise. In Rowell LB, Shepherd JT, eds. Handbook of Physiology Exercise: Regulation and Integration of Multiple Systems. Bethesda, MD: American Physiological Society, 1966;720–838.

3. White S, Higgins CB, Vatner SF, et al. Effects of altering ventricular rate on blood flow distribution in conscious dogs. Am J Physiol 1971;221:H1402–H1407.

4. Sheriff DD, Nelson CD, Sundermann RK. Does autonomic blockade reveal a potent contribution of nitric oxide to locomotion-induced vasodilation? Am J Physiol 2000;279:H726–H732.

5. Sheriff DD, Van Bibber R. Flow-generating capability of the isolated skeletal muscle pump. Am J Physiol 1998;274:H1502–1508.

6. Victor RG, Pryor SL, Secher NH, et al. Effects of partial neuromuscular blockade on sympathetic nerve responses to static exercise in humans. Circ Res 1989;65:468–476.

7. Victor RG, Secher NH, Lyson T, et al. Central command increases muscle sympathetic nerve activity during intense intermittent isometric exercise in humans. Circ Res 1995;76:127–131.

8. Bristow JD, Brown EB Jr, Cunningham DJC, et al. Effect of bicycling on the baroreflex regulation of pulse interval. Circ Res 1971;28:582–592.

9. Melcher A, Donald DE. Maintained ability of carotid baroreflex to regulate arterial pressure during exercise. Am J Physiol 1981;241:H838–H849.

10. McIlveen SA, Hayes SG, Kaufman MP. Both central command and exercise pressor reflex reset carotid sinus baroreflex. Am J Physiol 2001;280:H1454–1463.

11. Ogoh S, Fadel PJ, Nissen P, et al. Baroreflex-mediated changes in cardiac output and vascular conductance in response to alterations in carotid sinus pressure during exercise in humans. J Physiol (Lond) 2003;500:317–324.

12. O'Leary DS, Seamans DP. Effect of exercise on autonomic mechanisms of baroreflex control of heart rate. J Appl Physiol 1993;75:2251–2257.

13. Potts JT, Shi XR, Raven PB. Carotid baroreflex responsiveness during dynamic exercise in humans. Am J Physiol 1993;265:H1928–1938.

14. Ogoh S, Fadel PJ, Monteiro F, et al. Haemodynamic changes during neck pressure and suction in seated and supine positions. J Physiol (Lond) 2002;540:707–716.

15. Potts JT, Shi XR, Raven PB. Cardiopulmonary baroreceptors modulate carotid baroreflex control of heart rate during dynamic exercise in humans. Am J Physiol 1995;268:H1567–H1576.

16. Pawelczyk JA, Raven PB. Reductions in central venous pressure improve carotid baroreflex responses in humans. Am J Physiol 1989;257:H1389–H1395.

17. Iellamo FM, Massaro JM, Legramante G, et al. Spontaneous baroreflex modulation of heart rate during incremental exercise in humans. FASEB J 1998;12:A692.

18. Remensnyder JP, Mitchell JH, Sarnoff SJ. Functional sympatholysis during muscular activity. Circ Res 1962;11:370–380.

19. O'Leary DS. Regional vascular resistance versus conductance: which index for baroreflex responses? Am J Physiol 2001;260:H632–H637.

20. Collins HL, Augustyniak RA, Ansorge EJ, et al. Carotid baroreflex pressor responses at rest and during exercise: cardiac output vs. regional vasoconstriction. Am J Physiol 2001;280:H642–H648.

21. Alam M, Smirk FH. Observations in man upon a blood pressure raising reflex arising from the voluntary muscles. J Physiol (Lond) 1938;89:372–383.

22. Sheriff DD, O'Leary DS, Scher AM, et al. Baroreflex attenuates pressor response to graded muscle ischemia in exercising dogs. Am J Physiol 1990;258:H305–H310.

23. O'Leary DS, Sheriff DD. Is the muscle metaboreflex important in control of blood flow to active skeletal muscle. Am J Physiol 1995;268:H980–H986.

24. Wallin BG, Victor RG, Mark AL. Sympathetic outflow to resting muscles during static handgrip and postcontraction muscle ischemia. Am J Physiol 1989;256:H105–H110.

25. Hayes SG, Kaufman MP. Gadolinium attenuates exercise pressor reflex in cats. Am J Physiol 2001;280:H2153–2161.

26. Waldrop TG, Mitchell JH. Effects of barodenervation on cardiovascular responses to static muscular contraction. Am J Physiol 1985;249:H710–H714.

27. Hammond RL, Augustyniak RA, Rossi NF, et al. Heart failure alters the strength and mechanisms of the muscle metaboreflex. Am J Physiol 2000;278:H818–H828.

28. Levine BD, Buckey JC, Fritsch JM, et al. Physical fitness and cardiovascular regulation: mechanisms of orthostatic intolerance. J Appl Physiol 1991;70:112–122.

29. Raven PB, Rohm-Young D, Blomqvist CG. Physical fitness and cardiovascular responses to lower body negative pressure. J Appl Physiol 1984;56:138–144.

30. Smith ML, Graitzer HM, Hudson DL, Raven PB. Baroreflex function in endurance- and static exercise-trained men. J Appl Physiol 1988;65:1789–1795.

31. Raven PB, Pawelczyk JA. Chronic endurance exercise training: a condition of inadequate blood pressure regulation and reduced tolerance to LBNP. Med Sci Sports Exerc 1993;25:713–721.

32. Shi X, CG Crandall, JT Potts, et al. A diminished aortic-carotid reflex during hypotension in aerobically fit young men. Med Sci Sports Exerc 1993;251:1024–1030.

33. Mack GW, Convertino VA, Nadel ER. Effect of exercise training on cardiopulmonary baroreflex control of vascular-resistance in humans. Med Sci Sports Exerc 1993;25:722–728.

34. DiCarlo SE, Stahl LK, Bishop VS. Daily exercise attenuates the sympathetic nerve response to exercise by enhancing cardiac afferents. Am J Physiol 1997;273:H1606–H1610.

35. Kramer JM, Beatty JA, Little HR, et al. Chronic exercise alters caudal hypothalamic GAD regulation of the cardiovascular system in hypertensive rats. Am J Physiol 2001;280:R389–R397.

CHAPTER 13

The Cardiovascular System: Cardiac Function

RUSSELL L. MOORE

Introduction

Physical activity covers a large portion of a continuum of normal physiological states in man. For successful existence in this continuum, significant alterations must occur in cardiac output and central cardiac function to accommodate the systemic demands imposed on an organism by physical activity. The autonomic nervous system (ANS) is primarily responsible for the integrated control of the cardiovascular system and has central importance in enabling an organism to match oxygen supply with the metabolic demands of physical activity (see Chapter 14). While the ANS is critical to the integrated control of the cardiovascular system and its responses to physical activity, significant elements of pump function control are intrinsic to the heart. These intrinsic control elements are critical to the overall systemic response of an organism to acute exercise, and some respond adaptively to exercise training. Training-induced improvements in maximal and submaximal work capacity are accompanied by several central cardiovascular adaptations that are regarded as signatures of the trained state. These fundamental adaptive changes, which have been documented in man and all mammalian species examined, include bradycardia during rest and submaximal exercise, increased maximal stroke volume (SV), an increase in left ventricular end-diastolic dimension, improved myocardial contractile function, and subtle to moderate increases in myocardial mass.

General Cardiovascular Adjustments to Acute Exercise

During exercise, systemic oxygen consumption ($\dot{V}O_2$) increases in response to the increase in metabolic demand of active muscle. The cardiovascular system is responsible for increasing the delivery of blood and oxygen to working skeletal muscle and the pulmonary vasculature. The attendant increase in cardiac output is accomplished via increases in heart rate, stroke volume, systolic blood pressure, and myocardial contractile activity, a general reduction in systemic vascular resistance, and only small changes in mean arterial and diastolic blood pressure (1–3). In quantitative terms, the increased demands for oxygen consumption that occur during physical exercise are met according to the following relationship: $\dot{V}O_2$ = heart rate (HR) × stroke volume (SV) × arteriovenous oxygen content difference (Δ a-v O_2). Two components of the product describing $\dot{V}O_2$, heart rate and stroke volume, are directly attributable to the performance of the heart. As the demands for systemic blood flow increase, both heart rate and stroke volume increase (Fig. 13.1). Over the continuum of dynamic aerobic work intensity, the adjustment in stroke volume occurs early on and is virtually complete at 40 to 50% $\dot{V}O_{2max}$ whereas heart rate increases continuously from rest until $\dot{V}O_{2max}$ is achieved. With the onset of exercise, key events at the level of the heart that contribute to augmented heart rate, stroke volume, and

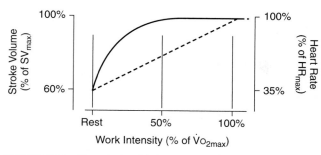

FIGURE 13.1 The relationship between work intensity and heart rate (HR) and stroke volume (SV). In general, between the resting state and $\dot{V}O_{2max}$, HR increases approximately linearly as a function of work intensity. The adjustment in stroke volume across the same continuum is curvilinear, with most of the increase occurring at the lower work intensities (< 50% $\dot{V}O_{2max}$).

pump function include an increase in sympathetic drive, venous return, and as the work bout proceeds, changes in the ion composition of the extracellular milieu (4). The overall consequence is that cardiac contractile activity increases concomitantly with the demand on the processes involved in excitation and contraction.

Myocardial Mechanisms for Heart Rate Control

$$\dot{V}O_2 = HR \times SV \times \Delta\, a - v\, O_2$$

Under normal circumstances, heart rate is governed in large part by the cardiodepressant and cardioaccelerator influences of the parasympathetic and sympathetic nervous systems, respectively. Across the continuum from rest to $\dot{V}O_{2max}$, adjustments in heart rate occur as a result of alterations in the relative magnitudes of parasympathetic and sympathetic input into the heart (see Chapter 14). Specifically, the parasympathetic and sympathetic arms of the ANS control heart rate by modulating the intrinsic pacemaker activity of the heart. To understand the cellular basis for this type of chronotropic modulation, it is necessary to understand the ionic basis for intrinsic pacemaker activity of the heart and how both arms of the ANS influence specific ionic events.

Heart rate is controlled via the primary pacemaker activity of cardiocytes in the sinoatrial node (SAN). The spontaneous cyclic depolarization of primary pacemaker cells in the SAN that establish intrinsic heart rate arises from the unique time-dependent characteristics of a variety of depolarizing and hyperpolarizing currents. Over the past 5 to 10 years, the number of candidate currents (and intracellular mechanisms) that contribute to the primary pacemaker activity of SAN myocytes has markedly increased, as have the theoretical descriptions of the mechanisms by which cardiac pacemaker activity occurs (5–8). The classical description of the ionic basis of SAN pacemaker activity is that action po-

tential configuration is determined by two outward hyperpolarizing K^+ currents, IK and IK1, and two depolarizing inward currents, I_{Ca} and I_f, that are carried primarily by Ca^{2+} and Na^+, respectively. During diastole, the membrane potential of SAN pacemaker cells exhibits a depolarizing drift until such time as a threshold potential is achieved. The gradual membrane depolarization that precedes the threshold activation of an action potential has been attributed to an overall decline in the net conductance of hyperpolarizing K^+ currents and a prominent increase in I_f in the latter diastolic phase of the pacemaker potential. Once a threshold potential is reached, I_{Ca} (an L-type current) markedly increases, and the rapid upstroke phase of the action potential ensues. Action potential repolarization occurs as a result of the net increase in the magnitudes of the hyperpolarizing K^+ currents.

One version of an emerging and more contemporary (simplified) view of SAN pacemaker activity is this: In addition to the diminution in hyperpolarizing K^+ currents and the increase in I_f, the slow membrane depolarization that leads to the triggered action potential is due to an increase in a transient (T-type) inward Ca^{2+} current ($I_{Ca,T}$), a progressive filling of the sarcoplasmic reticulum (SR) with Ca^{2+} during diastole. This leads to an increase in the magnitude of leak of Ca^{2+} from the SR into a confined space close to the sarcolemma and an increase in a forward sodium–calcium exchange current (I_{NaCa}) (Fig 13.2, *A* and *B*). During the earliest phase of the diastolic pacemaker potential, slow membrane depolarization begins to occur as a result of a reduction in the magnitude of hyperpolarizing K^+ currents and an increase in the magnitude of I_f. This initial depolarization leads to the activation of I_{Ca},T, a depolarizing current, which leads to further membrane depolarization and activation of I_{Ca},T during the latter depolarization phase. During diastole, several other key events also contribute to late-phase membrane depolarization. Not only does the progressive increase in I_{Ca},T have a depolarizing effect on the membrane, but there is evidence to support the idea that the inward Ca^{2+} current is also sufficient to increase the occurrence of small focal Ca^{2+} releases from the SR (Ca^{2+} sparks). The frequency of Ca^{2+} sparks increases in the latter phase of the diastolic depolarization and results in an increase in $[Ca^{2+}]$ in a confined space between the SR and the sarcolemma. This increase in subsarcolemmal $[Ca^{2+}]$ ($[Ca^{2+}]ss$) elicits the activation of forward sodium–calcium exchange that mediates an exchange of Ca^{2+} out and Na^+ in, in an attempt to normalize $[Ca^{2+}]ss$. Since the stoichiometry of the exchange is three Na^+ for one Ca^{2+}, the exchange is electrogenic and mediates a net inward current, I_{NaCa}, that leads to further depolarization of the cell membrane. The interrelated actions of $I_{Ca,T}$, SR Ca^{2+} sparks, and I_{NaCa} creates a positive feedback loop that culminates in a progressive membrane depolarization to a threshold potential. Once threshold is achieved, an L-type current rapidly activates, and an action potential is triggered.

The intrinsic pacemaker activity of cardiocytes in the SAN is powerfully modulated by the actions of the autonomic

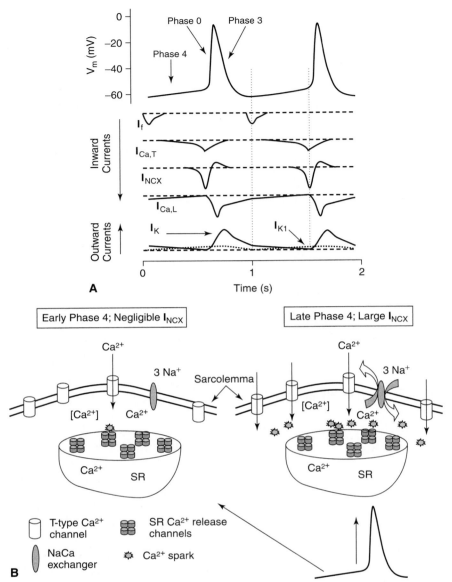

FIGURE 13.2 A more contemporary view (simplified) of the currents and intracellular processes responsible for the pacemaker activity of cells in the SAN. The principles underlying the genesis of pacemaker activity are similar to those described in Figure 13.3. However, in this scheme, I_f plays a prominent role in the part of phase 4 of the action potential. **A.** The increase in I_f elicits an initial membrane depolarization that leads to the activation of a T-type Ca^{2+} current ($I_{Ca,T}$) and the subsequent activation of a forward (depolarizing) sodium-calcium exchange current (I_{NCX}). This is thought to be a prominent late phase 4 current that ultimately brings the membrane potential V_m to a threshold value. **B.** The activation of T-type Ca^{2+} channels results in Ca^{2+} influx into a confined space between the sarcolemma and the SR, and $[Ca^{2+}]$ in the space begins to increase. This triggers the focal release of Ca^{2+} (sparks) from SR Ca^{2+} release channels, further increasing $[Ca^{2+}]$ in the space. This in turn leads to the activation of I_{NCX} and further membrane depolarization toward a threshold potential. Increased vagal stimulation slows the pacemaker activity of the SAN. **C.** See page 329: At lower levels of vagal input, depolarizing currents (e.g., I_f) are suppressed. This leads to a decrease in the slope of phase 4 of the action potential, an increase in the time required to reach threshold, and a slowing of heart rate. **D.** See page 329: When vagal input is more robust, ACh-sensitive K^+ channels are activated, and this leads to membrane hyperpolarization. This effect, in combination with the effect described in C, contributes to a further slowing of heart rate.

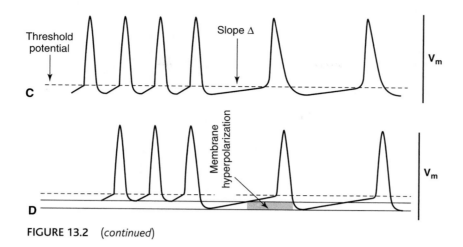

FIGURE 13.2 *(continued)*

nervous system. Heart rate across the physiological range is determined by the combined influences of the sympathetic and parasympathetic nervous systems. Increased vagal (parasympathetic) input into the SAN decreases the frequency at which pacemaker cells spontaneously depolarize (Fig 13.2, *C* and *D*). Classically, this is thought to occur via combinations of three mechanisms that include the following:

1. A reduction in the rate of diastolic depolarization
2. Action potential hyperpolarization
3. A upward shift in action potential threshold

Of these three mechanisms, the former two are probably the most prominent. The events that give rise to the slowing of pacemaker activity with vagal stimulation are quite complex (5). These events can be simplified in concept by describing them as being modifications of depolarizing and hyperpolarizing currents, particularly during the diastolic phase of the action potential. Vagal stimulation results in the release of acetylcholine (ACh) from nerve endings at the SAN. Released ACh binds to muscarinic receptors (M2) on SAN myocytes, activating or modulating several important processes. First, ACh can directly activate a specific class of K^+ channels (K_{ACh}) in SAN myocytes. Activation of K_{ACh} channels in the SAN produces a hyperpolarizing current that opposes the effects of depolarizing currents during the diastolic phase of the action potential. Second, several depolarizing diastolic currents are suppressed by ACh. The latter mechanism is thought to occur at lower levels of vagal activation and can provide a conceptual explanation for a reduction in the rate of diastolic depolarization without prominent membrane hyperpolarization (Fig. 13.2*C*). The former mechanism is more prominent at higher levels of vagal activation and explains ACh-mediated action potential hyperpolarization (Fig. 13.2*D*). The net effect of both mechanisms is to prolong the time required for diastolic depolarization to proceed to an action potential threshold.

The release of ACh onto SAN myocytes can also slow heart rate by suppressing membrane-bound adenylate cy-

clase activity (AdC) via a G protein–coupled M2-AdC mechanism. This mechanism is relevant to more contemporary theories of intrinsic SAN pacemaker activity, in which processes involved in diastolic membrane depolarization are strongly influenced by cyclic adenosine monophosphate (cAMP) dependent protein kinases. For example, both inward Ca^{2+} current activity and SR Ca^{2+} spark frequency can be increased by cAMP-dependent processes. These contribute to the acceleration of diastolic membrane depolarization via the actions of I_{NaCa}, whereas suppression of these processes would result in a reduction in the rate of membrane depolarization.

Sympathetic stimulation accelerates pacemaker activity of SAN myocytes. This manifests as a marked increase in the rate of diastolic depolarization and an increase in the amplitude of the pacemaker action potential (Fig 13.3). The increase in the rate of diastolic depolarization probably results from an increase in the magnitude of I_f and a cAMP-mediated increase in SR Ca^{2+} spark frequency. The latter occurs as a result of a phosphorylation-induced increase in the open probability of the SR Ca^{2+} release channel (direct) and to an increase in SR Ca^{2+} pump activity and Ca^{2+} load (indirect). The net effect would be to increase $[Ca^{2+}]ss$ more rapidly, which would in turn lead to augmentation of I_{NaCa} and further membrane depolarization to an action potential threshold. Once the threshold is achieved, the amplitude of the ensuing action potential is augmented. Explanations for this phenomenon include cAMP-mediated increases in the open probability of L-type Ca^{2+} channels and an augmentation in I_{Ca}, as well as an augmentation in I_{NaCa} that occurs secondary to a greater release of Ca^{2+} from SR with greater Ca^{2+} loads.

Overall, in the transition from rest to exercise of increasing intensity, heart rate initially increases as a result of withdrawal of vagal input to the SAN. As work intensity increases, further increases in heart rate are produced via the concomitant withdrawal of parasympathetic drive and increase in sympathetic drive to the pacemaker cells in the SAN.

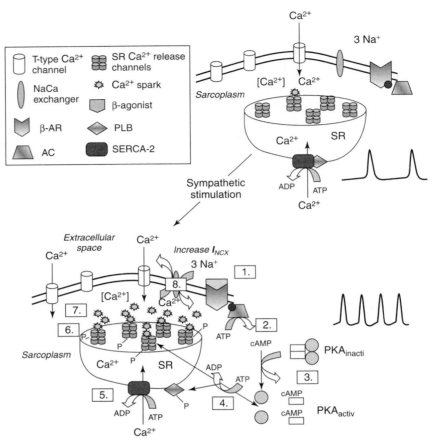

FIGURE 13.3 Increased sympathetic stimulation of SAN myocytes leads to an increase in heart rate via a variety of mechanisms. Part of the effect of β-agonist on SAN pacemaker activity is thought to be secondary to modulation of intracellular Ca^{2+} handling. The binding of β-agonist to β-adrenergic receptors (β-AR) (*1*) leads to the G protein–mediated activation of a membrane-bound adenylate cyclase (AC), the formation of cAMP (*2*), and subsequent activation of a cAMP-dependent protein kinase (PKA) (*3*). The active catalytic subunits of PKA are thought to lead to the phosphorylation of a variety of proteins that include phospholamban (PLB) and SR Ca^{2+} release channels (*4*). This elicits an increase in SR Ca^{2+} pump (SERCA-2) activity (*5*) and SR Ca^{2+} loading as well as the Ca^{2+} spark frequency (*6*). These events culminate in a faster increase in $[Ca^{2+}]$ in the confined space between the SR and sarcolemma (*7*) and a more robust activation of a depolarizing I_{NCX} (*8*). The acceleration of processes *6* to *8* results in a shortening of phase 4 of the pacemaker action potential and an increase in heart rate.

Myocardial Mechanisms for Heart Rate Control: Adaptations to Training

A hallmark of the exercise-trained state is bradycardia at rest and during submaximal exercise. Based on the observation that resting bradycardia persists under conditions of sympathetic and parasympathetic blockade in both humans and animals (4,9), it appears that the intrinsic pacemaker activity of the heart is altered by training. However, no data are available regarding whether and how the various pacemaker currents (or associated processes) respond adaptively to training. Finally, it is likely that training-induced alterations

in the autonomic control of the cells in the SAN play a more pronounced role in the bradycardia that occurs during submaximal exercise than during rest. This issue is addressed in detail in Chapter 14.

Some work, however, has been devoted to determining whether or not training bradycardia is a result of intrinsic changes in atrial adrenergic and cholinergic muscarinic receptor systems. Hammond and associates (9) found that chronic exercise elicited a decrease in β-adrenergic receptor number and no changes in muscarinic cholinergic receptor number in right atrial membranes isolated from endurance-trained pigs. In this porcine model of training, it was also found that the heart rate response to adrenergic stimulation was attenuated in trained animals. These data strongly implicate a training-induced down-regulation of the right atrial β-adrenergic system as being a contributing factor to training bradycardia in the porcine model of exercise training. In a subsequent study, Hammond and associates (10) found that the training-induced reduction in right atrial β-adrenergic receptor number was accompanied by an increase in stimulatory G protein ($G_{s\alpha}$) content. The increase in $G_{s\alpha}$ was associated with a training-induced reduction in the dose of isoproterenol required to elicit 50% of a maximal heart rate response even though training elicited a marked reduction in the maximal isoproterenol-stimulated heart rate response (10). In addition to the effect of training on heart rate and the right atrial β-adrenergic receptor system, it was also demonstrated that intrinsic heart rate in the presence of β-adrenergic and muscarinic cholinergic blockade was reduced (10). Schaefer and associates (11) clearly demonstrated in the running rat model that intrinsic atrial firing frequency was reduced by training and that this atrial bradycardia was due to factors other than those associated with receptor-mediated signal transduction mechanisms. The idea that training bradycardia is also due at least in part to intrinsic atrial adaptations independent of sympathetic and parasympathetic mechanisms is also supported by other work in rat and human models of endurance training (4).

Myocardial Mechanisms Influencing Stroke volume During Exercise

$$\dot{V}O_2 = HR \times SV \times \Delta a\text{-}v\,O_2$$

Left ventricular stroke volume is the amount of blood that is ejected from the left ventricle (LV) during a single cardiac cycle and is described as the difference between LV end diastolic volume (EDV) and end systolic volume (ESV). At rest, stroke volume is typically about 70 mL in a normal healthy adult. Maximal stroke volume values range from about 100 to 200 mL, varying as a function of a person's maximal cardiac output and aerobic capacity. Factors that influence LV-EDV include the size of the heart, LV filling pressure, and the compliance of LV during the diastolic filling phase of the cardiac cycle. Factors that influence ESV include afterload and LV myocardial contractile force. In the transition from rest to exercise, LV-EDV increases and LV-ESV decreases, both phenomena contributing to the increase in stroke volume as exercise intensity increases (1,12). The increase in LV-EDV with the onset of exercise has been associated with increases in venous return and LV filling pressure. The progressive decrease in LV-ESV with increasing exercise intensity is attributable to augmented myocardial contractile function. The latter results from increased sympathetic drive to the heart and second messenger–mediated modulation of contractile function and from intrinsic length-dependent (heterometric)

and length-independent (homeometric) mechanisms. During exercise, all of these mechanisms work in concert to optimize LV diastolic and systolic function. An appreciation of the elegant integration of these processes requires a basic understanding of the cellular processes of myocardial excitation, contraction, and relaxation (13).

In the heart, an action potential that originates in the SAN is propagated through the atria and into both ventricles of the heart. This membrane depolarization is the triggering event in the excitation-contraction (EC) coupling process (Fig. 13.4). Action potential conduction into the t-tubular system elicits the voltage-dependent opening of L-type Ca^{2+} channels and the generation of a small inward Ca^{2+} current (I_{Ca}). Many of the L-type Ca^{2+} channels in the t-tubular membrane are found to be in a highly ordered association with and in close proximity to large-conductance SR Ca^{2+} release channels in the terminal cisternal face of the SR. SR Ca^{2+} release channels act as highly specific receptors for the plant alkaloid ryanodine. Ryanodine alters SR Ca^{2+} channel function, and at high concentrations it suppresses SR Ca^{2+} release. For this reason, SR Ca^{2+} release channels are often referred to as ryanodine receptors, or RyRs. Different SR Ca^{2+} release channel–ryanodine receptor isoforms exist in cardiac, skeletal, and smooth muscle; the cardiac isoform is RyR2.

A very small confined space exists between the t-tubular membrane (containing L-type channels) and the terminal cisternal face of the SR membrane (containing RyRs). This is significant because when a small I_{Ca} is triggered by an action potential, the Ca^{2+} entering the small confined space produces an increase in $[Ca^{2+}]$ in the space to the extent that Ca^{2+} can bind to specific Ca^{2+}-binding sites on RyRs. The binding of Ca^{2+} to RyRs promotes the opening of these channels and facilitates the focal release of Ca^{2+} from small, spatially organized clusters of RyRs. Initially, SR Ca^{2+} release appears as discrete, spatiotemporally organized Ca^{2+} release, or Ca^{2+} sparks. While it was once thought that a single spark represented the release of Ca^{2+} from a single RyR, it is now known that a spark is the result of the simultaneous release of Ca^{2+} from clusters (about 10 to 20) of RyRs. With multiple Ca^{2+} sparks, $[Ca^{2+}]$ in the confined space and around other RyRs elicits a rapid and explosive opening of more RyRs, and a massive release of Ca^{2+} from the SR ensues. This general process of I_{Ca}-triggered release of Ca^{2+} from the SR is referred to as Ca^{2+}-induced Ca^{2+} release (CICR). Once CICR begins, Ca^{2+} rapidly diffuses from the confined space into the myofibrillar space of each sarcomere. The subsequent elevation in $[Ca^{2+}]$ around the contractile apparatus elicits Ca^{2+} to troponin C, the release of the steric inhibition of actin-myosin interactions by the troponin-tropomyosin complex, and the activation of crossbridge cycling and cardiac muscle contraction. These are the events of EC coupling (13–16).

The relaxation phase of the cardiac cycle occurs when $[Ca^{2+}]$ around the contractile apparatus is reduced. This occurs primarily via the actions of the 2A isoform of the

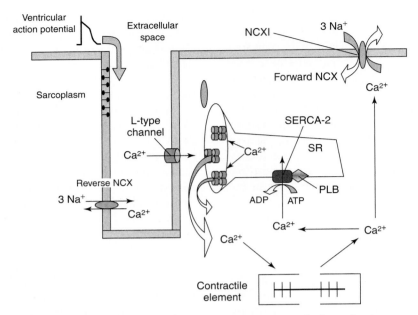

FIGURE 13.4 The basic processes of excitation-contraction (EC) coupling in ventricular myocardium.

sarco(endo)plasmic reticulum Ca^{2+} adenosine triphosphatase (ATPase) (SERCA 2A) and the cardiac sarcolemmal sodium-calcium exchanger (NCX1). On a beat-to-beat basis, Ca^{2+} removal by the SR is quantitatively the most important; depending upon animal species, it accounts for about 70 to 85% of the reduction in sarcoplasmic $[Ca^{2+}]$. While NCX1-mediated Ca^{2+} extrusion from the cell is quantitatively less important in the beat-to-beat regulation of sarcoplasmic $[Ca^{2+}]$, it does play a critical role in providing a mechanism to regulate cardiocyte Ca^{2+} content by quantitatively balancing the Ca^{2+} influx into the cell that occurs via I_{Ca}. Transient imbalances between cardiocyte Ca^{2+} influx and efflux over several beats can markedly influence cellular Ca^{2+} content, SR Ca^{2+} load, and the amount of Ca^{2+} that is released from the SR during a single EC coupling cycle. The NCX1 is an electrogenic exchanger (three Na^+ for one Ca^{2+}), and under physiological conditions, operation in the forward (Ca^{2+} out, Na^+ in) mode is favored at membrane potentials more negative than about −35 mV. This is relevant to the discussion of rate-dependent modulation of cardiac contractile force later in the chapter.

Sarcomere Length–Tension Relationship

With the onset of exercise, the increase in LV-EDV and decrease in LV-ESV are not independent phenomena. Starling's law of the heart is that myocardial contractile force increases in proportion to increases in myocardial muscle fiber length, such as would occur with increases in LV-EDV. Functionally, this provides for quantitative homeostatic control of venous return and cardiac output to en-

sure that the blood presented to the left ventricle is pumped from the left ventricle. Several cellular mechanisms contribute to Starling's law of the heart. The effect of myocardial fiber length on myocardial contractile force can be explained in part in the context of the sliding filament theory: maximal muscle contractile force is directly proportional to the degree of overlap of thin and thick filaments in the sarcomere (17). This is manifest as the classic length–tension relationship that is exhibited in all striated muscle (Fig. 13.5A). In the heart, the physiologically operational sarcomere length range is between about 1.85 and 2.20 μ, and in this range, there is a very steep length–tension relationship (18). With the onset of exercise, an increase in LV-EDV forces average sarcomere lengths toward the apex of the length–tension relationship and optimizes myocardial contractile force during systole, resulting in an increase in stroke volume.

[Ca²⁺]–Tension Relationship

Myocardial contractile force varies as a function of the amount of Ca^{2+} that is presented to the contractile element (19) (Fig. 13.5B). In normal myocardium, sarcoplasmic diastolic $[Ca^{2+}]$ is in about the 100 to 200 nM range and during contraction, it approaches μM concentrations. The sensitivity of the myocardial contractile element to activation by Ca^{2+} is greater than that observed in skeletal muscle. Factors that influence the amount of Ca^{2+} released by the SR during EC coupling have a direct effect on the extent of thin filament–mediated contractile element activation and therefore of myocardial contractile force. In addition, the [Ca^{2+}]–tension relationship is not static. Rather, it is subject to regulation by several factors. It varies as a function of muscle (sarcomere) length (Fig. 13.6, *A* and *B*). Increasing muscle length within the physiologically relevant range of sarcomere lengths causes a leftward shift in the [Ca^{2+}]–tension relationship (20,21). This results in a sensitization of the contractile element to activation by Ca^{2+}. The molecular basis for the length dependence of the pCa versus tension relationship is thought to involve simple alterations in the geometry of the sarcomere. If one considers the sarcomere to be a constant-volume entity, it follows that when length increases, cross-sectional dimension must decrease. The consequence of the latter is that thick filaments are closer to thin filaments, which increases the probability of force-generating actin-myosin encounters when myosin-binding domains on actin become exposed. Conversely, the pCa versus tension relationship moves rightward when sarcomere length is decreased. This property of the [Ca^{2+}]–tension relationship makes good

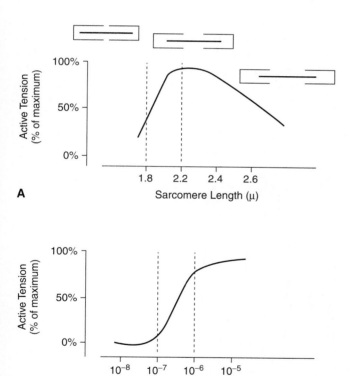

FIGURE 13.5 **A.** The cardiac muscle length–tension relationship. Note the very steep increase in tension between sarcomere lengths of 1.8 and 2.2 μ (the ascending limb). The decline in tension on the descending limb of the relationship is more gradual. The descending limb is rarely encountered physiologically except in severely pathological conditions. **B.** A representation of the cardiac muscle [Ca^{2+}]–tension relationship. The vertical broken lines denote the theoretical intracellular [Ca^{2+}] boundaries between diastole (*left*) and systole (*right*). The relationship is presented in a semilogarithmic fashion.

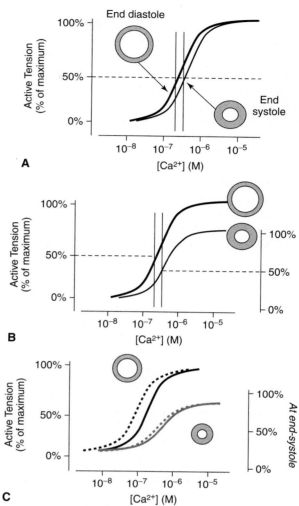

FIGURE 13.6 The length-dependence of the cardiac muscle [Ca^{2+}]–tension relationship. **A.** During end diastole, when chamber volume is large and muscle length is long, the [Ca^{2+}]–tension relationship lies to the left of that occurring during end systole, when chamber volume is small and muscle length is short. Maximal forces occurring at long and short sarcomere lengths are scaled to illustrate the length-dependent shift in sensitivity of the contractile element to activation by Ca^{2+}. **B.** In reality, at shorter sarcomere lengths, not only is there a rightward shift in the [Ca^{2+}]–tension relationship, but maximal force-generating capabilities are diminished as a result of a movement to the left on the length–tension relationship (compare part A). Both phenomena optimize the system for relaxation. **C.** Training alters the length dependence of the [Ca^{2+}]–tension relationship. Diffee and Nagle (21) found that the sensitivity of the cardiac contractile element to activation by Ca^{2+} was altered by training only at long (e.g., end diastolic) sarcomere lengths. The hypothetical consequences of this type of adaptation are illustrated here. At long sarcomere lengths, during end diastole (*black lines*) the sensitivity of the myocardial contractile element to activation by Ca^{2+} is greater in myocardium from the trained (*broken lines*) than in the sedentary (*solid lines*) state. Contractile force development is favored in the trained state under these conditions. However, at end systole (gray lines), when sarcomere lengths are short, relaxation is similarly favored in both the trained and sedentary states.

sense in that at long sarcomere lengths, such as those that occur during end diastole, the contractile element is sensitized to activation by Ca^{2+}. This would provide for a more forceful contraction at the beginning of systole. As blood is ejected from the heart, sarcomere length decreases and the $[Ca^{2+}]$–tension relationship moves back to the right, rendering the contractile element less sensitive to activation by Ca^{2+}. Desensitization of the contractile element at the end of the ejection phase of the cardiac cycle also makes good sense because this would favor myocardial relaxation and filling of the ventricle with blood during diastole. This dynamic length-dependent modulation of the $[Ca^{2+}]$–tension relationship provides another mechanism that contributes to Starling's law of the heart.

A third length-dependent mechanism may also contribute to Starling's law of the heart. There is evidence that the amount of Ca^{2+} released from the SR during an EC coupling cycle is proportional to myocardial segment length (22,23). This may be a result of an augmentation in the magnitude of I_{Ca}, SR Ca^{2+} load, and release of Ca^{2+} from the SR. Collectively, the increase in myocardial segment length that occurs during the filling phase of the cardiac cycle sets up conditions that are ideal for the generation of myocardial contractile force: the degree of overlap of thick and thin filaments is optimized and the sensitivity of the contractile element to activation by Ca^{2+} is increased, as is the amount of Ca^{2+} delivered to the contractile element.

Rate-Dependent Regulation of Myocardial Contraction

For more than 100 years (24,25), it has been well known that an increase in heart rate is accompanied by a progressive increase in contractile force of the myocardium, or the staircase phenomenon (25) (Fig. 13.7). There is good evidence to indicate that this rate-dependent augmentation in cardiac contractile force results from a progressive increase in Ca^{2+} content of the SR and in the amount of Ca^{2+} that is released from it on a beat-to-beat basis (13). The progressive increase in SR Ca^{2+} content with an increase in contraction frequency is thought to be due to a transient imbalance between Ca^{2+} influx via I_{Ca} and Ca^{2+} efflux via sodium-calcium exchange (NaCa exchange). As mentioned earlier, NaCa exchange is electrogenic, and its operation in the forward Ca^{2+} out–Na^+ in mode is favored at hyperpolarized membrane potentials whereas during membrane depolarization (i.e., the action potential), reverse Ca^{2+} in–Na^+ out exchange is favored. A simple explanation for the heart rate–dependent increase in SR Ca^{2+} load is as follows. In any given window of time, when heart rate is increased, the frequency of I_{Ca} increases, and this contributes to an increase in Ca^{2+} influx into the cell. In addition, the time between EC coupling events is decreased, resulting in less time for Ca^{2+} extrusion from the cell. In combination with the increase in Ca^{2+} influx, this can result in an increase in the amount of Ca^{2+} that is taken up

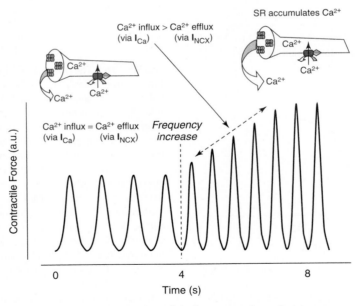

FIGURE 13.7 A representation of the heart rate–dependent increase in cardiac contractile force development, or the staircase (or treppe) phenomenon. As heart rate increases, muscle contractile force increases to a new steady-state plateau. The increase in force is secondary to a transient imbalance in cellular Ca^{2+} influx and efflux (favoring influx), an increase in SR Ca^{2+} content, and a larger SR Ca^{2+} release during each EC coupling cycle.

by the SR during diastole. Finally, when heart rate is increased, the myocardial membrane is depolarized for a greater fraction of time in the cardiac cycle, a condition that is not conducive to forward NaCa exchange. The net effect is that when heart rate is increased, the delicate and dynamic equilibrium that exists between cellular Ca^{2+} influx and efflux transiently shifts in favor of influx, and the excess Ca^{2+} is retained by and subsequently released from the SR. (An exception to the general observation that myocardial contractile force increases in direct proportion to heart rate is seen in hearts from smaller rodents [rat, mouse]. In these species, a negative staircase is typically observed, related to a rate-dependent depletion of Ca^{2+} from the SR [13]. Species-dependent differences in the relative durations of the cardiac action potential and the intracellular $[Ca^{2+}]$ transient are thought to contribute to this difference.)

β-Adrenergic Modulation of Myocardial Contraction

The increase in sympathetic drive that occurs with the onset of exercise not only affects heart rate via effects on pacemaker cells in the SAN, it also affects the myocardial contractile force (Fig. 13.8A). Hallmark alterations in cardiac contractile function resulting from β-adrenergic stimulation include a marked increased in peak contractile force and acceleration in myocardial relaxation. Overall, this culminates in a contraction that is larger but shorter. This adaptation is ideal to accommodate the generation of large stroke volumes at high frequencies (e.g., heart rates). The cellular basis for the effects of β-adrenergic agonists on the characteristics of cardiac contractile force has been characterized in good detail.

In cardiocytes of the ventricular myocardium, the binding of agonists (epinephrine, norepinephrine) to $β_1$-adrenergic receptors (β-AR) results in the G protein–mediated activation of adenylate cyclase, the formation of cAMP and subsequent activation of cAMP-dependent protein kinase (PKA) (Fig. 13.8C). While the active catalytic subunit of PKA has numerous intracellular targets, at least four are thought to contribute to augmented myocardial pump function during exercise (13–16). Myocardial contractile force is known to be modulated by the PKA-mediated phosphorylation of the L-type Ca^{2+} channel, the SR proteins phospholamban and RyR2, and troponin I on the thin filament. Phosphorylation of troponin I produces a rightward shift in the $[Ca^{2+}]$–tension relationship. This desensitization of the contractile element to activation by Ca^{2+} would promote myocardial relaxation. Phospholamban is a SR protein that acts to suppress the activity of the SR Ca^{2+} pump. Phosphorylation of phospholamban by PKA acts to release the inhibitory effects of phospholamban on SR Ca^{2+} pump activity, and this increases in the rate of Ca^{2+} clearance from the sarcoplasm by the SR and promotes relaxation. With respect to the PKA-mediated mechanisms that augment myocardial relaxation, the phospholamban phosphorylation probably has greater quantita-

tive significance than the troponin I phosphorylation. Phosphorylation of L-type Ca^{2+} channels by PKA increases L-type channel open probability and open time, and the physiological consequence is that I_{Ca} is markedly increased. There is also evidence that I_{Ca} can be increased by β-adrenergic agonists via a more direct β-AR/G protein–mediated process (26). Since I_{Ca} is the trigger for CICR, one consequence of an increase in I_{Ca} would be that the magnitude of Ca^{2+} release from the SR would increase (27). In addition, β-adrenergic stimulation leads to an increase in the amount of Ca^{2+} available to be released from the SR (Fig. 13.8B). The augmentation in SR Ca^{2+} load occurs via two mechanisms. First, the increase in I_{Ca} magnitude that occurs on a beat-to-beat basis increases the influx of Ca^{2+} into the cell. Since NaCa exchange is not directly influenced by β-adrenergic stimulation, a transient imbalance between cellular Ca^{2+} influx and efflux would occur, and the Ca^{2+} retained by the cell would be taken up into the SR. Second, since β-adrenergic stimulation markedly increases SR Ca^{2+} pump activity, a greater fraction of the Ca^{2+} that is removed from the sarcoplasm by the combined actions of SR pump activity and NaCa exchange would be removed via the SR mechanism. In other words, the sarcoplasmic Ca^{2+} clearance pathway that favors cellular Ca^{2+} retention (e.g., the SR Ca^{2+} pump activity) competes more effectively with the NaCa exchange, the Ca^{2+} extrusion pathway. Again, the net effect is that SR Ca^{2+} load increases and more Ca^{2+} is available for release when CICR is triggered by I_{Ca}. An increase in SR Ca^{2+} load also has the powerful effect of increasing the sensitivity of SR Ca^{2+} release from the SR by I_{Ca}.

Finally, under the influence of β-adrenergic stimulation, the sensitivity of the cardiac SR Ca^{2+} release mechanism to the triggering effects of I_{Ca} is increased via two mechanisms. First, the sensitivity of the SR Ca^{2+} release channel opening by I_{Ca} is powerfully (about geometrically) influenced by SR Ca^{2+} load. Very small increases in SR Ca^{2+} load produce very large changes in probability of the SR Ca^{2+} release channel opening. The link between SR Ca^{2+} load and probability of the SR Ca^{2+} release channel opening occurs via a physical coupling of RyRs with the intraluminal SR protein calsequestrin (via the proteins junctin and triadin). Calsequestrin is a high-capacity Ca^{2+} binding protein, and increased Ca^{2+} binding to calsequestrin (i.e., when SR Ca^{2+} load increases) exerts a strong influence on SR Ca^{2+} release channel sensitivity to triggered opening by I_{Ca}. Second, RyRs exist as complex multimeric protein complexes that include both the catalytic and regulatory subunits of PKA. Under the influence of β-adrenergic stimulation, RyRs are directly phosphorylated by PKA, and this phosphorylation elicits a direct increase in the sensitivity of the SR Ca^{2+} release mechanism to the triggering effects of I_{Ca}.

Overall, β-adrenergic stimulation promotes myocardial relaxation and diastolic filling via the phosphorylations of phospholamban and troponin I. Once the heart fills with blood, systolic function is increased via augmented SR Ca^{2+} release that occurs both directly and indirectly from the phosphorylations of L-type Ca^{2+} channels, RyRs, and phospholamban.

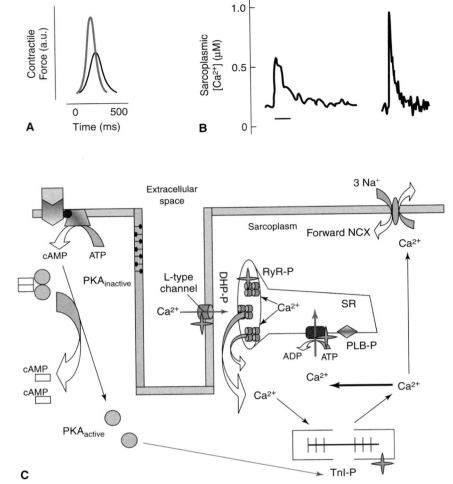

FIGURE 13.8 β-Adrenergic stimulation increases cardiac contractile force and accelerates myocardial relaxation. **A.** With β-adrenergic stimulation, cardiac contractile force markedly increases (gray tracing). In addition, the duration of the force transient is abbreviated. The former effect favors more powerful systolic ejection, whereas the latter effect favors diastolic filling, as would be required at high heart rates. **B.** The mechanical effects depicted in part A are associated with similar alterations in the magnitude and duration of the intracellular [Ca²⁺] transient. [Ca²⁺] transients occur in the same cell prior to (*left*) and after (*right*) exposure to β-agonist. (Representative data acquired from our laboratory for purposes of illustration only.) **C.** The effects of β-agonist on the intracellular [Ca²⁺] transient and myocardial contractile force are secondary to the effects of PKA-mediated phosphorylations of phospholamban, RyR, Tn-I, and the L-type of Ca²⁺ channels. The scheme and symbols used in this panel are consistent with those in Figures 13.3 and 13.4.

Integration of Mechanisms to Improve Cardiac Contractile Function During Exercise

In the transition from rest to exercise, parasympathetic drive is reduced and sympathetic drive is increased as a response to increase systemic cardiac output. At the level of the SAN, this results in an increase in the frequency of pacemaker activity and a subsequent increase in heart rate. Since cardiac output (CO) = HR × SV, the effect of this adjustment in pacemaker activity on cardiac output is obvious. In addition, independent of the direct effects of sympathetic input on the ventricular myocardium, the rate-dependent augmentation in SR Ca²⁺ may also increase myocardial contractile force and affect stroke volume.

At the level of the ventricular myocardium, the onset of exercise brings about several important changes. An increase in venous return to the heart elicits an increase in LV-EDV and an increase in end-diastolic sarcomere length. In addition, increased sympathetic β-adrenergic stimulation acts on processes that improve both the lusitropic and inotropic function of the heart (Fig. 13.9). During EC coupling, the magnitude of SR Ca^{2+} release is markedly increased by β-adrenergic stimulation. The resulting increase in sarcoplasmic $[Ca^{2+}]$ that occurs during EC coupling is easily sufficient to overcome any desensitization of the contractile element that occurs via troponin I phosphorylation. In addition, in a normal cardiac cycle, EC coupling is initiated when diastolic volume is maximal and sarcomere lengths are near the apex of the length–tension curve. This not only optimizes the degree of thick and thin filament overlap at the beginning of systole, but this length increase also acts to sensitize the contractile element to activation by Ca^{2+} by eliciting a leftward shift in the $[Ca^{2+}]$–tension relationship, thus opposing any desensitization caused by troponin I phosphorylation. The net result is that all of these processes act to optimize contractile force upon the initiation of systole. This is the basis for the observation that end-systolic volume decreases in the transition from rest to exercise.

Following the ejection phase of the cardiac cycle, myocardial relaxation and ventricular filling are required to sustain effective myocardial pump function. This is particularly important during exercise, when elevated heart rates are achieved primarily via the abbreviation of diastole as opposed to systole. Two primary mechanisms contribute to improved relaxation during the abbreviated diastolic filling period during exercise. First, the marked acceleration in sarcoplasmic Ca^{2+} clearance by the SR that occurs secondary to phospholamban phosphorylation profoundly accelerates the relaxation of the heart. Second, relaxation is further facilitated via the length-dependent rightward shift that occurs in the $[Ca^{2+}]$–tension relationship when LV-ESV is small and sarcomeres are short. The net result of these processes is that myocardial relaxation and ventricular filling can occur rapidly and optimal LV-EDV be achieved prior to the onset of another EC coupling event, even when exercise heart rates are high. These lusitropic processes begin to fail to compensate for the extreme shortening in diastolic filling times that occur at extremely high heart rates (e.g., more than about 200 beats/min). This failure manifests as a reduction in LV-EDV at extremely high heart rates.

Training-induced Adaptations to Stroke Volume During Submaximal and Maximal Dynamic Exercise

The fundamental systemic characteristics of the trained state include an increased organismic maximal oxygen consumption ($\dot{V}O_{2max}$), where $\dot{V}O_{2max} = HR_{max} \times$ maximal stroke volume (SV_{max}) × maximal arteriovenous oxygen content difference (Δ a-v O_{2max}) [18] and bradycardia during rest and submaximal exercise [22]. Adaptations in HR_{max} do not contribute to training-induced increases in $\dot{V}O_{2max}$. As a rule, at least 50% of the training-induced increase in $\dot{V}O_{2max}$ can be attributed to an increase in SV_{max} and the remainder to an increase in Δ a-v O_{2max} [2,28,29]. It can generally be stated that training-induced increases in SV_{max} are virtually always associated with increases in LV-EDV, whereas the contribution of augmented myocardial contractile function (and a decrease in LV-EDV) to SV_{max} varies [2,29]. Training-induced increases in maximal LV-EDV (LV-EDV$_{max}$) may be achieved by a variety of mechanisms that include (a) an increase in the intrinsic compliance of the myocardium, (b) an increase in end-diastolic filling pressure, and/or (c) an increase in LV chamber dimension secondary to myocyte growth.

Augmentation of LV-EDV With Training

Exercise training is generally thought to increase the intrinsic compliance of normal, healthy myocardium. From a methodological perspective, there is no absolute clarity on this issue. In the normal heart, training has been found to increase or leave unaltered myocardial compliance in diastole [4,30]. These discrepant findings may be due in part to the different techniques used in interpretive assumptions associated with making compliance determinations in a dynamic system. Diastolic compliance of the heart is determined by both passive and active tissue properties. In certain disease states, the decreased compliance of the heart

Myocardial Relaxation Optimized
- Ca^{2+} desensitized contractile element
  - length, TnI phosphorylation
- on ascending limb of length-tension relationship
- increased SR Ca^{2+} pump activity (PLB phosphorylation)

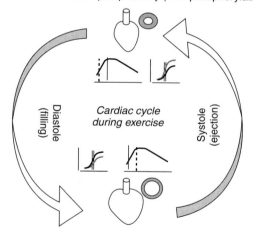

Contractile Force Development Optimized
- Resensitization of contractile element to activation by Ca^{2+}
  - Length effect
- Near apex of length-tension relationship
- Increased SR Ca^{2+} release
  - increased I_{Ca}
    - L-type Ca^{2+} channel phosphorylation
  - Increased SR Ca^{2+} load
    - Heart rate
    - Increase SR Ca^{2+} pump activity (PLB phosphorylation)

FIGURE 13.9 The mechanisms activated to improve cardiac function during exercise. The processes that favor both systole and diastole are listed in the context of the cardiac cycle.

is associated with changes in the amount and composition of interstitial connective elements, which have a marked effect on the passive compliance of the myocardial material. In a dynamically contracting and relaxing system, active properties certainly affect the compliance of the heart and influence its ability to relax and fill during diastole. An example of an active property that affects diastolic compliance is sarcoplasmic Ca^{2+} handling. In animal models of advanced age and diabetes mellitus, diminished sarcoplasmic Ca^{2+} clearance and alterations in the sensitivity of the contractile element to activation by Ca^{2+} have been shown to contribute to increased diastolic stiffness (31). It has been clearly demonstrated that in pathological settings, exercise training can increase the compliance of the heart during diastole. Furthermore, this type of improvement in diastolic compliance has been clearly shown to be associated with active rather than passive properties of the heart. Blood and plasma volume expansion occurring as a result of exercise training may also contribute to increases in $LV\text{-}EDV_{max}$. Such a phenomenon has been observed in normal healthy subjects, and it provides an attractive mechanism for improved diastolic filling during maximal exercise (1).

An important mechanism for training-induced augmentation of $LV\text{-}EDV_{max}$ is myocardial growth that produces an intrinsic increase in the LV chamber dimension. Exercise training has been shown to elicit small to modest (0–25%) increases in the mass of the heart. Since cardiac myocytes are terminally differentiated, training-induced increases in myocardial mass must be accomplished via hypertrophy of individual myocytes. In a variety of studies on animal models of exercise training, it has been demonstrated that increases in mean myocyte dimension can account for all of the increase in ventricular mass that is produced by training. Myocyte growth has been shown to occur in both the longitudinal and cross-sectional dimensions (4,30). Importantly, with exercise training longitudinal myocyte growth occurs in the absence of intrinsic alterations in sarcomere length. This type of cardiocyte growth in the LV would have several very important consequences. Since LV dimension can be approximated as a surface of revolution around a longitudinal axis, a 5% increase in mean LV myocyte length would produce a 5% increase in mean circumferential dimension as well as about a 5% increase in the length of the axis of revolution. The net result would be that longitudinal myocyte growth of 5% would elicit about a 16% increase in LV chamber volume. In addition, according to La Place's law of the heart, this type of increase in chamber volume would elicit only a small (not more than 5%) increase in ventricular wall stress, which is likely offset by a commensurate increase in myocyte cross-sectional dimension.

This type of increase in intrinsic LV chamber volume would have several important consequences for function. First, an increase in stroke volume would be expected to occur even if the contractility and fractional shortening of myocytes in the LV myocardium were unaltered by training. Second, an increase in LV-EDV resulting purely from longitudinal myocyte growth would allow EDV to be increased independent of increases in mean sarcomere length. This elegantly simple mechanism would leave the Frank-Starling mechanism intact to improve cardiac function further via an optimization of the "sarcomere length–tension" relationship and other length-dependent mechanisms. This mechanism also provides a simple cellular basis to explain the observation that a training-induced increase in LV-EDV produces a rightward but parallel shift in the ventricular pressure–volume relationship (4,30).

In summary, exercise training–induced increases in SV_{max} are virtually always associated with increases in LV-EDV. The latter almost certainly results from intrinsic alterations in LV chamber geometry that result from cardiac hypertrophy accompanied by longitudinal myocyte growth. There is also evidence that LV-EDV increases associated with training may be in part due to increased LV filling pressures that result from training-induced plasma volume expansion and to increased compliance of the myocardium.

Finally, relative bradycardia during rest and submaximal exercise is a classic marker of the trained state. Since the relationship between cardiac output, systemic oxygen consumption, and the absolute amount of external work performed within a species is highly invariant, it follows that stroke volume at rest and during fixed, absolute submaximal workloads is augmented by training. The mechanisms identified in the preceding paragraphs to explain the effect of training on SV_{max} are also applicable to the effect of training on submaximal stroke volume. In addition, however, it is probable that increased diastolic filling time secondary to training-induced bradycardia contributes to augmented stroke volume during rest and submaximal work in the trained state.

Intrinsic Alterations in Contractile Function With Training

The body of evidence supportive of the concept that chronic dynamic exercise can invoke adaptive changes in intrinsic myocardial contractile function is substantial (4,28,30). Interestingly, attempts to elucidate the cellular mechanisms that underlie these functional changes have not yet produced clear and unified ideas about what systems respond adaptively to training and how these adaptations actually contribute to training-induced improvements in the contractile performance of the heart. Over the past 30 years, much effort has been focused on determining how training influences contractile element composition and intrinsic function (18), the complex events that are involved in sarcoplasmic [Ca^{2+}] regulation during the cardiac cycle (22), the metabolic processes that are responsible for defending the tight coupling between ATP supply and demand that must be maintained in support of normal contractile activity (32), and systems that can modulate cardiocyte energy metabolism and mechanical function (14).

THE EFFECT OF TRAINING ON MYOCARDIAL ENERGY METABOLISM

In general, it can be stated that unlike skeletal muscle, in which training can produce dramatic increases in oxidative metabolic potential, the adaptive response of myocardial energy metabolism to exercise training is at best subtle. The observation that the activities of the key oxidative enzymes in rat heart are two to four times higher than those seen in skeletal muscle (32) suggest that the pathways of oxidative metabolism are already well adapted to support the energy demands imposed by daily bouts of exercise. This is not surprising in view of the fact that even at rest, the heart exhibits mechanical activity around the clock, whereas skeletal muscle is largely quiescent. This is not to say, however, that the heart does not exhibit the potential for metabolic adaptations. It is known that the activities of key enzymes of myocardial oxidative energy metabolism can be increased in response to sustained increases in heart rate and mechanical work that are brought about by electrical pacing (4,30). It is also clear, however, that the stimulus imposed by intermittent and relatively brief (about 1 to 2 hours) daily bouts of exercise is not sufficient to elicit significant changes in these enzymatic markers of myocardial energy production (33). Overall, the normal healthy heart is well adapted to meet the metabolic demands that are placed on it on a daily basis, and the metabolic potential of the heart is not markedly influenced by training. (A significant and complex body of literature addresses the adaptive effects of exercise training on myocardial energy metabolism, and in-depth reviews on the subject can be found elsewhere [4,30].)

THE EFFECT OF TRAINING ON THE MYOCARDIAL CONTRACTILE ELEMENT

Considerable attention has been devoted to characterizing the effects of chronic exercise on contractile element protein composition. In small rodents, training elicits compositional change in myosin that is reflected as a shift in myosin isoform composition toward the native V1 form (an isoform possessing a higher ATPase activity). However, it is now clear that changes in ventricular myosin ATPase activity and/or isoform composition are not obligatory for improved ventricular performance secondary to chronic exercise.

There is some evidence from animal models that training may increase the sensitivity of the contractile element to activation by Ca^{2+}. This idea is supported by the observation that paced myocytes isolated from trained and sedentary rats shortened to the same extent even though the cytosolic $[Ca^{2+}]$ achieved during contraction was lower in the myocytes from the trained animals (30). In addition, it has been recently demonstrated that in chemically skinned cardiocytes subjected to strict sarcomere length control, endurance training produced a leftward shift in the $[Ca^{2+}]$–tension relationship (34). It was also demonstrated that this training-induced sensitization of the contractile element to activation by Ca^{2+} was apparent at long (diastolic) sarcomere lengths but not at short (systolic) sarcomere lengths (35). This is also consistent with the recent observation in intact cardiocytes

that the steepness of the length–tension relationship is increased by training (36) (Fig. 13.6C). This type of adaptation would provide for a training-induced optimization of contractile element activation at the beginning of the ejection phase of the cardiac cycle, whereas the effect would be lost at short sarcomere lengths and therefore would not contribute to impaired myocardial relaxation at initiation of chamber filling. This adaptation has not been confirmed in species other than the rat, and whether this type of adaptation occurs in larger mammals is not known.

THE EFFECT OF TRAINING ON EC COUPLING AND SARCOPLASMIC $[Ca^{2+}]$ REGULATION

Since myocardial contractile force is governed in large part by the amount of Ca^{2+} presented to the contractile element, it is not surprising that considerable effort has been spent on determining whether or not training alters cardiocyte EC coupling and/or Ca^{2+} regulation. Critical examination of the extensive literature in the field (4,30) reveals two safe conclusions in this regard. First, in normal healthy myocardium, training does not appear to elicit striking effects on EC coupling and/or cellular Ca^{2+} regulation. In this regard, it must be recognized that cardiocyte Ca^{2+} homeostasis and control during EC coupling is delicately balanced by a myriad of processes. It is unlikely that profound alterations in any of these processes would be conducive to fine control of myocardial contractile force. In addition, seemingly subtle alterations in points of Ca^{2+} control may in fact elicit physiologically significant adjustments in control that contribute to improved cardiac function in the trained state. Second, in pathological settings when aberrant Ca^{2+} regulation can be readily detected, training has been shown to be effective in normalizing cardiocyte Ca^{2+} regulation. For example, age- and diabetes-related deficits in myocardial relaxation have been attributed to slowed sarcoplasmic Ca^{2+} clearance by the SR, and training has been shown to be particularly effective in ameliorating these deficits.

THE EFFECT OF TRAINING ON β-ADRENERGIC SIGNALING IN THE HEART

A significant number of processes involved in the control of cardiac function can be modulated by β-adrenergic receptor agonists via the actions of PKA. The effect of aerobic exercise training on various aspects of the β-adrenergic system have been examined in a variety of training models. One clear characteristic of the trained state is that at a given absolute submaximal work load, sympathetic drive as reflected by circulating catecholamine levels is attenuated relative to that observed in untrained subjects (see Chapter 14). At the level of the heart, however, whether training influences the inotropic sensitivity of the heart to β-agonists is not clear. Following training, the contractile responsiveness of the heart to catecholamines has been reported to increase, decrease, or remain unchanged (4,30). The adaptive responsiveness of key elements of the β-adrenergic signaling cascade to exercise training have also been examined in considerable detail, and no clear consensus has been reached.

However, at present it would appear that training-induced alterations in β-adrenergic signaling in ventricular myocardium are minimal, whereas at the level of the right atrium, β-adrenergic receptor number is probably down-regulated, perhaps contributing to the bradycardia that occurs following exercise training (9).

The Effect of Training on the Coronary Vasculature

The regulation of cardiac function cannot be fully appreciated without acknowledging the important contribution of coronary vasculature in matching oxygen delivery with myocardial oxygen demand. Training-induced alterations in cardiocyte dimension produce significant consequences with respect to the coronary vasculature and its ability to service the working myocardium. For example, if training-induced cardiocyte growth is not accompanied by angiogenesis and/or adaptations in the mechanisms regulating myocardial perfusion, the heart may be exposed to energetic risk during periods of increased mechanical activity. Clearly, cardiocyte growth without parallel adaptations in the coronary vasculature is maladaptive. In most circumstances, exercise training–induced cardiocyte growth is accompanied by parallel (at least) growth of the coronary vasculature (30,37,38). Exercise train-

ing has been shown to elicit structural changes in the vasculature of the heart, including growth of the larger proximal coronary arteries such that arterial size increases are commensurate with or greater than the relative increase in myocardial mass that is produced by training. Overall, training usually elicits adaptation in the coronary vasculature such that at a minimum microvasculature development occurs in parallel with the modest myocyte hypertrophy that is often observed in response to exercise training (4). In severe models of training, cardiac hypertrophy is not accompanied by sufficient growth and restructuring of the coronary microvasculature; normalization of capillary to mid myocyte diffusion distances does not appear to occur (4). An analogous mismatch in microvascular growth is observed in pressure overload models of ventricular hypertrophy, in which myocyte cross-sectional area is increased dramatically and capillarity is decreased. Finally, training elicits robust effects on the reactivity of the coronary vasculature to humoral and mechanical stimuli. In a variety of animal models of exercise training, both the coronary smooth muscle and vascular endothelium appear to respond adaptively to training, and in most cases these adaptations are vasodilatory (37–43). These types of adaptations likely represent physiological mechanisms to preserve adequate regional coronary blood flow during periods of increased cardiac work.

A MILESTONE OF DISCOVERY

With the caveat that singling out specific milestones of discovery risks a disservice to many giant contributions to the field of muscle physiology, I present a point of view on two works that have added significantly to our understanding of how cardiac contractile force is dynamically regulated in the cardiac cycle.

The cellular basis for Starling's law of the heart is often described in the context of the classic work of Gordon and associates (17) in which they elegantly demonstrated that in frog skeletal muscle, the length–tension relationship could be attributed to the degree of thin and thick filament overlap in the sarcomere. However, in cardiac muscle, while the same principles of sarcomere geometry certainly apply, Allen and associates (18) observed that the steepness of the ascending limb of the length–tension relationship of cardiac muscle was much greater than that observed in skeletal muscle. This observation defied explanation solely by the principles of the sliding filament theory, and it was proposed that activation processes of some sort contributed to this difference. Subsequent to this key observation, Hibberd and Jewell (20) demonstrated a marked length dependence in the cardiac [Ca^{2+}]–tension relationship. Specifically, at longer (end diastolic) sarcomere lengths, the sensitivity of the contractile element to activation by Ca^{2+} was significantly greater than at shorter (end systolic) sarcomere lengths. In addition, Allen and Kurihara (22) conducted experiments demonstrating that in the physiological sarcomere length range, there was a direct re-

lationship between the magnitude of the intracellular [Ca^{2+}] transient and sarcomere length.

Collectively, these observations were important for several key reasons. First, it is now clear that across sarcomere lengths that occur physiologically (i.e., between end-systole and end-diastole), less than about 50% of the length-dependent regulation of cardiac contractile force can be explained in the context of the sliding filament theory. Second, the marked length dependencies of Ca^{2+} release to the contractile element and the sensitivity of the contractile element to activation by Ca^{2+} provide viable explanations for the steepness of the ascending limb of the cardiac muscle length–tension relationship. Third, and most important, this also provides for an elegant and powerful scheme of regulation whereby cardiac contractile force development is optimized once the heart fills with blood, and the processes favoring relaxation are optimized after blood has been ejected.

Allen DG, Kurihara S. The effects of muscle length on intracellular calcium transients in mammalian cardiac muscle. J Physiol (Lond) 1982;327:79–94.

Hibberd, MB, Jewell BR. Calcium- and length-dependent force production in rat ventricular muscle. J Physiol (Lond) 1982;329: 527–540.

ACKNOWLEDGMENTS

I thank Drs. Douglas R. Seals and Robert Mazzeo for their useful and insightful discussions. I also thank David A. Brown for his useful editorial input and Dr. Lisa Mace for help with illustrations.

REFERENCES

1. Rowell LB. Human Cardiovascular Control. New York: Oxford University, 1993;162–479.
2. Saltin B, Blomqvist G, Mitchell JH, et al. Response to exercise after bed rest and after training. A longitudinal study of adaptive changes in oxygen transport and body composition. Circulation 1968;38(Suppl VII):1–78.
3. Saltin B, Rowell LB. Functional adaptations to physical activity and inactivity. Fed Proc 1980;39:1506–1513.
4. Moore R, Korzick D. Cellular adaptations of the myocardium to chronic exercise. Prog Cardiovasc Dis 1995;37:371–396.
5. Demir SS, Clark JW, Giles WR. Parasympathetic modulation of sinoatrial node pacemaker activity in rabbit heart: a unifying model. Am J Physiol 1999;276:H2221–H2244.
6. Katz AM. Physiology of the Heart. 2nd ed. New York: Raven, 1992;687.
7. Lipsius SL, Huser J, Blatter LA. Intracellular Ca^{2+} release sparks atrial pacemaker activity. NIPS 2001;16:101–106.
8. Brown HF. Electrophysiology of the Sinoatrial node. Physiol Rev 1982;62:505–530.
9. Hammond HK, White FC, Brunton LL, et al. Association of decreased myocardial β-receptors and chronotropic response to isoproterenol and exercise in pigs following chronic dynamic exercise. Circ Res 1987;60:720–726.
10. Hammond HK, Ransas LA, Insel PA. Noncoordinate regulation of cardiac Gs protein and β-adrenergic receptors by a physiological stimulus, chronic dynamic exercise. J Clin Invest 1988;82:2168–2171.
11. Schaefer ME, Allert JA, Adams HR, et al. Adrenergic responsiveness and intrinsic sinoatrial automaticity of exercise-trained rats. Med Sci Sports Exerc 1992;24:887–894.
12. Poliner LR, Dehmer GJ, Lewis E, et al. Left ventricular performance in normal subjects: a comparison of the responses to exercise in the upright and supine positions. Circulation 1980;62:528–534.
13. Bers DM. Excitation-contraction Coupling and Cardiac Contractile Force. 2nd ed. Dordrecht, Netherlands: Kluwer Academic, 2001;427.
14. Bers DM. Cardiac excitation-contraction coupling. Nature 2002;415:198–205.
15. Korzick DH. Regulation of cardiac excitation-contraction coupling: a cellular update. Adv Physiol Educ 2003;27:92–200.
16. Marks AR. Cardiac intracellular calcium release channels: role in heart failure. Circ Res 2000;87:8–11.
17. Gordon AM, Huxley AF, Julian FJ. The variation in isometric tension with sarcomere length in vertebrate muscle fibres. J Physiol (Lond) 1966;184:170–192.
18. Allen DG, Jewell BR, Murray JW. The contribution of activation processes to the length tension relation in cardiac muscle. Nature 1974;248:606–607.
19. Solaro RJ, Wise RM, Shiner JS, et al. Calcium requirement for cardiac myofibrillar activation. Circ Res 1974;34:525–530.
20. Hibberd MG, Jewell BR. Calcium- and length-dependent force production in rat ventricular muscle. J Physiol (Lond) 1982;329:527–540.
21. Kentish JC, ter Keurs HE, Ricciardi L, et al. Comparison between the sarcomere length-force relations of intact and skinned trabeculae from rat right ventricle. Circ Res 1986;58:755–768.
22. Allen DG, Kurihara S. The effects of muscle length on intracellular calcium transients in mammalian cardiac muscle. J Physiol (Lond) 1982;327:79–94.
23. Fabiato A. Calcium release in skinned cardiac cells: variations with species, tissues, and development. Fed Proc 1982;41:2238–2244.
24. Bowditch HP. Über die Eigenthumlichkeiten der Reizbarkeit, welche die Muskelfasem des Herzens zeigen. Ber Sachs Ges Wiss 1871;23:652–689.
25. Woodworth RS. Maximal contraction, "staircase" contraction, refractory period, and compensatory pause, of the heart. Am J Physiol 1902;8:213–249.
26. Yatani A, Codina J, Imoto Y, et al. A G protein directly regulates mammalian cardiac calcium channels. Science 1987;238:1288–1292
27. Fabiato A. Stimulated calcium current can both cause calcium loading in and trigger calcium release from the sarcoplasmic reticulum of a skinned canine Purkinje cell. J Gen Physiol 1985;85:291–320.
28. Schaible TF, Scheuer J. Cardiac adaptations to chronic exercise. Prog Cardiovasc Dis 1985;27:297–324.
29. Scheuer J, Tipton CM. Cardiovascular adaptations to physical training. Ann Rev Physiol 1977;39:221–251.
30. Moore RL, Palmer BM. Exercise training and cellular adaptations of normal and diseased hearts. Exerc Sport Sci Rev 1999;27:285–315.
31. Lakatta EG. Cardiovascular regulatory mechanisms in advanced age. Physiol Revs 1993;73:413–467.
32. Baldwin KM, Cooke DA, Cheadle WG. Time course adaptations in cardiac and skeletal muscle to different running programs. J Appl Physiol 1977;42:267–272.
33. Laughlin MH, Hale CC, Novela L, et al. Biochemical characterization of exercise-trained porcine myocardium. J Appl Physiol 1991;71:229–235.
34. Diffee GM, Seversen EA, Titus MM. Exercise training increases the Ca^{2+} sensitivity of tension in rat cardiac myocytes. J Appl Physiol 2001;91:309–315.
35. Diffee GM, Nagle DF. Exercise training alters the length dependence of contractile properties in rat myocardium. J Appl Physiol 2003;94:1137–1144.
36. Natali AJ, Wilson LA, Peckham M, et al. Different regional effects of voluntary exercise on the mechanical and electrical properties of rat ventricular myocytes. J Physiol (Lond) 2002;541:863–875.
37. Laughlin MH, Oltman CL, Bowles DK. Exercise training-induced adaptations in the coronary circulation. Med Sci Sports Exerc 1998;30:352–360.

38. Laughlin MH, Oltman CL, Muller JM, et al. Adaptation of coronary circulation to exercise training. In Fletcher GF, ed. Cardiovascular Response to Exercise. Mount Kisco, NY: Futura, 1994;175–205.

39. Bowles DK, Woodman CR, Laughlin MH. Coronary smooth muscle and endothelial adaptations to exercise training. Exerc Sport Sci Rev 2000;28:57–62.

40. Laughlin MH, McAllister RM. Exercise training-induced coronary vascular adaptation. J Appl Physiol 1992;73: 2209–2225.

41. Laughlin MH, Overholser KA, Bhatte MJ. Exercise training increases coronary transport reserve in miniature swine. J Appl Physiol 1989;67:1140–1149.

42. Laughlin MH, Rubin LJ, Rush JW, et al. Short-term training enhances endothelium-dependent dilation of coronary arteries, not arterioles. J Appl Physiol 2003;94: 234–244.

43. Laughlin MH, Tomanek RJ. Myocardial capillarity and maximal capillary diffusion capacity in exercise-trained dogs. J Appl Physiol 1987;63:1481–1486.

CHAPTER 14

Organization and Control of Circulation to Skeletal Muscle

STEVEN S. SEGAL AND SHAWN E. BEARDEN

Introduction

Blood flow to skeletal muscle is dictated by the perfusion pressure across the vascular bed and the total resistance presented by vessel branches. With arterial and venous pressures maintained, changes in muscle blood flow are governed through changes in vascular resistance, which resides primarily in the precapillary vasculature (Milestone of Discovery). Through relaxation of vascular smooth muscle, the magnitude of blood flowing through skeletal muscle can increase from 5 to 10 mL · min · 100 g^{-1} at rest to more than 250 mL · min · 100 g^{-1} during exercise. This functional, or exercise, hyperemia represents a dynamic range of 25- to 50-fold (1,2). The positive relationships among muscle contraction, oxygen consumption ($\dot{V}O_2$), and blood flow indicate that the convection and diffusion of oxygen from the vasculature are related intimately to energy expenditure. Moreover, the elevation of blood flow in response to contractile activity demonstrates the intrinsic coupling between skeletal muscle and its vascular supply.

Blood flow to skeletal muscle is also determined by the activity of the sympathetic nervous system and the need to maintain systemic blood pressure. Indeed, sympathetic vasoconstriction diverts flow from inactive tissues to redistribute (as well as enhance) cardiac output to active skeletal muscle (3). Considerable knowledge has been gained in understanding the regulation of muscle blood flow during ex-

ercise and its adaptations to physical training (2). The goal of this chapter is to illustrate the functional organization of the vascular supply to skeletal muscle and explore how muscle blood flow is controlled in light of the physical determinants of oxygen delivery to active muscle fibers during exercise.

Organization of the Vascular Supply

The Microcirculation Is a Highly Branched Network

Understanding how the peripheral vasculature is organized anatomically is integral to understanding the nature of blood flow control to skeletal muscle. Vascular resistance to blood flow begins with the small muscular arteries that are external to the muscle. These feed arteries arise from larger conduit vessels (e.g., brachial and femoral arteries) that are designed for rapidly conveying blood from the heart to peripheral tissues. Feed arteries, which can present half of the total resistance to blood flow, are positioned to control the total amount of blood entering the muscle (4). When maximally dilated, the diameter of feed arteries ranges from 100 to several hundred micrometers. Because feed arteries are external to the muscle, they are physically removed from vasoactive stimuli produced by skeletal muscle fibers.

Upon entering skeletal muscle, feed arteries give rise to primary arterioles, which typically branch into second- and third-order arterioles (Fig. 14.1). These intermediate branches distribute blood throughout the muscle and thereby control regional tissue perfusion. In some muscles, anastomoses between branches provide alternative pathways for the delivery of blood. Arising from the distributing arterioles are the fourth-order and terminal branches of the arteriolar network, which control the perfusion of capillaries with red blood cells (RBCs) (5). The effluent blood from capillaries drains into collecting venules, which converge into progressively larger branches that often course along arterioles as they carry blood back toward the heart (Fig. 14.1). The maximal (dilated) diameter of arterioles ranges from more than 100 μm in proximal branches to 10 to 15 μm in distal branches (6). The highly branched arrangement of the resistance network implies that proximal, intermediate, and distal branches must coordinate their responses for effective control of the magnitude and distribution of blood flow to exercising muscle. The mechanisms and signaling pathways underlying this behavior are considered later in this chapter.

Resistance Vessels Are Composed of Smooth Muscle Lined by Endothelium and Surrounded by Sympathetic Nerves

The primary physiological mechanism for controlling blood flow is through changes in the diameter of resistance vessels, which is governed by the contractile status of smooth muscle

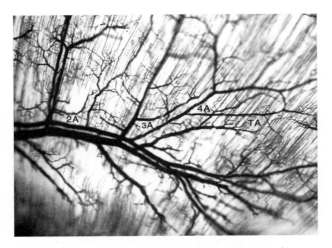

FIGURE 14.1   Arteriolar and venular networks are paired in skeletal muscle. A vascular cast of the mouse gluteus maximus muscle begins with the second-order arterioles (*2A*) to illustrate network branching into third-order (*3A*) and fourth-order (*4A*) arterioles. The primary arteriole and feed artery, which are proximal to 2A, are not shown. Venules (not labeled) are often paired with arterioles, particularly in the larger proximal branches. Distal arterioles diverge from venules and form microvascular units (Fig. 14.5).

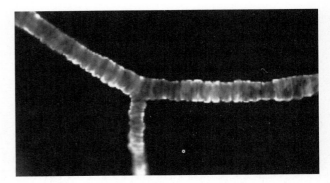

FIGURE 14.2   A continuous monolayer of arteriolar smooth muscle cells. A third-order arteriole (resting diameter, 25 μm) gives rise to a fourth-order daughter branch in the mouse gluteus maximus muscle. Smooth muscle cells are visualized by immunolabeling for α-actin. Note how each cell wraps completely around the vessel and abuts its neighbor to form a continuous monolayer surrounding the vessel lumen.

cells. In arterioles and feed arteries, each smooth muscle cell is wrapped circumferentially around the vessel wall and perpendicular to the underlying endothelial cells. Individual smooth muscle cells are about 5 μm in diameter and when fully relaxed can exceed 100 μm in length. Individual smooth muscle cells can wrap completely around the lumen of smaller arterioles (Fig. 14.2) but do not completely encircle the larger proximal arterioles or feed arteries. Nevertheless, each smooth muscle cell circumscribes multiple endothelial cells around the vessel lumen, and this physical association is integral to vasomotor control (discussed later). The media of arterioles typically contains a single layer of smooth muscle cells, though it can be two or three cells thick in proximal arterioles and feed arteries. Adjacent smooth muscle cells form a continuous layer along feed arteries and throughout much of the arteriolar network but can become discontinuous in distal arteriolar branches (6). In capillaries, only the endothelium is present, which minimizes the barrier for exchange of solutes between the blood and muscle fibers. Though individual capillaries are the smallest of all vessels, their total number far exceeds that of all other branches, resulting in the lowest total resistance (and greatest surface area) of the entire vascular system. Beyond the capillaries, smooth muscle cells return in the venules, which serve as key sites of regulating vascular capacitance through changes in diameter and volume. Capillaries and venules are also the primary loci for regulating vascular permeability and inflammation, which are not considered further here.

As with all blood vessels, the intimal surface of the resistance vasculature is lined by a continuous monolayer of endothelial cells that are oriented along the vessel axis and in direct contact with blood flowing within the vessel lumen (Fig 14.3). Smooth muscle and endothelium are separated by the internal elastic lamina, which is penetrated by projections

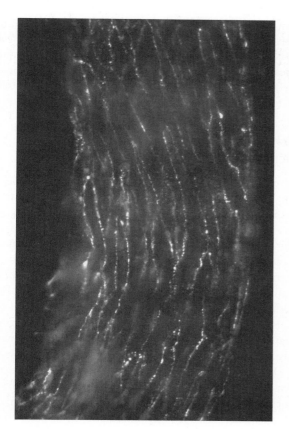

FIGURE 14.3   A continuous monolayer of endothelial cells lines the lumen of all blood vessels. Shown is a feed artery (resting diameter, 75 μm) of the hamster retractor muscle following immunolabeling for connexin 43, a protein that is integral to the formation of gap junction channels at the borders of endothelial cells in feed arteries and arterioles. Cell-to-cell coupling via gap junction channels enables electrical signals to travel rapidly along the vessel wall.

Capillaries Are Organized Into Microvascular Units

The functional unit of blood flow control can be defined as the smallest volume of tissue to which oxygen delivery can be independently controlled (9). In skeletal muscle, this functional entity is the microvascular unit (MVU), which consists of all of the capillaries arising from a common terminal arteriole (TA). The TAs typically run perpendicular to muscle fibers, giving off capillaries that course between and along muscle fibers for a distance of about 1 mm and then empty into a collecting venule (Fig. 14.5). A group of about 20 individual capillaries arise from the TA and course along the muscle fibers, often with a similar group of capillaries originating in the opposite direction from the same TA. The volume of muscle tissue within a MVU is about 0.1 mm³, with average dimensions of 1 to 2 mm long, 0.5 mm wide, and 0.2 mm thick. These dimensions result in 10 to 20 MVUs per cubic millimeter (or milligram) of intact skeletal muscle. The volume of muscle supplied by each MVU contains segments of 20 to 30 muscle fibers. Because the individual

from respective cells to form myoendothelial contacts (6). Individual endothelial cells are 50 to 100 μm long, about 5 to 10 μm wide, and less than 1 μm thick. Each endothelial cell spans multiple smooth muscle cells along the vessel wall. Such spatial arrangements between respective cell layers are integral to blood flow control. A rich plexus of perivascular sympathetic nerve fibers surrounds feed arteries and arterioles (Fig. 14.4). Although venules in skeletal muscle are not directly innervated, spillover of neurotransmitter (e.g., norepinephrine) released around nearby arterioles can diffuse to and constrict venular smooth muscle cells, which promotes venous return of blood towards the heart (7). Resistance vessels assume a smooth and cylindrical shape when fully dilated. However, longitudinal ridges and folds form along the intima during smooth muscle cell shortening and vasoconstriction (8). This inward deformation of endothelial and smooth muscle cells amplifies the reduction in vessel caliber during vasoconstriction.

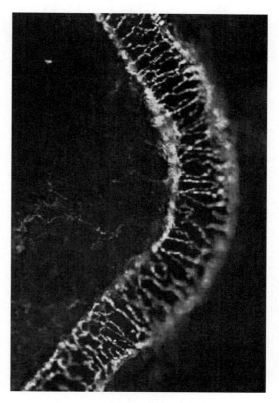

FIGURE 14.4   Resistance vessels are surrounded by sympathetic nerves. A feed artery (resting diameter, 75 μm) of the hamster retractor muscle is shown following histochemical staining for glyoxylic acid to reveal catecholamine-containing nerve fibers in the adventitia surrounding the smooth muscle cell layer. This rich nerve plexus extends throughout the arteriolar network but not into capillaries or venules.

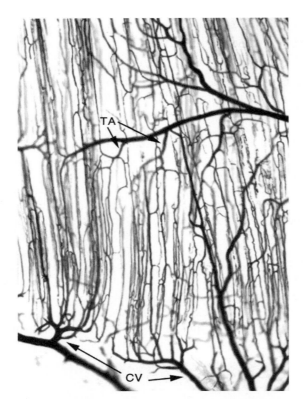

FIGURE 14.5 Capillaries are organized into microvascular units along skeletal muscle fibers. Microscopic examination of a vascular cast near a thin edge of the mouse gluteus maximus muscle shows terminal arterioles giving rise to groups of capillaries that extend for about 1 mm and converge on collecting venules. A terminal arteriole (TA) typically gives rise to capillaries in both directions along muscle fibers. Furthermore, collecting venules (CV) typically receive blood from capillaries that originate from more that one terminal arteriole. As muscle thickness increases, MVUs stack on top of and next to each other, making it difficult to resolve capillaries associated with individual MVUs.

muscle fibers within a motor unit are dispersed throughout a muscle rather than lying side by side, the adjacent fiber segments within the tissue volume perfused by each MVU are typically derived from different motor units. Thus, a particular capillary or MVU may have any number of adjacent muscle fibers consuming oxygen at a given moment, according to the pattern of motor unit recruitment (10).

Perfusion with blood flow is not controlled at the level of individual capillaries. Instead, each TA serves as the functional equivalent of a precapillary sphincter by being the last branch of the arteriolar network that still contains smooth muscle and thereby can actively control vessel diameter. Thus, constriction of a TA prevents the entire group of capillaries within an MVU from receiving blood flow, whereas dilation of a TA results in perfusion of the entire MVU (5). However, the distribution of RBCs within a MVU is not uni-

form among capillaries; it is determined passively by differences in the physical determinants of RBC entry into each capillary (11) and variations in the hemodynamic resistance of respective capillary segments, attributable to corresponding differences in their lengths and branching characteristics (12).

Each Muscle Fiber Spans Multiple Microvascular Units

Individual muscle fibers are typically several centimeters long, which contrasts with the 1- to 2-mm distance spanned by each MVU. Because metabolic demand increases along the entire length of an active muscle fiber, the perfusion of multiple MVUs is required to deliver oxygen and nutrients to each fiber. In turn, the muscle fibers of each motor unit are dispersed through the muscle. Thus, the firing of a motor neuron will result in perfusion of far more capillaries than needed to supply only the active fibers, particularly at low levels of motor unit recruitment (10). This functional organization precludes any selective increase in blood flow to only active muscle fibers.

Within the muscle, individual MVUs are stacked next to each other (5). This arrangement results in blood flow being concurrent between some capillaries (e.g., those arising in the same direction from neighboring TAs) while being countercurrent between capillaries arising in the opposite direction along muscle fibers. This proximity of neighboring MVUs promotes oxygen diffusion between capillaries of neighboring MVUs that can offset heterogeneities in oxygen delivery between capillaries.

Oxygen Is Transported From Microvessels to Muscle Fibers

Capillary Density Is a Primary Determinant of Oxygen Diffusion

Early in the twentieth century, August Krogh proposed that each capillary supplies oxygen to a cylindrical region of muscle fibers surrounding it (13). This Krogh cylinder model of oxygen diffusion has dominated much of the thinking about the supply and utilization of oxygen in skeletal muscle. Krogh based many of his conclusions upon spatial relationships determined in muscle cross-sections, which remains a common practice today. Thus, the ability of the microcirculation to present oxygen to muscle fibers is typically evaluated in terms of capillary density (number of capillaries per square millimeter) or as the capillary-to-fiber ratio in cross-sections of whole muscles or muscle biopsies (14). Human skeletal muscle fibers typically have one or two capillaries in contact at each point along their length (14). Although it is well established that the capillary supply and vascular transport capacity of skeletal muscle are enhanced in response to physical training (2), it has not yet been resolved whether the arteriolar network responds in a similar fashion. Thus, in terms of the control of capillary perfusion discussed earlier, an important issue for future research is to resolve whether individual MVUs increase in size, total number, or both.

The capillary-to-fiber ratio can be remarkably consistent among muscles (or muscle regions) in the presence of large differences in capillary density. This is explained by corresponding differences in the diameter of muscle fibers. For example, the distance between capillaries will be less for type I muscle fibers (slow oxidative), which have a small diameter, than for type IIB muscle fibers (fast glycolytic), which have a larger diameter (14). The capillary supply of skeletal muscle considered in three dimensions is more accurately expressed in terms of volume density, that is, the total volume of capillaries per volume of muscle (15), as this estimate accounts for capillary tortuosity and branching that are not apparent in individual tissue cross-sections.

According to the Krogh cylinder model, an increase in metabolic rate will lower intracellular P_{O_2} in myocytes and increase the gradient for oxygen diffusion from the capillary to respiring mitochondria within muscle fibers. Once capillary P_{O_2} falls below a critical level, $\dot{V}_{O_2}$ becomes limited by blood flow through the capillary (16). The occurrence of flow-limited $\dot{V}_{O_2}$ can be delayed by perfusing additional capillaries (i.e., recruiting MVUs) as metabolic demand increases. This early response reduces the distance and increases the surface area for oxygen diffusion. The ability to increase capillary perfusion is augmented by capillary proliferation in response to physical conditioning (14). Furthermore, with smaller diffusion distances, capillary P_{O_2} can decrease and still maintain myocyte P_{O_2} above limiting values. This explains why an increase in capillary density enhances oxygen flux from blood to muscle fibers and supports the production of adenosine triphosphate (ATP) through aerobic metabolism. Nevertheless, structural indices alone cannot fully describe the physiological properties of capillary networks or the diffusion of oxygen from blood to muscle fibers. In part, this is because these indices assume that the oxygen content of capillary blood is homogeneous and that the capillary is the only source of oxygen to the muscle fibers. The following discussion illustrates why this fundamental assumption of the Krogh cylinder model is not correct.

Red Blood Cell Transit Time in Capillaries Is a Determinant of Oxygen Extraction

The time that RBCs remain within the capillaries is known as the RBC capillary transit time. It is proportional to the length of the path taken by a RBC from TA to collecting venule and inversely proportional to flow velocity (12). Intuitively, transit time affects the degree to which the oxygen content of the

capillary blood can be lowered; that is, longer transit times should facilitate oxygen extraction. At any given level of blood flow, transit time is also influenced by the total number (volume) of capillaries perfused. Acutely, this can be altered through MVU recruitment and over time by physical training (14). Thus, increasing the total number (volume density) of perfused capillaries will prolong transit times as a result of the greater cross-sectional area in which blood flow is distributed.

Measurements of total muscle blood flow and the estimated capillary density per unit volume of biopsied tissue have led to calculated mean capillary transit times of several seconds at rest to less than 1 second during heavy exercise. However, the idea of a mean capillary transit time is misleading, as it treats the flow of RBCs through capillaries as homogeneous. Direct observations using intravital microscopy have revealed both temporal and spatial heterogeneity in the flow of RBCs through capillary networks. Indeed, actual flow path lengths taken by RBCs (e.g., through interconnecting capillary branches) can be considerably greater than direct anatomical path lengths, resulting in a broad distribution of values for capillary transit time as well as for RBC flux (cells per second) and capillary flow path length (12). These dynamic rheological properties of blood flow suggest that individual capillaries are not uniform in their ability to supply oxygen to the surrounding tissue, though such heterogeneity can be offset by diffusional interactions within and among MVUs.

The RBC Content of Capillaries Increases During Hyperemia

The volume fraction of a capillary that is occupied by RBCs varies with the vasomotor state of resistance vessels and with the metabolic demand of muscle fibers (16). Capillary tube hematocrit is calculated from the number of RBCs per unit of capillary length based upon the volume of individual RBCs and the volume of the capillary. As the amount of oxygen dissolved in plasma is negligible compared to that bound to hemoglobin, tube hematocrit provides an index of capillary oxygen content at any given moment. Capillary hematocrit can be less than 20% of systemic hematocrit in resting muscle, but during hyperemia it increases rapidly to approximate that of the systemic circulation (16). Thus, the oxygen content of a capillary will increase with the number of RBCs it contains, which has the effect of maintaining a higher P_{O_2} along the capillary at a given level of $\dot{V}_{O_2}$. Further, by reducing plasma gaps between RBCs, an increase in capillary hematocrit during high $\dot{V}_{O_2}$ can augment the effective capillary surface for oxygen diffusion to myocytes even with no change in the total number of capillaries perfused.

Changes in capillary hematocrit are explained by the presence of a glycocalyx on the luminal surface of the capillary that can change its thickness according to the level of capillary blood flow. At rest (i.e., with low tube hematocrit), the endothelial cell glycocalyx results in a layer of stabilized plasma adjacent to the capillary wall that is nearly a micrometer thick and excludes RBCs. Remarkably, the thickness of this cell-free layer is diminished during hyperemia, when the flux of RBCs and capillary hematocrit increase during vasodilation. In addition to enabling more of the capillary volume to fill with RBCs, the diffusion distance between RBCs and muscle fibers is reduced, as the RBCs are closer to the capillary wall. Although capillary diameter is typically not considered to be a variable during exercise, this dynamic and reversible expansion of the capillary lumen can augment oxygen transport during exercise hyperemia. Thus, the ability of individual capillaries to deliver oxygen to muscle fibers is enhanced in response to an increase in metabolic demand.

Oxygen Diffuses out of Arterioles and Between Microvessels

Inherent to the idea that the capillary is the only source of oxygen delivery to the tissue is the assumption that the oxygen content of blood decreases progressively along the capillary. However, studies of the living microcirculation reveal this to be an oversimplification (17). For example, countercurrent flow of RBCs in overlapping diffusion fields from adjacent MVUs may lead to mixing of capillary P_{O_2} rather than a progressive arterial-to-venous P_{O_2} gradient along each capillary. Indeed, mean P_{O_2} within individual capillaries, as well as arterioles and venules, can increase as well as decrease within 1 second, attributable to the gain and loss of oxygen to and from neighboring microvessels by diffusion. Further, the findings indicate that RBCs can release substantive amounts of oxygen before reaching the capillaries (17). This should not be surprising, as smooth muscle cells surrounding the endothelium present little barrier to the diffusion of oxygen across the arteriolar wall.

While the P_{O_2} of venous blood reflects the extraction of oxygen within the muscle, it does not provide an accurate index of the local gradients driving oxygen diffusion from RBCs to mitochondria. For example, any variation in the flux of oxygen from individual capillaries (e.g., due to changes in velocity, flux, or spacing of RBCs) would be masked in a time-averaged blood sample. In turn, when capillaries supplied from different TAs empty into a collecting venule, the returning blood mixes from respective MVUs and reaches some intermediate level of P_{O_2}. This homogenization is cumulative as venules converge and carry blood back toward the heart. Superimposed upon the temporal and spatial mixing of postcapillary blood is the diffusion of oxygen from capillaries and arterioles in proximity to venules, which may set a lower limit on the amount of oxygen that can actually be extracted from the blood. Nevertheless, these diffusive interactions between microvessels help to offset local heterogeneities in oxygen content and P_{O_2}.

The focus on regulating blood flow through the peripheral circulation in terms of oxygen transport raises the question whether oxygen delivery or tissue P_{O_2} is actually regulated. In skeletal muscle, arteriolar diameter changes with ambient oxygen tension, constricting with an increase in P_{O_2} and dilating with a fall in P_{O_2}. This interaction demonstrates that the resistance vasculature is indeed sensitive to the balance between oxygen supply and demand. Remarkably, rather than changes in tissue P_{O_2} providing the vasoactive stimulus, the RBC itself may act as the oxygen sensor. Through this mechanism, as RBCs enter a region of increased metabolic demand relative to supply, the fall in hemoglobin oxygen saturation evokes the release of a vasodilator substance (e.g., ATP) to reduce arteriolar tone (18). In contrast to being tightly regulated (i.e., within a few torr), tissue P_{O_2} in skeletal muscle has a broad distribution (19) that can shift according to local changes in oxygen supply and consumption. Within myocytes, particularly those adapted to endurance exercise, the presence of myoglobin serves to buffer intracellular P_{O_2} above the level required to support mitochondrial respiration. Nevertheless, with respect to whether the peripheral circulation can support aerobic metabolism, the critical issue is whether (and if so, how much of) the distribution of muscle P_{O_2} falls below that which supports the aerobic production of ATP.

Blood Flow Is Controlled in Response to the Metabolic Demand of Skeletal Muscle Fibers

We now explore how blood flow is controlled in response to the metabolic demand of muscle fibers. These regulatory mechanisms are intrinsic to skeletal muscle and its vascular supply. We then consider how the sympathetic nervous system exerts extrinsic control over the vascular supply in the context of redistribution of cardiac output and maintenance of arterial blood pressure during exercise (3). Figure 14.6 illustrates the multiple dimensions of blood flow control at rest and during activity.

Muscle Blood Flow Increases With Oxidative Capacity

Blood flow to exercising muscle is proportional to the oxidative capacity of its constituent fibers. In rats, blood flow during exercise is highest in muscles and muscle regions that are composed primarily of oxidative fibers and lowest where fibers are primarily glycolytic (2). Differential control of blood flow in accord with muscle fiber type may be ex-

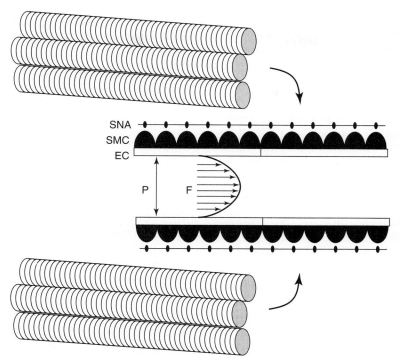

FIGURE 14.6 Multiple stimuli determine vasomotor tone in resistance vessels of skeletal muscle. Summary illustration depicts a segment of an arteriole embedded in muscle fibers (not to scale). The vessel is sectioned along its axis to show endothelial cells (EC) lining the lumen and circumscribed by smooth muscle cells (SMC), which are therefore in cross-section. In resting skeletal muscle, basal vasomotor tone reflects the interplay between two hemodynamic forces: transmural distending pressure (P), which promotes myogenic vasoconstriction, and blood flow (F) through the lumen, which exerts shear stress on the endothelium (indicated by parabolic flow profile; *arrows* indicate relative velocity) to stimulate the production of vasodilator autocoids (e.g., prostacyclin and NO). Perivascular sympathetic nerve activity (SNA) increases vasomotor tone, whereas contraction of muscle fibers leads to the production of vasodilator stimuli (*arrows*) that reduce vasomotor tone.

plained not only by the pattern of motor unit recruitment but also by complementary adaptations in the architecture and reactivity of resistance vessels that supply muscles or muscle regions containing a predominance of a particular fiber type. Although human skeletal muscle characteristically lacks such regional differences in fiber type (14), this property does not preclude the ability of the vascular network to direct flow to particular muscles or muscle regions according to their capacity for oxidative metabolism and the organization of their vascular supply.

Motor Unit Recruitment Promotes Capillary Perfusion

The greater distances spanned by muscle fibers (several centimeters) as compared to MVUs (1–2 mm) implies that for capillary perfusion to increase along the fiber, a mechanism is required whereby the perfusion of multiple MVUs is coordinated in some manner. Further, the dispersion throughout a muscle of the individual muscle fibers belonging to each motor unit implies that perfusion to regions of inactive muscle must increase to increase the perfusion of capillaries associated with active fibers (10). While such perfusion of inactive fibers may appear wasteful, this initial response can effectively provide a feed-forward mechanism of oxygen supply, because the perfusion of MVUs precedes the activation of most muscle fibers in a given MVU (10). Hence, upon the recruitment of additional motor units, capillaries already contain RBCs, which would help to minimize any delay in elevating aerobic metabolism (20). Indeed, this relationship explains how prior warmup activity can facilitate ensuing performance at higher intensity.

Further, rapidly increasing the functional capillary surface area facilitates the extraction of oxygen until substantial increases in total muscle blood flow occur (1). We now consider the coordination of vasodilation among branches of the resistance network.

Vasodilation Ascends the Resistance Network as Metabolic Demand Increases

The determinants of $\dot{V}O_2$ are expressed by the Fick relationship, which states that the oxygen consumed by a tissue is the product of its convective delivery through the peripheral circulation and its extraction through diffusion into muscle fibers. In resting skeletal muscle, the resistance vasculature maintains a high level of vasomotor tone, and the removal of oxygen from the blood is only a few of its (typically) 20 vol% (1). In response to metabolic stress, the initial response is to increase the extraction of available oxygen. This is accomplished through a fall in myocyte PO_2, which increases the gradient for oxygen diffusion, along with the increase in capillary perfusion (i.e., dilation of TAs and recruitment of MVUs). These initial responses account for the large fall in venous PO_2 at the onset of exercise and during mild activity (1). Greater total delivery of oxygen through the peripheral circulation is necessary to prevent a fall in tissue PO_2 below levels necessary to sustain oxidative metabolism.

Once a TA dilates and MVUs are perfused, the volume of blood delivered into capillaries is governed by dilation of proximal vessel branches. As metabolic demand increases, vasodilation progressively ascends from the distal arterioles into larger arterioles and their feed arteries (21). Remember that these proximal branches govern the total amount of blood flowing into the muscle. The contributions of proximal and distal resistance vessels to the control of muscle blood flow can be represented using a simple model of resistance elements connected in series (Milestone of Discovery). With high levels of resting tone throughout the resistance network, dilation of distal branches would increase blood flow, but this response would be restricted by proximal segments. In contrast, when proximal vessels dilate in concert with distal vessels, major increases in muscle blood flow are obtained.

The coordination of vasodilation between distal and proximal branches is intrinsic to the resistance vasculature and is essential to achieving maximal perfusion of skeletal muscle as the intensity of exercise increases. Consistent with this relationship, dilation of feed arteries as well as arterioles increases progressively with duty cycle and with motor unit recruitment (21). The integrated response of the resistance vasculature is reflected by the large increase in oxygen extraction at exercise onset and during light activity, leading to a progressive increase in total flow as workload increases (1).

Multiple Signaling Pathways Govern Functional Hyperemia

Muscular activity produces a multitude of signals that contribute to functional hyperemia. No single stimulus or signaling pathway can explain the complex physiological response of muscle blood flow to contracting muscle fibers. Rather, the initiation and maintenance of functional hyperemia reflects the integration of multiple stimuli that vary temporally as well as spatially through the resistance network. Furthermore, the effectiveness of a given stimulus can vary among vessel branches. These relationships are illustrated in Figure 14.7. The intent here is not to define the mechanism or site of action for each known stimulus but to use examples that illustrate how vascular resistance may be governed in response to a variety of signaling events. Therefore, in describing regulatory pathways, examples are intended to be conceptual rather than highly detailed.

Contraction and Relaxation of Vascular Smooth Muscle Controls Vascular Resistance

Blood flow control reflects changes in vessel diameter that result from the contraction or relaxation of smooth muscle cells. The contraction of smooth muscle typically results from an increase in the free (i.e., unbound) concentration of intracellular Ca^{++}. The influx of Ca^{++} through the plasma membrane is controlled largely by voltage-operated L-type Ca^{++} channels (LTCC). The conductance of these channels increases with depolarization and decreases with hyperpolarization. In turn, the entry of Ca^{++} through LTCC is modulated largely through the activity of K^+ channels, which hyperpolarize cells as their conductance increases (22). Free intracellular Ca^{++} is also derived internally from the endoplasmic reticulum. The release of Ca^{++} from internal stores is largely independent of membrane potential and is affected via second messengers (e.g. inositol triphosphate, IP_3) generated by receptor-mediated signaling events at the plasma membrane. Thus, events that suppress the production of IP_3 also promote vasodilation. Unlike skeletal or cardiac muscle, vascular smooth muscle can alter its contractile activity independent of changes in Ca^{++} through changes in the phosphorylation state of regulatory proteins and the sensitivity of contractile proteins to Ca^{++}. Stimulation of endothelial cells can also produce smooth muscle cell hyperpolarization through K^+ channel activation. For example, metabolites of arachidonic acid released by the endothelium stimulate calcium-activated K^+ channels in the smooth muscle membrane to produce hyperpolarization and relaxation (23). The endothelium-dependent vasodilator acetylcholine also acts through this signaling pathway. Because many of these regulatory events have been defined in isolated vessel and vascular cell preparations, a considerable amount of additional research is required before their role in controlling the peripheral circulation during exercise can be estab-

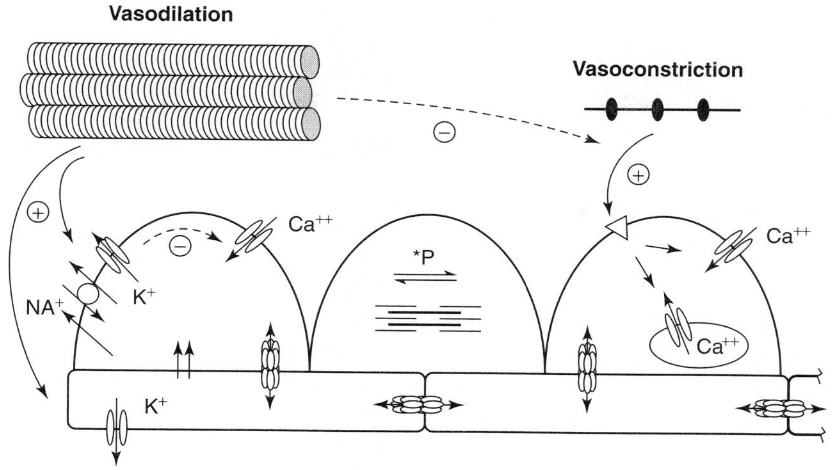

FIGURE 14.7 Multiple signaling pathways interact to determine whether vasodilation or vasoconstriction prevails during exercise. Summary illustration depicts the production of vasodilator stimuli from the contractile activity of muscle fibers and vasoconstriction through sympathetic nerve activity (SNA). Three smooth muscle cells (SMCs) are shown above a pair of adjacent endothelial cells (ECs; not to scale). On the left, vasodilation results from hyperpolarization of the SMC through the activation of K^+ channels and/or stimulation of the Na^+/K^+ pump in the plasma membrane. Alternatively, activation of K^+ channels in ECs can produce smooth muscle hyperpolarization by current flow through myoendothelial gap junctions (vertical bidirectional channels). Hyperpolarization of SMCs inhibits the influx of Ca^{++} across their plasma membrane through L-type Ca^{++} channels (LTCC) (*broken line*). Relaxation of SMC can also be effected via stimulation of EC to produce vasodilator autocoids (*double arrow*). Cell-to-cell coupling along ECs through gap junctions (horizontal bidirectional channels) enables hyperpolarization to travel along the vessel wall and thereby coordinate relaxation of SMCs within and between vessel branches. As shown on the right, SNA during exercise releases norepinephrine that diffuses to its receptors on nearby SMC to promote the opening of LTCC in the plasma membrane and release of Ca^{++} from internal stores to produce vasoconstriction. Sympathetic vasoconstriction is antagonized (*broken line*) by products of muscle fiber contraction. The middle SMC indicates that contractile status can also be altered independently of changes in membrane potential or intracellular $[Ca^{++}]$, for example through modulation of regulatory kinase and phosphatase activities (**P*) and alterations in the sensitivity of the contractile machinery to intracellular $[Ca^{++}]$.

lished. Nevertheless, vasodilator signals can act directly on the smooth muscle cell or indirectly via the endothelium.

Transmural Pressure and Luminal Shear Stress Interact to Determine Vasomotor Tone

The vasculature is continually exposed to transmural pressure (tangential wall stress) and luminal shear stress. These mechanical forces give rise to myogenic (24) and flow-mediated (25) mechanisms of vasomotor control, respectively. In the absence of sympathetic nerve activity (SNA, discussed later), these regulatory processes interact to establish the resting contractile state, or spontaneous vasomotor tone, of vascular smooth muscle cells throughout the resistance network (Fig. 14.6). Resistance vessels sup-

plying skeletal muscle typically rest at 50 to 70% of their maximal diameter (21).

Myogenic Autoregulation Is Governed by Smooth Muscle Cells

Smooth muscle cells of resistance vessels are inherently responsive to changes in transmural pressure. Through this mechanism, an increase in circumferential wall stress (proportional to the product of transmural pressure and lumen radius; inversely proportional to vessel wall thickness) stimulates smooth muscle contraction. This response is explained by mechanical transduction (e.g., through integrins) leading to depolarization and the activation of LTCC (24). Thus, with an increase in transmural pressure (and wall stress), the influx of Ca^{++} into smooth muscle cells produces vasoconstriction, which restores wall stress. With chronic elevation of pressure (days to weeks, such as occurs in hypertension), the vessel remodels around a smaller lumen and with a thicker media. In skeletal muscle, as observed in the cerebral and renal circulations, myogenic autoregulation of vasomotor tone acts to maintain the constancy of tissue blood flow throughout the physiological range of perfusion pressures. With skeletal muscle contraction, the increase in tissue pressure can reduce transmural pressure (upon muscle relaxation) throughout the arteriolar network and result in vasodilation. In this manner, myogenic vasodilation can provide a transient increase in muscle blood flow following a vigorous contraction until the initial transmural pressure and myogenic tone are restored.

Flow-mediated Vasodilation Is Governed by Endothelial Cells

The flow of blood exerts shear stress (proportional to the product of blood flow velocity and blood viscosity, related inversely to luminal diameter) on the endothelial cells lining the vessel lumen. The endothelium responds by releasing autacoids (e.g., nitric oxide and metabolites of arachidonic acid) that induce relaxation of adjacent smooth muscle cells. Shear stress also hyperpolarizes endothelial cells by activating K^+ channels in the plasma membrane; this electrical signal can be transmitted directly to smooth muscle (Fig. 14.7), where hyperpolarization will inhibit LTCC and produce relaxation. The following example of autoregulation illustrates how pressure and flow interact dynamically to establish a prevailing level of vasomotor tone. An increase in perfusion pressure will produce myogenic vasoconstriction and increase luminal shear stress, which in turn stimulates the endothelium to promote smooth muscle relaxation and restore the initial diameter. Conversely, with a fall in perfusion pressure, myogenic relaxation reduces shear stress and diminishes the production of autacoids by the endothelium, which reduces the magnitude of vasodilation. In this manner, flow-mediated vasodilation can provide negative feedback to both myogenic vasoconstriction and vasodilation.

When blood flow remains elevated, vessels remodel over days to weeks to form an enlarged lumen through arteriogenesis (26). This mechanism can increase the conductance of supplying vessels and is especially important in the development of collateral circulation when the primary vascular supply is insufficient or interrupted. Signaling events underlying arteriogenesis include macrophage infiltration along with the release of growth factors and proteolytic enzymes essential to remodeling of the extracellular matrix. Complementary signaling events result in sprouting and proliferation of capillary endothelial cells (angiogenesis) in response to elevated shear stress as well as mechanical stretch (27). Taken together, these adaptations of the pe-

ripheral vasculature contribute to the enhanced vascular transport capacity of skeletal muscle in response to exercise conditioning (2).

Metabolic Vasodilators Initiate and Sustain Vasodilation

The metabolic theory of blood flow control is based upon the release of vasodilator substances from active muscle fibers in proportion to their energy expenditure (Fig. 14.6). These substances then diffuse to relax the arteriolar smooth muscle cells, producing vasodilation (28). The ensuing increase in blood flow removes vasoactive metabolites as they diffuse into capillaries and are carried away in the venous effluent. Through such negative feedback, hyperemia is maintained during activity at a level that is commensurate with the intensity of metabolic demand. Research into the regulation of the peripheral circulation has increasingly focused on the role of ion channels as sites of action for metabolic vasodilators (Fig. 14.7). For example, extracellular K^+ concentration ($[K^+]_o$) increases at the onset of muscle contraction. From a resting ($[K^+]_o$) of about 5 mM, a 5- to 10-mM increase in ($[K^+]_o$) will activate inward-rectifying K^+ channels to promote K^+ efflux and hyperpolarization. The elevation in ($[K^+]_o$) can also stimulate Na^+-K^+ ATPase to hyperpolarize the smooth muscle cell membrane. However, the increase in ($[K^+]_o$) from active skeletal muscle cells is transitory, and it is unlikely that K^+ mediates sustained elevations in muscle blood flow.

Steady-state contractions are associated with a sustained reduction in P_{O_2} and corresponding elevation of P_{CO_2} in the venous blood. Both of these signals have long been implicated in the maintenance of functional hyperemia, and recent studies have shown both gases to modulate the activity of ion channels in vascular smooth muscle. For example, in addition to the effect of changing P_{O_2} on the metabolic production of vasodilators (e.g., adenosine), a more direct effect involves modulating the activation of LTCC (e.g., depolarization and Ca^{++} influx with elevated P_{O_2}; hyperpolarization and relaxation as P_{O_2} falls). In a complementary manner, activation of ATP-sensitive K^+ channels with a fall in P_{O_2} would promote vasodilation through hyperpolarization and inactivation of LTCC (Fig. 14.7). As discussed earlier, local reductions in tissue P_{O_2} may act indirectly by stimulating RBCs to release ATP and promote vasodilation, thereby increasing oxygen delivery according to increases in metabolic demand. Indeed, recent findings in humans are consistent with such a mechanism for governing exercise hyperemia, particularly during steady-state activity (29).

Venules also serve an important though often unrecognized role in the metabolic control of peripheral resistance. Adhesive junctions between endothelial cells of the venular wall are not as tight as those in arterioles or capillaries. This difference results in greater permeability of venular endothelium, which allows vasoactive metabolites carried in the effluent blood (e.g., adenosine) to pass readily into the interstitium. Thus, where venules run across or countercurrent to arterioles, metabolites can diffuse down their concentration gradients to influence the contractile status of arteriolar smooth muscle (30). Venular endothelial cells can also release dilator autacoids in response to chemical or physical stimuli. Thus, vasodilator stimuli arising from venules provide concerted feedback for governing arteriolar diameter and local blood flow in accord with the metabolic status and oxygen consumption of dependent muscle fibers (30).

Conducted Vasodilation Coordinates Vasomotor Control

Up to this point, we have focused on vasomotor responses of smooth muscle cells directly or indirectly (via endothelial cells) exposed to a stimulus. However, with vascular resistance distributed among proximal as well as distal branches of the precapillary network, vasodilation constrained to the vicinity of a local stimulus has little effect on local blood flow. In contrast, when vasodilation spreads from the local stimulus to encompass proximal branches, blood flow into the affected region readily increases (31). We now consider how vasoactive signals initiated at distinct sites within a muscle can travel rapidly along resistance networks over considerable distances.

The conduction of vasodilation is enabled through gap junction channels in the vessel wall, particularly those expressed at the cell borders of endothelial cells (Fig. 14.3). The strong electrical coupling and the axial orientation of endothelial cells promote signal transmission along and between vessel branches. Gap junction channels are also expressed between smooth muscle cells and between smooth muscle cells and endothelial cells. Analogous to the spread of electrical activity in the heart, electrical signals initiated in one location can thereby travel rapidly from cell to cell along the vessel wall. Indeed, conduction along the endothelium and into smooth muscle underlies the ability of feed arteries to dilate in concert with arterioles and thereby attain peak levels of muscle blood flow during contractile activity (31). Conduction can also be initiated from capillaries and possibly venules (18), with vasoactive signals traveling upstream into corresponding TAs and their parent branches. This signaling pathway provides an explanation of how MVU perfusion may be coordinated along (and among) active muscle fibers to increase the functional capillary surface area discussed earlier. Further, responses initiated in separate MVUs or arteriolar branches can be summed and integrated in their parent vessels. In this manner, vasomotor response of parent vessels reflects the integration of input from daughter branches along with vasoactive metabolites released in the vicinity of arteriolar smooth muscle cells (Fig. 14.7). This concerted behavior is consistent with vasodilation progressively ascending from distal into proximal vessels as the intensity of metabolic demand increases (21), resulting in greater blood flow and oxygen delivery.

The physiological stimulus (or stimuli) for conducted vasodilation with muscle fiber contraction has yet to be established. Indeed, multiple signals could produce an electrical signal that can travel from cell to cell along the vessel wall. Under experimental conditions, the nature of conduction has been studied extensively using acetylcholine for its consistency in triggering conducted responses. In skeletal muscle, the end plate of motor nerves is the apparent physiological source of this neurotransmitter. Although it remains controversial whether spillover of acetylcholine from neuromuscular junctions can trigger conducted vasodilation on nearby capillary or arteriolar endothelial cells, growing evidence points to rapid vasodilation that is initiated with the onset of muscle fiber recruitment. This rapid response may serve in the initial stages of matching MVU perfusion with metabolic demand and in coordinating the dilation of feed arteries with arterioles as the hyperemic response fully develops. Also, vasodilation initiated on distal arterioles will increase blood flow through their parent arterioles and feed arteries. In turn, the elevated shear stress in these proximal vessels can further promote and sustain vasodilation, albeit with a slower time course than for conduction. Thus, flow-mediated vasodilation may further contribute to maintaining a sustained increase in muscle blood flow during exercise.

Sympathetic Vasoconstriction Interacts With Functional Vasodilation to Establish Peripheral Vascular Resistance

Sympathetic nerve activity (SNA) increases with the mass of muscle recruited during exercise in accordance with the intensity of muscular contractions (3). Understanding the interaction between functional vasodilation and sympathetic vasoconstriction has long been a subject of intense study of the peripheral circulation, with controversial findings. On one hand, sympathetic vasoconstriction can restrict blood flow to exercising muscle; this effect is particularly apparent when another large mass of muscle is active simultaneously and demands a substantial portion of cardiac output (3). On the other hand, sympathetic vasoconstriction is impaired during muscle contractions. To address this dichotomy, recognize that the interaction between muscle contraction and SNA in controlling vessel diameter is graded with the intensity of respective stimuli and with the location of vessel branches within the resistance network (32).

When an isolated muscle group is exercising, muscle blood flow may be "excessive," as indicated by oxygen extraction across the leg of 12 to 15 vol% at maximal $\dot{V}O_2$ (1). The extraction of oxygen by active muscle increases when its blood flow is restricted, indicating that muscle fibers are more effective in removing oxygen from the blood as flow becomes limiting. Thus, as SNA increases, vasodilation prevails in distal arterioles to promote capillary perfusion and the extraction of oxygen, while the total increase of blood flow into the muscle is restricted progressively through constriction of feed arteries and primary arterioles (32). Because feed arteries are external to the muscle, they are not directly exposed to the products of metabolism. In such manner, these vessels serve as a key site for maintaining total peripheral resistance and arterial pressure during peak demands on cardiac output (3).

The inhibition of sympathetic vasoconstriction may occur presynaptically by preventing neurotransmitter release as well as postsynaptically by interfering with intracellular signaling pathways activated by norepinephrine on vascular smooth muscle. In addition, the conduction of vasodilation can attenuate sympathetic vasoconstriction, providing a complementary signaling pathway for antagonizing the effect of SNA on arteriolar resistance. Another mechanism for inhibiting the vasoconstrictor effect of SNA occurs as a result of increasing Ca^{++} in smooth muscle subsequent to the activation of α-adrenoreceptors. This response establishes a diffusion gradient for Ca^{++} into endothelial cells through myoendothelial gap junctions. As Ca^{++} enters the endothelium, it stimulates production of nitric oxide and activation of K^+ channels, both of which counter the vasoconstriction (33). Thus, multiple mechanisms can inhibit sympathetic vasoconstriction during muscular activity.

The Muscle Pump Promotes Exercise Hyperemia

Muscle blood flow is typically evaluated as a mean value over time and is proportional to exercise intensity and the oxidative capacity of active muscle fibers (2). However, with each contraction, the rhythmic changes in length and tension produce cyclic oscillations in intramuscular pressure. With venous valves preventing backflow, the squeezing and emptying of veins propels blood away from the muscle and back to the heart. Thus, in the presence of constant arterial pressure, the reduction in venous pressure during relaxation increases the pressure gradient for capillary perfusion. As vasodilation ensues, the volume of blood within the muscle increases during the period of filling between contractions. Thus ejection of blood from active muscle during each contraction increases until a steady level of hyperemia is attained (34). In addition, this pumping action of skeletal muscle on the peripheral vasculature imparts substantial kinetic energy to the blood, thereby reducing stress on the heart. Indeed, as much as half of the total energy required for circulating the blood during exercise may be generated by the muscle pump, and this kinetic energy is essential to achieving the high blood flows that accompany maximal aerobic exercise (2).

SUMMARY: VASOMOTOR RESPONSES ARE INTEGRATED AND COORDINATED DURING BLOOD FLOW CONTROL TO SKELETAL MUSCLE

This chapter describes the organization and control of peripheral circulation to skeletal muscle in the context of exercise hyperemia. We consider the functional anatomy of the resistance network, the cellular signaling pathways within and between smooth muscle and endothelium, how the activity of muscle fibers gives rise to vasomotor responses that encompass progressively greater portions of the resistance network, and how (as well as where) sympathetic innervation competes with functional vasodilation. It is apparent that the response of the peripheral circulation to the activity of skeletal muscle requires coordination among a diverse array of vasoactive signals. At each level of the resistance network, vascular smooth muscle serves as an integrator of signals that arise from muscle fiber contraction. This occurs against the background of hemodynamic forces acting on the vessel wall, the activity of perivascular sympathetic nerves, and the mechanical effects of rhythmic muscle contractions.

At rest, in the absence of SNA, vasomotor tone and peripheral vascular resistance manifest the interaction between myogenic contraction of vascular smooth muscle cells and its modulation by the endothelium in response to luminal shear stress. Functional hyperemia has long been attributed to the production and release of vasodilator substances from active muscle fibers (28). However, metabolic vasodilation requires at least 5 to 6 seconds for substances to be produced by skeletal muscle fibers and diffuse to arteriolar smooth muscle cells in sufficient concentration to elicit vasodilation. In practice, these processes are too slow to account for the rapid onset (within 1 or 2 seconds) of functional hyperemia (35). While the muscle pump rapidly promotes venous return and increases the driving pressure for capillary perfusion, it is not fully effective until vasodilation has ensued. Thus, the rapid onset of vasodilation, together with the coordinated increase in capillary perfusion, may best be explained by the initiation and conduction of vasodilation coincident with motor unit recruitment, with metabolic and flow-mediated vasodilation governing steady-state components of the hyperemic response, which is further enhanced by the muscle pump.

Vasodilation triggered by muscle fiber activation ascends from terminal arterioles into proximal arterioles and feed arteries as metabolic demand increases. Indeed, dilation of these proximal resistance vessels is integral to the full expression of functional hyperemia. The location of feed arteries external to the muscle physically removes them from the direct influence of the vasoactive products of muscular activity. It is at this level of the peripheral circulation where sympathetic vasoconstriction effectively limits blood flow during exercise. Under such conditions, the volume of blood flow to active muscle (and thereby its oxygen consumption) is restricted while extraction is optimized by dilation of arterioles within the muscle.

A MILESTONE OF DISCOVERY

Where and how is muscle blood flow actually controlled? Through the 1960s, it was recognized that different segments of the vasculature varied in their responses to vasoactive stimuli. In the mesenteric microcirculation, the sensitivity to humoral stimuli increased from proximal resistance vessels to the precapillary sphincters, yet these distal vessels appeared to be less responsive to sympathetic vasoconstriction. Others found that the functional capillary surface area of skeletal muscle remained high despite flow restriction during SNA.

Folkow and coworkers tested the hypothesis that the site of flow restriction to skeletal muscle during SNA would vary over time and with metabolic demand. The nerve and vascular supply to calf muscles were isolated in anesthetized cats, and total blood flow into the muscle was measured with a flowmeter. Blood pressure was measured at three key sites: upstream from the muscle in the femoral artery (Pa), downstream from the muscle in the femoral vein (Pv), and at an intermediate site (Pi) represented by the sural artery. The contributions of proximal resistance arteries (Rp) and distal precapillary arterioles (Rd) to total vascular resistance (Rt) were evaluated according to a model of resistive segments arranged in series, where Rt = Rp + Rd (Fig. 14.8). Relative to control conditions, an increase in Rd/Rt indicated that distal vessels had constricted more than proximal vessels. Conversely, a fall in Rd/Rt indicated that the proximal vessels were constricted more than distal vessels.

Blood flow decreased as Rt increased in resting muscle during SNA, while the ratio of Rd to Rt increased transiently and then

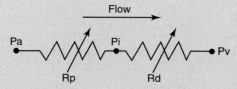

FIGURE 14.8 The contributions of proximal resistance arteries (Rp) and distal precapillary arterioles (Rd) to total vascular resistance (Rt) were evaluated according to a model of resistive segments arranged in series, where Rt = Rp + Rd.

declined as SNA was maintained. This behavior indicated that distal vessels were initially the primary site of constriction and then reversed to dilation over time, while constriction of the proximal vessels accounted for the sustained increase in Rt. In response to rhythmic muscle contractions, Rt decreased over time, with two characteristic components to the response: Rd fell rapidly over about the first 30 seconds and was attributed to the action of vasodilator metabolites on precapillary arterioles. This was succeeded by a decline in Rp over several minutes, indicating that vasodilation progressively ascended into the resistance arteries as exercise continued. When SNA was performed during steady-state muscle contractions, the increase in Rt was much lower than in resting muscle, and Rd/Rt declined. Thus, sympathetic vasoconstriction appeared to be inhibited in distal branches but sustained in proximal branches.

These insightful experiments resolved distinct components of the integrated vasomotor response to SNA, to muscle contraction, and to the nature of interaction between these opposing stimuli. Remarkably, another decade would elapse before the role of the endothelium in governing vasodilation was ascertained. Entire journals and books are now dedicated to research on this cellular monolayer that lines the entire cardiovascular system.

The predictions of vascular function that were made from the classic whole-organ experiments of Folkow and coworkers have been confirmed and extended using intravital microscopy. Complementary studies have demonstrated regional differences in the expression and inhibition of adrenoreceptor subtypes that mediate sympathetic vasoconstriction. The expression and regulation of ion channels and signaling pathways that govern and coordinate the contractile status of vascular smooth muscle cells are also now known to display regional variations in the peripheral vasculature. Furthering our understanding of the role of exercise in modifying the cellular, molecular, and genomic regulation of vascular smooth muscle and endothelium has broad implications for ameliorating such widespread diseases of the peripheral vasculature as atherosclerosis, diabetes, and hypertension.

Folkow B, Sonnenschein RR, Wright DL. Loci of neurogenic and metabolic effects on precapillary vessels of skeletal muscle. Acta Physiol Scand 1971;81:459–471.

ACKNOWLEDGMENTS

Support for this work was provided by the National Institutes of Health, grants RO1-HL56786, RO1-HL41026 and R21-AG19347. S.E.B. was supported by NIH T32-NS07455.

REFERENCES

1. Andersen P, Saltin B. Maximal perfusion of skeletal muscle in man. J Physiol 1985;366:233–249.

2. Laughlin MH, Korthius RJ, Duncker DJ, et al. Control of blood flow to cardiac and skeletal muscle during exercise. In Rowell LB, Shepherd JT, eds. Handbook of Physiology, Section 12: Exercise: Regulation and Integration of Multiple Systems. New York: Oxford University, 1996;705–769.

3. Rowell LB, O'Leary DS, Kellog DLJ. Integration of cardiovascular control systems in dynamic exercise. In Rowell LB, Shepherd JT, eds. Handbook of Physiology, Section 12: Exercise: Regulation and Integration of Multiple Systems. New York: Oxford University, 1996;770–838.

4. Christensen KL, Mulvany MJ. Location of resistance arteries. J Vasc Res 2001;38:1–12.

5. Delashaw JB, Duling BR. A study of the functional elements regulating capillary perfusion in striated muscle. Microvasc Res 1988;36:162–171.

6. Rhodin JA. The ultrastructure of mammalian arterioles and precapillary sphincters. J Ultrastruct Res 1967;18:181–223.

7. Marshall JM. The venous vessel within skeletal muscle. NIPS 1991;6:11–15.

8. Greensmith JE, Duling BR. Morphology of the constricted arteriolar wall: physiological implications. Am J Physiol 1984;247:H687–698.

9. Bloch EH, Iberall AS. Toward a concept of the functional unit of mammalian skeletal muscle. Am J Physiol 1982; 242:R411–420.

10. Fuglevand AJ, Segal SS. Simulation of motor unit recruitment and microvascular unit perfusion: spatial considerations. J Appl Physiol 1997;83:1223–1234.

11. Klitzman B, Damon DN, Gorczynski RJ, et al. Augmented tissue oxygen supply during striated muscle contraction in the hamster: relative contributions of capillary recruitment, functional dilation, and reduced tissue Po_2. Circ Res 1982; 51:711–721.

12. Sarelius IH. Cell flow path influences transit time through striated muscle capillaries. Am J Physiol 1986;250:H899–907.

13. Krogh A. The number and distribution of capillaries in muscles with calculations of the oxygen pressure head necessary for supplying the tissue. J Physiol 1918;52:409–415.

14. Saltin BG, Gollnick PD. Skeletal muscle adaptability: significance for metabolism and performance. In Peachey LD, ed. Handbook of Physiology, Section 10: Skeletal Muscle. Bethesda, MD: American Physiological Society, 1983;555–631.

15. Weibel ER. Scaling of structural and functional variables in the respiratory system. Annu Rev Physiol 1987;49:147–159.

16. Duling BR, Desjardins C. Capillary hematocrit: what does it mean? NIPS 1987;2:66–69.

17. Tsai AG, Johnson PC, Intaglietta M. Oxygen gradients in the microcirculation. Physiol Rev 2003;83:933–963.

18. Ellsworth ML. Red blood cell-derived ATP as a regulator of skeletal muscle perfusion. Med Sci Sports Exerc 2004;36: 35–41.

19. Lund N, Jorfeldt L, Lewis DH. Skeletal muscle oxygen pressure fields in healthy human volunteers: a study of the normal state and the effects of different arterial oxygen pressures. Acta Anaesth Scand 1980;24:272–278.

20. Bearden SE, Moffatt RJ. $\dot{V}o_2$ and heart rate kinetics in cycling: transitions from an elevated baseline. J Appl Physiol 2001; 90:2081–2087.

21. VanTeeffelen, JW, Segal SS. Effect of motor unit recruitment on functional vasodilatation in hamster retractor muscle. J Physiol 2000;524:267–278.

22. Jackson WF. Ion channels and vascular tone. Hypertension 2000;35:173–178.

23. Busse R, Edwards G, Feletou M, et al. EDHF: bringing the concepts together. Trends Pharmacol Sci 2002;23:374.

24. Davis MJ, Hill MA. Signaling mechanisms underlying the vascular myogenic response. Physiol Rev 1999;79:387–423.

25. Davies PF. Flow-mediated endothelial mechanotransduction. Physiol Rev 1995;75:519–560.

26. Schaper W, Scholz D. Factors regulating arteriogenesis. Arterioscler Thromb Vasc Biol 2003;23:1143–1151.

27. Haas TL. Molecular control of capillary growth in skeletal muscle. Can J Appl Physiol 2002;27:491–515.

28. Haddy FJ, Scott JB. Metabolic factors in peripheral circulatory regulation. Fed Proc 1975;34:2006–2011.

29. Gonzalez-Alonso J, Olsen DB, Saltin B. Erythrocyte and the regulation of human skeletal muscle blood flow and oxygen delivery: role of circulating ATP. Circ Res 2002;91: 1046–1055.

30. Hester RL, Hammer LW. Venular-arteriolar communication in the regulation of blood flow. Am J Physiol 2002;282: R1280–1285.

31. Segal SS, Jacobs TL. Role for endothelial cell conduction in ascending vasodilatation and exercise hyperaemia in hamster skeletal muscle. J Physiol 2001;536:937–946.

32. VanTeeffelen JW, Segal SS. Interaction between sympathetic nerve activation and muscle fibre contraction in resistance vessels of hamster retractor muscle. J Physiol 2003;550: 563–574.

33. Yashiro Y, Duling BR. Integrated Ca^{++} signaling between smooth muscle and endothelium of resistance vessels. Circ Res 2000;87:1048–1054.

34. Anrep GV, Von Saalfeld E. The blood flow through the skeletal muscle in relation to its contraction. J Physiol 1935;85:375–399.

35. Tschakovsky ME, Rogers AM, Pyke KE, et al. Immediate exercise hyperemia in humans is contraction intensity dependent: evidence for rapid vasodilation. J Appl Physiol 2004;96:639–644.

CHAPTER 15

The Gastrointestinal System

ROBERT MURRAY AND XIAOCAI SHI

Introduction

During exercise, the loss of water and minerals in sweat and the oxidation of carbohydrate by active skeletal muscle can lead to early fatigue due to a combination of dehydration, hyperthermia, and carbohydrate depletion. Consuming fluid during exercise replaces water and solute, a practice that benefits performance, sustains cardiovascular and thermoregulatory function, and reduces the risk of heat-related problems and other injuries. In addition, disturbances in gastrointestinal function, such as stomach upset, bloating, nausea, and diarrhea are neither uncommon nor trivial problems for many exercisers. Even though sustained heavy exercise is in part dependent on efficient gastrointestinal function, the gastrointestinal tract has received relatively little attention from exercise scientists. After all, the gut is rarely thought of as athletic organ, and compared to the volume of literature detailing the involvement of other organ systems in exercise, comparatively little research has been conducted on gastrointestinal function. In fact, Gisolfi (1) emphasized that in the past 150 years, few scientists have demonstrated more than just a passing interest in the effects of exercise on gastrointestinal function. However, to the athlete engaged in vigorous training or competition, the gastrointestinal tract is key to attenuating fluid losses and providing the exogenous energy required for sustained activity.

The knowledge base on gastrointestinal function during exercise can best be characterized as a patchwork quilt of information. Although there is a large and robust body of literature on general gastrointestinal physiology, only a small portion of this research deals with the effects of exercise, and those studies have been published in fits and spurts over the past century and a half. Fortunately, much of the exercise-related work is quite instructive, and this chapter relies upon that body of knowledge to address what we know, what we think we know, and what we do not know about gastrointestinal function during exercise. In so doing, the chapter focuses on the effects of dynamic sustained exercise on gastrointestinal function. Keep that in mind whenever the term *exercise* or *exercise training* is used.

Functional Anatomy of the Gastrointestinal System

There is at least one certainty about the gastrointestinal system: it is large. From mouth to anus, the gastrointestinal system in an adult can be 6 to 10 meters (about 20–33 feet) long. This chapter focuses on the function of the stomach and small intestine in determining the rates of water and solute absorption during exercise. Although the oropharyngeal region, esophagus, and large intestine play critical roles in gastrointestinal function, only passing attention will be paid to them, either because the exercise-related literature is sparse or because, as in the case of thirst and drinking, it is a topic better addressed in another chapter.

Fundamentals of Neuromuscular Control of Gut Function

The gastrointestinal system effectively has its own nervous system, the enteric nervous system, extending from esophagus to anus. The enteric nervous system contains more than 100 million efferent and afferent neurons, roughly the same number as in the spinal cord (2). The primary purpose of the enteric nervous system is to ensure efficient absorption of water and solute by controlling muscular contraction, secretion, and blood flow. Interestingly, the gastrointestinal system is endowed with as many afferent as efferent fibers, if not more. For example, in the vagus nerve, 80% of the fibers are afferent (2). The preponderance of afferent output from the gut reflects the importance of signals from gut chemoreceptors, osmoreceptors, and mechanoreceptors to the brain and spinal cord.

The enteric nervous system has two primary plexuses, the myenteric plexus and the submucosal plexus; the activity of both plexuses can be modified by sympathetic and parasympathetic input. In general, parasympathetic fibers from the vagus nerve provide excitatory input for secretion and motility via acetylcholine release, while sympathetic fibers have an inhibitory effect. Sympathetic activation causes contraction of vascular smooth muscle, vasoconstriction of intestinal blood vessels, inhibition of wall contractions, and decreased sphincter activity. Norepinephrine and circulating epinephrine are the neurotransmitters that cause the reductions in gut blood flow and smooth muscle activity during exercise. Interestingly, although the reduction in gut (splanchnic) blood flow is an important compensatory response during dynamic exercise that helps maintain central blood volume (3), water and solute absorption are usually not affected (4).

The stomach and small intestine are surrounded by an outer longitudinal layer and an inner circular layer of smooth muscle. The smooth muscle of the gastrointestinal system functions as a syncytium that allows action potentials to travel in all directions, helping facilitate the peristaltic contractions that churn and transport food and fluid in the gut. Ease of depolarization among smooth muscle cells occurs as a result of each cell having more than 200 gap junction connections with adjacent cells (2). In resting humans, rhythmic contractions occur in the stomach and small intestine approximately 3 to 12 times each minute. The type and strength of contractions change upon eating and drinking, such that stronger and more frequent contractions and peristaltic movements help empty the stomach and sweep the chyme along the small intestine.

Fundamentals of Gut Vascular Response

The splanchnic circulation supplies blood to the gastrointestinal system, including the stomach, pancreas, spleen, liver, and the small and large intestines. The celiac artery, part of the splanchnic circulation, provides blood to the stomach and spleen, while the mesenteric arteries serve the intestinal tract. The general anatomical scheme is that blood flowing from the stomach, intestines, spleen, and pancreas flows to the liver and then through the hepatic veins to the vena cava and the general circulation.

Dynamic exercise has a profound effect on splanchnic blood flow. Rowell (3) notes that regional vasoconstrictor outflow is proportional to the severity of exercise, as reflected by the close relationship between heart rate and plasma norepinephrine at heart rates above 100 beats per minute; in brief, splanchnic blood flow decreases as heart rate increases. The decrease in splanchnic blood flow that occurs during exercise is a critical compensatory response to ensure the maintenance of adequate central blood volume and pressure, although how this affects blood flow to the intestinal mucosa via the superior and inferior mesenteric arteries is less clear. In theory, a substantial drop in mesenteric blood flow could impair absorption, because flowing blood removes water and solute and maintains the concentration gradient between the intestinal lumen and the intestinal epithelial cell (enterocyte). Diminished blood flow to the microvilli would reduce both the concentration gradient and speed of absorption. In support of this thinking is the fact that when mesenteric blood flow declines to less than 50% of normal, both glucose absorption and oxygen uptake are reduced (4). This could result in local accumulation of water and solute in the gut, reduced absorption, and increased gastrointestinal discomfort. A counterpoint to this notion is that because of its length, the small intestine has such a large reserve capacity for absorption that it is easy to compensate for a local reduction in blood flow and absorption. In summary, although reduced splanchnic blood flow plays an important role in cardiovascular control during exercise, it appears to do so without impairment of water and solute absorption (1).

However, should mesenteric blood flow to the intestinal epithelium be severely compromised for a sufficient period, the resultant ischemia can alter barrier function and cause cellular necrosis. This is a possibility during prolonged dynamic exercise in the heat, when the combination of dehydration and hyperthermia can severely limit splanchnic blood flow. In fact, some endurance-trained athletes have developed such severe ischemic colitis during races that surgery was required to remove infarcted tissue (5).

Fundamentals of Gut Immune Properties

The gastrointestinal epithelium is only one cell thick, creating an enormous yet extremely thin interface between the body and the outside world. The intestinal epithelium is constantly exposed to a wide variety of nutrients, antigens, and microbes, any one of which could provoke an adverse reaction or inflammatory immune response. In addition to the pathogens and foreign proteins ingested in foods and beverages, the gastrointestinal system is home to more than 400 types of bacteria (6), so it should not be surprising that the gut has robust immune response capabilities. The healthy gut is endowed with effective barriers and a rich array of innate and adaptive immune response options that identify and destroy pathogens and other antigens while allowing for the selective absorption of macronutrients, micronutrients, and water (7).

The intestinal barrier is formed by numerous components including the surface mucus layer, the absorptive brush border cell membrane of the enterocytes (the intestinal epithelial cells), the tight junctions between cells, the epithelial and subepithelial immune defense mechanisms, and the intestinal lymph nodes. The intent of the intestinal barrier is to exclude potentially harmful antigenic, toxic, viral, bacterial, or carcinogenic compounds from provoking local inflammatory responses and from entering the body. As will be addressed later in the chapter, gut barrier function can be compromised by prolonged heavy exercise and likely exacerbated by the accompanying dehydration and hyperthermia.

Gastric Emptying of Foods and Fluids During Exercise

The stomach is a semi-isolated holding tank for ingested foods and fluids, and with the exception of small amounts of alcohol and vitamin B_{12}, water and nutrients are not absorbed from the stomach into the bloodstream. For that reason, rapid gastric emptying is an essential prelude for the rapid absorption of water and nutrients required to sustain vigorous exercise. For example, many athletes sweat at rates exceeding $2 \text{ L} \cdot \text{h}^{-1}$, necessitating an aggressive fluid replacement regimen and unimpeded absorption if significant dehydration is to be avoided. Ingestion of foods and beverages that are not optimally formulated for the exercise occasion will invariably result in delayed gastric emptying. This reduces the rate at which ingested fluid can be absorbed across the epithelium of the small intestine, increasing the risk of gastric discomfort and slowing nutrient absorption.

Measurement of Gastric Emptying Rate

Gisolfi (1) credits the first report on gastric function during exercise to surgeon and physiologist William Beaumont, who in 1833 observed stomach function compliments of an amazingly cooperative patient with an abdominal shotgun wound. Beaumont observed that exercise sufficient to produce modest perspiration was accompanied by an accumulation of fluid in the stomach and concluded that exercise retarded digestion. Subsequent research proved Beaumont correct; any-

thing that induces sympathetic discharge, such as exercise, fear, anxiety, or pain, will decrease gastric emptying rate.

Gastric emptying rate during rest and exercise is often assessed by means of a nasogastric tube that allows for serial measurements of the change in gastric volume based upon changes in the concentration of a nonabsorbable marker such as phenol red (8). Other methods, such as magnetic resonance imaging, scintigraphy, electrical impedance, ultrasonography, and radiography, have also been used to study gastric emptying, but the nasogastric tube is often the method of choice because subjects can engage in a variety of exercise modalities of varying intensities, and the presence of the tube does not affect gastric emptying (9).

Determinants of Gastric Emptying Rate

The stomach is the most distensible part of the gastrointestinal system, and its unfilled volume is small, about 50 mL, yet it can quickly expand to 1000 mL without much change in intragastric pressure. In fact, the very act of swallowing causes reflex relaxation of the stomach, so that the initial intake of food or fluid does not result in a substantial rise in intragastric pressure (2).

Control of gastric motility occurs via efferent and afferent sympathetic and parasympathetic nerves, spinal feedback reflexes, and hormones released from the intestinal mucosa. This control is essential during both rest and dynamic exercise because unrestricted emptying of gastric contents into the duodenum and jejunum results in osmotic diarrhea and nutrient wasting. For this reason, gastric emptying is tightly controlled to ensure that the intestine receives fluid and nutrients at rates that are less than its absorptive capacity and therefore compatible with efficient digestion and absorption. Vasoactive intestinal peptide, γ-aminobutyric acid, substance P, gastrin, cholecystokinin, serotonin, nitric oxide, gastric inhibitory polypeptide, and glucagon-like peptide are examples of hormones and neurotransmitters released by gastric and intestinal nerve and endocrine cells that influence gastric emptying, gastrointestinal motility, and secretions from the pancreas and gallbladder in response to a meal.

Three layers of muscles surround the stomach, arrayed as an outer longitudinal layer, a middle circular layer, and an inner oblique layer. The frequency and strength of contraction of the muscles determines gastric emptying rate by altering the pressure in the antrum of the stomach (Figure 15.1), the space closest to the pyloric sphincter. When pressure in the antrum exceeds the pressure in the duodenal bulb, the pylorus opens and stomach contents (chyme) enter the small intestine.

The gastric emptying rate varies widely among individuals; some empty test meals and solutions twice as rapidly as others. In general, the rate of gastric emptying follows an exponentially declining pattern regardless of the average rate of emptying. In other words, the most rapid gastric emptying rates occur in the first minutes after consumption, when

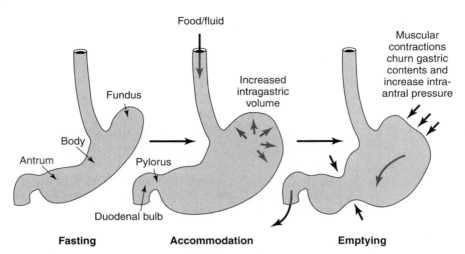

FIGURE 15.1 The rate at which the stomach empties is proportional to the frequency and strength of contractions of the musculature surrounding the stomach. In brief, gastric emptying occurs when pressure in the antrum of the stomach exceeds that in the duodenal bulb, resulting in chyme passing through the pylorus. In the fasting state, the volume of the stomach is small (about 50 mL), but it increases via reflex relaxation of the proximal stomach (fundus), providing the ingested contents with a reservoir and enabling an increase in gastric volume without a rise in intragastric pressure. The gastric contents are emptied from the stomach at a rate that does not exceed the absorptive capacity of the proximal small intestine.

gastric volume is high, and then the rate declines over time, reaching low values when most of the test meal or solution has left the stomach. Mean gastric emptying rates of 15 to more than 20 mL · min^{-1} are common during both rest and dynamic exercise when water or a dilute carbohydrate solution is ingested. Sustaining emptying rates greater than 20 mL · min^{-1} is possible but requires repeated ingestion of water or a dilute carbohydrate beverage to maintain high gastric volume (9).

Gastric emptying can be maintained at a high rate by maintaining a high gastric volume and therefore a high antral pressure. For example, saline pumped continuously into the stomach was shown to empty at 75 mL · min^{-1} (4.5 L · h^{-1}) (2). A wide variety of factors influence gastric emptying rate, with gastric volume topping the list (i.e., the larger the gastric volume, the faster the rate of emptying). In addition to gastric volume, energy content, body position, exercise intensity, gastric pH, the osmolality of the gastric contents, and heat stress have all been shown to affect gastric emptying (10). Of these, the two most important factors are the energy content and volume of the gastric residue.

It is well established that the gastric emptying rate of a carbohydrate solution varies with the energy content of the ingested beverage, such that an increase in carbohydrate content results in slower gastric emptying (11). In general, the ingestion of a relatively dilute carbohydrate solution (e.g., 6% carbohydrate; 60 g · L^{-1}) has been shown to result in a gastric emptying rate that is statistically indistinguishable from that of an equal volume of water (8). However, some investigators have reported delayed gastric emptying

rates (compared to water) for carbohydrate solutions less than 6% (12), while others have found that gastric emptying is unimpeded even with solutions containing 10% carbohydrate (13,14). These inconsistent results are likely due to differences in the volume of fluid consumed, the frequency of fluid intake, measurements taken at rest versus during exercise, the use of solutions containing different types of carbohydrate with varying osmolalities, and differences in the methods used to measure gastric emptying.

Gastric volume has a much greater influence on gastric emptying than does beverage osmolality (9). All things considered, athletes with slow gastric emptying rates and those who sweat profusely can benefit from maintaining a large yet comfortable gastric volume to help maximize gastric emptying rate. This can be achieved by drinking water or a sports drink within 15 minutes before starting exercise and continuing to drink at frequent intervals (e.g., every 10–15 min).

Effects of Dynamic Exercise on Gastric Emptying Rate

The current consensus is that exercise at intensities above 75% $\dot{V}O_{2max}$ slows gastric emptying (9), although this is another area ripe for additional research. Because sporting activities require intermittent high-intensity efforts such as those seen in basketball and soccer, delayed gastric emptying may be unavoidable. However, such sports also include periods of relatively low-intensity exercise and rest, so there is likely ample opportunity for rapid gastric emptying to occur at those times. Drinking strategies can be adjusted to take advantage of occasions when rapid gastric emptying is most likely to occur.

Interestingly, there is a dearth of scientific evidence regarding the mechanisms by which heavy exercise delays gastric emptying. Dehydration, hyperthermia, overall sympathetic discharge, and rising catecholamine levels are all possible candidates, and research demonstrates that each can result in reduced gastric emptying (9,10).

Effects of Dehydration and Hyperthermia on Gastric Emptying Rate

Many individuals who engage in long-duration running, cycling, and triathlon training and competition have experienced the unfortunate chain of gastrointestinal events that often begins with dehydration. Dehydration reduces gastric emptying, which in turn induces bloating and gastrointestinal discomfort, which limits voluntary fluid intake, resulting in greater dehydration, hyperthermia, and fatigue if dynamic exercise continues. The only solution to the problem appears to be avoiding dehydration and limiting the ingestion of foods and fluids with high energy content; that is, taking the steps necessary to maintain a high rate of gastric emptying.

The effect of dehydration and hyperthermia on gastric emptying is another area of exercise science that deserves further attention. There is little doubt that these factors impede gastric emptying (1,9,10), yet we can only speculate that the mechanism may involve inhibition of gastric motility induced by enhanced sympathetic discharge.

Effects of Training on Gastric Emptying Rate

As Leiper (9) emphasizes, anecdotal evidence suggests that athletes can learn to tolerate the ingestion of larger volumes of fluid at more frequent intervals, yet there is little scientific evidence to confirm this observation. The overall composition of the athlete's normal diet and even the composition of the previous meal may influence gastric emptying, another area where research is lacking. The best that can be said on the basis of the existing literature is that active individuals should avoid abrupt changes in diet during critical phases of training or prior to competition.

Absorption of Water and Solute During Exercise: Role of the Small Intestine

In the simplest characterization, the intestine functions as an absorbing surface for water and nutrients (solutes) and as a barrier to prevent harmful substances from entering the body. In those regards, three fundamental concepts are worth remembering: (*a*) Water absorption from hypoosmotic solutions can occur rapidly, especially in the duodenum, as a result of simple osmosis. (*b*) Water absorption from isosmotic

and hyperosmotic solutions is secondary to solute absorption because solute absorption establishes an osmotic gradient that results in water absorption. (*c*) Alterations in the osmotic gradient across the intestinal epithelium can occur with the ingestion of inappropriate foods and fluids during exercise or as a result of the presence of noxious microorganisms (e.g., *Escherichia coli, Vibrio cholera*) and can quickly change net fluid absorption into net fluid secretion, with resulting gastrointestinal discomfort and profuse diarrhea.

From a functional standpoint, it is easiest to think of the epithelium of the small intestine as having two separate components (Fig. 15.2): the brush border lipid membrane of the enterocytes, which is exposed to the intestinal lumen, and the vast paracellular space between the enterocytes, namely the tight junctions. Each are capable of allowing water and solute to pass into the bloodstream and so play critical roles in regulating absorption at rest and during dynamic exercise.

From an anatomical standpoint, the small intestine is superbly designed for the absorption of water and solute. The first 25 cm past the pylorus is the duodenum, an area characterized by a leaky epithelium. This characteristic allows for rapid osmotic equilibration of the gastric effluent because water freely flows across the epithelium in response to the prevailing osmotic gradient. As a result, a hypertonic effluent, such as a concentrated carbohydrate solution (e.g., a regular soft drink or fruit juice), will provoke secretion of water into the duodenum to reduce osmolality as a preface to net water absorption further down the small intestine. Hypotonic fluids such as water are quickly absorbed in the duodenum, as water molecules are free to pass across the duodenal epithelium into the higher-osmolality environment of the intracellular and extracellular fluid.

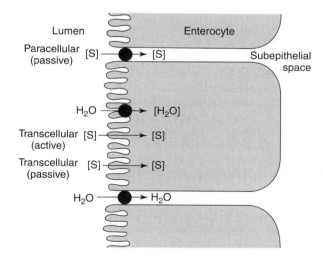

FIGURE 15.2 The structure of intestinal epithelial cells allows water and solute ([S]) to be absorbed by both paracellular (via tight junctions between cells) and transcellular active and passive processes mediated by transport proteins in the epithelial membrane.

The next 250 cm (about 8 feet) of the small intestine is the jejunum, a microvilli-covered section rich in membrane-bound transport molecules and cellular junctions that open and close in response to the prevailing luminal environment. (The presence of mucosal folding and microvilli in the small intestine creates an absorptive surface area about the size of a doubles tennis court, 20 times the surface area of a smooth tube of like length.) The ileum is the final 300 cm (about 10 feet) of the small intestine, but its function is not covered in this chapter because its role in water and solute absorption during exercise is usually minimal; the ileum provides reserve absorptive capacity for water and solutes that escape absorption in the upper small intestine.

Measurement of Water and Solute Absorption

The absorption of water and solute in the proximal small intestine can be studied using a variety of *in vitro* techniques (e.g., Ussing chamber, tissue incubation, oocyte expression of transport proteins), tracer techniques (most often with D_2O), and perfusion methods using double- and triple-lumen perfusion tubes. Among these methods, the triple-lumen perfusion technique, also called steady-state perfusion, is arguably the gold standard for studying regional water and solute absorption in the resting or exercising human. One limitation of the perfusion technique is that it measures only the absorptive characteristics of the segment of intestine that is perfused, usually about 35 to 40 cm. However, this is an acceptable limitation for studying the absorption of water and carbohydrate and electrolyte beverages, because most absorption occurs within that length of the proximal small intestine. The perfusion technique requires a triple-lumen tube to be placed via the mouth into the subject's small intestine under fluoroscopic guidance. Once proper tube placement is verified, a test solution containing a nonabsorbable marker such as polyethylene glycol is infused into the small intestine through one lumen of the tube, and samples are collected from the proximal and distal ports of the tube for analysis of the nonabsorbable marker and solutes, such as carbohydrates and electrolytes. The change in the concentration of the nonabsorbable marker and solutes from the proximal and distal sampling sites allows calculation of the absorption rates of water and solutes.

Principles of Solute and Water Absorption

Solute absorption refers to the movement of nutrients, such as carbohydrates, amino acids, and small peptides, and minerals, such as sodium and potassium, from the intestinal lumen into the bloodstream either transcellularly (across the epithelial cell membrane and out of the cell into the bloodstream) or paracellularly (between the epithelial cells via the tight junctions).

Solute and fluid absorption are primarily linked by the activity of the sodium- and glucose-linked transporter molecule (SGLT1) that is found in abundant quantities in the jejunal epithelium. SGLT1 plays the pivotal role in water absorption, and for this reason has been the subject of considerable research attention over the past 50 years. In fact, the discovery in the late 1950s and early 1960s that sodium and glucose transport were linked had enormous public health implications because it paved the way for the formulation of the simple oral rehydration solutions (ORS) that continue to save the lives of millions of people stricken with diarrheal disease. In the 1960s, the first sports drink was developed, based in part on the principle that water molecules quickly follow solute across the intestinal epithelium. An ORS formulated to replace diarrheal fluid loss typically contains about 2% carbohydrate and high levels of sodium (45–75 mEq $\cdot$ L^{-1}) and potassium (20 mEq $\cdot$ L^{-1}), whereas sports drinks contain more carbohydrate (e.g., 6–7% carbohydrate) and less electrolytes (e.g., 20–40 mEq $\cdot$ L^{-1} Na^+ and 3–5 mEq $\cdot$ L^{-1} K^+). The differences in formulation are due to differences in the intended benefits. Diarrheal electrolyte losses are usually considerably higher than electrolyte losses in sweat, so more electrolytes are needed in an ORS to offset those loses. In terms of carbohydrate concentration, the 2% glucose concentration of an ORS will stimulate water absorption but will not provide the amount of exogenous carbohydrate required for improved performance (11).

Carbohydrate Digestion and Absorption

In the intestinal lumen and at the brush border, disaccharides and oligosaccharides are digested to their monomer components. Pancreatic amylases in the intestinal lumen begin the process of starch digestion. At the brush border, lactase phlorizin hydrolase digests lactose, the primary carbohydrate in milk. (Lactose intolerance occurs when the activity of this enzyme declines to low levels, as can happen during childhood.) Sucrase digests sucrose into glucose and fructose. Isomaltase and α-glucosidase digest starches and other polymers of glucose into individual glucose monomers. These brush border enzymes are transcriptionally regulated, and their abundance in the cell membrane is influenced by diet (15).

Glucose and galactose are absorbed across the brush border membrane by SGLT1. The concentration of SGLT1 in the membrane is primarily influenced by dietary carbohydrate content. For example, the presence of glucose and galactose in the gut can rapidly increase the trafficking of SGLT1 from intracellular storage sites to the brush border membrane (15). Such rapid response is an important functional characteristic of the small intestine because it ensures that the absorptive capacity of the intestine always exceeds nutrient intake, a critical balance if osmotic diarrhea is to be avoided. In this regard, the plasticity of the small intestine is quite remarkable. Stevens (16) noted that reversible increases in absorptive capacity can occur within hours or days as a result of (*a*) mucosal hyperplasia and increased villus height, (*b*) up-regulation of specific transporters in response to the ingestion of specific solutes, and (c) local regulation of transporter kinetics.

The GLUT5 transporter molecule shuttles fructose across the brush border membrane into the intestinal epithelial cell. Fructose is absorbed by facilitated transport, a mechanism that allows for faster absorption rates than that of passively absorbed carbohydrates, such as rhamnose. However, GLUT5-facilitated transport of fructose is slower than that of actively transported carbohydrates, such as glucose and galactose, via SGLT1. Interestingly, the turnover of GLUT5 protein occurs in diurnal fashion in the rat, even in the absence of dietary fructose (15). Whether the same is true in humans is not yet known. Once inside the epithelial cell, glucose, galactose, and fructose exit the basolateral membrane of the intestinal epithelial cell into the portal blood via the GLUT2 transporter (15).

It is hypothesized but still unproved that sucrose is absorbed via a distinct transport system, the disaccharidase-related transport system (DRTS) (17). This transport mechanism appears to be associated with sucrose hydrolysis, but it is unclear whether the enzyme (sucrase) transfers the products of hydrolysis (glucose and fructose) to DRTS or whether the carrier is an integral part of the enzyme itself.

Another proposed solute transport mechanism is paracellular transport (18). SGLT1 solute transport triggers contraction of perijunctional actomyosin to open tight junctions between jejunal cells and thereby stimulate solvent drag. For example, in addition to transport via GLUT5, fructose can be absorbed paracellularly, carried along by the solvent drag created by active glucose absorption.

Amino Acid Absorption

There are a number of amino acid transporters in the gut (16). Some depend upon cotransport of sodium; others do not. Some transporters are specific to cationic amino acids, others to anionic amino acids, yet others to dipolar amino acids. Even some dipeptides and tripeptides can be absorbed by enterocytes. How dynamic exercise or exercise training influences amino acid absorption is unknown.

Because some amino acids are actively transported, there has been interest in determining whether the addition of certain amino acids can augment water absorption from a carbohydrate-electrolyte beverage. To date the results have been disappointing. For example, the amino acid glutamine is the preferred energy substrate for intestinal epithelial cells (although enterocytes will also use glucose for energy when it is available in high concentrations), but there appears to be no absorption-related advantage of providing glutamine in a beverage formulated for consumption during exercise.

Mineral Absorption

There is no doubt that sodium is the mineral that plays the most pivotal role in water absorption in the small intestine.

Sodium is always present in the intestinal lumen. In addition to sodium supplied by food and drink, luminal sodium is derived from extracellular fluid, from sodium bicarbonate, and from bile salts. In the fasting human, sodium concentration in the duodenum (about 60 mEq $\cdot$ L^{-1}) is about half of that in the jejunum (about 140 mEq mEq $\cdot$ L^{-1}). There is evidence that sodium absorption is influenced by the type of carbohydrate in the ingested beverage. For example, maltodextrin (glucose polymers) appear to produce a faster rate of sodium absorption than glucose and maltose; maltose is superior to glucose, and glucose and oligosaccharides are better than sucrose (19). Perfusion of a fructose solution initially results in sodium secretion and slower absorption than with a glucose solution (19). The practical ramifications of these differences have yet to be elucidated, but the principle is that fast sodium (solute) absorption is an indispensable characteristic of an ORS. Additional research is required to assess the effect on sodium and water absorption of ingesting solutions containing blends of different carbohydrates and electrolytes in varying concentrations and osmolalities.

Chloride and potassium are largely transported by solvent drag through paracellular channels, while other minerals, such as calcium, iron, and zinc, rely on yet other solute-specific transport mechanisms. However, there is no evidence that water or solute absorption is augmented with the addition of common minerals other than sodium chloride to an ORS.

The effect of dynamic exercise or exercise training on mineral absorption has not been well studied. One supposition is that because sodium absorption does not appear to be influenced by dynamic exercise (20), it is unlikely that the absorption characteristics or other minerals are affected.

Water Absorption

Although the athlete's requirements for water, carbohydrate, and electrolytes during training and competition can be impressively high (e.g., sweat rates above 2 L $\cdot$ hour^{-1}, carbohydrate oxidation rates above 3 g $\cdot$ minute^{-1}, and sodium losses above 1 g $\cdot$ L^{-1} of sweat), those demands fall well below the capacity of the gastrointestinal system to absorb water and solute. For example, the V_{max} of glucose and amino acid transport is estimated to exceed typical dietary intake by a factor of 2 (15). However, that is not to say that the small intestine has an unlimited capacity for water and solute absorption. That is clearly not the case and is one reason feedback inhibition from intestinal osmoreceptors and chemoreceptors is needed to ensure that the gastric emptying rate does not exceed the absorptive capacity of the proximal small intestine.

During the course of a normal day, more than 10 L of water crosses the intestinal epithelium of physically active adults (Fig. 15.3). This daily water recycling is sometimes referred to as the enterosystemic cycle. Reflecting the changing

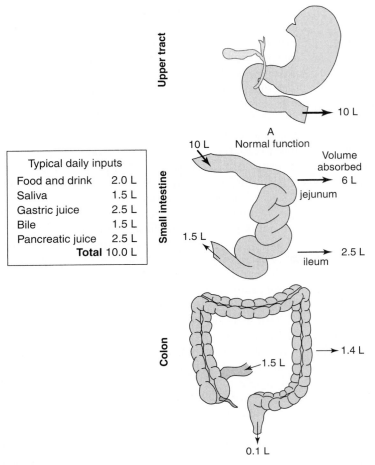

Typical daily inputs	
Food and drink	2.0 L
Saliva	1.5 L
Gastric juice	2.5 L
Bile	1.5 L
Pancreatic juice	2.5 L
Total	10.0 L

FIGURE 15.3 The enormous capacity of the gastrointestinal tract to absorb water. Under normal conditions, only about 1% of ingested fluid is lost in feces. Athletes, workers, and soldiers who are physically active in a hot environment may ingest more than 12 L of fluid per day. Rarely does such large fluid intake result in diarrhea.

permeability characteristics of the gastrointestinal tract as it extends from pylorus to anus, the upper small intestine is estimated to absorb more than 70% of ingested and secreted fluids, with 20% being absorbed by the ileum and only about 5% from the colon.

Water molecules cross the enterocyte membrane via SGLT1 or by transcellular and paracellular diffusion driven by the osmotic gradient (Figure 15.4). Considerable research and scientific debate have been devoted to quantifying the proportion of water absorption that occurs via paracellular versus transcellular transport. Suffice to say that although the tide of evidence favors greater transcellular absorption, both mechanisms are critical in ensuring the water and solute absorption required during exercise.

SGLT1 is a 290-kDa molecule composed of four 73-kDa subunits (16). The activity of SGLT1 is energized by the transmembrane electrical potential that is maintained by active sodium-potassium transport in the basolateral mem-

brane by Na$^+$-K$^+$-ATPase and by facilitated transport of Cl$^-$ from adjacent epithelial cells or from the intestinal lumen. The SGLT1 molecule is thought to function in the following way: When two sodium ions bind to the active site of SGLT1, a conformational change allows glucose to bind. Once glucose is bound, another conformational shift occurs, and the sodium ions and glucose molecule are transported across the membrane and released. SGLT1 then undergoes yet another conformational change back to its original position, ready to bind additional sodium and glucose.

In the absence of glucose or galactose, SGLT1 serves as a sodium uniporter and a passive water channel. An important feature of SGLT1 is that in its active state it also serves as a molecular pump for water, accounting for up to 70% of total daily water absorption in the jejunum. Each time that SGLT1 transports glucose and sodium into the enterocyte, approximately 225 water molecules follow (15). Assuming a rotation rate of 25 times per second, each SGLT1 molecule

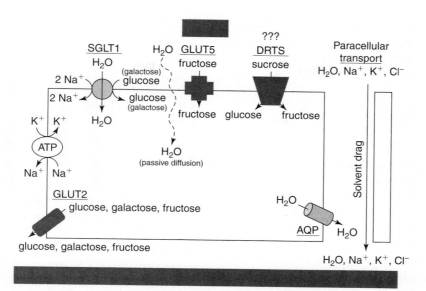

FIGURE 15.4 Proposed mechanisms of water and solute absorption. Active sodium and glucose cotransport by the SGLT1 transporter in the enterocyte brush border membrane and extrusion of sodium and glucose across the basolateral membrane stimulate water and solute absorption through both transcellular and paracellular routes. The roles of GLUT5, GLUT2, DRTS, Na^+-K^+ ATPase, and aquaporins (AQP) are also depicted. Following activation of SGLT1, solutes such as monosaccharides, minerals, and perhaps even small peptides and oligosaccharides can be absorbed via the paracellular pathway.

could be responsible for the absorption of 5625 water molecules per second. This impressive figure is an obvious reason an effective ORS and a properly formulated sports drink can take advantage of this fundamental characteristic of the intestinal epithelium.

DETERMINANTS OF THE RATE OF WATER ABSORPTION

A handful of factors influence the rate of water absorption in the proximal small intestine. Gastric emptying rate has an obvious influence on absorption: delayed gastric emptying results in delayed absorption. In addition to gastric emptying rate, the primary factors influencing the rate of water absorption are beverage osmolality, the concentration of carbohydrate, the type of carbohydrate, and the number of transportable solutes in the beverage. The sheer number of interactions among these variables complicates the study of how beverage composition affects water absorption, although a partial and instructive picture has emerged.

EFFECT OF BEVERAGE OSMOLALITY ON THE RATE OF WATER ABSORPTION

The proximal small intestine, especially the duodenum, functions as an osmotic equilibrator that rapidly adjusts the osmolality of the gastric effluent toward isosmolality. For example, a hyperosmotic effluent will be diluted in the duodenum by water secretion, whereas a hypo-osmotic effluent will promote solute secretion (primary sodium and chloride). As would be expected, the rate of water absorption in the proximal small intestine tends to be inversely related to the osmolality of the perfused solution (4,9). However, this relationship may not always hold true. For example, in two studies, an isosmotic carbohydrate-electrolyte solution promoted greater water absorption than distilled water (21,22). In addition, Shi and associates (23) and Gisolfi and associates (24) reported no significant differences in water absorption at rest or during dynamic exercise from carbohydrate-electrolyte beverages that varied in osmolality from hypoosmotic (186–197 mOsm · kg^{-1}), isosmotic (283–295 mOsm · kg^{-1}), to hyperosmotic (403–414 mOsm · kg^{-1}). It may be that the effect of beverage osmolality is modified by the concentration and types of carbohydrates in the beverage, a possibility addressed later in this chapter.

Effect of Carbohydrate Concentration on the Rate of Water Absorption

The rate of water absorption is influenced by carbohydrate concentration, in part because carbohydrate concentration often determines the osmolality of the beverage. The inverse relationship between the glucose concentration of a test solution and water absorption is commonly observed in the literature (21,22). Generally speaking, too much carbohydrate in the beverage slows the rate of water absorption. For example, Ryan and colleagues (25) reported slower water absorption from 8 and 9% carbohydrate beverages than with water or from a 6% carbohydrate beverage.

Although the beverages differed in osmolality, carbohydrate type, and electrolyte content, it is possible that beverages with more than 6% carbohydrate saturate the absorption process for glucose in the jejunum. In support of this possibility, Rolston and Mathan (26) estimated that the SGLT1 transporter process in the jejunum is saturated at approximately 200 mM glucose (about 35 g · L⁻¹, the equivalent of a 3.5% glucose solution).

EFFECT OF CARBOHYDRATE TYPE ON THE RATE OF WATER ABSORPTION

There is little doubt that the type of carbohydrate can influence the rate of water absorption because of the differences in solution osmolality conferred by carbohydrate type (e.g., equal concentrations of glucose, sucrose, and maltodextrins have widely varying osmolalities) and differences in the rates at which the carbohydrates are absorbed (e.g., glucose more than fructose). For example, ORS typically contains 2% glucose (about 120 mM) because decades of studies have demonstrated that such solutions stimulate rapid water absorption and save lives. In contrast, carbohydrate-electrolyte beverages (sports drinks) usually contain a blend of carbohydrates at concentrations around 60 g · L⁻¹ (i.e., a 6% carbohydrate solution; about 350 mM). The higher amount of carbohydrate provides the palatability required for consumption during exercise and supplies enough exogenous substrate to improve performance (11). If such beverages are properly formulated, high rates of water absorption can be maintained. However, if the wrong blend of carbohydrate is used (e.g., too much fructose) or if the carbohydrate concentration is too high (more than 6–7%), the rate of water absorption will be reduced.

A study by Shi and colleagues (27) (Fig. 15.5) demonstrated how water absorption in resting humans is influenced by the number of transportable carbohydrates and solution osmolality. The effect of solution osmolality on water absorption was attenuated by enhanced solute absorption when more than one transportable carbohydrate was present in the test solution. In other words, even slightly hyperosmotic beverages (e.g., 300–400 mOsm · kg⁻¹) can be rapidly absorbed if more than one transportable carbohydrate is present (23,24). However, as Figure 15.5 illustrates, the obvious tendency is for solutions of lower osmolality to be absorbed at directionally faster rates.

EFFECT OF DYNAMIC EXERCISE ON THE RATE OF WATER ABSORPTION

Does exercise affect the rate at which water is absorbed? Evidence on this important question is conflicting. In 1967, Fordtran and Saltin (28) (Milestone of Discovery) reported no consistent effect of exercise on glucose, water, or electrolyte absorption during treadmill running for 1 hour at 64 to 78% V̇O₂max. This finding was supported by Gisolfi and colleagues (20) using segmental perfusion to study intestinal absorption during 1-h bouts of cycle exercise at 30, 50, and 70% V̇O₂max. However, there is evidence that higher exercise intensities may delay absorp-

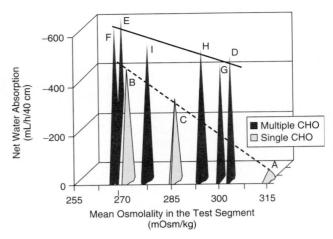

FIGURE 15.5 The relationship between water absorption and luminal osmolality of solutions containing single- and multiple-transportable carbohydrates. The broken line represents the regression line for single carbohydrates (A, B, and C), while the solid line does the same for multiple carbohydrates (D, E, F, G, H, and I). Two important features: the presence of multiple carbohydrates increases net water absorption, and the presence of multiple carbohydrates diminishes the effect of osmolality. Negative values indicate net water absorption. (Solution carbohydrate composition and mean osmolality in the test segment of the jejunum: A, 8% glucose, 314 mOsm · kg⁻¹; B, 6% maltodextrin, 271 mOsm · kg⁻¹; C, 8% maltodextrin, 286 mOsm · kg⁻¹; D, 4% glucose + 4% fructose, 304 mOsm · kg⁻¹; E, 4% sucrose + 2% glucose, 269 mOsm · kg⁻¹; F, 3% glucose + 2% sucrose + 1% maltodextrin, 268 mOsm · kg⁻¹; G, 3% glucose + 3% fructose + 2% sucrose, 300 mOsm · kg⁻¹; H, 8% sucrose, 296 mOsm · kg⁻¹; I, 4% sucrose + 2% glucose + 0.4% glycine, 276 mOsm · kg⁻¹.) The figure is based on the data of Shi X, Flanagan S, Summers RW, et al. Effects of carbohydrate type and concentration and solution osmolality on water absorption. Med Sci Sports Exerc 1995;27:1607–1615.)

tion (9). Whether this finding is consistent remains to be determined. Part of the difficulty in quantifying the effects of intense exercise on absorption is that very few subjects can sustain intense exercise long enough to allow for segmental perfusion measurements to be made.

EFFECTS OF DEHYDRATION AND HYPERTHERMIA ON THE RATE OF WATER ABSORPTION

Dehydration during exercise results in plasma hyperosmolality, reduced skin and splanchnic blood flow, decreased sweat rate, and hyperthermia. The combination of dehydration, hyperthermia, and heavy exercise has been linked to increased intestinal permeability, ostensibly as a result of reduced mesenteric blood flow and local ischemia. How these changes affect water and solute absorption is not well understood. Ryan and colleagues (25) investigated the effect of hypohydration (loss of 2.7% body mass prior to the commencement of exercise) on water absorption during 85-min cycle exercise at 65% V̇O₂max in a cool environment. This study compared fluid absorption from 6, 8, and 9% carbohydrate-electrolyte beverages and water and also compared absorption rates between hypohydrated and euhydrated states (water trial only). The results indicated that hypohydration did not affect absorption. Additional research is necessary to corroborate and extend these findings, to determine whether greater levels of dehydration affect absorption, and to investigate the interaction between dehydration and hyperthermia on water and solute absorption.

EFFECT OF DIET ON THE RATE OF WATER ABSORPTION   Absorption of water in the small intestine follows the establishment of a favorable osmotic gradient due either to ingestion of a hypo-osmotic beverage or secondary to the osmotic gradient established by solute absorption. In the latter regard, glucose is the solute that provokes the most robust stimulation of water absorption. The rate of carbohydrate absorption in the small intestine is related to the concentration and activity of SGLT1, GLUT5, and GLUT2 in the enterocyte membrane. Consequently, anything that affects the regulation of carbohydrate transporters may affect water absorption. Animal studies have shown that SGLT1 and GLUT5 transporter activity and site density are up-regulated by consumption of a high-carbohydrate diet (15). In fact, within 4 hours of fructose exposure, GLUT5 mRNA protein levels rise (15). When animals are on a carbohydrate-free diet, levels of sucrase-isomaltase and SGLT1 decline (15).

Low-sodium diets decrease glucose transport by decreasing the number of brush border glucose transporters, whereas a high-sodium diet does not appear to effect SGLT1 trafficking. Aside from these findings, there is a dearth of evidence regarding the effects of changes in the macronutrient composition of the diet on water and solute absorption. Individuals in training typically ingest diets high in carbohydrate and sodium, providing the nutritional impetus for the maintenance of an ample quantity of membrane transporters. However, it would be useful to know more about how water and solute absorption are influenced by short-term changes in diet and by fasting.

EFFECT OF AGING ON THE RATE OF WATER ABSORPTION   The effect of aging on water absorption has not been extensively studied. However, carbohydrate malabsorption has been demonstrated in about one-third of healthy individuals over age 65 (29), and altered carbohydrate absorption could retard water absorption. Impaired carbohydrate absorption with age may be due to a reduction in the effective absorptive surface of the small intestine and/or a reduction in splanchnic blood flow, but little is known about how dynamic exercise and exercise training affect water and solute absorption in older, physically active individuals. There is no reliable evidence that the intestine changes in length, weight, or permeability with aging.

Gastrointestinal Transit and Intestinal Motility During Dynamic Exercise

Gastrointestinal transit and intestinal motility during exercise in humans are relatively neglected areas of investigation. Accelerated gastrointestinal transit time can reduce nutrient absorption, cause gastrointestinal discomfort, and increase the risk of diarrhea. Delayed transit time can increase the risk of gastrointestinal discomfort. Based upon the existing literature, it is impossible to determine the effect of exercise on gastrointestinal transit time because the results show accelerated, slowed, or unchanged gastrointestinal transit time (30,31). The effect of exercise on intestinal motility in humans is similarly difficult to discern because the available evidence is also equivocal.

Intestinal Barrier Function During Dynamic Exercise

Can exercise affect gut barrier function? Yes. The most obvious example of impaired gut barrier function is the intestinal bleeding sometimes seen in marathon runners (30,31). Heavy exercise can cause mucosal lesions, such as hemorrhagic gastritis and ischemic colitis (32), and increased intestinal permeability to macromolecules and/or bacteria (33). As a counterpoint to these changes in gut barrier function, there is evidence of improved gut barrier function with exercise training in animals (1).

Nonsteroidal anti-inflammatory drugs (NSAIDs) are commonly used by active individuals to relieve pain during training and competition. Use of NSAIDs, such as aspirin and ibuprofen, increases intestinal permeability, yet there is also evidence that NSAID use decreases the frequency of gastrointestinal bleeding (30).

Gastrointestinal Discomfort During Dynamic Exercise

Gastrointestinal discomfort is commonly observed before, during, and after prolonged heavy exercise, mainly in long-distance running, cycling, and triathlons. Many gastrointestinal symptoms may be related to factors such as psychological stress; the mode, duration, and intensity of exercise; and the type, amount, and timing of food and drink ingested before and during exercise. Common symptoms include upper gastrointestinal discomfort, such as bloating, heartburn, upset stomach, nausea, and vomiting, and lower gastrointestinal discomfort, such as diarrhea, bleeding, and side stitch (30,31). Research indicates that the incidence of gastrointestinal discomfort varies widely, ranging from 1 to 81% of race participants (30,31).

Endotoxemia is sometimes evident after strenuous prolonged exercise because of the translocation of endotoxins from the gut into the bloodstream (30,31,34). Endotoxin, also known as lipopolysaccharide (LPS), is present in the walls of gut bacteria. LPS initiates an immune reaction as it translocates through the gut epithelium and into the portal and systemic circulations. This can lead to various gastrointestinal symptoms, such as nausea, vomiting, diarrhea, and even fever and a systemic inflammatory response. These problems all can increase the risk of heat-related injury.

SUMMARY

Gastrointestinal function during exercise is an area much in need of additional research. Although the fundamental mechanisms of gastric emptying and intestinal water and solute absorption are well established, there is much to be learned about how the body responds to fluid and nutrient ingestion during dynamic exercise and how training and diet may affect those responses. The gastrointestinal system is the primary limiting factor in an active individual's ability to replace enough fluid, carbohydrate, and minerals to prevent dehydration, hyperthermia, hypoglycemia, hyponatremia, cramping, and premature fatigue. Additional research is necessary to reveal how water and solute delivery can be maximized and gastrointestinal disturbances minimized by the ingestion of an optimal combination of water and solute.

The effect of dynamic exercise and training on gastrointestinal function is similarly an incomplete picture. Water and solute absorption have been reported to be unaffected by dynamic exercise at 70% $\dot{V}O_{2max}$, and water absorption appears uninfluenced by dehydration up to at least −3% body mass. Dynamic exercise greater than 70 to 80% $\dot{V}O_{2max}$ appears to slow gastric emptying rate, but it is less clear whether such heavy exercise affects water and solute absorption in the proximal small intestine. How dehydration, hyperthermia, and heavy exercise may combine to affect the function of the gastrointestinal system also remains to be elucidated. Little is known about how exercise training and diet influence gastrointestinal responses to water and nutrient absorption. For example, does exercise training have any effect on the membrane-bound solute transporters, or do acute or chronic dietary habits have an overriding influence? Can the stomach be trained to accommodate larger volumes of fluid consumed during dynamic exercise to improve hydration? How much can the small intestine improve its capacity for solute and therefore fluid absorption? What combination of nutrients optimizes solute and water absorption? What range of beverage osmolality promotes the greatest water absorption during dynamic exercise? Much remains to be learned about gastrointestinal function during dynamic exercise and training. The value of pursuing research along these lines is that new knowledge not only will benefit scientists interested in this area of study but will also generate information of practical value for individuals who regularly engage in dynamic exercise activities.

A MILESTONE OF DISCOVERY

Does heavy exercise affect gastrointestinal function? Specifically, does exercise interfere with the athlete's ability to replace sweat loss and ingest carbohydrate during exercise? In the 1960s, there were only suggestions in the scientific literature that gut function might be adversely affected during exercise, and those suggestions were derived from studies on gastric emptying published in 1928 and 1934. A few studies in the early 1960s reported that exercise reduced blood flow to the gut, a further indication that water and solute absorption might be impaired. This led John Fordtran and Bengt Saltin to combine their formidable scientific talents to conduct a study directly measuring gastric emptying and intestinal absorption during treadmill exercise. They speculated that "were it possible to replace sweat losses and to maintain a sufficient supply of glucose during exercise, performance might be improved." They also noted that some Olympic-caliber cross-country skiers believed that drinking a glucose solution during competition was a key to improved performance. To address the conflicting evidence, Fordtran and Saltin designed a study that required their subjects to run at 70% $\dot{V}O_{2max}$ while gastric emptying measurements were made on one day and absorption measurements on another. The test beverages were a 13.3% glucose solution, a 0.3% saline solution, and water. The results showed a clear reduction in gastric emptying with the concentrated glucose solution but no effect of exercise on gastric emptying. Exercise also had no effect on water and solute absorption. Glucose absorption in both the jejunum and ileum were unaffected by exercise, and the same was true for water, sodium, potassium, chloride, and bicarbonate absorption. From these results, the authors surmised that it would be possible for active individuals to replace sweat loss and to supply carbohydrate and electrolytes "during heavy exercise, even in hot environments." This hallmark study by Fordtran and Saltin not only set the stage for all future research along this line but also established the scientific rationale for the subsequent formulation of effective sports drinks.

Fordtran JS, Saltin B. Gastric emptying and intestinal absorption during prolonged severe exercise. J Appl Physiol 1967;23:331–335.

ACKNOWLEDGMENTS

We are eternally grateful to the late Dr. Carl V. Gisolfi of the University of Iowa for the expertise, guidance, mentoring, patience, and friendship he freely gave and for his many contributions to the area of gastrointestinal function during exercise. We are also indebted to Drs. Robert W. Summers of the University of Iowa, Harold P. Schedl of the University of Iowa, Ronald J. Maughan of the University of Loughborough, and John B. Leiper of the University of Aberdeen for their astute tutelage and numerous contributions to this area of science. Finally, we acknowledge our colleagues at The Gatorade Company for their unwavering support of our research and for encouraging us to engage in scholarly activities such as this.

REFERENCES

1. Gisolfi CV. The gastrointestinal system. In Tipton CV, ed. Exercise Physiology: People and Ideas. New York: Oxford University, 2003;475–495.

2. Davenport HW. Physiology of the Digestive Tract. Chicago: Year Book, 1982.

3. Rowell LB. Human Circulation During Physical Stress. New York: Oxford University, 1986.

4. Gisolfi CV, Summers RW, Schedl HP. Intestinal absorption of fluids during rest and exercise. In Gisolfi CV, Lamb DR, eds. Perspectives in Exercise Science and Sports Medicine, vol 3. Fluid Homeostasis During Exercise. Indianapolis: Benchmark, 1990;129–180.

5. Lucas W, Schroy PC. Reversible ischemic colitis in a high endurance athlete. Am J Gastroenterol 1998;93:2231–2234.

6. Baumgart DC, Dignass AU. Intestinal barrier function. Curr Opin Clin Nutr Metab Care 2002;5:685–694.

7. Nagler-Anderson C. Man the barrier! Strategic defences in the intestinal mucosa. Nature Rev 2001;1:59–67.

8. Murray R, Eddy DE, Bartoli WP, et al. Gastric emptying of water and isocaloric carbohydrate solutions consumed at rest. Med Sci Sports Exerc 1994;26:(6)725–732.

9. Leiper JB. Gastric emptying and intestinal absorption of fluids, carbohydrates, and electrolytes. In Maughan RJ, Murray R, eds. Sports Drinks: Basic Science and Practical Aspects. Boca Raton: CRC Press, 2001;89–128.

10. Costill DL. Gastric emptying of fluids during exercise. In Gisolfi CV, Lamb DR, eds. Perspectives in Exercise Science and Sports Medicine, vol 3. Fluid Homeostasis During Exercise. Indianapolis: Benchmark, 1990;97–128.

11. Murray R. The effects of consuming carbohydrate-electrolyte beverages on gastric emptying and fluid absorption during and following exercise. Sports Med 1987;4:322–351.

12. Vist GE, Maughan RJ. Gastric emptying of ingested solutions in man: effect of beverage glucose concentration. Med Sci Sports Exerc 1994;26:1269–1273.

13. Owen MD, Kregel KC, Wall PT, et al. Effects of ingesting carbohydrate beverages during exercise in the heat. Med Sci Sports Exerc 1986;18:568–575.

14. Zachwieja JJ, Costill DL, Beard GC, et al. The effect of a carbonated carbohydrate drink on gastric emptying, gastrointestinal distress, and exercise performance. Int J Sports Nutr 1992;2:239–250.

15. Thomson ABR, Keelan M, Thiesen A, et al. Small bowel review: normal physiology part 1. Dig Dis Sci 2001;46:2567–2587.

16. Stevens BR. Vertebrate intestine apical membrane mechanisms of organic nutrient transport. Am J Physiol 1992;263:R458–R463.

17. Ugolev A, Zaripov B, Lezuitova N, et al. A revision of current data and views on membrane hydrolysis and transport in the mammalian small intestine based on a comparison of techniques of chronic and acute experiments: experimental reinvestigation and critical review. Comp Biochem Physiol 1986;85A:593–612.

18. Madara JL, Pappenheimer JR. Structural basis for physiological regulation of paracellular pathways in intestinal epithelia. J Membrane Biol 1987;100:149–164.

19. Fordtran JS. Stimulation of active and passive sodium absorption by sugars in the human jejunum. J Clin Invest 1975;55:728–737.

20. Gisolfi CV, Spranger KJ, Summers RW, et al. Effects of cycle exercise on intestinal absorption in humans. J Appl Physiol 1991;71:2518–2527.

21. Gisolfi CV, Summers RW, Schedl HP, et al. Human intestinal water absorption: direct vs indirect measurements. Am J Physiol 1990;258:G216–G222.

22. Leiper JB, Maughan RJ. Absorption of water and electrolytes from hypotonic, isotonic and hypertonic solutions. J Physiol (Lond) 1986;373:90P.

23. Shi X, Summers RW, Schedl HP, et al. Effects of solution osmolality on absorption of select fluid replacement solutions in human duodenojejunum. J Appl Physiol 1994;77:1178–1184.

24. Gisolfi CV, Summers RW, Lambert GP, et al. Effect of beverage osmolality on intestinal fluid absorption during exercise. J Appl Physiol 1998;85:1941–1948.

25. Ryan AJ, Lambert GP, Shi X, et al. Effect of hypohydration on gastric emptying and intestinal absorption during exercise. J Appl Physiol 1998;84:1581–1588.

26. Rolston DDK, Mathan VI. Jejunal and ileal glucose-stimulated water and sodium absorption in tropical enteropathy: implications for oral rehydration therapy. Digestion 1990;46:55–60.

27. Shi X, Flanagan S, Summers RW, et al. Effects of carbohydrate type and concentration and solution osmolality on water absorption. Med Sci Sports Exerc 1995;27:1607–1615.

28. Fordtran JS, Saltin B. Gastric emptying and intestinal absorption during prolonged severe exercise. J Appl Physiol 1967;23:331–335.

29. Beaumont DM, Cobdent L, Sheldon WL, et al. Passive and active carbohydrate absorption by the aging gut. Age Ageing 1987;16:294–300.

30. Gil SM, Yazaki E, Evans DF. Aetiology of running-related gastrointestinal dysfunction. Sports Med 1998;26:365–378.

31. Peters HPF, Akkermans LMA, Bol E, et al. Gastrointestinal symptoms during exercise. Sports Med 1995;20:5–76.

32. Moses FM. The effect of exercise on the gastrointestinal tract. Sports Med 1990;9:159–172.

33. Oktedalen O, Lunde OC, Opstad PK, et al. Changes in the gastrointestinal mucosa after long-distance running. Scand J Gastroenterol 1992;27:270–274.

34. Ryan AJ. Heat stroke and endotoxemia: sensitization or tolerance to endotoxins? In Gisolfi CV, Lamb DR, Nadel ER, eds. Perspectives in Exercise Science And Sports Medicine, vol 6. Exercise, Heat, and Thermoregulation. Indianapolis: Benchmark, 1993;335–386.

CHAPTER 16

The Metabolic Systems: Control of ATP Synthesis in Skeletal Muscle

RONALD A. MEYER AND ROBERT W. WISEMAN

Introduction

The transition from rest to tetanic contraction imposes a unique burden on the metabolism of skeletal muscle compared to most other tissues. During this transition, which can occur within 30 ms in a fast muscle, the adenosine triphosphate (ATP) utilization rate can increase from about $0.01\,\mu mol$ $ATP \cdot g^{-1} \cdot s^{-1}$ at rest to nearly $10\,\mu mol$ $ATP \cdot g^{-1} \cdot s^{-1}$, a 1000-fold increase! The ATP content of mammalian fast skeletal muscles is 7 to $8\,\mu mol \cdot g^{-1}$. Thus, the entire ATP content of a fast muscle fiber could in principle be depleted after a 1-second contraction. In reality, however, net depletion of muscle ATP is observed only during the most intense heavy exercise regimens and even then rarely exceeds 30 to 40% of the available muscle ATP content. This chapter explains how this tight coupling of ATP synthesis to ATP utilization in skeletal muscle emerges from the integrated response of the metabolic system to changes in work intensity. It is only by considering the response of the system as whole that one can understand phenomena such as the oxygen deficit at the onset of exercise and the dependence of lactate production on exercise intensity.

Many excellent textbooks and monographs, for example Hochachka (1), provide introductions to exercise biochemistry. Therefore, we assume you are already familiar with basic aspects of metabolism, such as the pathways of glycolysis, the citric acid cycle, and the principles of enzyme kinetics. This chapter focuses on intracellular control mechanisms. The importance of adequate oxygen and carbon substrate delivery to muscle cells during exercise is considered in other chapters of this book.

The Rate of ATP Use During Contraction

The ATP hydrolysis rate during a muscle contraction and ultimately during repetitive exercise depends on two factors: (a) fiber type, or more specifically, the myosin and SERCA (sarcoplasmic-endoplasmic reticulum calcium ATPase) isoform types, and (b) the peak force and mechanical nature of the contraction. Myosin ATPase accounts for 70% of contractile ATP use, and SERCA activity accounts for most of the remaining 30%. Thus, variations in the kinetic properties of these two enzymes are the major source of the variation in the intrinsic ATP cost of muscle contraction, both within a species and across species. Of course, differences in myosin and SERCA isoform expression, along with differences in metabolic profile, are also the key features distinguishing the mammalian fiber types (see Chapters 5 and 6). Mammalian fibers with the fastest myosin kinetics (fast-twitch white fibers with type IIB/IIX myosin heavy chain [MHC]) and fastest SERCA (type 1) develop force quickly, shorten at the highest velocity, and relax most rapidly after a contraction. At the other extreme, slow-twitch red fibers (type I MHC, type 2A SERCA) develop force, shorten, and relax relatively slowly.

The profound effect of fiber type on contractile ATP cost (ATP used divided by force times time integral) or economy (the reciprocal of ATP cost) is not subjectively apparent to an exercising human, first because intact human muscles are generally composed of a mix of fiber types and second because the fastest fibers are organized in large motor units recruited only during the heaviest efforts. However, the limbs of rodents and some other quadrupeds have muscles with relatively uniform fiber type. For example, the soleus muscle of mice, rats, and cats consists of predominantly slow-twitch fibers, whereas the anterior tibialis or biceps brachii muscles consist of predominantly fast fiber types. Studies of these animal muscles demonstrate that slow fibers can maintain isometric force with more than three times the economy of fast fibers (2). For example, the ATP cost of a fused isometric tetanus is 2.4 μmol $\cdot$ (g muscle)$^{-1}$ $\cdot$ (kg force)$^{-1}$ $\cdot$ s^{-1} in intact cat soleus muscle (95% slow twitch) versus 8.0 in cat biceps brachii muscle (>70% fast twitch white, 20% fast twitch red). Analogous measurements have not been performed in human muscles; for example, no one has made a study of subjects with genetically diverse fiber compositions. However, based on studies of ATP turnover during activation of glycerinated, skinned single human fibers (i.e., fibers from which the sarcolemma and all internal cell membranes are removed by glycerin treatment), the difference in contractile economy between human fiber types is similar (3). This difference in contractile economy between fiber types has important implications for understanding the energetic cost of locomotion (4) and also for understanding individual differences in performance. For example, the association between elite performance in endurance sports and a high percentage of slow fibers may be largely due to the greater economy of slow fibers rather than to differences in mitochondrial content between human fiber types. In fact, the mitochondrial contents of human fast red and slow fibers are not substantially different. Endurance training can dramatically increase mitochondrial content in all the fibers recruited by a training regimen (see Chapter 21), but there is little evidence that exercise training alone can significantly change an individual's fiber type distribution. Of course, the downside to the high economy of slow fibers is their slower shortening velocity, hence lower peak mechanical power output (power equals force times velocity). Thus, individuals endowed with the slow fiber type predominance appropriate for low-power activities, such as long-distance running, are necessarily at a disadvantage for events requiring a high power output, such as sprinting.

The second major determinant of contractile ATP cost is the force and mechanical nature (e.g., isometric vs. isotonic) of the contraction. For isometric contractions lasting several seconds, contractile ATP use increases linearly with force times time integral, and for series of twitch contractions, steady-state ATPase rate is proportional to peak twitch force times twitch rate (5). To a first approximation these relationships hold during fatigue; that is, as peak force decreases during a series of fatiguing contractions, the ATP rate decreases, sometimes disproportionately. Finally, contractile ATP cost varies with the type of contraction. For example, ATPase rate of isolated muscles or skinned fibers is up to twice as high during shortening contractions than during isometric contractions, which is consistent with models of the kinetics of myosin crossbridge cycling at various velocities (3). Conversely, the ATPase rate in isolated muscles decreases during lengthening (eccentric) compared to isometric contractions, although this effect was not apparent in a recent study of ATP cost in human muscles during voluntary contractions (6).

In intact rat fast-twitch skeletal muscle the *peak cellular* ATPase rate during a fused tetanus has been estimated to exceed 10 μmol g^{-1} $\cdot$ s^{-1} (5). This estimate is based on gated phosphorus nuclear magnetic resonance (NMR) studies that were validated by comparison to steady-state measurements of muscle oxygen consumption at lower contraction intensities. Unfortunately, analogous measurements during maximal activation in intact human muscles are not easy to obtain. The estimated ATP cost of maximum voluntary contractions in human muscle ranges from 0.5 to 2 μmol $\cdot$ g^{-1} $\cdot$ s^{-1}. Unfortunately, these measurements are the average from an unknown mixed fiber population, and there is no assurance that all motor units are recruited or that all units are maximally active during a maximum voluntary contraction. Electrical stimulation of motor nerves at rates sufficient to achieve a fused tetanus would be quite painful, and the force generated from synchronous discharge of all motor units in a human muscle could be damaging. Therefore, the peak cellular ATPase rate in fast human muscle fibers can at present be estimated only by comparison with animal studies. For example, extrapolating from comparison of the ATP cost of a twitch in human mixed versus rat fast muscle (0.15 vs. 0.26 μmol $\cdot$ g^{-1} for human and rat, respectively [5,7]), the maximal ATP turnover in tetanized human fast fibers must be at least 5 μmol $\cdot$ g^{-1} $\cdot$ s^{-1}. Of course, this maximal rate, which would correspond to an oxygen consumption of over 1000 mL oxygen (kg muscle)$^{-1}$ $\cdot$ min^{-1}, cannot be continuously sustained for long (discussed later). During realistic repetitive exercises, the average rate of muscle ATP turnover is somewhat less. For example, the rate of oxygen consumption during heavy cycling exercise in well-trained subjects is around 3600 mL oxygen per minute. Assuming 10 kg of active leg muscle and assuming six muscle ATPs produced per oxygen consumed, this corresponds to an average muscle ATP turnover of around 1.6 μmol (g muscle)$^{-1}$ $\cdot$ s^{-1}.

The Capacity of ATP Synthesis Pathways in Muscle

The pathways for ATP production in vertebrate skeletal muscle are the same as in most other tissues: (*a*) direct rephosphorylation of ADP by phosphocreatine (PCr), (*b*) glycolytic ATP production, and (*c*) mitochondrial ATP production. Exercise physiology books traditionally present these pathways in a hierarchy from the most rapidly activated but shortest-lasting source of ATP (PCr utilization) to the most slowly activated but longest-lasting source (mitochondrial ATP production). Although this hierarchy correctly characterizes the relative total capacities of the three pathways for ATP generation, it obscures the key feature of the integrated metabolic response at the onset of exercise. In fact, fluxes through all three pathways occur simultaneously, and the *control* of each depends on the *regulated* response of the whole system to a change in ATPase rate. Nonetheless, it is useful to summarize this traditional hierarchy.

High-energy Phosphate (ATP and PCr) Stores

Direct rephosphorylation of ADP to ATP occurs via the reactions catalyzed by creatine kinase (CK):

$$PCr + ADP \leftrightarrow ATP + creatine$$

and adenylate kinase:

$$ADP + ADP \leftrightarrow ATP + AMP$$

(For simplicity, we largely omit the important dependence of these and the subsequent reactions on pH, cation concentration, hence on the ionic distribution of the substrates. For an example, consult Harkema and Meyer [8].) In skeletal muscle the total cytoplasmic activities of these enzymes are quite large, and so these reactions are typically assumed to be near equilibrium during contraction. In fact, calculations suggest that the CK reaction is significantly displaced from equilibrium during tetanic contractions (5). However, equilibrium is reestablished within less then a second after a tetanus, so the equilibrium assumption is reasonable when averaged over a repetitive exercise regimen.

The well-known consequence of these near-equilibrium reactions is that even in the absence of other ATP-regenerating pathways, adenosine diphosphate (ADP) accumulation is limited, first by PCr depletion and ultimately by adenosine monophosphate (AMP) accumulation. Furthermore, in skeletal muscle AMP accumulation is limited by its deamination to inosine monophosphate (IMP), catalyzed by AMP deaminase:

$$AMP \rightarrow IMP + NH_3$$

Thus, in the absence of any other source of ATP regeneration, hydrolysis of ATP results in discharge of the energy stored as PCr and ATP and ultimately in partial depletion of the adenine nucleotide pool to IMP. This occurs with minimal drop in energy *potential*, because the increase in ADP is minimized, and the free energy of ATP hydrolysis is largely preserved at 37°C, pH 7 (Fig. 16.1):

$$\Delta G_{ATP} = \Delta G'_{ATP} + RT \ln\left([ADP][Pi]/[ATP]\right)$$
$$= -32 \, kJ/mol + 2.58 \ln\left([ADP][Pi]/[ATP]\right)$$
$$[Equation \; 16.1]$$

The total capacity of this high-energy phosphate system in a fast muscle, assuming complete depletion of PCr (about 25–

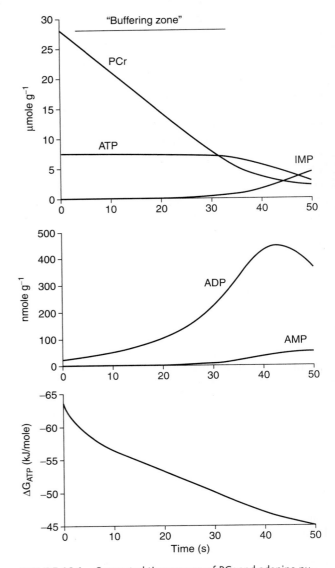

FIGURE 16.1 Computed time course of PCr and adenine nucleotide depletion in a fast-twitch skeletal muscle hydrolyzing ATP at a steady-state rate of 1 $\mu mol \cdot g^{-1} \cdot s^{-1}$, assuming there is no source for ATP resynthesis except high energy phosphate stores. Metabolite contents were computed using a kinetic model for CK and adenylate kinase fluxes (25). AMP deaminase flux assumed a simple Michaelis-Menten type of dependence on substrate AMP concentration with Km = 0.7 mM and $\dot{V}_{max}$ = 5 mM $\cdot s^{-1}$. The maximum contents of PCr, ATP, and IMP (top panel, in $\mu mol \cdot g^{-1}$) are much greater than the maximum contents of ADP and AMP (middle panel, in $nmol \cdot g^{-1}$). The buffering zone is the operating region before substantial net ATP depletion, when both PCr and ΔG_{ATP} (bottom panel) decrease nearly linearly with time or with net high energy phosphate depletion. This is range of muscle metabolite levels observed during steady-state submaximal exercise.

30 μmol · g^{-1}) and ATP (7.5 μmol · g^{-1} × 2, assuming depletion to AMP and IMP) is around 40 μmol · g^{-1}, or in principle enough to sustain a maximal contraction for about 4 seconds.

Glycolytic ATP Synthesis

The net reaction of anaerobic glycolysis from glycogen-stored glucose to lactate is

$$(glucose)_n + 3\,ADP + 3\,P_i \rightarrow (glucose)_{n-1} + 3\,ATP + 2\,lactic\ acid$$

Assuming only stored glycogen as substrate (50–100 μmol glucose units · g^{-1}), the total capacity for ATP generation by this pathway alone is thus around 150 to 300 μmol ATP g^{-1}, or enough to sustain maximal contraction for up to 30 seconds. Despite the low yield of ATP, this pathway is not thermodynamically inefficient, because as emphasized by Brooks (9), most of the available free energy remains in lactate, which can be further oxidized in the muscle or in other tissues.

Surprisingly, some authors have suggested that lactic acid production via glycolysis is not the cause of muscle acidosis, because hydrogen ion release actually occurs earlier in the pathway and ATP hydrolysis also produces hydrogen ions. However, with respect to its effect on pH balance in the muscle, all that matters is the net reaction. Because glycolytic ATP production is balanced by ATP utilization so that the net change in ATP is minor (and as illustrated in Fig. 16.1, any significant ATP depletion is largely balanced by IMP and ammonia production, not ADP accumulation), the net glycolytic reaction in an active muscle is just glucose → 2 lactic acid. Therefore, lactic acid production is the major cause of muscle acidosis during exercise.

The functional consequences of intracellular lactic acidosis are complex and not necessarily deleterious. For example, although acidosis does slow muscle relaxation rate after contractions, the idea that muscle fatigue is caused by direct effects of lactic acidosis on myofibrillar actin-myosin interaction and force generation has been largely abandoned (10). Certainly acidosis inhibits many enzymes and ion channels and may decrease the maximum rate of mitochondrial ATP production in intact muscle. On the other hand, acidosis actually appears to increase the mitochondrial energy potential for ATP synthesis (8). One might naively assume that acidosis lowers the cytosolic free energy of ATP hydrolysis, because net ATP hydrolysis yields a fractional hydrogen ion above pH 6.5:

$$ATP \rightarrow ADP + Pi + \alpha H^+$$

Where α = the molar fraction of hydrogen ions released per mole of ATP hydrolyzed.

However, if ATP hydrolysis is thermodynamically coupled to PCr hydrolysis via the CK reaction, acidosis has the opposite net effect on ATP free energy. Assuming equilibrium of the CK reaction, the free energy of ATP hydrolysis must equal that of PCr hydrolysis, and the free energy of PCr

hydrolysis increases (i.e., is more negative) as pH falls (8). Stated another way, the pH dependence of the CK reaction over the physiological range is as follows:

$$PCr + ADP + \beta H^+ \leftrightarrow ATP + creatine$$

Where β = the molar fraction of hydrogen ion consumed per mole of PCr hydrolyzed ranging from about 0.9 to 0.6 from pH 7 to pH 6. This tends to lower ADP as a muscle becomes acidic. For example, assuming equilibrium of the CK reaction, constant muscle [PCr]/[Cr] = 1, and [P$_i$] = 15 mM (reasonable values during moderately heavy exercise) (where P$_i$ = inorganic phosphate), a decrease in pH from 7.1 to 6.5 increases the free energy of PCr and ATP hydrolysis from −55.8 to −57.7 kJ · mole^{-1} (8). Thus, in the presence of the CK system, lactic acidosis actually blunts the decline in ATP free energy that would otherwise occur with depletion of PCr.

Oxidative Phosphorylation

Finally, the net reaction for complete oxidation of glycogen-derived pyruvate (including the reduced nicotinamide adenine dinucleotide (NADH) yield from glycolysis) is as follows:

$$2C_3H_5O_3 + 6O_2 + 2NADH + 33ADP + 33P_i \rightarrow 6CO_2 + 6H_2O + 2NAD + 33ATP$$

The corresponding net reaction for complete oxidation of the 16-carbon saturated fatty acid palmitate is thus:

$$C_{16}H_{32}O_2 + 23O_2 + 129ADP + 129P_i \rightarrow 16CO_2 + 16H_2O + 129ATP$$

Clearly mitochondrial oxidative phosphorylation is the only source of ATP production with the capacity to support prolonged exercise, and in this respect the traditional presentation is correct.

The tempting inference from this traditional hierarchy is that these pathways are controlled independently and that their relative importance at the onset of exercise is related to the speed at which they can be activated and how long they can last. This inference is *not* correct. For example, although it is correct that net PCr hydrolysis accounts for most of the ATP used during the first seconds at the onset of contractions, this fact does not demonstrate that there is any intrinsic delay or inertia for activation of either glycolysis or mitochondrial ATP production. On the contrary, these pathways respond simultaneously and in an integrated fashion to the same initiating events: calcium release and hydrolysis of ATP.

Control Versus Regulation in Muscle Metabolism

It is important to distinguish between metabolic *control* and metabolic *regulation*. Control is the effect of a signal on the flux through an enzyme or pathway. Regulation is the maintenance of some parameter in a relatively constant state despite changes in external signals or pathway flux. By these definitions, the central external controlling element in muscle metabolism is the input from the motor neuron, reflected intracellularly by release of calcium from the sarcoplasmic reticulum (SR), and by activation of myosin and SERCA ATPases. The central *regulated* parameter is not the ATP hydrolysis rate or pathway fluxes *per se* but rather the cytoplasmic free energy of ATP hydrolysis. This regulation arises from the entire network behavior of the ATP synthesizing pathways and the main ATPases, that is, myosin and SERCA. Its effectiveness is illustrated by the fact that the maximum drop in ATP free energy observed in human muscle even during the heaviest exercise is only 14 kJ · mole^{-1} (to −50 kJ · mole^{-1} from near −64 kJ · mole^{-1} at rest) (J. A. L. Jeneson, personal communication, January 2004).

The physiological importance of regulating cytoplasmic ATP free energy can be appreciated by considering the energy required to maintain ion gradients across the sarcolemma and SR. For example, ignoring electrical effects and assuming a stoichiometry of two calcium ions pumped per ATP hydrolyzed by the SERCA pump, the maximum cytoplasmic to SR luminal calcium gradient that can be developed depends on ΔG_{ATP}:

$$\left[Ca^{++}\right]_{SR}/\left[Ca^{++}\right]_{CYTO} = \exp\left[\left(-\Delta G_{ATP}/\left(2 \times RT\right)\right)\right]$$
[Equation 16.2]

where RT = the gas constant times absolute temperature (2.58 kJ · mole^{-1} at 37°C). Thus, a 14 kJ · mole^{-1} drop in ATP free energy would reduce this maximum gradient by more than 93%. If ΔG_{ATP} were to fall to less than −48 kJ · mole^{-1}, there would not be sufficient energy to sequester calcium against the normal 10,000-fold gradient after a contraction (11), and the muscle might fail to relax, with obviously disastrous effects on locomotion. Similarly, the maximum sodium gradient that can be maintained across the cell membrane by Na-K ATPase, assuming three sodium ions pumped per ATP hydrolyzed, depends on ΔG_{ATP}:

$$\left[Na^{+}\right]_{out}/\left[Na^{+}\right]_{in} = \exp\left(\left(-\Delta G_{ATP}/3 - F \times Em\right)/RT\right)$$
[Equation 16.3]

where Em = the membrane potential (−80 mV) and F = Faraday's constant and ignoring the small additional energy needed to cotransport potassium, which is near electrochemical equilibrium across the membrane. Thus, failure of the sarcolemmal Na-K ATPase to maintain the normal 20-fold sodium gradient across the sarcolemma would also occur near −48 kJ · mole^{-1}, with equally disastrous consequences for the muscle.

The concept that muscle ATPase rate controls the rate of ATP production is easy to apply to the direct production of ATP from PCr and ADP. In this case it is obvious that no other control mechanism is required, because the CK and adenylate kinase near-equilibrium reactions simply respond by mass action to the change in adenine nucleotide concentrations when ATP is hydrolyzed.

It may appear impossible to apply the same concept to control of glycogenolysis and glycolysis because of the entrenched view that control of this pathway must reside at the rate-limiting or irreversible reactions catalyzed by glycogen phosphorylase (GP), phosphofructokinase, and pyruvate kinase. However, no enzymatic reaction is irreversible on the molecular level, although the thermodynamic drive for the reaction might point very heavily in one direction *in vivo*. Lambeth and Kushmerick (12) recently exploited this basic consideration in a simulation of glycogenolysis and glycolysis in skeletal muscle. The simulation assumed that all of the reactions between glycogen and lactate production were reversible, that glycogen concentration was constant, and that lactate removal equaled lactate production, so that pH effects were not considered. The simulation was run to steady-state at three ATPase activities corresponding to rest, moderate exercise, and heavy exercise (up to 1 mM ATP · second^{-1}, equivalent to 224 mL of oxygen per kilogram of muscle per minute), and the steady-state sensitivities of glycolytic flux to each enzyme's activity were computed. Sensitivity is the ratio of percent change in a pathway's steady-state flux to percent change in an enzyme's activity, and in the formalism of metabolic control analysis it is also known as the flux control coefficient (13) (discussed later). The main conclusion from these computations was that flux control over glycolysis resided almost entirely (>95%) in the ATPase over the entire range considered. At the highest ATPase rate, the small proportion of flux control contributed by glycolytic enzymes was widely distributed over the whole pathway, whereas at rest it was confined to GP and phosphofructokinase. Increasing the percentage of GP in the active (a) form from 1 to 40% (similar to the activation observed at the onset of exercise in human muscle) had no effect on the overall flux but did shift the minor flux control exerted by glycolytic enzymes to include greater contributions from enolase and pyruvate kinase. The latter result explains some previously puzzling experimental results, for example the observations that the inactivation of GP after a few minutes of exercise does not decrease glycolytic flux and that activation of GP by administration of epinephrine does not necessarily increase glycolytic flux. If a pathway is tightly coupled to ATP synthesis, pathway flux cannot increase unless ATPase rate increases or the contribution from some other ATP producing pathway decreases. On the other hand, this modeling does not yet explain another puzzling aspect of glycolysis in muscle: flux stops within seconds after the end of a series of anoxic contractions, even though the products of net high-energy phosphate hydrolysis (ADP, creatine, AMP, IMP and phosphate) are presumably still elevated (14).

The concept that calcium-activated ATPases are central to the control of muscle mitochondrial ATP production was examined by Jeneson and associates (15) using the principles of metabolic control analysis. Metabolic control analysis is a quantitative method for analyzing the distribution of flux control within a steady-state network of reactions (13).

The relative contribution to control of each enzyme or functional element of a pathway's flux is characterized by its sensitivity or flux control coefficient, as defined earlier. The effects of a shared substrate on each element's activity are characterized by elasticity coefficients. Elasticity is analogous to a reaction's order with respect to a substrate. For example, the elasticity of a simple Michalis-Menten type of enzymatic reaction to a saturating substrate is zero, since the reaction's rate does not increase with further increases in the substrate. Finally, the concentration control coefficient of an enzyme on a pathway's shared substrate is just the relative change in that substrate's concentration with a change in the enzyme's activity. These coefficients are related by several algebraic constraints, for example that the sum of control coefficients for a pathway flux must equal one and the sum of concentration control coefficients for a substrate must equal zero. In practice, the mathematics of metabolic control analysis becomes formidable for networks with more than a few elements, and calculation of elasticity coefficients *in vivo* from enzyme kinetic data *in vitro* is not always straightforward. Nonetheless, Jeneson and associates (15) solved this algebraic problem for a three-element network of myosin ATPase, SERCA, and mitochondrial ATP production, assuming ATP and ADP as the only common substrates and using flux estimates derived from studies of human muscle during twitch stimulation. As might be expected, all three elements exerted some concentration control over the ATP/ADP ratio. However, over the range from mild to moderate stimulation intensities, *flux control* over the mitochondria (the only ATP-generating element in the model) resided almost entirely within the myosin and SERCA ATPases. Only when the calculations

were extrapolated to very high stimulation rates did control over mitochondrial ATP generation shift to the mitochondrial element itself. The conceptual result is that the entire system adapts to increased flux with minimal perturbation in ATP free energy.

The Control of Muscle Respiration

The argument that mitochondrial ATP production and respiration rate are controlled by muscle ATPases is not likely to satisfy many readers because it does not specify any distinct biochemical signaling mechanism acting at the mitochondria. Mitochondrial ATP production occurs in a complicated membrane-bound organelle and involves the coordinated activity of dozens of nonvectorial and vectorial reaction steps. (Vectorial reactions are those that occur with a spatial orientation, such as ion transport.) Therefore, the idea that specific signals are required to control mitochondria is appealing, and enormous effort been spent to determine what controls muscle respiration. Consideration of the candidates requires a summary of the mechanism and energetics of mitochondrial ATP production.

   Mitochondria are small organelles (0.5–1 μm across) composed of two lipid bilayers (Fig. 16.2). The outer membrane is smooth and permeable to the free diffusion of substrates such as carbon fuels, ADP, ATP, P_i, creatine, PCr, and ions (including hydrogen ions) and dissolved gases. The inner membrane is relatively impermeable and highly invaginated, essential properties for mitochondrial function. The invaginations, termed cristae, vary with the oxidative capacity of

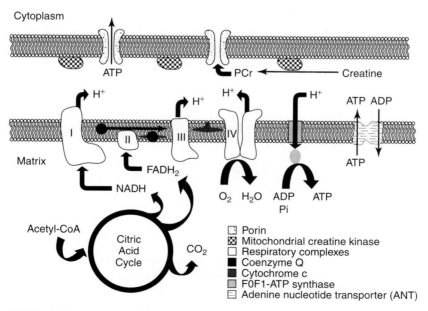

FIGURE 16.2 Locations of the major respiratory components in the mitochondrial membranes and matrix.

the mitochondrion because of the high density of respiratory complexes and specific transporters embedded within this membrane. Thus, energetically important metabolites such as ATP, ADP, and P_i freely diffuse through the outer membrane but require carriers for their transport across the inner membrane, as do the monocarboxylic and dicarboxylic acid carbon substrates. The inner membrane encompasses the mitochondrial matrix, a lumen that contains all the enzymes, substrates and cofactors necessary for the function of the citric acid cycle (CAC). Mitochondria produce ATP by converting the energy in chemical bonds from the oxidation of carbohydrates and fats into NADH, which is used by the electron transport system to create a hydrogen ion electrochemical gradient. This gradient is generated across the inner membrane by pumping hydrogen ions out of the matrix and into the inner membrane space using the respiratory complexes. The flow of hydrogen ions back down this energy gradient into the matrix rapidly alters the conformation of F0/F1 ATP synthase, thus transferring the energy from the gradient into the terminal phosphate bond of ATP. Finally, the exchange of cytoplasmic ADP for matrix ATP via the ade-nine nucleotide transporter is in effect driven by the energy of the hydrogen ion gradient.

The conceptual flux and energetic relationships through mitochondria are depicted in Figure 16.3 by a sequence of pipes and reservoirs. Each element of the overall mechanism has an associated flux (illustrated by the size of the black arrows in the pipes) and a maximum flux capacity (illustrated by the diameters of the pipes). The energetic state of the system is characterized by several free energy potentials, depicted by the relative heights of the shaded areas in each potential reservoir. For, example, the redox potential is the free energy available in oxidation of NADH to nicotinamide adenine dinucleotide (NAD); that is:

$$\Delta G_{REDOX} = \Delta G^{\circ}_{REDOX} + RT \ln([NAD]/[NADH])$$
$$[Equation\ 16.4]$$

The standard free energy, ΔG°_{REDOX}, is about -218 kJ · mole^{-1}, so even at an NAD/NADH ratio of 1, there is more than enough potential energy to synthesize three ATPs at a cytoplasmic ATP free energy of -60 to -65 kJ · mole^{-1}. The hydrogen ion electrochemical potential depends on the hydrogen

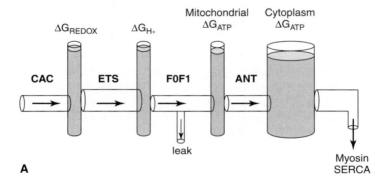

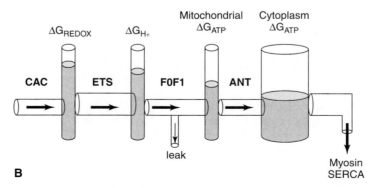

FIGURE 16.3 The steady-state relationship between intramitochondrial and extramitochondrial energy potentials and the pathway conductances connecting them under various conditions. **A.** State 4, or resting skeletal muscle. **B.** Skeletal muscle during submaximal exercise. **C.** Effect of mitochondrial dehydrogenase activation during submaximal exercise. **D.** Effect of hypoxia during submaximal exercise.

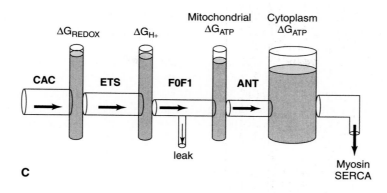

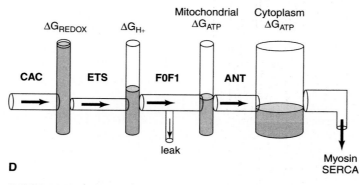

FIGURE 16.3   *(continued)*

ion gradient across the inner membrane and membrane potential according to the following:

$$\Delta G_{H+} = 2.303 \times RT \left(pH_{matrix} - pH_{cyto} \right) + F \times Em$$

[Equation 16.5]

The ATP free energy inside and outside the mitochondria can be computed as in Equation 16.1.

(In this conceptual diagram we have ignored the fact that the ATP/ADP ratio and therefore the free energy of ATP hydrolysis are lower in the matrix of mitochondria than in the cytoplasm. The additional potential in the cytoplasm is gained by the exchange of ATP^{4-} for ADP^{3-} in the adenine nucleotide transporter, energetically driven by the hydrogen electrochemical potential gradient.) These various potentials are coupled but can change relative to each other depending on the magnitude of the connecting fluxes relative to their maximum flux capacities. In the steady state, the flux into and out of each element is equal, and the steady-state flux through the system could in principle be limited at any element.

Figure 16.3A depicts the situation in skeletal muscle at rest, or in isolated mitochondria near the classic state 4, that is, with unlimited carbon fuel and oxygen but relatively little drain on the system by cytoplasmic ATP hydrolysis. In state 4, all of the potentials are charged, and the only drain on the system is the uncoupled leak of hydrogen ions back

into the mitochondrial matrix. (By leak we mean any dissipation of the hydrogen ion gradient that is not coupled to ATP synthesis and export.) The situation in a skeletal muscle at rest approximates the situation in state 4 except that the basal resting ATP synthesis rate is normally much greater than the leak, and the ratio of ATP synthesized to oxygen consumed approaches the optimal coupling ratio of 6.

Now consider the effect on this system if the cytoplasmic ATP hydrolysis rate is increased (Fig. 16.3B), for example to 50% of the muscle cell's maximum possible oxidative capacity. The cytoplasmic ΔG_{ATP} will fall, ADP and P_i concentrations will increase, the transport of these substrates into the matrix will increase, and the rate of ATP synthase will increase. This will in turn lower the hydrogen ion potential and flux through the electron transport chain will increase, and so on back through the entire sequence. The potential energy at every step will decrease to an extent determined by the kinetic properties and maximum capacity of the flux elements into and out of those potentials. Ultimately a new steady state with equally higher flux into and out of each element will be established. Of course, each element will behave in a fashion consistent with its kinetic properties. For example, the steady-state transport of nucleotides by adenine nucleotide transporter will be consistent with its binding affinities for ADP and ATP, and the synthesis of ATP by F1/F0 ATP synthase will be consistent with its affinities for ADP and P_i. Thus, under some specific set of experimental conditions (e.g., isolated mitochondria saturated with all other substrates), a plot of ADP concentration versus steady-state respiration rate might yield a simple Michalis-Menten type of first-order (hyperbolic) relationship, with the apparent Michaelis constant near that of the adenine nucleotide transporter binding constant for ADP. Under some other set of conditions, the relationship between ADP and respiration rate might be higher order (sigmoidal), reflecting kinetic elasticity to ADP at more than one site, for example at both adenine nucleotide transporter and ATP synthase (16). If phosphate is initially low, there might be a satisfying relationship between phosphate concentration and steady-state respiration rate. The key point is that measurement of the relationship between a single factor and the overall steady-state flux under some set of conditions does not establish its preeminence as the controlling or limiting factor under all conditions.

Now consider the effect of calcium activation on this system (Fig. 16.3C). In addition to the activation of cytoplasmic ATPases, calcium has effects at four possible sites within the mitochondria: pyruvate dehydrogenase (PDH), α-ketoglutarate dehydrogenase, isocitrate dehydrogenase, and ATP synthase (17). Of these, the evidence is most complete for PDH, so for simplicity we consider only the effect of calcium at that site. PDH (actually a 3-megadalton complex of enzymes) catalyzes the following net reaction:

$$Pyruvate + NAD + CoA \rightarrow acetyl\text{-}CoA + NADH + CO_2$$

Thus, this reaction both contributes to the redox potential and provides input of acetyl-coenzyme A (CoA) to the citric acid cycle. Calcium-stimulated dephosphorylation of the complex effectively increases the maximum flux capacity, an effect illustrated in Figure 16.3C by increased diameter of the flux connection into the redox potential. *Ignoring* the effect of increased calcium on cytoplasmic ATPases, the result is a new steady state with higher redox potential and higher hydrogen ion and ATP free energy potentials (assuming constant leak) and with no change in the steady-state rate of ATP production. *Including* the parallel effect of calcium on cytoplasmic ATPases, the result would be a new steady state with higher flux throughout the system. In that case, the changes in potential accompanying the increased flux would depend on the balance between calcium's effects at the various sites. For example, in a tightly coupled system with densely packed mitochondria operating at high flux rates (e.g., cardiac muscle) flux control might reside predominantly in the calcium-sensitive dehydrogenases. In that case, changes in respiratory flux can occur with little or no change in cytoplasmic ATP free energy (18).

Finally, consider the effect of low oxygen concentration on this system (Fig. 16.3D). The result is restriction of flow in the electron transport chain. The system might still be able to support the same steady-state flux, but the upstream redox potential would increase, and the downstream hydrogen ion and ATP potentials would fall. Therefore, changes in oxygen

concentration can alter the steady-state relationship between cytoplasmic phosphate metabolites and respiratory rate (19).

Thus, we arrive by a different route to the view presented in the previous section: over the submaximal range the steady-state rate of skeletal muscle respiration is largely controlled by the rate of cytoplasmic ATP hydrolysis, signaled to the mitochondria primarily by the increase in ADP and to some extent by P_i. Under the conditions prevalent in mammalian fast muscle over the submaximal range of exercise intensities, these signaling mechanisms translate into the experimentally observed quasi-linear relationship between respiratory rate and cytoplasmic ΔG_{ATP} (Fig. 16.4). Other factors, such as oxygen or carbon substrate availability, activation of PDH, and altered mitochondrial content after exercise training or deconditioning, can effectively alter the maximum flux capacity or change the overall thermodynamic drive for mitochondrial ATP synthesis and thereby modulate the steady-state relationship between cytoplasmic nucleotides and respiratory flux. Nonethe-less, in skeletal muscle the control resides primarily in the ATPases.

The Limit to Muscle Respiratory Response Time

The response time for the increase in oxygen consumption to a new steady state in human skeletal muscle at the onset

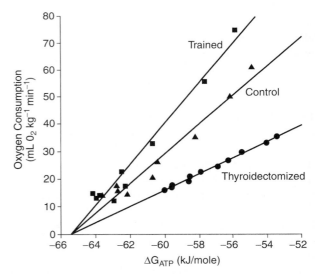

FIGURE 16.4 Relationships between cytoplasmic ΔG_{ATP} and estimated oxygen consumption during recovery after submaximal stimulation in gastrocnemius muscles from trained (highest muscle mitochondrial content), control, and chemically thyroidectomized (lowest mitochondrial content) rats. (Redrawn with permission from Paganini AT, Foley JM, Meyer RA. Linear dependence of muscle phosphocreatine kinetics on oxidative capacity. Am J Physiol 272 [Cell Physiol 41] 1997;C501–C510. Assuming resting oxygen consumption of 12.5 mL oxygen per kilogram per minute in all groups.)

of submaximal exercise is 30 seconds or more (20). In contrast, at 37°C the response time of isolated mitochondria to a step increase in external ADP or P_i concentration is less than 3 seconds (17), an order of magnitude faster. What accounts for this difference?

The main part of the answer is implicit in Figure 16.3. Any transition from one respiratory rate to another (e.g., from rest, as in Fig. 16.3A, to submaximal exercise, as in Fig. 16.3B) is accompanied by a change in the height of one or more of the potential reservoirs. The speed with which these changes can occur depends on the volume, or *capacitance,* of the reservoirs, and on the maximum flow capacity, or *conductance,* of the connecting pipes. Thus, each metabolic potential has an associated capacitance that influences how fast that potential, and therefore the net flux through the whole pathway, can change. If all of the potentials change, the response time of the whole system will be dominated by the potential with the largest capacitance.

The concept of metabolic capacitance can be quantitatively applied to each of the potentials depicted in Figure 16.3. In the presence of the CK reaction, the capacitance of the cytoplasmic ΔG_{ATP} potential over most of the submaximal range (the buffering zone of Fig. 16.1) just depends on the total creatine content (PCr + creatine). Total creatine is about 35 to 45 μmol $\cdot$ g^{-1} in mammalian fast muscle and somewhat less in slow-twitch muscle. This greatly exceeds the total capacitance associated with all of the other intramitochondrial potentials depicted in Figure 16.3, because all of these capacitances are restricted to the relatively small volume of the mitochondrial matrix (at most 8% of skeletal muscle cell volume). For example, the capacitance of the mitochondrial matrix adenine nucleotide pool is not augmented by a CK system. Therefore, its maximum capacitance is just equal to the total intramitochondrial adenine nucleotide content, or at most 1.6 μmol $\cdot$ g^{-1} of muscle, assuming 20 mM total nucleotide concentration in the matrix compartment. Similarly, the capacitance associated with the mitochondrial redox potential just depends on total mitochondrial NAD and NADH content. Even assuming the entire NAD and NADH content in skeletal muscle is in the matrix, this is less than 1 μmol $\cdot$ g^{-1} of muscle. The capacitance associated with the hydrogen ion electrochemical potential just depends on the pH buffering capacity of the matrix (again limited by the small matrix volume) plus a very minor contribution from the electrical capacitance of the inner membrane. Finally, the capacitance associated with the PDH reaction itself is trivial, because the total content of CoA in skeletal muscle is less than 0.02 μmol $\cdot$ g^{-1}.

Because the metabolic capacitance of the cytoplasmic CK system so greatly exceeds all other potential capacitances associated with mitochondria ATP production, the time-dependent behavior of the system in Figure 16.3, and therefore of muscle respiration, can be shown by collapsing all the intramitochondrial potentials and conductances into single elements. To a good approximation, the time dependence can

be modeled by a three-element circuit composed of a single lumped mitochondrial potential (represented by a battery), a single mitochondrial conductance, and a single parallel capacitance representing the cytoplasmic CK system (Fig. 16.5A). The main feature of this circuit is that after a step increase in load (i.e., increased cytoplasmic ATP hydrolysis rate), the flux through the conductance (mitochondrial ATP production) and the flux from the capacitance (PCr hydrolysis) both approach a new steady state along exponential time courses, with time constant just equal to capacitance divided by conductance (21). Therefore, this model explains the observation that the kinetics of PCr and oxygen consumption at the onset of and after submaximal exercise are mirror images

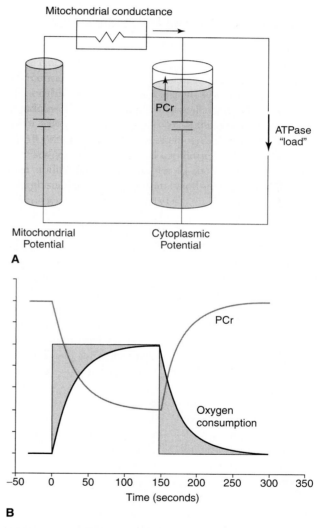

FIGURE 16.5   **A.** Collapsed three-element potential, conductance, and capacitance model of respiratory kinetics with an overlaid electrical circuit analogue. **B.** Relationships between muscle PCr (gray line), muscle oxygen consumption rate (black line), and the associated muscle oxygen deficit (initial shaded area) and recovery oxygen debt (second shaded area) at the onset of and after exercise requiring a steady-state increase in muscle ATPase rate.

(Fig. 16.5*B*). The model also explains the fact that increased mitochondrial content (increased conductance) shortens the time constant for both PCr and oxygen consumption kinetics during submaximal exercise, in addition to increasing the maximum respiratory rate and increasing the slope of the relationship between cytoplasmic ΔG_{ATP} and respiratory rate (Fig. 16.4). Interestingly, increased mitochondrial content appears to have no effect on the lumped mitochondrial potential in rat fast muscle. As shown in Figure 16.4, extrapolations of the relationships between estimated respiratory rate and ΔG_{ATP} to zero respiratory rate yield the same potential independent of mitochondrial content. This no-load potential is an estimate of the lumped intramitochondrial potential for ATP synthesis in this muscle type (-65 kJ $\cdot$ mole^{-1}).

The Oxygen Deficit and Metabolic Inertia

Inasmuch as the circuit model of Figure 16.5*A* explains the coincidence of PCr and oxygen consumption kinetics at the onset of submaximal exercise, it also explains the oxygen deficit at the onset of submaximal exercise and the oxygen debt after it (the shaded areas in Figure 16.5*B*). According to this view, the oxygen deficit results from the time dependence of the whole system and does not represent "the period when the energy demand of contraction *cannot* [emphasis added] be met solely by mitochondrial ATP generation" (22). This explanation for the oxygen deficit suggests that some intrinsic delay or inertia must be overcome before mitochondrial ATP production can be activated and that PCr hydrolysis just makes up the deficit caused by the slow mitochondrial response. The inertial delay in mitochondrial activation has variously been attributed to delayed oxygen delivery, to a need to prime the Krebs cycle with substrates (anaplerosis), and most recently to a delay in activation of the PDH complex and production of acetyl-CoA (22).

In fact, the observation that PCr and oxygen consumption kinetics are both faster in muscles with higher mitochondrial content provides *prima facie* evidence that this alternative explanation for the oxygen deficit must be largely incorrect. If there was a long *intrinsic* delay in mitochondrial activation, then all other things being equal, having more mitochondria would have no effect on the delay, although it still would increase maximum steady-state oxygen consumption. Clear evidence against this explanation comes from the effect of depleting total creatine content on muscle PCr kinetics. If PCr and oxygen consumption kinetics were both determined by an intrinsic delay in mitochondrial activation, partial depletion of total creatine content would have no effect on the time constant for PCr depletion, provided that sufficient PCr remained to make up the deficit. In contrast, if the kinetics are determined by mitochondrial conductance and CK capacitance together, as argued earlier, then decreasing total creatine content, and hence the capacitance of the system, should hasten the kinetics of both PCr and oxygen consumption. This experiment was performed

over a decade ago (23). The result was that the time constant for PCr changes decreased nearly linearly with depletion of total creatine. Similarly, inhibition of CK shortens the time constant for changes in oxygen consumption with increased workload in isolated hearts (24). A dramatic decrease in respiratory response time may occur in skeletal muscle of mice with genetic knockout of cytoplasmic CK (25). However the kinetics of skeletal muscle oxygen consumption have not yet been reported in muscles of these animals.

Of course, the simplified model of Figure 16.5 omits important modulating effects considered in the previous section, such as the effects of hypoxia or PDH activation. For example, if acetyl-CoA production via PDH were the conductance element limiting maximum oxygen consumption in muscle, then pharmacological activation of PDH with a drug such as dichloroacetate would effectively hasten the kinetics of oxygen consumption at the onset of submaximal exercise. However, recent evidence indicates that dichloroacetate does not alter the kinetics of either PCr or oxygen consumption in human muscle (26). Instead, the reported effects of PDH activation (decreased net PCr hydrolysis and lactate accumulation during exercise in some [22] but not all [27] studies) are most likely related to an effect on mitochondrial redox potential. Higher redox potential would drive the same steady-state respiration with less decrease in cytoplasmic ΔG_{ATP} and therefore relatively less drive on the PCr and glycogenolysis pathways.

In summary, the response time of mitochondrial ATP production at the onset of submaximal exercise is determined by the muscle's mitochondrial content or maximum respiratory capacity *and* by the capacitance of the cytoplasmic CK system. Evidence that other "inertial" factors significantly limit respiratory kinetics in well-oxygenated skeletal muscle is scanty. In any case, use of the term *inertia* to describe metabolic kinetics should be discouraged. Inertia refers to the property of a mass to continue in constant motion unless some energy is applied or dissipated to alter that motion. The electrical analogue of inertia is inductance; that is, energy must be applied or dissipated to *change* the current in coil of wire. It is difficult to imagine how a metabolic flux could have inertia or inductance, because metabolic flux always dissipates some energy and must cease when there is no driving free energy potential.

The Limits to Maximum Sustainable ATP Turnover Rate in Muscle

As described earlier, the maximum *instantaneous* rate of ATP utilization during contraction depends on the muscle's myosin and SERCA isoform types and on the extent of their activation by calcium. Of course, in the absence of any balancing ATP production, this rate cannot be sustained for long. Because of fatigue processes, force generation and therefore the ATP hydrolysis rate will decrease, attenuating the drop in cytoplasmic ΔG_{ATP}. Fatigue therefore plays a crucial role in the regulation of ΔG_{ATP} in healthy skeletal muscle. If fatigue processes did not limit ATP hydrolysis, a muscle cell could work itself to death. The precise mechanism or mechanisms of muscle cell fatigue are not fully understood. However, most recent evidence suggests that decreased force during heavy repetitive exercise regimens (for example, weightlifting) is largely due to decreased SR calcium release (see Chapter 8).

It follows that the maximum *sustainable* rate of ATP utilization in muscle cells depends on the maximum flux capacity of the pathways for ATP production, along with the duration over which the rate must be sustained. For contraction regimens of relatively short duration, the sustainable rate can be highest, because all three pathways for ATP production can contribute significantly to the total. In that case, the balance between the three pathways is determined by their maximum flux capacities relative to each other (which varies with fiber type and training status) *and* by the interplay between their differing elasticities to calcium and/or net ATP hydrolysis. Thus, PCr hydrolysis contributes the most to muscle ATP synthesis during the first seconds of exercise *at any intensity* because the response of the CK reaction to the initial change in ATP/ADP ratio is the greatest, not because the response times of glycolysis and oxidative respiration are intrinsically slow. The contribution of glycolysis to ATP production is greatest during short-duration heavy exercises, both because the maximum oxidative capacity of recruited fibers is limited *and* because the type IIB and IIX fibers recruited at high intensities have the greatest complement of glycolytic enzymes. On the other hand, for prolonged exercise, which must rely on the high *total* ATP-producing capacity of mitochondria, the maximum sustainable rate depends directly on mitochondrial content, or more specifically on the activity of inner mitochondrial membrane complexes (28).

Of course, maximum sustainable ATPase rate might be reduced further if oxygen or carbon substrate supply is limited, for example by poor blood flow or by limited diffusion of these substances to the muscle cells. While these possibilities are beyond the scope of this chapter, there is a related question about intracellular energy. Does the intracellular diffusion of ATP and ADP between sites of ATP use (e.g., myofibrils and SERCA) and ATP production (e.g., mitochondria) limit the maximum sustainable ATPase rate?

Intracellular Diffusion as a Limit to Maximum Sustainable ATPase Rate

Assuming no specific diffusion barrier for adenine nucleotides compared to other similar-sized molecules, this question can be answered by considering the nature of molecular diffusion. Diffusion is just the statistical result of random molecular motions. From this it can be shown that on average, the time (t) it takes an individual molecule to randomly move some distance (d) increases with the *square* of the distance:

$$t = d^2/2D \text{ (for one dimensional diffusion).}$$
$$[\text{Equation 16.6}]$$

Therefore, the effectiveness of diffusion as a transport mechanism depends critically on the diffusion distance. The diffusion coefficient, D, depends on the effective radius of the diffusing molecule, and on the medium in which it is diffusing. For example, the diffusion coefficient of P_i in solution at 37°C (about 1×10^{-6} cm$^2 \cdot$ s^{-1}) is higher than that of ATP (about 0.5×10^{-6} cm$^2 \cdot$ s^{-1}). Both molecules diffuse more slowly in muscle cells than in water, presumably because of the tortuosity of the diffusion path around myofilaments and other intracellular structures. The familiar Fick law of steady-state diffusion also follows directly from the statistical average of random molecular motions. In one dimension, Fick's law is as follows:

$$J = D \times dC/dx \qquad [\text{Equation 16.7}]$$

Where J = the diffusive flux across some plane and dC/dx = the concentration gradient perpendicular to that plane. Thus, the concentration gradient required to maintain some steady-state flux depends on the diffusion coefficient. For example, for any steady-state flux, the phosphate gradient from myofibrils to mitochondria is less than the ADP gradient (and also less than the ATP gradient in the opposite direction).

It seems plausible that ADP would be the metabolite limiting intracellular flux between myofibrils or SERCA and mitochondria, because the concentration of ADP is much lower than the concentration of ATP and P_i. If a substantial gradient for ADP was required, ADP would have to be substantially higher at the myofibrils and SERCA than at the mitochondria, which might inhibit calcium uptake and slow shortening velocity. However, despite the intuitive plausibility of this notion, the truth depends critically on the actual diffusion distance between the organelles. Calculations show that for distances less than several micrometers (e.g., the axial distance across several myofibrils), the required ADP gradient could not be energetically significant. On the other hand, over longer distances (e.g., in a 50-µm-diameter muscle fiber with mitochondria clustered in the periphery) the gradient could become significant to energy (5). However, in both of these cases, the CK reaction actually decreases the required ADP diffusion gradients to insignificance. Because specific CK isozymes are localized in mitochondria and in myofibrils (in addition to the soluble CK in between), the CK system provides an additional path for metabolite diffusion: the creatine shuttle (29,30).

The Creatine Shuttle

The fact that most of the diffusive flux of high-energy phosphate between sites in muscle cells is actually carried by creatine and PCr rather than by ADP and ATP is now widely accepted. However, the *reason* the creatine shuttle works so effectively is sometimes misunderstood. Certainly the concentration of free creatine in muscle (up to 20 μmol $\cdot$ g^{-1} at the upper end of the submaximal buffering range illustrated in Fig. 16.1) is much higher than the concentration of ADP (less than 0.2 μmol $\cdot$ g^{-1} over the submaximal range). Therefore, development of the same absolute diffusion gradient requires a much smaller percent difference in creatine. Furthermore, the diffusion coefficient of creatine is about twice as large as that of the larger-molecular-weight nucleotides, so the creatine gradient required to support the same diffusive flux would be less. The product of diffusion coefficient times concentration is sometimes called diffusivity, and clearly the diffusivity of creatine is much higher than that of ADP in skeletal muscle. However, this difference in diffusivity does not fully convey the key underlying factor that determines the effectiveness of the creatine shuttle. In fact, most of its effectiveness arises from the high apparent equilibrium constant of the CK reaction. It has been shown (30) that assuming near equilibrium of the CK reaction, the ratio of steady-state diffusive fluxes carried by creatine versus ADP (and PCr vs. ATP) across any surface between sites of ATP hydrolysis and ATP synthesis varies according to

$$J_{Cr}/J_{ADP} = \left(D_{Cr}/D_{ADP}\right) \times \left(\text{total creatine/total nucleotide}\right)$$
$$\times K_{CK} \times \left[(R+1)/(R+K_{CK})\right]^2 \quad \text{[Equation 16.8]}$$

where D = the diffusion coefficients, K_{CK} = the CK equilibrium constant in the direction shown above, and R = the ATP/ADP ratio. The ratio of diffusion coefficients is approximately 2, and the ratio of total creatine to total adenine is about 4. In contrast, K_{CK} is approximately 100. Therefore, this is by far the dominant term as long as the ATP/ADP ratio is high. Stated another way, the creatine shuttle is extremely effective because small spatial *differences* in ADP concentration translate into much larger *differences* in creatine concentration via the CK equilibrium. The CK system does not simply add another diffusing pair of metabolites; it greatly amplifies the effective diffusion gradient.

The importance of considering K_{CK} rather than just diffusivity in the effectiveness of the creatine shuttle can be illustrated by considering the expected result of increasing muscle total creatine content, for example by creatine supplementation. Creatine supplementation can increase muscle total creatine content in some individuals by up to 30%. If one considered only the effect of this increase on creatine diffusivity, one might imagine that this could in principle increase the shuttle's effectiveness by 30% and (assuming diffusion limits aerobic capacity) increase aerobic power by 30%. However, because K_{CK} is so dominant, a 30% increase in total creatine would not significantly add to the shuttle's already overwhelming effectiveness. Therefore, even if creatine supplementation did increase aerobic capacity, this effect could not be attributed to enhancement of the creatine shuttle. In fact, there is no convincing evidence that creatine supplementation increases muscle aerobic capacity. On the contrary,

chronic creatine depletion or genetic ablation of cytoplasmic CK results in increased skeletal muscle mitochondrial content and aerobic capacity, presumably because of an adaptive response to the increased pulsatility of nucleotide levels that must occur in the absence of CK buffering (25).

All of this assumes that there is no specific barrier to nucleotide diffusion to the inner mitochondrial membrane. Although no such barrier is evident in isolated mitochondria, it has been suggested that the outer membrane is much less permeable to nucleotides *in vivo* than *in vitro*. This view is largely based on studies of respiration in permeabilized muscle fibers or bundles of fibers, whose sarcolemma is made permeable to small molecules but not to larger molecules, such as proteins, after treatment with a mild detergent (34). The experimental observation is that addition of creatine to the bath surrounding the fiber bundles enhances the respiration rate at submaximal ADP concentrations, increasing the apparent affinity of the mitochondria for ADP. Conversely, addition of PCr suppresses respiration and decreases the apparent affinity for ADP in this experimental situation. Thus, it is proposed that PCr and creatine traverse the outer mitochondrial membrane more freely than the nucleotides and are the metabolites that actually control muscle respiration (31). Unfortunately, there is now good evidence (32) that the diffusion barrier in permeabilized fiber experiments lies not at the outer membrane but is instead simply due to the relatively long path from the bath to the core of the fibers in these experiments (50 μm or more). This is exactly the situation in which ADP diffusion alone is likely to become rate limiting.

SUMMARY

The main message of this chapter is that cytoplasmic ATPases control muscle ATP production at work rates below the maximal sustainable rate. As exercise intensity approaches the maximum sustainable rate, control increasingly depends on the limited maximum capacity of the ATP generating pathways themselves. Of course, many important questions remain to be answered. For example, although it is unlikely that the intracellular diffusion of small molecules such as ADP limits metabolic rate, it is quite possible that the spatial arrangement of large metabolic enzymes and enzyme complexes is important for flux control. For example, more than 20 years ago it was suggested that glycogen particles and associated glycogenolytic enzymes may be in close proximity to SR ATPases, which may explain the observed coupling between glycogenolysis and contraction (33). With the tools of modern molecular biology, it should now be possible to test this idea *in vivo* by genetically mutating the interacting domains of these enzyme complexes. Similarly, the possibility that energy-related signals, such as AMP, are important for control of muscle gene expression and the adaptations to exercise training has just begun to be explored (34). These are exciting times for those interested in muscle metabolism.

The First Phosphorus NMR Spectra of Skeletal Muscle

Researchers now routinely use NMR spectroscopy to measure the time course of many metabolic events in exercising human skeletal muscle. The first phosphorus NMR spectra of intact skeletal muscle (reproduced nearby) were published by David Hoult and his colleagues at the University of Oxford in 1974. At that time there were no NMR magnets large enough to accommodate a human subject or even a whole rat. This paper reported the time course of metabolic changes in ischemic hindlimb muscles freshly excised from anesthetized rats and placed in a magnet designed for spectroscopy of organic chemicals in small test tubes. Nonetheless, many future applications of phosphorus NMR to exercise physiology were clearly foreshadowed in this paper. For example, the faster depletion of PCr (peak III in the figure) than ATP (peaks IV, V, and VI are the γ-, α-, and β-phosphates of ATP, respectively) was evident over time, and the extent of muscle acidification (from pH 7.1 in the freshly excised muscle down to pH 6.2 after 160 minutes

of ischemia at 20°C) was determined from the changing position of the inorganic phosphate peak (peak II). Furthermore, the authors correctly deduced that the breadth of the phosphate peak compared to the PCr peak was due to pH heterogeneity within the muscle and hinted that this pH heterogeneity might be used to characterize the fiber compartments of the muscle.

As exciting as these first results were to researchers interested in muscle metabolism, it is not likely that by themselves they would have led to the widespread availability of human-sized NMR magnets. Fortunately, the paper describing the principle of magnetic resonance imaging (MRI) had been published just a year earlier (35), and within 10 years human MRI magnets were available at most major medical centers. Hoult and his colleagues at Oxford went on to make many important contributions to MRI, as well as to muscle spectroscopy.

Hoult DI, Busby SJW, Gadian DG, et al. Observation of tissue metabolites using 31P nuclear magnetic resonance. Nature 1974;352: 285–287.

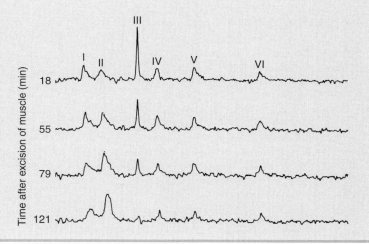

REFERENCES

1. Hochachka PW. Muscles as Molecular and Metabolic Machines. Boca Raton, FL: CRC Press, 1994.
2. Harkema SJ, Adams GR, Meyer RA. Acidosis has no effect on the ATP cost of contraction in cat fast- and slow-twitch skeletal muscles. Am J Physiol 272 (Cell Physiol 41) 1997; C485–C490.
3. He ZH, Bottinelli R, Pellegrino MA, et al. ATP consumption and efficiency of human single muscle fibers with different myosin isoform composition. Biophys J 2000;79:945–961.
4. Taylor CR. Relating mechanics and energetics during exercise. Adv Vet Sci Comp Med 1994;38A:181–215.
5. Meyer RA, Foley JM. Cellular processes integrating the metabolic response to exercise. In Rowell LB, Shepherd JT, eds.

Handbook of Physiology, Section 12: Exercise: Regulation and Integration of Multiple Systems. New York: Oxford University, 1996;841–869.
6. Ryschon TW, Fowler MD, Wysong RE, et al. Efficiency of human skeletal muscle in vivo: comparison of isometric, concentric, and eccentric muscle action. J Appl Physiol 1997;83:867–874.
7. Blei ML, Conley KE, Kushmerick MJ. Separate measures of ATP utilization and recovery in human skeletal muscle. J Physiol (Lond) 1993;465:203–222.
8. Harkema SJ, Meyer RA. Effect of acidosis on control of respiration in skeletal muscle. Am J Physiol 272 (Cell Physiol 41)1997;C491–C500.
9. Brooks GA. The lactate shuttle during exercise and recovery. Med Sci Sports Exerc 1986;18:360–368.

10. Brooks GA. Lactate doesn't necessarily cause fatigue: why are we surprised? J Physiol (Lond) 2001;536:1.

11. Chen W, London R, Murphy E, et al. Regulation of the Ca^{++} gradient across the sarcoplasmic reticulum in perfused rabbit heart: A 19F nuclear magnetic resonance study. Circ Res 1998;83:898–907.

12. Lambeth MJ, Kushmerick MJ. A computational model for glycogenolysis in skeletal muscle. Ann Biomed Eng 2002;30: 808–827.

13. Cornish-Bowden A. Fundamentals of enzyme kinetics. London: Portland, 1995.

14. Hsu AC, Dawson MJ. Muscle glycogenolysis is not activated by changes in cytosolic P-metabolites: a 31P and 1H MRS demonstration. Magn Reson Med 2003;49:626–631.

15. Jeneson JAL, Westerhoff HV, Kushmerick MJ. A metabolic control analysis of kinetic controls in ATP free energy metabolism in contracting skeletal muscle. Am J Physiol (Cell Physiol 279) 2000;C813–C832.

16. Jeneson JAL, Wiseman RW, Westerhoff HV, et al. The signal transduction function for oxidative phosphorylation is at least second order in ADP. J Biol Chem 1996;271:27995–27998.

17. Territo PR, French SA, Dunleavy MC, et al. Calcium activation of heart mitochondrial oxidative phosphorylation: Rapid kinetics of mVO2, NADH, and light scattering. J Biol Chem 2001;276:2586–2599.

18. Balaban RS, Kantor HL, Katz LA, et al. Relation between work and phosphate metabolite in the in vivo paced mammalian heart. Science 1986;232:1121–1123.

19. Hogan MC, Richardson RS, Haseler LJ. Human muscle performance and PCr hydrolysis with varied inspired oxygen fractions: a 31P-MRS study. J Appl Physiol 1999;86:1367–1373.

20. Rossiter HB, Ward SA, Doyle VL, et al. Inferences from pulmonary O2 uptake with respect to intramuscular phosphocreatine kinetics during moderate exercise in humans. J Physiol (Lond) 1999;518:921–932.

21. Meyer RA. A linear model of muscle respiration explains monoexponential phosphocreatine changes. Am J Physiol 254 (Cell Physiol 23) 1988;C548–C553.

22. Greenhaff PL, Campbell-O'Sullivan SP, Constantin-Teodosiu D, et al. An acetyl group deficit limits mitochondrial ATP production at the onset of exercise. Biochem Soc Trans 2002;30:275–280.

23. Meyer RA. Linear dependence of muscle phosphocreatine kinetics on total creatine content. Am J Physiol 257 (Cell Physiol 26) 1989;C1149–C1157.

24. Harrison GJ, van Wijhe MH, de Groot B, et al. CK inhibition accelerates transcytosolic energy signaling during rapid workload steps in isolated rabbit hearts. Am J Physiol 276 (Heart Circ Physiol 45) 1999;H134–H140.

25. Roman BB, Meyer RA, Wiseman RW. Phosphocreatine kinetics at the onset of contractions in skeletal muscle of MM creatine kinase knockout mice. Am J Physiol Cell Physiol 2002;283:C1776–C1783.

26. Rossiter HB, Ward SA, Howe FA, et al. Effects of dichloroacetate on VO2 and intramuscular 31P metabolite kinetics during high-intensity exercise in humans. J Appl Physiol 2003;95:1105–1115.

27. Savasi I, Evans MK, Heigenhauser GJF, Spriet LL. Skeletal muscle metabolism is unaffected by DCA infusion and hyperoxia after the onset of intense aerobic exercise. Am J Physiol Endocrinol Metab 2002;283:E108–E115.

28. McAllister RM, Terjung RL. Acute inhibition of respiratory capacity of muscle reduces peak oxygen consumption. Am J Physiol 259 (Cell Physiol 28) 1990;C889–C896.

29. Bessman SP, Geiger PJ. Transport of energy in muscle: the phosphorylcreatine shuttle. Science 1981;211:448–452.

30. Meyer RA, Sweeney HL, Kushmerick MJ. A simple analysis of the "phosphocreatine shuttle." Am J Physiol 246 (Cell Physiol 15) 1984;C365–C377.

31. Walsh B, Tonkonogi M, Soderlund K, et al. The role of phosphorylcreatine and creatine in the regulation of mitochondrial respiration in skeletal muscle. J Physiol (Lond) 2001;537:971–978.

32. Kongas O, Yuen TL, Wagner MJ, et al. High km of oxidative phosphorylation for ADP in skinned muscle fibers: where does it stem from? Am J Physiol (Cell Physiol 283) 2002;C743–C751.

33. Entman ML, Keslensky SS, Chu A, et al. The sarcoplasmic reticulum-glycogenolytic complex in mammalian fast twitch skeletal muscle: proposed in vitro counterpart of the contraction-activated glycogenolytic pool. J Biol Chem 1980;255:6245–6252.

34. Zong H, Ren JM, Young LH, et al. AMP kinase is required for mitochondrial biogenesis in skeletal muscle in response to chronic energy deprivation. Proc Natl Acad Sci USA 2002;99:15983–15987.

35. Lauterbur PC. Image formation by induced local interactions: examples using nuclear magnetic resonance. Nature 1973;242:190–191.

CHAPTER 17

The Metabolic Systems: Carbohydrate Metabolism

MARK HARGREAVES

Introduction

Carbohydrate (CHO) is the preferred substrate for contracting skeletal muscle during strenuous exercise, and the importance of available CHO for endurance exercise performance has been recognized since the early 1900s. In the ensuing years, considerable experimental effort has further characterized the effects of exercise on CHO metabolism and the systemic and cellular factors that regulate CHO mobilization and utilization. In animal tissues CHO is stored as glycogen, a branched polymer of glucose with a mixture of α-1,4 and α-1,6 linkages between glucose units. The liver has the highest concentration of glycogen, but by virtue of its mass, skeletal muscle contains the largest store of glycogen (Table 17.1). The size of both the liver and muscle glycogen reserves is influenced by interactions between habitual levels of exercise and dietary CHO intake. Since the endogenous CHO stores are relatively low and are utilized to a large extent during athletic competition and training, adequate dietary CHO intake is essential to ensure optimal CHO availability before, during, and after exercise. A focus on CHO intake, together with energy and fluid balance, is a cornerstone of performance and sports nutritional programs.

During exercise, liver and muscle glycogen stores are mobilized, and muscle glycogen use and glucose uptake increase along with increasing intensity of exercise. At exercise intensities greater than 50 to 60% $\dot{V}O_{2max}$, muscle glycogen is the major substrate for oxidative metabolism (1,2) (Fig. 17.1). As exercise duration is extended, liver and muscle glycogen levels decrease and uptake of glucose increases progressively until in the absence of CHO supplementation, falling blood glucose levels limit glucose uptake. Reduced intramuscular glycogen availability and hypoglycemia are associated with the development of fatigue during prolonged strenuous exercise, and nutritional strategies to enhance endurance performance focus on increasing CHO availability prior to (3) and during (4) such exercise. This chapter briefly describes the effects of exercise on CHO mobilization and utilization, the important regulatory mechanisms, and aspects of CHO metabolism during the recovery period post exercise. In most instances, reference will be made to studies undertaken in human subjects, and the focus is on dynamic exercise. Although relatively less studied, muscle glycogen and blood glucose are also utilized during resistance exercise, especially at high loads, when increased intramuscular pressure can occlude blood supply, thereby reducing oxygen delivery and increasing muscle glycogenolysis.

Muscle Glycogen Utilization During Exercise

The utilization of muscle glycogen is most rapid at the onset of exercise and increases exponentially with increasing exercise intensity (Fig. 17.1). During supramaximal exercise, the

TABLE 17.1	Sites and Amount of CHO Stored in a Rested, Moderately Active 70-kg Man With 40% of Body Mass as Skeletal Muscle		
Tissue	Weight or volume (kilograms or liters)	Concentration (mmol · kg⁻¹ or · *L⁻¹)	CHO store (g)
Liver	1.8	250 (0–500)	80 (0–160)
ECF	10.0	5*	9
Muscle	28.0	100 (0–200)	500 (300–700)

Numbers in parentheses represent possible range depending upon exercise, training, and dietary CHO intake.

rate of muscle glycogenolysis is as high as 40 mmol · kg⁻¹ · min⁻¹ of wet mass, while during prolonged submaximal exercise it can be as low as 1 to 2 mmol · kg⁻¹ · min⁻¹ (5,6). Thus, the regulation of glycogenolysis is exquisitely sensitive to the metabolic rate of skeletal muscle during exercise. With exercise rapid activation of glycogen phosphorylase, the enzyme that catalyzes the rate-limiting step in muscle glycogenolysis, results from covalent modification, allosteric regulation, and changes in intramuscular concentrations of substrates. As exercise duration increases, the rate of muscle glycogenolysis declines as glycogen availability and phosphorylase activity decrease, intramuscular [H⁺] increases (during intense exercise), and the availability of other substrates for oxidative metabolism, such as glucose and free fatty acids (FFA), increases. During prolonged exercise at power outputs eliciting 60 to 75% V̇O₂max, muscle glycogenolysis occurs predominantly in type I muscle fibers, with increasing glycogen degradation in type II fibers as the type I fibers are depleted of glycogen. Fatigue during such exercise is often associated with muscle glycogen depletion (5,6). With increasing exercise intensity there is a greater rate of glycogenolysis in type I fibers, together with recruitment of type II fibers, such that at exercise intensities approaching and exceeding V̇O₂max,

glycogenolysis occurs in all muscle fiber types but at a higher rate in type II fibers.

In addition to intensity and duration of exercise, major factors influencing the rate of muscle glycogenolysis during dynamic exercise are preceding diet and training status. Increased dietary CHO intake is associated with greater muscle glycogen utilization, while increased fat intake results in a lower muscle glycogen use during subsequent exercise. These effects are mostly related to changes in intramuscular glycogen availability, although alterations in plasma hormone and substrate concentrations may also contribute. However, 5 days on a high-fat diet resulted in reduced muscle glycogen use during dynamic exercise, compared with 5 days on a high-CHO diet, despite muscle glycogen levels before exercise being similar following consumption of a high-CHO diet for 24 hours prior to exercise in both trials (7). This suggests that metabolic adaptations to a high-fat diet, independent of muscle glycogen availability, result in an attenuation of muscle glycogenolysis during exercise following such a diet. Muscle glycogenolysis during dynamic exercise is reduced following a period of endurance training, despite an increase in resting muscle glycogen levels. The well-described increase in muscle oxidative capacity is generally believed to be responsible for this alteration in muscle glycogen metabolism (8).

Morphological studies have characterized a heterogeneous intramuscular distribution of glycogen and its association with the sarcolemma, sarcoplasmic reticulum, mitochondria, and myofibrils. Furthermore, glycogen granules, or glycosomes, are physically associated with a number of proteins, including glycogen phosphorylase, phosphorylase kinase, glycogen synthase, glycogenin, protein phosphatases, and adenosine monophosphate (AMP) activated protein kinase, that are involved in the metabolism of glycogen itself and other substrates, such as glucose. This implies that glycogen not only is a substrate for oxidative metabolism during dynamic exercise but may also have a role in metabolic regulation. The chemical association of protein with glycogen results in differential acid solubility of glycogen within skeletal muscle: an acid-soluble species with a high ratio of CHO to protein and a molecular mass of up to about 10,000 kDa is termed macroglycogen; and an acid-insoluble species with a lower ratio of CHO to protein and a mass up to 400 kDa is called proglycogen. The functional significance of these biochemically

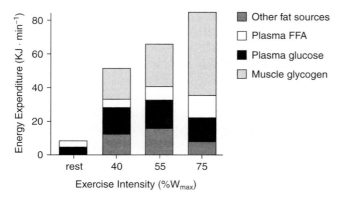

FIGURE 17.1 Contributions from muscle glycogen and plasma glucose to total energy expenditure during 20-min dynamic exercise bouts of increasing intensity, expressed as %Wmax. *(Reprinted with permission from Van Loon LJC, Greenhaff PL, Constantin-Teodosiu D, et al. The effects of increasing exercise intensity on muscle fuel utilisation in humans. J Physiol [Lond] 2001;536:301.)*

determined glycogen species remains to be fully elucidated; however, recent studies have observed a greater use of proglycogen during exercise, suggesting the possibility of differential metabolic regulation.

Regulation of Muscle Glycogenolysis

The activity of glycogen phosphorylase is regulated by the interplay between intramuscular factors related to muscle contractile activity and metabolism and by systemic hormonal and substrate availability. This dual control (9) ensures that muscle glycogenolysis is closely matched to the energetic demands of dynamic exercise. In the resting state, glycogen phosphorylase exists primarily in the inactive b form. With the onset of dynamic exercise phosphorylase kinase phosphorylates the b form to the active a form in response to elevated calcium levels and binding of epinephrine to β-adrenergic receptors on the sarcolemma. The activity of both forms of the enzyme can be increased allosterically by AMP and adenosine diphosphate (ADP) and by increases in inorganic phosphate (P_i). Since the rate of muscle glycogenolysis is not always closely associated with the percent phosphorylase a (10), these latter so-called posttransformational factors enhance glycogenolytic rate during exercise of increasing intensity and following reversal of phosphorylase transformation during prolonged exercise.

Local Factors

The increase in sarcoplasmic calcium during excitation-contraction coupling results in conversion of phosphorylase b as a result of calcium binding to the calmodulin subunit of phosphorylase kinase and to troponin C. The increase in percent phosphorylase a is rapidly reversed (9) despite ongoing contractile activity, and this may be partly related to the decline in muscle glycogen, conformational changes in glycogen phosphorylase and/or phosphorylase kinase, and/or decreased muscle pH, which inhibits enzyme activity. The maintenance of glycogenolytic activity during ongoing dynamic exercise, especially at high intensities, is due to increased intramuscular concentrations of P_i, a substrate for phosphorylase, and AMP and ADP, which allosterically activate both phosphorylase a and b.

Substrate Availability

The availability of P_i and glycogen, the substrates for glycogen phosphorylase, has been shown to affect glycogen phosphorylase activity and glycogenolysis during dynamic exercise. Increases in intramuscular [P_i] during muscle contractions stimulate glycogen phosphorylase activity and contribute to enhanced glycogenolysis during exercise. Glycogen can bind to glycogen phosphorylase, thereby increasing its activity, and this explains the linear relationship between muscle glycogen levels before exercise and its utilization during submaximal exercise. Despite the greater glycogenolysis, increased muscle glycogen availability prior to dynamic exercise

enhances performance in endurance events lasting more than 90 minutes (3). The influence of muscle glycogen is less apparent during supramaximal exercise, and results in the literature are conflicting. Increased blood glucose availability may reduce glycogenolysis, since increases in glucose 6-phosphate have the potential to inhibit glycogen phosphorylase activity; however, this does not occur during prolonged, strenuous cycling exercise (4,11), and there are conflicting data on the effect of CHO ingestion on muscle glycogen use during treadmill running. The ergogenic effects of CHO ingestion appear to be due to elevated blood glucose levels, which contribute to maintenance of skeletal muscle CHO oxidation (4) and cerebral glucose supply and energy turnover. Reduced blood glucose levels may increase reliance on muscle glycogen use, although this has not been tested directly. Hyperinsulinemia before exercise results in a fall in blood glucose with the onset of dynamic exercise, and this has sometimes been associated with increased muscle glycogen use (11); however, since hyperinsulinemia also inhibits lipolysis, this effect could equally be due to reduced plasma FFA levels, which also increases reliance on muscle glycogen during exercise. In contrast, elevated plasma FFA levels are associated with reduced muscle glycogenolysis, an effect that appears to be due to lower glycogen phosphorylase activity secondary to attenuated increases in ADP, AMP, and P_i during dynamic exercise.

Hormonal Regulation

In addition to local intramuscular factors, glycogen phosphorylase is also subject to regulation by epinephrine, which binds to sarcolemmal β-adrenergic receptors and results in cyclic AMP-mediated activation of glycogen phosphorylase kinase. Increased epinephrine is associated with greater glycogen phosphorylase activity and glycogenolysis during muscle contraction in the perfused rat hindlimb (9) and with greater glycogenolysis during moderate exercise in humans (12). During heavy dynamic exercise, epinephrine infusion does not further increase muscle glycogenolysis, probably because of sufficient activation of glycogenolysis by endogenous epinephrine secretion and increases in intramuscular concentrations of ADP, AMP, and P_i.

Muscle Glucose Uptake During Dynamic Exercise

During exercise skeletal muscle glucose uptake can increase several fold, depending upon exercise intensity and duration (13,14) (Fig. 17.1). This is a consequence of enhanced glucose delivery to contracting skeletal muscle as a result of increased muscle blood flow and capillary recruitment and increased glucose extraction as measured by a greater arteriovenous glucose difference. Glucose extraction is increased by enhanced sarcolemmal glucose transport and activation of the glycolytic and oxidative pathways responsible for glucose metabolism. Sarcolemmal glucose transport is increased following translocation of the glucose transporter isoform 4 (GLUT4) from intracellular sites to the plasma membrane with exercise (15) (Fig. 17.2). The importance of GLUT4 is demonstrated by the almost complete abolition of contraction-stimulated glucose uptake in transgenic mice with selective deletion of GLUT4 from skeletal muscle (16). In addition to translocation to the sarcolemma, it is possible that exercise also increases the intrinsic activity of GLUT4, but this is more contentious. Once inside the cell, glucose is rapidly phosphorylated by hexokinase and further metabolized in the glycolytic and oxidative pathways. There is little if any intracellular accumulation of glucose during exercise except at power outputs close to or at $\dot{V}O_{2max}$, when glucose utilization may be less than glucose transport (13). One possible explanation for reduced glucose utilization is an increase in concentration of muscle glucose 6-phosphate, an inhibitor of hexokinase, as a result of enhanced muscle glycogenolysis (11). With increasing exercise duration, there is a progressive increase in muscle glucose uptake associated with increased sarcolemmal GLUT4 (15) (Fig. 17.2) and reduced muscle glycogen levels (11). During prolonged heavy exercise in the absence of CHO supplementation, blood glucose levels decline and become limiting for muscle glucose uptake, which is then reduced. If CHO is ingested, blood glucose levels and CHO oxidation are maintained (4), exercise duration is increased (4), and glucose uptake increases continuously to the point of volitional fatigue.

Increased dietary CHO and fat intakes are generally associated with enhanced and reduced muscle glucose uptake, respectively, secondary to changes in plasma glucose and insulin levels. When muscle glycogen levels are equalized after such dietary intakes, the effect of preceding diet on glucose uptake is negligible (7). Dynamic endurance exercise training results in a lower muscle glucose uptake during exercise at the same absolute power output (17), an effect that is less apparent during exercise at the same relative exercise intensity. In fact, with exercise intensity approaching $\dot{V}O_{2max}$, there may even be an increased muscle glucose uptake after training. This enhanced glucose uptake capacity is partly due to increased skeletal muscle GLUT4 protein expression after training, an adaptation that also contributes to greater insulin-stimulated skeletal muscle glucose uptake in trained subjects.

Regulation of Skeletal Muscle Glucose Uptake

Increased skeletal muscle blood flow and capillary recruitment enhance glucose supply to contracting skeletal muscle, but local factors within muscle have the major role. In particular, sarcolemmal glucose transport is thought to be rate limiting for glucose uptake in most circumstances. Glucose transport is regulated by signals related to excitation-contraction coupling, most notably the increase in sarcoplasmic calcium, and by feedback signals that reflect the metabolic state of the muscle cell, including AMP, phosphocreatine, and glycogen levels (18). Calcium has long been recognized as a stimulator of muscle glucose transport (19), although the downstream events that ultimately increase glucose transport have not been fully described. It is possible that calcium interacts directly with proteins involved in the trafficking of GLUT4 vesicles to the sarcolemma. Alternatively or in addition, calcium may act via calcium-sensitive signaling pathways such as the conventional isoforms of protein kinase C (PKC α, β, γ) and the calcium- and calmodulin-dependent kinase (18). Muscle contractions increase PKC activity in the membrane fraction and intracellular levels of diacylglycerol (DAG), an activator of both the conventional and novel (δ, ε, θ, η) isoforms of PKC. Furthermore, the PKC inhibitor calphostin C partially inhibits contraction-stimulated glucose transport, suggesting a role for the DAG-sensitive conventional and novel isoforms (18). In addition, it has recently been demonstrated that treadmill running increases atypical (ζ, ι/λ) PKC activity in mouse skeletal muscle. Collectively, these results implicate PKC activation in the contraction-induced stimulation of muscle glucose transport, although additional studies are required to better define the importance of the various PKC isoforms.

There has been considerable interest in the possible role of AMP-activated kinase (AMPK) in the regulation of muscle glucose uptake during dynamic exercise. This enzyme is

GLUT4

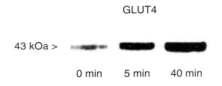

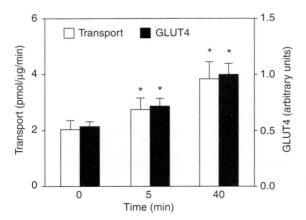

FIGURE 17.2 Representative GLUT4 immunoblot (*top*) and the mean glucose transport and GLUT4 protein content (*bottom*) in sarcolemmal vesicles from human muscle obtained before and after 5 and 40 min of moderate exercise. Values are means + SEM, n = 9. * denotes different from 0; P < .05. (*Reprinted with permission from Kristiansen S, Hargreaves M, Richter EA. Progressive increase in glucose transport and GLUT4 in human sarcolemmal vesicles during moderate exercise. Am J Physiol 1997;272:E386.*)

activated by decreases in the ratios of ATP to ADP and phosphocreatine to creatine, indicators of metabolic stress within skeletal muscle during moderate to heavy dynamic exercise, and with hypoxia. Pharmacological activation of the enzyme by aminoimidazole-4-carboxamide-1-β-D-riboside (AICAR) increases sarcolemmal GLUT4 and muscle glucose uptake via an insulin-independent mechanism. Furthermore, exercise increases AMPK activity, in particular the α_2-isoform, although during very intense exercise the α_1-isoform is also activated. These observations have led to the suggestion that AMPK is responsible for the exercise-induced increase in muscle glucose uptake. However, mice expressing a dominant negative (inactive) form of AMPK in skeletal muscle retained 60 to 70% of their contraction-stimulated glucose transport despite abolition of hypoxia- and AICAR-stimulated glucose transport. Furthermore, contraction-stimulated glucose transport was not affected in muscle from either α_2-AMPK or α_1-AMPK knockout mice, suggesting that neither isoform is essential for glucose transport during muscle contractions (18). Thus, while activation of AMPK increases muscle glucose uptake, the importance of this protein in regulating muscle glucose uptake during dynamic exercise remains to be fully clarified.

Other stimuli that potentially regulate muscle glucose transport during exercise include the mitogen-activated protein kinases (MAPK) and nitric oxide. Muscle contraction increases the activities of MAPK pathways including the extracellular regulated kinases (ERK) and the stress-activated protein kinases JNK and p38. Inhibition of an upstream kinase from ERK does not affect glucose transport during muscle contraction, casting some doubt on the importance of these kinases. It has been demonstrated that while p38 MAPK has no effect on GLUT4 translocation, it increases GLUT4 activity following insulin stimulation, although whether exercise increases GLUT4 activity is still debated. More research is required to elucidate the importance of the MAPK pathways in the activation of glucose transport during dynamic exercise. Contracting skeletal muscle produces nitric oxide, and some studies have shown that inhibition of nitric oxide synthase attenuates the contraction-induced increase in glucose transport *in vitro* and the exercise-induced increase in muscle glucose uptake in humans. Since contrary results have also been obtained, the importance of nitric oxide for muscle glucose uptake during exercise is somewhat equivocal (20).

Hormonal Regulation of Muscle Glucose Uptake During Dynamic Exercise

The increase in muscle glucose uptake during exercise occurs via a mechanism that involves some or all of the signaling pathways identified earlier but does not require activation of the insulin signaling pathway. Despite early suggestions that a "permissive" level of insulin was required for muscle glucose transport to increase with contractions, it is now clear that insulin is not required for the contraction-induced increase in muscle glucose transport. Indeed, the effects of insulin and muscle contractions on GLUT4 translocation and glucose transport in skeletal muscle are additive (19). The preservation of the exercise-sensitive pathway in insulin-resistant states, such as type 2 diabetes and obesity, provides a rationale for the promotion of regular physical activity in the management of patients with these metabolic disorders. Furthermore, the additive nature of the exercise and insulin stimuli on muscle glucose uptake accounts for the observations of increased muscle glucose uptake and premature hypoglycemia when exercise is commenced with an elevated plasma insulin (e.g., after a high-CHO meal or insulin injection in a type 1 diabetic) and increased glucose uptake and oxidation when CHO is ingested during prolonged heavy dynamic exercise (4).

Increased epinephrine inhibits muscle glucose uptake during exercise (12), an effect that appears to be due to its stimulatory effect on muscle glycogenolysis and the consequent increase in muscle glucose 6-phosphate, an inhibitor of hexokinase and glucose phosphorylation. However, the inhibitory effect of epinephrine during exercise is still present when muscle glycogen levels are low before exercise, which results in a blunted increase in glucose 6-phosphate. This implies a potential direct effect on sarcolemmal glucose transport, and there are data suggesting that epinephrine, via cyclic AMP, may inhibit GLUT4 intrinsic activity. β-Adrenergic blockade results in enhanced glucose disposal during dynamic exercise, consistent with removal of the inhibitory effect of epinephrine.

Substrate Availability

Since muscle glucose uptake occurs by facilitated diffusion, increases and decreases in blood glucose availability have the expected effects on muscle glucose uptake. During prolonged low-intensity exercise in the absence of CHO supplementation, the decline in blood glucose results in reduced muscle glucose uptake (14,21). When blood glucose levels are maintained or increased by CHO ingestion during exercise, muscle glucose uptake and oxidation are increased. There are data demonstrating that hyperglycemia can enhance sarcolemmal GLUT4 translocation, but factors unrelated to glucose also contribute to the increased muscle glucose uptake under these conditions, most notably the higher plasma insulin. There is an inverse relationship between muscle glycogen availability and glucose uptake during exercise (20,22). This is due to effects on both intramuscular glucose metabolism, mediated via glucose 6-phosphate, and membrane glucose transport, since sarcolemmal GLUT4 translocation in response to muscle contraction is greater with low muscle glycogen (20). Low muscle glycogen before exercise also results in greater activation of AMPK during exercise, which may also partly contribute to the enhanced muscle glucose uptake (22). Plasma FFA availability may also influence muscle glucose uptake during exercise, although the weight of evidence in human exercise studies supports a conclusion that plasma FFA has a relatively minor influence on muscle glucose uptake during dynamic exercise. The classical glucose–fatty acid cycle hypothesis proposed by Randle and colleagues predicts an inhibitory effect of elevated plasma FFA on muscle glucose uptake. While this has been observed in one human study, there are several in the literature demonstrating reduced muscle glycogen use but no effect of increased FFA on glucose uptake. Similarly, although inhibition of adipose tissue lipolysis by nicotinic acid has been shown to increase glucose disposal slightly, the major effect was to increase muscle glycogenolysis, which accounted for almost all of the observed increase in CHO oxidation during exercise under conditions of reduced FFA availability.

Liver Glucose Output During Dynamic Exercise

The maintenance of blood glucose during exercise in the face of large increases in muscle glucose uptake is achieved by a concomitant increase in liver glucose output. The increase in liver glucose output is also dependent upon exercise intensity and duration (Fig. 17.3) in a manner very similar to muscle glucose uptake; however, at higher exercise intensities, liver glucose output may exceed muscle glucose uptake, resulting in hyperglycemia. The early increase in liver glucose output is due to stimulation of liver glycogenolysis, and analysis of liver biopsy samples obtained before and after 1 hour of heavy exercise demonstrated a decline in liver glycogen from the normal postabsorptive value of 270 to 125 mmol · kg · kg^{-1} (6). As exercise duration increases, the liver glycogen level decreases, and its contribution to liver glucose output is reduced (Fig. 17.3). There is enhanced uptake of gluconeogenic precursors, such as lactate, pyruvate, glycerol and alanine (14,21), and activation of liver gluconeogenic enzyme activity. The result is that the contribution of gluconeogenesis to total liver glucose output increases from about 25% in the resting state to 45 to 50% after 4 hours of low-intensity exercise (14,21) (Fig. 17.3). Despite the increase in gluconeogenesis, it cannot completely compensate for decreased liver glycogen availability, and liver glucose output is reduced, resulting in a falling blood glucose level and muscle glucose uptake. Nevertheless, the importance of gluconeogenesis, at least in exercising rodents, is demonstrated by the observation that inhibition of liver gluconeogenesis reduces endurance capacity by about 30%. Given that endogenous liver glucose output cannot sustain glucose availability during prolonged strenuous exercise, endurance athletes ingest CHO to enhance performance, and under these circumstances gut-derived glucose augments and may completely replace endogenous liver glucose output. Following endurance training, liver glucose output during dynamic exercise at the same absolute power output is reduced in parallel with the decrease in muscle glucose uptake and oxidation (17).

Regulation of Liver Glucose Output

The regulation of liver glucose output involves complex, interactive, and redundant mechanisms, and it is highly unlikely

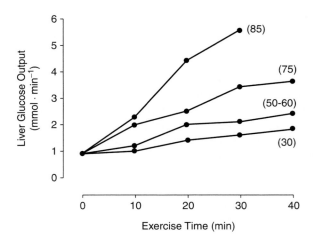

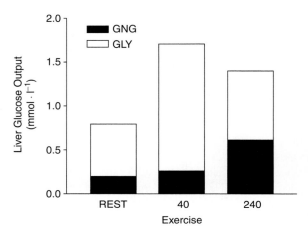

FIGURE 17.3 Liver glucose output during cycling exercise at varying exercise intensities (*top*) and during prolonged exercise at about 30% V̇o$_{2max}$ (*bottom*), with estimated contributions from either glycogenolysis (GLY) or gluconeogenesis (GNG). Parenthetical numbers in top panel refer to exercise intensity, expressed as percent V̇o$_{2max}$. (*Top panel redrawn from Hultman E, Harris RC. Carbohydrate metabolism. In Poortmans JR, ed. Principles of exercise biochemistry. Basel: Karger, 1988;78–119. Data for bottom panel from Ahlborg G, Felig P, Hagenfeldt L, et al. Substrate turnover during prolonged exercise in man. J Clin Invest 1974;53:1080–1090.*)

that a single factor is responsible for the stimulation of liver glucose output during dynamic exercise. Rather, neural and hormonal factors function together to ensure that it increases in an attempt to maintain glucose supply to active skeletal muscle and to the central nervous system. The close association between liver glucose output and muscle glucose uptake during moderate exercise raised the possibility of intricate feedback from contracting skeletal muscle, mediated by small decreases in blood glucose, afferent nerve activity, or even a circulating factor released from active muscle. In contrast, during heavy dynamic exercise the increase in liver glucose output often precedes and is greater than the increase in muscle glucose uptake, which suggests a so-called feed-forward regulation. The neuroendocrine pathways responsible for enhanced liver glucose output are activated in parallel with motor cortical activation of skeletal muscle (central command) in a manner similar to that described for the cardiovascular and respiratory responses to exercise. One piece of evidence in support of this is the exaggerated liver glucose output during dynamic exercise under conditions of relative muscle weakness and enhanced central command (23). This does not diminish the importance of feedback control; rather, both mechanisms work together to ensure that liver glucose output is appropriate for the prevailing exercise intensity and duration and glucose availability. Indeed, when both central command and afferent nerve feedback are abolished by electrically induced cycling in the presence of complete epidural blockade, plasma glucose levels are lower than during voluntary dynamic exercise at the same oxygen uptake. There is also interaction between feed-forward and feedback regulation; for example, increased blood glucose blunts the rise in liver glucose output to a lesser extent during high-intensity exercise than during exercise of low to moderate intensity.

Pancreatic Hormones

Insulin and glucagon are important regulators of liver glucose output in the resting state, but their essential role during exercise is less clear. The decline in plasma insulin levels probably allows liver glucose output to increase, while elevated plasma glucagon levels late in prolonged exercise stimulate gluconeogenesis. Liver glucose output increases early in exercise without any major change in plasma glucagon. Prevention of the changes in the pancreatic hormone levels during exercise has produced conflicting results, suggesting that they are not absolutely required for liver glucose output to increase and/or that other stimuli compensate for their absence. It may be difficult to assess the role of these hormones in human subjects, given the difficulty in accessing the portal vein, where levels are higher than those measured peripherally. On balance, while plasma insulin and glucagon levels can influence liver glucose output during dynamic exercise, other factors must also be involved in stimulating the liver to increase glucose output (24).

Sympathoadrenal Activity

In many exercise situations (e.g., intense exercise, with hypoxia, exercise in the heat, with addition of arm exercise to leg exercise), the increase in liver glucose output is often closely correlated with enhanced sympathoadrenal activity, as reflected by increases in plasma epinephrine and norepinephrine. However, in many studies in which sympathoadrenal activity has been inhibited (adrenergic blockade, adrenalectomy, liver nerve resection), there has been no significant attenuation of the exercise-induced increase in liver glucose output. Exogenous infusion of epinephrine can stimulate liver glucose output, either directly or by increasing plasma lactate, a gluconeogenetic precursor, secondary to enhanced muscle

glycogenolysis. However, increased sympathoadrenal activity does not appear to be absolutely required for the increase in liver glucose output during dynamic exercise (25). Again, these results suggest complex redundancy in the regulation of liver glucose output and the interactions between sympathoadrenal activity, pancreatic hormones, and other as yet unidentified mediators of liver glucose output during dynamic exercise.

CHO Availability

Liver glucose output during dynamic exercise is higher after a CHO-rich diet than after a CHO-poor diet, consistent with marked differences in liver glycogen availability prior to exercise (6). Similarly, after a prolonged fast (60 hours) liver glucose output during exercise was about 65% lower than after an overnight fast, with gluconeogenesis contributing 78 and 13% to total liver glucose output, respectively (6). During intense exercise exogenous glucose infusion at a rate that equaled the average liver glucose output in a previous control trial abolished the normal exercise-induced increase in liver glucose output (26). Similar results have been obtained with CHO ingestion during dynamic exercise. Thus, blood glucose availability provides powerful feedback regulation of liver glucose output during exercise.

Regulation of CHO Oxidation During Dynamic Exercise

The degradation of glucosyl units, derived from either muscle glycogen or blood glucose, in glycolysis yields pyruvate, which can be either oxidized or converted to a number of other metabolites, such as lactate and alanine. For pyruvate to be oxidized, it must be first converted to acetyl coenzyme A (CoA) in a reaction catalyzed by pyruvate dehydrogenase (PDH), a multienzyme complex within the mitochondrial matrix. Thus, PDH regulates the entry of CHO into the tricarboxylic acid cycle and its subsequent oxidation. The PDH complex comprises three enzymes and a kinase (PDH kinase, or PDK) and a phosphatase (PDH phosphatase) that catalyze phosphorylation (inhibition) and dephosphorylation (activation) of the PDH enzyme, respectively. Increased ratios of ATP to ADP, acetyl CoA to CoASH, and NADH to NAD^+ activate PDH kinase, and increased pyruvate inhibits it, while increased sarcoplasmic calcium activates PDH phosphatase (27). During exercise, the major activators of PDH are increased calcium and ADP, both of which also stimulate glycolysis and the production of pyruvate, another activator of PDH (27). These changes account for the close agreement between greater PDH activation and CHO oxidation with increasing exercise intensity (10) (Fig. 17.4). Increasing glycolytic flux and the rate of pyruvate production during exercise, either by increasing muscle glycogen prior to exercise or by infusing epinephrine (12), results in greater PDH activation and CHO oxidation. Conversely, increased FFA

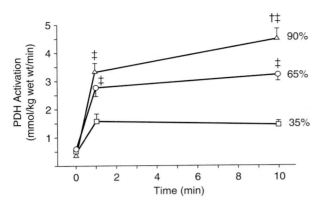

FIGURE 17.4 PDH activation at rest and during 10 minutes of exercise at varying power outputs, expressed as percent $\dot{V}O_{2max}$. *(Reprinted with permission from Howlett RA, Parolin ML, Dyck DJ, et al. Regulation of skeletal muscle glycogen phosphorylase and PDH at varying exercise power outputs. Am J Physiol 1998;275:R420.)*

availability and a high-fat diet, together with glycogen-depleting exercise, reduced PDH activation during exercise (28). During exercise lasting several hours, reduced pyruvate production secondary to diminished glycolytic flux as muscle glycogen and glucose uptake are reduced is the most likely explanation for the observed decreases in PDH activation and CHO oxidation under these conditions. Collectively, these results indicate that PDH activation is the major determinant of CHO oxidation during dynamic exercise.

PDH activation is also important at the onset of exercise. During the transition from rest to exercise there is a lag in oxygen uptake, and the energy demands of exercise are met by increased phosphocreatine degradation and glycolytic adenosine triphosphate (ATP) production. The lag in oxidative energy production has traditionally been attributed to the slow increase in oxygen delivery to contracting skeletal muscle. Recent findings suggest that a delay in PDH activation may also partly contribute, since pharmacological activation of PDH by dichloroacetate resulted in reduced phosphocreatine degradation and lactate production (27).

Lactate Metabolism During Dynamic Exercise

Perhaps one of the most studied responses to exercise is blood lactate during incremental exercise. The exponential increase in blood lactate closely follows the increased glycolytic flux and reliance on muscle glycogenolysis during exercise of increasing intensity. There has been ongoing debate in the exercise physiology literature on the underlying cause of lactate production during exercise at intensities well below maximal oxygen uptake and on the possible links between muscle hypoxia, blood lactate, and ventilatory con-

trol, as articulated in the anaerobic threshold hypothesis. Irrespective of underlying mechanisms, measurement of blood lactate during dynamic exercise has become widespread in the physiological evaluation of endurance athletes, and indeed, lactate variables, such as lactate threshold, onset of blood lactate accumulation, and maximal lactate steady state, are often better predictors of endurance exercise performance than maximal oxygen uptake. This reflects the close associations between lactate threshold, muscle oxidative capacity and the rate of CHO utilization during dynamic exercise (28). Furthermore, the right shift in the blood lactate–power output curve is the classical marker of metabolic adaptation to endurance training. During prolonged dynamic exercise above the lactate threshold, there is a continuous rise in blood lactate, indicating a sustained rate of lactate production and a greater reliance on CHO and/or reduced lactate removal. In contrast, below the lactate threshold a steady-state blood lactate level is achieved as a result of a balance between the rates of lactate production and release into the bloodstream and lactate removal, and the level may even approach resting levels during prolonged exercise.

Although for many years lactate was considered simply a metabolic byproduct of glycolysis, there are now convincing data that lactate is an important metabolic intermediate during and after exercise, being a substrate for oxidative metabolism in contracting skeletal and cardiac muscle and a gluconeogenic precursor. The concept of a lactate shuttle has been developed (29), and there is evidence in support of exchange of lactate between active and inactive muscles during exercise. Contracting skeletal muscle is a major site of lactate oxidation during exercise, which contributes as much as 30% of the total CHO oxidation (30). Thus, lactate can be simultaneously released and taken up by contracting skeletal muscle during exercise, with uptake closely linked with delivery. There is also evidence that noncontracting muscle releases lactate, particularly during the latter stages of prolonged dynamic exercise, thereby providing a mechanism for supplying additional carbon for oxidation and/or gluconeogenesis. It has been suggested that increases in epinephrine stimulate glycogenolysis in and lactate release from inactive muscle.

The transport of lactate across the sarcolemma is mediated by proton-linked monocarboxylate transporters (MCT), and as many as eight isoforms have been identified (31). In human skeletal muscle, the most abundant isoform is MCT1, followed by MCT4. MCT1 expression correlates closely with muscle oxidative capacity and appears to be responsible for lactate uptake, while MCT4 is more abundant in type II fibers and may be important for lactate efflux from muscles with a greater reliance on glycolysis (31). Endurance training increases MCT1 expression in skeletal muscle, and together with the increase in muscle oxidative capacity, it contributes to enhanced lactate uptake and oxidation.

As mentioned earlier, there has been debate on the regulation of lactate production during exercise and the role of oxygen availability (32). In many situations in which oxygen delivery to contracting skeletal muscle is reduced (hypoxia, anemia, carbon monoxide exposure) during exercise, blood and muscle lactate levels are increased. It has been suggested that this is a necessary consequence of increases in ADP, P_i and NADH that not only act to stimulate mitochondrial respiration but also activate glycolysis and conversion of pyruvate to lactate in the lactate dehydrogenase reaction (32). Since this reaction is stimulated by pyruvate via a mass action effect, lactate is produced whenever there is a mismatch between the rate of pyruvate production in the glycogenolytic–glycolytic pathway and the ability of PDH and mitochondrial shuttle systems to remove pyruvate and NADH, respectively, from the cytosol for oxidation (33). During the transition from rest to exercise or from a lower power output to a higher one, insufficient oxygen delivery and/or inadequate PDH activation results in a greater reliance on phosphocreatine and glycolytic ATP and lactate production. Similarly, manipulations that increase glycogenolytic–glycolytic flux and pyruvate production at a given level of oxygen consumption during exercise (e.g., epinephrine infusion, increased muscle glycogen availability, heat stress) result in higher muscle and blood lactate accumulation (12).

Post-Exercise CHO Metabolism

The period post exercise is characterized by the need to replenish muscle glycogen stores. Although exercise-induced glycogen depletion activates glycogen synthase (34), significant resynthesis of muscle glycogen is dependent upon ingestion of CHO, which increases blood glucose and insulin levels. In particular, insulin stimulates GLUT4 translocation to the sarcolemma and further activates glycogen synthase. Studies in transgenic mice overexpressing either GLUT4 or glycogen synthase in skeletal muscle have demonstrated that both are critical for muscle glycogen synthesis, although the enhanced muscle glycogen storage observed in trained athletes appears to be more related to increased skeletal muscle GLUT4 expression (19). An increase in both GLUT4 gene and protein expression has been observed immediately post exercise, and this appears to be linked to the restoration of muscle glycogen (19). Glycogen synthase activity is increased after exercise, the increase in activity being greater with more extensive glycogen depletion (34). Interestingly, exercise commenced with very low muscle glycogen levels that resulted in no further glycogen degradation did not increase glycogen synthase activity over the already elevated basal level (34). The mechanisms responsible for this association between muscle glycogen and glycogen synthase activity remain to be fully elucidated, but they may be related to the intracellular location of glycogen synthase within muscle and/or the activity of protein phosphatase 1 (PP1), an enzyme that dephosphorylates glycogen synthase, thereby increasing its activity (34). There is evidence that this

enzyme may be bound to glycogen, and particular interest has focused on the GM targeting subunit. The exercise-induced increase in glycogen synthase activity is critically dependent on GM-PP1 activity, and it has been suggested that the activity of this complex is inhibited by high muscle glycogen levels.

The period post exercise is also characterized by enhanced insulin sensitivity that may persist for up to 2 days. This enhanced insulin action partly arises from enhanced sarcolemmal GLUT4 and activation of glycogen synthase, and it allows for restoration of muscle glycogen to levels above the normal resting levels, a phenomenon known as glycogen supercompensation that was first reported in humans in 1966 (Milestone of Discovery). Enhanced insulin sensitivity is closely linked to glucose availability post exercise, since glucose deprivation prolongs the time course of elevated insulin action, while CHO feeding speeds the reversal of enhanced insulin action, an observation made in both rodents (19) and humans (35). These changes in insulin action are linked with muscle glycogen availability, since there is an association between muscle glycogen use during exercise and the increment in muscle glucose uptake during physiological hyperinsulinemia 3 hours after exercise (20) (Fig. 17.5). Low muscle glycogen enhances glycogen synthase activity (34) and insulin-stimulated muscle glucose transport (20). The cellular mechanisms responsible for this latter observation are not completely understood, but GLUT4 translocation to the sarcolemma in response to insulin stimulation is enhanced by prior muscle glycogen depletion (19,20). However, enhanced insulin action persists after restoration of muscle glycogen stores (19), implying that other factors must contribute to the effects of exercise on insulin action. Taken together, these various results provide a biochemical rationale for regular exercise in the prevention and management of metabolic disorders characterized by insulin resistance.

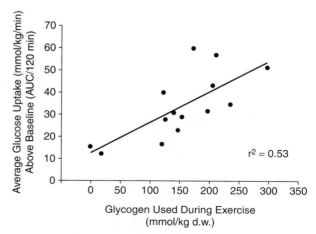

FIGURE 17.5 Relationship between glucose uptake during hyperinsulinemia 3 hours after exercise and the amount of glycogen used during exercise. *(Reprinted with permission from Richter EA, Derave W, Wojtaszewski JFP. Glucose, exercise and insulin: emerging concepts. J Physiol [Lond] 2001;535:317.)*

SUMMARY

Muscle glycogen and blood glucose derived from liver glycogenolysis and gluconeogenesis are the major oxidative substrates for contracting skeletal muscle during heavy exercise, and fatigue often coincides with depletion of these CHO stores. The rates of muscle glycogen utilization, muscle glucose uptake, and liver glucose output are determined primarily by exercise intensity and duration, but they can be modified by the preceding diet and training status. Key regulatory mechanisms include local control by intramuscular levels of calcium and metabolic intermediates; alterations in glycogen, glucose, and FFA availability; and neural and hormonal control. In the period post exercise, restoration of muscle glycogen stores, which takes precedence, is dependent upon the ingestion of CHO. Enhanced muscle glycogen synthesis and sarcolemmal glucose transport, along with increased GLUT4 expression, in the period post exercise contribute to enhanced insulin action and

---

A MILESTONE OF DISCOVERY

The Swedish scientists Jonas Bergström and Eric Hultman (Fig. 17.6) pioneered the use of the percutaneous needle biopsy in studies of muscle metabolism during exercise in human volunteers. In the late 1960s, they published a number of papers in which they examined aspects of phosphocreatine and glycogen metabolism in human skeletal muscle during exercise and the effects of various nutritional interventions. They collaborated with Lars Hermansen and Bengt Saltin on further exercise studies that verified and extended the classic studies of Christensen and Hansen and established the theoretical basis of dietary regimens for increasing muscle glycogen availability and enhancing endurance exercise performance.

For their 1966 *Nature* paper, Bergström and Hultman conducted an elegant experiment on themselves in which they were placed on either side of a cycle ergometer and performed single-leg exercise to deplete the muscle glycogen stores of one leg as the other leg rested. Muscle samples were obtained from both legs at the end of exercise and after 1, 2, and 3 days of recovery and consumption of a high-CHO diet. The muscle glycogen values (millimoles per kilogram wet mass) obtained from analysis of these samples are summarized in Table 17.2.

The data clearly show the utilization of muscle glycogen during exercise, rapid resynthesis of glycogen to preexercise levels within 24 hours in the previously exercised leg, and glycogen supercompensation when a high CHO intake was continued for

TABLE 17.2	Muscle Glycogen Levels Before and After Select Days on a High Carboyhydrate Intake Following Single Leg Exercise				

		Time (day)			
Subject	Leg	0	1	2	3
JB	Rested	72.3	94.5	83.4	111.2
	Exercised	5.6	116.8	177.9	216.8
EH	Rested	77.8	94.5	94.5	100.1
	Exercised	5.6	116.8	189.0	205.7

Units are mmol · kg⁻¹ wet mass.

another 2 days. These results provided the theoretical basis for future studies on muscle glycogen loading and exercise performance and initial insights into the possible influence of muscle glycogen on substrate metabolism and insulin action post exercise. The authors concluded:

> Exercise with glycogen depletion enhances the resynthesis of glycogen. The factor operates locally in the exercised muscle and the effect persists for at least 3 days. The nature of the mechanisms involved is unknown. It could be that a stimulation of one or more of the factors directly involved in glycogen synthesis takes place or that an effect is provided on the cell membrane, stimulating glucose uptake. It is possible that some of the beneficial effects of exercise in normal and diabetic subjects are mediated by this factor, thus promoting the storage of carbohydrate as glycogen instead of fat.

In the years since this study, many investigators have further characterized glycogen metabolism post exercise and elucidated the important role for muscle glycogen in the activation of glycogen synthase, insulin- and contraction-stimulated GLUT4 translocation and glucose uptake, skeletal muscle GLUT4 expression, and enhanced insulin sensitivity (24).

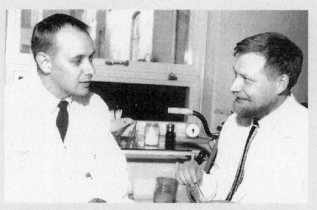

FIGURE 17.6 The late Jonas Bergström (*left*) and Eric Hultman in their laboratory at St. Erik's Hospital, Stockholm, in 1967. (*Reproduced with permission from Professor Eric Hultman.*)

Bergström J, Hultman E. Muscle glycogen synthesis after exercise: an enhancing factor localized to the muscle cells in man. Nature 1966;1210: 309–310.

partly account for the beneficial effects of acute and chronic exercise in insulin-resistant states.

ACKNOWLEDGMENTS

My research work has been supported by the Australian Research Council, the National Health and Medical Research Council of Australia, and the Deakin University Priority Research Area scheme.

REFERENCES

1. Romijn JA, Coyle EF, Sidossi LS, et al. Regulation of endogenous fat and carbohydrate metabolism in relation to exercise intensity and duration. Am J Physiol 1993;265:E380–E391.
2. Van Loon LJC, Greenhaff PL, Constantin-Teodosiu D, et al. The effects of increasing exercise intensity on muscle fuel utilisation in humans. J Physiol (Lond) 2001;536:295–304.
3. Hawley JA, Schabort EJ, Noakes TD, et al. Carbohydrate-loading and exercise performance: an update. Sports Med 1997;24:73–81.
4. Coyle EF, Coggan AR, Hemmert MK, et al. Muscle glycogen during prolonged strenuous exercise when fed carbohydrate. J Appl Physiol 1986;61:165–172.
5. Gollnick PD, Piehl K, Saltin B. Selective glycogen depletion pattern in human muscle fibres after exercise of varying intensity and at varying pedalling rates. J Physiol (Lond) 1974; 241:45–57.
6. Hultman E, Harris RC. Carbohydrate metabolism. In Poortmans JR, ed. Principles of Exercise Biochemistry. Basel: Karger, 1988;78–119.
7. Burke LM, Angus DJ, Cox GR, et al. Effect of fat adaptation and carbohydrate restoration on metabolism and performance during prolonged cycling. J Appl Physiol 2000;89:2413–2421.
8. Chesley A, Heigenhauser GJF, Spriet LL. Regulation of muscle glycogen phosphorylase activity following short-term endurance training. Am J Physiol 1996;270:E328–E335.
9. Richter EA, Ruderman NB, Gavras H, et al. Muscle glycogenolysis during exercise: dual control by epinephrine and contractions. Am J Physiol 1982;242:E25–E42.
10. Howlett RA, Parolin ML, Dyck DJ, et al. Regulation of skeletal muscle glycogen phosphorylase and PDH at varying exercise power outputs. Am J Physiol 1998;275:R418–R425.
11. Hargreaves M. Interactions between muscle glycogen and blood glucose during exercise. Exerc Sport Sci Rev 1997; 25:21–39.
12. Watt MJ, Howlett KF, Febbraio MA, et al. Adrenaline increases skeletal muscle glycogenolysis, PDH activation and carbohydrate oxidation during moderate exercise in humans. J Physiol (Lond) 2001;534:269–278.
13. Katz A, Broberg S, Sahlin K, et al. Leg glucose uptake during maximal dynamic exercise in humans. Am J Physiol 1986; 251:E65–E70.
14. Wahren J. Glucose turnover during exercise in man. Ann NY Acad Sci 1977;301:45–55.
15. Kristiansen S, Hargreaves M, Richter EA. Progressive increase in glucose transport and GLUT4 in human sarcolemmal vesicles during moderate exercise. Am J Physiol 1997;272:E385–E389.
16. Zisman A, Peroni AD, Abel ED, et al. Targeted disruption of the glucose transporter 4 selectively in muscle causes insulin resistance and glucose intolerance. Nat Med 2000;6:924–928.
17. Coggan AR, Kohrt WM, Spina RJ, et al. Endurance training decreases plasma glucose turnover and oxidation during moderate-intensity exercise in men. J Appl Physiol 1990; 68:990–996.
18. Richter EA, Nielsen JN, Jörgensen SB, et al. Signalling to glucose transport in skeletal muscle during exercise. Acta Physiol Scand 2003;178:329–335.
19. Holloszy JO. A forty-year memoir of research on the regulation of glucose transport into muscle. Am J Physiol 2003; 284:E453–E467.
20. Richter EA, Derave W, Wojtaszewski JFP. Glucose, exercise and insulin: emerging concepts. J Physiol (Lond) 2001;535: 313–322.
21. Ahlborg G, Felig P, Hagenfeldt L, et al. Substrate turnover during prolonged exercise in man. J Clin Invest 1974;53: 1080–1090.
22. Wojtaszewski JFP, MacDonald C, Nielsen JN, et al. Regulation of 5′AMP-activated protein kinase activity and substrate utilization in exercising human skeletal muscle. Am J Physiol 2003;284:E813–E822.
23. Kjaer M, Secher NH, Bach FW, et al. Role of motor center activity for hormonal changes and substrate mobilisation in humans. Am J Physiol 1987;253:R687–R695.
24. Coker RH, Wasserman DH, Simonsen L, et al. Stimulation of splanchnic glucose production during exercise in humans contains a glucagon-independent component. Am J Physiol 2001;280:E918–E927.
25. Kjaer M, Engfred K, Fernandes A, et al. Regulation of hepatic glucose production during exercise in humans: role of sympathoadrenergic activity. Am J Physiol 1993;265:E275–E283.
26. Howlett KF, Angus DJ, Proietto J, et al. Effect of increased blood glucose availability on glucose kinetics during exercise. J Appl Physiol 1998;84:1413–1417.
27. Spriet LL, Heigenhauser GJF. Regulation of pyruvate dehydrogenase (PDH) activity in human skeletal muscle during exercise. Exerc Sport Sci Rev 2002;30:91–95.
28. Coyle EF, Coggan AR, Hopper MK, et al. Determinants of endurance in well-trained cyclists. J Appl Physiol 1988;64: 2622–2630.
29. Brooks GA. Intra-and extra-cellular lactate shuttles. Med Sci Sports Exerc 2000;32:790–799.
30. Van Hall G, Jensen-Urstad M, Rosdahl H, et al. Leg and arm lactate and substrate kinetics during exercise. Am J Physiol 2003;284:E193–E205.
31. Juel C, Halestrap AP. Lactate transport in skeletal muscle: role and regulation of the monocarboxylate transporter. J Physiol (Lond) 1999;517:633–642.
32. Katz A, Sahlin K. Regulation of lactic acid production during exercise. J Appl Physiol 1988;65:509–518.
33. Spriet LL, Howlett RA, Heigenhauser GJF. An enzymatic approach to lactate production in human skeletal muscle during exercise. Med Sci Sports Exerc 2000;32:756–763.
34. Nielsen JN, Richter EA. Regulation of glycogen synthase in skeletal muscle during exercise. Acta Physiol Scand 2003; 178:309–319.
35. Bogardus C, Thuillez P, Ravussin E, et al. Effect of muscle glycogen depletion on in vivo insulin action in man. J Clin Invest 1983;72:1605–1610.

CHAPTER 18

The Metabolic Systems: Lipid Metabolism

LAWRENCE L. SPRIET

Introduction

It is now accepted that lipid is an important substrate for the aerobic production of energy in human skeletal muscle during mild, moderate, and even heavy dynamic exercise. However, it was not until the work of Christensen and Hansen was published in 1939 that the controversy over whether lipid (fat) could be used as a substrate for exercise was finally solved (1). They demonstrated, through a series of elegant studies, that both fat and carbohydrate (CHO) could be used as substrate for muscular contractions and that the amount of fat and CHO used depended on several factors. The preceding diet was the main factor during short-duration dynamic exercise of low to moderate intensity. As exercise increased in intensity, the proportion of fat oxidation decreased and CHO oxidation increased such that fat use was virtually absent at a power output that elicited 100% $\dot{V}O_{2max}$. However, during prolonged moderate dynamic exercise, the relative fat contribution increased because of the increasing availability of plasma free fatty acids (FFA) and decreasing CHO stores. Later studies used more direct experimental approaches to demonstrate the importance of plasma FFA and FFA derived from stores inside the muscle as substrates for oxidation during dynamic exercise (2,3).

Fat is often the dominant fuel for skeletal muscle at rest and during mild to moderate exercise. In absolute terms, the contribution of fat to the total energy production increases from low-power outputs to a maximum of about 50 to 65% $\dot{V}O_{2max}$ and then decreases as the exercise intensity increases to about 85% $\dot{V}O_{2max}$ and above (4–6) (Fig. 18.1). Consequently, as a substrate, fat is less important than CHO during heavy dynamic exercise. While CHO can provide all of the substrate required for dynamic exercise at about 100% $\dot{V}O_{2max}$ when no fat is available, fat can provide substrate only at a rate to sustain about 60 to 75% $\dot{V}O_{2max}$ when no CHO is available. However, fat is an energy-dense fuel with a high yield per unit mass and is stored in large quantities in the body. Therefore, fat can provide a substantial and increasing amount of energy during prolonged dynamic exercise at low to moderate intensities. Aerobic training also increases the maximal rate at which fat oxidation can produce energy in skeletal muscle and increases the proportion of energy produced from fat oxidation at any absolute power output (7). Also, fat metabolism is not activated as quickly as CHO metabolism at the onset of exercise, and it cannot be used to generate anaerobic energy during heavy exercise above 100% $\dot{V}O_{2max}$ (sprint exercise).

Large quantities of fat are stored as triglyceride or triacylglycerol (TG) in numerous adipose tissues in the body. Smaller amounts of fat are also stored directly in muscle cells. Because of the high energy density of fat, the fat stored in muscle can provide almost as much fuel as muscle glycogen (about 67–100%). Therefore, the intramuscular TG (IMTG) store is not trivial. Fat is also found in numerous forms in the circulation. However, it appears that the FFA bound to albumin is the predominant source of circulatory fat that is

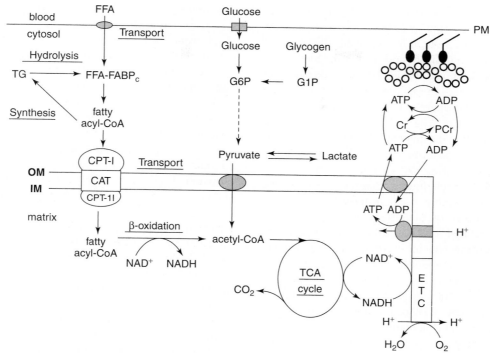

FIGURE 18.1   Overview of fat metabolism in skeletal muscle. PM, plasma membrane; OM, IM, outer and inner mitochondrial membranes; FFA, free fatty acid; FABP$_c$, cytoplasmic fatty acid–binding protein; TG, triacylglycerol; CoA, coenzyme A; CPT I & II, carnitine palmitoyltransferase I & II; CAT, carnitine-acylcarnitine translocase; NAD$^+$, NADH, oxidized and reduced nicotinamide adenine dinucleotide; G6P, G1P, glucose 6- and 1-phosphate; PCr, phosphocreatine; Cr, creatine; TCA, tricarboxylic acid; ETC, electron transport chain. *(Adapted with permission from Spriet LL. Regulation of skeletal muscle fat oxidation during exercise in humans. Med Sci Sports Exerc 2002;34:1477–1484.)*

readily available for uptake and oxidation by skeletal muscle during dynamic exercise. Circulating TG in the form of chylomicrons and very low density lipoproteins appear to contribute less than 5 to 8% of the fat oxidized during dynamic exercise (3,8). At rest, when the need for FFA uptake is low, circulating TG can be degraded and provide FFA for storage and oxidation in the muscle.

Historically, the regulation of fat metabolism in skeletal muscle has not been studied as thoroughly as CHO metabolism. It was initially believed that skeletal muscle fat metabolism was not heavily regulated. Many textbooks still claim that the only sites of control are the release of FFA into the blood from adipose tissue and the transport of FFA across the mitochondrial membranes of the muscle cell. However, it is now clear that the regulation of fat metabolism is more complex and involves additional sites of control in adipose tissue and skeletal muscle. This chapter outlines what is known regarding the regulation of fat metabolism in skeletal muscle. The bias is toward the events that lead to the production of energy from the oxidation of fat in human skeletal muscle during dynamic exercise, although numerous citations of research in skeletal muscle of other species are made. The chapter begins with an overview of the pathways involved in the control of fat metabolism. Subsequent sections

provide more detail regarding the putative sites of regulation and other issues related to fat metabolism.

Overview of Fat Metabolism

A major source of fat for the working muscle during exercise is the delivery of long-chain FFA to the muscle from adipose tissue (9). The degradation of FFA from adipose tissue TG and the release and removal of FFA from adipose tissue are regulated processes. The FFA bind to albumin in the blood, and the bulk transport of FFA to the muscle (flow × [FFA]) plays a role in the ability of muscle to take up FFA (Fig. 18.1). A common theme with the transport of FFA is the need to provide a protein chaperone. Unbound FFA interfere with electrical activity, act as a detergent, and are indiscriminate enzyme inhibitors. Therefore, at every step involved in the transport and metabolism of FFA, proteins bind the so-called free fatty acids. While the fat is free from its stored or esterified form, most of it is always coupled to a binding protein. Only a small fraction of the FFA are truly free, to promote binding to albumin in adipose tissue and possibly the removal from albumin in skeletal muscle.

Recent evidence suggests that most of the FFA that enter muscle cells are transported or assisted across the muscle membrane by transport proteins, most notably the fatty acid translocase protein (FAT/CD36) and the plasma membrane fatty acid binding protein (FABP$_{pm}$) (10). A smaller portion appears to diffuse across the membrane. Once inside the muscle, FFA must be chaperoned by cytoplasmic fatty acid binding proteins (FABPc). The FFA destined for storage as IMTG or for oxidation in the mitochondria must first be activated via binding with coenzyme A (CoA) through the activity of fatty acyl-CoA synthase (9). This may occur at several sites in the cytoplasm, including the plasma membrane, the outer mitochondrial membrane, and near the IMTG droplet. A second major source of fat is the release of FFA from IMTG. The evidence that IMTG contributes substrate for energy production during dynamic exercise is now convincing, but the quantitative importance at varying intensities and durations of exercise remains somewhat controversial (11). There appear to be several steps involved in muscle lipolysis, including activation of TG or hormone sensitive lipase (HSL), movement of the HSL complex to the lipid droplet, and possibly the removal of a protective protein layer around the lipid droplet.

All of the cytoplasmic FABPc FFA, whether derived from outside the cell (plasma FFA) or inside the muscle cell (IMTG), must be transported to the outer mitochondrial membrane. It is then activated with CoA, if not already activated, and converted to fatty acyl carnitine by carnitine fatty acyltransferase I, commonly called carnitine palmitoyltransferase (CPT) I (12). This compound is moved across the mitochondrial membranes via a translocase while carnitine moves in the opposite direction. Inside the mitochondria, the carnitine is removed and the CoA is rebound to the long-chain fatty acid by the action of another distinct enzyme, CPT II. The fatty acyl-CoA molecules are then metabolized in the β-oxidation pathway with the production of acetyl-CoA and the reducing equivalents reduced nicotinamide adenine dinucleotide and (NADH) and reduced flavin adenine dinucleotide (FADH$_2$). The reducing equivalents are directly used in the electron transport chain, while the acetyl-CoA is further metabolized in the tricarboxylic acid pathway with the production of additional reducing equivalents. The electron transport chain accepts the reducing equivalents to generate a proton motive force, which provides the chemical energy to synthesize adenosine triphosphate (ATP) from inorganic phosphate (P$_i$) and adenosine diphosphate (ADP) while consuming oxygen in the process of oxidative phosphorylation.

The sites that may control skeletal muscle fat metabolism and oxidation during dynamic exercise appear to include (a) adipose tissue lipolysis, FFA release from adipose tissue, and FFA delivery to the muscle; (b) FFA movement across the muscle membrane; (c) regulation of muscle HSL activity; (d) binding and transport of FFA in the cytoplasm; (e) regulation of FFA movement across the mitochondrial membranes; and (f) the mitochondrial volume of proteins (i.e., β-oxidation enzymes) available to metabolize fat.

It would be expected that the regulation of fat metabolism during an acute dynamic exercise bout lasting several minutes would involve control by both hormonal signals and signals originating inside the muscle. The blood catecholamine and insulin concentrations are major hormonal regulators. Inside the muscle, three classes of signals are generally associated with the acute activation of energy producing metabolic pathways: (a) Ca^{++}, released to initiate muscle contraction and the early warning signal for the activation of metabolic processes; (b) feedback from byproducts related to ATP use—often called the energy state of the muscle—including the free concentrations of ATP, ADP, adenosine monophosphate (AMP) and P$_i$; (c) feedback from the involvement of the reduction-oxidation (redox) couple (NAD$^+$/NADH) at many sites in the mitochondria.

These signals and regulators have been well studied and heavily implicated in controlling the cytoplasmic pathways involved in the metabolism of CHO and the tricarboxylic acid cycle in the mitochondria, which accepts acetyl-CoA as a substrate from both CHO and fat metabolism. However, until recently, there has not been the same interest or level of success in linking these putative regulators with the regulation of fat metabolism.

Adipose Tissue Lipolysis

The ability of adipose tissue to respond to dynamic exercise by activating TG hydrolysis and releasing FFA into the blood is important for increasing and maintaining the delivery of FFA to the working muscle. The regulation of adipose tissue lipolysis has been well studied and reviewed (9,13,14). The current understanding of the regulation of adipose tissue lipolysis centers on the control of HSL activity. HSL appears to be the rate-limiting enzyme in the degradation of TG to 3 FFA and glycerol (Fig. 18.2). It exists in an active phosphorylated form and an inactive dephosphorylated form. The exact amount of active and inactive HSL at any time is controlled by the relative activities of protein kinase A (PKA), which phosphorylates the enzyme and a phosphatase, which dephosphorylates the enzyme. HSL catalyzes the breakdown of TG to diacylglycerol (DG) and FFA, and DG to monoacylglycerol (MG) and FFA. The enzyme DG lipase also degrades DG to MG and FFA (as does HSL), and MG lipase degrades MG to FFA and glycerol. However, the DG and MG lipases are near-equilibrium enzymes and are not externally regulated. They simply respond to changing concentrations of substrates and products. Therefore, when HSL activity increases the availability of DG and MG, they respond by cleaving another FFA from the remaining lipid molecule.

It was believed for some time that regulating HSL activity was the only control step in the degradation of TG, but it

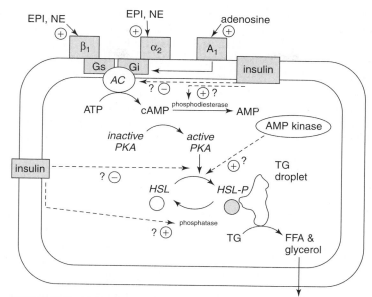

FIGURE 18.2   The major regulation of adipose tissue lipolysis during exercise. EPI, epinephrine; NE, norepinephrine; G_s and G_i, stimulatory and inhibitory G proteins; cAMP, cyclic AMP; PKA, protein kinase A; TG, triacylglycerol, HSL, hormone sensitive lipase; FFA, free fatty acid. *(Reprinted with permission from Spriet LL. Regulation of skeletal muscle fat oxidation during exercise in humans. Med Sci Sports Exerc 2002;34:1477–1484.)*

does not appear to be the sole site of control. Recent evidence suggests that regulation also exists at steps distal to HSL. These may include the migration of the activated HSL to the vicinity of the lipid droplets (15) and/or the removal of a protective outer layer of protein (perilipin) on the lipid droplet (16) to enable lipolysis. These processes have not been clarified in detail but do appear to have potential as sites of control.

Resting Lipolysis

While the body is at rest, adipose tissue lipolysis is maintained at a low rate through the inhibitory influences by several hormones (9,14,17). The plasma catecholamines norepinephrine and epinephrine exert an inhibitory effect on lipolysis at low concentrations through a cascade of events ending in the maintenance of HSL, predominantly in the dephosphorylated or inactive form. Low NE and epinephrine levels activate the α_2-adrenergic receptor, which stimulates the inhibitory G protein (G_i) and decreases the activity of adenylate cyclase and the production of cyclic AMP (cAMP). A low cAMP level in turn decreases the activation of PKA and HSL activities, ultimately reducing the degradation of TG. Adenosine also contributes to the resting inhibition of lipolysis by binding to adenosine receptors and activating the G_i protein. This process can be antagonized by caffeine in the blood, as caffeine competes for the adenosine binding sites, prevents the activation of G_i, and often leads to increased lipolysis and plasma FFA levels at rest. This drug has been

used experimentally to increase the availability of FFA to the muscles during rest and exercise. Nicotinic acid also affects adipose tissue lipolysis and has been commonly used to examine the effects of reduced plasma FFA availability on skeletal muscle metabolism. Nicotinic acid inhibits adipose tissue lipolysis by binding to HM74 receptors that are coupled to G_i proteins. Subsequent decreases in cAMP levels prevent the PKA-induced activation of HSL, leading to decreased systemic FFA release.

The presence of insulin in the blood can also inhibit lipolysis and may be the most important regulator at rest. Insulin exerts a strong antilipolytic effect following a meal containing significant amounts of CHO, as the body attempts to reduce the use of fat while storing and oxidizing the ingested CHO. Insulin binds to insulin receptors and is believed to inhibit lipolysis through a cascade of signaling metabolites at several sites: (*a*) via direct inhibition of adenylate cyclase activity, (*b*) through activation of phosphodiesterase activity and the removal of cAMP, (*c*) via direct inhibition of PKA, which reduces the activation of HSL, and (*d*) via activation of phosphatase, which deactivates HSL.

Lipolysis During Dynamic Exercise

Dynamic exercise is associated with an increase in sympathetic nervous system activity resulting in an accumulation of epinephrine and norepinephrine in the blood. Epinephrine originates mainly from the adrenal medulla, while norepinephrine originates mainly from spillover from sympathetic nerve terminals. The increased catecholamine concentrations during exercise exert powerful effects to increase lipolysis and override the combined inhibitory influences that dominate at rest. The increases in plasma norepinephrine and epinephrine during exercise bind to β-adrenergic receptors and activate the G stimulatory protein (G_s). This antagonizes and overrides the effects of the G_i protein to increase adenylate cyclase activity, cAMP production, PKA activity, HSL activity, and ultimately the potential for lipolysis. The effects of the catecholamines are also powerful enough to negate the inhibitory effects of insulin, especially if plasma insulin levels decrease during exercise. The net result is the activation of HSL and ultimately TG degradation to FFA and glycerol. The FFA are then either reesterified to TG, or preferably, during exercise, released from the adipose tissue into the blood. The escape of the FFA into the blood is dependent on the availability of albumin. This process does not appear to be limiting during most dynamic exercise, but it may be limiting during heavy exercise, as discussed next.

FFA Release From Adipose Tissue and Delivery to Muscle

The delivery of FFA to contracting muscle is a function of the plasma [FFA] and muscle blood flow. Since muscle blood flow increases as a function of the dynamic exercise power output, even the maintenance of a constant blood [FFA] means that muscle FFA delivery increases several fold during exercise. During prolonged mild to moderate exercise, the blood [FFA] increases within 10 to 30 minutes and also contributes to the increased FFA delivery, as FFA release from adipose tissue slightly exceeds its removal from the plasma. Increased FFA delivery to the muscle correlates with increased muscle FFA uptake and oxidation during dynamic exercise, although the relationship is not linear during all exercise. The movement of FFA across the muscle membrane appears to be a saturable process in both rodent and human skeletal muscle and will be discussed in the following section.

Adipose Tissue Lipolysis and FFA Release During Mild, Moderate, and Heavy Dynamic Exercise

To study of the importance of adipose tissue lipolysis and FFA release, simultaneous measurements of plasma [FFA] and estimations of adipose tissue lipolysis and muscle oxidation of plasma FFA have been made during dynamic exercise at increasing power outputs in well-trained cyclists (4,6). Lipolysis increased as a function of the power output at 25 and 65% $\dot{V}_{O_2max}$ and the plasma [FFA] remained high during exercise at these two intensities (FFA before exercise were already high at about 0.8–1.0 mM as a result of an overnight fast). Therefore, FFA delivery to the contracting

muscles increased from rest to exercise at 25% $\dot{V}_{O_2max}$ and again from 25 to 65% $\dot{V}_{O_2max}$ and correlated with the maintenance of high plasma FFA uptake and oxidation rates at these two intensities.

These same relationships did not hold during dynamic exercise at 85% $\dot{V}_{O_2max}$ (4). Adipose tissue lipolysis was not decreased during 30 minutes of exercise at 85% $\dot{V}_{O_2max}$, but was maintained at the same rate as exercise at 65% $\dot{V}_{O_2max}$.

However, the oxidation rate of plasma FFA decreased at 85% $\dot{V}_{O_2max}$. The prediction from these results would be an increase in plasma FFA, but the FFA concentration actually decreased by about 50%. To explain these results, it was proposed that in spite of the maintained lipolytic rate at 85% $\dot{V}_{O_2max}$, a decrease in adipose tissue blood flow prevented much of the liberated FFA from reaching the blood. A reduced blood flow decreased the availability of albumin, which is necessary to bind the FFA and permit transport in the blood. Therefore, the uptake of FFA by the muscles continued at a higher rate than the release from adipose tissue and accounted for the lower blood [FFA].

It is likely that the large fall in [FFA] during dynamic exercise from 65 to 85% $\dot{V}_{O_2max}$ outweighed the increase in muscle blood flow, resulting in a decrease in FFA delivery to the contracting muscles at 85% $\dot{V}_{O_2max}$. This correlated with a significant decrease in plasma FFA uptake and oxidation at 85% $\dot{V}_{O_2max}$. However, these results do not exclude changes related to muscle membrane or metabolism from contributing to the reduced fat oxidation at the higher power output.

To assess the importance of FFA delivery to the contracting muscles during dynamic exercise, the plasma [FFA] at 85% $\dot{V}_{O_2max}$ was artificially maintained at the higher 65% $\dot{V}_{O_2max}$ level by infusing a TG emulsion and heparin solution (18). The plasma FFA uptake and oxidation rates were increased at 85% $\dot{V}_{O_2max}$ when FFA delivery was maintained but did not reach the same rates as at 65% $\dot{V}_{O_2max}$. These findings implied that other factors, related to the muscle membrane or metabolism inside the muscle, also play an important role in determining the rate of plasma FFA uptake and oxidation at higher intensities of dynamic exercise.

FFA Transport Across the Muscle Membrane

Until recently, it was believed that FFA simply diffused through the bipilid layer of the muscle membrane into the muscle cell. The plasma [FFA] and/or the rate of FFA delivery to the muscles were believed to be the only controlling factors. While it remains controversial, there is now strong evidence that a major portion of the FFA that enter muscle do so via protein-mediated mechanisms (10,19). This may involve actual transport of FFA across the muscle membrane by carrier proteins and/or facilitation of their movement across the membrane by initial binding to transport proteins.

The presence of proteins that transport or assist the movement of FFA into muscle cells implies that this is a major site of regulation for fat metabolism (Fig. 18.3).

Three possible fat transport proteins have been identified: the $FABP_{pm}$, the FAT/CD36, and the fatty acid transport protein (FATP). Research has attempted to measure the gene expression (messenger RNA), protein abundance, and functional significance of these proteins in response to a variety of physiological stimuli that alter the uptake of FFA in skeletal muscle. Much of the pioneering research has been done in red and white rodent skeletal muscle; investigators have tried to determine whether there is a strong relationship between the expression and protein content of the putative transporters and actual FFA uptake (10,20). The giant sarcolemmal vesicle technique has also been very useful to measure pure FFA transport in a controlled environment. The skeletal muscle vesicles are entirely right side out and contain ample FABPc to sequester incoming FFA during the uptake measurements. Direct measurements of FFA uptake have shown that all of the FFA moved into the vesicle are bound to FABPc. None of the incoming FFA are metabolized in this preparation, such that FFA uptake can be measured without the confounding influence of ongoing metabolism. The abundance of muscle membrane transporter protein on the vesicles can also be measured to correlate with actual transport rates. It has been reported that mRNA abundance and protein content of the FFA transporters in the plasma membrane and FFA transport capacity were several fold higher in red oxidative rodent muscle (high capacity for fat metabolism) versus white glycolytic muscle (20). The transport of FFA also appeared to

be a saturable process in sarcolemmal vesicles prepared from both red and white rat muscles. This correlated with similar findings in rat hindlimb and human skeletal muscle exposed to high FFA availability (21,22).

There is an increase in FFA uptake and oxidation during dynamic exercise as both FFA and CHO metabolism increase to meet the demand for ATP. There is also a well-documented increase in the capacity to oxidize plasma FFA following dynamic exercise training (7,22). Chronic electrical stimulation has been shown to increase the expression of FAT/CD36 mRNA and protein, vesicle fatty acid transport, and fatty acid oxidation in rodent red and white muscle (23). Dynamic exercise training in humans has also been reported to increase muscle $FABP_{pm}$ protein content (24). An exciting finding was the recent report that the FAT/CD36 protein was acutely translocated from an intracellular pool to the muscle membrane (25) during a single bout of muscle contractions, in a manner similar to that reported for the GLUT4 transporter. The increased FAT/CD36 content in the membrane correlated with increased fatty acid transport into vesicles prepared from the contracted muscle. These data strongly suggest that the ability to translocate FAT/CD36 to the muscle membrane is part of a complex and highly regulated system for promoting fat uptake during dynamic exercise.

Recent studies have reported that insulin can also translocate FAT/CD36 to the muscle membrane and that membrane FAT/CD36 transport protein is more abundant in obese than in lean rats without an increase in total protein content (10). This underscores the importance of measuring fatty acid transporter abundance directly in the muscle

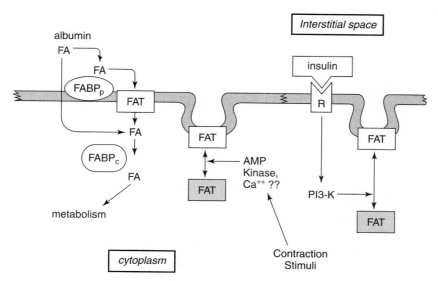

FIGURE 18.3   Potential mechanisms for long-chain fatty acid uptake across the muscle membrane. *Dark squares.* Vesicles where FAT protein is stored. *Open squares.* FAT protein at the surface of the membrane. FA, fatty acid; $FABP_p$, plasma membrane fatty acid binding protein; FAT, fatty acid translocase; $FABP_c$, cytoplasmic fatty acid binding protein; R, receptor; PI3-K, PI3-kinase. *(Courtesy of Dr. Arend Bonen of the University of Guelph, Guelph, Ontario.)*

plasma membrane and not simply in the whole muscle homogenate.

To date there has been little research to identify the factors that activate the translocation of fat transporter proteins to the membrane during exercise. It might be expected that Ca^{++} and the factors related to the energy status of the cell (e.g., free ADP, P_i, and AMP-activated protein kinase [AMPK] activity) would be involved, as they are important in activating the pathways that metabolize CHO in the cytoplasm. However, the time course of the changes involved in up-regulating FFA uptake and oxidation appears to be slower than the activation of glucose uptake, glycogen breakdown, and CHO metabolism during exercise. There has been a significant amount of research examining the importance of AMPK in activating both CHO and fat metabolism. It appears to function as an energy sensor, being sensitive to decreases in muscle phosphocreatine content and increases in free AMP (26). Activation of AMPK with AMP analogues has been repeatedly demonstrated to correlate with activated CHO metabolism and increased fat oxidation in resting skeletal muscle, suggesting that AMPK may be the key energy sensor in skeletal muscle at rest. Its role during exercise in the presence of powerful additional signals for stimulating metabolism is less clear. It may be that AMPK plays a more powerful role in activating fat metabolism than CHO metabolism during dynamic exercise. Increases in Ca^{++} and reductions in the energy state of the cell during the onset of exercise activate CHO metabolism in a more direct and rapid manner.

Binding and Transport of FFA in the Cytoplasm

Once inside the muscle cell, FFA are bound to FABPc, which functions as an intracellular chaperone in a manner similar to the function of albumin in the plasma (27). The FABPc bind with high affinity to saturated and unsaturated FFA and appear responsible for transferring FFA to cytoplasmic (for storage as IMTG) and mitochondrial (for oxidation) sites for further processing. The content of FABPc is proportional to the oxidative capacity of the muscle fiber in rodent skeletal muscle but similar in most human skeletal muscles. This is likely due to the reasonably high aerobic capacity of the two dominant fiber types in human skeletal muscles, types I and IIA, and the low abundance of type IIB fibers. FABPc content is also sensitive to physiological stimuli, and it increases following aerobic training and a high-fat diet (27).

The role of FABPc in the regulation of fat transport appears to be necessary but permissive (27). Experiments with knockout animals have shown that skeletal muscle FABPc can be decreased by about 67% without altering fat transport as measured in giant sarcolemmal vesicles. If FABPc is completely removed, fat transport is severely reduced. This argues that FABPc are in great excess in the cytoplasm and play a permissive role in fat transport. Estimates suggest that only 2% of the total FABPc are bound to FFA at any time.

The FABPc-FFA complex is activated by the addition of a CoA group through the action of the enzyme fatty acyl-CoA synthase, most likely at several sites in the cell. The resultant fatty acyl-CoA appears to attach to an additional binding protein, the aptly named acyl-CoA binding protein. This new complex is the suitable substrate for either esterification into IMTG in the cytoplasm or transport into the mitochondria for oxidation.

Synthesis of Muscle Triacylglycerol

FFA that has been transported into the cell or was previously released from IMTG in the cell can be reesterified to IMTG. The substrates to complete reesterification include glycerol 3-phosphate and ultimately three moieties of fatty acyl-CoA. There are four reactions in the synthesis pathway, with glycerol 3-phosphate acting as a backbone in the first step to accept one fatty acyl-CoA to produce acylglycerol-3-phosphate (9). Additional fatty acyl-CoA moieties are added at steps 2 and 4. The enzymes that add fatty acyl-CoA to the structure are acyltransferases, and the process is acylation. The phosphatidic acid produced at step 2 is the substrate for the final acylation step, but it can also be a substrate for phospholipid production in the cell. The enzymes involved in this pathway were originally thought to have no external regulators and simply be controlled by substrate and product concentrations. However, recent evidence suggests that the enzymes at steps 1 and 4, glycerol-phosphate acyltransferase and DG acyltransferase, are externally regulated. Insulin appears to play a role in activating these enzymes.

There has also been interest in the extent of the cycling that might occur between IMTG breakdown and reesterification in skeletal muscle both at rest and during dynamic exercise. While the existence of this TG–fatty acid cycle has been demonstrated many times in a variety of muscle preparations at rest, it is not clear how significant FFA reesterification is during dynamic exercise when there is net utilization of IMTG as an energy substrate. A recent study using a dual tracer approach reported that FFA reesterification was only about 7% of IMTG breakdown during moderate dynamic exercise (13).

The Use of IMTG as a Substrate During Dynamic Exercise

There has been considerable controversy regarding whether IMTG actually contributes a significant amount of energy during dynamic exercise when FFA oxidation provides a major portion of the energy. However, recent studies using new techniques for measuring IMTG and examining the variability of direct assessments of IMTG appear to have resolved this controversy. There now appears to be a consensus that IMTG is an important substrate during prolonged moderate dynamic exercise and up to about 85% $\dot{V}_{O_2max}$ in well-trained athletes (11).

Estimating IMTG Use During Dynamic Exercise

Four approaches have been used to study the use of IMTG in muscle (11). Two direct approaches use muscle sampled with a biopsy needle followed by either extraction of the lipid from the sample and biochemical measurement of TG or histochemical staining of the sampled muscle for lipid. A third approach has been to estimate the whole-body fat oxidation rate (RER) and also measure the rate of disappearance of plasma FFA with a tracer. Assuming that skeletal muscle metabolism is dominating whole-body metabolism during moderate dynamic exercise, an indirect estimation of IMTG use is the difference between whole-body fat oxidation and that provided from the plasma. Recently a fourth approach that is direct and noninvasive uses ^{1}H-magnetic resonance spectroscopy (MRS) on the surface of muscle to distinguish between TG within and outside the muscle (28).

Many laboratories measured [IMTG] before and after dynamic exercise with direct biochemical analyses on needle biopsy samples taken from the vastus lateralis muscles of men and reported that IMTG was not an important substrate during exercise lasting 90 to 120 minutes at a power output of 50 to 65% $\dot{V}_{O_2max}$. Meanwhile, there were fewer studies reporting a net IMTG use during dynamic exercise in men and women (11). A major criticism of the biopsy work was the possibility that the samples were contaminated by the presence of adipose tissue TG, making any estimation of true IMTG use inaccurate. The fact that the between-biopsy (three biopsies) variation of this measurement was as high as about 20 to 26% in a group of untrained and active individuals supported this contention (29). At the same time, almost all of the studies that estimated the use of IMTG with measurements of whole body RER and plasma FFA oxidation reported a significant use of IMTG during prolonged dynamic exercise. In addition, many studies employing histochemical IMTG staining techniques also reported that IMTG was reduced following dynamic exercise (11). Third, with the emergence of the MRS technique, more reports of significant IMTG use in a variety of upper and lower leg muscles during prolonged dynamic exercise appeared.

In response to the divergent findings, the issue of IMTG use during exercise, when measured biochemically, was reassessed by taking two biopsies from a group of well-trained cyclists at each time point throughout dynamic exercise. The between-biopsy variation was lower in the trained subjects (about 12%) than previously reported in the untrained and active subjects (about 24%), and this allowed for detection of a significant decrease in IMTG content during 2 hours of cycling at 57% $\dot{V}_{O_2max}$ (30). Therefore, it has been argued that

much of the controversy regarding IMTG use during dynamic exercise in the studies employing biochemical analyses of muscle biopsy samples was a function of two things: (a) A significant variability between muscle biopsy samples in human skeletal muscle; however, this is less in trained subjects. (b) Because of the high energy density of fat, the amount of IMTG used during 90 to 120 minutes of cycling at 50 to 65% $\dot{V}_{O_2max}$ is not large (about 2–4 mmol per kilogram of dry muscle, or only 10–15% of the total TG store) and can be less than the between-biopsy variation in untrained active subjects.

It also seems apparent from these recent studies that adipose tissue contamination of the biochemical estimates of IMTG is either not present or minimal, as the measured values are in the same range or lower than the estimated IMTG values reported using the 1H-MRS technique. A final point is that the few studies that have examined this issue in well-trained females all suggest that IMTG is a significant source of substrate during prolonged dynamic exercise. Interestingly, this includes studies that have measured IMTG content directly with the biochemical and ^{1}H-MRS techniques and indirectly from the RER and plasma FFA oxidation estimates (11).

In summary, it appears that there is a consensus that IMTG is a significant source of substrate during moderate dynamic exercise in active and trained individuals. This may extend to heavy exercise (about 85% $\dot{V}_{O_2max}$) in well-trained individuals. However, there still exists some controversy over the accuracy of the various methods used to estimate IMTG use during dynamic exercise and therefore the magnitude of the IMTG contribution to total substrate use.

Is Lipid Ingestion Post Exercise Important?

Of late, a series of experiments examining the replenishment of IMTG following exercise have raised a new concern regarding lipid ingestion post exercise. If IMTG is used during dynamic exercise sessions, it must be replenished during the recovery period. It is not known whether beginning a dynamic exercise session with an IMTG store that is less than normal will actually limit the ability to perform exercise of moderate intensity. However, it seems clear that an inability to replenish this store over repeated dynamic exercise sessions could lead to such a situation, as has been documented for muscle glycogen. The few studies that have examined the replenishment of IMTG following prolonged dynamic exercise reported that high levels of fat intake (35–57% of total energy intake) will replete IMTG stores more quickly than low levels of fat (10–24%). The amount of ingested fat needed to produce complete IMTG repletion has been estimated to be about 2 g · kg^{-1} body mass per day (31). However, the high fat intake may compromise the ability to replete muscle glycogen and impair dynamic exercise performance. Additional studies examining fat intake following exercise in the range of 20 to 30% of the total energy intake are needed to clarify this issue. It may be that when 2 days are available for recovery, a diet of 25 to 30% fat, 15% protein, and 55 to 60% CHO of the total energy intake will be optimal. If prolonged dynamic exercise occurs nearly every day, it has been recommended that the diet in the initial 6 to 8 hours post exercise should be high in CHO and low in fat (31). Following this time period, fat can be added in the form of regular meals.

Regulation of Muscle Lipolysis and Hormone Sensitive Lipase Activity

A significant amount of fat is stored in human skeletal muscle, usually in the range of 20 to 40 mmol per kilogram dry muscle or enough energy to account for about 67 to 100% of the energy stored as glycogen in a well-fed person. Three reactions lead to the degradation of IMTG to three FFA and glycerol. However, HSL can degrade IMTG to DG and FFA and also degrade DG to MG and FFA, and this appears to be the regulatory step, as it is the only site of external regulation in this pathway (9). The additional enzymes (DG and MG lipase) responsible for removing the final two FFA are near equilibrium in nature and continue to degrade the DG and MG as a function of increasing substrate concentrations. (Both HSL and DG lipase contribute to the degradation of DG to MG and FFA.)

A skeletal muscle version of HSL has been identified, and it is distinct from the other lipases in muscle. It has a neutral pH optimum and is covalently activated by the action of kinases (PKA and extracellular signal-regulated kinase, or ERK) that add a phosphate and deactivated by phosphatases that remove a phosphate at the activating sites (Fig. 18.4). Kinases also phosphorylate the enzyme at different or inhibitory sites (AMPK and calcium-calmodulin kinase II) than PKA and ERK and make phosphorylation at the activating PKA and ERK sites more difficult (32–34).

Very little is known regarding the regulation of this important enzyme, as several factors have delayed research in this area. The first problem with studying muscle HSL has been the possibility of contamination with the two other lipases in skeletal muscle, a lysosomal lipase with an acidic pH optimum, and a lipoprotein lipase with an alkaline pH optimum. Lipoprotein lipase is produced in vesicles and secreted to the outside of the muscle cell, ultimately to reside on the endothelial surface of the muscle blood vessels. It is important in regulating the degradation of circulating TG in the blood during rest. A second problem has been the controversy regarding whether IMTG is actually utilized as a substrate during dynamic exercise, as discussed earlier. A third problem delaying work on the regulation of muscle TG degradation was the lack of a viable analytical technique for trapping and measuring the activity of HSL in the inactive and active fractions during dynamic exercise. These techniques exist for other covalently regulated enzymes that metabolize CHO, such as glycogen phosphorylase and pyruvate dehydrogenase. Recently a series of experiments established

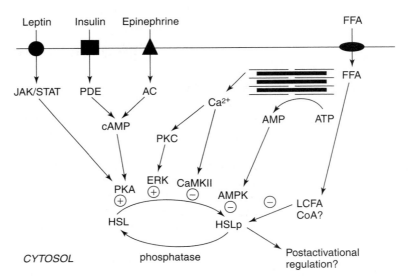

FIGURE 18.4 Potential mechanisms for control of skeletal muscle hormone-sensitive lipase (HSL). PKA and ERK phosphorylate HSL at activator sites to make the enzyme more active. CaMKII and AMPK are believed to phosphorylate the enzyme at inhibitory sites, as they make phosphorylation at the activator sites difficult. PDE, phosphodiesterase; AC, adenylate cyclase; cAMP, cyclic AMP; PKA, protein kinase A; PKC, protein kinase C; LCFA CoA, long chain fatty acyl CoA; ERK, extracellular signal regulated kinase; CaMKII, Ca^{2+}/calmodulin-dependent protein kinase II; AMPK, 5'-AMP-activated protein kinase.

a viable method for measuring the active form of HSL in mammalian skeletal muscle and reported activities of the inactive and active fractions of muscle HSL in a variety of conditions (32–34).

In human skeletal muscle at rest, there is a high constitutive level of HSL activity. The combination of low epinephrine and calcium concentrations and resting levels of insulin appear to determine the levels of HSL activity measured at rest. During the initial minute of mild and moderate dynamic exercise, HSL is activated by contractions in the apparent absence of increases in circulating epinephrine. However, epinephrine may contribute to the early activation of HSL during heavy dynamic exercise. The contraction-induced activation appears related to increased protein kinase C and ERK activity by calcium and/or other unknown activators. As mild or moderate dynamic exercise continues beyond a few minutes, activation by epinephrine through the cAMP cascade and PKA also appears to occur. With moderate dynamic exercise beyond 1 to 2 hours and sustained heavy dynamic exercise, HSL activity decreases in spite of continuing increases in epinephrine, possibly because of increasing accumulations in free AMP, activation of AMPK, and phosphorylation of inhibitory sites on HSL. Taken together, the data on human muscle suggest that intramuscular factors dominate the control of HSL activity, with hormonal factors playing a smaller role. Therefore, the muscle lipase may be more aptly named contraction-induced lipase rather than HSL.

The existing work in human skeletal muscle also supports the idea of numerous levels of regulation involved in the degradation of IMTG, with control points downstream from HSL activation also playing important roles. Phosphorylation of HSL (activation), the first step, is essential for IMTG degradation. However, factors distal to this step are also important in fine-tuning the actual rate of IMTG degradation. HSL activation can be thought of as a gross level of regulation, setting the stage for downstream control by other factors. For example, actual flux (IMTG lipolysis) through HSL may be allosterically inhibited during prolonged exercise by the accumulation of long chain fatty acyl-CoA (LCFA-CoA) (Fig. 18.4). In addition, it has been proposed that the actual movement of HSL in the cytosol to the lipid droplet and phosphorylation of a phosphoprotein coat encapsulating the lipid droplet (perilipin, or adipose differentiation-related protein) are also necessary steps to permit the physical docking of HSL with the lipid droplet. However, these steps have not been studied in human skeletal muscle.

FFA Transport Across the Mitochondrial Membranes

The CPT complex, consisting of CPT I, acylcarnitine translocase, and CPT II, plays a regulatory role in the transport of long chain fatty acids into the mitochondria for β-oxidation in skeletal muscle (Fig. 18.5) (12).

CPT I, which appears to span the outer mitochondrial membrane, catalyses the transfer of a variety of long-chain fatty acyl groups from CoA to carnitine. The generated acylcarnitine can then permeate the inner membrane via

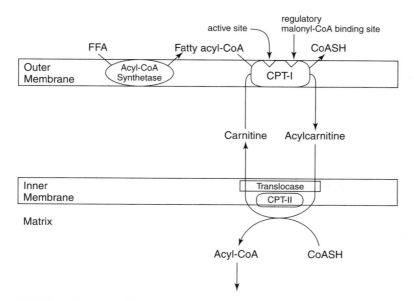

FIGURE 18.5 Proposed regulation of long-chain free fatty acid transport into the mitochondria. CPT I and II, carnitine palmitoyltransferase I and II. *(Reprinted with permission from Spriet LL. Regulation of skeletal muscle fat oxidation during exercise in humans. Med Sci Sports Exerc 2002;34:1477–1484.)*

the acylcarnitine/carnitine translocase. The fatty acyl-CoA is then reformed in the matrix of the mitochondria by CPT II. This enzyme on the inner mitochondrial membrane catalyses the transfer of the acyl group from carnitine to CoA, and the re-formed acyl-CoA enters the β-oxidation pathway.

Regulation of Mitochondrial FFA Transport by Malonyl-CoA

CPT I is considered the rate-limiting step in the oxidation of long-chain fatty acids, as it is regulated by external factors. It is reversibly inhibited by malonyl-CoA (M-CoA), the first committed intermediate in fatty acid synthesis (35,36). Thus, there has been considerable interest in the potential role of M-CoA in regulating mitochondrial FFA uptake and oxidation in skeletal muscle. Research in rodent skeletal muscle suggests that muscle M-CoA levels are highest at rest to inhibit CPT I activity and maintain low rates of mitochondrial fatty acid transport. During exercise, when increased mitochondrial FFA transport and oxidation are needed, M-CoA levels decrease and release the inhibition of CPT I (37).

Another line of research has proposed that fat metabolism is regulated by the level of glycolytic activity in the muscle (38). Increases in glycolytic flux rates, as the aerobic exercise intensity increases, correlate with decreasing rates of FFA oxidation. It was proposed that signals related to the increased glycolytic flux down-regulate FFA metabolism inside the muscle cell and that increases in [M-CoA] could be the regulator that inhibits mitochondrial FFA uptake and oxidation during heavy dynamic exercise.

However, recent studies have demonstrated that M-CoA levels in human skeletal muscle do not change during mild to moderate dynamic exercise of varying duration despite large increases in fatty acid oxidation rates (39). In addition, increasing the dynamic exercise intensity from 65 to 90% $\dot{V}O_{2max}$ was not associated with an increase in muscle [M-CoA] despite large decreases in FFA oxidation. Therefore, the conclusion at present appears to be that M-CoA is not involved in the up-regulation of mitochondrial FFA transport from rest to mild and moderate dynamic exercise and also not responsible for down-regulating mitochondrial FFA transport when dynamic exercise becomes heavy.

Other Mechanisms Regulating Mitochondrial FFA Transport?

These findings in human muscle suggest that the regulation of CPT I activity is more complex than control by only [M-CoA]. Research using isolated and intact subsarcolemmal and intermyofibrillar mitochondria from human skeletal muscle determined that CPT I is also inhibited by small, physiologically relevant decreases in pH (7.0 to 6.8) (35). This sensitivity to pH may also explain the decrease in mitochondrial FFA transport and metabolism that occurs during a move from moderate to heavy dynamic exercise.

However, other regulators of metabolism, including calcium, free ADP, and AMP, were without effect on CPT I activity. Other metabolites that accumulate (acetyl-CoA, acetyl carnitine) or decrease (CoA) during dynamic exercise were also without effect. Other factors, including substrate–enzyme interactions, structural changes in the binding of M-CoA to CPT I and/or the presence of other unknown regulators may be important for increased mitochondrial FFA transport during exercise.

One interesting recent development is the report of a CPT I isoform that is insensitive to M-CoA in rodent skeletal muscle (40). It may be that a control system independent of M-CoA accounts for the up-regulation of mitochondrial FFA transport and oxidation during exercise. A second very recent development is research demonstrating the presence of FAT/CD36 in the membrane of both subsarcolemmal and intermyofibrillar mitochondria of rodent and human skeletal muscle (41). The mitochondrial FAT/CD36 content increased in rodent muscle in response to acute muscle contractions, which suggests that it may translocate to the membrane as proposed at the plasma membrane. The FAT/CD36 content in the membrane also increased in response to chronic muscle contractions, and inhibition of the protein with an antibody decreased the oxidation of FFA. These findings suggest that FAT/CD36 is involved in the movement of FFA across the mitochondrial membranes. If confirmed, such a finding would not be surprising, as this appears to be a common theme in the handling of FFA.

It has also been proposed that the level of free carnitine may regulate mitochondrial FFA uptake during heavy dynamic exercise, as it is a substrate for the CPT I reaction (6). The carnitine content decreases as a function of increasing intensity of dynamic exercise and increased glycolytic flux. The decreasing free carnitine level may limit the ability to transport FFA into the mitochondria and ultimately limit FFA oxidation during dynamic exercise when glycolytic flux is high. However, no experimental model has been able to test whether this is a causal relationship. It is also not known how much free carnitine is needed in the cytoplasm to maintain the CPT I–mediated FFA transport into the mitochondria. However, the highest rates of FFA oxidation occur when the carnitine levels are already substantially lower than resting levels, and carnitine is not consumed in the transport process but recycled into the cytoplasm. These factors make it unlikely that free carnitine availability limits FFA oxidation.

β-Oxidation

The fatty acyl-carnitine that is moved into the matrix of the mitochondria is reconverted to fatty acyl-CoA via CPT II, and the released carnitine is free to move out of the mitochondria. The fatty acyl-CoA then passes through the β-oxidation pathway, where a series of four reactions remove two carbons to form one molecule of acetyl-CoA with the production of reducing equivalents (one NADH and one $FADH_2$) along the way (9). The NADH and $FADH_2$ are immediate substrates for the electron transport chain, where they ultimately produce about 3ATP/NADH and 2 ATP/$FADH_2$. The remaining fatty acyl-CoA, now two carbon atoms shorter, repeatedly passes through the pathway until totally degraded. Therefore, an 18-carbon fatty acyl-CoA (i.e., stearic acid) provides 9 acetyl-CoA, 8 NADH, and 8 $FADH_2$ in the β-oxidation pathway. Since each acetyl-CoA goes on to provide additional reducing equivalents (3 NADH, 1 $FADH_2$) and 1 guanosine triphosphate (GTP) in the tricarboxylic acid cycle, the energy density of each fatty acyl-CoA molecule becomes very clear.

There do not appear to be any external regulators of the enzymes in the β-oxidation pathway. This suggests that the acute rate of β-oxidation is regulated by the availability of pathway substrates (fatty acyl-CoA, water, NAD^+, FAD, and free CoA) and products (NADH, FADH2, and acetyl-CoA) (5). It is likely that the provision of fatty acyl-CoA, NAD^+ and FAD are the dominant regulators and the products are not, as NADH, FADH2, and acetyl-CoA are, quickly used in the electron transport chain and tricarboxylic acid cycle, respectively. In addition, acetyl-CoA, which is a product of the pathway, increases during exercise, and the flux in the β-oxidation pathway increases several fold. The implication of substrate control is that β-oxidation will proceed when fatty acyl-CoA is delivered to the mitochondrial matrix. It also moves the site of β-oxidation regulation and ultimately the regulation of fat oxidation upstream to the movement of fatty acyl-CoA across the mitochondrial membranes.

The other manner in which to regulate the β-oxidation pathway is chronically (days) to increase or decrease the content of the pathway enzymes, as occurs with dynamic exercise training and disuse or detraining, respectively. It is common to measure the maximal activity of the third enzyme in the pathway, β-hydroxyacyl-CoA dehydrogenase, to assess the adaptation to dynamic exercise training programs.

SUMMARY

Lipid is an important substrate for the aerobic production of energy in human skeletal muscle during mild and moderate dynamic exercise in most individuals and even heavy dynamic exercise in well-trained individuals. FFA released from adipose tissue and delivered to contracting muscles is a major source of substrate for the muscle during dynamic exercise. Fat is also stored inside the muscle as TG and can be degraded to FFA during exercise to provide substrate for oxidation. While CHO can provide all of the substrate required for dynamic exercise at about 100% $\dot{V}O_{2max}$ when no fat is available, fat can provide substrate only at a rate to sustain about 60 to 75% $\dot{V}O_{2max}$ when no CHO is available. However, fat is an energy-dense fuel with a high yield per unit mass and is stored in large quantities in the body. Therefore, fat can provide a substantial and increasing amount of energy during prolonged dynamic exercise at low to moderate intensities. Aerobic training also increases the maximal rate at which fat oxidation can produce energy in skeletal muscle, and it increases the proportion of energy produced from fat oxidation at any absolute power output. Also, fat metabolism is not activated as quickly as CHO metabolism at the onset of exercise, and it cannot be used to generate anaerobic energy during heavy exercise above 100% $\dot{V}O_{2max}$ (sprint exercise).

Unlike CHO metabolism, the regulation of fat metabolism in human skeletal muscle during exercise has not been well studied. Traditionally it was believed that the regulation of fat metabolism was mainly at the level of FFA provision to the muscle (adipose tissue lipolysis) and transport of long-chain fatty acids into the mitochondria (CPT I activity). It is now known that the regulation of fat metabolism is complex and that it involves additional sites of control, including the transport of FFA into the muscle cell, the binding and transport of FFA in the cytoplasm, and the regulation of muscle HSL activity within the cell.

A MILESTONE OF DISCOVERY

In the 1960s Havel and coworkers published a series of papers designed to examine the importance of plasma FFA as a substrate source for skeletal muscle at rest and during dynamic exercise. Their findings also had large implications for the importance of fat stored inside the muscle as a substrate for exercise. It was already quite clear that plasma FFA accounted for a significant portion of the oxidative metabolism both at rest and during mild to moderate dynamic exercise. This study took a more direct approach to assessing substrate use during leg exercise in four active men. The subjects reported to the laboratory following a 13- to 15-hour overnight fast, and catheters were placed in the brachial artery of one arm and the brachial vein of the other arm. A catheter was also placed in the femoral vein to sample the blood draining the contracting muscles of the leg. A constant infusion of ^{14}C-palmitate allowed for the estimation of FFA uptake, oxidation, and release from the leg region during dynamic exercise. Expired air was sampled to measure the content of $^{14}CO_2$ and for the estimation of pulmonary oxygen uptake. Arterial and femoral venous blood samples were analyzed for oxygen and carbon dioxide content using the classic Van Slyke method. Subjects then exercised for 90 to 120 minutes at low

(continued)

A MILESTONE OF DISCOVERY

dynamic intensities. The increase in oxygen uptake measured at the mouth from rest to exercise was assumed to originate entirely from the region drained by the femoral vein. Leg blood flow was then estimated using the Fick equation: leg blood flow equals increase in pulmonary oxygen uptake divided by arterial minus venous femoral oxygen.

The fraction of FFA extracted by the leg decreased during exercise, but the influx of FFA into the leg increased. A net uptake of FFA by the leg was constantly observed during dynamic exercise. The output of ^{14}C in the blood carbon dioxide almost equaled the FFA input from the plasma following 1 hour of exercise. The pulmonary RER was 0.81 + 0.03, and the leg RQ averaged 0.80 + 0.11 during the exercise, suggesting that fat provided about 60 to 65% of the total oxidized substrate. The authors suggested that the large standard deviation for leg RQ was a function of the dependence on four measurements. This underscored the problems that researchers still face today when making these same measurements. Plasma FFA accounted for about 50% and plasma TG less than 8% of the FFA oxidized during dynamic exercise. This provided strong evidence that other fat sources accounted for the remainder of the oxidized FFA. It

led the authors to suggest that "either local stores of triglyceride in fat cells which deliver fatty acids directly to muscle without traversing the general circulation, or lipids within muscle cells (i.e., IMTG) are utilized for oxidative metabolism of working skeletal muscle." Research in the intervening years has supported the latter contention, that IMTG is degraded and oxidized during mild and moderate dynamic exercise. This study presented the strongest data at the time to demonstrate that FFA derived from both outside and inside the muscle cell could be oxidized during dynamic exercise, as had been shown for CHO. It was also interesting to note that the subjects in this study fasted overnight and began exercise with high resting FFA concentrations of about 0.6 mM, which would bias metabolism toward using more fat and less CHO. Therefore, the results must be examined in this light, and as a result, controversy continues as to whether subjects for metabolic research should be studied in a fed or fasted state.

Havel RJ, Pernow B, Jones NL. Uptake and release of free fatty acids and other metabolites in the legs of exercising men. J Appl Physiol 1967;23:90–99.

REFERENCES

1. Asmussen E. Muscle metabolism during exercise in man. A historical survey. In Pernow B, Saltin B, eds. Muscle Metabolism During Exercise. New York: Plenum, 1971;1–11.
2. Froberg SO, Mossfeldt F. Effect of prolonged strenuous exercise on the concentration of triglycerides, phospholipids and glycogen in muscle of man. Acta Scand Physiol 1971;82: 167–171.
3. Havel RJ, Pernow B, Jones NL. Uptake and release of free fatty acids and other metabolites in the legs of exercising men. J Appl Physiol 1967;23:90–99.
4. Romijn JA, Coyle EF, Sidossis LS, et al. Regulation of endogenous fat and carbohydrate metabolism in relation to exercise intensity and duration. Am J Physiol 1993;265:E380–E391.
5. Schulz H. Beta-oxidation of fatty acids. Biochim Biophys Acta 1991;1081:109–120.
6. VanLoon LJ, Greenhaff PL, Constantin-Teodosiu D, et al. The effects of increasing exercise intensity on muscle fuel utilization in humans. J Physiol (Lond) 2001;536:295–304.
7. Kiens B, Essen-Gustavsson B, Christensen NJ, et al. Skeletal muscle substrate utilization during submaximal exercise in man: effect of endurance training. J Physiol (Lond) 1993; 469:459–478.
8. Mackie BG, Dudley GA, Kaciuba-Uscilko H, et al. Uptake of chylomicron triglycerides by contracting skeletal muscle of rats. J Appl Physiol 1980;49:851–855.
9. VanderVusse GJ, Reneman RS. Lipid metabolism in muscle. In Rowell LB, Shepherd JT, eds. Handbook of Physiology, Section 12. Exercise: Regulation and Integration of Multiple Systems. New York: Oxford University, 1996;952–994.
10. Bonen A, Luiken JJ, Glatz JF. Regulation of fatty acid transport and membrane transporters in health and disease. Mol Cell Biochem 2002;239:181–192.
11. Watt MJ, Heigenhauser GJF, Spriet LL. Intramuscular triacylglycerol utilization in human skeletal muscle during exercise: Is there a controversy? J Appl Physiol 2002;93:1185–1195.
12. McGarry JD, Brown NF. The mitochondrial carnitine palmitoyltransferase system: from concept to molecular analysis. Eur J Biochem 1997;224:1–14.
13. Guo Z, Burguera B, Jensen MD. Kinetics of intramuscular triglyceride fatty acids in exercising humans. J Appl Physiol 2000;89:2057–2064.
14. Hodgetts V, Coppack SW, Frayn KN, et al. Factors controlling fat mobilization from human subcutaneous adipose tissue during exercise. J Appl Physiol 1991;71:445–451.
15. Holm C, Osterlund T, Laurell H, et al. Molecular mechanisms regulating hormone-sensitive lipase and lipolysis. Ann Rev Nutr 2000;20:365–393.
16. Mottagui-Tabar S, Ryden M, Lofgren P, et al. Evidence for an important role of perilipin in the regulation of human adipocyte lipolysis. Diabetologia 2003;46:789–797.
17. Carey G. Mechanisms regulating adipocyte lipolysis. In Richter EA et al., eds. Skeletal Muscle Metabolism in Exercise and Diabetes. New York: Plenum, 1998;157–170.
18. Romijn JA, Coyle EF, Sidossis LS, et al. Relationship between fatty acid delivery and fatty acid oxidation during strenuous exercise. J Appl Physiol 1995;79:1939–1945.
19. Turcotte LP. Muscle fatty acid uptake during exercise: Possible mechanisms. Exer Sport Sci Rev 2000;28:4–9.
20. Bonen A, Luiken JJFP, Liu S, et al. Palmitate transport and fatty acid transporters in red and white muscles. Am J Physiol 1998;275:E471–E478.

21. Turcotte L, Kiens B, Richter EA. Saturation kinetics of palmitate uptake in perfused skeletal muscle. FEBS Lett 1991;279: 327–329.

22. Turcotte L, Richter EA, Kiens B. Increased plasma FFA uptake and oxidation during prolonged exercise in trained vs. untrained humans. Am J Physiol 1992;262:E791–E799.

23. Bonen A, Dyck DJ, Ibrahimi A, et al. Muscle contractile activity increases fatty acid metabolism and transport and FAT/CD36. Am J Physiol 1999;276:E642–E649.

24. Kiens B, Kristainsen S, Jensen P, et al. Membrane associated fatty acid binding protein (FABPpm) in human skeletal muscle is increased by endurance training. Biochem Biophys Res Comm 1997;231:463–465.

25. Bonen A, Luiken JJFP, Arumugam Y, et al. Acute regulation of fatty acid uptake involves the cellular redistribution of fatty acid translocase. J Biol Chem 2000;275:14501–14508.

26. Winder WW. Energy-sensing and signaling by AMP-activated protein kinase in skeletal muscle. J Appl Physiol 2001;91: 1017–1028.

27. Glatz JFC, Schapp FG, Binas B, et al. Cytoplasmic fatty acid-binding protein facilitates fatty acid utilization by skeletal muscle. Acta Physiol Scand 2003;178:367–372.

28. Szczepaniak LS, Babcock EE, Schick F, et al. Measurement of intracellular triglyceride stores by 1H spectroscopy: validation in vivo. Am J Physiol 1999;276:E977–E989.

29. Wendling PS, Peters SJ, Heigenhauser GJF, et al. Variability of triacylglycerol content in human skeletal muscle biopsy samples. J Appl Physiol 1996;81:1150–1155.

30. Watt MJ, Heigenhauser GJF, Dyck DJ, et al. Intramuscular triacylglycerol, glycogen and acetyl group metabolism during 4 hours of moderate exercise. J Physiol (Lond) 2002;541: 969–978.

31. Decombaz J. Nutrition and recovery of muscle energy stores after exercise. Sportmedizin Sporttraumatologie 2003;51: 31–38.

32. Langfort J, Ploug T, Ihlemann J, et al. Expression of hormone-sensitive lipase and its regulation by adrenaline in skeletal muscle. Biochem J 1999;340:459–465.

33. Langfort J, Ploug T, Ihlemann J, et al. Stimulation of hormone-sensitive lipase by contractions in rat skeletal muscle. Biochem J 2000;351:207–214.

34. Watt MJ, Heigenhauser GJF, Spriet LL. Effects of dynamic exercise intensity on the activation of hormone-sensitive lipase in human skeletal muscle. J Physiol (Lond) 2003;547: 301–308.

35. Bezaire V, Heigenhauser GJF, Spriet LL. Regulation of CPT I activity in intermyofibrillar and subsarcolemmal mitochondria from human and rat skeletal muscle. Am J Physiol 2004; 286:E85–E91.

36. McGarry JD, Mills SE, Long CS, et al. Observations on the affinity for carnitine, and M-CoA sensitivity, of carnitine palmitoyltransferase I in animal and human tissues: demonstration of the presence of malonyl-CoA in nonhepatic tissues of the rat. Biochem J 1983;214:21–28.

37. Winder WW, Arogyasami J, Barton RJ, et al. Muscle malonyl-CoA decreases during exercise. J Appl Physiol 1989;67: 2230–2233.

38. Coyle EF, Jeukendrup AE, Wagenmakers AJM, et al. Fatty acid oxidation is directly regulated by carbohydrate metabolism during exercise. Am J Physiol 1997;273:E268–E275.

39. Odland LM, Howlett RA, Heigenhauser GJF, et al. Skeletal muscle malonyl-CoA content at the onset of exercise at varying power outputs in humans. Am J Physiol 1998;274: E1080–1085.

40. Kim JY, Koves TR, Yu GS, et al. Evidence of a malonyl-CoA-insensitive carnitine palmitoyltransferase I activity in red skeletal muscle. Am J Physiol 2002;282:E1014–E1022.

41. Campbell SE, Tandon NM, Woldegiorgis G, et al. A novel function for fatty acid translocase (fat)/CD36: involvement in long chain fatty acid transfer into the mitochondria. J Biol Chem 2004;279:36235–36241.

CHAPTER 19

The Metabolic Systems: Interaction of Lipid and Carbohydrate Metabolism

Lawrence L. Spriet and Mark Hargreaves

Introduction

The previous chapters have outlined the regulation of lipid and carbohydrate (CHO) metabolism and established that both fuels are important substrates for oxidative phosphorylation. Of course, the oxidation of any one fuel at rest or during exercise rarely occurs in isolation. Skeletal muscle, like other systems in the body, is an integrative organ, and many aspects of metabolism are simultaneously active at any time. It has long been known that both CHO and lipid are oxidized at rest to provide the energy required for basal metabolic processes in skeletal muscle. It is also known that there is a reciprocal relationship between the oxidation of CHO and lipid such that the availability of CHO and fat can influence the proportions of fuels that are oxidized. At rest, these shifts in fuel use are typically in the face of a low and largely unchanged metabolic demand. For example, increasing the availability of CHO in the blood increases the uptake and oxidation of CHO and decreases the availability and oxidation of fat in skeletal muscle, with little change in metabolic demand.

During the onset of exercise the situation is quite different, as the need for energy increases several fold and the metabolic pathways that oxidize both fat and CHO must be activated simultaneously. However, once aerobic exercise of a given intensity and metabolic demand has been established, there is some room for reciprocal shifts in the proportion of CHO and lipid oxidized. This is largely dependent on the rate at which energy is needed and the availability of fuels. Given the demands of exercise, how is skeletal muscle able to regulate the proportion of fuel that is provided from the two main fuel sources? In other words, how does the muscle communicate information between the pathways

such that a given amount of energy is provided from each of the fuel sources? This chapter attempts to answer these questions. The focus is on information obtained in human skeletal muscle, but findings from other mammalian models are cited where human information is lacking. While descriptive studies documenting changes in the proportion of fat and CHO utilization are numerous, the mechanisms regulating these shifts in fuel use have not been thoroughly elucidated.

Exercise and Substrate Selection

Many factors can influence the proportions of fat and CHO use during exercise. They may be loosely categorized as dietary interventions, exercise intensity, exercise duration, intermittent bouts of exercise, aerobic training, and pharmacological interventions. Classic experiments have established the importance of dietary intake on substrate availability and ultimately substrate selection. The intake of CHO in the days and hours before exercise, during exercise, and post exercise can influence exercise fuel selection. The ingestion of fat in the days and hours before exercise and during exercise has less of an influence on substrate selection. However, as is the case with CHO, recent evidence suggests that adequate fat consumption following exercise is critical for replenishment of the intramuscular triacylglycerol (IMTG) store. It has also been demonstrated that artificially increasing availability of plasma free fatty acid (FFA) can increase the oxidation of fat and decrease CHO oxidation, and increasing availability of CHO can do the opposite.

The classic experiments of Christensen and Hansen established that independent of dietary manipulations, the reliance on CHO increased as the exercise intensity increased (1). This is interpreted as a positive shift in fuel selection, as the rate of energy provision from the oxidation of CHO is faster than from fat and the amount of energy provided per liter of oxygen consumed is about 10% greater than fat. However, this situation reverses during prolonged moderate or intense exercise, when the availability of CHO wanes. The availability of muscle glycogen is finite and can be exhausted following 1–2 hours of moderate to intense exercise. The muscle glycogen content before exercise has also been correlated with exercise performance (2). The liver glycogen store is also limited and may be depleted during prolonged exercise. While liver can make new glucose, the rate of gluconeogenesis does not match the demand for hepatic glucose output during exercise (3). At the same time, an increase in the provision of fat from adipose tissue triacylglycerol and IMTG may also down-regulate CHO oxidation. Therefore, this shift toward fat and away from CHO during prolonged exercise may spare CHO. This is advantageous, assuming that the ultimate goal of prolonged exercise is to slow the use of CHO and delay the depletion of the muscle and liver glycogen stores to maintain performance.

A key adaptation in skeletal muscle following repeated bouts of exercise over days and months is the increase in mitochondrial volume and the accompanying increase in the capacity for fat oxidation (see Chapter 20). This is another example of a shift in fuel use in which the increased fat oxidation in effect spares the use of CHO. Following aerobic training, fat oxidation represents a greater proportion of the required energy at any given absolute exercise intensity. The maximal rate of energy provision from fat also increases, as does the maximal rate of CHO-derived energy production. These higher rates of fat and CHO-derived energy production translate into the attainment of higher power outputs and increased endurance at a given aerobic power output.

The ingestion of pharmacological agents has also been used to either promote or decrease the use of fat during exercise and to probe the mechanisms regulating this shift in fuel utilization. Caffeine has been commonly used in an attempt to increase fat mobilization and oxidation, but the response to this procedure has been variable between subjects, limiting what can be concluded on a group basis. When effective, caffeine appears to antagonize the normal inhibitory effects of adenosine on adipose tissue lipolysis at rest, resulting in measurable increases in plasma FFA concentrations and subsequent increases in FFA delivery to and oxidation by the working muscles during exercise. Nicotinic acid has also been administered to decrease the availability of plasma FFA, as binding with receptors on adipose tissue leads to powerful and rapid inhibition of lipolysis. Again, the response to this drug varies. Some subjects respond with large decreases in fat oxidation and increases in CHO oxidation during exercise, and others are seemingly able to replace the "missing" fat

from adipose tissue with fat from the IMTG store, resulting in no shift in the proportional use of fat and CHO.

Classic Carbohydrate–Fatty Acid Interaction Studies

The pioneering work by Randle and associates in the early 1960s introduced the concept of a reciprocal relationship between fat and CHO oxidation in muscle (4,5). They termed this relationship the glucose–fatty acid cycle (G-FA) and used it to explain the interaction between CHO and lipid metabolism in disease states (Milestone of Discovery). Their early experiments examined the regulation of fuel interaction in muscle using perfused contracting heart muscle and incubated resting diaphragm muscle from rodents (Fig. 19.1). Increasing the FFA availability to the muscles increased fat oxidation and reduced CHO oxidation. It also increased the muscle acetyl-coenzyme A (CoA), citrate and, glucose 6-phosphate (G-6-P) contents. Previous work *in vitro* established that acetyl-CoA inhibited the activity of the mitochondrial enzyme pyruvate dehydrogenase (PDH) by activating PDH kinase, the enzyme that phosphorylates PDH to its less active form. Additional work *in vitro* identified citrate as a potent inhibitor of the cytoplasmic enzyme phosphofructokinase (PFK), predicting an *in vivo* effect. This assumed that the FFA-induced increase in mitochondrial citrate escaped to the cytoplasm. Lastly, G-6-P had also been shown to inhibit hexokinase (HK) *in vitro*. By combining the findings from their isolated muscle experiments with the enzyme studies *in vitro*, Randle and associates (4,5) established the mechanistic basis for their G-FA cycle, which explained the reciprocal relationship between fat and CHO oxidation. Increased availability of FFA increased muscle acetyl-CoA and citrate, leading to down-regulation of PDH and PFK activities. The reduced flux through the glycolytic pathway caused an accumulation of G-6-P, which inhibited HK activity and ultimately decreased the uptake of glucose, presumably by increasing the free glucose concentration, hence leading to a decreased transsarcolemmal glucose gradient.

As mentioned earlier, most of the early support for the G-FA cycle was obtained from rodent contracting heart or resting diaphragm muscle bathed in or perfused with a medium either low or high in FFA. Heart and diaphragm muscles have regular contraction duty cycles, which ultimately dictates that most oxidizable substrate must be delivered from outside the cell. Conversely, in most skeletal muscles other than diaphragm, especially in human skeletal muscle, the higher energy demands of moderate and high-intensity aerobic exercise dictate that most oxidizable fuel originates from fuel stores inside the cells, most notably the glycogen store.

Hickson and associates (6) and Rennie and Holloszy (7) advanced this work to examine the existence and regulation

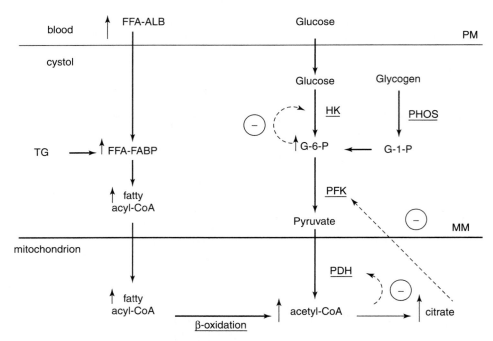

FIGURE 19.1 The glucose-fatty acid cycle in muscle. Increasing availability of plasma free fatty acid (FFA) increases fat oxidation and elevates mitochondrial contents of acetyl-CoA and citrate, which feed back to inhibit pyruvate dehydrogenase (PDH) and phosphofructokinase (PFK) activities (-). Decreased glycolytic activity then leads to increased glucose 6-phosphate content and inhibition of hexokinase (HK) activity (-), decreased glucose phosphorylation, and ultimately decreased glucose uptake. ALB, albumin; FABP, fatty acid binding protein; PHOS, glycogen phosphorylase; G-1-P, glucose 1-phosphate; PM, plasma membrane; MM, mitochondrial membranes.

of the G-FA cycle in skeletal muscle of exercising rats and isolated perfused rat hindlimbs. Animals were fed corn oil followed by infusions of heparin to increase [FFA] before exercise to about 1 mM versus 0.2 mM in the control group (6). Fat-fed rats ran longer, used less glycogen in the soleus (SOL), red vastus lateralis (RVL), and red gastrocnemius (RG) muscles and in the liver. They also had a smaller decrease in blood glucose during exercise than the control animals. In all cases, citrate contents were elevated during exercise in the muscles exposed to high fat. Rennie and Holloszy (7) perfused rat hindlimbs with a mixture of rejuvenated human red blood cells and a Krebs-Henseleit solution containing either 1.8 mM oleate or no fat. Hindlimb glucose uptake and lactate release were decreased with high fat perfusion during 10 minutes of electrical stimulation of the hindlimb muscles. Muscle glycogen utilization was reduced by 33 to 50% and lactate accumulation by 50% in the SOL and RG muscles perfused with high fat. The reduction in muscle CHO use coincided with elevations in G-6-P and citrate contents in SOL and RG muscles. These results suggested that the G-FA cycle did operate in contracting red skeletal muscle and that the citrate arm of the cycle functioned as originally proposed for contracting heart and resting diaphragm muscles.

However, a number of other perfusion studies could not demonstrate the existence of the G-FA cycle in contracting red skeletal muscle. For example, Richter and associates (8) re-

ported no effect of perfusion with 1.6 mM palmitate on hindlimb glucose uptake or muscle glycogen breakdown and citrate content in the SOL, RG and white gastrocnemius muscles during 20 minutes of stimulation. A more recent attempt employed a series of stimulation intensities (0.4–4 Hz) that produced a wide range of hindlimb oxygen uptakes and glycogenolytic rates in the SOL, RG, and plantaris (PL) muscles (9). The results for the RG muscle demonstrated that high fat (1.5–1.9 mM FFA) perfusions did not produce glycogen sparing across most stimulation frequencies. Muscle glycogen use with high fat was significantly reduced only at a stimulation frequency of 0.7 Hz. In the SOL, high fat perfusion had no effect on glycogen use at any stimulation intensity, and in the PL, a significant reduction was found only at 1 Hz.

Interestingly, similar work in human skeletal muscle has produced more consistent results demonstrating a clear reciprocal relationship between CHO and fat oxidation during exercise.

Increased Lipid Availability and Exercise

Dietary attempts at increasing the availability of circulating or endogenous fat to the working muscles in humans immediately prior to exercise or during exercise have been largely unsuccessful. Because fat is not digested quickly and substantial alterations in the normal diet are needed to alter the IMTG store, these practices are not in use by athletes. Most of what we know regarding the ability of fat to down-regulate CHO metabolism has been derived from studies that use experimental manipulations to acutely increase or decrease availability of plasma FFA without affecting many other processes. While many models, including high-fat meals and diets, short- and long-term aerobic training, caffeine ingestion, fasting, and prolonged aerobic exercise, have been used with varying success, the acute infusion of a triacylglycerol solution coupled with periodic heparin administration has been most commonly and effectively used. This technique has the advantage of acutely (about 30 min) increasing the plasma [FFA] without significant alterations in other fuels, metabolites, and hormones (10–12) (Fig. 19.2).

It would be expected that any fat-induced down-regulation of CHO oxidation would target the key sites (transport, enzymatic reactions) regulating CHO metabolism and oxidation. In the muscle, these include glucose uptake and the glucose transporters (GLUT1, GLUT4), glucose phosphorylation (HK), glycogenolysis (glycogen phosphorylase [PHOS]), glycolysis (PFK), and conversion to acetyl-CoA (PDH).

Effects of Increased Exogenous FFA on Carbohydrate Metabolism

The experiments examining the interaction between fat and CHO in human skeletal muscle suggest that it is possible to alter the proportions of fat and CHO oxidation during exercise, but the mechanisms controlling these shifts are largely

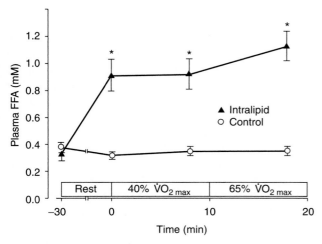

FIGURE 19.2 Plasma FFA during 10 min of cycling at 40% and 10 min at 65% $\dot{V}O_{2max}$ with intralipid (and heparin) infusion or control. Values are means ± SE. *, significant main effect between trials. (Data reprinted with permission from Odland LM, Heigenhauser GJF, Wong D, et al. Effects of increased fat availability on fat-carbohydrate interaction during prolonged exercise in men. Am J Physiol 1998;275:R894–R902.)

different from those originally proposed in the G-FA cycle. The original work by Randle and associates (4,5) did not involve the regulation of muscle glycogen degradation, as contracting heart is less reliant on this fuel than skeletal muscle.

During exercise at about 80% $\dot{V}O_{2max}$, increased FFA availability decreased net glycogen use by about 50% in the initial 15 minutes of exercise and increased fat oxidation by about 15% during 30 minutes of exercise (12,13). The muscle contents of free adenosine monophosphate (ADP) and adenosine monophosphate (AMP), important activators of glycogen PHOS, were significantly reduced in the high-FFA condition, and this appeared to explain the decreased glycogen use. There were no effects on muscle citrate, acetyl-CoA, or G-6-P content or the proportion of PDH in the active form (PDHa) (10,13). To date, no one has examined the effects of elevated [FFA] on glucose uptake at this intensity. Therefore, at this intense aerobic power output, the fat-induced down-regulation of CHO oxidation was regulated at the level of glycogen PHOS (Fig. 19.3).

When the same experiments were repeated at lower exercise power outputs (about 40% and 65% $\dot{V}O_{2max}$), high fat provision appeared to down-regulate CHO oxidation at more sites. Based on respiratory exchange ratio (RER) measurements, fat oxidation increased and CHO oxidation decreased at both power outputs (14). Muscle glycogen use was reduced with high FFA provision, but to a smaller extent than at the higher power output, and muscle glucose uptake was unaffected during whole-body cycle exercise. However, another study reported no effect of high FFA provision on muscle glycogen use but found a reduced glucose uptake during knee extension exercise (11). Muscle measurements revealed no effect of high fat on acetyl-CoA and G-6-P contents but a small increase in citrate and a lower PDHa (15) (Fig. 19.3). These experiments suggested that fat-induced down-regulation of CHO metabolism occurs at multiple sites during moderate aerobic exercise, including PHOS, PFK, and PDH (Fig. 19.3). However, test tube work examining the inhibitory effects of citrate on PFK activity suggested that the small increase in citrate in the high-fat trials would have minimal effect in contracting human skeletal muscle (16).

Recent work taking the opposite approach decreased the availability of plasma FFA during exercise at about 60% $\dot{V}O_{2max}$ by ingestion of nicotinic acid and reported increased RER, glycogen use, and PDHa (17). However, there were no effects on muscle citrate, acetyl-CoA, or pyruvate content.

These experiments measured the decreases in PHOS and PDH activities in the presence of more circulating fat or the opposite effects when FFA availability was reduced, but what are the signals that cause these changes in the muscle?

Mitochondrial NADH Regulates Fuel Preference During Exercise

An interesting finding of the studies that increased exogenous FFA availability was that the fall in the energy charge

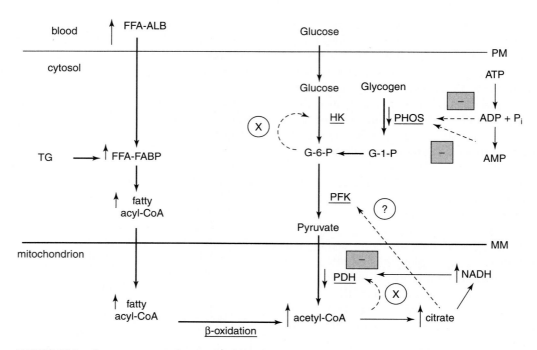

FIGURE 19.3 Contemporary and summary view of reciprocal relationship between carbohydrate and fat oxidation during exercise at power outputs of 40%, 65%, and ~80% $\dot{V}O_{2max}$. Increasing the availability of plasma free fatty acids (FFA) has no effect on acetyl-CoA and glucose-6-phosphate (G-6-P) contents (X) at any power outputs and increased citrate content only at 40 and 65% $\dot{V}O_{2max}$. Reduced FFA availability did reduce PDH activity at 40 and 65% $\dot{V}O_{2max}$ and the flux through glycogen phosphorylase (PHOS) at all power outputs. The effect of PHOS flux was dominant at ~80% $\dot{V}O_{2max}$ and less important at 40 and 65% $\dot{V}O_{2max}$ (see text). The accumulation of free ADP, AMP, and inorganic phosphate (P$_i$) was reduced during exercise (–) in the presence of increased FFA availability. One theory suggests that mitochondrial NADH is more abundant with high fat provision during the onset of exercise, increasing the aerobic production of ATP and reducing the mismatch between ATP demand and supply and accounting for the reduced accumulation of ADP, AMP, and P$_i$. PFK, phosphofructokinase; FABP, fatty acid binding protein; ALB, albumin; G-1-P, glucose-1-phosphate; HK, hexokinase.

of the muscle that normally occurs during exercise was reduced. This was assessed by measuring muscle phosphocreatine, creatine, adenosine triphosphate (ATP) and lactate (to predict [hydrogen ion]) and calculating muscle free ADP, AMP, and inorganic phosphate (P$_i$) content. As P$_i$ is a substrate for PHOS and ADP and AMP are direct allosteric regulators of the active form of PHOS, the noted reductions in these regulators could account for the decreased glycogenolysis with high fat provision (10). Less free ADP accumulation would also make it more difficult for PDH to convert to the active form during exercise at 40 and 65% $\dot{V}O_{2max}$, as a high ATP/ADP ratio activates PDH kinase (PDK) activity and decreases PDHa (Figs. 19.3). However, a key question is what accounts for a more favorable energy charge during exercise with increased fat availability. It has been proposed that increased fat availability in the minutes prior to exercise and early in exercise increases fat oxidation, resulting in an increased provision of reduced nicotinamide adenine dinucleotide (NADH) from fat and a higher NADH concentration in the mitochondria (15). The major

inputs for aerobic ATP production in the mitochondria are ADP and P$_i$, oxygen, and NADH (reducing equivalents). It has been suggested that an increase in NADH at a given energy demand (power output) may allow for the blunted accumulation of free ADP and P$_i$ during exercise while maintaining a constant drive for mitochondrial respiration (18).

Unfortunately, this hypothesis has been difficult to test, as mitochondrial NADH is not easy to measure in intact human skeletal muscle, and much controversy surrounds the various techniques that have been employed. When NADH was estimated using the whole-muscle homogenate technique, it was elevated at rest and at 1 minute of exercise at 40% $\dot{V}O_{2max}$ when extra fat was provided (15). However, following 10 min at 40% $\dot{V}O_{2max}$ and again after 10 min at 65% $\dot{V}O_{2max}$, NADH was no longer higher than the control condition. When the opposite approach was taken and FFA provision was reduced by nicotinic acid administration, CHO use and muscle PDHa were increased and fat use was decreased. However, the decreased FFA

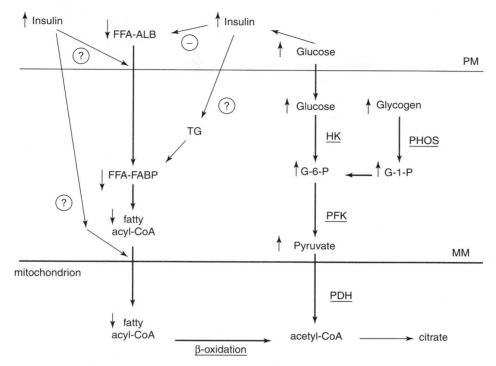

FIGURE 19.4 Schematic representation of potential effects of carbohydrate ingestion before dynamic exercise in decreasing plasma free fatty acid (FFA) concentration and down regulating fat metabolism in skeletal muscle. Ingested glucose increases the release of insulin, which inhibits adipose tissue lipolysis and reduces the plasma [FFA]. Increased insulin may also inhibit FFA transport across the plasma (PM) and mitochondrial (MM) membranes and decrease triacylglycerol (TG) breakdown in the muscle. Carbohydrate oxidation, possibly from plasma glucose and/or muscle glycogen, is increased. ALB, albumin; FABP, fatty acid binding protein; HK, hexokinase; G-6-P and G-1-P, glucose 6- and 1-phosphate; PFK, phosphofructokinase; PDH, pyruvate dehydrogenase.

availability (expected decrease in NADH) did not exacerbate the fall in the muscle energy status (free ADP and AMP) during exercise (17). Therefore, while the mitochondrial NADH theory for explaining the reciprocal control of fuel use when fat availability is increased or decreased during exercise is attractive, there are many unexplained findings, and a more thorough testing of this theory awaits improved techniques for measuring mitochondrial NADH content.

Increased FFA Availability During Prolonged Exercise

When exercise of moderate intensity is prolonged beyond 1–2 hours, the availability of plasma FFA increases to high levels and the availability of muscle glycogen decreases (19). Not surprisingly, fat oxidation rises and CHO oxidation falls. This scenario provides another opportunity to study the reciprocal control of fat and CHO oxidation during exercise. PDHa decreases during prolonged exercise, in keeping with the decreased reliance on CHO, but surprisingly, no changes in the energy status of the cell or de-

creases in pyruvate content accompanied the decrease in PDHa and glycogenolysis (19). It is possible that a reduction in the availability of substrate was responsible for the decreased PHOS and PDHa activities, as the glycogen content was low and the production of pyruvate was decreased, even though it did not translate into a decreased content in the muscle. However, an alternative possibility to explain the decreased PDHa involves the rapid up-regulation of PDK activity.

High Fat Availability Up-Regulates PDK Activity and Decreases PDHa

Situations that chronically decrease CHO availability and increase the reliance of skeletal muscle on fat produce increases in the mRNA and protein contents of the PDK-4 isoform and the activity of PDK (20). This ultimately leads to a decreased fraction of PDH in the active form at rest and decreased whole-body CHO oxidation. While these changes occurred over hours and days, the question arose whether more rapid fat-induced up-regulation of PDK activity could occur during prolonged exercise and explain the down-regulation of PDH that occurred during 4 h of moderate exercise. Recent work examined this question and demonstrated that PDK activity was increased after 4 h of moderate exercise, but without increases in PDK-2 and PDK-4 protein contents (21). This suggested that incorporation of existing PDK protein loosely associated with the PDH complex was incorporated into the complex to increase the intrinsic PDK activity. In summary, the increased PDK activity appeared to contribute to the down-regulation of PDH during prolonged exercise. It is not clear what regulates these changes, although activation of signals secondary to the increasing FFA concentrations and/or diminishing CHO (glycogen store and insulin concentration) supply may be involved.

Increased Availability of Intramuscular Fat

The most common method to alter availability of IMTG is via dietary manipulation. IMTG can be increased by 50 to 80% following the consumption of a high-fat diet (22,23), that is, when fat supplies 50 to 70% of the total energy intake. IMTG can also be decreased when dietary fat intake is reduced from 22% to 2% of caloric intake (24). It is possible that the IMTG content in muscle exerts an inhibitory effect on CHO metabolism during exercise. Muscle glycogen use and CHO oxidation rates were reduced during moderate exercise following a long-term high-fat diet, although muscle glucose uptake was similar (25). On the other hand, whole-body CHO oxidation and muscle glycogen utilization were lower, and whole-body glucose uptake was unchanged with reduced dietary fat intake (24). These data suggest that IMTG has no effect on muscle glucose uptake during exercise but does influence muscle glycogen utilization. However, this conclusion is confounded by the reciprocal changes in muscle glycogen availability that occur as a consequence of these perturbations, which likely also contributed to the altered patterns of fat utilization. Clearly, to elucidate the possible interaction between the IMTG store and CHO fuel metabolism, studies must employ interventions that induce acute changes in IMTG independent of alterations in the availability of other substrates (e.g., muscle glycogen, plasma FFA). Burke and associates (26) moved in this direction and demonstrated that the effects of a high-fat diet on reducing glycogen use during exercise persisted even when CHO availability was returned to normal for 1 day to restore muscle glycogen stores. When CHO was also given both prior to and during exercise, the CHO-sparing effects of the high-fat diet were still present. The subjects in this study and others by the same authors were well trained and continued to exercise while ingesting the high-fat, low-CHO diets. The mechanisms responsible for these persistent effects of the high fat diet are not known.

Increased Carbohydrate Availability and Exercise

Several studies have demonstrated that increasing the availability of exogenous CHO before and during exercise and the availability of endogenous CHO (glycolytic flux) during exercise increases CHO and decreases fat oxidation (27–29). However, less work has been done to examine the mechanisms underlying these shifts in fuel selection.

Increased Availability of Exogenous Glucose

CHO ingestion before exercise reduces fat oxidation during a subsequent bout of mild to moderate exercise, and accumulating evidence supports a direct inhibitory role of increased exogenous glucose availability on fat utilization during exercise. The reduction in fat metabolism following glucose ingestion appears to be due to the combined effects of decreased FFA availability secondary to decreased adipose lipolysis and to direct effects on fatty acid oxidation in the muscle.

Researchers have measured the effects of CHO ingestion on adipose tissue lipolysis during mild to moderate exercise (27,28). During exercise in the fasted state adipose tissue lipolysis exceeded skeletal muscle fat oxidation, whereas CHO ingestion resulted in elevated plasma insulin, reduced adipose tissue lipolysis, and decreased fat oxidation. CHO ingestion before exercise also increased glycolytic flux and CHO oxidation and reduced oxidation of both plasma-derived FFA and IMTG (Table 19.1). The magnitude of the decreased fat oxidation equaled the reduction in lipolysis, suggesting a limitation of FFA availability for fat oxidation. However, when plasma FFA availability was restored by intravenous triacylglycerol and heparin infusion, FFA oxidation was increased but not fully restored (12). This suggested that CHO ingestion also exerted an inhibitory effect on fat oxidation directly in the muscle. In addition, increasing the exercise intensity from 40 to 80% $\dot{V}_{O_{2max}}$ reduced long-chain FFA uptake and oxidation (dependent on membrane transport) but not medium-chain fatty acid octanoate oxidation (independent of membrane transport) (30). This suggested an inhibitory effect of CHO oxidation on the transport of FFA across the muscle membrane and/or the mitochondrial membranes and ultimately the oxidation of fat.

Increased Endogenous Glucose Availability

Increasing exercise power output increases the availability of endogenous CHO (glycogen breakdown) and results in decreased fat oxidation. Fat oxidation increases from rest during mild to moderate exercise (40–65% $\dot{V}_{O_{2max}}$) but decreases at power outputs above about 75% $\dot{V}_{O_{2max}}$ (31). Blood glucose levels, muscle glycogenolysis, glycolytic

TABLE 19.1	Effect of Glucose Ingestion (Glc) Compared to Fasting (Fast) on Various Aspects of Fat Metabolism During Exercise					
		umol/kg/min				
Trial	Time, min	Total fat oxidation	Ra FFA	Rd FFA	Plasma FFA oxidation	FA oxidation from intramuscular TG
Fast-palmitate	20–30	30.9 ± 2.1	12.2 ± 1.0	12.0 ± 1.0	10.5 ± 0.8	20.4 ± 2.1
	30–40	32.1 ± 1.6	12.8 ± 1.0	12.7 ± 1.0	10.9 ± 0.8	21.2 ± 1.9
Glc-palmitate	20–30	19.7 ± 1.5*	8.3 ± 0.8*	8.2 ± 0.8*	5.7 ± 0.4*	14.0 ± 1.8*
	30–40	21.1 ± 1.6*	8.2 ± 0.6*	8.1 ± 0.5*	5.7 ± 0.4*	15.4 ± 1.8*

Values are means + SE for 6 subjects. [1-^{13}C]palmitate was intravenously infused during both trials. R_a and R_d are rates of appearance and disappearance of free fatty acids (FFA), respectively. Plasma FFA oxidation is calculated as the product of R_d FFA and % of infused palmitate tracer oxidized. Fatty acid oxidation from intramuscular triglyceride (TG) is calculated as the difference between total fat oxidation and plasma FFA oxidation. *, Glc-palmitate trial significantly lower than Fast-palmitate trial at that time, $P < 0.05$. Table has been redrawn from reference 27 with permission from the American Physiology Society.

flux, PDH activation, and CHO oxidation are increased during exercise at high than at moderate exercise power outputs (32,33). The same results occur when epinephrine is infused to high physiological levels to stimulate muscle glycogenolysis (34).

Potential Mechanisms for Carbohydrate-Induced Down-Regulation of Fat Oxidation

It would be expected that any CHO-mediated down-regulation of fat metabolism and oxidation would target the following sites: (*a*) triacylglycerol degradation and release of FFA from adipose tissue, (*b*) transport of FFA into the cell (plasma membrane fatty acid binding protein (FABPpm) and fatty acid translocase [FAT/CD36]), (*c*) release of FFA from IMTG (hormone-sensitive lipase [HSL] activity), and (*d*) transport of FFA into the mitochondria (carnitine palmitoyl transferase I [CPT I] activity).

Increased Insulin Concentration

The reduction in fat metabolism following glucose ingestion appears to be due to the combined effects of decreased FFA availability secondary to decreased adipose tissue lipolysis and to direct effects on fatty acid oxidation in the muscle. Both effects may be the result of increased plasma insulin levels.

Elevated plasma insulin levels exert a powerful inhibitory effect on HSL in adipose tissue, reducing the breakdown of triacylglycerol and decreasing circulating plasma FFA concentrations. This translates into a reduced delivery of FFA to the muscles during exercise and a documented decrease in FFA uptake and oxidation. It is also possible that increased plasma insulin has direct effects on several regulatory sites of fat metabolism and oxidation in the muscle (Fig. 19.4). Insulin has been shown to increase the content of fat transporter proteins in the muscle membrane to facilitate transport. While at first this seems to support increased fat oxidation, insulin may also stimulate esterification of FFA and decrease IMTG lipolysis in skeletal muscle and direct incoming FFA toward storage and away from oxidation, as occurs in adipose tissue. There is also the finding that HSL activity is reduced when CHO is ingested during exercise (35), but there has generally been little done in human skeletal muscle. While an elevated insulin concentration may exert these effects following glucose ingestion, it would not explain the decrease in fat oxidation that occurs when the power output increases from 40 to 80% $\dot{V}O_{2max}$, for example.

CHO-Induced Decrease of Fat Oxidation via Malonyl-CoA?

It is also well known that an abundant CHO supply and high insulin levels cause an elevation of malonyl-CoA (M-CoA) content in lipogenic tissues via stimulation of acetyl-CoA carboxylase (ACC) (36,37). The M-CoA inhibits CPT I activity and the transport of lipid into the mitochondria. M-CoA has been detected in human skeletal muscle (38,39), and a muscle isoform of ACC, which appears to be regulated differently from hepatic ACC, has also been discovered in skeletal muscle. Because skeletal muscle is not a lipogenic tissue, it is not clear what role M-CoA plays in regulating the entry of FFA into the mitochondria at rest and during exercise. The unique challenge that skeletal muscle faces during exercise is the need to greatly increase the production of energy from both fat and CHO oxidation, not simply switch between fuels. This is quite different from the reciprocal changes in CHO and fat oxidation that occur in resting skeletal muscle and other tissues that do not undergo large increases in metabolic demand.

The M-CoA theory, extended to the findings in rodent skeletal muscle, suggests that resting M-CoA levels are high enough to limit FFA transport into the mitochondria. It is clear that M-CoA levels decrease during muscle contractions in rodent skeletal muscle, when energy production from fat oxidation is increasing (37). This suggests that the decrease in M-CoA may be important in relieving the inhibition of CPT I that is normal in resting skeletal muscle and in increasing FFA transport into the mitochondria during aerobic exercise.

Measurements of M-CoA contents in human skeletal muscle during exercise demonstrated that M-CoA was largely unaffected by exercise at varying power outputs (35–100% $\dot{V}_{O_{2max}}$) and rates of fat oxidation (38,39). These results do not support a regulatory role for M-CoA in fat oxidation during exercise in human skeletal muscle; they suggest that the regulation of CPT I activity during the onset of exercise is more complex.

Decreased Fat Oxidation by Metabolic Regulators Important for Carbohydrate Regulation?

Aerobic power outputs of moderate to high intensity result in small but measurable decreases in muscle pH (33). Studies in mitochondria isolated from resting human skeletal muscle showed that decreases in pH from 7 to 6.8 caused large reductions in CPT I activity (40). In view of the lowered pH at moderate and intense exercise power outputs, this could lead to decreased CPT I activity and decreased fatty acid oxidation. Future studies are necessary to clarify the regulation of CPT I activity during exercise and to determine the mechanisms whereby increasing glycolytic activity could down-regulate fat oxidation at this step. Surprisingly, increasing concentrations of calcium and free ADP, AMP, and P_i, which occur with increasing exercise intensities and increased CHO use, did not down-regulate CPT I activity in mitochondria isolated from human skeletal muscle.

Long-Chain FFA-CoA Inhibition of IMTG Lipolysis?

If increasing glycolytic activity causes decreased mitochondrial FFA uptake, it is possible that long-chain fatty acyl (LCFA)-CoA accumulates in the cytoplasm of skeletal muscle cells. This may lead to allosteric inhibition of HSL and reduced IMTG hydrolysis, as has been shown in adipose tissue (41). Indeed, glycerol released from the muscle (an index of IMTG hydrolysis) was reduced during hyperinsulinemia (42) and insulin-suppressed IMTG hydrolysis and fatty acid oxidation in the isolated contracting rodent soleus muscle (43). These data suggest that the elevated insulin associated with increased CHO availability may decrease IMTG hydrolysis secondary to increased LCFA-CoA accumulation and fatty acid oxidation. Alternatively, the carbohydrate-induced increase in insulin may offset any LCFA-CoA accumulation in the muscle by simply reducing the availability of FFA. These suggestions have not been directly tested in human skeletal muscle.

Increased Muscle Glycogen Availability

In contrast to the numerous studies that have demonstrated a regulatory role of skeletal muscle glycogen content on both muscle glycogenolysis and glucose uptake, there is little information pertaining to the influence of muscle glycogen on FFA uptake, IMTG metabolism, and FFA oxidation. One study reported similar rates of FFA uptake between exercising legs 12 hours after glycogen-depleting exercise in one leg (44). In the same study, glycerol release from the low-glycogen leg was about 60% greater than the control leg, suggesting a possible increase in IMTG hydrolysis with low muscle glycogen. These data are consistent with decreased muscle glycogen use and increased whole-body fat metabolism following a 12-hour high-fat diet (23). However, in another study leg FFA uptake increased when muscle glycogen was low, but FFA clearance was similar, which suggests that dietary or hormonal effects on plasma [FFA] were probably the main factor (45). However, they also observed greater AMP kinase activity and ACC phosphorylation with low glycogen content, which may play a role in enhancing FFA uptake and mobilization of FFA from the IMTG store. Therefore, muscle glycogen may play a role in fuel selection through interaction with modulators and key enzymes of fat metabolism. These possibilities should be examined in future studies.

SUMMARY

Carbohydrate and fat are the primary metabolic substrates oxidized during aerobic exercise. The notions that increasing the availability of CHO can increase the oxidation of CHO and increasing the exogenous FFA availability can increase fat oxidation are well supported. There are data to suggest that increasing fat availability decreases CHO oxidation. However, the classic glucose–fatty acid cycle does not explain this interaction during exercise. Instead, increasing fat availability down-regulates muscle glycogenolysis and PDH activity, possibly by increasing mitochondrial NADH availability and ultimately buffering the fall in the cellular energy charge. During prolonged exercise, increased plasma [FFA] may up-regulate PDK activity and thereby attenuate the activation of PDH. There is also evidence indicating that altering exogenous CHO availability can decrease fat oxidation, possibly via an increase in plasma insulin and decreased FFA availability and also by decreasing the rate of fat transport into the muscle and/or the mitochondria. Increasing the exercise intensity stimulates a greater reliance on CHO as a fuel and appears to down-regulate fat metabolism through mechanisms based in the muscle. Future studies examining membrane fat transport, muscle TG lipolysis (HSL activity), and mitochondrial fat transport (CPT I activity) in human skeletal muscle and the effects of altered endogenous fuel availability (IMTG, muscle glycogen content) on the interaction between CHO and fat metabolism during exercise are clearly warranted.

A MILESTONE OF DISCOVERY

In the 1960s the English scientists Randle, Garland, Newsholme, and Hales published a series of papers on examination of the regulation of glucose uptake and carbohydrate metabolism in muscle and the abnormalities that accompanied changes in insulin sensitivity and diabetes mellitus. They noticed that abnormalities of carbohydrate metabolism were often accompanied by increases in the concentrations of plasma FFA and ketone bodies. Interestingly, many of these abnormalities were the same ones that we are still studying and attempting to explain today—diabetes, starvation, carbohydrate deprivation, and obesity. They wished to determine whether these high levels of circulating FFA and ketone bodies could produce the same abnormalities as reported in these diseases—decreased glucose uptake, glycolysis, and pyruvate oxidation in muscle. A series of studies *in vitro* and *in vivo* led to the formation of the idea of the glucose–fatty acid cycle. Philip J. Randle outlined his recollection of the essential components of the glucose–fatty acid cycle in the CIBA Medal Lecture in London in December 1985 (46):

> (1) [T]he relationship between glucose and fatty acid metabolism is reciprocal and not dependent; (2) in vivo, the oxidation of fatty acids and ketone bodies released into the circulation in diabetes or starvation may inhibit the catabolism of glucose in muscle; (3) in vitro, the oxidation of fatty acids released from muscle triglyceride may play a similar role; (4) the effects of fatty acid and ketone body oxidation are mediated by inhibition of the pyruvate dehydrogenase (PDH) complex, phosphofructokinase-1 (PFK) and hexokinase (HK); (5) the essential mechanism is an increase in the mitochondrial ratio of [acetyl-CoA]/[CoA], which inhibits the PDH complex and by indirect means leads to inhibition of PFK by citrate and of HK

by glucose 6-phosphate (G-6-P); (6) the effect of low concentrations of insulin to accelerate glucose transport is inhibited by oxidation of fatty acids or ketone bodies.

These authors combined the results from studies *in vivo* using perfused contracting heart muscle and incubated resting diaphragm muscle from rodents with *in vitro*, or test tube, experiments using muscle homogenates. To form their theory they examined the ability of certain modulators to affect the activity of the key glycolytic enzymes. When the FFA availability to the muscles was increased, fat oxidation increased, CHO oxidation decreased, and muscle acetyl-CoA, citrate, and G-6-P contents increased. The work *in vitro* had already established that acetyl-CoA inhibited the activity of PDH by activating PDH kinase, the enzyme that phosphorylates PDH to its less active form; that citrate was a potent inhibitor of PFK; and that G-6-P inhibited HK.

These experiments were performed with heart and diaphragm muscles that have regular contraction cycles and derive most of the required oxidizable substrate from outside the cell. This situation is different from the working conditions of most skeletal muscles, especially human skeletal muscle, in which the higher energy demands of moderate and high-intensity aerobic exercise dictates that most oxidizable substrate must come from stores inside the cells. However, these landmark experiments provided a testable theory for future experimenters to study and attempt to explain the relationship between carbohydrate and fat use in contracting skeletal muscle at various exercise intensities and durations and nutritional states.

Randle PJ, Garland PB, Hales CN, Newsholme EA. The glucose fatty-acid cycle: its role in insulin sensitivity and the metabolic disturbances of diabetes mellitus. Lancet 1963;1:785–789.

REFERENCES

1. Asmussen E. Muscle metabolism during exercise in man: a historical survey. In Pernow B, Saltin B, eds. Muscle Metabolism During Exercise. New York: Plenum, 1971;1–11.
2. Bergstrom J, Hermansen L, Hultman E, et al. Diet, muscle glycogen and physical performance. Acta Physiol Scand 1967;71:140–150.
3. Ahlborg G, Felig P, Hagenfeldt L, et al. Substrate turnover during prolonged exercise in man: splanchnic and leg metabolism of glucose, free fatty acids, and amino acids. J Clin Invest 1974;3:1080–1090.
4. Randle PJ, Hales CN, Garland PB, et al. The glucose fatty-acid cycle: its role in insulin sensitivity and the metabolic disturbances of diabetes mellitus. Lancet 1963;I:785–789.
5. Randle PJ, Newsholme EA, Garland PB. Regulation of glucose uptake by muscle: 8. Effects of fatty acids, ketone bodies and pyruvate, and of alloxan-diabetes and starvation, on the uptake and metabolic fate of glucose in rat heart and diaphragm muscles. Biochem J 1964;93:652–665.
6. Hickson RC, Rennie MJ, Conlee RK, et al. Effects of increased plasma fatty acids on glycogen utilization and endurance. J Appl Physiol 1977;43:829–833.
7. Rennie MJ, Holloszy JO. Inhibition of glucose uptake and glycogenolysis by availability of oleate in well-oxygenated perfused skeletal muscle. Biochem J 1977;168:161–170.
8. Richter EA, Ruderman NB, Gavras H, et al. Muscle glycogenolysis during exercise: dual control by epinephrine and contractions. Am J Physiol 1982;242:E25–E32.
9. Dyck DJ, Peters SJ, Wendling PS, et al. Effect of high FFA on glycogenolysis in oxidative rat hindlimb muscles during twitch stimulation. Am J Physiol 1996;270:R766–R776.
10. Dyck DJ, Peters SJ, Wendling PS, et al. Regulation of muscle glycogen phosphorylase activity during intense aerobic cycling with elevated FFA. Am J Physiol 1996;270:E116–E125.
11. Hargreaves M, Kiens B, Richter EA. Effect of plasma free fatty acid concentration on muscle metabolism in exercising men. J Appl Physiol 1991;70:194–210.
12. Romijn JA, Coyle EF, Sidossis LS, et al. Relationship between fatty acid delivery and fatty acid oxidation during strenuous exercise. J Appl Physiol 1995;79:1939–1945.

13. Dyck DJ, Putman CT, Heigenhauser GJF, et al. Regulation of fat-carbohydrate interaction in skeletal muscle during intense aerobic cycling. Am J Physiol 1993;265:E852–E859.

14. Odland LM, Heigenhauser GJF, Wong D, et al. Effects of increased fat availability on fat-carbohydrate interaction during prolonged exercise in men. Am J Physiol 1998;275: R894–R902.

15. Odland LM, Heigenhauser GJF, Spriet LL. Effects of high fat availability on muscle PDH activation and malonyl-CoA content during moderate exercise. J Appl Physiol 2000;89: 2352–2358.

16. Peters SJ, Spriet LL. Skeletal muscle phosphofructokinase activity examined under physiological conditions *in vitro*. J Appl Physiol 1995;78:1853–1858.

17. Stellingwerff T, Watt MJ, Heigenhauser GJF, et al. Effects of reduced free fatty acid availability on skeletal muscle PDH activation during aerobic exercise. Am J Physiol 2003;284: E583–E588.

18. Wilson DF. Factors affecting the rate and energetics of mitochondrial oxidative phosphorylation. Med Sci Sports Exerc 1994;26:37–43.

19. Watt MJ, Heigenhauser GJF, Dyck DJ, et al. Intramuscular triacylglycerol, glycogen and acetyl group metabolism during 4 hours of moderate exercise in man. J Physiol (Lond) 2002;541:969–978.

20. Peters SJ, Harris RA, Wu P, et al. Human skeletal muscle PDH kinase activity and isoform expression during three days of a high fat/low carbohydrate diet. Am J Physiol 2001; 281:E1151–E1158.

21. Watt MJ, Heigenhauser GJF, Leblanc PJ, Spriet LL, Inglis JG, Peters SJ. Rapid upregulation of pyruvate dehydrogenase kinase activity in human skeletal muscle during prolonged exercise. J Appl Physiol 2004;97:1261–1267.

22. Kiens B, Essen-Gustavsson B, Gad P, et al. Lipoprotein lipase activity and intramuscular triglyceride stores after long-term high-fat and high-carbohydrate diets in physically trained men. Clin Physiol 1987;7:1–9.

23. Starling RD, Trappe TA, Parcell AC, et al. Effects of diet on muscle triglyceride and endurance performance. J Appl Physiol 1997;82:1185–1189.

24. Coyle EF, Jeukendrup AE, Oseto MC, et al. Low-fat diet alters intramuscular substrates and reduces lipolysis and fat oxidation during exercise. Am J Physiol 2001;280:E391–E398.

25. Helge JW, Watt PW, Richter EA, et al. Fat utilization during exercise: adaptation to a fat-rich diet increases utilization of plasma fatty acids and very low density lipoprotein-triacylglycerol in humans. J Physiol (Lond) 2001;537: 1009–1020.

26. Burke LM, Angus DJ, Cox GR, et al. Effect of fat adaptation and carbohydrate restoration on metabolism and performance during prolonged cycling. J Appl Physiol 2000;89:2413–2421.

27. Coyle EF, Jeukendrup AE, Wagenmakers AJM, et al. Fatty acid oxidation is directly regulated by carbohydrate metabolism during exercise. Am J Physiol 1997;273:E268–E275.

28. Horowitz JF, Mora-Rodriguez R, Byerley LO, et al. Lipolytic suppression following carbohydrate ingestion limits fat oxidation during exercise. Am J Physiol 1997;273:E768–E775.

29. Sidossis LS, Stuart CA, Shulman GI, et al. Glucose plus insulin regulate fat oxidation by controlling the rate of fatty acid entry into the mitochondria. J Clin Invest 1996;98: 244–2250.

30. Sidossis LS, Gastaldelli A, Klein S, et al. Regulation of plasma fatty acid oxidation during low- and high-intensity exercise. Am J Physiol 1977;272:E1065–E1070.

31. Romijn JA, Coyle EF, Sidossis LS, et al. Regulation of endogenous fat and carbohydrate metabolism in relation to exercise intensity and duration. Am J Physiol 1993;265:E380–E391.

32. Gollnick PD, Piehl K, Saltin B. Selective glycogen depletion pattern in human muscle fibres after exercise of varying intensity and at varying pedalling rates. J Physiol (Lond) 1974;241:45–57.

33. Howlett RA, Parolin ML, Dyck DJ, et al. Regulation of skeletal muscle glycogen phosphorylase and pyruvate dehydrogenase at varying power outputs. Am J Physiol 1998;275: R418–R425.

34. Watt MJ, Howlett KF, Febbraio MA, et al. Adrenaline increases skeletal muscle glycogenolysis, pyruvate dehydrogenase activation and carbohydrate oxidation during moderate exercise in humans. J Physiol (Lond) 2001;534.1:269–278.

35. Watt MJ, Krustrup P, Secher NH, et al. Glucose ingestion blunts hormone-sensitive lipase activity in contracting human skeletal muscle. Am J Physiol 2004;286:E144–E150.

36. McGarry JD, Brown NF. The mitochondrial carnitine palmitoyltransferase system: from concept to molecular analysis. Eur J Biochem 1997;244:1–14.

37. Winder WW, Arogyasami J, Barton RJ, et al. Muscle malonyl-CoA decreases during exercise. J Appl Physiol 1989;67: 2230–2233.

38. Dean D, Daugaard JR, Young ME, et al. Exercise diminishes the activity of acetyl-CoA carboxylase in human muscle. Diabetes 2000;49:1295–1300.

39. Odland LM, Heigenhauser GJF, Lopaschuk GD, et al. Human skeletal muscle malonyl-CoA at rest and during prolonged submaximal exercise. Am J Physiol 1996;270:E541–E544.

40. Starritt EC, Howlett RA, Heigenhauser GJF, et al. Sensitivity of CPT I to malonyl-CoA in trained and untrained human skeletal muscle. Am J Physiol 2000;278:E462–E468.

41. Jepson CA, Yeaman SJ. Inhibition of hormone-sensitive lipase by intermediary lipid metabolites. FEBS Lett 1992; 310:197–200.

42. Enoksson S, Degerman E, Hagstrom-Toft E, et al. Various phosphodiesterase subtypes mediate the in vivo antilipolytic effect of insulin on adipose tissue and skeletal muscle in man. Diabetologia 1998;41:560–568.

43. Dyck DJ, Steinberg G, Bonen A. Insulin increases FA uptake and esterification but reduces lipid utilization in isolated contracting muscle. Am J Physiol 2001;281:E600–E607.

44. Blomstrand E, Saltin B. Effect of muscle glycogen on glucose, lactate and amino acid metabolism during exercise and recovery in human subjects. J Physiol (Lond) 1999;514: 293–302.

45. Wojtaszewski JFP, MacDonald C, Nielsen JN, et al. Regulation of 5′AMP-activated protein kinase activity and substrate utilization in exercising human skeletal muscle. Amer J Physiol 2003;284:E813–E822.

46. Randle PJ. Fuel selection in animals. Biochem Soc Trans 1986;14(5):799–806.

CHAPTER 20

The Metabolic Systems: Protein and Amino Acid Metabolism in Muscle

Anton J. M. Wagenmakers

Introduction

The ability of humans to walk, run, and perform physical work is critically dependent on the presence and maintenance of an appropriate muscle mass. In a lean young adult 70-kg male, skeletal muscle mass is 28 to 35 kg, and his body contains 12 kg of protein, of which at least 7 kg is in the skeletal muscles. Most of the muscle protein is accounted for by the myofibrils, the contractile elements that enable the muscle to contract and thus generate movement and work. The higher the myofibrillar protein mass, the greater the maximal force that the muscle can develop. For maintenance of the myofibrillar mass and therefore of maximal force, it is essential that the rate of protein synthesis of the constituent myofibrillar proteins is equal to the rate of protein degradation. Heavy-intensity resistance training is known to lead to an increase in the number of myofibrils per muscle fiber and muscle hypertrophy. During hypertrophy, protein synthesis must be higher than protein degradation. In many chronic diseases (e.g., heart failure, pulmonary obstruction, liver failure, kidney disease, cancer, and AIDS) and also during the aging process, there is a slow progressive loss of muscle mass (sarcopenia) that leads to muscle weakness and reduced mobility. In the elderly this condition frequently leads to accidental and fatal falls. This chapter first describes the biochemical pathways and regulatory mechanisms that control muscle protein synthesis and degradation. Then it relates them to changes in muscle protein synthesis and degradation rates that have been observed in humans.

In the 1960s it was shown that endurance training both in rats (1) and humans (2) substantially increases the content of the mitochondrial enzymes with a role in oxidative metabolism and of proteins with a role in substrate transport and mobilization. High concentrations of these oxidative enzymes also are intrinsically related to high insulin sensitivity. On the other hand, inactivity and chronic disease reduce the content of the oxidative enzymes (3) and reduce insulin sensitivity in parallel. It is quite clear today that changes in gene expression play an important role in the adaptation of the protein profile to dynamic exercise (see Chapter 30). This chapter explains the potential role of qualitative and quantitative changes in protein synthesis and degradation.

In the 1840s the German physiologist Von Liebig hypothesized that muscle protein was the main substrate used to achieve muscular contraction. After this view was invalidated by experimental data (4), many exercise physiologists took the opposite stand and disregarded the amino acid pool in muscle as having any significance in exercise and energy metabolism. Therefore, the final section of this chapter gives an overview of the role of muscle in the handling and metabolism of amino acids in the overnight fasted state and following ingestion of protein-containing meals. Finally, the chapter discusses the effects of exercise on these conditions.

Biochemical Pathways and Basal Regulatory Mechanisms of Protein Synthesis and Degradation

The Importance of Protein Turnover

Amino acids occur in nature in the form of proteins (amino acid polymers connected by peptide linkages) and free amino acids. There are 20 amino acids that can be charged to an aminoacyl-tRNA and used for protein synthesis. The body of a 70-kg man contains 12 kg of protein and 200 to 230 g of free amino acids (4). Approximately 120 g of the free amino acids is within skeletal muscle cells. There is a continuous exchange of amino acids between the free amino acid pool and the protein pool, as proteins are constantly being synthesized and degraded (this cyclic exchange process is called protein turnover). Protein turnover at the whole-body level amounts to 280 g per day in man (4) and requires approximately 20% of the resting energy expenditure. Protein turnover is a prerequisite for survival, as otherwise proteins damaged by toxic compounds, free radicals, peroxidation, exposure to UV light, or extreme contraction forces would not be replaced with new, functionally intact proteins.

Mechanisms to Alter Muscle Protein Content and Protein Composition

A net gain in the total protein content of a muscle fiber can be achieved by an increase in protein synthesis or a decrease in protein degradation and by any combination of changes in which the protein balance is positive (protein synthesis > protein degradation). A net gain of the total protein content by definition also leads to hypertrophy of muscle cells and gain of muscle mass. A negative protein net balance (protein synthesis < protein degradation) will lead to a net loss of the protein content and muscle fiber atrophy and sarcopenia.

A change in the protein composition of a muscle cell in response to a physiological stimulus, such as exercise or nutrition, on a theoretical base can be achieved by the following mechanisms:

- A change of the gene expression profile leading to the appearance of a different set of mRNAs or a change in the relative concentration of mRNAs in the expressed profile
- A change in the breakdown rate of specific mRNAs leading to a change in the relative concentration of mRNAs in the expressed profile
- A selection of specific mRNAs for translation initiation and protein synthesis
- A selection of specific proteins for preferential degradation by the proteolytic systems that operate in muscle

This implies that part of the control of the proteins that are ultimately present in muscle is at the DNA transcription level, part at the level of the stability and turnover of the expressed mRNAs, and part at the level of protein synthesis and of protein degradation. The first two levels are addressed in Chapter 30. This chapter describes the latter two levels.

The Pathways and General Control Mechanisms of Muscle Protein Synthesis

The biochemical pathways by which mRNAs are translated into proteins have primarily been investigated in a large variety of established eukaryotic cell lines (5–7). Kimball and colleagues (8) investigated these pathways and their regulation by hormones, amino acids, and exercise in rat skeletal muscle both in vitro and in vivo and as such have contributed most to our present insight in the control of muscle adaptation at the translation level. Today very little research has been performed on the pathways and their control in human skeletal muscle, but as the pathways appear to be universal and conservative, we can safely assume that they are basically the same.

Translation of mRNA into proteins can be divided into three phases: initiation, elongation, and termination. Initiation and elongation are the main regulatory sites. Together they control the translation rate in response to most physiological stimuli. Initiation of translation (Fig. 20.1) occurs via a series of discrete steps and is mediated by a dozen proteins referred to as eukaryotic initiation factors (eIFs). The end result of the process is the assembly of a translationally competent ribosome at the AUG start site near the 5′ end of the mRNA. Translation initiation can be functionally divided into three stages: (a) the binding of initiator methionyl-tRNA (met-tRNA$_i$) to the 40S ribosomal subunit to form the 43S preinitiation complex, (b) the binding of the mRNA capped with eIF4E, eIF4A, eIF4G to the 43S preinitiation complex to form the 48S preinitiation complex, and (c) the binding of the 60S ribosomal subunit to the 48S preinitiation complex to form the active 80S initiation complex (Fig. 20.1). In each of these steps some of the involved eIFS can be phosphorylated by regulatory kinases, leading to either an increased or a decreased formation rate of translationally competent ribosomes.

In the elongation phase of mRNA translation the polypeptide is assembled. This phase consumes a substantial amount of metabolic energy, with at least four high-energy bonds being consumed for each amino acid added to the nascent peptide chain (5). Elongation is mediated by a set of nonribosomal proteins called eukaryotic elongation factors or eEFs. Several of the eEFS can also be phosphorylated. Among them are eEF1A and eEF1B, which are activated by phosphorylation and are involved in the recruitment of amino acyl-tRNAs to the ribosome, and eEF2, which mediates ribosomal translocation along the mRNA and is inhibited by phosphorylation (5).

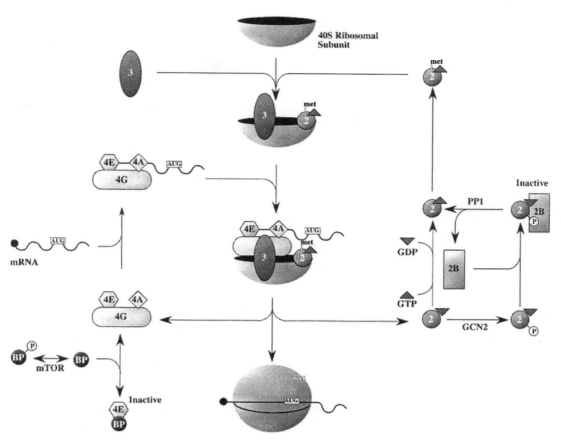

FIGURE 20.1   The biochemical pathways of translation initiation: the three stages of translation initiation (binding of methionyl-tRNA$_i$ (met) to the 40S ribosomal subunit followed by binding of the mRNA, and finally binding of the 60S ribosomal subunit). The translation initiation factors that participate in the individual stages are depicted as geometric shapes and are labeled with a number or number and letter on the basis of the identity of the factor. For example, eukaryotic initiation factor (eIF) eIF4E is depicted as a hexagon with the label 4E in the center. In addition, the regulation of eIF2B activity by phosphorylation of the α-subunit of eIF2 and the sequestration of eIF4E by eIF4E binding protein-1 (4E-BP1) are illustrated. eIF2B is the protein that recharges the eIF2-GDP complex with GTP, such that the eIF2B-GTP complex can bind to a new molecule of met-tRNA$_i$ and start a new initiation cycle. Phosphorylation of 4E-BP1 by the mTOR (mammalian target of rapamycin) signaling pathway prevents its binding to eIF4E and thus enhances capping of the mRNA with the relevant eIF4s. AUG, the nucleoside triplet adenosine, uridine, guanosine, is encoding for the start site of translation of the mRNA; GCN2, general control nonderepressing eIF2a protein kinase 2. *(Reprinted with permission from Kimball SR, Farrell PA, Jefferson LS. Invited review: role of insulin in translational control of protein synthesis in skeletal muscle by amino acids and exercise. J Appl Physiol 2002;93:1169.)*

Role of Nutrients and Hormones in the Translational Control of Protein Synthesis in Skeletal Muscle

Hormones and amino acids are among the major signals that modulate the involved kinases and phosphatases. Insulin and insulinlike growth factor (IGF) 1 were first shown to stimulate protein synthesis via their action on key signaling molecules downstream of phosphatidylinositol 3-kinase (PI-3 kinase) and protein kinase B (PKB) in the insulin-signaling cascade. An important recent finding is that the rapamycin-sensitive mTOR (mammalian target of rapamycin) signaling pathway plays an important role further downstream in the control of translation by insulin and IGF-1. Insulin and

IGF-1 via mTOR activation among others stimulate the phosphorylation state of the eIF 4E-binding protein 1 (4E-BP1) and of ribosomal protein S6 kinase (p70S6K). 4E-BP1 binds to eIF4E, thereby reducing its availability for the capping of the mRNA with two other eIF4s and formation of the 48S preinitiation complex. Phosphorylation of 4E-BP1 prevents its binding to eIF4E and thereby enhances formation of the mRNA-eIF4F complex and accelerates the formation of translationally competent ribosomes and polyribosomes. p70S6k is a kinase that acts upon protein S6 of the small ribosomal subunit. Phosphorylation of S6 has been shown to switch on a mechanism that allows the preferential initiation and translation of a set of mRNA termed the 5′-TOP (tract of oligopyrimidine) (6), which among others includes those encoding for each of the ribosomal proteins and for eEF1A and eEF2 (6,9). Via this mechanism refeeding of fasted rats (8) rapidly increases the concentration of rRNA and eEFs and thus regenerates the capacity of the protein synthetic machinery that is reduced during prolonged fasting. Insulin-stimulated and IGF-1-stimulated phosphorylation of p70S6k also results in suppression of the activity of the kinase that phosphorylates eEF2 (5) and via this mechanism increases elongation rates independently of increases in the capacity of the protein synthetic machinery.

The next important observation was that amino acids, particularly leucine, also can activate mTOR via an insulin-independent mechanism. Amino acids can thus directly cause phosphorylation of 4E-BP1 and p70S6K; but in muscle this seems to require the presence of a minimal amount of insulin (8). It has also been shown that activation of PKB and insulin cannot phosphorylate and activate mTOR in muscle cells that are deprived of amino acids (8). Therefore, phosphorylation of mTOR seems to be an important point of integration of the signals arising from insulin, IGF-1, and amino acids (Fig. 20.2). This seems to be the point where fine-tuning of control of the rate of initiation (which determines the proportion of ribosomes attached to mRNAs), the rate of elongation (efficiency of translation), and the rate of synthesis of ribosomal proteins and eEFs (upgrading the capacity of the protein synthetic machinery) occurs.

Role of Exercise in the Translational Control of Protein Synthesis in Skeletal Muscle

ACUTE EFFECTS OF RESISTANCE EXERCISE Bylund-Fellenius and colleagues (10) subjected rat hindleg muscles to electrical stimulation via the sciatic nerve for 10 minutes. The procedure led to maximal isometric contractions and resulted in substantial decreases both in the muscle adenosine triphosphate (ATP) and creatine phosphate (CrP) content and in the muscle protein synthesis rate compared to the resting situation. Compelling evidence in many cultured cell types shows that an acute energy deficit down-regulates the activity of several kinases with a crucial role in both translation initiation (6,7) and elongation (5). AICAR (5-aminoimidazole-4-carboxamide 1–β-D-ribonucleoside) is an organic compound that is taken up by most cell types and converted to an analogue of adenosine monophosphate (AMP), thereby mimicking an energy deficit. Addition of AICAR to hepatocytes (5) gave rise to a rapid and robust increase in the phosphorylation state of eEF2, implying that the elongation rate is acutely down-regulated. Bolster and colleagues (9) injected rats with AICAR and thus increased the activity of the AMP-activated protein kinase (AMPK) in skeletal muscle by 51%. This change reduced the muscle protein synthesis rate in the rats to less than half. Substantial parallel reductions were seen in the phosphorylation status

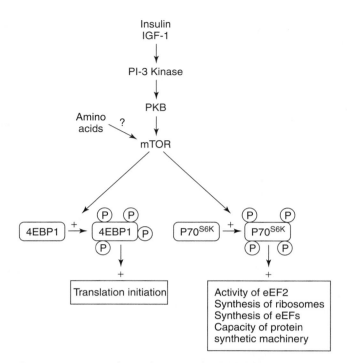

FIGURE 20.2 Signal transduction pathways leading to hyperphosphorylation of 4E-BP1 and p70S6k. Hyperphosphorylation of 4E-BP1 leads to increased formation rates of translationally competent polyribosomes (Fig. 19.1). Hyperphosphorylation of p70S6k activates this kinase and leads to phosphorylation of the ribosomal protein S6. As a consequence, S6 will select the mRNAs encoding for the ribosomal proteins and for elongation factors (eEFs) for preferential translation, increasing the synthesis of ribosomes, the capacity for recruitment of aminoacyl tRNAs to the mRNA, and translocation of ribosomes along the mRNA. This increase in the overall capacity of the protein synthetic machinery is estimated to take at least 1 or 2 h, as these proteins first have to be synthesized. Hyperphosphorylation of p70S6k also suppresses the activity of the kinase that phosphorylates and inactivates eEF2 and via this mechanism increases elongation rates instantaneously, independent of time-dependent increases in the capacity of the protein synthetic machinery.

of PKB, mTOR, p70S6k, and 4E-BP1. (Fig. 20.3). Together these experiments indicated that activation of AMPK leads to acute reductions of both the initiation and elongation steps of protein synthesis. High-intensity contractions in rat, therefore, apparently acutely down-regulate the activity of the energy-demanding protein synthetic machinery in skeletal muscle via a mechanism controlled by the energy status and the AMPK signaling route, shutting down the signaling route that mediates the anabolic effects of hormones and amino acids.

EFFECTS OF RESISTANCE EXERCISE IN THE PERIOD POST EXERCISE Using different rat models of resistance exercise, several laboratories (8,11–14), have presented data indicating that it is again the PKB–mTOR pathway that is activated by

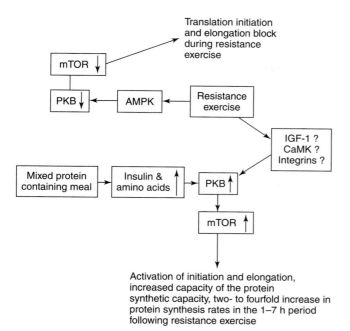

FIGURE 20.3 The dual effect of resistance exercise on the anabolic PKB/mTOR signaling pathway and muscle protein synthesis. During resistance exercise this pathway is inhibited by AMPK, leading to a fall in muscle protein synthesis, but 10–20 minutes after resistance exercise this inhibition is relieved and is changing into an activation. The largest increases in protein synthesis after resistance exercise are seen in the 2- to 7-h period when a mixed-protein–containing meal is ingested.

resistance exercise in the hours following its cessation. The exact nature of the exercise signal that leads to this activation is not known. Among the likely candidates are integrin signaling pathways, the muscle-specific IGF-1 isomers that are locally produced in response to heavy-intensity contractions, and the calcium/calmodulin–dependent protein kinases (CaMK). Baar and Esser (11) used electrical stimulation of rat hindlegs to create heavy-intensity lengthening contractions of the extensor digitorum longus and tibialis anterior muscle. They found that 6 h after a single exercise bout, much more of the muscle RNA was present in the polyribosome fraction, indicating that more translationally competent (poly)ribosomes had been formed. The phosphorylation of p70S6k in the muscles was maximal (similar to that seen following insulin stimulation) 3 and 6 h after exercise and remained increased above resting control levels for 36 h. In the same exercise model it was more recently (13) shown that the mRNA encoding for elongation factor EF1A (one of the 5′-TOP mRNAs) was preferentially translated 6 h after exercise. Kimball and colleagues (8), Bolster and colleagues (12), and Hernandez and colleagues (14) have used another model of resistance exercise in which rats repeatedly lift a weight that they carry in a backpack while standing on their hindlegs. The time course of changes in PI3-kinase activity, in p70S6k activity, and in protein syn-

thesis rates, was originally studied by Hernandez and colleagues (14). No changes were seen 1 and 3 h after exercise. PI3-kinase activity and p70S6k activity were significantly increased 6 h after exercise and remained elevated until 24 h. However, protein synthesis rates were increased by only approximately 30% 12 and 24 h after exercise. Hernandez and colleagues (14) therefore concluded that there is an exercise effect on protein synthesis but with a delay of at least 12 h before it becomes effective. However, as protein synthesis rates were routinely made in this study after 5 h of fasting, the data may also imply that a minimal period of food intake is required following resistance exercise to switch on the exercise signals or keep them active and thus increase the capacity of the protein synthetic machinery and protein synthesis rates. Because of the nutritional design chosen, the animals that were studied 1 and 3 h after exercise did not receive food before and after exercise, while the 6-h animals had free access to food until the first hour after exercise. The animals, studied 12 and 24 h after exercise, received food both before exercise and for 7 and 19 h after exercise. In another recent study of the same group (12), using the same exercise model, the rats were fasted for 5–8 h before exercise and in the h after exercise. A brief transient increase was seen in the first hour after exercise in the phosphorylation state of PKB, mTOR, 4E-BP1, p70S6k, and ribosomal protein S6. The increase was not present immediately after exercise, was maximal in the 10- to 20-min period, and had returned for most variables to control levels after 60 min. The difference in time course of activation between this study and those of Baar and Esser (11) is striking. Differences in exercise intensity and in the feeding status of the animals are the factors most likely to explain the apparent controversy. In the study of Baar and Esser (11) the rats had free access to food both before and after exercise. As the effects of exercise, nutrients, and amino acids seem to operate in concert on the same signaling routes and kinases, these discrepant findings raise important questions that have not been answered today: Can translation initiation and elongation be chronically (for 6 h or more) activated? Can the capacity of the protein synthetic machinery be up-regulated by an increased synthesis of ribosomes and eEFs when the rats are not fed immediately after exercise?

EFFECTS OF FUNCTIONAL OVERLOAD AND DISUSE Bodine and associates (15) provided clear evidence that the PKB–mTOR pathway also plays a major role in the muscle hypertrophy that is caused by chronic functional overload and that repression of the pathway will lead to muscle atrophy. They created a functional overload of the plantaris muscle in rats by synergist ablation. The amount of PKB and the phosphorylation status of PKB, 4E-BP1, and p70S6k were markedly increased after 14 days. The effects were achieved via the mTOR signaling pathway, as rapamycin could reverse the increase in phosphorylation status of 4E-BP1 and p70S6k and severely blunt the hypertrophy. Unloading of the plantaris via hindlimb suspension (a model of disuse) after 14 days caused decreased phosphorylation of PKB and p70S6k and an increase in 4E-BP1–eIF4E complex assembly, which inhibited capping of the mRNA with the relevant eIF4s. The importance of the PKB–mTOR signaling route in the development of muscle hypertrophy was also demonstrated by the overexpression of PKB by plasmid DNA injection. Such treatment caused muscle hypertrophy in adult mice and blunted the atrophy observed during hindlimb suspension.

EFFECTS OF DYNAMIC ENDURANCE EXERCISE Knowledge about the translation initiation regulatory mechanisms in rats during and after acute endurance exercise and training is limited (reviewed by Kimball and associates [8]). An hour following 2 h of moderate endurance exercise by rats on a treadmill was associated with a 26% down-regulation of the mixed muscle protein synthesis rate in rats that were not fed immediately after exercise. This decrease was attended by a fourfold increase in the amount of eIF4 that was bound to 4E-BP1. Feeding a meal containing both carbohydrate and protein prevented the down-regulation of protein synthesis and reversed the increased binding of eIF4 to 4E-BP1. A 100% carbohydrate meal could not prevent the down-regulation of protein synthesis and the binding of eIF4 to 4E-BP1. There are no indications that the PKB–mTOR signaling route is activated in the hour following endurance exercise, as observed with resistance exercise. It is not known today whether the mRNAs encoding for the mitochondrial enzymes or fat metabolism can be selected for preferential translation to increase their protein content. However, evidence shows that the transcription rate of several genes encoding for mitochondrial enzymes is up-regulated for periods of 6 h or more following acute endurance exercise bouts both in rats and humans (see Chapters 21 and 30). This leads to transient increases in the concentration of the mRNA's encoding for these enzymes and therefore is expected to lead to transient periods of increased rates of the oxidative enzymes following each bout of dynamic exercise.

To date, the general literature lacks direct evidence to support this claim. This is because the methodology involved in measuring the synthesis rates of individual mitochondrial proteins or of GLUT4 is difficult to perform and to date has not been undertaken in animals or humans under appropriate conditions after endurance exercise. In support of this claim are findings indicating that young and adult trained animals have higher synthesis rates for mitochondrial proteins than old and untrained animals (older rats tend to be less active as well [16]). A single bout of acute exercise apparently does not provide a large enough stimulus to produce a measurable increase in the concentration of oxidative enzymes. However, it is well documented that the additive effect of repeated exercise bouts during train-

ing durations of 6–12 wk will significantly increase mitochondrial density and the oxidative capacity of skeletal muscle (1,2).

The Pathways and General Control Mechanisms of Muscle Protein Degradation

Proteins in skeletal muscle undergo a continuous cycle of synthesis and degradation (protein turnover), which regulates both the overall protein mass and the levels of specific proteins. Increased rates of protein degradation, among others, contribute to the muscle wasting seen with fasting and in many disease states. Despite potentially being equal in importance in the control exerted on protein quantity and quality, we are just beginning to unravel the pathways, signal routes, and mechanisms that regulate protein degradation (17–20).

Like other mammalian tissues, skeletal muscle contains multiple proteolytic systems. The lysosomal, Ca++-activated and ubiquitin-proteasome–dependent pathways have the highest enzyme activities (17–20); are quantitatively the most important in the daily response to nutrients, hormones and exercise; and also seem to control the selection of proteins for degradation (18).

The Lysosomal Pathway

The best-known proteolytic system is the lysosomal pathway. Lysosomes are small vacuolar organelles surrounded by a membrane. They are particularly abundant in liver and are able to create an internal milieu with a low pH. In addition, they contain a variety of enzymes with maximum activity at low pH and are active in the clearance of proteins and macromolecules such as glycogen, RNA, and DNA. Skeletal muscle contains only few lysosomes, and the major lysosomal proteinases (cathepsins B, H, L, and D) do not contribute significantly to bulk protein breakdown in muscle and to the breakdown of the myofibrillar proteins (17). The pathway has been suggested to be primarily responsible in muscle for the breakdown of some long-lived membrane and endocytosed proteins (plasma proteins, virus proteins, infiltrating macrophages).

Calcium-Activated Proteinases

The two major Ca++-activated proteinases are μ-calpain and m-calpain (17). The activity of both of these ubiquitous cysteine proteinases is regulated by Ca++ and by an endogenous inhibitor called calpastatin. In skeletal muscle a third calpain, p94, is expressed abundantly (17). The calcium-dependent proteolysis also does not contribute significantly to the bulk of protein breakdown in muscle in normal conditions, and the activity of the calpains is not up-regulated in most muscle-wasting conditions, the exception being the muscular dystrophies. However, the Ca^{++}-dependent proteinases may have an important function in the selection of proteins for proteolysis. Many short-lived proteins contain negatively charged PEST (Pro, Glu, Ser, Thr) sequences that may bind Ca^{++} and thus create a microenvironment of higher Ca^{++} concentration that is favorable to calpain-mediated proteolysis. Among suggestions is that the insulin receptor substrate (IRS-1) has such a PEST sequence that is susceptible to calpain degradation and that the processing of protein kinase C is controlled by calpains. This effect implies that the programmed activation of calpains has a role in modulating the activity of important signaling pathways. Calpains have important functions in the disassembly of sarcomeric proteins (nebulin, titin, troponin, and tropomyosin) and in Z-band disintegration. Unfortunately, our knowledge of the physiological role of the calpains and their control by nutrients and hormones is still in its infancy, and the effects of exercise and training remain unknown. Proteins that have undergone limited proteolysis by calpains most likely subsequently undergo complete hydrolysis in muscle by the ubiquitin–proteasome system (18).

The Ubiquitin-Proteasome System

The ubiquitin–proteasome pathway is primarily responsible for bulk protein breakdown in muscle and also for the breakdown of the myofibrillar proteins actin and myosin. The pathway is activated in most diseases and conditions characterized by muscle wasting and cachexia. These among others include fasting, protein deficiency, glucocorticoid treatment, and the acute response to cancer, kidney failure, trauma, and sepsis (17–20). In more chronic wasting conditions such as aging, Cushing's syndrome (chronic high levels of glucocorticoids), progressive stages of renal failure, and the muscular dystrophies, the pathway is not up-regulated (anymore). These changes suggest that the ubiquitin–proteasome pathway is especially involved in acute and rapid changes in bulk protein content of skeletal muscle.

The proteolytic machinery of the ubiquitin–proteasome pathway consists of several hundreds of proteins. These include the ubiquitination/deubiquitination enzymes (200–300), the proteasome subunits (about 50), and endogenous proteasome activators and inhibitors. The pathway is performing housekeeping functions in basal protein turnover and in the elimination of miscoded, misfolded, mislocalized, or damaged abnormal proteins. Schematically there are two main steps in the pathway: (*a*) covalent attachment of a polyubiquitin chain to the protein substrate under the control of ubiquitination and deubiquitination enzymes to tag proteins that should be broken down and (*b*) specific recognition of proteins tagged with a polyubiquitin chain and degradation of the tagged proteins by the 26S proteasome (Fig. 20.4).

Ubiquitination of proteins has both proteolytic and nonproteolytic functions. Monoubiquitinated, diubiquitinated, or triubiquitinated proteins usually are not degraded but are targeted for other fates. For example, monoubiquitination is a signal of endocytosis of a number of receptors (18). A polyubiquitin chain of four or more is a signal for proteolysis. Polyubiquitination is a complex multiple-step process explained in Figure 20.4. Molecular details of the involved ubiquitination enzymes (E1 and the superfamilies of E2 and E3), the DUB superfamily, the proteasome subunits, and the complex structural and functional organization of the proteasome multienzyme complex (containing specific and multiple subunits and sites for recognition, unfolding, a cylindrical proteolytic core, and regulation by specific activator and inactivator proteins) have been reviewed by Attaix and colleagues (18).

Regulation of the Proteolytic Pathways by Hormones and Nutrients

Insulin and amino acids have a well-known antiproteolytic effect in incubated muscle preparations (17–20) and *in vivo* both at the whole-body level and in muscle. However, neither all of the tissues nor the proteolytic pathways that are affected have been well characterized. There is no clear evidence in the literature that insulin and/or amino acids acutely down-regulate the activity or expression of lysosomal proteolytic enzymes or calpains. Refeeding of rats after prolonged starvation with carbohydrates and amino acids down-regulated the expression of several enzymes of the ubiquitin–proteasome system (18), but it takes more than 12 h to adjust the protein concentration of the involved enzymes. As the antiproteolytic response in incubated muscles to insulin is much faster, part of the control may also involve phosphorylation and dephosphorylation or alternative acute allosteric activation mechanisms. Whatever the situation, the involved kinases and phosphorylation sites have yet to be identified.

Regulation of the Proteolytic Pathways by Exercise, Disuse, and Chronic Overloading

EFFECTS OF ACUTE RESISTANCE AND ENDURANCE EXERCISE Research in animal models has demonstrated that eccentric exercise will stimulate muscle proteolysis. Moreover, several studies in humans (e.g., 21) have shown that eccentric exercise has resulted in increased levels of free ubiquitin and ubiquitin conjugates and in increased proteasome activities with repeated exercise. On the other hand, endurance exercise by rats for 5 consecutive days resulted in down-regulation of the rate of proteolysis and a parallel reduction in proteasome activity (22). Results from human studies have also shown that the expression of the components of the ubiquitin–proteasome system is down-regulated by regular dynamic exercise. It is not known

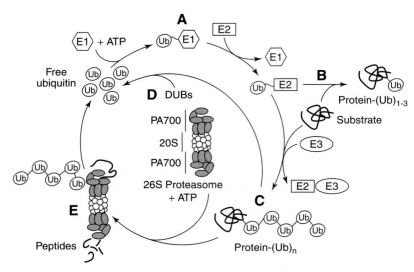

FIGURE 20.4 The ubiquitin-proteasome pathway. *A.* Ubiquitin (Ub) is a 76–amino acid marker polypeptide. It is first activated by a single enzyme called the ubiquitin-activating enzyme (E1) and then transferred to one of the ubiquitin-conjugating enzymes (E2s). *B.* An E2 covalently attaches one to three ubiquitin moieties to a selected protein [Protein-(Ub)1–3]. The first ubiquitin molecule is attached via an isopeptide bond between the activated C-terminal glycine residue of ubiquitin and the ε-amino group of a lysine residue in the substrate. Protein molecules carrying an ubiquitin chain of one to three molecules are not targeted for protein breakdown. *C.* With (and in some cases without) the help of one of the ubiquitin protein ligases (E3s), the E2 can form a polyubiquitinated protein [Protein-(Ub)n] carrying four or more ubiquitin moieties. E3s also have an important function in recognizing and selecting proteins that should be broken down. *D.* Protein-(Ub)n can either be deubiquitinated by the deubiquitinating enzymes (DUBs) to be safe from proteolysis, or (E) is recognized by the proteasome multienzyme complex, unfolded, injected into the 26S proteasome proteolytic subunit unit, and degraded into peptides. The pathway consumes ATP both in step A and E. In man about 10% of resting energy is used to drive the ubiquitin-proteasome pathway at the whole-body level. *(Reprinted with permission from Attaix D, Combaret L, Kee AJ, et al. Mechanism of ubiquitination and proteasome-dependent proteolysis in skeletal muscle. In: Zempleini J, Daniel H, eds. Molecular Nutrition, Wallingford, UK: CABI, 2003:220.)*

whether this down-regulation leads to a reduced global protein degradation rate or is a response of specific muscle proteins that are involved in the adaptations to endurance exercise.

EFFECTS OF IMMOBILIZATION, DENERVATION AND DISUSE Immobilization, denervation and hindlimb suspension in rodents are highly catabolic treatments and are attended by a massive parallel up-regulation of most components of the ubiquitin–proteasome system, The mRNAs encoding for the ubiquitin–proteasome system are preferentially translated in these conditions. More recently two muscle-specific ubiquitin protein ligases (E3s) that are overexpressed in immobilization, denervation, and hindlimb suspension have been identified (23). These E3s appear to have an important function in the rapid muscle wasting that occurs in these conditions.

ROLE OF THE UBIQUITIN–PROTEASOME SYSTEM IN THE REMODELING OF SKELETAL MUSCLE Changes in functional load and in pattern of contractile activity are known to lead to a muscle remodeling that involves the increased expression of select proteins and the disappearance of others (e.g., the well-known shifts in myosin heavy chain isomer expression). Also involved in the remodeling process are protein breakdown and the proteasome. Ordway and associates (24) observed a marked and coordinated increase in mRNA and protein levels of the proteasome subunits and in proteasome activity in rabbit tibialis anterior muscle that had been subjected to chronic electrical stimulation for up to 28 days. Taillandier and colleagues (25) investigated the adaptations that occur when unweighted rats are reloaded. They found that after 8 h of reloading, the components of the ubiquitin–proteasome system were actively expressed and translated, as demonstrated by an analysis of the polyribosome fraction. Both protein synthesis and protein degradation *in vitro,* as measured in incubated muscles from these animals, were increased. Following 7 days of reloading there still was an increased amount of ubiquitin conjugates in the myofibrillar fraction. Presumably, the upregulation of the proteasome pathway in these cases is required to tag or to target specific proteins (e.g., damaged proteins or the myosin heavy chain isomers that were present before the reloading) for rapid elimination and/or replacement.

Muscle Protein Synthesis and Degradation in Human Studies

Methods to Measure Rates of Protein Synthesis and Degradation *in Vivo*

The methodology used to measure protein synthesis and degradation rates at the whole-body level and in individual tissues and proteins has been described in detail (16,26). In brief, the most accurate, reliable, and direct method to measure the synthesis rate of mixed muscle protein or of individual proteins is the amino acid incorporation technique. In most human studies a continuous infusion for 3–6 h is required of an amino acid with a stable isotope label ($^{13}C^-$, $^{15}N^-$ or $^{2}H^-$). The increase in enrichment with time is divided by the enrichment of the amino acid precursor pool and the incorporation time to give the fractional synthesis rate (FSR) in percent per day or per hour. The method has successfully been used to measure the synthesis rate of mixed muscle protein and to investigate the control of protein synthesis by fasting and refeeding and by hormones (16,26).

However, very few laboratories worldwide are technically able to apply the method to muscle protein subfractions, especially individual proteins. This is the primary reason insights on the time course of the increases in the synthesis rate of myofibrillar proteins, mitochondrial proteins, and important transport proteins, such as GLUT4, after various modes of exercise are still limited today. The net balance approach across a forearm or a leg has been developed to measure muscle protein synthesis and degradation rates simultaneously. In brief, a tracer amino acid is given by a primed continuous infusion until the plasma concentration and enrichment are constant (in tracer steady state), and then a set of replicates is obtained from both arterial and venous blood from the forearm or the leg. In most cases, researchers use an amino acid that is not transaminated or oxidized in muscle, so that the amino acid can disappear from the muscle compartment only via incorporation into muscle protein and release to the blood and can appear in the muscle compartment only via uptake from the blood and

protein degradation. Equations are then used to calculate the net balance of the traced amino acid and of the tracer. The process yields protein synthesis and degradation as unknowns, and these can be calculated. However, other tissues than muscle (skin, bone, and adipose tissue) are present in arms and legs and significantly contribute to the indicated net balances. A limitation of the method is that the calculation of protein synthesis depends on the measurement of at least four variables, each with a confidence limit. The estimate of protein synthesis therefore tends to be less accurate and have a greater variance than with the incorporation method. Also, the tissue net balance approach can only examine the total protein pool (muscle and other tissue) in the sampled compartment and not the synthesis and degradation rates of individual muscle proteins. The methodological and technical limitations of the tissue net balance and of later modifications (e.g., the three-pool model of Biolo and colleagues (27) have been previously discussed in great detail (16).

Despite their known limitations, both methods have made significant contributions to our present knowledge on the control of muscle protein synthesis and degradation *in vivo* in humans (16,26).

Human Skeletal Muscle Proteins Have a Slow Turnover

Mixed muscle protein in overnight-fasted humans has a turnover rate of 1.15% per day (Table 20.1). This is much lower than in liver and gut tissues and only 0.25% of the value of very low density lipoprotein (VLDL) apo-B100, the protein with the highest reported turnover rate in humans. Subfractionation of muscle protein has shown that the myofibrillar proteins have the lowest turnover rates, close to 1% per day, while mitochondrial proteins and the cytosolic

TABLE 20.1	Fractional Protein Synthesis Rates in Humans[a]	
	FSR (% per day)	Percent of Qwb
Mixed muscle protein	1.15	29.00
Mitochondrial protein	2.50	—
Mixed liver protein	12.1	11.00
Plasma albumin	5–6	2.40
VLDL apo-B100	425	0.12

[a]Measured as the incorporation of a tracer-labeled amino acid in the indicated protein fraction during a continuous intravenous infusion and calculated contributions of individual tissues to whole-body protein turnover.
Qwb, whole-body protein turnover, assumed to be 280 g of protein per day.
Data from Wagenmakers AJM. Tracers to investigate protein and amino acid metabolism in human subjects. Proc Nutr Soc 1999;58:987–1000.

enzymes generally have slightly higher turnover rates (16) (Table 20.1). It has been speculated that important key enzymes have higher protein turnover rates, as relatively small changes in either protein synthesis or degradation can lead to a rapid adjustment of the concentration of that enzyme in response to a physiological stimulus. This in return can contribute to metabolic regulation. A mean turnover rate of 1.15% per day for mixed muscle protein implies that in a 70-kg man with 7 kg of muscle protein, 70 g of muscle protein is being synthesized and degraded daily. This rate also implies that muscle, despite its enormous protein mass, contributes only approximately 30% to whole-body protein turnover (estimated at 280 g per day; Table 20.1).

Effects of Feeding and Fasting

In a person in energy and protein balance there will be no change with time in the size of the muscle and whole-body protein pool. In muscle, as with other tissues, there is a diurnal cycle to consider with the size of the protein pool. This is because some protein is being deposited during the daylight feeding period and the same amount is being lost during overnight fasting. The high plasma insulin concentration in the postprandial state, especially following ingestion of a mixed-protein–containing meal, in combination with increases in the intracellular concentration or arterial availability of the essential amino acids, both stimulates protein synthesis and reduces protein degradation in liver and muscle tissues (16,26). During the feeding period, muscle protein synthesis is increased by about 10 to 20% and protein degradation is reduced by 20%. These changes mean that only 7 to 14 g of protein is deposited within the skeletal muscles, or that only 0.1 to 0.2% of the total amount of muscle protein was involved. Whole-body protein level estimates indicated that 35 g of protein is deposited during the feeding period on a normal protein intake ($0.7 \text{ g} \cdot \text{kg}^{-1}$ per day) and 90 g on a high-protein intake ($2.5 \text{ g} \cdot \text{kg}^{-1}$ per day). Thus, diurnal cycling is increased with protein intake. It is generally assumed that gut and liver are the main sites where these proteins are temporarily deposited following ingestion of protein-containing meals. Breakdown of these splanchnic proteins in the overnight fasting period will in the 24-h period make the meal-derived amino acids more evenly available to other tissues like heart, kidney, brain, and muscle, such that these tissues will show only minimal changes in the size of the protein pool during the night.

Acute Effects of Exercise

The methodology in use to measure protein synthesis in humans allows detection only of changes that are prolonged (>1 hour) and do not involve rapid changes in pool size,

amino acid enrichment, and protein turnover rates (16,26). This is the reason that no attempts have been made to quantitate muscle and whole-body protein synthesis and degradation during acute bouts of resistance exercise in man. However, a large number of studies have investigated the effect of dynamic exercise.

Nineteenth Century Nitrogen Balance Studies Did Not Show Net Protein Breakdown

In the 1840s the German physiologist Von Liebig hypothesized that muscle protein was the main substrate used to achieve muscular contraction, which, of course, would imply that protein oxidation and net protein breakdown (degradation minus synthesis) would substantially increase during exercise. As early as the 1870s this hypothesis was invalidated, as nitrogen balance studies failed to show an increase in nitrogen losses during and following prolonged periods of heavy exercise (16). Also, in recent literature most of the carefully controlled nitrogen balance studies in trained athletes show that the increase in nitrogen losses during prolonged dynamic exercise lasting 1–4 h at intensities between 30 and 75% $\dot{V}O_{2max}$ is minimal or nonexistent. Minor increases in nitrogen excretion (reflecting the net breakdown of maximally g amounts of muscle protein) have been observed only when the glycogen stores were deliberately emptied before the start of exercise.

Stable Isotope Tracer Studies Do Not Show Decreases in Muscle Protein Synthesis or Increased Urea Production During Prolonged Exercise

With the introduction of stable-isotope amino acids, new techniques became available to investigate protein metabolism during exercise in man. Wolfe and colleagues (28) in 1982 used L-[1–^{13}C]-leucine as a tracer to follow whole-body protein metabolism. Leucine flux and whole-body protein degradation were similar at rest and during 1 hour of exercise at 30% $\dot{V}O_{2max}$, but leucine oxidation increased nearly threefold. As flux equals synthesis plus oxidation in the mathematical whole-body tracer model used (for details see Wagenmakers [16]), protein synthesis decreased during exercise. However, there was a discrepancy with a second method used in this study. Whole-body urea production estimated from the dilution of isotopically labeled urea, which should increase when protein oxidation is increased, was exactly similar at rest and during exercise. Since 1982 many laboratories have used various tracer techniques and not found evidence of increased amino acid oxidation and a reduction in muscle or whole-body protein synthesis during treadmill running and cycling at intensities between 30 and 70% $\dot{V}O_{2max}$ for 1–6 h. Direct measurements of the FSR in mixed-muscle protein did not show changes from rest. This result was independent of the feeding status of the subjects (overnight fasted or during ingestion of carbohydrate drinks) and of the training status. The increased $^{13}CO_2$ production from L-[1–^{13}C]-leucine has been confirmed by many laboratories in the meantime (16). The increase in leucine oxidation seems to be specific for leucine only and does not seem to point at a general increase in protein oxidation, as originally assumed (28).

Knee Extensor Exercise and Exercise in Patients With McArdle's Disease

There are a few exceptions to the rule that prolonged endurance exercise does not lead to an imbalance between muscle protein synthesis and protein degradation. Van Hall and associates (29) have investigated the exchange of amino acids during 90 min of one-leg knee extensor exercise in trained human subjects and observed a 10-fold increase in the release of amino acids (phenylalanine, tyrosine, threonine, lysine, methionine, and glycine) that are not transaminated or oxidized in muscle. This indicates that protein synthesis must fall far below protein degradation. Another condition with an even larger imbalance between protein synthesis and degradation is normal bicycling exercise in patients with McArdle's disease (4). These patients do not have access to muscle glycogen during exercise, as they lack an active form of glycogen phosphorylase in muscle. During one-leg knee-extensor exercise the workload and oxygen consumption per kilogram of muscle is twofold to threefold higher than during normal cycling, which implies that the energy status is more likely to be disturbed. There is ample evidence in the literature that in patients with McArdle's disease the energy disturbance is large and leads to excessive increases in both AMP concentration and AMP-activated protein kinase activity. As explained earlier, activation of AMPK down-regulates the mTOR pathway and blocks both the initiation and elongation phase of protein synthesis (5,9,10).

Effects of Exercise and Nutrition on Protein Synthesis and Degradation in the Period Following Resistance Exercise

Using the amino acid incorporation technique, two groups (30,31) have investigated the time course of muscle FSRs after a single bout of resistance exercise in untrained subjects. Both observed substantial increases in protein synthesis for periods of more than 24 h. In one of the studies (30), the fractional protein synthesis rates were measured during ingestion of a mixed-protein–containing meal (in repeated boluses to ensure maintenance of a tracer steady state), and in the other (31) the rates were measured in the fasted state. The highest increase in both studies was seen in the first 2–6 h after exercise, with the maximal values of fractional protein synthesis being approximately twofold to threefold higher than in the basal period before exercise. Phillips and associates (31) also reported increases in fractional protein degradation rates

for more than 24 h, confirming that protein degradation may contribute to the remodeling of muscle induced by resistance exercise (18,21).

Several attempts have also been made to investigate in placebo-controlled studies whether amino acid ingestion or infusion or carbohydrate ingestion can further increase muscle protein anabolism post resistance exercise. The results of studies using the amino acid incorporation technique to measure FSRs of mixed muscle protein are summarized. Roy and colleagues (32) investigated the effect of glucose ingestion (1 g · kg^{-1}) immediately and 1 h after resistance exercise in comparison to a placebo control and observed only a 36% increase over basal control values in muscle FSRs measured over the first 10 h following exercise when glucose had been ingested. Biolo and colleagues (27) infused a balanced amino acid mixture (0.15 g · kg · h^{-1}) in the 1- to 4-h period following either rest or resistance exercise. In the basal postabsorptive state muscle FSR was 1.58% per day. This value increased to 2.40% per day and to 3.45% per day during the amino acid infusion in the rest trial and after performing resistance exercise. Tipton and colleagues (33) have measured muscle FSRs over a 24 h in a study with a complex design involving two trials. In the first trial the subjects rested throughout the day; in the second trial they performed a bout of resistance exercise at noon (6 h after the start of the study) and ingested 15 g of an essential amino acid supplement both immediately before and after the exercise. In both trials they also ingested a mixed protein–containing meal 2–3 h before the time of the exercise and a second mixed protein–containing meal in repeated boluses (to assure a tracer steady state) in a 2-h period about 5–7 h after exercise. FSRs of mixed muscle protein were found to be higher in the exercise trial in three periods: (a) in the period involving the first meal, the exercise bout and the intake of the essential amino acid supplements (1.40 vs. 1.14% per day); (b) during the 2-h period of ingestion of the second meal (4.51 vs. 1.82% per day); and (c) during the night following ingestion of the second meal (1.70 vs. 1.32% per day).

Most of these studies seem to suggest that the ingestion of a mixed-protein–containing meal is required to increase fractional protein synthesis rates to maximal values, which can increase to 200–400% of the normal postabsorptive control value of 1.15% per day. This conclusion was confirmed by a number of leg balance studies by the Wolfe group (34). However, there is uncertainty about some of these conclusions because they investigated the effect of the oral ingestion of boluses of solutions containing glucose, amino acids, or amino acid–carbohydrate mixtures. The use of bolus feedings implies that there are no proper steady-state conditions, and in such cases failure to correct for changes in the concentration or enrichment of amino acids in the blood and muscle pool will bias the results. For this reason, the messages and conclusions from these studies on the optimal timing and composition of the solutions of amino acid, protein, and carbohydrate consumed after exercise for an optimal anabolic effect are waiting confirmation by studies using more appropriate methodology.

The conclusion that a mixed meal should be ingested to reveal the anabolic effect of resistance exercise may also explain why Hernandez and associates (14) did not observe increases in protein synthesis rates in fasted rats in the first 6 h after resistance exercise. Modest 30% increases were seen in the 12- to 24-h period, but as explained earlier, may have been related to the ingestion of food in that period. Maximal rates of protein synthesis in the previously mentioned human studies were observed in the time window between 1 and 7 h after resistance exercise, which coincides with the maximal increases in the phosphorylation state of p70S6k and the maximal amount of RNA in the polyribosomal fraction in the rat study of Baar and Esser (11). Together the rat and human studies suggest that the continued activation of the PKB–mTOR pathway following resistance exercise requires the ingestion of a mixed-protein–containing meal in the period after exercise and that maximal (twofold to fourfold) increases of protein synthesis are reached in that case in the 1- to 7-h period after resistance exercise. The effect of amino acids and insulin on protein synthesis is substantially larger after exercise than in the resting condition, suggesting that exercise potentiates the anabolic effect of insulin and amino acids.

Effects of Exercise and Nutrition on Protein Synthesis and Degradation Rates Following Dynamic Exercise

The researchers who measured muscle FSR during recovery from endurance exercise in humans did not observe changes in comparison to the periods before or during exercise (16,26). However, there may be two reasons for the absence of an effect. The first is that the measurements were made without ingestion of a mixed meal or without ingestion or infusion of an amino acid–glucose mixture. The second is that in no published studies did the researchers measure the synthesis rates of individual mitochondrial proteins or oxidative enzymes. A potential up-regulation of the synthesis rate of these proteins may well have been hidden by the absence of an effect or even a compensatory decrease in the synthesis rate of other muscle proteins after endurance exercise.

Age- and Disease-Related Changes in the Regulation of Muscle Protein Metabolism by Exercise and Nutrients

It is quite clear that regular exercise is necessary to maintain muscle mass and muscle quality in all stages the human life and in pathological conditions, which by definition are attended by extended periods of bedrest and inactivity (1–4,16,35,36). Some of the changes that occur in these conditions simply are the consequence of disuse, but some also are clearly related to aging or to disease-specific changes (36).

Myofibrillar FSRs measured in the postabsorptive state are approximately 30% lower in muscles of men and women of over 60 years of age than in young adults (16), and 3 months of resistance training did not reverse this decrease. In the recent literature many suggestions have been made that the anabolic PKB–mTOR pathway is not as easily activated in old as in young muscles by insulin, IGF-1, and amino acids (particularly leucine). It has also been suggested that to achieve an anabolic effect from resistance exercise, elderly humans should take food sooner after exercise than should young adults (35). It has been suggested that older muscles have a reduced capacity to produce the muscle-specific isomer of IGF-1 in response to heavy-intensity contractions; a local humoral regulation mechanism may have an important function in achieving an anabolic effect from resistance exercise and have a reduced capacity for regeneration after damage or periods of disuse. Unfortunately, to date it is not known whether and which of these muscle-specific factors can be corrected by regular exercise and training. However, it is known that with old mice, a single bout of aerobic exercise is enough to restore the responsiveness of the muscle to infusions of IGF-1.

In many chronic diseases the losses of muscle mass and function are much more prominent than can be expected on the basis of bedrest and disuse alone. In several disease processes, acute and chronic inflammation has been shown to lead to a decrease of the membrane potential of muscle and nerve (36), hence to a functional denervation of the muscle or at least to changes in the 24-h profile of the afferent and efferent signals that travel between the central nervous system and muscle. (Reflex loops have roles in muscle coordination, and in the regulation of muscle gene expression and metabolism.) In patients with trauma and sepsis this among others has been shown to lead to very low expression rates of myosin, low ratios of myosin to actin, acute down-regulation of the mitochondrial content and a massive up-regulation of the ubiquitin–proteasome system (36). In patients with cancer, chronic obstructive pulmonary disease, chronic heart failure, and chronic kidney failure we simply do not know what the molecular and electrophysiological changes are and how they explain the extreme fatigability of the peripheral muscles of these patients (36). It is quite likely, though, that there are abnormalities in both gene expression and mRNA translation and that these abnormalities lead to chronic changes in protein content and composition that impair muscle contractile function, insulin sensitivity, and metabolism.

Muscle Amino Acid Metabolism

Not only are amino acids in muscle the precursor for protein synthesis and the product of protein degradation, but muscle is also actively involved in the metabolism of some amino

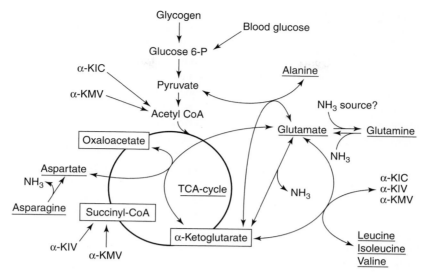

FIGURE 20.5 Schematic presentation of muscle amino acid metabolism and of the interactions of amino acids with the tricarboxylic acid (TCA) cycle. The transamination products of leucine, isoleucine, and valine are α-ketoisocaproic acid (α-KIC), α-ketomethylvaleric acid (α-KMV) and α-ketoisocaproic acid (α-KIV). Glucose 6-P, glucose-6-phosphate. *(Reprinted with permission from Van Hall G, Saltin B, Wagenmakers AJM. Muscle protein degradation and amino acid metabolism during prolonged knee-extensor exercise in humans. Clin Sci 1999;97:565.)*

acids. A detailed review is given in (4), hence only a brief summary follows here. Figure 20.5 shows the major pathways of muscle amino acid metabolism.

Only six amino acids are substantially metabolized in resting and exercising skeletal muscles. These are the branched-chain amino acids (leucine, isoleucine, and valine), asparagine, aspartate, and glutamate. These amino acids together provide the amino groups and ammonia for synthesis of glutamine and alanine, which are released in excessive amounts both in the postabsorptive state and during ingestion of protein-containing meals. Only leucine and part of the isoleucine molecule are converted to acetyl-CoA in muscle and can therefore be oxidized and contribute to the synthesis of ATP. The other carbon skeletons are used solely for *de novo* synthesis of tricarboxylic acid (TCA) cycle intermediates and glutamine. Stable isotope tracer studies have shown that the carbon atoms of the released alanine originate primarily from glycolysis of blood glucose and from muscle glycogen breakdown followed by glycolysis. In resting conditions these processes contribute each about half of the required amount of pyruvate, while glycogen breakdown is the main source during exercise at intensities above 50% $\dot{V}O_{2max}$. After consumption of a protein-containing meal most amino acids are taken up and metabolized in the splanchnic area (gut and liver). However, the branched-chain amino acids and glutamate escape from the splanchnic area and are primarily taken up by muscle to be converted to glutamine. About half of the glutamine released from muscle originates from glutamate taken up from the blood after over-

night fasting, prolonged starvation, or consumption of a mixed-protein–containing meal, while the remainder of the glutamine is generated by *de novo* synthesis from the six amino acids that are metabolized in muscle. Glutamine produced by muscle is an important substrate for mucosa cells and immune system cells and provides the nitrogen for synthesis of DNA and RNA in all rapidly dividing cells. Glutamine in several cells is also able to activate the mTOR pathway and therefore has an important function in the signal routes and regulation mechanisms discussed in this chapter. Conditions in which the muscle is not able to keep up glutamine production are often characterized by a weakened immune function and wasting of muscle mass.

The alanine aminotransferase reaction functions to establish and maintain high concentrations of TCA cycle intermediates in muscle during the first few minutes of exercise and during subsequent work rate increments. Pyruvate, primarily originating from glycogen breakdown and glycolysis, and glutamate in the muscle pool and taken up from the blood are both used to generate the carbon skeletons of TCA cycle intermediates (pyruvate + glutamate ↔ alanine + α-ketoglutarate). The increase in concentration of TCA cycle intermediates probably is needed to increase the flux of the TCA cycle and meet the increased energy demand of exercise. However, many other reactions control the flux into and through the TCA cycle, and there is a continuing debate on the relative importance of the TCA cycle anaplerosis via conversion of amino acids. In glycogen-depleted muscles (29) and in muscles of patients with

McArdle's disease (muscle glycogen phosphorylase deficiency [4]) deamination of the six aforementioned amino acids and glutamine synthesis present alternative anaplerotic mechanisms but only allow exercise at intensities of 40 to 50% of $\dot{V}O_{2max}$. Collectively, these observations indicate that the metabolism of amino acids in muscle serves a number of important roles in the regulation of energy metabolism both at rest and during exercise and in the support of mucosa and immune system cells with a continuous supply of glutamine.

SUMMARY

Resistance training leads to muscle hypertrophy and an increase in the number of myofibrils per muscle fiber. Elderly subjects and patients with chronic diseases, on the other hand, show a slow progressive muscle atrophy, which makes them immobile and weak, leading to social isolation and a dramatic reduction in their quality of life. Dynamic exercise training leads to an increase in the number of mitochondria per muscle volume, while immobility and disuse have the opposite effect. Therefore, the trained athlete has an enhanced endurance performance, but many elderly humans cannot walk for more than 500 m. This chapter identifies the most important pathways and signaling routes that can lead to the anabolism of strength training and to the atrophy of disuse. This knowledge opens the way for the development of new therapeutic approaches based on a combination of feasible exercise programs and well-timed high quality nutrition and on the development of new pharmaceutical strategies or a combination of the two. Though we know little today about the enzymes that control muscle proteolysis, it is evident that they also make important contributions to changes in muscle mass and in the protein profile. Our knowledge about the role of protein synthesis and degradation in the control of the molecular adaptation to endurance training and the loss of the mitochondrial oxidative enzymes in disuse, aging, and disease is still is in its infancy. In any case, we do know that chronic exercise and training (preferably a mixture of resistance and endurance exercise) can prevent most of the muscle function losses seen with aging and chronic disabling diseases; greatly improve health, well-being, and quality of life; and reduce the frequency of chronic age-related diseases (cardiovascular disease, obesity, and type 2 diabetes). So the final message is that all human beings of all ages should exercise as frequently as possible to keep the protein composition of their muscles optimal, and they will be rewarded with immense performance and health benefits.

A MILESTONE OF DISCOVERY

David Halliday in 1975 was the first to combine a continuous intravenous infusion of L-[α-^{15}N]-lysine in five human subjects with serial biopsies of the vastus lateralis muscle using the percutaneous Bergstrøm needle. Serial samples of plasma were also used for purification of albumin. The infusion solution contained the tracer amino acid and also a mixture of essential and nonessential amino acids. The subjects ingested carbohydrate drinks every 2 hours during the infusions, which lasted for 21 to 30 hours, and therefore they were in an artificial state of continuous feeding. This design enabled Halliday and McKeran to make the first simultaneous estimates of skeletal muscle protein synthesis, plasma albumin synthesis, and whole-body protein turnover. This early study was one of the most thorough and complete amino acid incorporation studies yet performed, despite the fact that the required analytical techniques were very complex and labor intense and required great analytical skills, both in the chemical and in the mass spectrometry laboratory. Also, the sensitivity of the isotope ratio mass spectrometer (IRMS) was much lower than it is today and gas chromatography–combustion–IRMS systems, which combine the separation of amino acids online with the generation and analysis of nitrogen, did not yet exist. A separation was made between the myofibrillar protein fraction, which constitutes the bulk of the muscle protein, and the sarcoplasmic proteins, the soluble enzymes in the cytosol of muscle fibers. The main result of the study was that in continuously fed humans the fractional synthetic rate was 1.46% per day in the myofibrillar protein fraction, 3.80 % in the sarcoplasmic protein fraction, and 13.2% in plasma albumin, and whole-body protein turnover was 250 g per day. This paper set the scene for more detailed investigations of the regulation of muscle protein synthesis by feeding, fasting, hormones and by (prior) exercise. Halliday and coworkers in 1985 (37) also were the first to report a simultaneous estimate of muscle protein synthesis and protein degradation in man by combining the use of a continuously infused L-[1–^{13}C, ^{15}N]-leucine tracer with deep venous and arterialized blood sampling of the forearm. Similar tracer methodologies today still are the only available technique to make estimates of muscle protein degradation in humans and laboratory animals and as such are essential to further our understanding of the role of muscle protein degradation in the protein adaptation to exercise and training. David Halliday and his collaborators not only made important contributions to the development of stable isotope tracer methodologies but also have made a major contribution to the current insight in the regulation of muscle amino acid and protein metabolism in man.

Halliday D, McKeran RO. Measurement of muscle protein synthetic rate from serial muscle biopsies and total body protein turnover in man by continuous intravenous infusion of L-[α-^{15}N] lysine. Clin Sci Mol Med 1975;49:581–590.

ACKNOWLEDGMENTS

I acknowledge the helpful discussions with Didier Attaix (Human Nutrition Research Centre of Clermont-Ferrand and National Institute of Agricultural Research, Nutrition and Protein Metabolism Unit, Ceyrat, France) and with Luc van Loon, Matthijs Hesselink and the doctoral students of Maastricht University who have contributed to the integrative view presented in this chapter. Thanks also to the students in Birmingham for proofreading.

REFERENCES

1. Holloszy JO. Biochemical adaptations in muscle. J Biol Chem 1967;242:2278–2282.
2. Saltin B, Henriksson J, Nygaard E, et al. Fiber types and metabolic potentials of skeletal muscles in sedentary man and endurance runners. Ann NY Acad Sci 1977;301:3–29.
3. Wagenmakers AJM, Coakley JH, Edwards RHT. The metabolic consequences of reduced habitual activities in patients with muscle pain and disease. Ergonomics 1988;31:1519–1527.
4. Wagenmakers AJM. Muscle amino acid metabolism at rest and during exercise: role in human physiology and metabolism. Ex Sport Sci Rev 1998;26:287–314.
5. Browne GJ, Proud CG. Minireview: regulation of peptide-chain elongation in mammalian cells. Eur J Biochem 2002;269:5360–5368.
6. Proud CG. Minireview: Regulation of mammalian translation factors by nutrients. Eur J Biochem 2002;269:5338–5349.
7. Sonenberg N, Hershey JWB, Mathews MB, eds. Translational Control of Gene Expression, vol. 39. New York: Cold Spring Harbor Laboratory, 2000.
8. Kimball SR, Farrell PA, Jefferson LS. Invited review: role of insulin in translational control of protein synthesis in skeletal muscle by amino acids and exercise. J Appl Physiol 2002;93:1168–1180.
9. Bolster DR, Crozier SJ, Kimball SR, et al. AMP-activated protein kinase suppresses protein synthesis in rat skeletal muscle through down-regulated mammalian target of rapamycin (mTOR) signaling. J Biol Chem 2002;277:23977–23980.
10. Bylund-Fellenius AC, Ojamaa KM, Flaim KE, et al. Protein synthesis versus energy state in contracting muscles of perfused rat hindlimb. Am J Physiol 1984;246:E297–E305.
11. Baar K, Esser K. Phosphorylation of p70S6k correlates with increased skeletal muscle mass following resistance exercise. Am J Physiol 1999;276:C120–C127.
12. Bolster DR, Kubica N, Crozier SJ, et al. Immediate response of mTOR-mediated signaling following acute resistance exercise in rat skeletal muscle. J Physiol (Lond) 2003;553:213–220.
13. Chen YW, Nader GA, Baar KR, et al. Response of rat muscle to acute resistance exercise defined by transcriptional and translational profiling. J Physiol (Lond) 2002;545:27–41.
14. Hernandez JM, Fedele MJ, Farrell PA. Time course evaluation of protein synthesis and glucose uptake after acute resistance exercise in rats. J Appl Physiol 2000;88:1142–1149.
15. Bodine SC, Stitt TN, Gonzalez M, et al. AKT/mTOR pathway is a crucial regulator of skeletal muscle hypertrophy and can prevent muscle atrophy in vivo. Nat Cell Biol 2001;3:1014–1019.
16. Wagenmakers AJM. Tracers to investigate protein and amino acid metabolism in human subjects. Proc Nutr Soc 1999;58:987–1000.
17. Attaix D, Taillandier D. The critical role of the ubiquitin-proteasome pathway in muscle wasting in comparison to lysosomal and Ca++-dependent systems. In Bittar EE, Rivett AJ, eds. Intracellular protein degradation. Greenwich, CT: JAI Press Inc. Adv Mol Cell Biol 1998;27:235–266.
18. Attaix D, Combaret L, Kee AJ, et al. Mechanisms of ubiquitination and proteasome-dependent proteolysis in skeletal muscle. In Zempleni J Daniel H, eds. Molecular nutrition. Wallingford, UK: CABI, 2003, 219–235.
19. Hasselgren PO, Wray C, Mammen J. Molecular regulation of muscle cachexia: it may be more than the proteasome. Biochem Biophys Res Comm 2002;290:1–10.
20. Lecker SH, Solomon V, Mitch WE, et al. Muscle protein breakdown and the critical role of the ubiquitin-proteasome pathway in normal and disease states. J Nutr 1999;129:227S–237S.
21. Stupka, N, Tarnopolsky MA, Yardley NJ, et al. Cellular adaptation to repeated eccentric exercise-induced muscle damage. J Appl Physiol 2001;91:1669–1678.
22. Kee AJ, Taylor AJ, Carlsson AR, et al. IGF-1 has no effect on postexercise suppression of the ubiquitin-proteasome system in rat skeletal muscle. J Appl Physiol 2002;92:2277–2284.
23. Bodine SC, Latres E, Baumhueter S, et al. Identification of ubiquitin ligases required for skeletal muscle atrophy. Science 2001;294:1704–1708.
24. Ordway GA, Neufer PD, Chin ER, et al. Chronic contractile activity upregulates the proteasome system in rabbit muscle. J Appl Physiol 2000;88:1134–1141.
25. Taillandier D, Aurousseau E, Combaret L, et al. Regulation of proteolysis during reloading of the unweighted soleus muscle. Int J Biochem Cell Biol 2003;35:665–675.
26. Liu Z, Barrett EJ. Human protein metabolism: its measurement and regulation. Am J Physiol 2002;283:E1105–E112.
27. Biolo G, Tipton KD, Klein S, et al. An abundant supply of amino acids enhances the metabolic effect of exercise on muscle protein. Am J Physiol 1997;273:E122–E129.
28. Wolfe RR, Goodenough RD, Wolfe MH, et al. Isotopic analysis of leucine and urea metabolism in exercising humans. J Appl Physiol 1982;52:458–466.
29. Van Hall G, Saltin B, Wagenmakers AJM. Muscle protein degradation and amino acid metabolism during prolonged knee-extensor exercise in humans. Clin Sci 1999;97:557–567.
30. Chesley A, MacDougall JD, Tarnopolsky MA, et al. Changes in human muscle protein synthesis after resistance exercise. J Appl Physiol 1992;73:1383–1388.
31. Phillips SM, Tipton KD, Aarsland A, et al. Mixed muscle protein synthesis and breakdown after resistance exercise in humans. Am J Physiol 1997;273:E99–E107.

32. Roy BD, Tarnopolski MA, MacDougall JD, et al. Effect of glucose supplement timing on protein metabolism after resistance training. J Appl Physiol 1997;82: 1882–1888.

33. Tipton KD, Borsheim E, Wolf SE, et al. Acute response of net muscle protein balance reflects 24–h balance after exercise and amino acid ingestion. Am J Physiol 2003;284: E76–E89.

34. Miller SL, Tipton KD, Chinkes DL, et al. Independent and combined effects of amino acids and glucose after resistance exercise. Med Sci Sports Exerc 2003;35:449–455.

35. Esmarck B, Andersen JL, Olsen S, et al. Timing of postexercise protein intake is important for muscle hypertrophy with resistance training in elderly humans. J Physiol (Lond) 2001;535:301–311.

36. Wagenmakers AJM. The primary target of nutritional support: body composition or muscle function? Nestlé Nutr Workshop Ser Clin Perform Programme 2002;7:219–234.

37. Cheng KN, Dworzak F, Ford GC, et al. Direct determination of leucine metabolism and protein breakdown in humans using L-[1–13C, 15N]-leucine and the forearm model. Eur J Clin Invest 1985;15(6):349–354.

CHAPTER 21

Mitochondrial Biogenesis Induced by Endurance Training

DAVID A. HOOD AND ISABELLA IRRCHER

Introduction

Research over the past decade has provided us with a remarkable increase in our understanding of the relevance of structure, function, and biogenesis of mitochondria. Mitochondria, long known for their vital roles in cellular energy production, are now established participants in cell signaling events leading to apoptosis (programmed cell death). Moreover, it is now recognized that mitochondrial dysfunction, brought about by either nuclear or mitochondrial DNA (mtDNA) mutations, can lead to a bewildering array of pathophysiological conditions affecting the nervous system, the heart, and/or skeletal muscle. Thus, cell biologists and clinicians alike have become keenly interested in how mitochondrial function and dysfunction contribute to cell signaling and maladaptation. In skeletal muscle, the term *muscle plasticity* was coined (1) to describe the remarkable capability of this tissue to alter its gene expression profile and phenotype in response to changes in functional demand. The first convincing demonstration that mitochondrial content in muscle had the potential to increase in response to a change in functional demand (endurance training) was provided by John Holloszy (2) (See Milestone of Discovery). Contractile-activity–induced adaptations in muscle are highly specific and depend upon the type of exercise (i.e., dynamic or resistance), as well as

its frequency, intensity, and duration. It is now well established that repeated bouts of endurance exercise interspersed with recovery periods result in altered expression of a wide variety of gene products, leading to an altered muscle phenotype and improved fatigue resistance (3–5). This improved endurance is highly correlated with the increase in muscle mitochondrial density and enzyme activity. In addition, it has been established for many years that conditions of muscle disuse (e.g., microgravity, denervation, immobilization, sedentary lifestyle, and aging) lead to diminished mitochondrial content and compromised energy production. These findings are very important for exercise physiologists interested in the cellular basis of endurance performance and are of practical importance for athletes in training programs. Perhaps more important, this adaptive mitochondrial content permits us to be optimistic about the role of training in ameliorating the functional capacity of previously sedentary individuals, in altering processes that lead to cell death and myonuclear decay, and in reversing the pathophysiology of mitochondrial disease in skeletal muscle. Thus, the synthesis of mitochondria induced by chronic exercise is now recognized to have implications for a broader range of health issues than the enhancement of athletic performance. In addition, the process itself can serve as a valuable cellular model of organelle assembly within eukaryotic cells. Our understanding of the mechanisms of mitochondrial adaptation, broadly termed *mitochondrial biogenesis,* has progressed rapidly in recent years. This is because of the following:

1. The remarkable advances in molecular biology
2. The increased use of animal and cell culture models to study mitochondrial adaptations
3. Improvements in microscopy techniques, which permit better resolution of organelle structure and function
4. The development of techniques that permit measures of mitochondrial function and gene expression in single cells or in homogeneous cell populations (3)

This chapter describes the established cellular mechanisms involved in mitochondrial biogenesis and their physiological relevance.

Physiology of Muscle Mitochondrial Biogenesis

Mitochondrial biogenesis can be induced by dynamic exercise (endurance training). Skeletal muscle falls into three classes of fibers based on metabolic and contractile properties:

1. Slow-twitch red (STR) fibers containing largely the myosin heavy chain (MHC) type I isoform
2. Fast-twitch red (FTR) fibers containing mainly MHC type IIA isoforms
3. Fast-twitch white (FTW) fibers, possessing mainly MHC type IIB or IIX isoforms, depending on the species

Each of these muscle fiber types has a varying steady-state mitochondrial content that contributes to the intensity of their red appearance and their endurance capacity. In humans, the STR fibers have the largest-volume fraction of mitochondria, followed by FTR and FTW fibers, respectively (4). Although considerable overlap exists, there is an approximate threefold to fourfold difference in the capacity for oxidative metabolism between red and white muscle. Repeated bouts of dynamic exercise in the form of endurance training can induce increases in the mitochondrial content of all three muscle fibers types (6), provided that the training program has been tailored toward the recruitment of fast motor units containing the type IIA and IIX muscle fibers. Mitochondrial adaptations will not occur in muscle fibers that are not recruited during the exercise bout, consistent with the idea that mitochondrial biogenesis produced by exercise is initiated by stimuli within the contracting muscle, independent of humoral influences.

Endurance training in humans and other mammals can produce an increase in mitochondrial content usually ranging from 30 to 100% within about 4–6 wk. This results in improved endurance performance that is largely independent of the much smaller 10–20% training-induced changes in $\dot{V}O_{2max}$ (7). The extent of the increase in mitochondrial content in muscle cells depends upon the initial mito-

chondrial content. A muscle fiber with a low-oxidative white phenotype (FTW, type IIB or IIX fiber) will increase its mitochondrial content by a greater amount than a FTR (type IIA) muscle fiber (8). The conversion of phenotype from a white muscle to one with a visibly red appearance is brought about by enhanced synthesis of the red pigment heme and its incorporation into myoglobin and mitochondrial cytochromes.

Mitochondrial biogenesis can be replicated using models of simulated exercise, such as chronic contractile activity produced by electrical stimulation of the motor nerve. This model has the advantage of producing relatively large changes in mitochondrial biogenesis that can occur in a shorter time (1–4 wk) (8). Thus, both chronic endurance exercise training and chronic stimulation are commonly used to study the cellular processes involved in mitochondrial biogenesis. In addition, recently developed culture models of muscle contraction can provide insight. Chronically stimulated cardiac (9) or skeletal muscle myocytes (10) have more recently been used to advantage in describing some of the gene expression responses which precede mitochondrial biogenesis. In this chapter, the term *chronic contractile activity* describes the role and effects of exercise in all of these experimental models with an appreciation for the limitations and advantages of each technique.

Mitochondrial Subfractions Exist in Skeletal Muscle

Electron microscopic views of both cardiac cells and skeletal muscle fibers has revealed that the mitochondrial reticulum is distributed primarily in two distinct geographic locations: concentrated under the sarcolemma, termed subsarcolemmal (SS) mitochondria, and interspersed throughout the myofibrils, called intermyofibrillar (IMF) mitochondria (Fig. 21.1, *A* and *B*) (35).

Although fiber types and species differ, the relative proportion of IMF mitochondria is usually at least 75% of the total mitochondrial volume. The functional role of these subfractions in delivering adenosine triphosphate (ATP) for compartmentalized energy utilization continues to remain speculative. However, these subfractions differ in their adaptability to a stimulus (e.g., training), suggesting that their location within the cell makes them differentially sensitive to a common cellular signal. Variations in chronic muscle use and disuse have revealed that SS mitochondria consistently adapt to a greater degree, or sooner, than IMF mitochondria. When isolated from cells and studied *in vitro,* these subfractions exhibit an inherent difference in the rate of oxygen consumption (34). In isolated mitochondria, oxygen consumption is usually measured in the absence of adenosine diphosphate (ADP) (resting respiration, termed state 4) and in the presence of nonlimiting amounts of ADP (activated respiration, termed state 3). State 3 and 4 respiration rates are approximately 2.5 times greater in IMF than in SS mito-

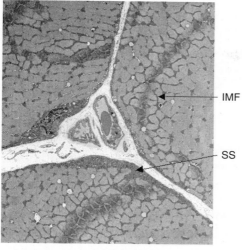

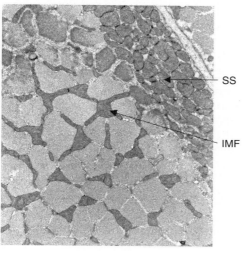

FIGURE 21.1 Electron micrograph of a cross-section of human skeletal muscle. Mitochondria are divided into two separate subfractions in skeletal muscle. **A.** Lower magnification of three muscle fibers adjoining a capillary. **B.** Higher magnification of a single muscle fiber. Note the different cellular locations and shapes of subsarcolemmal (SS) and intermyofibrillar (IMF) mitochondria. SS mitochondria are concentrated below the sarcolemma; IMF mitochondria are distributed between myofibrils. *(Modified with permission from Hoppeler H. Kraft- und Ausdauertraining: funktionelle und strukturelle Grundlagen. In Der Muskel. Medizinisch Literarische Verlagsgesellschaft. Uelzen: MBH (Medical Literary), 1989;9–17.)*

myonuclei and to a differential capacity of each mitochondrial subfraction for protein synthesis and import (discussed later in the chapter).

Mitochondrial Composition Can Change in Response to Contractile Activity

Mitochondrial content can be measured directly, using morphometric estimates of organelle volume in relation to total cellular volume. More commonly, and with much less effort, mitochondrial content is estimated by the change in maximal activity of a typical marker enzyme such as citrate synthase or by the change in content of a protein like cytochrome *c*. This is valid under most conditions because changes in mitochondrial volumes estimated morphometrically parallel the changes in enzyme $\dot{V}_{max}$ values (8). The measurement of single proteins or enzyme activities has been useful for determining rates of mitochondrial turnover, assuming that the behavior of the protein resembles that of the organelle as a whole. The caveat in this approach is the recognition that mitochondrial protein composition can be altered in response to chronic exercise, particularly during the imposition of additional confounding situations, such as iron deficiency or mitochondrial disease.

Mitochondrial proteins turn over with a half-life of about 1 wk following the onset of a new level of muscle contractile activity (e.g., greater intensity, duration, or frequency per week) (12). Mitochondrial phospholipid content changes occur with an even shorter half-life (about 4 days), suggesting that the assembly and/or degradation of the organelle could be initiated by changes in phospholipid composition. In the absence of normal rates of cytochrome synthesis and incorporation into the inner membrane during iron deficiency, imposed contractile activity appears to lead to continued membrane lipid synthesis, producing an increased mitochondrial volume with a markedly reduced and abnormal protein content. These data point to the independent synthesis of proteins and phospholipids during contractile-activity–induced mitochondrial biogenesis.

Mitochondrial Content Can Influence Metabolism During Dynamic Exercise

The increased endurance performance that results from mitochondrial biogenesis is a consequence of changes in muscle metabolism during exercise. At the onset of exercise, the calcium-induced activation of myosin adenosine triphosphatase (ATPase) results in an elevated concentration of free ADP (ADP_f; Fig. 21.2). This molecule serves to activate the following:

1. The creatine phosphokinase (CPK) reaction toward the formation of ATP and creatine
2. Glycolysis
3. State 3 mitochondrial respiration

chondria. The resulting ATP concentration inside the organelle is about twofold greater in IMF mitochondria (11). The reasons for this difference in respiration rate may be related to their divergent enzyme and lipid compositions. In turn, these biochemical and physiological differences may be due to the local proximity of SS mitochondria to peripheral

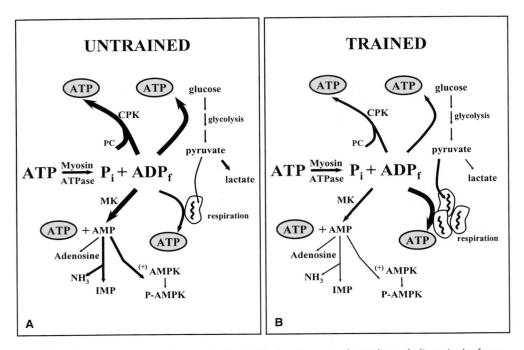

FIGURE 21.2 **A.** Acute exercise in untrained individuals triggers accelerated metabolism via the formation of ADP_f by the myosin ATPase reaction. ADP_f simultaneously activates the creatine phosphokinase (CPK) reaction, glycolytic flux, and mitochondrial respiration to maintain ATP levels constant. Two molecules of ADP_f can be converted to ATP and AMP in the myokinase (MK) reaction. In fast-twitch muscle fibers, AMP is metabolized to inosine monophosphate (IMP) and ammonia (NH_3) by AMP deaminase. In slow-twitch muscle fibers, AMP is largely converted to adenosine. The increase in AMP and the drop in PC activate AMP kinase (AMPK) activity. **B.** Acute exercise elicits the same response in an endurance-trained individual. However, the trained muscle has a greater mitochondrial content as a result of organelle biogenesis, with very little change in the V_{max} of key reactions in other pathways. Thus, more ATP can be provided via mitochondrial respiration. This reduces the consumption of phosphocreatine (PC), attenuates the rate of glycolysis and lactic acid production, reduces the formation of AMP and NH_3, and decreases the activation of AMPK. This, along with the concomitant training-induced increase in mitochondrial fatty acid oxidation enzymes, promotes carbohydrate sparing and enhances endurance performance. Line thicknesses illustrate approximate shifts from one pathway to another with training.

Since endurance training increases the mitochondrial content of skeletal muscle without effects on CPK or glycolytic enzymes, the result is that a greater fraction of the energy required at a given exercise intensity will be derived from mitochondrial metabolism, and a lower concentration of ADP_f will be required to attain the same level of oxygen consumption. This lower ADP_f concentration at a given $\dot{V}O_2$ will reduce the rates of glycolysis and lactic acid formation, lower rates of adenosine monophosphate (AMP) formation, and phosphocreatine sparing (13). Reduced synthesis of AMP should lead to lower allosteric activation of phosphorylase and spare glycogen. In addition, the activation of AMP kinase should be attenuated, reducing signal transduction that mediates the translocation of GLUT4 to the plasma membrane. These adaptations, along with increased activities of mitochondrial β-oxidation enzymes, predispose the individual toward greater lipid and less carbohydrate oxidation during exercise and enhance endurance performance.

Overview of the Cellular Events in Mitochondrial Biogenesis

The morphological manifestation of mitochondrial biogenesis produced by multiple exercise bouts performed over several weeks can be visualized by electron microscopy as an expansion of the mitochondrial reticulum in both subsarcolemmal and intermyofibrillar regions of each muscle fiber. However, the requirement for weeks of training to achieve this new steady-state mitochondrial content is not a reflection of the early molecular events that ultimately lead to those measurable morphological changes. The final phenotypic adaptation is the cumulative result of a complex series of events that begins with the first bout of exercise in a training program. The time between the onset of the first exercise bout and the ultimate mitochondrial adaptation is characterized by intermittent contraction-induced signaling events. These signals are known to activate protein kinases and phosphatases that modify the activity of transcription factors within the nucleus and mRNA stability factors within the cytosol, resulting in an increase in the mRNA expression of nuclear-encoded mitochondrial proteins (NEMPs) (Fig. 21.3).

Following translation, the NEMPs are chaperoned to the mitochondria and imported into the different compartments, such as the matrix space or the inner or outer membrane. A small subgroup of NEMPs are transcription factors that act directly on mtDNA to increase the mRNA expression of mitochondrial gene products and mtDNA copy number. mtDNA is tiny by genomic standards (16.6 kb), but it is critical because it encodes vital proteins involved in the mitochondrial respiratory chain. Because mtDNA contains no introns (intervening, noncoding DNA sequences within a gene), point mutations within the genome have severe consequences. Thus, to

produce an organelle that is functional in providing cellular ATP, contractile-activity–induced mitochondrial biogenesis requires (*a*) the integration of a multitude of contraction-induced cellular signals and (*b*) the cooperative and timely expression of the nuclear and mitochondrial genomes.

Cellular Mechanisms of Mitochondrial Biogenesis

Contractile Activity Initiates Cell Signaling Events

The molecular signals linking acute exercise responses to subsequent long-term increases in mitochondrial content are beginning to be defined. The intensity and duration of the

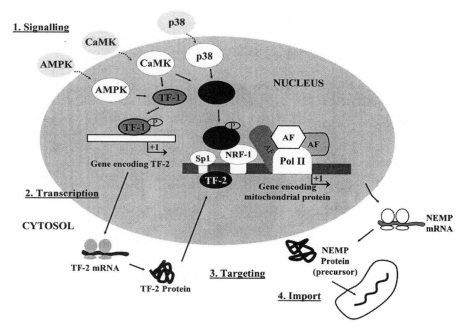

FIGURE 21.3　Muscle contraction initiates cell signals, which activate protein kinases, such as p38, AMPK, and calmodulin kinase (CaMK). Once activated, these kinases can translocate to the nucleus to phosphorylate transcription factors. In a hypothetical example, transcription factor-1 (TF-1) is activated by phosphorylation, which enhances its DNA binding activity. TF-1 subsequently affects the rate of transcription of other transcription factors (e.g., TF-2). Once TF-2 mRNA is produced, it is exported and translated into TF-2 protein in the cytosol. It can then be targeted to the nucleus to modify the rate of transcription of genes which encode mitochondrial proteins. In a more specific case, exercise is known to affect the expression of the transcription factors Specificity protein 1 (Sp1) and nuclear respiratory factor-1 (NRF-1), as well as the coactivator peroxisome proliferator–activated receptor (PPAR) γ-coactivator-1α (PGC-1α). These alter the transcription rates of nuclear genes encoding mitochondrial proteins by directly interacting with the basal transcription machinery. This multi-subunit enzyme complex consists of the RNA polymerase II (Pol II) and a number of associated factors (AF). The mRNA representing the nuclear-encoded mitochondrial protein (NEMP) is translated into protein in the cytosol and targeted to the mitochondria via molecular chaperones, followed by import into the organelle (Fig. 21.5).

contractile effort determines the magnitude of the signal or signals. This signaling can affect the following:

1. The activation or inhibition of transcription factors
2. The activation or inhibition of mRNA stability factors that mediate changes in mRNA degradation
3. Alterations in translational efficiency
4. The posttranslational modification of proteins
5. Changes in the kinetics of the transport of newly made proteins from the cytosol into the mitochondria (protein import)
6. Alterations in the rate of folding or assembly of proteins into multi-subunit complexes

Signaling to these cellular events likely occurs via a variety of enzymatic processes, but the most commonly studied ones are those mediated by the activation of protein kinases and phosphatases, which covalently modify proteins by phosphorylation and dephosphorylation, respectively. Exercise is now known to be a potent activator of these enzymes (14). Among those discussed later in the chapter that appear to be involved in mitochondrial biogenesis include protein kinase C (PKC), calcium/calmodulin-dependent protein kinase (CaMK), p38 mitogen-activated protein (MAP) kinase, and AMP-activated protein kinase (AMPK) (Fig. 21.3).

There is now strong evidence for the participation of intracellular Ca^{++} fluxes and ATP turnover as interacting triggers of mitochondrial biogenesis at the onset of exercise (discussed later in the chapter). Despite the evidence favoring these two stimuli, much research remains to be done within the context of exercise or contractile activity models. This is because the experimental models used to produce mitochondrial biogenesis are limited by the fact that they typically involve not exercise but other methods (e.g., transgenic animals or overexpression studies in cell culture) in which changes in ATP turnover or Ca^{++} levels can be elicited in a dramatic fashion. Nonetheless, these studies have provided valuable insight into the contribution of these signals to mitochondrial biogenesis.

ATP Turnover

Exercise increases the rate of ATP turnover within muscle cells. This alters the ratio of ATP to ADP_f and stimulates muscle metabolic rate. A similar change in energy status can be achieved without exercise through the uncoupling of the mitochondrial respiratory chain, by mtDNA depletion, with iron deficiency, by genetic disruption of the creatine phosphokinase system, or with prolonged use of the agent β-guanadinopropionic acid (β-GPA). The rise in muscle AMP levels and the decreases in phosphocreatine and ATP concentrations associated with these conditions lead to the activation of AMPK. AMPK can also be activated pharmacologically using the adenosine analogue 5-aminoimidazole-4-carboxamide-1-β-D-ribofuranoside (AICAR). This drug is frequently used to mimic the metabolic effects of chronic exercise in muscle. AMPK activation via AICAR treatment of animals increased mitochondrial enzyme activities, while activation of the enzyme using chronic β-GPA increased the expression of downstream targets, including cytochrome c and δ-aminolevulinic acid synthase (ALAs). Cytochrome c is an important component of the electron transport chain, while ALAs is the rate-limiting enzyme in the synthesis of heme, the cytochrome prosthetic group. These downstream effects are probably mediated by an increase in activation of the transcription factor nuclear respiratory factor-1 (NRF-1) (discussed later) and its subsequent binding to a DNA sequence in the promoter regions of these genes.

Calcium

Ca^{++} is released from the sarcoplasmic reticulum (SR) as a result of motor neuron–induced depolarization. Ca^{++} then mediates actin and myosin interaction and muscle contraction. It also acts as a second messenger to couple the initial electrical events to subsequent alterations in gene expression. Disturbances in mitochondrial ATP production, evident from studies of mtDNA depletion or in mitochondrial myopathy patients, also result in elevated intracellular Ca^{++} levels. These Ca^{++} changes modify the activities of a multitude of calcium-dependent protein kinases and phosphatases, including CaMK, PKC, and calcineurin, among others. In the early 1980s it was noted that treatment of muscle cells in culture with the drug A23187 could produce an increase in mitochondrial enzyme activities. A23187 is an ionophore, an agent that increases the permeability of membranes to specific ions. In this case, A23187 specifically increases the intracellular concentration of Ca^{++}. In contrast to this, a reduction of extracellular Ca^{++}, which may ultimately have affected intracellular Ca^{++} stores, resulted in lowered mitochondrial enzyme levels. More recently it was shown that an increase in the mRNA and protein expression of mitochondrial enzymes, the electron transport chain component cytochrome c, and the important transcriptional coactivator PGC-1α (15) could be produced in muscle cells using continuous exposure of muscle cells to A23187. Furthermore, the intermittent exposure of muscle cells to ionomycin, another Ca^{++} ionophore, or to caffeine, which stimulates the release of Ca^{++} from the SR, also produced mitochondrial biogenesis. Finally, transgenic mice selectively expressing a constitutively active form of CaMK IV in muscle showed an increase in mtDNA copy number and expression of a wide variety of genes involved in mitochondrial biogenesis. These included gene products directly involved in oxidative phosphorylation, fatty acid metabolism, and PGC-1α (16). These data imply that Ca^{++} released from the SR during each action potential could serve as an important second messenger leading to mitochondrial biogenesis. However, the amplitude, duration, and temporal pattern of the Ca^{++} signals necessary to provoke such changes must be established under more physiological conditions.

In summary, the findings to date suggest that alteration of the energy status of the muscle cell (e.g., contractile activity) simultaneously brings about activation of AMPK and modifies intracellular Ca^{++} levels. It is likely that both of these signaling pathways are instrumental in producing mitochondrial biogenesis, likely via the transcriptional coactivator PGC-1α.

Contractile Activity Affects Transcription of Nuclear Genes Encoding Mitochondrial Proteins

The regulation of gene expression is a highly dynamic process involving alterations in gene transcription (the synthesis of mRNA from DNA) or posttranscriptional events. Central to the basis of gene transcription, which is initiated in the nucleus, is the activity and expression of proteins known as transcription factors (Fig. 21.3). Transcription factors regulate transcription by interacting and binding directly to specific DNA sequences within the regulatory regions of target genes the promoter region), generally found upstream of the transcription start site. Most eukaryotic protein-coding genes, including those involved in mitochondrial biogenesis, are encoded by the nuclear genome and transcribed by the RNA polymerase II multi-subunit enzyme complex. Recruitment of this enzyme complex to the promoter DNA sequences, along with interaction of transcription factors that also bind DNA and modify RNA polymerase activity, forms the basic transcriptional platform from which a change in gene expression can occur.

Numerous transcription factors have been implicated in mediating the physiological and metabolic adaptations associated with adaptations to contractile activity. Those involved in mitochondrial biogenesis include nuclear respiratory factors 1 and 2 (NRF-1, NRF-2), peroxisome proliferator–activated receptor-α and receptor-γ (PPAR-α and PPAR-γ), specificity protein 1 (Sp-1) and the products of the immediate early genes c-jun and c-fos (3,17). This variety of transcription factors appears to be required to satisfy the diverse nucleotide composition found in the upstream region of nuclear genes encoding mitochondrial proteins. Contractile activity has been shown to induce increases in the mRNA and/or protein levels of several transcription factors, consistent with their roles in mediating phenotypic changes as a result of chronic exercise. The fact that these transcription factors are sequentially activated in response to contractile activity supports their involvement in the cellular adaptations that result. For example, both contractile activity in vitro (9) and exercise in vivo have been shown to induce NRF-1 mRNA expression. This precedes the expression of cytochrome c mRNA, a NRF-1 target gene often used as an indicator of mitochondrial adaptations (discussed later in the chapter).

Within mitochondria are several hundred NEMPs that contribute to organelle function. Inspection of the promoter regions of several genes encoding NEMPs reveals that they have considerable sequence variability, meaning that they do not all bind the same transcription factors. This variability suggests that a coordinated up-regulation of nuclear gene transcription in response to a stimulus like exercise could potentially be difficult to achieve in the absence of a universal regulatory protein. One element that appears to be common to many promoters is the binding site for Sp-1, and contractile activity increases the level of Sp-1 and its binding to that site within the cytochrome c promoter (10). However, other evidence suggests that Sp-1 may be a negative regulator of transcription in some but not all genes. Thus, the expression of NEMPs in response to contractile activity could not possibly be coordinately up-regulated if Sp-1 acted alone to produce the transcriptional effect. Neither is the dilemma solved by the action of NRF-1, since many but not all nuclear genes encoding mitochondrial proteins possess NRF-1 sites within their promoters.

An alternative molecular mechanism by which a coordinated up-regulation of NEMPs could be achieved is by the action of proteins that act as coactivators of gene transcription. These proteins do not bind DNA directly but affect gene transcription through protein–protein interactions with DNA-binding transcription factors such as NRF-1. In this respect, the recently discovered coactivator of transcription factors termed PPARγ coactivator-1α (PGC-1α) (Fig. 21.3) has emerged as an important regulator of numerous cellular processes, including adaptive thermogenesis in adipocytes, gluconeogenic capacity in hepatocytes, and skeletal muscle fiber specialization (18,19). In addition, it appears to be vital for the orchestration of mitochondrial biogenesis in a variety of tissues. Several studies in which PGC-1α has been artificially overexpressed have documented the potential role of PGC-1α to coordinate the expression of both the nuclear and the mitochondrial genomes, leading to mitochondrial biogenesis in muscle, heart, and adipocytes. This effect appears to be mediated in part by its strong coactivation of a variety of transcription factors, including NRF-1. This leads to increased levels of several NEMPs, including mitochondrial transcription factor A (Tfam). This protein is vital for expression of the mitochondrial genome, and its induction provokes an increase in mtDNA transcription and replication (discussed later in the chapter). The result is that PGC-1α overexpression can produce an overall increase in mitochondrial content and cellular oxygen consumption (20).

What role does PGC-1α have with increased contractile activity? Several recent studies have reported that PGC-1α mRNA and protein are increased as a relatively early event in skeletal muscle as a result of increased contractile activity. The increase in PGC-1α expression is coincident with enhanced levels of NRF-1 and Tfam, and prior to increases in cytochrome c oxidase (COX) activity in contracting muscle

(15). Surprisingly, PGC-1α protein expression was also increased in response to 5 days of thyroid hormone treatment in a variety of tissues, including both slow- and fast-twitch muscle fiber types (15). This result suggests that PGC-1α may be a common link between these two divergent stimuli that lead to organelle biogenesis.

Contractile Activity Affects mRNA Stability

The stability of mRNA, or its resiliency to degradation by cytosolic RNAses, has emerged as an important regulatory component of gene expression. This cellular mechanism can be as effective as alterations in gene transcription in mediating increases in specific mRNA levels. However, it generates much less scientific attention than the events of gene transcription, in part because the methods for its assessment are less familiar. mRNA levels are a function of the rate of production (i.e., gene transcription) and the rate of degradation (i.e., mRNA stability). The stability of mRNA is usually mediated by protein factors that interact at the 3′ end of the transcript to either stabilize or destabilize the mRNA. These are expressed in a tissue-specific fashion, leading to wide variations in the stability of mRNA across tissues. In general, nuclear transcripts encoding mitochondrial proteins appear to be least stable in liver and most stable in skeletal muscle. For example, the mRNA encoding ALAs, the heme metabolism enzyme, has a very short half-life ($t_{1/2}$) of 22 minutes in liver but has a $t_{1/2}$ of approximately 14 hours in skeletal muscle. Thus, mRNA stabilization may have the greatest consequence for mitochondrial biogenesis in liver, since modest increases in stability can have a marked effect on mRNA levels in this tissue.

A unique finding was obtained several years ago by Chrzanowska-Lightowlers and associates (21). Using a liver-derived cell line, they demonstrated that inhibition of mitochondrial protein synthesis led to a widespread increase in the stability of nuclear-derived mRNAs encoding mitochondrial proteins, while no effect was observed on transcripts that were mitochondrially encoded. This suggested that a reduction in mitochondrial protein synthesis, which disrupts the assembly of the respiratory chain, leads to enhanced activity of cytosolic RNA binding proteins, which protect nuclear transcripts from degradation, and results in increased mRNA levels. Interestingly, a marked up-regulation of mRNAs derived from multiple nuclear genes encoding mitochondrial proteins is also observed in cells with respiratory impairment brought about by mtDNA depletion and in patients with mtDNA mutations. The common feature of these diverse conditions is probably the reduced energy status of the cell or possibly the increase in reactive oxygen species (ROS) produced when the electron transport chain is inhibited. The data suggest that deleterious modifications in respiratory chain structure leading to reduced function (i.e., decreased ATP supply) relative to normal may be a signal for the up-regulation of nuclear-encoded mRNAs encoding mi-

tochondrial proteins. The data lend further support to the idea that a metabolically derived signal related to ATP turnover is involved in mediating mitochondrial biogenesis.

Contractile Activity–Induced Increases in Cytochrome C Expression Are Mediated by Changes in Transcription and mRNA Stability

Cytochrome *c* has long been used as an indicator of muscle mitochondrial adaptations. Its expression is decreased by muscle disuse and increased by thyroid hormone during development and by variations in exercise intensity and duration. The rat cytochrome *c* promoter has been shown to contain NRF-1 and Sp-1 binding elements and a site resembling a cyclic AMP response element (CRE) that binds the CRE-binding protein CREB (Fig. 21.4). These appear to be the most important determinants of cytochrome *c* transcription (17).

Experiments in cell culture and *in vivo* have revealed insights into the regulation of cytochrome *c* expression during contractile activity. Electrical stimulation of neonatal cardiac myocytes in culture resulted in an increase in cytochrome *c* mRNA after 48 hours. This was preceded by an increase in transcriptional activation at about 12 hours of stimulation. The stimulation effect was markedly attenuated if the NRF-1 site or the CRE was mutated. Both basal transcription and the magnitude of the stimulation response were also reduced if the Sp-1 site was mutated (9). These data illustrate the importance of NRF-1, Sp-1 and c-Jun (which binds to the CRE in this case) in the transcriptional activation of cytochrome *c* in heart cells.

Additional studies *in vivo* have examined cytochrome *c* expression in skeletal muscle and have revealed roles for contractile-activity–induced changes in both gene transcription and mRNA stability. Gene transcription *in vivo* has often been assessed using direct injection of plasmid DNA. A plasmid is a circular DNA molecule normally found in bacteria. Using conventional molecular biology techniques, it is possible to isolate plasmid DNA, cut the DNA at specific sites using restriction endonuclease enzymes, and insert a fragment of DNA encoding a foreign gene (e.g., a reporter gene). Reporter genes encode enzymes, such as firefly luciferase, that are not normally expressed in the tissue being studied. These genes are typically inserted into the plasmid at a site distal to the promoter of the gene of interest (i.e., cytochrome *c*). Thus, when this recombined plasmid is injected into a tissue such as muscle, endogenous transcription factors bind to the promoter and increase the expression of the reporter enzyme, whose activity can be easily measured as an index of transcriptional activity in the cell.

Such a cytochrome *c* promoter–reporter DNA construct was injected into tibialis anterior muscles of animals undergoing unilateral chronic electrical stimulation (3 h to days) for 1–7 days (22). This technique, along with an mRNA decay assay *in vitro,* revealed time-dependent changes in

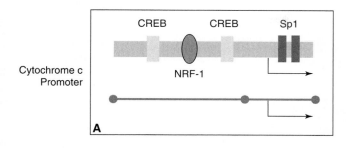

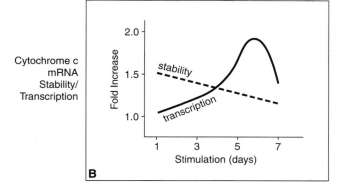

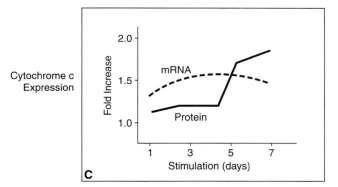

FIGURE 21.4 Regulation of cytochrome *c* expression. **A.** Important DNA sequence elements for the binding of transcription factors NRF-1, cAMP response element binding protein (CREB), and Sp1 in the regulatory region of the cytochrome *c* gene. The numbers indicate the general location of the sites relative to the transcription start site (+1). The Sp1 site is within the first intron of the gene, while the other sites are within the promoter region, upstream of the gene. **B.** Effect of 7 days of chronic stimulation–induced contractile activity (3 hours per day) on the relative changes (-fold above unstimulated) in cytochrome *c* mRNA stability and gene transcription. **C.** Effect of events in B on cytochrome *c* expression at the mRNA and protein levels. *(Data in B and C are reprinted with permission from Freyssenet D, Connor MK, Takahashi M, et al. Cytochrome c transcriptional activation and mRNA stability during contractile activity in skeletal muscle. Am J Physiol 1999;277: E26–E32.)*

both transcriptional activity and mRNA stability. The results indicated that the increase in cytochrome *c* mRNA observed as a result of chronic contractile activity was initially due to an induced increase in mRNA stability (2–4 days) and that this was followed by transcriptional activation leading to an increase in cytochrome *c* mRNA and protein (Fig. 21.4). Whether this sequence of events holds for other proteins of the mitochondrial inner membrane remains to be determined, but the data indicate that the cellular processes of transcription and mRNA stability have to be considered when contractile-induced changes in gene expression are observed.

Contractile Activity Affects Mitochondrial Protein Import

Description of the Protein Import Machinery

Of the hundreds of mitochondrial proteins within the organelle, only 13 are encoded by mtDNA. Therefore, an elaborate system transports nuclear-derived proteins from the cytosol into mitochondria (23) (Fig. 21.5), and this process is absolutely vital for organelle synthesis. The targeting pathway of these proteins depends on their ultimate location in the organelle (i.e., matrix, outer or inner membrane, intermembrane space). Many proteins are fabricated as precursor proteins with a signal sequence, often at the N-terminus. The most established and widely studied pathway is the one that directs proteins to the matrix space. In this case, the positively charged N-terminal signal sequence of the precursor interacts with a cytosolic molecular chaperone that unfolds it and directs it to the outer membrane import receptor complex, termed the translocase of the outer membrane (Tom complex) (Fig. 21.5). Cytosolic chaperones include heat shock protein 70 kDa (HSP70), mitochondrial import–stimulating factor (MSF), and possibly Tom34. Precursors are directed via these chaperones to either the Tom20 and Tom22 receptors or to the Tom70–Tom37 heterodimer. They are then transferred to Tom40 and the small Tom proteins 5, 6, and 7, which form an aqueous channel through which the precursor protein passes to be sorted to the outer membrane, the inner membrane, or to the translocase of the inner membrane (Tim complex). The key Tim complex proteins include Tim17, Tim23, and Tim44. Tim17 and Tim23 span the inner membrane and have domains associated with both the matrix and intermembrane space. In a manner analogous to the Tom complex, Tim17 and Tim23 bind the precursor protein and form a pore through which the precursor can travel. Upon emerging on the inner face of the inner membrane, the precursor is pulled into the matrix by the ratchetlike action of mitochondrial Hsp70 (mtHsp70). This protein is anchored to the inner membrane through its interaction with Tim44, a peripheral inner membrane protein. Along with these essential protein components of the

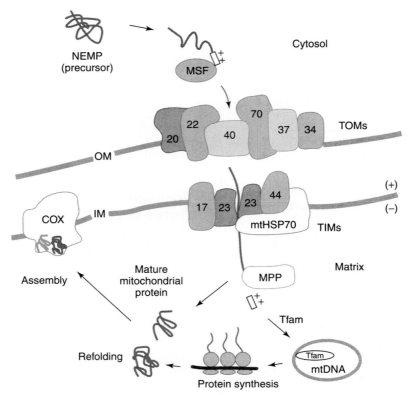

FIGURE 21.5 Nuclear-encoded mitochondrial proteins (NEMPs) synthesized in the cytosol are imported into mitochondria and can combine with mtDNA-encoded gene products to form multi-subunit complexes like cytochrome *c* oxidase (COX). Precursor proteins destined for the matrix of the mitochondria are made with a positively charged N-terminal presequence to which molecular chaperones bind. Chaperones such as mitochondrial import–stimulating factor (MSF) guide the precursor protein to the outer membrane translocase complex (Tom complex). The precursor protein is unfolded and directed through the outer membrane aqueous pore mainly consisting of Tom40. The precursor then interacts with the inner membrane phospholipid cardiolipin (not shown) and the translocase of the inner membrane (Tim complex). The matrix chaperone mitochondrial heat shock protein 70 (mtHSP70) pulls in the precursor, and the signal sequence is cleaved by the mitochondrial processing peptidase (MPP), forming the mature protein in the matrix. It is refolded by chaperonins heat shock protein 60 (HSP60) and chaperonin 10 (not shown). ATP is required for multiple steps during the import process, including cytosolic unfolding and mtHSP70-directed movements. The number within each import machinery component refers to its size in kilodaltons. Chronic contractile activity accelerates the import process, in part via the induction of important components of the import machinery, including MSF, Tom20, mtHSP70, and the refolding proteins HSP60 and chaperonin 10. An adaptive increase in the rate of transcription and translation within a muscle cell could also increase the rate of import by providing more precursor substrate for the translocation process. mtDNA transcription is initiated by mitochondrial transcription factor A (Tfam) binding to a DNA sequence in the regulatory D-loop region. mRNA transcripts are translated within the organelle (protein synthesis) to form a total of 13 proteins. These are incorporated directly into the respiratory chain as single proteins, or they combine with nuclear-encoded imported proteins to form multi-subunit complexes such as COX.

import machinery, the inner membrane phospholipid cardiolipin appears to be important for the protein translocation process. Its role is less well defined, but it seems to orient the precursor in the correct position for interaction with the Tim44–mtHsp70 complex. Once in the matrix, the N-terminal signal sequence of the precursor is cleaved by a mitochondrial processing peptidase to form the mature protein. It is then folded into its active conformation by the chaperonins heat shock protein 60 kDa (HSP60) and chaperonin 10 kDa (cpn10) (24).

Apart from the import machinery itself, the translocation process into the matrix requires the presence of an intact membrane potential ($\Delta\Psi$, negative inside) across the inner membrane to help pull the positively charged presequence into the matrix. In addition, ATP is required for cytosolic unfolding in the cytosol and for the action of mtHsp70 in the matrix. Thus, uncoupling agents that dissipate the membrane potential, or ATP depletion, reduce the rate of protein import. Conceivably, reductions in muscle cell ATP levels such as those produced by severe contractile activity or defects in ATP production that might be encountered in cells with mtDNA mutations could affect the rate of protein import into mitochondria.

Import Studies in Skeletal Muscle Mitochondria

Most of the pioneering work on the mitochondrial protein import pathway began in the late 1970s, mainly though the efforts of the laboratories of G. Schatz (Basel) and W. Neupert (Munich) using the yeast *Saccharomyces cerevisiae* and the fungus *Neurospora crassa*. More recently, this work has been extended to mammalian tissues, such as skeletal muscle and heart. The first studies performed with isolated muscle mitochondria indicated that the kinetics of precursor protein import into the matrix of skeletal muscle SS and IMF mitochondrial subfractions differed by about twofold. IMF mitochondria import precursor proteins more rapidly than SS mitochondria, and there is a close relationship between the rate of mitochondrial respiration and ATP production and the rate of protein import (11). This may contribute to the established differences in the biochemical characteristics of these mitochondrial subfractions.

Adaptations in the protein import machinery have relevance for mitochondrial biogenesis in both heart and skeletal muscle. In response to chronic contractile activity, a number of protein import machinery components are induced, up to approximately twofold. These include the cytosolic chaperones MSF and HSP70, the intramitochondrial proteins mtHSP70, HSP60, and cpn10, and the import receptors Tom20 and Tom34. Coincident with these changes are parallel contractile-activity–induced increases in the rate of import into the matrix (25). Tom20 appears to be particularly important in this respect, since experiments in muscle cells in which this outer membrane protein was artificially overexpressed and underexpressed led

to parallel concomitant changes in the rates of protein import. Interestingly, the contractile-activity effect that enhanced the rate of protein import into the matrix had no effect on import of proteins into the outer membrane. This differential targeting to mitochondrial compartments is likely an important factor in determining the compositional changes that occur in mitochondria in response to training (discussed earlier in the chapter). A very similar adaptation in the protein import pathway has been observed in cardiac mitochondria as result of thyroid hormone treatment. This indicates that the adaptive response is not unique to a contractile stimulus. Rather, it is common to other stimuli that increase mitochondrial biogenesis. What is the physiological value of this adaptation? First, the import step is critical to the synthesis of mitochondria. Second, the contractile-activity–induced increases in the capacity for protein import produce a population of mitochondria that is more sensitive to changes in precursor protein concentration. This could arise if upstream events such as transcription and translation were accelerated, a situation that would be advantageous for mitochondrial biogenesis at any given upstream production rate of cytosolic precursor proteins.

Recently, the first disease that can be solely attributed to a mutation in a component of the protein import machinery was identified. The protein closely resembles Tim8p, an intermembrane space protein involved in the import process (26). The mutation results in a neurodegenerative disorder characterized by muscle dystonia, sensorineural deafness, and blindness. Further progress in the study of protein import will be substantial as additional mammalian homologues of the import machinery are identified. The recent cloning of Tom22, Tom40, and members of the Tim machinery will be helpful in determining the functional roles of individual import machinery components during mitochondrial biogenesis, the relevance of import in additional mitochondrial diseases, and the possible role of increased contractile activity in improving protein import defects.

Contractile Activity Affects the Expression and Copy Number of mtDNA

One of the most fascinating aspects of mitochondrial synthesis is that it requires the cooperation of the nuclear and mitochondrial genomes (Figs. 21.5 and 21.6). Mitochondria are unique in the fact that they house multiple copies of a small circular DNA molecule (mtDNA) comprising 16,569 nucleotides. While mtDNA is minuscule in comparison to the 3 billion nucleotides found in the nuclear genome, it nonetheless contributes 13 mRNA, 22 tRNA, and 2 rRNA molecules that are essential for mitochondrial biogenesis and function. The 13 mRNA molecules all encode protein components of the respiratory chain, responsible for electron transport and ATP synthesis. The import of nuclear-encoded

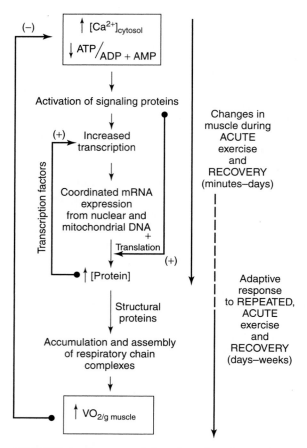

FIGURE 21.6 Summary of time-dependent changes in muscle cell signaling, gene expression, and assembly of multi-subunit proteins (e.g., COX), resulting in functional (increased $\dot{V}O_2$ per gram of muscle) and phenotypic (white to red) adaptations in muscle. Acute exercise increases intracellular calcium and accelerates the turnover of ATP. The magnitude of these signals depends on the intensity and duration of the exercise stimulus. Within minutes, these changes can activate signaling proteins (e.g., CaMK, AMPK) which covalently modify proteins involved in transcription, translation, or mRNA stability (not shown). The altered rates of transcription of nuclear and mitochondrial DNA result in the coordinated expression of mRNAs derived from both genomes. Over time, the mRNAs accumulate and are translated to protein, which becomes detectable after several days to weeks. The resulting proteins can contribute further to the adaptive changes in the pathway of gene expression (e.g., if they are synthesized as nuclear-encoded transcription factors), or they can be assembled into components of metabolic pathways within the organelle, such as Krebs cycle enzymes, cytochromes, or multi-subunit complexes of the respiratory chain. The resulting increased capacity for oxygen consumption (after several weeks of training) leads to the metabolic and performance alterations described in Fig. 21.2 and attenuates the exercise stress signal as mitochondrial biogenesis proceeds.

mtDNA maintenance proteins is necessary to transcribe and replicate this genome. These proteins include Tfam, mtRNA polymerase, DNA polymerase (POL-γ), single-stranded binding protein (mtSSB), RNA processing enzymes, and mitochondrial transcription factor B. Tfam has been studied most extensively because of its importance in both mtDNA transcription and replication. The level of Tfam correlates well with mtDNA abundance, and its loss, either in patients with mitochondrial myopathies or produced by experimental disruption of the Tfam gene, results in partial or total depletion of mtDNA. Homozygous Tfam knockout animals die prior to birth, and they are characterized by abnormal mitochondria and low rates of oxidative phosphorylation (27). Animals possessing heart- and muscle-specific disruptions of Tfam exhibit reduced levels of mtDNA and mtRNA, and they display characteristics found in the mitochondrial disease Kearns-Sayre syndrome, such as dilated cardiomyopathy, abnormal mitochondrial morphology, and atrioventricular conduction block. These data provide evidence for the importance of Tfam in normal cardiac function, perhaps because the heart possesses the highest amount of mitochondria of all tissues.

The pioneering work of Williams and associates (28) showed that chronic contractile activity induces increases in mtDNA copy number, mtRNA transcripts, and the proportion of triplex DNA structure in the D-loop region. These data suggest that the replication of mtDNA into multiple copies regulates the level of mitochondrial gene expression in skeletal muscle cells. However, there is no universal agreement on this issue, since in some conditions (e.g., altered thyroid status) the copy number of mtDNA is not changed but the level of mRNA transcripts increases (29). In any event, the increase in mtDNA copy number observed as a result of chronic contractile activity is accompanied by the augmented expression of SSB, the RNA subunit of RNAse MRP, but not POL-γ. These data suggest that POL-γ is sufficiently abundant and not limiting for the transcription of mtDNA. In addition, contractile activity induces an early and rapid increase in Tfam mRNA and protein expression in muscle. This is followed by an accelerated rate of Tfam import into mitochondria, accompanied by an increase in Tfam-mtDNA binding. This leads to an enhanced transcription of mtRNA and increased activity of enzymes possessing mtDNA-encoded subunits (e.g., COX) (30). When combined with the actions of PGC-1α and NRF-1 on the nuclear genome, these changes are largely responsible for the observed coordination between nuclear and mitochondrial mRNA responses to chronic contractile activity. This serves to maintain the correct stoichiometry between nuclear-encoded and mitochondrially encoded subunits during the assembly of respiratory chain complexes.

Deletions or mutations of mtDNA leading to defective or absent gene products result in impaired respiration and mitochondrial disease, of which a large number have now been documented (31). These are largely tissue-specific diseases, and they predominate in organs with high energy demands, such as brain, heart, and muscle. In skeletal muscle, the result of a mtDNA abnormality is termed mitochondrial myopathy, and it is characterized by exercise intolerance, fatigue, and exaggerated lactic acid production. An important, emerging question is whether exercise training can improve—or worsen—this situation in mitochondrial myopathy patients? Recent studies on patients have begun to shed some light on the adaptive potential of exercise training. Most mtDNA-induced mitochondrial myopathy patients have a mixture of wild-type and mutant mtDNA, a situation known as mtDNA heteroplasm. The extent of the pathophysiology is dependent upon the ratio of mutant to normal, wild-type mtDNA copies per cell. It has recently been shown that aerobic training can induce increased levels of respiratory enzymes in mitochondrial myopathy patients (32). This increase led to an improvement in oxidative capacity. However, the endurance training protocol also produced an increase in the relative fraction of mutated mtDNA in most of the patients. Although an improvement in work capacity was noted, the long-term implications of an expanded mutant mtDNA pool could not be determined. Thus, it was suggested that further examination and study are necessary before implementation of an aerobic training program with symptomatic patients with heteroplasmic mtDNA. Interestingly, in a case study reported by the same group, a mitochondrial myopathy patient was subject to resistance training, as opposed to endurance training. The result was a dramatic increase in the proportion of wild-type mtDNAs. It was hypothesized that this would occur, because resistance training promotes the activation and fusion of satellite cells to muscle cells. In contrast to muscle cells, satellite cells do not possess mutated mtDNA, and the fusion of the two cell types would produce a cell in which the proportion of wild-type mtDNA could potentially increase. Thus, it is clear that more work using different training regimens and in a greater number and variety of mitochondrial myopathy patients is necessary to establish the utility of this approach for improving the quality of life for patients with mitochondrial disease.

Intramitochondrial Protein Synthesis Is Essential for the Mitochondrial Adaptations to Contractile Activity

Since an impairment of mitochondrial protein synthesis can lead to disease, it is not surprising to learn that the process is vital for normal organelle adaptation to exercise. mRNA transcripts derived from mtDNA are employed along with the rRNAs and tRNAs in mitochondrial translation. Unfortunately, this process is not widely studied in any tissue, and very little information is available on its physiological regulation. In skeletal muscle, measurements using

isolated mitochondrial subfractions have revealed that IMF mitochondria synthesize protein at a greater rate than SS mitochondria, consistent with their greater oxidative capacity. When animals are treated with the mitochondrial protein synthesis inhibitor chloramphenicol during chronic stimulation-induced mitochondrial biogenesis, reduced adaptive increases in the activities of COX but not citrate synthase were observed (36). This is because citrate synthase is entirely nuclear encoded, whereas COX contains three essential catalytic subunits derived from mtDNA that are translated within the organelle.

In response to acute (5 min), intense contractile activity, protein synthesis within SS mitochondria decreases, possibly as a result of the contraction-induced reduction of ATP within the organelle. Rates of protein synthesis are restored to normal during the recovery period. These data indicate that intramitochondrial protein turnover is influenced by acute contractile activity. To evaluate whether chronic contractile activity altered the rates of protein synthesis or degradation, skeletal muscle was chronically stimulated for 14 days to produce a significant increase in COX activity. Surprisingly, no adaptive increases in protein synthesis or degradation were observed. Thus, either the changes in protein turnover which occur as a result of exercise happen relatively early in the adaptation process or they remain unaffected and ultimately do not limit the mitochondrial biogenesis response to contractile activity.

Exercise-induced Changes in Gene Expression Are Most Evident During Recovery

It has long been suspected that adaptive responses to exercise manifest during the recovery phase following the exercise period. A wealth of evidence shows that the most pronounced changes occur during this time. This may be because when exercise stops, the energy required for processes such as gene expression and protein synthesis are redirected from serving contractile activity purposes to those that are more anabolic. The augmented gene expression during recovery is evident with respect to key events involved in mitochondrial biogenesis, such as the induction of ALAs (33) and the transcription factor NRF-1. Other events related to muscle adaptation that increase during the recovery period include total muscle protein synthesis and degradation, increased activity of a variety of kinases involved in translation and cell signaling, and increases in mRNAs encoding important proteins involved in transcription (e.g., *c-jun, c-fos*) and glucose metabolism (e.g., GLUT4, glycogenin), among others. These changes appear to be preceded by increased rates of gene transcription (5). Thus, the data support these ideas:

1. The final adaptations to various forms of contractile activity are a result of an accumulation of adaptive responses that originate with an acute exercise bout

but that are not manifest until the recovery period, when the muscle is at rest.
2. The recovery period is an important component of the adaptation phase of gene expression leading to mitochondrial biogenesis.

SUMMARY

Chronic exercise training produces a well-established adaptation in skeletal muscle termed mitochondrial biogenesis. The physiological benefit of this is enhanced endurance performance. This is advantageous for athletic endeavors, and it improves the quality of life and functional independence of previously sedentary individuals. This chapter reviews the benefits of this adaptation with respect to metabolism and the underlying molecular basis for mitochondrial biogenesis

in skeletal muscle subjected to models of endurance training, notably electrical stimulation–induced chronic contractile activity. This includes a discussion of the following:

1. The initial signals arising in contracting muscle
2. The transcription factors involved in mitochondrial and nuclear DNA transcription
3. The posttranslational import mechanisms required for organelle synthesis

A summary of our understanding of the molecular and cellular mechanisms that govern the increases in mitochondrial volume with repeated bouts of exercise is shown in Fig. 21.6.

Further insights into the mechanisms involved may lead us to therapeutic interventions that will benefit those with mitochondrial diseases and those unable to withstand regular physical activity.

A MILESTONE OF DISCOVERY

Does endurance exercise training improve respiratory enzyme activity and result in enhanced oxygen uptake of skeletal muscle? Until 1967, properly designed studies using an appropriate duration per day, frequency per week, and intensity per exercise bout to test this hypothesis had not been completed. Limited evidence from comparative studies of birds and mammals indicated a relationship between the activity of a muscle and the content of respiratory enzymes. In addition, it was known that mitochondrial content in skeletal muscle could be increased by administration of thyroid hormone. In light of this, Holloszy hypothesized that the improvement in endurance performance observed with training could be due to an adaptive process of mitochondrial synthesis. At the time, only two studies had addressed the adaptability of mitochondrial enzyme activity and oxidative capacity to an exercise stimulus. Examination of the exercise intensities used in those investigations suggested that although a daily exercise program lasting 5 to 8 weeks should have been sufficient to provoke an adaptive response, the intensity and duration (daily 30-minute bout of swimming) were insufficient to provoke an adaptive response. Therefore, Holloszy used a treadmill training program that progressively increased in intensity and duration over 12 weeks. Muscles were then removed from the animals, and homogenates and isolated mitochondrial fractions were prepared for oxygen consumption and enzyme activity measurements. One of the key findings of this study is shown in the table below. Oxygen uptake, expressed as microliters of oxygen per hour per gram, in mitochondria isolated from 1 g fresh muscle was twice

as high in the trained (exercising) group as in comparable samples from sedentary muscles.

Increases in oxygen uptake also coincided with 60% increases in the yield of total mitochondrial protein and a remarkable sixfold improvement in run time to exhaustion compared to the sedentary group. Holloszy was the first to predict that this improved performance could be a result of lower concentrations of ADP in the cytoplasm due to the greater rate of oxidative phosphorylation, which reduced lactate formation during exercise. This prediction was subsequently confirmed experimentally, and this idea is now central to our understanding of the adaptations associated with endurance training. The novelty of the training program and the insight and interpretation provided by Holloszy in this study led to a remarkable advance in our knowledge of muscle adaptations to exercise. This work set the stage for literally hundreds of subsequent investigations on muscle plasticity, phenotype differences among muscle fiber types, and alterations in gene expression as a result of exercise. It also provided a new experimental model for the study of mitochondrial biogenesis. Finally, it shed light on the potential contributions of muscle adaptations to changes in whole body $\dot{V}O_{2max}$ and ultimately on the role of these adaptations in the overall health of the individual.

Holloszy JO. Biochemical adaptations in muscle: effects of exercise on mitochondrial oxygen uptake and respiratory enzyme activity in skeletal muscle. J Biol Chem 1967;242:2278–2282.

Group	Oxygen Uptake ($\mu L \cdot g^{-1}$)	Respiratory Control Index	P:O Ratio
Sedentary	506 ± 53	14.7 ± 2.6	2.7 ± 0.2
Exercising	1022 ± 118	16.1 ± 2.2	2.6 ± 0.1

ACKNOWLEDGMENTS

We are grateful to Dr. Hans Hoppeler (University of Berne, Berne, Switzerland) for the provision of the electron micrographs of muscle mitochondria. Research in our laboratory is supported by the Natural Science and Engineering Research Council of Canada (NSERC) and the Canadian Institutes for Health Research (CIHR). Isabella Irrcher is the recipient of a NSERC Post-Graduate Fellowship. David A. Hood is the holder of a Canada Research Chair in Cell Physiology.

REFERENCES

1. Pette D, ed. Plasticity of Muscle. Berlin: Walter de Gruyter, 1980.
2. Holloszy JO. Biochemical adaptations in muscle. J Biol Chem 1967;242:2278–2282.
3. Hood DA. Invited review: contractile activity-induced mitochondrial biogenesis in skeletal muscle. J Appl Physiol 2001;90:1137–1157.
4. Hoppeler H. Exercise-induced ultrastructural changes in skeletal muscle. Int J Sports Med 1986;7:187–204.
5. Pilegaard H, Ordway GA, Saltin B, et al. Transcriptional regulation of gene expression in human skeletal muscle during recovery from exercise. Am J Physiol 2000;279:E806–E814.
6. Baldwin KM, Klinkerfuss GH, Terjung RL, et al. Respiratory capacity of white, red, and intermediate muscle: adaptive response to exercise. Am J Physiol 1972;222:373–378.
7. Henriksson J, Reitman JS. Time course of changes in human skeletal muscle succinate dehydrogenase and cytochrome oxidase activities and maximal oxygen uptake with physical activity and inactivity. Acta Physiol Scand 1977;99:91–7.
8. Reichmann H, Hoppeler H, Mathieu-Costello O, et al. Biochemical and ultrastructural changes of skeletal muscle mitochondria after chronic electrical stimulation in rabbits. Pflügers Arch 1985;404:1–9.
9. Xia Y, Buja LM, Scarpulla RC, et al. Electrical stimulation of neonatal cardiomyocytes results in the sequential activation of nuclear genes governing mitochondrial proliferation and differentiation. Proc Natl Acad Sci USA 1997;94:11399–11404.
10. Connor MK, Irrcher I, Hood DA. Contractile activity-induced transcriptional activation of cytochrome c involves Sp1 and is proportional to mitochondrial ATP synthesis in C2C12 muscle cells. J Biol Chem 2001;276:15898–15904.
11. Takahashi M, Hood DA. Protein import into subsarcolemmal and intermyofibrillar skeletal muscle mitochondria. J Biol Chem 1996;271:27285–27291.
12. Terjung RL. The turnover of cytochrome c in different skeletal-muscle fibre types of the rat. Biochem J 1979;178:569–574.
13. Dudley GA, Tullson PC, Terjung RL. Influence of mitochondrial content on the sensitivity of respiratory control. J Biol Chem 1987;262:9109–9114.
14. Sakamoto K, Goodyear LJ. Invited review: intracellular signaling in contracting skeletal muscle. J Appl Physiol 2002;93:369–383.
15. Irrcher I, Adhihetty PJ, Sheehan T, et al. PPARγ coactivator-1α expression during thyroid hormone- and contractile activity-induced mitochondrial adaptations. Am J Physiol 2003;248:C1669–C1677.
16. Wu H, Kanatous SB, Thurmond FA, et al. Regulation of mitochondrial biogenesis in skeletal muscle by CaMK. Science 2002;296:349–352.
17. Scarpulla RC. Nuclear activators and coactivators in mammalian mitochondrial biogenesis. Biochim Biophys Acta 2002;1576:1–14.
18. Lin J, Wu H, Tarr PT, et al. Transcriptional co-activator PGC-1α drives the formation of slow-twitch muscle fibres. Nature 2002;418:797–801.
19. Puigserver O, Spiegelman BM. Peroxisome proliferator-activated receptor-γ coactivator-1α (PGC-1α): transcriptional coactivator and metabolic regulator. Endocr Rev 2003;24:78–90.
20. Lehman JJ, Barger PM, Kovacs A, et al. Peroxisome proliferator-activated receptor γ coactivator-1 promotes cardiac mitochondrial biogenesis. J Clin Invest 2000;106:847–856.
21. Chrzanowska-Lightowlers ZMA, Preiss T, Lightowlers RN. Inhibition of mitochondrial protein synthesis promotes increased stability of nuclear-encoded respiratory gene transcripts. J Biol Chem 1994;269:27322–27328.
22. Freyssenet D, Connor MK, Takahashi M, et al. Cytochrome c transcriptional activation and mRNA stability during contractile activity in skeletal muscle. Am J Physiol 1999;277:E26–E32.
23. Pfanner N, Meijer M. Mitochondrial biogenesis: the Tom and Tim machine. Curr Biol 1997;7:R100–R103.
24. Stojanovski D, Johnston AJ, Streimann I, et al. Import of nuclear-encoded proteins into mitochondria. Exp Physiol 2003;88:57–64.
25. Takahashi M, Chesley A, Freyssenet D, et al. Contractile activity-induced adaptations in the mitochondrial protein import system. Am J Physiol 1998;274:C1380–C1387.
26. Koehler CM, Leuenberger D, Merchant S, et al. Human deafness dystonia syndrome is a mitochondrial disease. Proc Natl Acad Sci USA 1999;96:2141–2146.
27. Larsson N-G, Wang J, Wilhelmsson H, et al. Mitochondrial transcription factor A is necessary for mtDNA maintenance and embryogenesis in mice. Nature Gen 1998;18:231–236.
28. Williams RS. Genetic mechanisms that determine oxidative capacity of striated muscles: control of gee transcription. Circulation 1990;82:319–331.
29. Wiesner RJ. Adaptation of mitochondrial gene expression to changing cellular energy demands. News Physiol Sci 1997;12:178–183.
30. Gordon JW, Rungi AA, Inagaki H, et al. Effects of contractile activity on mitochondrial transcription factor A expression in skeletal muscle. J Appl Physiol 2001;90:389–396.
31. Wallace DC. Mitochondrial defects in cardiomyopathy and neuromuscular disease. Am Heart J 2000;139:S70–S85.

32. Taivassalo T, Shoubridge EA, Chen J, et al. Aerobic conditioning in patients with mitochondrial myopathies: physiological, biochemical, and genetic effects. Ann Neurol 2001;50:133–141.

33. Holloszy JO, Winder WW. Induction of δ-aminolevulinic acid synthetase in muscle by exercise or thyroxine. Am J Physiol 1979;236:R180–R183.

34. Cogswell AM, Stevens RJ, Hood DA. Properties of skeletal muscle mitochondria isolated from subsarcolemmal and intermyofibrillar regions. Am J Physiol 1993;264: C383–C389.

35. Hoppeler H. Kraft- und Ausdauertraining: funktionelle und strukturelle Grundlagen. In Der Muskel. Medizinisch Literarische Verlagsgesellschaft. Uelzen: MBH (Medical Literary Publishing), 1989;9–17.

36. Willams RS, Harlan W. Effects of inhibition of mitochondrial protein synthesis in skeletal muscle. Am J Physiol 1987;253:C866–C871.

CHAPTER 22

The Endocrine System: Integrated Influences on Metabolism, Growth, and Reproduction

ANNE B. LOUCKS

Introduction

The endocrine response to exercise depends upon the nutritional status of the individual. The physiological consequences of that response also depend upon the nutritional status of the individual. This is true acutely in response to a single exercise bout and chronically in response to exercise training. In essence, that is the theme of this chapter. The development of this theme for the chapter draws attention to the immaturity of endocrinology as a subdiscipline of exercise physiology. The exercise endocrinology literature includes inconsistent experimental results and conflicting interpretations, and in some areas basic descriptive studies have yet to lay a firm foundation for mechanistic experiments; therefore, this chapter raises as well as answers questions.

Consciously, intentionally, and intelligently or not, all athletes are bodybuilders. Exercise remodels the body, and athletes maximize their performance in part by managing that remodeling process to acquire a sport-specific (and in some team sports, position specific) optimum body size, body composition, and mix of energy stores. The endocrine system integrates the influences of diet and exercise on the remodeling process and on the resulting athletic performance. The endocrine system also regulates fluid and electrolyte balance and other physiological functions discussed elsewhere in this book. This chapter describes how hormones regulate the mobilization and replenishment of energy stores to meet the metabolic demands of exercise and how they regulate the remodeling of body proteins to cope with repetitions of those demands. In doing so, this chapter assumes a familiarity with the basic endocrinology of hormone classification, chemistry, synthesis, secretion, transport, feedback, and intracellular signaling. Students should also seek more detailed information in other chapters about the physiological aspects of systems and processes whose regulation is discussed here.

Exercise imposes demands on the body in two ways. First, mechanical loads impose stress, strain, and sometimes damage on working muscle and connective tissue; and second, exercising muscle requires a supply of metabolic fuels from which to extract the energy to overcome these mechanical loads. Physical activities differ greatly in the intensity, duration, and frequency with which they impose these two types of demands, and they stimulate specific responses to meet these demands.

Despite the responsiveness of the endocrine system, when the metabolic demands of exercise exceed the availability of metabolic fuels, the eventual result is fatigue, and when the demands of exercise training persistently exceed the supply of nutrients in the diet, the eventual result is disease. Dietary energy is used in five fundamental physiological functions: basal metabolism, thermoregulation, growth, locomotion, and reproduction. Energy consumed in one of these functions is not available for the others. In athletes, the amount of energy habitually consumed in locomotion can so exceed the amount provided in the diet that the other processes cannot operate normally. Under such conditions, the body minimizes the allocation of energy to basal metabolism and thermoregulation and defers growth and reproduction.

Undernutrition is especially common in endurance, esthetic, and weight class sports. Since undernutrition damages the reproductive and skeletal health of female athletes, the American College of Sports Medicine published a position stand in 1997 warning athletes, coaches, and parents about the female athlete triad, a syndrome in which undernutrition leads to amenorrhea and osteoporosis (1). To prevent adverse effects on the competitive performance, physical health, and normal growth and development of wrestlers, the ACSM published another position stand in 1996 recommending measures to educate coaches and wrestlers about sound nutrition and weight control behavior, to curtail weight cutting, and to enact rules limiting weight loss (2). The National Collegiate Athletic Association adopted such rules (3) after three wrestlers collapsed and died in 1997 in the presence of coaches as the wrestlers were cutting weight to qualify for competition.

Regulation of the Storage and Mobilization of Metabolic Fuels

Glucose Homeostasis

Compared to other mammals, the human brain has an extremely high, nearly constant rate of energy consumption, accounting for about 20% of basal metabolism in adults and about 50% in children, even though it constitutes only about 2% of body weight. The brain depends almost exclusively on glucose as a metabolic fuel for energy, and because it has virtually no glucose storage capacity, it depends on a constant supply of glucose from the bloodstream. At a normal plasma glucose concentration of about 5 mM, brain glucose uptake is about twice the rate of brain glucose utilization (about 100 g · day^{-1}), so that as much glucose is recycled to the bloodstream as is oxidized and otherwise utilized. Since brain glucose uptake is proportional to plasma glucose concentration, however, a declining plasma glucose concentration eventually limits brain metabolism, and this occurs at about 3.6 mM.

Plasma glucose falls during prolonged dynamic exercise, the magnitude of the drop being directly related to the absolute intensity of the work and the duration of the exercise bout. Furthermore, the fall in blood glucose is more extreme during successive bouts of exercise, even when the duration and workload are identical (4). For example, five times as much glucose had to be infused to maintain plasma glucose concentrations during the second of two 90-min exercise bouts at 50% $\dot{V}O_{2max}$ on the same day, even though glycogen stores were replenished after the first bout (5).

Between meals, the brain relies on the mobilization of glucose by the liver for its supply of glucose, because skeletal muscle lacks the enzyme to return glucose from muscle glycogen stores to the bloodstream. Since liver glycogen stores (about 50 g · kg^{-1} tissue ≈ 90 g) can supply the brain energy requirement for less than a day, however, and since liver glycogen stores are also used to meet the metabolic demands of working muscle, working muscle competes directly with the brain for glucose, and it competes very aggressively. During a 2-h marathon race, for example, working muscle consumes as much glucose as the brain consumes in a week.

In this metabolic peril, human beings have survived because we have evolved multifaceted, redundant (i.e., highly reliable) endocrine mechanisms for preventing hypoglycemia, including rapidly responsive mechanisms activated between meals and during exercise and more slowly responding mechanisms activated by chronic dietary carbohydrate deficiency that reduce demands from tissues competing with the brain.

Glucose Counterregulation

With use of a stepped hypoglycemic clamp technique, the defenses against the isolated influence of hypoglycemia have been found to be triggered at so-called glycemic thresholds (i.e., arterialized venous plasma glucose concentrations) (6). Insulin secretion is suppressed as a first line of defense at 4.5 mM. Glucagon, epinephrine, and growth hormone (GH) secretion are stimulated at about 3.7 mM and cortisol secretion at about 3.6 mM as a second line of defense, triggered when brain glucose uptake becomes limiting on brain metabolism. If the plasma glucose concentration falls further, neural glucose deprivation causes perceptible neurogenic symptoms (sweating, hunger, tingling, tremor, heart pounding, and anxiety) and neuroglycopenic symptoms (warmth, weakness, confusion, drowsiness, faintness, dizziness, difficulty speaking, and blurred vision) to stimulate eating as a third line of defense at about 3.0 mM. Cognitive dysfunction occurs at about 2.6 mM.

The plasma glucose concentration is the primary determinant of insulin secretion by pancreatic islet β-cells, with increases in plasma glucose increasing secretion and vice versa. This responsiveness of β-cells to the plasma glucose concentration is suppressed by α$_2$-adrenergic sympathetic stimulation by epinephrine from the adrenal medulla and by norepinephrine from sympathetic nerve terminals. Thus, the rise in catecholamines during exercise suppresses insulin secretion even when the plasma glucose concentration is maintained at 5.3 mmol · L^{-1} by an exogenous glucose infusion (Fig. 22.1) (7).

The plasma glucose concentration is also the primary determinant of glucagon secretion by pancreatic islet α-cells, with increases in plasma glucose reducing secretion and vice versa. Whether catecholamines directly stimulate glucagon

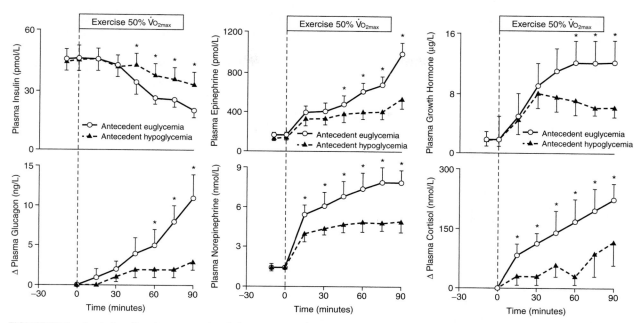

FIGURE 22.1 Acute insulin, glucagon, epinephrine, norepinephrine, growth hormone, and cortisol responses to 90 min of exercise at 50% $\dot{V}o_{2max}$ under clamped euglycemic conditions after clamped euglycemia (5.3 mM) and after two 90-min bouts of clamped hypoglycemia (3.0 mM) on the previous day. Exercise responses occurred despite clamped euglycemia. Antecedent hypoglycemia blunted all the responses. *(Reprinted with permission from Davis SN, Galassetti P, Wasserman DH, et al. Effects of antecedent hypoglycemia on subsequent counterregulatory responses to exercise. Diabetes 2000;49:76,77.)*

secretion in humans is a matter of dispute. Because glucagon secretion is inhibited by the paracrine tonic influence of insulin within the islet, however, the rise in catecholamines during exercise appears to act indirectly via insulin to raise glucagon concentrations even when euglycemia is maintained by exogenous glucose infusion (Fig. 22.1) (7).

The plasma glucose concentration also regulates the secretion of epinephrine by the adrenal medulla, GH by the pituitary, and cortisol by the adrenal cortex, in all cases mediated by glucose sensors in the central nervous system, with increases in plasma glucose decreasing secretion and vice versa. Exercise also activates these hormones, even when euglycemia is maintained by exogenous glucose infusion (7) (Fig. 22.1).

Even though increases in GH and cortisol are part of the counterregulatory response to exercise and contribute to the prevention of hypoglycemia, their contribution is of secondary importance (6,8). Prolonged hypoglycemic insulin clamp experiments have demonstrated that the rapid mobilization of metabolic fuels that prevents acute hypoglycemia is accomplished by increases in sympathetic activity and glucagon secretion, whereas GH and cortisol responses do not begin to affect glucose production or plasma glucose levels until 4 h later, long after the increased metabolic demands of most exercise bouts have ceased. Nor is either GH or cortisol necessary for recovery from hypoglycemia, since plasma glucose concentrations rise equally rapidly after several hours of insulin-induced hypoglycemia in patients with hypopituitarism (but normal pancreatic function) and in normal con-

trol subjects. Thus, when insulin and glucagon responses are operative, GH and cortisol are not involved in the correction of brief hypoglycemia or in the prevention of hypoglycemia during an exercise bout, and they contribute in only a minor way to the defense against slowly developing hypoglycemia during the overnight fast and in chronic undernutrition.

While there is consensus about the primacy of insulin and the relative unimportance of GH and cortisol in the prevention of severe hypoglycemia and the recovery of euglycemia, the importance of catecholamines for glucoregulation during exercise in humans continues to be a matter of dispute. Experiments that prevent the action of sympathoadrenal mechanisms by severing nerves or pharmacologically blocking receptors have been interpreted as implying that these mechanisms make little contribution to glucose production during exercise until after at least 90 min of moderate exercise (9) (Fig. 22.2). Recently, however, in other investigations of the effects of prolonged hypoglycemia and prolonged exercise on glucose counterregulation, researchers have left sympathoadrenal mechanisms intact, and these findings seem to imply that sympathoadrenal mechanisms operate in a subtle manner almost from the onset of exercise.

Hypoglycemia-Associated Autonomic Failure

It is evident that these glycemic thresholds are dynamic, shifting to higher levels following sustained hyperglycemia and to lower ones following episodes of hypoglycemia or prolonged

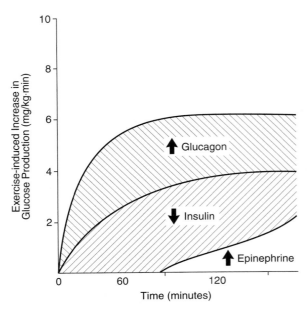

FIGURE 22.2 Rise in glucose production during moderate exercise and the contributions to it of the fall in insulin and the rises in glucagon and epinephrine. Epinephrine becomes increasingly important as exercise is prolonged. *(Reprinted with permission from Wasserman DH, Cherrington AD. Regulation of extra muscular fuel sources during exercise. In LB Rowell, JT Shephard, eds. Handbook of physiology, Section 12: Exercise: Regulation and Integration of Multiple Systems. Oxford: Oxford University, 1996;1051.)*

exercise (10). As Figure 22.1 illustrates, two 90-min episodes of insulin-induced hypoglycemia on a single day lower glycemic thresholds in response to prolonged exercise the next day, thereby blunting glucose counterregulatory hormone responses, hepatic glucose production, and lipolysis by 50% and impairing the ability to maintain normal plasma glucose levels (7). This effect is reciprocal in that two 90-min bouts of 50% $\dot{V}O_{2max}$ exercise on a single day have the same effects on insulin-induced hypoglycemia the following day (11). Aside from their academic interest for the insight they offer into glucose counterregulation, these experiments have practical relevance for endurance athletes who may do two-a-day workouts during an intensive training regimen.

Because the threshold for neurogenic and neuroglycopenic symptoms is reduced along with those for the counterregulatory hormones, the affected individual is unaware of the hypoglycemia on the second day. Consequently, a vicious circle may ensue: the absence of symptoms leads to episodes of more severe hypoglycemia, which further lower glycemic thresholds, and so on. The hazard in progressively reducing glycemic thresholds is that eventually further hypoglycemia elicits symptoms too late for behavioral or medical intervention. This hazard is especially serious in type I diabetics, who lack both the first (insulin) and second (glucagon) lines of defense against hypoglycemia.

The mechanism of this effect, termed hypoglycemia-associated autonomic failure (HAAF), involves a decline in adrenomedullary and sympathetic activation, which is reflected in lower plasma catecholamine concentrations and reduced skeletal muscle sympathetic nerve activity (12). In Figure 22.1, the suppression of plasma norepinephrine after antecedent hypoglycemia appears to affect some other counterregulatory hormones as early as 15 min after the onset of exercise.

Although it is associated with hypoglycemia, HAAF is not caused by hypoglycemia, for it occurs even when plasma glucose concentrations are maintained by the exogenous infusion of glucose during antecedent prolonged exercise (13). The factor suppressing sympathetic activity is the stimulation of corticosteroid receptors in the brain. HAAF does not occur in patients with Addison's disease, who lack the ability to secrete cortisol (10), and it can be induced in rats by infusing a low dose of cortisol into the paraventricular nucleus (PVN) of the brain under euglycemic systemic conditions and prevented by infusing a corticosteroid antagonist during antecedent episodes of hypoglycemia (10).

This appears to explain why HAAF occurs only in men (11) and in postmenopausal women (14); these women lack estrogen, which accentuates cortisol responses to stress (15) and stimulates corticotropin-releasing hormone (CRH) gene expression in the PVN (16). In postmenopausal women, estrogen replacement prevents the blunting of counterregulatory responses to hypoglycemia (14). By suppressing adrenomedullary and sympathetic activity, HAAF blunts the mobilization of lactate, glycerol, and free fatty acids, thereby impairing gluconeogenesis and the conversion of skeletal muscle fuel selection from glucose to free fatty acids. Thus, HAAF causes men to require a much greater exogenous supply of glucose than do premenopausal women to maintain normal plasma glucose levels during the late stages of prolonged exercise (11). This effect lasts as long as cortisol remains bound to PVN corticosteroid receptors, which may be several days (10).

Effects of Dynamic Exercise Training

Besides raising a new caution about intensive endurance training programs, the discovery of HAAF raises some new questions about the mechanisms associated with effects of endurance exercise training. It has been known but not understood for almost 30 years that the exercise-induced decreases in insulin and increases in counterregulatory hormones are all blunted by exercise training. Basal and glucose-stimulated insulin levels are also reduced in trained individuals as a result of decreased insulin secretion. Because sensitivity to insulin is increased while sensitivity to the counterregulatory hormones is not, the reduced counterregulatory responsiveness is probably due to the reduction in insulin concentration (17). Training effects on insulin are essentially complete less than 2 wk after the onset of training and lost

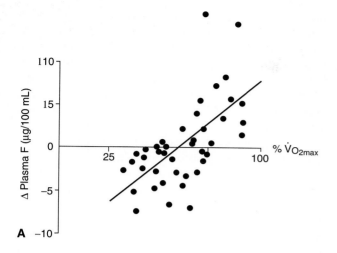

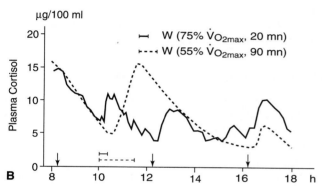

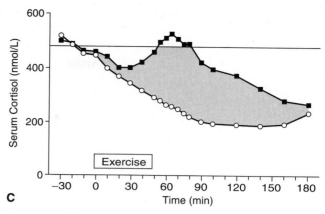

FIGURE 22.3 (*continued*)

FIGURE 22.3 **A.** Serum cortisol responses to 60 min of aerobic exercise, calculated by subtracting concentrations before exercise from postexercise concentrations. Responses appear to be more or less than zero in proportion to the degree to which exercise intensity is more or less than 60% $\dot{V}_{O_{2max}}$. *(Reprinted with permission from Davies CT, Few JD. Effects of exercise on adrenocortical function. J Appl Physiol 1973;35:889.)* **B.** Serum cortisol concentrations measured at 10-min intervals for 10 h on separate days when a subject performed 75% $\dot{V}_{O_{2max}}$ exercise for 20 min and 55% $\dot{V}_{O_{2max}}$ exercise for 90 min beginning at 10 h. The response to 55% $\dot{V}_{O_{2max}}$ exercise appears to be much greater than zero and the response to 75% $\dot{V}_{O_{2max}}$ exercise. *(Reprinted with permission from Brandenberger G, Follenius M. Influence of timing and intensity of muscular exercise on temporal patterns of plasma cortisol levels. J Clin Endocrinol Metab 1975;40:848.)* **C.** Serum cortisol concentrations before, during and after 50 min of 70% $\dot{V}_{O_{2max}}$ exercise at 8 in the morning (**solid squares**) and at the same times of another day at rest (*open circles*). The baseline before exercise is drawn as a horizontal line through the mean of samples drawn before exercise. The shaded portion of the cortisol response to exercise was not detected by calculating the response relative to concentrations before exercise. *(Reprinted with permission from Thuma JR, Gilders R, Verdun M, et al. Circadian rhythm of cortisol confounds cortisol responses to exercise: implications for future research. J Appl Physiol 1995;78:1660.)*

less than 2 wk after training stops. Since removal of the adrenal medulla blocks the effect of training on insulin in rats (18), questions arise about whether effects of endurance exercise training and HAAF are related. From a practical perspective, it would be interesting to learn whether training effects suppress the awareness of hypoglycemia and thereby create a hazard, as some endurance athletes are unaware of lower and lower plasma glucose concentrations. It would also be interesting to learn whether athletic performance could be improved if such effects could be prevented or reduced.

Cortisol Responses to Exercise

If it were desirable to minimize HAAF, one way to do so might be to consume carbohydrates during exercise. Exogenous glucose administration reduces the responses to exercise of all glucoregulatory hormones, including cortisol (19,20). Infusion of glucose to establish and maintain a hyperglycemic 12 mM plasma glucose concentration entirely abolishes the cortisol response to 120 min of 70% $\dot{V}_{O_{2max}}$ exercise (19), but the same effect was achieved during 50% $\dot{V}_{O_{2max}}$ exercise to exhaustion by infusion of only enough glucose to maintain the preexercise glucose concentration (20). Glucose infusions were used in these experiments to achieve precise control of plasma glucose concentrations and to avoid limitations and variations in the absorption of orally administered glucose, but the same effect was also achieved during a 21-km hill walk by increasing the consumption of biscuits, chocolate bars, flapjacks, and cheese sandwiches (21).

Anyone taking a quantitative interest in cortisol responses to exercise will want to measure those responses accurately. The first successful effort to explain prior inconsistent assessments of cortisol responses to exercise found these responses to be roughly proportional (R = .62) to the relative rather than absolute exercise workload (22). After 60 min of exercise, Davies and Few (22) found cortisol levels to be higher or lower than levels before exercise in proportion to the extent to which relative workloads were greater or less than 60% of $\dot{V}_{O_{2max}}$, respectively (Fig. 22.3A).

As might have been expected from a finding that explained only $R^2 = 38\%$ of the observed variance, however, this insight did not bring an end to inconsistencies in measurements of cortisol responses to exercise. Brandenberger and Follenius soon demonstrated what appeared to be very large cortisol responses to 90 min of exercise at 55% $\dot{V}O_{2max}$ by making measurements every 10 min for 10 h (Fig. 22.3B) (23). Nevertheless, for the next 20 years, many exercise physiologists continued to assess cortisol responses to exercise as Davies and Few had done, by comparing a single measurement after exercise to a single measurement before exercise. Then the magnitude of the errors by this method were shown to be as much as 93% when compared to responses calculated relative to the diurnal rhythm of cortisol on another day at rest (24) (Fig. 22.3C). Even the sign of the response could be wrong (appearing to indicate a reduction in cortisol secretion rather than an increase) if the post-exercise measurement was taken in the morning as the diurnal rhythm is declining rapidly—when Davies and Few performed their experiment.

Thus, cortisol and other counterregulatory hormone responses to exercise have yet to be comprehensively quantified. Acquiring this basic descriptive information will require a series of experiments spanning a wide range of exercise durations and intensities, at various times of day, in various nutritional states, with and without antecedent exercise or hypoglycemia, in trained and untrained men and women, with responses calculated by reference to the diurnal rhythm on another resting day long enough to capture the entire response. With that research as a foundation, better advice may be developed to help athletes mobilize and extend endogenous supplies of metabolic fuels to maximize performance in endurance events.

Glucose Production

The effectiveness of insulin and glucagon in maintaining glucose homeostasis by regulating hepatic glucose production benefits from the pancreas and liver being anatomically in series (25). Although changes in each of these hormones are correlated with changes in hepatic glucose production, the ratio between glucagon and insulin has the strongest correlation (8), because the fall in insulin sensitizes the liver to the effects of glucagon. Indeed, in the absence of glucagon the fall in insulin does not stimulate hepatic glucose production (26). Conversely, the rapid postprandial rise in insulin quickly lowers the glucagon-to-insulin ratio to inhibit glucose production.

The rate of hepatic glycogenolysis is determined by the activity of the enzyme phosphorylase a, which is stimulated by two mechanisms, one involving glucagon and the other involving α-adrenergic stimulation. The regulation of hepatic gluconeogenesis is more complicated because it depends upon the mobilization of gluconeogenic precursors, their extraction by the liver, and the efficiency of their conversion to

glucose within the liver. Dynamic exercise stimulates all three of these processes. The accelerated proteolysis, lipolysis, and glycolysis during exercise increase amino acid, glycerol, lactate, and pyruvate precursors, and the rise in glucagon increases the fractional extraction of these precursors and the efficiency of their conversion into glucose. The endocrine mediation of proteolysis and lipolysis are discussed later in the chapter.

During prolonged dynamic exercise, gluconeogenesis increases the supply of glucose beyond the capacity of liver glycogen stores. Glycogenolysis precedes gluconeogenesis. During the first hour of exercise or hypoglycemia, glycogenolysis predominates, accounting for about 85% of glucose production. Later, as glycogen stores are depleted and gluconeogenic precursors become available, gluconeogenesis predominates and accounts for about 85% of glucose production after about 6 hours (27). Gluconeogenesis also occurs in every individual every day in intervals between meals and during sleep to maintain glucose availability to the brain.

Skeletal Muscle Glucose Uptake

The rate-limiting step for glucose uptake by skeletal muscle is the rate of glucose transport across the cell membrane. Insulin stimulates the active transport of glucose into muscle cells. Insulin mediates its action through a membrane receptor and a complicated series of protein kinases (28). Despite extensive studies, the mechanism by which insulin elicits its various intracellular effects is not yet completely understood (29) (Fig. 22.4).

The homodimer insulin receptor in the cell membrane is the hormone-activated protein tyrosine kinase, which catalyzes the transfer of phosphate groups from adenosine triphosphate (ATP) to tyrosine residues of proteins. Insulin binding stimulates autophosphorylation and activation of the receptor kinase, and the activated receptor then phosphorylates several endogenous cellular substrate proteins. The best characterized of these is a family of cytosolic proteins including IRS-1 (insulin-receptor substrate-1), IRS-2, IRS-3, and IRS-4.

Most of the downstream partners of the IRS proteins contain specific recognition sequences called SH2 domains that promote protein–protein interaction between the partner protein and the sites of tyrosine phosphorylation. The three best-studied SH2 domain proteins involved in insulin signaling are a lipid-metabolizing enzyme, phosphatidylinositol 3-kinase (PI3-kinase); a phosphotyrosine phosphatase called SHP2; and an adapter molecule called GRB2, which links insulin signaling to a pathway involving Ras and a cascade of intracellular serine kinases centering on an enzyme called microtubule-associated protein (MAP) kinase. Most current studies indicate that the PI3-kinase is the critical pathway for most metabolic events, including stimulation of glucose transport.

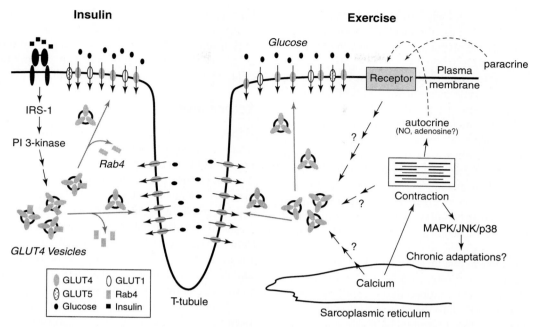

FIGURE 22.4   Incompletely understood mechanisms by which insulin and exercise stimulate glucose uptake by skeletal muscle. Acting via a PI3-kinase pathway, insulin causes GLUT4 glucose transporters to translocate from the cytosol to the plasma membrane. Exercise also causes GLUT4 transporters to translocate to the plasma membrane by an independent paracrine/autocrine or intracellular mechanism. *(Reprinted with permission from Goodyear LJ. AMP-activated protein kinase: a critical signaling intermediary for exercise-stimulated glucose transport? Exerc Sport Sci Rev 2000;28:116.)*

A major component of the mechanism of insulin-stimulated glucose transport is a temperature- and energy-dependent translocation of intracellular vesicles containing glucose transporter proteins to the cell membrane. The effect is reversible, so that the glucose transporters return to the intracellular pool when insulin is removed. The most important glucose transporter for insulin action is GLUT4. Exactly how receptor kinase activation is coupled to transporter translocation is unknown.

Dynamic exercise also stimulates GLUT4 translocation to the cell membrane and glucose transport independently by different, as yet unknown, intracellular, autocrine, or paracrine mechanisms, thereby increasing insulin sensitivity (i.e., glucose uptake for a given insulin concentration) during and for a period after exercise.

Fat Metabolism

Fatty Acid Cycling by Adipose Tissue

Adipose tissue plays an important role in whole-body energy metabolism, because it is the only tissue able to release non-esterified fatty acids (NEFA) into the circulation. During prolonged exercise, plasma NEFA are the major energy source of working muscle. In almost all physiological circumstances, all of the fatty acids released by adipose tissue were previously taken up from circulating chylomicrons carrying di-etary fat and very low density lipoproteins (VLDL) carrying triglycerides secreted by the liver. The energy equivalent of this cycling of fatty acids between adipose tissue and the circulation amounts to about 1200 kcal · day^{-1} in normal human subjects. This includes substantial reesterification of released NEFA, the regulation of which makes possible the rapid amplification of adipose tissue NEFA output in response to metabolic demand. This regulation is achieved by the integrated effects of blood flow through the tissue, autonomic nervous system activity, and the levels of hormones and substrates circulating in the blood (30,31).

Unless it is unavailable, the energy source of adipose tissue is glucose. Glucose availability is also rate limiting for the synthesis of triglycerides, because adipocytes lack the enzyme glycerokinase and cannot reesterify the glycerol released by lipolysis. Therefore, the glycerol-3-phosphate used in esterifying triglycerides is obtained by glycolysis. This is not an important glucose disposal pathway, however, accounting for only about 4% of an oral glucose load compared to about 35% accounted for by skeletal muscle. Considering the small amount of energy in the form of glucose required to control such a large amount of energy in the form of NEFA, therefore, adipose tissue is the most efficient energy storage tissue in the body. Glucose uptake by adipocytes is accomplished by insulin-dependent GLUT4 transporters and insulin-independent GLUT1 transporters, but insulin has no physiologically important effect on adipose tissue glucose uptake, because the insulin concentration for half-maximal stimulation of glucose uptake in adipose tissue is only about 13 pM (32).

Thus, the major function of adipose tissue is the storage and release of chemical energy in the form of NEFA. The direction of this energy flow is determined by the coordinated regulation of the enzymes hormone-sensitive lipase and lipoprotein lipase. Insulin inhibits and the counterregulatory hormones stimulate hormone-sensitive lipase, which catalyzes the hydrolysis of stored triglycerides to release NEFA and glycerol. Since half-maximal suppression of hormone-sensitive lipase by insulin occurs at a concentration of only about 120 pM, the release of NEFA is substantially suppressed within 30 min and is essentially zero within 60–90 min after a mixed meal.

By contrast, a rise in insulin stimulates and a rise in catecholamines inhibits lipoprotein lipase, which hydrolyses VLDL triglycerides in the adipose tissue capillary bloodstream and releases NEFA into the plasma, from where they are available for uptake by adipocytes. Synthesized in and secreted by adipocytes, lipoprotein lipase migrates to the adipose tissue capillary lumen, where it attaches to endothelial cells by proteoglycan chains so that it comes into contact with circulating chylomicrons and VLDL triglycerides. Since insulin also stimulates the esterification of fatty acids in adipose tissue (33), the precipitous postprandial rise in insulin after a mixed meal raises the plasma concentration and lowers the intracellular adipocyte NEFA concentration, creating a concentration gradient down which NEFA flow from the bloodstream into adipocytes for esterification. The gradual fall in insulin after a meal slowly releases the inhibition of hormone-sensitive lipase and suppresses esterification and lipoprotein lipase activity, thereby gradually reversing the concentration gradient and the direction of NEFA flow.

Coordination of NEFA release with the sudden increase in metabolic demand at the onset of exercise is mediated by β-adrenergic effects of sympathetic activation (34). Norepinephrine released from sympathetic nerves is the important stimulus, since the effect is retained after adrenomedullation (35). As exercise continues, adrenergic stimulation of lipolysis and inhibition of VLDL hydrolysis is reinforced by the gradual decline in insulin and rise in GH and cortisol (36). These stimuli also reduce the reesterification of NEFA to approximately zero within 60 min during exercise at 50–60% of $\dot{V}_{O_{2max}}$, further increasing the concentration gradient driving NEFA output. By contrast, muscular contractions and catecholamines stimulate muscle lipoprotein lipase to promote lipid uptake during exercise and postabsorptive conditions.

Adipose tissue blood flow responds rapidly to nutrient ingestion, facilitating triglyceride disposal (37), and β-adrenergic stimulation has vasodilator effects in adipose tissue. Nevertheless, during exercise adipose tissue blood flow is insufficient to absorb all of the NEFA released, and the rate of appearance of NEFA in the bloodstream declines as exercise intensity increases despite the associated increase in β-adrenergic drive (38). As a result, at the end of exercise an accumulated backlog of NEFA in adipose tissue is suddenly released into the circulation (36).

Ketogenesis

Hepatic ketogenesis is a reflection of the energy state of the liver. As a marker of hepatic fat oxidation, a key source of energy for gluconeogenesis, ketogenesis occurs in acute and chronic circumstances that require high rates of gluconeogenesis. The rate of ketogenesis is determined by the mobilization of NEFA by adipose tissue, by the uptake of NEFA by the liver, and by the efficiency with which NEFA are converted to ketone bodies in the liver. Therefore, by regulating the mobilization of NEFA, the exercise responses of insulin and the glucose counterregulatory hormones also contribute to the regulation of ketogenesis.

Insulin also inhibits the fractional extraction of NEFA from the bloodstream by the liver. Therefore, the fall in insulin during exercise further contributes to ketogenesis by increasing hepatic NEFA uptake (39). Meanwhile, the rise in glucagon increases the activity of carnitine acyltransferase, the key enzyme in ketone production. The ratio of ketone body output to NEFA uptake is an index of NEFA-to-ketone conversion efficiency. During 60 min of moderate exercise, this ratio increases from 20 to 40% in normal healthy subjects and from 60 to 100% in poorly controlled insulin-dependent diabetics (40).

Initially, ketones in the liver are taken up from the blood and metabolized by the heart, kidney, and skeletal muscle so that circulating levels in the blood remain low. If glucose deficiency continues for only a few days, however, glucose and ketone utilization by these tissues decline, and plasma ketone concentrations rise to levels exceeding those of plasma glucose, making substantial amounts of ketones available as an alternative metabolic fuel for the brain. Hepatic ketone production capacity is uniquely high in human beings, and this is what maintains brain metabolism in human beings during chronic dietary carbohydrate deficiency. Conveniently, when plasma ketone levels begin to rise, some ketones pass through the kidneys into the urine, in which they can be readily detected.

Regulation of Muscle Plasticity

Protein Turnover

Of the three macronutrients, protein is unique in that there is no pool of stored protein not serving important physiological purposes. As might be expected, therefore, protein is the least oxidized of the three metabolic fuels for meeting daily energy requirements. Nevertheless, even though the energy required to synthesize protein is twice as great as that required to synthesize glycogen or triglycerides, the daily turnover of protein (about 37 mmol · kg · day⁻¹) greatly exceeds the turnover of carbohydrates (about 15 mmol · kg · day⁻¹) and triglycerides (about 24 mmol · kg · day⁻¹) (41) and is equivalent to the protein content of 1–1.5 kg of muscle. Individual proteins turn over at widely different rates, with half-lives as short as 15 min for some regulatory proteins, about 2 wk for actin and myosin, and as long as 3 months for hemoglobin.

In muscle protein turnover, many factors associated with genetics, age, exercise, nutrition, and hormonal regulation influence the intracellular signaling pathways that control gene transcription; mRNA translation; posttranslational modification and degradation of myofibrillar, mitochondrial, cytosolic, membrane, and extracellular proteins; and the proliferation and differentiation of muscle satellite cells. Muscle growth and atrophy result from small differences in the rates of protein synthesis and breakdown that constitute the daily turnover of muscle protein. Protein synthesis and breakdown both occur all the time, and they are different, separately regulated processes, not simply the reverse of one another. Both processes are selective with respect to the muscles and fiber types as well as the particular fibers and proteins involved at any given time. Protein breakdown is a necessary part of fiber type transformation and muscle remodeling generally. Indeed, since proteolysis is performed by proteins, an increase in protein breakdown depends upon the increased synthesis of proteolytic proteins.

The rates of protein synthesis and breakdown in muscle depend in part on the intracellular availability of amino acids, including those derived from the breakdown of intracellular proteins and those transported in both directions across the cell membrane. In addition to supplying amino acids from old proteins as raw materials for the synthesis of new proteins, proteolysis supplies amino acids for gluconeogenesis and other important physiological functions. Thus, by imposing huge demands for glucose, prolonged exercise is a leak draining the pool of amino acids available for protein synthesis. Of course, the intracellular availability of amino acids is directly affected by the protein content of the diet. As described earlier, it is also indirectly affected by the carbohydrate content of the diet and by exercise through their influence on glucoregulatory hormones that also affect amino acid transport and protein synthesis and breakdown.

Proteolysis

In the past 15 years there has been an explosion of research into the mechanisms of protein breakdown, motivated by the clinical consequences of muscle atrophy in various catabolic conditions, including cancer, metabolic acidosis, AIDS, sepsis, starvation, diabetes, trauma, surgery, paralysis, and space flight, and by the discovery that most proteolysis occurs in a highly selective, tightly regulated, and therefore controllable process. This research has revealed that there are at least four proteolytic processes in skeletal muscle, each of which targets different proteins and is regulated differently.

The Ubiquitin–Proteosome System

The ATP-dependent ubiquitin–proteosome system (42) accounts for about 80% of total protein breakdown, including myofibrillar proteins, which constitute 50–70% of muscle protein content. In this system, proteins selected for degradation are first conjugated to many molecules of the protein ubiquitin and then transported to large, complex cytosolic enzyme bodies called proteasomes for unfolding and breaking into small peptides and amino acids. Myofibrillar proteins in intact myofibrils are not accessible for polyubiquitination, however. Therefore, one or more other proteolytic systems must first release the constituent proteins of actomyosin before this system can act upon them.

Lysosomes

The ATP-independent lysosomal system isolates acid proteases, including cathepsins and other hydrolases, from cellular proteins within the lysosomal membrane. This system degrades mainly endocytosed extracellular and membrane-associated proteins, such as hormone receptors, but also certain endocytosed cytosolic proteins, into peptides.

Calpains

A Ca⁺⁺-dependent system involving several proteases known as calpains and several calpain inhibitors known as calpastatins (43) are found in the cytosol but concentrated in the Z-disk. Calpains initiate digestion of myofibrillar proteins except actin and myosin heavy chain (MHC). They are activated by the release of calcium from the sarcoplasmic reticulum during muscular contractions and by calcium influx through the sarcolemma during injury.

Caspases

A family of apoptotic cytosolic proteases known as caspases (44) clip proteins, including actomyosin complexes, into peptides at aspartic acid. Possibly activated by reactive oxygen species and/or intracellular Ca⁺⁺, caspases can cleave actomyosin complexes and cytoskeleton proteins, DNA and myonuclei, and ultimately can disintegrate the cell into membrane-bound bodies that are phagocytosed by surrounding cells and macrophages.

Hormone Effects on Protein Turnover
Goldberg's Rats

During the late 1960s and early 1970s, Alfred Goldberg conducted a series of experiments investigating the mechanism of work-induced hypertrophy of skeletal muscle in rats (45). In these experiments Goldberg severed the insertion of the gastrocnemius muscle from the Achilles tendon in one hindlimb to eliminate its usual synergistic assistance to the soleus and plantaris muscles in extending the ankle. After only 5 days, the overloaded soleus and plantaris muscles had grown by a surprising 40% and 20%, respectively, compared to the corresponding muscles in the sham-operated contralateral limb. What was especially remarkable, however, was that the same growth occurred in hypophysectomized, diabetic, and starving rats. Goldberg concluded that work-induced hypertrophy of skeletal muscle is mediated by mechanisms intrinsic to the particular working muscles, unlike developmental growth, which was known to depend on circulating pituitary axis hormones (GH, insulinlike growth factor-1 [IGF-I], testosterone, thyroxine), insulin, and nutrients. These findings inspired a stream of experiments that continues to this day to elucidate the mechanism by which the autocrine expression of IGF-I mediates the hypertrophy of working muscle.

Wolfe's Men

Over the past 10 years Robert Wolfe's laboratory has conducted another series of experiments investigating the mechanism of work-induced hypertrophy of skeletal muscle in men (46). Employing different methods, he comes to different conclusions from Goldberg's. Using a combination of stable isotope infusion, arterial and venous blood sampling, and muscle biopsy, Wolfe calculates rates of protein synthesis and breakdown and the rates of inward and outward amino acid transmembrane transport in the quadriceps muscle at a particular point in time.

Figure 22.5 summarizes Wolfe's findings on the effects of dietary intake and resistance exercise on protein synthesis and breakdown in men (46). After a 12-h fast, protein breakdown exceeds protein synthesis. Under such catabolic conditions, resistance exercise increases the rates of both protein synthesis and breakdown 3 hours later so that breakdown still exceeds synthesis (#2). By contrast, consuming amino acids at rest establishes anabolic conditions by selectively increasing protein synthesis (#3). When amino acids are consumed within 3 hours after a resistance exercise bout, the effects of the two treatments are additive: synthesis exceeds breakdown, and both processes are accelerated (#4). Consuming glucose as well as amino acids at rest further accelerates both synthesis and breakdown (#5), and then exercise selectively accelerates protein synthesis to magnify the anabolic effect (#6). Thus, Wolfe's results appear to indicate that circulating supplies of nutrients, and the hormone responses to them, are what determine whether working muscle grows or atrophies and that exercise magnifies the anabolic response only when sufficient glucose and presumably insulin are available.

Of course, there are substantial differences between Goldberg's and Wolfe's experiments that may eventually be

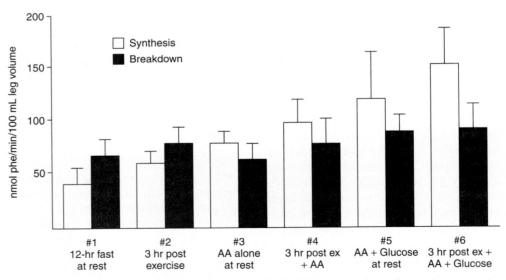

FIGURE 22.5 The influence of exercise, amino acids, and glucose on mixed muscle protein turnover in young volunteers. Under postabsorptive conditions, protein breakdown exceeds synthesis at rest (1), and exercise accelerates both processes (2). A meal of amino acids increases protein synthesis and suppresses protein breakdown at rest, so that synthesis exceeds breakdown (3), and exercise accelerates both processes (4). Adding glucose to the meal further increases synthesis and breakdown at rest (5), and again exercise accelerates both processes to increase net protein synthesis (6). Thus, nutritional status determines whether exercise is anabolic or catabolic. *(Reprinted with permission from Rasmussen BB, Phillips SM. Contractile and nutritional regulation of human muscle growth. Exerc Sport Sci Rev 2003;31:131.)*

shown to account for their apparently inconsistent findings. There are profound species differences between rats and humans. For example, plasma glucose and insulin levels and metabolic rates are substantially higher in rats. Wolfe's and Goldberg's resistance exercise treatments were also different. Goldberg's was applied constantly for 5 days, whereas Wolfe's was applied only once. Their outcome variables were also different. Wolfe calculated rates of protein synthesis and breakdown at a particular point in time 3 h after an exercise bout, whereas Goldberg measured the integrated effects of synthesis and breakdown on muscle size and mass over several days. While not nearly the complete story about work-induced muscle hypertrophy in humans, Wolfe's men show that the story is not as simple as Goldberg's rats appeared to indicate.

Insulin

Insulin has a major influence on protein turnover, and the regulation of protein turnover by insulin and amino acids differs between splanchnic and skeletal muscle beds (47). This can lead to substantial discrepancies between estimates of whole body and skeletal muscle protein turnover. The action of insulin is mostly on skeletal muscle, whereas amino acids act on both skeletal muscle and the splanchnic bed.

The most consistently observed effect of insulin on protein metabolism is to suppress protein degradation (48). This effect is independent of blood glucose levels (49). Since methyl-histidine fluxes across the leg and the forearm do not change when insulin is administered, however, it is clear that insulin deficiency alone does not break down myofibrillar proteins (50).

All four protein degradation pathways in skeletal muscle are insulin dependent. Insulin deficiency activates the ubiquitination of proteins (51) and stabilizes the lysosomal membrane, thereby reducing free cathepsin activity and limiting protein breakdown (52). Insulin also inhibits caspase (53) and calpain activity (54) by reducing PI3-kinase activity. Only modest increases in plasma insulin are necessary to diminish skeletal muscle protein breakdown. As Figure 22.6A illustrates, the suppressive effect of insulin on proteolysis in forearm muscles of fasting humans is saturated at about 150 pM (about 25 uU · mL^{-1}) (48).

Observations of the effects of insulin on protein synthesis are less consistent. Insulin increases the rate of amino acid uptake by skeletal muscle (55). Insulin signaling also regulates protein synthesis at both transcription and translation initiation steps. Insulin increases mRNA for selected proteins, including MHC-α in rat skeletal muscle. Peptide chain initiation in muscle is reduced in insulin deficiency and restored by insulin treatment. As a result, decreasing insulin availability through experimental diabetes or starvation reduces the rate of protein initiation by 40 to 50% (41). On the other hand, hyperinsulinemia can also suppress protein synthesis. Without concurrent amino acid infusion or con-

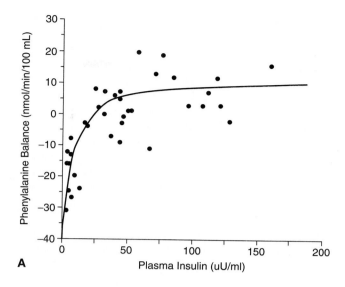

A

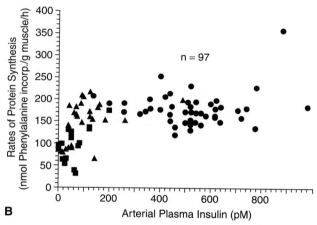

B

FIGURE 22.6   **A.** Dose-response relationship between plasma insulin and net forearm skeletal muscle amino acid (phenylalanine) balance during postabsorptive rest. Proteolysis occurs below about 150 pM (about 25 uU/mL). Above about 150 pM insulin has no effect on protein breakdown. (1 uU/mL = 6 pM). *(Reprinted with permission from Louard RJ, Fryburg DA, Gelfand RA, et al. Insulin sensitivity of protein and glucose metabolism in human forearm skeletal muscle. J Clin Invest 1992;90:2353.)* **B.** Dose-response relationship between arterial plasma insulin and rates of protein synthesis after acute resistance exercise in 97 rats. Below about 80 pM, insulin deficiency limited exercise-stimulated protein synthesis. *(Reprinted with permission from Fedele MJ, Hernandez JM, Lang CH, et al. Severe diabetes prohibits elevations in muscle protein synthesis after acute resistance exercise in rats. J Appl Physiol 2000;88:105.)*

sumption, insulin administrations can lower amino acid concentrations in the blood, reducing the supply of substrate for skeletal muscle protein synthesis and thereby lowering the protein synthesis rate.

Peter Farrell's laboratory has investigated the effects of insulin on protein synthesis, employing an experimental model that has features in common with those of both Goldberg and Wolfe. Farrell's experimental animal is also a rat, and his resistance exercise treatment is also applied constantly for several days, but to both hindlegs as the rat lifts a progressively more heavily weighted vest by standing on its hindlegs to reach an overhead bar that it is trained to press 50 times a day. After several days, Farrell measures protein synthesis rates in the gastrocnemius muscle. He also measures insulin levels. As Figure 22.6B shows, the stimulation of skeletal muscle protein synthesis under physiological conditions in Farrell's rats is saturated at a fasting insulin concentration of only about 80 pM, corresponding to levels seen in severely diabetic rats after 5 h of fasting (56). Below this level, insulin deficiency limited the stimulation of protein synthesis by resistance exercise. Thus, Farrell's data indicate that insulin does affect protein synthesis in working skeletal muscle of the rat, but only below what is a very low concentration for a rat. Above 80 pM, protein synthesis increases with amino acid availability and with stimulation by resistance exercise. Were insulin levels higher in Goldberg's diabetic and starving rats? Maybe, but we'll never know, because he didn't measure them. We do not yet know whether insulin's stimulation of protein synthesis in working muscle is also saturated at about 80 pM or at some other concentration in humans.

These thresholds, above which insulin's stimulation of protein synthesis in the working muscle of rats (about 80 pM) and its inhibition of protein breakdown in the resting muscle of humans (about 150 pM) are saturated, are much lower than the concentration at which the insulin's stimulation of skeletal muscle glucose uptake in humans is saturated (>600 pM). Thus, insulin's effects on protein turnover occur in the lower part of its physiological range. To put these thresholds into a human physiological perspective, Figure 22.7A shows them in relation to the variations in insulin levels in normal healthy, sedentary individuals eating three meals a day at 8:00 A.M., 2:00 P.M., and 8:00 P.M. Insulin levels are almost always below 150 pM, and they fall below 80 pM within 4 h after the most recent meal. These data illustrate the challenge posed by the need of athletes to manage their diet to keep up their insulin levels for avoiding unnecessary protein breakdown and perhaps also to avoid limiting protein synthesis. The decline in insulin during prolonged exercise further increases this challenge. These data also emphasize the importance of the carbohydrate content of the diet for optimizing protein turnover.

Cortisol

Cortisol is often credited with being the principal catabolic hormone because of its central role in proteolysis. Since proteolysis increases the availability of amino acids for gluconeogenesis, the proteolytic and glucoregulatory roles of cortisol are often regarded as two sides of the same coin. While this is true, the coin is a strange one, because it has different val-

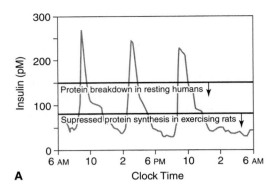

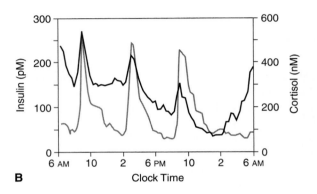

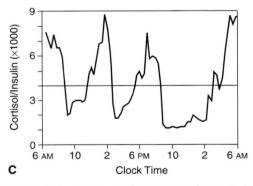

FIGURE 22.7 **A.** Mean insulin concentrations over 24 h in eight men and women who consumed three standardized meals at 8:00 A.M., 2:00 P.M., and 8:00 P.M. Horizontal lines indicate the insulin concentrations at which insulin's suppression of protein breakdown in resting humans and stimulation of protein synthesis in exercising rats are saturated. **B.** Mean insulin and cortisol concentrations over 24 h in the same men and women. **C.** Cortisol-to-insulin ratios over 24 h in the same men and women. Proteolysis is accelerated when the cortisol-to-insulin ratio is above the horizontal line at 4 (×1000). *(Adapted with permission from Van Cauter E, Shapiro ET, Tillil H, et al. Circadian modulation of glucose and insulin responses to meals: relationship to cortisol rhythm. Am J Physiol 1992;262:E470.)*

TABLE 22.1	Postabsorptive Hormone and Glucose Concentrations and Amino Acid Appearance Rates[a]		
	Before	12–16 h	60–64 h
Hormones			
Cortisol (nM)	280 ± 30	890 ± 120	990 ± 40
Insulin (pM)	68 ± 7	100 ± 4	129 ± 9
Cortisol/insulin (×1000)	4.1	8.9	7.7
Glucose (mM)	4.6 ± 0.1	5.9 ± 0.2	5.6 ± 0.1
Amino acid appearance rates			
Leucine (%)	100	117	113
Phenylalanine (%)	100	114	118
Glutamine (%)	100	139	139
Alanine (%)	100	138	229

[a]Before and during 64 h of hydrocortisone infusion in six healthy young men. Modified with permission from Darmaun D, Matthews DE, Bier DM. Physiological hypercortisolemia increases proteolysis, glutamine, and alanine production. Am J Physiol 1988;255: E366–E373.

ues on its two sides. On one side the daily turnover of protein is much greater than the turnover of carbohydrates and fats, while on the other side protein is the least oxidized of the three metabolic fuels. That is, cortisol's importance for protein turnover exceeds its importance for glucoregulation.

Elevated physiological levels of cortisol are necessary but not sufficient to accelerate muscle protein breakdown by the ubiquitin–proteosome system. Cortisol and other glucocorticoids increase the capacity of this system by stimulating the expression of ubiquitin, ubiquitin carrier, and proteosome genes, resulting in increases in ubiquitin, ubiquitin carrier, and proteosome subunit mRNAs and proteins, but a second factor must be present to activate ubiquitination. In exercise, muscle damage, the release of Ca^{++} into the cytosol from the sarcoplasmic reticulum, and elevated reactive oxygen species in the form of incompletely oxidized metabolic fuels are factors inherent in exercise that activate lysosomal, calpain, and caspase proteases to make myofibrillar proteins available for ubiquitination. In type I diabetes, fasting, and some other catabolic conditions, the second factor is low insulin levels (49). In type II diabetes, uremia, sepsis, and metabolic acidosis, the second factor is impaired responsiveness to insulin. Thus, over and above the inherent mechanisms by which exercise stimulates proteolysis, undernutrition and the energy cost of exercise drive proteolysis by raising the ratio of cortisol to insulin.

Table 22.1 shows the results of infusing hydrocortisone into six healthy young men for 64 h (57). Measurements were made under resting conditions immediately before the infusion began 16 h after their last meal, as well as 12–16 h and 60–64 h after the infusion started. By mobilizing amino acids and promoting gluconeogenesis, the elevation of cortisol concentrations into the upper part of the physiological range increased plasma glucose levels, which raised insulin

levels in response. Nevertheless, because the rise in insulin was not as great as the rise in cortisol, the ratio of cortisol to insulin rose from 4.1 (×1000) to more than 7 (×1000), increasing the rates of appearance of amino acids beyond the initial postabsorptive rates.

With that experiment in mind, consider Figure 22.7B, which shows daily variations in cortisol in relation to insulin concentrations in individuals consuming three meals a day. The resulting daily variations in the ratio of cortisol to insulin are shown in Figure 22.7C. The ratio exceeds 4 (×1000) for about 6 h during sleep. This is largely unavoidable and may be beneficial. Eating only three meals per day, however, doubles the number of hours each day during which an elevated ratio of cortisol to insulin accelerates proteolysis.

Figure 22.8 shows the effect of an intravenous infusion of glucose on the ratios of cortisol to insulin occurring during a prolonged exercise bout under postabsorptive conditions at 70% $\dot{V}O_{2max}$ (19). Exercising for 2 h without the glucose infusion raised the postabsorptive ratio of cortisol to insulin from about 10 (×1000) to more than 30 (×1000)! By contrast, glucose infusion suppressed the ratio to less than 4 (×1000). These data demonstrate how strongly proteolysis is stimulated during prolonged exercise in the postabsorptive state.

Growth Hormone

Postnatal somatic growth and especially peripubertal and postpubertal growth depend on the normal pulsatile secretion of GH from the pituitary. GH administration substantially reverses the impaired growth that occurs in hypophysectomized animals, and chronic administration of recombinant human

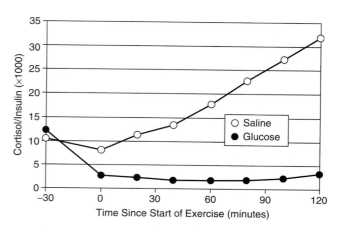

FIGURE 22.8   Cortisol-to-insulin ratios in eight men during 2 h of exercise in the post-absorptive state at 70% $\dot{V}O_{2max}$ with glucose and saline infusions. The glucose infusion maintained plasma glucose at 12 mM and suppressed the cortisol-to-insulin ratio to less than 4 (×1000). *(Adapted with permission from data in MacLaren DP, Reilly T, Campbell IT, et al. Hormonal and metabolic responses to maintained hyperglycemia during prolonged exercise. J Appl Physiol 1999;87:127,128.)*

GH (rhGH) restores growth in GH-deficient children and adolescents and increases lean body mass in GH-deficient adults and elderly patients. In such individuals GH, unlike insulin, stimulates protein synthesis without affecting proteolysis (58). In growing pigs, GH administration increases circulating insulin and IGF-I concentrations over and above the effect of feeding, making it ambiguous whether the actions of GH are direct or indirect via these other hormones (59). In skeletal muscle GH exerts its effect by increasing the efficiency of translation initiation, that is, the amount of protein synthesized per ribosome, rather than by increasing the number of ribosomes. This effect occurs over and above the effect of feeding on translation initiation, but it occurs only in the postprandial and not in the postabsorptive state (59).

In normal healthy adults, however, GH appears to play only a minor role in promoting muscle hypertrophy and strength (60). Of course, resistance exercise, like aerobic exercise, elicits an acute increase in GH concentrations that declines in the hour or so after exercise stops. The magnitude of this response is in proportion to the associated metabolic demand, but over the next 12 h GH concentrations are slightly suppressed (61). There is no evidence that these GH responses to resistance exercise have any effect on skeletal muscle growth. Acute local and systemic infusions of rhGH at pharmacological doses for 6 h have increased protein synthesis in adults, but when administered for several weeks in combination with resistance exercise training, supraphysiological doses of rhGH have only increased total body water, lean body mass, and whole-body protein synthesis in general without specifically increasing skeletal muscle protein synthesis or skeletal muscle mass, cross-sectional area, fiber size, strength, or power in untrained young men, experienced young weight lifters, or older men (60).

Insulinlike Growth Factor I

The anabolic influence of GH on somatic growth is probably mediated through IGF-I, since IGF-I knockout mice remain small despite markedly increased circulating GH levels resulting from the loss of IGF-I negative feedback (62). Three-quarters of circulating IGF-I is secreted by the liver in response to GH stimulation via exon-1 of the hepatic IGF-I gene. Although GH also stimulates IGF-I expression in type I fibers of skeletal muscle via exon-2, exercise-induced muscle hypertrophy does not depend on either circulating GH or circulating IGF-I. This is because increased mechanical loading leads to substantial compensatory hypertrophy in the overloaded skeletal muscles of hypophysectomized rats, in which both circulating GH and circulating IGF-I were drastically reduced (63). This occurs because type II skeletal muscle fibers have the intrinsic capacity to express IGF-I mRNA and IGF-I peptide via exon-1 of the IGF-I gene in response to mechanical loading, even in the absence of GH stimulation (64). Type II fibers express both a generalized form of IGF-I and a unique isoform of IGF-I known as

mechano growth factor (MGF). MGF is expressed only in response to stretch and loading (65) and is hardly detectable in muscle unless the muscle is exercised or damaged.

IGF-I stimulates protein synthesis and reduces protein breakdown in muscle fibers (66). GH-stimulated IGF-I expression maintains and expands slow-twitch type I fibers, while exercise-stimulated IGF-I expression maintains and expands fast-twitch type II fibers. Increased mechanical loading, stretch, and eccentric contraction all increase IGF-I and IGF-I mRNA expression in muscle cells (67), and pretreatment with IGF-I antiserum blocks the increase in muscle protein synthesis due to exercise (68). Even without mechanical stimulation, experimental manipulation of IGF-I levels in muscle, either by overexpression or direct infusion, induces hypertrophy, both *in vitro* and *in vivo*, and interference with intracellular IGF-I signaling prevents this response. Thus, it appears to be the paracrine/autocrine secretion and local action of IGF-I within working muscle cells, not the hepatic secretion and remote action of circulating IGF-I, that stimulates individual skeletal muscle fibers to adapt to the specific functional demands imposed by diverse physical activities.

Like insulin, IGF-I also reduces glucocorticoid-induced muscle proteolysis by inhibiting cathepsin, calpain, and proteasomal enzyme activities (69).

Beyond protein synthesis, sustained muscle hypertrophy requires contribution of additional nuclei to muscle fibers to maintain a relatively fixed ratio between the volume of muscle fibers and the volume of the nuclei that maintain them. This requirement is met by the proliferation and differentiation of muscle satellite cells and their fusion with enlarging muscle fibers. IGF-I is found in satellite cells (70) and facilitates all of these processes. The proportional and temporal expressions of IGF-I and its MGF isoform are very sensitive to the loading state of the muscle. Following muscle damage MGF is produced for about 24 h, whereas IGF-I production continues longer. MGF and IGF-I also differ greatly in their capacity to activate satellite cells. As a result, a 25% increase in muscle mass induced by local IGF-I administration over a period of 4 months was achieved by MGF administration in just 2 wk (71).

Androgens

A bout of high-volume resistance exercise lowers total and free testosterone concentrations by about 10% over the next 12 h (72), but regular high-volume resistance exercise training for several weeks does not affect basal testosterone concentrations (73). Hypertrophic responses to resistance exercise in women, in whom testosterone concentrations are only about 10% of those in men, appear to confirm Goldberg's findings in hypophysectomized rats (63) that the basal testosterone concentrations normally found in males are not necessary for hypertrophic responses to resistance training. Nevertheless, elevated basal testosterone concentrations do magnify these responses. Under anabolic dietary conditions, resistance training and supraphysiological exogenous doses of testosterone induce substantial similar and additive gains in fat-free mass, muscle size, and strength (Fig. 22.9) (74).

Testosterone acts by increasing muscle protein synthesis without having any effect on protein breakdown (75). Nor does testosterone have any effect on the transport of amino acids into muscle fibers (75). Acute elevations of testosterone for several hours do not increase protein synthesis, however, which indicates that testosterone acts via the genome by enhancing transcription and not by accelerating translation (76).

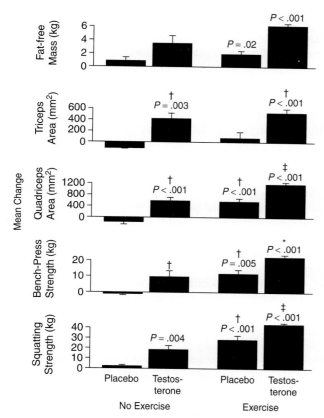

FIGURE 22.9 Changes from baseline mean (+SE) fat-free mass, triceps and quadriceps cross-sectional areas, and muscle strength in bench press and squatting exercises after 10 wk in a 2 × 2 design determining the independent effects of resistance exercise and supraphysiological testosterone treatments. P values indicate the detection of responses other than zero. Asterisks indicate significant (P < .05) differences between the indicated responses and the responses of the no-exercise groups; daggers, between the indicated responses and the response of the no-exercise placebo group; and double daggers between the indicated responses and the responses of all three other groups. Resistance exercise and supraphysiological testosterone independently increased muscle size and strength to a similar degree. (*Reprinted with permission from Bhasin S, Storer TW, Berman N, et al. The effects of supraphysiologic doses of testosterone on muscle size and strength in normal men. N Engl J Med 1996;335:6.*)

Testosterone exerts its effects by binding to the single receptor that binds all androgens in all androgen-sensitive tissues, with different androgen-dependent processes having different testosterone dose-response relationships. This androgen receptor regulates the transcription of androgen-sensitive target genes, and the concentrations of androgen receptor and androgen receptor mRNA reflect the degree of androgen responsiveness of a tissue. Testosterone administration has been shown to increase androgen receptor concentrations in skeletal muscle (77) and oxandrolone administration to increase androgen receptor mRNA concentrations in satellite cells (78). Electrical stimulation (79) and resistance exercise (80) also increase skeletal muscle androgen receptor mRNA concentrations, explaining, in part at least, how resistance exercise and testosterone have additive effects on muscle growth and strength (74).

Testosterone administration also increases IGF-I mRNA in skeletal muscle (49) and down-regulates IGF-I binding proteins (76), thereby further increasing IGF-I bioavailability. Conversely, testosterone suppression reduces muscle strength and IGF-I mRNA concentration and increases concentrations of IGF-I binding proteins, thereby reducing IGF-I bioavailability (81).

Dose-response effects of testosterone on several parameters of body and muscle size, strength, and power have been measured in subjects who were instructed to continue their usual diet and exercise habits (82). Increases in fat-free mass were related to testosterone concentrations from hypogonadal to supraphysiological levels, but with rapidly diminishing returns above the physiological range. Testosterone accounted for only about half ($100 \cdot R^2 = 53\%$) of the variance in the magnitudes of these effects, however (Fig. 22.10). Indeed, effects on every measured parameter of muscle size, strength, and power were as great in many individuals with physiological concentrations as they were in individuals with the highest supraphysiological concentrations.

Some of this variation may have been due to individual differences in physiological factors such as testosterone metabolism, polymorphisms of the androgen receptor, 5-α-reductase, and other muscle growth regulators, but given what we know about the similar additive effects of exercise and testosterone under anabolic conditions, much of the variance was probably due to the intentionally uncontrolled diet and exercise habits of the subjects. Clearly, even supraphysiological doses of testosterone do not in themselves enhance muscle growth in all individuals practicing their usual diet and exercise habits.

Thyroid Hormone, or Triiodothyronine

Triiodothyronine (T_3) has profound effects on protein turnover and thereby on metabolic rate. T_3 exerts its effects on gene expression at transcription, posttranscription, translation, and posttranslation levels (83). T_3 is transported into the nucleus, where it binds to T_3 receptors to affect transcription. These T_3-

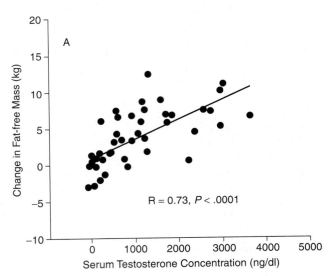

FIGURE 22.10 Changes in fat-free mass in relation to total serum testosterone concentrations in 61 healthy men after 16 wk of testosterone enanthate administration with uncontrolled diets and physical activity. Testosterone increased fat-free mass in a dose-dependent manner, but supraphysiological levels did not ensure increases greater than those in the normal physiological range (300–1000 ng · dL⁻¹). (*Adapted with permission from Figure 2A in Bhasin S, Woodhouse L, Casaburi R, et al. Testosterone dose-response relationships in healthy young men. Am J Physiol 2001;281:E1177.*)

bound receptors interact as monomers, as homodimers, as heterodimers with vitamin D and retinoic acid receptors, or in association with other auxiliary proteins in binding to the thyroid response elements of genes. The complexity of these combinations enables thyroid hormone to have diverse effects from tissue to tissue. Posttranscriptionally, T_3 appears to influence mRNA stability. T_3 also affects translation efficiency and proteolysis.

Although the responses of Goldberg's hypophysectomized rats indicated that T_3 is not necessary for the hypertrophy of overloaded muscles (63), T_3 does have a profound influence on muscle growth, with either an excess or a deficiency causing general muscle wasting. Moderate levels of T_3 stimulate protein synthesis and to a lesser extent proteolysis, but high levels selectively further stimulate proteolysis, and low levels suppress both proteolysis and synthesis. The effects of T_3 on proteolysis occur because of the dependence on ATP of the ubiquitin–proteosome system and because T_3 stimulates ATP production in mitochondria.

In addition to affecting muscle size, T_3 alters the distribution of fiber types in muscles, with slow muscles more sensitive to these effects than fast muscles. Differences in the contractile properties of slow and fast muscles derive in part from differences in their mix of MHC and myosin light chain (MLC) isoforms. Reductions in circulating T_3 increase the expression of the slow type I MHC isoform and decrease expression of the fast type IIB MHC isoform. In type IIA and IIX

isoforms, MHC expression shifts bidirectionally, depending on the muscle type. In slow muscles and in the red inner regions of fast muscles, reductions in T_3 cause some transformable type IIA and IIX fibers to express the type I MHC isoform, whereas in the white superficial regions of fast muscles, some transformable type IIB fibers revert to the type IIX MHC isoform. Hypothyroidism also up-regulates the expression of slow MLC isoforms in both slow and fast muscle and represses the expression of fast MLC isoforms in type IIA fibers in slow muscle. These effects on the interconversion of fiber types are similar to those of mechanical loading. Hyperthyroidism has the opposite effects, which are similar to those of chronic unloading. When they are in competition with one another, hyperthyroidism completely blocks MHC responses to mechanical loading, and hypothyroidism completely blocks MHC responses to mechanical unloading.

T_3 also has substantial effects on the sarcoplasmic reticulum, which performs three key functions (Ca^{++} release, uptake, and storage) in the contraction and relaxation cycle of working muscle. The uptake of Ca^{++} by the sarcoplasmic/endoplasmic reticulum Ca^{++}-ATPase pump (SERCA) expends one molecule of ATP for every two Ca^{++} taken up, an energy cost amounting to about 25% of metabolic energy expenditure during contractile activity. Like MHC and MLC isoforms, various mixes of both fast SERCA1 and slow SERCA2 mRNA isoforms are expressed in fibers of slow and fast muscle types. Like their effects on MHC and MLC isoforms, hypothyroidism reduces the rate of Ca^{++} uptake and hyperthyroidism increases it by regulating SERCA mRNA isoform expression in a fiber type–specific manner.

These influences of T_3 on myosin and Ca^{++}-ATPase pump expression have demonstrable effects on the mechanical properties of skeletal muscle. Hypothyroidism and hyperthyroidism have been shown to reduce and increase the maximum shortening velocity of soleus muscle, respectively. Thyroid hormone also influences the relationship between the frequency of stimulation and the force a muscle generates. Graphically, the relationship of force to frequency of slow muscle fibers lies to the left of that of fast fibers. By completely repressing the expression of fast fibers in the soleus muscle, hypothyroidism shifts this relationship further to the left. Conversely, by converting some slow type I fibers to fast type IIA and IIX fibers, hyperthyroidism shifts the relationship of soleus muscle to the right. By comparison, the force-frequency relationship of fast muscles is relatively insensitive to thyroid state. Muscle tension relaxation time is also sensitive to T_3 in a manner reflecting the fiber content of particular muscles. In the predominantly slow fiber soleus muscle, hyperthyroidism reduces relaxation time by about 50% and hypothyroidism increases it by about 100%. These effects are small in predominantly fast-fiber muscles and intermediate in mixed-fiber muscles. Thus, by reducing shortening velocity and extending relaxation time, the net effect of low thyroid hormone levels is to reduce the capacity of slow muscles to produce mechanical work and power.

Regulation of Mitochondrial Biogenesis and Coupling

Little is known about the endocrine regulation of the effects of endurance training on the transcriptional and translational processes involved in the biogenesis of mitochondria, the coordinated transcription of nuclear and mitochondrial DNA for mitochondrial proteins, the up-regulation of mitochondrial enzyme systems, the increased expression of fatty acid enzyme systems and glucose transporter proteins, and the transformation of MHC isoforms.

Mitochondrial Biogenesis

The replication of mitochondrial DNA (mtDNA) depends in part on mitochondrial transcription factor A (Tfam), the expression and function of which are modified by contractile activity (84). Recently a second transcription factor, p43, was found to bind to both mtDNA and T_3 and to regulate mtDNA independently of Tfam (85). This is of interest because it has been known for many years that mitochondrial biogenesis is also stimulated, independently of contractile activity, by T_3 (86) acting via nuclear and mitochondrial receptors. The response is fiber type specific, probably as a result of differences in the distribution of thyroid receptors (87).

Recently, sustained very high glucocorticoid levels were also shown to stimulate mitochondrial biogenesis in skeletal muscle, suggesting that glucocorticoids may contribute to the elevation in metabolic rate under chronically stressful conditions (88). Exogenous dexamethasone administration for 3 days at 1000 nM but not 100 nM elevated mtDNA-encoded transcripts for cytochrome *c* oxidase subunit III selectively in skeletal muscle and doubled the activity of cytochrome *c* oxidase, a marker of total oxidative phosphorylation capacity. These effects on ATP turnover suggesting an increase in mitochondrial mass were abolished by the administration of the antiglucocorticoid RU486, implying that they were mediated by glucocorticoid receptors. Dexamethasone had no effect on uncoupling protein-3 (UCP-3) mRNA expression, indicating that the glucocorticoid-induced increase in metabolic rate is independent of the coupling state of the respiratory chain. Whether repeated temporary elevations in cortisol in response to exercise training would have similar effects is unknown.

Regulation of Uncoupling Proteins

UCP-3 expression in skeletal muscle is induced by T_3, and this increases metabolic rate at rest (89). Uncoupling of the respiratory chain appears not to be the primary function of the uncoupling proteins, however, since their increased expression is not always associated with mitochondrial uncoupling. Rather, the primary function of UCP-3 appears to be to regulate the flux of lipid substrates across the mito-chondrial membrane in skeletal muscle, especially when glycolytic muscle is forced to shift substrate from glucose to lipids rather than in the basal utilization of lipids as fuel substrate (90). Specifically, UCP-3 is thought to export excess fatty acids out of the mitochondrial matrix when fatty acid oxidation predominates. Since fatty acid anions must be neutralized by protonation to pass through the inner mitochondrial membrane, the associated leak of protons reduces the proton gradient needed to drive ATP synthesis. This proton leak is the uncoupling of the respiratory chain.

UCP-3 expression is up-regulated by lipid infusion (91) and by the elevation of blood fatty acid levels during acute exercise (92). Even when they have a source of free fatty acids, however, mitochondria in the skeletal muscle of fasting rats do not show uncoupling, despite higher levels of UCP-3, until T_3 is administered (93). The resulting uncoupling is mediated by coenzyme Q, the levels of which are drastically reduced in fasting. T_3 prevents this reduction. Since T_3 levels are determined by glucose availability, T_3 shifts muscle substrate utilization away from fatty acids whenever glucose is available.

Reproduction

Regulation of Reproductive Function

Thirty years ago very high prevalences of menstrual disorders began to be reported in surveys of female athletes, with the highest prevalences in competitive endurance, aesthetic, and weight-class sports. This became a matter of clinical concern when it was discovered that the low estrogen levels in amenorrheic athletes were causing them to lose bone mass during the very years when they should be accumulating bone mass. As a result, some had the bone density of 60-year-old women.

Of course, virtually all causes of menstrual disorders in the general population occur among athletes. For this reason, all athletes with menstrual disorders should be differentially diagnosed by a qualified physician to ensure that they receive the appropriate medical care. Since many of these medical conditions are rare, however, no one expected them to explain the high prevalences of menstrual disorders found among athletes. Some medical conditions conveying competitive advantages in particular sports may lead to the affected women being overrepresented in those sports. For example, hyperandrogenism may lead women with polycystic ovary disease to self-select into sports in which increased muscle mass conveys a competitive advantage, and women with anorexia nervosa may disproportionately self-select into sports in which a low body weight is thought to convey a competitive advantage.

After all such medical conditions, as well as pregnancy and lactation, were excluded, however, early investigators were left with many athletes whose menstrual disorders were unexplained. Somehow athletic training itself appeared to disrupt reproductive function in otherwise apparently healthy young women. Many hypotheses were proposed. Since then, research has shown that these menstrual disorders are caused by low energy availability, defined as dietary energy intake minus exercise energy expenditure. Exercise has been shown to have no suppressive effect on reproductive function apart from its energy cost on energy availability. Athletes appear to be able to prevent or reverse menstrual disorders by dietary supplementation alone, with no moderation of their exercise regimen.

Regulation of the Female Reproductive System

The integrative center governing the hypothalamic-pituitary-ovarian axis is a cluster of cells in the arcuate nucleus of the hypothalamus in the brain. These cells secrete pulses of a peptide hormone, gonadotropin-releasing hormone (GnRH), into a network of portal blood vessels that transport these pulses directly to the pituitary. There gonadotrope cells in the anterior pituitary respond to the arrival of these pulses of GnRH by secreting pulses of follicle-stimulating hormone (FSH) and luteinizing hormone (LH) into the systemic bloodstream. Because the half-life of LH is so much shorter than that of FSH, the pulsatile pattern of GnRH secretion is more faithfully reflected in a corresponding pulsatile pattern of LH concentrations in the blood. Ovarian follicular development depends critically upon the frequency at which these pulses appear.

In response to the proper stimulation by LH and FSH in the early follicular phase, several clusters of ovarian cells ("ovarian follicles") begin to grow. Within the follicles, thecal cells respond to LH by converting increasing amounts of cholesterol to androgens, while granulosa cells respond to FSH by expressing increasing amounts of aromatase, which converts these androgens to estradiol. Gradually, the increasing negative feedback of estradiol carried in the blood to the pituitary constrains FSH secretion so that only the follicle most sensitive to FSH can continue developing. Eventually, the increasing amount of estradiol secreted into the blood by this dominant follicle exerts a positive feedback on LH secretion. In response, the pituitary gland secretes a surge of LH into the blood, resulting in the rupture of the dominant follicle and the release of an egg cell for fertilization. The remaining cells of the dominant follicle respond to the LH surge by undergoing rapid chemical and morphological changes to become the corpus luteum. LH receptors appear on granulosa cells, which reduce their aromatase activity as they accumulate large quantities of cholesterol and then synthesize and secrete a thousand times more progesterone than estradiol into the blood. The interval during which a dominant follicle develops, from menses until ovulation, is known as the follicular phase of the menstrual cycle, and the interval during which the corpus luteum is active from ovulation until the next menses is known as the luteal phase.

Estrogen and progesterone have profound influences on the uterine endometrium and on many other tissues in the body. Estrogen stimulates endometrial proliferation, and progesterone causes it to become highly vascularized. These are necessary hospitable conditions for the successful implantation of a fertilized egg. If no fertilization occurs within several days after ovulation, the capacity of the corpus luteum to secrete progesterone is exhausted, the structural integrity of the endometrium collapses, and menstruation ensues. Under normal circumstances, the secretory capacity of the corpus luteum is sustained long enough for the rapidly dividing cells derived from a fertilized egg to implant in the endometrium 6 or 7 days after fertilization. If the secretory capacity of the corpus luteum is exhausted too soon, the endometrium sloughs off before implantation can occur. The likelihood of this increases when the luteal phase is shorter than 10 days. Thus, infertility can result either from the failure of the ovary to release an egg for fertilization or from the failure of a fertilized egg to implant properly into the endometrium.

Characterization of the Ovarian Axis in Female Athletes

Secondary amenorrhea is the cessation of menstrual cycles sometime after they begin at menarche. Athletes with secondary amenorrhea produce low levels of estrogen and progesterone every day, indicating a complete absence of follicular development, ovulation, and luteal function (Fig. 22.11, AA) (94). By contrast, even the most eumenorrheic athletes display extended follicular phases and abbreviated luteal phases with blunted progesterone concentrations (Fig. 22.11, CA) compared to eumenorrheic sedentary women (Fig. 22.11, CS). Such observations have been made in eumenorrheic women running recreationally as little as 12 miles per week.

In a eumenorrheic sedentary young woman, the 24-h LH profile in the early follicular phase is characterized by regular high-frequency pulses of low amplitude (Fig. 22.12, Cyclic Sedentary) (94). During sleep, the frequency slows and the amplitude increases. Eumenorrheic athletes display a slower but still regular rhythm of larger pulses (Fig. 22.12, Cyclic Athlete). Amenorrheic athletes display even fewer pulses at irregular intervals (Fig. 22.12, Amenorrheic Athlete).

The prevalence of amenorrhea in endurance, esthetic, and weight-class sports can be as much as 10 times higher than in the general population. The less severe disorders of ovarian function (follicular and luteal suppression and anovulation) may display no menstrual symptoms at all, so that affected women are entirely unaware of their condition until they undergo an endocrine workup. Among eumenorrheic athletes, the incidence of follicular and luteal suppression and anovulation appears to be extremely high. Repeated endocrine workups have found that 79% of eumenorrheic female runners were luteally suppressed or anovulatory at least 1 month in 3 (95).

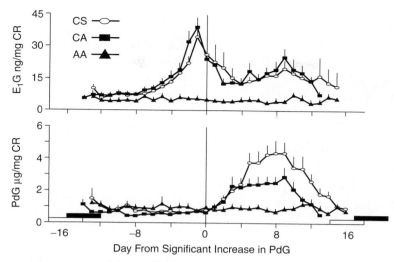

FIGURE 22.11   Mean (+SE) daily urinary excretion of the estrogen metabolite estrone glucuronide (E1G) (*top*) and the progesterone metabolite pregnanediol glucuronide (PdG) in cyclic sedentary women (CS), cyclic athletes (CA), and amenorrheic athletes (AA). Data are presented over one menstrual cycle for cyclic women and over 30 arbitrary days for amenorrheic women. Days are oriented from a significant increase in urinary PdG excretion, with day 1 being the day of the first significant increase. Filled bar, days of menses in CS; open bar, days of menses in CA. AA display no evidence of follicular development, ovulation, or luteal function. Luteal function is suppressed and abbreviated in CA. *(Reprinted with permission from Loucks AB, Mortola JF, Girton L, et al. Alterations in the hypothalamic-pituitary-ovarian and the hypothalamic-pituitary-adrenal axes in athletic women. J Clin Endocrinol Metab 1989;68:408.)*

Hypotheses About the Mechanism of Reproductive Disorders in Athletes

Testing the many competing hypotheses proposed to explain the menstrual disorders observed in athletes required several types of experiments. Some of these hypotheses proposed that acute endocrine responses to exercise itself might disrupt the female reproductive system. For example, it was proposed that androgen responses to exercise might masculinize women, that cortisol responses to exercise might indicate that the female reproductive system was suppressed by stress, and that the vibration of breasts during exercise might elicit a prolactin response like that which suppresses the reproductive system in nursing mothers. Instead, the acute androgen, cortisol, and prolactin responses to exercise turned out to be smaller in amenorrheic athletes than in eumenorrheic athletes.

The Body Fat Hypothesis

The most widely popularized hypothesis for explaining menstrual disorders in athletes proposed that the ovarian axis is disrupted when the amount of energy stored in the body as fat declines below a critical level. This amount of adipose tissue was first postulated to be necessary for the peripheral conversion of circulating androgens to estrogens, even though this conversion also takes place in skeletal muscle and athletes typically have more muscle mass than others. Observations of athletes did not consistently verify the association of menstrual status with body composition, however, and they did not find the appropriate temporal relationship between changes in body composition and menstrual function. Eumenorrheic and amenorrheic athletes were also found to span a common range of body composition leaner than most eumenorrheic sedentary women. Among women distance runners, energy balance was found to be a better predictor of estradiol levels than either body mass index or percent body fat. Furthermore, when the growth and sexual development of young animals was blocked by dietary restriction, normal LH pulsatility resumed only a few hours and ovulation only 3 to 4 days after *ad libitum* feeding was permitted, long before any change in body mass or composition occurred (96). And when surgical reduction of the stomachs of severely obese women (body weight about 130 kg; body mass index about 47) reduced the amount of food that they could eat, rapid weight loss and amenorrhea occurred while the patients were still overweight (body weight about 97 kg; body mass index about 35) (97).

Nevertheless, interest in the body composition hypothesis was rejuvenated in the mid-1990s with the discovery of the hormone leptin and the location of leptin receptors in the hypothalamus. Synthesized and secreted by adipose tissue,

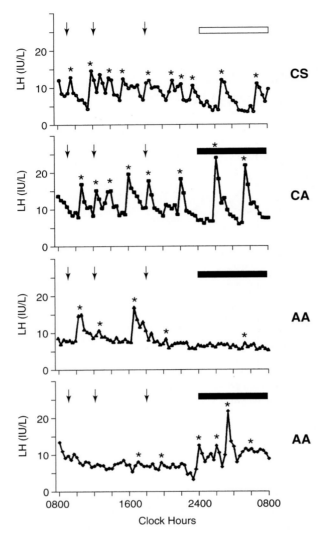

FIGURE 22.12 The 24-h rhythm of serum LH levels at 20-min intervals in a typical cyclic sedentary woman (CS), a typical cyclic athlete (CA), and two amenorrheic athletes. Asterisks indicate pulses detected by a computer program using objective pulse detection criteria. Arrows indicate mealtimes. Horizontal bars indicate sleep periods. The effects of LH on ovarian function were determined by the frequency of LH pulses, not the average LH concentration. *(Reprinted with permission from Loucks AB, Mortola JF, Girton L, et al. Alterations in the hypothalamic-pituitary-ovarian and the hypothalamic-pituitary-adrenal axes in athletic women. J Clin Endocrinol Metab 1989;68:407.)*

flux of glucose through the hexosamine biosynthesis pathway in muscle and adipose tissue. Then it was found that the diurnal rhythm of leptin actually depends not on energy intake but rather on energy availability (i.e., on the difference between dietary energy intake and exercise energy expenditure), or more specifically, on carbohydrate availability.

The Stress Hypothesis

The hypothesis that the stress of exercise activates the adrenal axis and thereby disrupts the GnRH pulse generator was supported by considerable animal research demonstrating that GnRH neurons are disturbed by activation of the hypothalamic-pituitary-adrenal axis via pathways involving corticotropin-releasing hormone and endogenous opioid and pro-opiomelanocortin-derived peptides and by increased cortisol negative feedback. Early experiments by Hans Selye and others induced anestrus and ovarian atrophy in rats by abruptly forcing them to run or swim for long periods, and elevated cortisol levels in such studies were interpreted as signs of stress. It was concluded that "exercise stress" had a counterregulatory influence on the female reproductive system.

These experiments induced extreme activations of the adrenal axis, however, raising cortisol concentrations by several hundred percent, in contrast to the mild 10 to 30% elevations seen in amenorrheic athletes and anorexia nervosa patients. Whether such mild elevations in cortisol influenced the GnRH pulse generator was entirely speculative. Only one experiment successfully employed exercise to induce menstrual disorders in eumenorrheic women (98). That experiment imposed a high volume of aerobic exercise abruptly in imitation of Selye. It caused a large proportion of menstrual disorders in the first month and an even larger proportion in the second. The disorders were more prevalent in a subgroup fed a controlled weight loss diet than in another subgroup fed for weight maintenance, but even the weight maintenance subgroup may have been underfed, because behavior modification and endocrine-mediated alterations in resting metabolic rate can counteract the potential influences of dietary energy excess or deficiency on body mass (99).

The first cracks in the stress hypothesis appeared when glucose administration during exercise was found to prevent the cortisol response to exercise in both rats and men. Since all previous animal and human investigations of the influence of the "activity stress paradigm" on reproductive function had confounded the stress of exercise with the stress of forcing animals to exercise (e.g., electroshock or fear of drowning) and/or with energy availability (requiring animals to run farther and farther for smaller and smaller food rewards), there was in fact no unconfounded experimental evidence that the stress of exercise, independent of its energy cost, disrupts reproductive function in voluntarily exercising women. Furthermore, since cortisol is a glucoregulatory hormone activated by low blood glucose levels, these elevated cortisol levels could also be interpreted as part of a multifaceted physiological response to chronic energy deficiency.

leptin was originally thought to communicate information about fat stores. Later leptin was found to vary profoundly in response to fasting, dietary restriction, refeeding after dietary restriction, and overfeeding before any changes in adiposity occurred. This led to the hypothesis that leptin signals information about dietary intake, particularly carbohydrate intake. Indeed, leptin was found to be regulated by the tiny

The Energy Availability Hypothesis

The energy availability hypothesis recognizes that the expenditure of energy in one physiological function, such as locomotion, makes it unavailable for others, including reproductive development and function. Specifically, this hypothesis holds that failure to provide sufficient metabolic fuels, especially glucose, to meet the energy requirements of the brain causes an alteration in brain function that disrupts the GnRH pulse generator. Thus, one can think of energy availability as the amount of dietary energy remaining for other physiological functions after subtracting the energy consumed by one particular function of interest.

Considerable data from biological field trials supported the hypothesis that mammalian reproductive function depends on energy availability, particularly in females. Anestrus has been induced in Syrian hamsters by food restriction, the administration of pharmacological blockers of carbohydrate and fat metabolism, insulin administration (which shunts metabolic fuels into storage), and cold exposure (which consumes metabolic fuels in thermogenesis) (100). Disruptive effects on the reproductive system were independent of body size and composition. Animal research also suggests that GnRH neuron activity and LH pulsatility are regulated by brain glucose availability via two separate mechanisms involving the area postrema in the caudal brainstem and the vagus nerve (101). Glucose-sensing neurons in the area postrema appear to transmit information to the GnRH pulse generator via neurons containing catecholamines, neuropeptide Y, and CRH. These glucose-sensing neurons are activated by fasting in part because of reductions in the inhibitory influences of insulin and leptin, as well as glucose.

In athletes, energy availability can be defined, quantified, and controlled as dietary energy intake minus exercise energy expenditure. Cross-sectional comparisons of estimated energy availability in amenorrheic and eumenorrheic athletes support the notion that their menstrual function is disrupted by low energy availability. Amenorrheic athletes were estimated to habitually self-administer an energy availability of only about 16 kcal $\cdot$ kg fat-free mass^{-1} per day, while eumenorrheic athletes habitually self-administered about 30 kcal $\cdot$ kg fat-free mass^{-1} per day (102). Surprisingly, amenorrheic and eumenorrheic athletes report their body weight to be stable despite dietary energy intakes similar to those of sedentary women.

Extensive observational data on the energy and carbohydrate intake of athletes in many sports indicate that with the notable exception of cross-country skiers, female athletes consume about 30% less energy and carbohydrate—normalized for body weight—than do male athletes (103). Not surprisingly, therefore, amenorrheic athletes display low levels of plasma glucose, insulin, IGF-I, IGF-I/IGFBP-1 (an index of IGF-I bioavailability), leptin, and T_3, as well as low resting metabolic rates. They also display elevated GH and mildly elevated cortisol levels. Compared to eumenorrheic sedentary women, luteally suppressed eumenorrheic athletes also display low levels of insulin, leptin, and T_3 and elevated levels of

GH and cortisol, but the magnitudes of these abnormalities were less extreme than in amenorrheic athletes. Thus, metabolic substrates and hormones in amenorrheic and eumenorrheic athletes tell a consistent story of chronic energy and carbohydrate deficiency resulting in mobilization of fat stores, slowing of metabolic rate, and reduction in glucose utilization, with more extreme abnormalities in amenorrheic athletes and less extreme abnormalities in eumenorrheic athletes.

Tests of the Exercise Stress and Energy Availability Hypotheses

The controversy over whether reproductive disorders in female athletes are caused by the stress of exercise or by low energy availability was resolved by an experiment that determined the independent effects of exercise stress and energy availability on LH pulsatility (104). Energy availability was defined, measured, and controlled operationally as dietary energy intake minus exercise energy expenditure, and exercise stress was defined as *everything* associated with exercise except its energy cost. Figure 22.13A shows the experimental design in which habitually sedentary women of normal body composition were assigned to sedentary (S) or exercising (X) groups and then administered balanced (B = 45 kcal $\cdot$ kg fat-free mass^{-1} per day) and deprived (D = 10 kcal $\cdot$ kg fat-free mass^{-1} per day) energy availability treatments in random order under controlled conditions in the laboratory.

Figure 22.13B shows the independent effects of exercise stress, determined by comparing the sedentary and exercising groups, and of energy availability, determined by comparing the balanced and deprived energy availability treatments: exercise stress had no suppressive effect on LH pulse frequency, and low energy availability suppressed LH pulse frequency whether or not the low energy availability was caused by dietary energy restriction alone or by exercise energy expenditure alone. Similar results (not shown) were obtained when half of the reduction in energy availability was caused by dietary energy restriction and half by exercise energy expenditure. Low energy availability also suppressed T_3, insulin, IGF-I, and leptin while increasing GH and cortisol (105) in a pattern very reminiscent of amenorrheic and luteally suppressed eumenorrheic athletes (102).

Since this experiment, the energy availability hypothesis has been confirmed through experimental disruptions of ovarian function. Amenorrhea was induced in monkeys by training them to run voluntarily on a motorized treadmill for longer and longer periods while their food intake remained constant (106). The monkeys became amenorrheic abruptly 7 to 24 months after one or two cycles of luteal suppression. When the diet of half of the monkeys was then supplemented without any moderation of their exercise regimen, their menstrual cycles were restored, while the rest of the monkeys remained amenorrheic (107). The rapidity of recovery was directly related to the number of calories consumed.

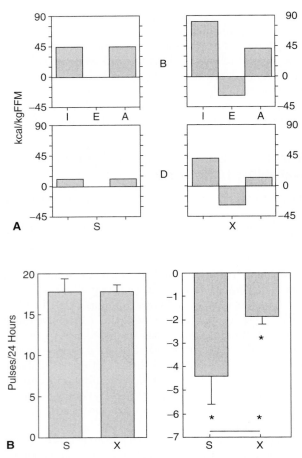

FIGURE 22.13 **A.** Experimental design for distinguishing the independent effects of exercise stress and energy availability on LH pulsatility in regularly menstruating, habitually sedentary women. In a sedentary group (S) balanced (B = 45 kcal · kg fat-free mass⁻¹ per day) and deprived (D = 10 kcal · kg fat-free mass⁻¹ per day) energy availabilities (A) were achieved by a dietary intakes (I) of 45 and 10 kcal · kg fat-free mass⁻¹ per day. The exercising group (X) expended 30 kcal · kg fat-free mass⁻¹ per day of energy in supervised exercise on a treadmill in the laboratory. Their balanced (B = 45 kcal · kg fat-free mass⁻¹ per day) and deprived (D = 10 kcal · kg fat-free mass⁻¹ per day) energy availabilities (A) were achieved by dietary intakes (I) of 75 and 40 kcal · kg fat-free mass⁻¹ per day. **B.** LH pulse frequency (*left*) and changes in LH pulse frequency due to low energy availability (*right*) in X and S. Exercise stress had no effect, and low energy availability suppressed LH pulse frequency. *(Reprinted with permission from Loucks AB, Verdun M, Heath EM. Low energy availability, not stress of exercise, alters LH pulsatility in exercising women. J Appl Physiol 1998;38,43.)*

Dose Dependence of LH Pulsatility on Energy Availability

The dose-response relationship between energy availability and LH pulsatility in exercising women has also been determined (105). LH pulse frequency was suppressed and pulse amplitude was increased below a threshold of energy avail-

ability at about 30 kcal · kg fat-free mass⁻¹ per day, suggesting that athletes may be able to prevent menstrual disorders by maintaining energy availabilities above 30 kcal · kg fat-free mass⁻¹ per day (Fig. 22.14). Figure 22.14 also shows that the disruption of LH pulsatility was substantially more extreme in women with short luteal phases. If the latter finding is confirmed through further investigations, the screening of women for luteal length may be a convenient way to identify those who need to take extra care to avoid falling below the threshold of energy availability needed to maintain normal LH pulsatility.

The maintenance of normal LH pulsatility in this experiment despite a restriction of energy availability to 30 kcal · kg fat-free mass⁻¹ per day demonstrated that the regulation of the reproductive system in women seems to be robust against reductions in energy availability as large as 33%. Since the exercise energy expenditure in this experiment was about 840 kcal, these results suggest that women may be able to maintain normal LH pulsatility while running up to 8 miles a day as long as they do not simultaneously reduce their dietary energy intake below 45 kcal · kg fat-free mass⁻¹ per day. If they do reduce their dietary energy intake, as many exercising women do, they risk falling below the threshold of energy availability needed to maintain normal LH pulsatility.

Figure 22.14 also shows the dose-response effects of energy availability on several metabolic hormones and substrates. Down to 30 kcal · kg fat-free mass⁻¹ per day, the effects of glucoregulatory hormone responses in mobilizing stored metabolic fuels were able to maintain plasma glucose concentrations to within a few percent of energy-balanced levels, but below that threshold glucose concentrations fall increasingly despite even larger hormone responses and steep increases in fat oxidation and gluconeogenesis as indicated by the rise in β-hydroxybutyrate. Because hepatic secretion of IGF-I in response to GH stimulation is limited by T_3, the fall in T_3, especially between 20 and 30 kcal · k fat-free mass⁻¹ per day, made the liver resistant to GH. Thus, as energy availability declines below 30 kcal · kg fat-free mass⁻¹ per day, we see progressively more extreme glucoregulatory responses being less and less effective at maintaining plasma glucose levels, and progressively more reliance on ketones as the alternative metabolic fuel for brain metabolism.

Reproductive Disorders in Male Athletes

Similar metabolic and reproductive disorders can occur in male athletes, especially those in endurance sports and sports with weight classes, but they are less obvious and less extreme than in women. They are less obvious because men do not present symptoms such as menstrual abnormalities, and they are less extreme in that reproductive development continues in males under conditions in which it is entirely blocked in females.

No 24-h studies of LH pulsatility in male athletes have been published to date. Shorter, less reliable studies have reported inconsistent results. Nor have any investigators re-

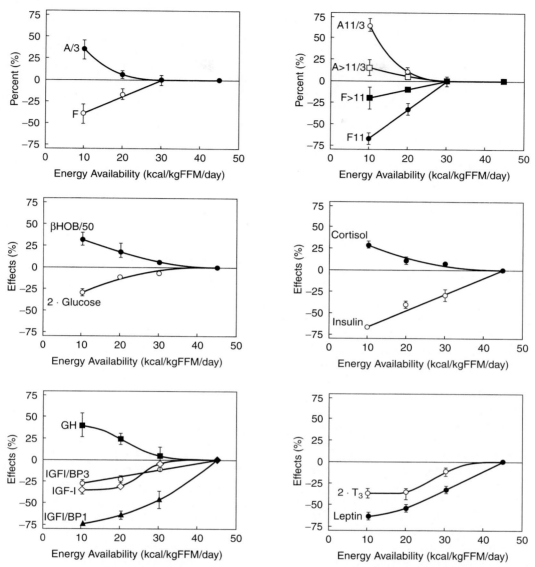

FIGURE 22.14 Incremental effects of energy availability on LH pulsatility and selected metabolic substrates and hormones in regularly menstruating, habitually sedentary women. All subjects expended 15 kcal · kg fat-free mass⁻¹ per day of energy in supervised exercise on a treadmill in the laboratory. Energy availabilities of 45, 30, 20, and 10 kcal · kg fat-free mass⁻¹ per day were achieved by dietary intakes of 60, 45, 35, and 25 kcal · kg fat-free mass⁻¹ per day. Effects are shown relative to 45 kcal · kg fat-free mass⁻¹ per day. *Top left.* Effects on LH pulse frequency (F) and amplitude (A/3) in all women at each energy availability treatment. Effects on LH pulsatility occurred below about 30 kcal · kg fat-free mass⁻¹ per day. *Top right.* Effects were larger in women with luteal phase lengths of 11 days (F11, A11/3) than in women with luteal phase lengths longer than 11 days (F >11, A >11/3). (Women with luteal lengths less than 11 days were excluded from study.) *Center left.* Incremental effects on the metabolic substrates β-HOB (βHOB/50) and plasma glucose (2 · Glucose). Effects on β-HOB have been divided by 50 and effects on glucose have been doubled for graphical symmetry. Effects on β-HOB and glucose became more extreme as energy availability decreased, despite more extreme responses of the metabolic hormones. *Center right.* Incremental effects on the metabolic hormones cortisol and insulin. Insulin declined linearly with energy availability, whereas effects on cortisol became increasingly extreme as energy availability decreased. *Bottom left.* Incremental effects on the somatotrophic metabolic hormones GH and IGF-I and on the ratios IGF-I/IGFBP-1 (IGFI/BP1) and IGF-I/IGFBP-3 (IGFI/BP3), which are indices of IGF-I bioavailability. GH resistance and elevated IGF-I binding proteins reduced IGF-I bioavailability as energy availability decreased. *Bottom right.* Incremental effects on the metabolic hormones T₃ (2 · T₃) and leptin. Effects on T₃ are doubled for clarity. The decline in T₃ accounts for the GH resistance. *(Reprinted with permission from Loucks AB, Thuma JR. Luteinizing hormone pulsatility is disrupted at a threshold of energy availability in regularly menstruating women. J Clin Endocrinol Metab 2003;88:304,306.)*

ported observations of semen quality outside the normal range. Reduced total and/or free testosterone levels have been reported by many but not all cross-sectional and prospective studies of endurance-trained male athletes, but only one has reported levels below the normal range. Where statistically significant reductions in reproductive hormones have been noted, these have been found in the most intensively training athletes. Consequently, the consensus is that reproductive dysfunction is uncommon in male athletes and that the long-term physiological consequences of the suppression of the hypothalamic-pituitary-testicular axis in male athletes probably has little clinical significance.

It was a prospective study of adolescent male wrestlers that found testosterone levels falling below the normal range during the wrestling season (108) along with reductions in body weight, fat mass, and strength (109). The wrestlers were consuming only half of their recommended energy intake before the season began, and they did not increase their energy intake during the season. As with female athletes, the failure of these male wrestlers to increase energy intake during the season induced GH resistance, with elevated GH and suppressed IGF-I levels. Levels of prealbumin, a classic biomarker of starvation, were also suppressed. As might be expected with reduced anabolic stimulation by testosterone and IGF-I, the wrestlers' fat-free mass and their mid arm and mid thigh cross-sectional areas all declined during the wrestling season. As a result, their arm and leg strength and power declined by an average of 13%, contradicting the belief that weight loss conveys a competitive advantage.

Proof that chronic low energy availability and not exercise stress disrupts reproductive function in men, as it does as in women, was reported in a study of young male soldiers participating in the 8-wk U.S. Army Ranger training course (110). This course was divided into four 2-wk phases in forest, desert, mountain, and swamp, during which trainees expended 4200 kcal · day^{-1} as they underwent daily military skill training, 8- to 12-km patrols carrying 32-kg rucksacks, and sleep deprivation (about 3.6 h of sleep per night), while consuming controlled diets providing about 2000 and about 5000 kcal · day^{-1} in alternate weeks (Fig. 22.15A). These rigors were so severe that only 30% of the trainees completed the course.

Trainees who completed the course lost about 12 kg of body weight. As Figure 22.15B shows, blood sampling at the ends of selected weeks revealed that T$_3$, IGF-I, and testosterone levels fell about 20%, about 50%, and about 70%, respectively, during weeks on diets of 2000 kcal · day^{-1} and returned to normal initial levels during alternate weeks on diets of 5000 kcal · day^{-1} despite continued exposure to all other training stresses.

SUMMARY

This chapter focuses on the main mechanisms by which the endocrine system integrates the influences of diet and exercise on the storage, mobilization, and utilization of metabolic

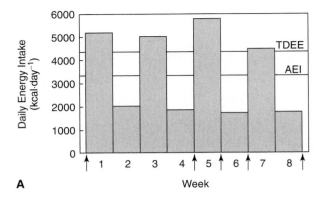

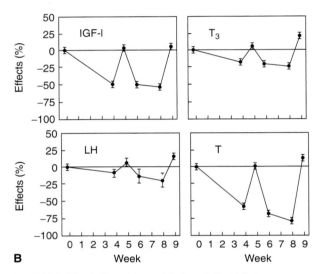

FIGURE 22.15 **A.** Experimental design of the U.S. Army Rangers experiment. Ranger candidates trained for 2 wk each in forest, mountain, desert, and swamp terrain working with a total daily energy expenditure (TDEE) of 4200 kcal · day^{-1} while consuming an average energy intake (AEI) of 3200 kcal · day^{-1} in controlled diets providing about 5000 and 2000 kcal · day^{-1} in alternate weeks. Blood was sampled at the beginning and after the fourth, fifth, sixth, and eighth weeks of training, and after 1 wk of ad libitum feeding after training. **B.** Effects of diet, exercise, and other training stresses on IGF-I, T$_3$, LH, and testosterone (T). One week of ad libitum refeeding after training (week 9) restored normal metabolic and reproductive hormone levels, and so did 1 wk of controlled refeeding in week 5, despite continued exercise and other training stresses. The restoration of metabolic and reproductive function in week 5 demonstrates that the disruption of reproductive function in men is caused by low energy availability, as it is in women, and not by exercise or other training stresses.

fuels, on the turnover and growth of skeletal muscle, and on reproductive function. A similar story could have been told about how the endocrine system integrates the influences of diet and trauma (or cold exposure or cancer and other processes that consume large amounts of energy) on the availability of metabolic fuels, on the turnover and growth of bone, and on immune function. All such stories about the endocrine system have in common the unique and extreme energy demand of the human brain, which requires strict tradeoffs between basal metabolism, thermoregulation, locomotion, growth, and reproduction when dietary energy is scarce. The endocrine mechanisms implementing these tradeoffs have made us survivors.

Exercise elicits acute glucoregulatory hormone responses to mobilize metabolic fuels for meeting the energy require-ments of working muscle. By restricting the supply of glucose to the brain, prolonged exercise training and dietary restriction, especially in combination, elicit chronic changes in these and other metabolic and reproductive hormones to reduce the metabolic demands of tissues competing against the brain. To optimize their performance and growth and to preserve their reproductive and skeletal health, athletes need to manage their diet and exercise programs to minimize the frequency and duration of such conditions.

A MILESTONE OF DISCOVERY

Does work-induced, that is, functional, hypertrophy of skeletal muscle depend on the presence of pituitary GH, as does the growth in muscle size that occurs during normal development? Until 1967, properly designed experiments measuring functional hypertrophy in the presence and absence of circulating GH had not been conducted. It was known that circulating GH is necessary for the growth process that increases all dimensions of body size during normal development. It was also known that individual muscles increase in size selectively in response to increased mechanical loading, while unloaded contralateral muscles do not. In a randomized 2 × 2 design, Goldberg assigned rats to be hypophysectomized or left intact, and he then surgically severed the gastrocnemius tendon of one hindlimb in half of the intact and half of the hypophysectomized rats to overload the synergistic soleus and plantaris muscles in those limbs. After 1, 3, 5, and 14 days, rats were killed, and the soleus and plantaris muscles from both hindlimbs were weighed. He also replicated this experiment in a second group of rats whose spinal cord was crushed just below the rib cage to paralyze and anesthetize the hind limbs. One of the key findings of this study is shown in Figure 22.16.

Overloading increased the sizes of the soleus and plantaris muscles by the same amounts in both hypophysectomized and intact rats. The mass of the soleus increased by about 40% and the plantaris by about 20%, and this process was complete in 5 days. In paralyzed rats, no increases in the sizes of soleus and plantaris muscles occurred in the limbs with a severed gastrocnemius tendon. This demonstrated that the observed hypertrophy had not been caused by the sectioning of the gastrocnemius but rather by the resulting increased loading of the intact soleus and plantaris muscles and that this hypertrophy does not depend on circulating GH or on any other circulating pituitary axis hormones, either. This experiment also demonstrated for the first time how rapidly skeletal muscle could undergo compensatory growth.

This experiment inspired decades of research into the mechanism by which the hypertrophy response is locally controlled by an intrinsic capability of skeletal muscles. Gradually it was learned that GH-dependent growth during normal development is mediated by IGF-I, that most circulating IGF-I is secreted by the liver in response to the combined stimulation of circulating GH and T_3, and that skeletal muscle has an intrinsic capability to express IGF-I in response to mechanical loading. Eventually a replication of

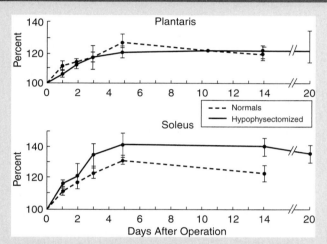

FIGURE 22.16 Comparison of the rate and extent of compensatory hypertrophy of the plantaris and soleus muscles in normal and hypophysectomized rats 5 days after tenotomy of the synergistic gastrocnemius muscle. Hypertrophy is expressed as the average ratios of the weight of the hypertrophied muscle to its contralateral control. In no instances are the responses of the two groups of animals statistically different, demonstrating that circulating GH, IGF-I, testosterone, and thyroid hormone are not necessary for exercise-induced hypertrophy.

Goldberg's experiment demonstrated that hypertrophy of the overloaded plantaris muscle is independent of circulating IGF-I and that the expression of IGF-I mRNA and peptide and the content of DNA reflecting satellite cell proliferation in the hypertrophying plantaris muscle all increase in a coordinated manner consistent with the hypothesis that locally expressed IGF-I mediates the hypertrophy response to mechanical loading. Since then, an isoform of IGF-I, MGF, which is expressed only in skeletal muscle in response to increased mechanical loading, has been found to be much more powerful than IGF-I in stimulating the hypertrophy response, and many details of intracellular and molecular signaling that mediate this response have been identified.

Goldberg AL. Work-induced growth of skeletal muscle in normal and hypophysectomized rats. Am J Physiol 1967;213:1193–1198.

ACKNOWLEDGMENTS

Research in my laboratory is supported in part by Grant DAMD 17-95-1-5053 from the U.S. Army Medical Research and Material Command (Defense Women's Health & Military Medical Readiness Research Program); the General Clinical Research Branch, Division of Research Resources, NIH Grant M01 RR00034; and by Ross Products Division, Abbott Laboratories. The content of the information reported in this paper does not necessarily reflect the position or the policy of the government, and no official endorsement should be inferred.

REFERENCES

1. Otis CL, Drinkwater B, Johnson M, et al. American College of Sports Medicine position stand: the female athlete triad. Med Sci Sports Exerc 1997;29:i–ix.

2. Oppliger RA, Case HS, Horswill CA, et al. American College of Sports Medicine position stand: weight loss in wrestlers. Med Sci Sports Exerc 1996;28:ix–xii.

3. Bubb RG. Rule 3. Weight certification, classification and weigh in. In Halpin T, ed. 2004 NCAA Wrestling Rules and Interpretations. Indianapolis: National Collegiate Athletic Association, 2003;WR-23–WR-35, WI-10–WI-11, WA-28-WA-33.

4. Kaciuba-Uscilko H, Kruk B, Szczpaczewska M, et al. Metabolic, body temperature and hormonal responses to repeated periods of prolonged cycle-ergometer exercise in men. Eur J Appl Physiol 1992;64:26–31.

5. Galassetti P, Mann S, Tate D, et al. Effect of morning exercise on counterregulatory responses to subsequent, afternoon exercise. J Appl Physiol 2001;91:91–99.

6. Cryer PE. The prevention and correction of hypoglycemia. In Jefferson LS, Cherrington AD, eds. Handbook of Physiology, Section 7. The Endocrine System. Vol 2. The Endocrine Pancreas and Regulation of Metabolism. Oxford: Oxford University, 2001;1057–1092.

7. Davis SN, Galassetti P, Wasserman DH, et al. Effects of antecedent hypoglycemia on subsequent counterregulatory responses to exercise. Diabetes 2000;49:73–81.

8. Wasserman DH, Lickley HL, Vranic M. Interactions between glucagon and other counterregulatory hormones during normoglycemic and hypoglycemic exercise in dogs. J Clin Invest 1984;74:1404–1413.

9. Wasserman DH, Cherrington AD. Regulation of extra muscular fuel sources during exercise. In LB Rowell, JT Shephard, eds. Handbook of Physiology, Section 12. Exercise: Regulation and Integration of Multiple Systems. Oxford, UK: Oxford Press, 1996;1036–1074.

10. Galassetti P. Reciprocity of hypoglycaemia and exercise in blunting respective counterregulatory responses: possible role of cortisol as a mediator. Diabetes Nutr Metab 2002;15:341–347; discussion 347–348, 362.

11. Galassetti P, Neill AR, Tate D, et al. Sexual dimorphism in counterregulatory responses to hypoglycemia after antecedent exercise. J Clin Endocrinol Metab 2001;86: 3516–3524.

12. Heller SR, Cryer PE. Hypoinsulinemia is not critical to glucose recovery from hypoglycemia in humans. Am J Physiol 1991;261:E41–E48.

13. Galassetti P, Mann S, Tate D, et al. Effects of antecedent prolonged exercise on subsequent counterregulatory responses to hypoglycemia. Am J Physiol 2001;280:E908–E917.

14. Sandoval DA, Ertl AC, Richardson MA, et al. Estrogen blunts neuroendocrine and metabolic responses to hypoglycemia. Diabetes 2003;52:1749–1755.

15. Young EA. The role of gonadal steroids in hypothalamic-pituitary-adrenal axis regulation. Crit Rev Neurobiol 1995;9:371–381.

16. Roy BN, Reid RL, Van Vugt DA. The effects of estrogen and progesterone on corticotropin-releasing hormone and arginine vasopressin messenger ribonucleic acid levels in the paraventricular nucleus and supraoptic nucleus of the rhesus monkey. Endocrinology 1999;140:2191–2198.

17. Tremblay A, Pinsard D, Coveney S, et al. Counterregulatory response to insulin-induced hypoglycemia in trained and nontrained humans. Metabolism 1990;39:1138–1143.

18. Richter EA, Galbo H, Sonne B, et al. Adrenal medullary control of muscular and hepatic glycogenolysis and of pancreatic hormonal secretion in exercising rats. Acta Physiol Scand 1980;108:235–242.

19. MacLaren DP, Reilly T, Campbell IT, et al. Hormonal and metabolic responses to maintained hyperglycemia during prolonged exercise. J Appl Physiol 1999;87:124–131.

20. Tabata I, Ogita F, Miyachi M, et al. Effect of low blood glucose on plasma CRF, ACTH, and cortisol during prolonged physical exercise. J Appl Physiol 1991;71: 1807–1812.

21. Ainslie PN, Campbell IT, Frayn KN, et al. Physiological, metabolic, and performance implications of a prolonged hill walk: influence of energy intake. J Appl Physiol 2003;94:1075–1083.

22. Davies CT, Few JD. Effects of exercise on adrenocortical function. J Appl Physiol 1973;35:887–891.

23. Brandenberger G, Follenius M. Influence of timing and intensity of muscular exercise on temporal patterns of plasma cortisol levels. J Clin Endocrinol Metab 1975;40:845–849.

24. Thuma JR, Gilders R, Verdun M, et al. Circadian rhythm of cortisol confounds cortisol responses to exercise: implications for future research. J Appl Physiol 1995;78:1657–1664.

25. Hirsch IB, Marker JC, Smith LJ, et al. Insulin and glucagon in prevention of hypoglycemia during exercise in humans. Am J Physiol 1991;260:E695–E704.

26. Zinker BA, Mohr T, Kelly P, et al. Exercise-induced fall in insulin: mechanism of action at the liver and effects on muscle glucose metabolism. Am J Physiol 1994;266:E683–E689.

27. Lecavalier L, Bolli G, Gerich J. Glucagon-cortisol interactions on glucose turnover and lactate gluconeogenesis in normal humans. Am J Physiol 1990;258:E569–E575.

28. Kahn CR. Glucose homeostasis and insulin action. In Becker KL, ed. Principles and Practice of Endocrinology and Metabolism. Baltimore: Lippincott Williams & Wilkins, 2001;1030–1307.

29. Goodyear LJ. AMP-activated protein kinase: a critical signaling intermediary for exercise-stimulated glucose transport? Exerc Sport Sci Rev 2000;28:113–116.

30. Frayn KN. Macronutrient metabolism of adipose tissue at rest and during exercise: a methodological viewpoint. Proc Nutr Soc 1999;58:877–886.

31. Frayn KN, Humphreys SM, Coppack SW. Fuel selection in white adipose tissue. Proc Nutr Soc 1995;54:177–189.

32. Taylor R, Husband DJ, Marshall SM, et al. Adipocyte insulin binding and insulin sensitivity in 'brittle' diabetes. Diabetologia 1984;27:441–446.

33. Leboeuf B. Regulation of fatty acid esterification in adipose tissue incubated *in vitro*. In Renold AE, Cahill GF, eds. Handbook of Physiology, Section 5. Adipose Tissue. Washington: American Physiological Society, 1965;385–391.

34. Arner P, Kriegholm E, Engfeldt P, et al. Adrenergic regulation of lipolysis in situ at rest and during exercise. J Clin Invest 1990;85:893–898.

35. Hoelzer DR, Dalsky GP, Schwartz NS, et al. Epinephrine is not critical to prevention of hypoglycemia during exercise in humans. Am J Physiol 1986;251:E104–E110.

36. Hodgetts V, Coppack SW, Frayn KN, et al. Factors controlling fat mobilization from human subcutaneous adipose tissue during exercise. J Appl Physiol 1991;71: 445–451.

37. Summers LK, Samra JS, Humphreys SM, et al. Subcutaneous abdominal adipose tissue blood flow: variation within and between subjects and relationship to obesity. Clin Sci (Lond) 1996;91:679–683.

38. Jones NL, Heigenhauser GJ, Kuksis A, et al. Fat metabolism in heavy exercise. Clin Sci (Lond) 1980;59:469–478.

39. Wasserman DH, Spalding JA, Lacy DB, et al. Glucagon is a primary controller of hepatic glycogenolysis and gluconeogenesis during muscular work. Am J Physiol 1989;257:E108–E117.

40. Wahren J, Sato Y, Ostman J, et al. Turnover and splanchnic metabolism of free fatty acids and ketones in insulin-dependent diabetics at rest and in response to exercise. J Clin Invest 1984;73:1367–1376.

41. Liu Z, Barrett EJ. Human protein metabolism: its measurement and regulation. Am J Physiol 2002;283: E1105–E1112.

42. Glickman MH, Ciechanover A. The ubiquitin-proteasome proteolytic pathway: destruction for the sake of construction. Physiol Rev 2002;82:373–428.

43. Goll DE, Thompson VF, Li H, et al. The calpain system. Physiol Rev 2003;83:731–801.

44. Phaneuf S, Leeuwenburgh C. Apoptosis and exercise. Med Sci Sports Exerc 2001;33:393–396.

45. Goldberg AL, JD Etlinger, DF Goldspink, et al. Mechanism of work-induced hypertrophy of skeletal muscle. Med Sci Sports 1975;7:185–198.

46. Rasmussen BB, Phillips SM. Contractile and nutritional regulation of human muscle growth. Exerc Sport Sci Rev 2003;31:127–131.

47. Nygren J, Nair KS. Differential regulation of protein dynamics in splanchnic and skeletal muscle beds by insulin and amino acids in healthy human subjects. Diabetes 2003;52:1377–1385.

48. Louard RJ, Fryburg DA, Gelfand RA, et al. Insulin sensitivity of protein and glucose metabolism in human forearm skeletal muscle. J Clin Invest 1992;90:2348–2354.

49. Mitch WE, Bailey JL, Wang X, et al. Evaluation of signals activating ubiquitin-proteasome proteolysis in a model of muscle wasting. Am J Physiol 1999;276:C1132–C1138.

50. Moller-Loswick AC, Zachrisson H, Hyltander A, et al. Insulin selectively attenuates breakdown of nonmyofibrillar proteins in peripheral tissues of normal men. Am J Physiol 1994;266:E645–E652.

51. Liu Z, Miers WR, Wei L, et al. The ubiquitin-proteasome proteolytic pathway in heart vs skeletal muscle: effects of acute diabetes. Biochem Biophys Res Commun 2000;276:1255–1260.

52. Kettelhut IC, Wing SS, Goldberg AL. Endocrine regulation of protein breakdown in skeletal muscle. Diabetes Metab Rev 1988;4:751–772.

53. Du J, Wang X, Miereles C, et al. Activation of caspase-3 is an initial step triggering accelerated muscle proteolysis in catabolic conditions. J Clin Invest 2004;113:115–123.

54. Pepato MT, Migliorini RH, Goldberg AL, et al. Role of different proteolytic pathways in degradation of muscle protein from streptozotocin-diabetic rats. Am J Physiol 1996;271:E340–E347.

55. Hedge GA, Colby HD, Goodman RI. Clinical Endocrine Physiology. Philadelphia: Saunders, 1987.

56. Fedele MJ, Hernandez JM, Lang CH, et al. Severe diabetes prohibits elevations in muscle protein synthesis after acute resistance exercise in rats. J Appl Physiol 2000;88: 102–108.

57. Darmaun D, Matthews DE, Bier DM. Physiological hypercortisolemia increases proteolysis, glutamine, and alanine production. Am J Physiol 1988;255:E366–E373.

58. Russell-Jones DL, Weissberger AJ, Bowes SB, et al. The effects of growth hormone on protein metabolism in adult growth hormone deficient patients. Clin Endocrinol (Oxf) 1993;38:427–431.

59. Bush JA, Kimball SR, O'Connor PM, et al. Translational control of protein synthesis in muscle and liver of growth hormone-treated pigs. Endocrinology 2003;144: 1273–1283.

60. Rennie MJ. Claims for the anabolic effects of growth hormone: a case of the emperor's new clothes? Br J Sports Med 2003;37:100–105.

61. Nindl BC, Hymer WC, Deaver DR, et al. Growth hormone pulsatility profile characteristics following acute heavy resistance exercise. J Appl Physiol 2001;91:163–172.

62. Liu JL, Grinberg A, Westphal H, et al. Insulin-like growth factor-I affects perinatal lethality and postnatal development in a gene dosage-dependent manner: manipulation using the Cre/loxP system in transgenic mice. Mol Endocrinol 1998;12:1452–1462.

63. Goldberg AL. Work-induced growth of skeletal muscle in normal and hypophysectomized rats. Am J Physiol 1967; 213:1193–1198.

64. Adams GR, Haddad F. The relationships among IGF-1, DNA content, and protein accumulation during skeletal muscle hypertrophy. J Appl Physiol 1996;81:2509–2516.

65. Yang S, Alnaqeeb M, Simpson H, et al. Cloning and characterization of an IGF-1 isoform expressed in skeletal muscle

subjected to stretch. J Muscle Res Cell Motil 1996;17:487–495.

66. Fryburg DA. Insulin-like growth factor I exerts growth hormone- and insulin-like actions on human muscle protein metabolism. Am J Physiol 1994;267:E331–336.

67. Adams GR. Invited Review: Autocrine/paracrine IGF-I and skeletal muscle adaptation. J Appl Physiol 2002;93: 1159–1167.

68. Fedele MJ, Lang CH, Farrell PA. Immunization against IGF-I prevents increases in protein synthesis in diabetic rats after resistance exercise. Am J Physiol 2001;280:E877–E885.

69. Li BG, Hasselgren PO, Fang CH, et al. Insulin-like growth factor-I blocks dexamethasone-induced protein degradation in cultured myotubes by inhibiting multiple proteolytic pathways: 2002 ABA paper. J Burn Care Rehabil 2004;25:112–118.

70. Wilson VJ, Rattray M, Thomas CR, et al. Effects of hypophysectomy and growth hormone administration on the mRNA levels of collagen I, III and insulin-like growth factor-I in rat skeletal muscle. Growth Horm IGF Res 1998;8:431–438.

71. Goldspink G. Method of treating muscular disorders. U.S. Patent 6,221,842 B1, 2001.

72. Nindl BC, Kraemer WJ, Deaver DR, et al. LH secretion and testosterone concentrations are blunted after resistance exercise in men. J Appl Physiol 2001;91:1251–1258.

73. McCall GE, Byrnes WC, Fleck SJ, et al. Acute and chronic hormonal responses to resistance training designed to promote muscle hypertrophy. Can J Appl Physiol 1999;24: 96–107.

74. Bhasin S, Storer TW, Berman N, et al. The effects of supraphysiologic doses of testosterone on muscle size and strength in normal men. N Engl J Med 1996;335:1–7.

75. Ferrando AA, Tipton KD, Doyle D, et al. Testosterone injection stimulates net protein synthesis but not tissue amino acid transport. Am J Physiol 1998;275:E864–E871.

76. Wolfe R, Ferrando A, Sheffield-Moore M, et al. Testosterone and muscle protein metabolism. Mayo Clin Proc 2000;75Suppl:S55–S59; discussion S59–S60.

77. Doumit ME, Cook DR, Merkel RA. Testosterone upregulates androgen receptors and decreases differentiation of porcine myogenic satellite cells in vitro. Endocrinology 1996;137:1385–1394.

78. Sheffield-Moore M, Urban RJ, Wolf SE, et al. Short-term oxandrolone administration stimulates net muscle protein synthesis in young men. J Clin Endocrinol Metab 1999;84: 2705–2711.

79. Inoue K, Yamasaki S, Fushiki T, et al. Rapid increase in the number of androgen receptors following electrical stimulation of the rat muscle. Eur J Appl Physiol 1993;66: 134–140.

80. Bamman MM, Shipp JR, Jiang J, et al. Mechanical load increases muscle IGF-I and androgen receptor mRNA concentrations in humans. Am J Physiol 2001;280:E383–E390.

81. Mauras N, Hayes V, Welch S, et al. Testosterone deficiency in young men: marked alterations in whole body protein kinetics, strength, and adiposity. J Clin Endocrinol Metab 1998;83:1886–1892.

82. Bhasin S, Woodhouse L, Casaburi R, et al. Testosterone dose-response relationships in healthy young men. Am J Physiol 2001;281:E1172–E1181.

83. Caiozzo VJ, Haddad F. Thyroid hormone: modulation of muscle structure, function, and adaptive responses to mechanical loading. Exerc Sport Sci Rev 1996;24:321–361.

84. Gordon JW, Rungi AA, Inagaki H, et al. Effects of contractile activity on mitochondrial transcription factor A expression in skeletal muscle. J Appl Physiol 2001;90:389–396.

85. Wrutniak-Cabello C, Casas F, Cabello G. Thyroid hormone action in mitochondria. J Mol Endocrinol 2001;26:67–77.

86. Winder W, Fitts R, Holloszy JO, et al. Effects of thyroid hormone on different types of skeletal muscle. In Pette D, ed. Plasticity of Muscle. Berlin: Walter de Gruyter, 1980; 581–591.

87. Schuler MJ, Pette D. Quantification of thyroid hormone receptor isoforms, 9–cis retinoic acid receptor gamma, and nuclear receptor co-repressor by reverse-transcriptase PCR in maturing and adult skeletal muscles of rat. Eur J Biochem 1998;257:607–614.

88. Weber K, Bruck P, Mikes Z, et al. Glucocorticoid hormone stimulates mitochondrial biogenesis specifically in skeletal muscle. Endocrinology 2002;143:177–184.

89. Clapham JC, Arch JR, Chapman H, et al. Mice overexpressing human uncoupling protein-3 in skeletal muscle are hyperphagic and lean. Nature 2000;406:415–418.

90. Dulloo AG, Samec S. Uncoupling proteins: their roles in adaptive thermogenesis and substrate metabolism reconsidered. Br J Nutr 2001;86:123–139.

91. Weigle DS, Selfridge LE, Schwartz MW, et al. Elevated free fatty acids induce uncoupling protein 3 expression in muscle: a potential explanation for the effect of fasting. Diabetes 1998;47:298–302.

92. Cortright RN, Zheng D, Jones JP, et al. Regulation of skeletal muscle UCP-2 and UCP-3 gene expression by exercise and denervation. Am J Physiol 1999;276:E217–E221.

93. Moreno M, Lombardi A, De Lange P, et al. Fasting, lipid metabolism, and triiodothyronine in rat gastrocnemius muscle: interrelated roles of uncoupling protein 3, mitochondrial thioesterase, and coenzyme Q. FASEB J 2003;17:1112–1114.

94. Loucks AB, Mortola JF, Girton L, et al. Alterations in the hypothalamic-pituitary-ovarian and the hypothalamic-pituitary-adrenal axes in athletic women. J Clin Endocrinol Metab 1989;68:402–411.

95. De Souza, MJ, Miller BE, Loucks AB, et al. High frequency of luteal phase deficiency and anovulation in recreational women runners: blunted elevation in follicle-stimulating hormone observed during luteal-follicular transition. J Clin Endocrinol Metab 1998;83:4220–4232.

96. Bronson FH. Food-restricted, prepubertal, female rats: rapid recovery of luteinizing hormone pulsing with excess food, and full recovery of pubertal development with gonadotropin-releasing hormone. Endocrinology 1986;118:2483–2487.

97. Di Carlo C, Palomba S, De Fazio M, et al. Hypogonadotropic hypogonadotropism in obese women after biliopancreatic diversion. Fert Steril 1999;72:905–909.

98. Bullen BA, Skrinar GS, Beitins IZ, et al. Induction of menstrual disorders by strenuous exercise in untrained women. N Engl J Med 1985;312:1349–1353.

99. Leibel RL, Rosenbaum M, Hirsch J. Changes in energy expenditure resulting from altered body weight. N Engl J Med 1995;332:621–628.

100. Wade GN, Schneider JE. Metabolic fuels and reproduction in female mammals. Neurosci Biobehav Rev 1992;16:235–272.

101. Wade GN, Schneider JE, Li HY. Control of fertility by metabolic cues. Am J Physiol 1996;270:E1–E19.

102. Thong FS, McLean C, Graham TE. Plasma leptin in female athletes: relationship with body fat, reproductive, nutritional, and endocrine factors. J Appl Physiol 2000;88:2037–2044.

103. Burke LM, Cox GR, Culmmings NK, et al. Guidelines for daily carbohydrate intake: do athletes achieve them? Sports Med 2001;31:267–299.

104. Loucks AB, Verdun M, Heath EM. Low energy availability, not stress of exercise, alters LH pulsatility in exercising women. J Appl Physiol 1998;84:37–46.

105. Loucks AB, Thuma JR. Luteinizing hormone pulsatility is disrupted at a threshold of energy availability in regularly menstruating women. J Clin Endocrinol Metab 2003;88: 297–311.

106. Williams NI, Caston-Balderrama AL, Helmreich DL, et al. Longitudinal changes in reproductive hormones and menstrual cyclicity in cynomolgus monkeys during strenuous exercise training: abrupt transition to exercise-induced amenorrhea. Endocrinology 2001;142: 2381–2389.

107. Williams NI, Helmreich DL, Parfitt DB, et al. Evidence for a causal role of low energy availability in the induction of menstrual cycle disturbances during strenuous exercise training. J Clin Endocrinol Metab 2001;86: 5184–5193.

108. Roemmich JN, Sinning WE. Weight loss and wrestling training: effects on growth-related hormones. J Appl Physiol 1997;82:1760–1764.

109. Roemmich JN, Sinning WE. Weight loss and wrestling training: effects on nutrition, growth, maturation, body composition, and strength. J Appl Physiol 1997;82:1751–1759.

110. Friedl KE, Moore RJ, Hoyt RW, et al. Endocrine markers of semistarvation in healthy lean men in a multistressor environment. J Appl Physiol 2000;88: 1820–1830.

CHAPTER 23

Exercise and the Immune System

Laurie Hoffman-Goetz and Bente Klarlund Pedersen

Introduction

The rationale for studying the effect of physical exercise on the immune system comes from pioneering work on the physiology of stress. Stress refers to the cluster of physiological responses arising from the perception of aversive or threatening situations, resulting in fight-or-flight reactions (1). Stress triggers activation of the neocortex, limbic system, and brainstem (with norepinephrine as the main neurotransmitter), stimulation of the sympathetic nervous system, and consequent secretion into the circulation of epinephrine, or adrenaline, and norepinephrine, or noradrenaline, from the adrenal medulla. Concurrent stimulation of the paraventricular nucleus of the hypothalamus results in release of corticotrophin-releasing hormone and adrenocorticotrophic hormone from the pituitary and secretion of glucocorticoids (GC) (cortisol and corticosterone) from the adrenal cortex. That lymphocytes and other immune cells should be responsive to stress hormones is not surprising, given the constitutive expression of adrenergic receptors and glucocorticoid receptors. Additional conceptual support for the idea that exercise affects the immune system comes from the general adaptation syndrome (2). Moreover, stressors that are perceived as arousing and challenging (e.g., participation in a 10-km race by a fit individual) lead to elevated catecholamine levels, whereas stressors that are overwhelming (e.g., participation in a marathon by an

unfit individual) lead to elevated GC levels. Thus, a variety of stimuli, including physical exercise, activate the hypothalamic-pituitary-adrenal axis and influence the number, function, and movement of lymphoid cells. Indeed, early twentieth century studies reported leukocytosis in men after a marathon run (3) and in acutely exercised infected rabbits a lower ability of neutrophils to opsonize and phagocytize bacteria (4). Over the past century, hundreds of studies have demonstrated the impact of exercise on the immune system. This chapter describes the effects of endurance and resistance exercise on major components of the innate and acquired immune systems, considers the underlying physiological mechanisms for the effects of exercise on immune cells, and places these responses within the context of physiological relevance.

Overview of the Immune System

The immune system is the primary physiological system that mediates resistance and response to noxious exogenous agents (e.g., endotoxin), endogenous agents (e.g., tumor cells) and pathogens (e.g., viruses). It is composed of a system of central and peripheral organs and tissues, cellular components, and soluble macromolecules. Traditionally, the immune system is divided into two functional divisions or systems, the natural host defenses (sometimes referred to as constitutive or innate) and acquired or adaptive host defenses, both of which interact and overlap in a coordinated fashion. See recent textbooks (5,6) for detailed coverage of immunology. This section is a brief overview of some of the key components of the immune system that are affected by exercise.

Innate Immune Responses

Constitutive host defenses include external and internal components. The external systems are the barriers—the skin and mucosa—and the various antimicrobial substances secreted onto the skin and mucous membranes. External factors, such as the low pH of the skin, provide resistance to penetration by parasites. Internal systems include a variety of circulating phagocytic cells, principally neutrophils and monocytes, and antimicrobial substances in blood and lymph (acute-phase proteins). The innate immune response is typically rapid and highly stereotyped.

Polymorphonuclear phagocytes (primarily neutrophils and eosinophils) arise from pluripotent stem cells in bone marrow and are characterized by the presence of cytoplasmic granules, which contain degradative enzymes such as acid hydrolases, neutral proteases, peroxidases, myeloperoxidase, cationic proteins, lysozyme, and lactoferrin (7). Mononuclear phagocytes (monocytes, macrophages) also develop from stem cells in bone marrow and lose their granules during successive differentiation.

The enzymes found in cytoplasmic granules of neutrophils are involved in oxygen independent (e.g., hydrolases, lysozyme) or oxygen dependent (e.g., myeloperoxidase) killing during phagocytosis. Some of these enzymes trigger complement cascades, which in turn facilitate and mediate cytolysis through pore formation at the target plasma membranes. Kinins are also activated by enzymes released from phagocytic granules, thereby indirectly enhancing vascular permeability and chemotaxis of phagocytic and other cells.

Oxygen-dependent killing by phagocytic cells is an important pathway for destruction of pathogens. During the respiratory burst, electron transfer from reduced nicotinamide-adenine dinucleotide phosphate (NADPH) to oxygen results in the production of superoxide, peroxide, and hydroxyl radicals within the phagosome of neutrophils (7). This reaction can be detected by chemoluminescence, a method often used in exercise immunology studies to measure neutrophil function. Generation of hypohalites via the myeloperoxidase-halide system also contributes to the killing of microorganisms within the phagosome, and oxidative decarboxylation of amino acids, generation of toxic aldehydes, and thiol group oxidation lead to loss of key microbial enzyme functions (7). When macrophages are activated, for example by exposure to lipopolysaccharide or by activation with interferon-γ (a cytokine produced by NK cells or T cells) nitric oxide synthetase is expressed, leading to the generation of nitric oxide and its metabolites nitrate and nitrite, which are toxic to microbes. Nitric oxide and reactive oxygen species interact to produce peroxy nitrite, which is harmful to microbial cell membranes (7).

Acquired Immune Responses

The acquired immune system is characterized by recognition of antigenic determinants or antigenic epitopes (the portion of the antigen molecule seen as foreign by the host's immune cells), specificity of antigen recognition (and resultant clonal expansion), and immunological memory. The cell type that mediates specific or acquired immune responses is the lymphocyte, which is identified by specific surface markers or surface antigens. The most important effector cells involved in specific immune responses are the T (thymus-derived) lymphocyte, the B lymphocyte, and the natural killer (NK) cell (Fig. 23.1).

Immune cells are identified by specific surface markers, referred to as CD (cluster of differentiation) antigens, and different subsets of lymphocytes express different CD antigens at the cell surface. For example, cells expressing the CD8 antigen are T lymphocytes with cytotoxic properties; CD19 cells are of the B cell lineage; and CD62L is an adhesion molecule that mediates lymphocyte homing to high endothelial venules and leukocyte rolling on activated endothelium during an inflammatory response. Lymphocytes may be further categorized within a given CD. Thus, CD45 cells (the marker that designates the common leukocyte antigen found on all white blood cells) are CD45RO$^+$ memory cells or CD45RA$^+$ naive cells. In phenotype assays using flow cytometry, lymphocytes are frequently identified by the presence of multiple CD antigens. For example, CD8$^+$CD56$^+$ lymphocytes are a group of unconventional T-NK cells. Lymphocytes can also be characterized by the absence of CD markers; for example, double positive T lymphocytes are CD4$^+$CD8$^+$ and indicate

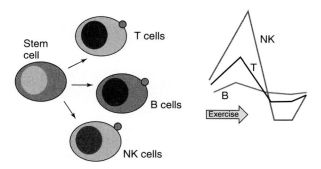

FIGURE 23.1 The major lymphocyte subpopulations involved in mediating specific immune responses. T lymphocytes are effector cells for cell-mediated reactions, and B lymphocytes are effector cells for humoral or antibody-mediated reactions. NK cells are involved in cytolysis of target cells. During dynamic exercise, the numbers of NK cells in blood increase more than T lymphocytes, which increase more than B lymphocytes.

an early phase of development of these cells in the thymus gland. Thus, the CD designations provide information about the structure, development, and function of leukocytes. Table 23.1 provides a summary of some of the CD antigens that have been characterized in relation to exercise. More than 200 CD antigens on lymphocytes and other cells have been identified, and many have not been studied in an exercise context; most immunology textbooks provide detailed descriptions of the known CD antigens.

Another important characteristic of lymphocytes is that they are not fixed within tissues but constantly recirculate from lymph nodes via efferent lymphatics into lymphatic vessels, lodge in other lymph nodes or specialized regions of secondary lymphoid tissues, or enter the circulation through the major lymphatic ducts. The implications of lymphocyte recirculation are twofold: First, up- or down-expression of cell adhesion molecules on the surface of lymphocytes is essential in the migration of lymphocytes (e.g., rolling, attachment, detachment from endothelium) Second, diverse physiological stimuli, including exercise, affect lymphocyte recirculation by altering the expression of cell adhesion molecules or by interaction with chemokines, a group of specialized cytokines with chemoattractant properties affecting cytoskeletal elements of cells. Rehman and colleagues (8) demonstrated the role of adhesion molecules by showing that circulating levels of intercellular adhesion molecule (ICAM) 1 in healthy individuals were significantly elevated after exhaustive exercise, and this effect could be mitigated by pretreatment with propranolol or metoprolol. Another consideration is that measurement of lymphocytes in one tissue compartment is an imperfect estimate of lymphocytes in other lymphoid tissues and organs. Although human stud-

ies use peripheral blood mononuclear cells or lymphocytes, circulating white blood cell responses to exercise may not be representative of white blood cell responses in tissue compartments (spleen, lymph nodes) where exposure to antigen occurs. Furthermore, inferences about the number and function of intraepithelial lymphocytes found in the gastrointestinal, pulmonary, and genitourinary tracts (5) based upon sampling of blood lymphocytes are even more problematic, since not all intraepithelial lymphocytes recirculate.

By convention, the specific immune response is described as cell mediated (involving T cells) or humoral mediated (involving B cells and antibody production). In cell-mediated responses, the first step is the processing of antigen by antigen-presenting cells, such as macrophages and dendritic cells. Upon internalization into a lysosomal vesicle within the antigen-presenting cells, antigen becomes fragmented into peptides, some of which are associated with specific cell membrane proteins known as MHC molecules. MHC refers to the major histocompatability complex–derived proteins found on the surface of cells, which are involved in the recognition of antigens by T lymphocytes. There are two types of MHC molecules, class I and class II. Class I molecules are found on all nucleated cells and are recognized by the cytolytic T cells (CD8). CD8 cells are also called MHC class I restricted T cells. Class II molecules have a more restricted cell distribution, being expressed constitutively only on antigen-presenting cells. Antigen-presenting cells take up the antigen, process or degrade the antigen, and present antigenic determinants to be seen at the surface by CD4 T lymphocytes. CD4 cells are also called MHC class II restricted T cells. In the case of antigen-presenting cells, vesicles return the processed antigen and MHC class II complex

TABLE 23.1	Cluster of Differentiation (CD) Antigens Found on Immune Cells Studied in Relation to Exercise	
CD Antigen	**Immune Cell Distribution**	**Major Function**
CD2	T cells, NK cells	Adhesion
CD3	T cells	T-cell receptor transduction
CD4	T helper cells	Differentiation marker; T-cell activation
CD8	T cytotoxic cells	T-cell activation
CD11a	Monocytes, macrophages, lymphocytes	Adhesion
CD11b	Neutrophils, monocytes, NK cells	Adhesion
CD18	Leukocytes	Adhesion
CD19	B cells, plasma cells	Signal transduction
CD28	T cells, plasma cells	T-cell proliferation; cytokine production
CD40	B cells	B-cell growth, differentiation
CD44	Many cells, including leukocytes	Adhesion
CD45	All leukocytes	T- and B-cell activation
CD56	NK cells; some T cells	?
CD62L	Peripheral B, T and NK cells; monocytes, macrophages	Adhesion
CD69	Activated T, B, NK cells, neutrophils	Early activation marker; role in NK-mediated lysis
CD86	Dendritic cells	Co-stimulation for T cells
CD95	Activated T and B cells	Apoptosis-inducing signal
CD103	Intraepithelial lymphocytes (intestine, bronchi)	Adhesion; accessory molecule for activation

See references 5 and 6 for extensive description of CD antigens on immune cells.

(together known as a T-cell epitope) to the cell surface, where it is presented to CD4 lymphocytes (9). Thus, the T cell epitope provides an induction signal for CD4 lymphocytes leading to mitosis, activation, and proliferation of memory and effector T cells. Effector CD4 T cells secrete growth factors that influence the behavior of various cells participating in the immune response. Naive CD4 lymphocytes are able to differentiate into type 1 helper (Th1) cells or type 2 helper (Th2) cells depending upon the types of stimuli and signals received. Naive CD8 lymphocytes have a more restricted array of cytokines, and the primary effector function of activated CD8 lymphocytes is the killing of target cells (5).

A crucial defining characteristic of CD4 type 1 and type 2 lymphocytes is the type of growth factors or cytokines produced. Cytokines are low-molecular-weight proteins that influence the direction, intensity, and duration of immune responses. Th1 cytokines, which include interferon-γ and interleukin (IL) 2, are associated with cell-mediated responses and down-regulation of Th2 responses. In contrast, Th2 cytokines, such as IL-4 and IL-10, are associated with humoral (antibody) responses and shift immune responses away from cell-mediated immunity. In general, type 1 T cells mediate protection against intracellular microorganisms, such as virus, whereas type 2 T cells are important in the defense against extracellular parasites, such as helminths. Figure 23.2 illustrates the cytokine profiles for CD4 Th1 and Th2 lymphocytes and the general effect of dynamic exercise on these cells.

What about CD8 lymphocytes? These cells, once activated, become cytotoxic T lymphocytes (CTLs), which are capable of lysing virally infected cells and tumor targets. Moreover, since CTLs recognize MHC class I molecules found on all nucleated cells, they are capable of eliminating almost any altered cell in the body. Similar to CD4 T lymphocytes, CD8 T lymphocytes require multiple signals for activation and proliferation into fully competent effector cells. The first signal is provided by antigenic peptides (for example, virus antigens) in the infected cell that are bound to MHC class I molecules; the T cell receptor of CD8 lymphocytes interacts with the class I molecule and antigen presented on the surface of the infected cell. A second co-stimulatory signal is normally necessary to activate naive CD8 lymphocytes into effector CTLs. This signal is transduced by the ligation of B7 (CD80 or CD86) on antigen-presenting cells with CD28 on CTLs. A third signal provided by IL-2, a classical Th1 cytokine produced by CD4 lymphocytes, may also be important in the generation of CTLs, since IL-2 knockout mice lack CTL-mediated target cell killing (10). Following activation, CTLs kill target cells by apoptosis, through insertion of a perforin-mediated pore in the target membrane and subsequent release of granzymes (serine proteases), which lead to DNA fragmentation. CTLs express membrane-bound Fas ligand (FasL), which interacts with the Fas receptor on the surface of target cells (see section on apoptosis for description of intrinsic and extrinsic pathways of apoptosis and the relation to dynamic exercise). CD8 T cells also produce cytokines, including IFN-γ, which enhance macrophage involvement as B7-bearing antigen-presenting cells (9,11).

B lymphocytes also require two signals to become activated by T-dependent antigens (most proteins are T-dependent antigens). First, the B-cell receptor (surface immunoglobulin [Ig]) must interact with antigen and be endocytosed, processed internally, and expressed on the plasma membrane in conjunction with a MHC class II molecule. Once this occurs, CD4 Th2 lymphocytes interact with the T-cell epitope and provide the first signal for antibody synthesis. A second signal is transmitted by the interaction of CD40 (present on B cells) and CD40L (present on T cells). Following activation and with stimulation from growth and differentiation cytokines (Th2 cytokines), B cells differentiate into plasma cells and secrete IgM, IgG, or IgA antibodies (IgE antibody is another isotype that plasma cells synthesize, although normally only in individuals with atopy or allergy). The primary antibody response (following initial exposure to an antigen) leads to a peak increase in antibody levels within about 2 wk; during this time both effector and memory cells are generated. A subsequent exposure to the antigen (e.g., through recall antigen testing) results in a shorter lag time for production of antibody and higher blood antibody concentrations (or titers), reflecting the expansion of existing memory B lymphocytes to active antibody producing plasma cells. Antibody mediates a number of effector functions. First,

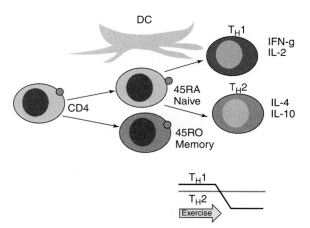

FIGURE 23.2 T_H1 and T_H2 subsets and their main cytokine profiles. Following presentation of antigen by dendritic cells (DC), CD4 helper T lymphocytes (45RA naive) differentiate into T_H1 or T_H2 cells. T_H1 cells produce the cytokines IFN-γ and IL-2, which enhance the cellular immune response. T_H2 cells produce the cytokines IL-4 and IL-10, which enhance the synthesis of antibody by B lymphocytes and humoral immunity. During dynamic exercise, there is a decrease in T_H1 cells, whereas numbers of T_H2 cells are relatively unchanged.

antibody can bind antigen through precipitation or agglutination reactions and neutralize the antigen. Second, antibody can promote phagocytosis of an antigen by opsonization. In opsonization, neutrophils and macrophages bind a portion of the antibody molecule (the Fc domain) at receptors (FcR) found on their surface, whereas the antibody molecule binds the antigen. The entire antibody-antigen complex is then taken up by the phagocytic cell. Third, some antibodies (notably IgM and IgG) activate the complement cascade, resulting in the nonspecific lysis of cells (such as red blood cells) with receptors for the C3b component of complement (5).

In summary, host defense entails physical and chemical barriers, stereotyped innate responses involving inflammatory cells, and an inducible immune response with the generation of, for example, T helper (Th1, Th2), T cytotoxic, and B lymphocytes. These cells provide the major pathway for recognizing and responding to infectious antigens, tumor antigens, and autoantigens.

Dynamic Exercise and the Immune Response

The largest body of evidence on exercise and immune responses comes from acute studies using aerobic exercise protocols in humans and animals. Using dynamic exercise protocols, the pattern of response is described for the various lymphocyte subpopulations in terms of number and function, NK cell activity, B cell responses, and immunoglobulin production.

Leukocyte and Lymphocyte Subpopulations

In response to acute exercise, blood leukocyte subpopulations react in a highly stereotyped fashion. Neutrophil concentrations increase during and post exercise, whereas lymphocyte concentrations increase during dynamic exercise and fall below pre-exercise values after physical work of prolonged duration (12). If the exercise has been of moderate intensity and/or short duration, lymphocytes are mobilized to the blood during the exercise and return to preexercise levels in the recovery phase of exercise. Several reports describe exercise-induced changes in subsets of blood mononuclear cells (BMNC) (13). The increased lymphocyte concentration observed early after the initiation of an exercise bout is likely due to the recruitment of all lymphocyte subpopulations to the vascular compartment: T cells, B cells, and NK cells. These numerical changes occur whether or not cells are analyzed as separated buffy-coat or whole-blood cultures. NK cells are more sensitive to dynamic exercise than T cells, which again are more sensitive than B cells (Fig. 23.1). During exercise the CD4/CD8 ratio decreases. This reflects the greater increase in CD8+ lymphocytes than CD4+ lymphocytes. CD4+ and CD8+ cells contain both CD45RO+ memory and CD45RA+ naive

cells, which are identified by the absence of 45RO and the presence of CD62L (14). Data show that the recruitment of T cells during exercise is primarily of CD45RO+ lymphocytes (15). Thus, the concentrations of CD45RO+ and CD45RO-CD62L increase during exercise, suggesting that memory but not naive lymphocytes are rapidly mobilized to the blood in response to physical exercise (16) (Fig. 23.3). This finding supports the idea that during exercise lymphocytes are recruited from peripheral compartments, such as the spleen, rather than from the bone marrow. In accordance, splenectomized individuals have an impaired ability to mobilize lymphocytes to the blood during stress.

As described in the overview section on the immune system, CD4 T helper (Th) and the CD8 T cytotoxic cells can be divided into type 1 and type 2 cells according to their cytokine profile, although CD8 lymphocytes have a more limited range of cytokines produced. Type 1 CD4 T cells produce, for example, interferon-γ and IL-2, whereas type 2 CD4 T cells produce IL-4, IL-5, IL-6, and IL-10. Type 1 T cell responses are stimulated by IL-12, and IL-6 has been shown to induce type 2-polarization by stimulating the initial production of IL-4. Type 1 T cells mediate protection against intracellular microorganisms such as virus, whereas type 2 T cells are important in the defense against extracellular parasites, such as helminths. The decrease in T lymphocyte number post exercise is accompanied by a more pronounced decrease in type 1 T cells (17). The more pronounced decrease in type 1 than in type 2 T cells in the recovery period may explain the increased sensitivity to infections following heavy dynamic exercise, as these infections are often caused by viruses.

Telomeres are the extreme ends of chromosomes that consist of TTAGGG repeats. After each round of cell division, telomeric sequence is lost because DNA polymerase cannot fully replicate the 5' end of the chromosome. Telomere

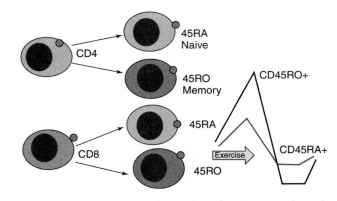

FIGURE 23.3   Generation of naive (45RA) and memory (45RO) CD4 and CD8 lymphocytes. In response to dynamic exercise, memory T cells increase more dramatically than naive T cells. The number of circulating naive and memory lymphocytes transiently fall below preexercise values after cessation of exercise, with recovery within 24 to 48 hours.

lengths have been used as a marker for replication history and the proliferation potential of the cells. In response to exercise, telomere lengths in CD4+ and CD8+ lymphocytes were shorter than in cells isolated at rest (16). Thus, the initial increase in CD4+ and CD8+ cells after exercise probably is not due to repopulation by newly generated cells but rather a redistribution of activated cells.

Natural Killer Cell Activity

NK cells mediate non–MHC-restricted cytotoxicity, with potential resistance to viral infections (18) and cytolysis of some malignant cells (19). The method frequently applied to measure NK cell activity is the 51Cr release assay, for which the percentage of lysed target cells is the end point. The cytolytic activity of NK cells is enhanced by IFN and IL-2, whereas certain prostaglandins and immune complexes down-regulate the function of NK cells. Dynamic exercise of various types, durations, and intensities induces recruitment to the blood of cells expressing characteristic NK cell markers (20). NK cell activity (lysis per fixed number of BMNC) increases consequent to the increased proportions of cells mediating non–MHC-restricted cytotoxicity. Following exercise, NK cell activity is suppressed on a per NK cell basis (21) if the exercise has been of heavy intensity and long duration (more than 45 min). Maximal reduction in NK cell concentrations, hence the lower NK cell activity, occurs 2–4 h after dynamic exercise. The NK cell activity is increased when measured immediately after or during both moderate and heavy exercise of a few minutes. The NK cell count and the NK cell activity are decreased following intense exercise of at least 1 hour's duration.

Immunoglobulins

Although IgA constitutes only 10–15% of the total immunoglobulin in serum, it is the predominant Ig class in mucosal secretions, and the level of IgA in mucosal fluids correlates more closely with resistance to upper respiratory tract infections than serum antibodies (22). Lower concentrations of the salivary IgA have been reported in cross-country skiers after a race (23). This finding was confirmed by a 70% decrease in salivary IgA, which persisted for several hours after completion of intense, prolonged ergometer cycling (24) (Milestone of Discovery). Decreased salivary IgA was found after intense swimming (25), after running (26), and after incremental treadmill running to exhaustion (27). Submaximal exercise had no effect on salivary IgA (27), and the percentage of B cells amongst BMNC did not change in relation to exercise (28).

Immune Responses *In Vivo*

In vivo impairment of cell-mediated immunity and specific antibody production could be demonstrated after intense exercise of long duration (triathlon race) (29). The cellular immune system was evaluated as a skin test response to seven recall antigens. A recall antigen is an antigen to which the individual has been previously exposed: the response reflects the activation of memory T or B lymphocytes. The humoral immune system was evaluated as the antibody response to pneumococcal polysaccharide vaccine, which is generally considered to be T cell independent, and tetanus and diphtheria toxoids, both which are T cell dependent. The skin test response was significantly lower in the group who performed a triathlon race than in triathlete controls and untrained controls, who did not participate in the triathlon. No differences in specific antibody titers were found between the groups.

Neutrophils and Phagocytosis

Neutrophils constitute 50–60% of the total circulating leukocyte pool. These cells are part of the innate immune system, are essential for host defense, and are involved in the pathology of various inflammatory conditions. The inflammatory involvement reflects tissue peroxidation resulting from incomplete phagocytosis. One of the more pronounced features of dynamic exercise on immune parameters is the prolonged neutrocytosis following acute and prolonged exercise bouts (12). A number of reports show that exercise triggers a series of changes in the neutrophil population and may affect certain subpopulations differentially. A reduction in the expression of L-selectin (CD62L) immediately after exercise followed by an increase during recovery has been reported (30). This supports that in response to the hormonal environment during exercise, neutrophils lose their ability to migrate into tissues (31). Increased expression of the cell adhesion molecules following exercise may contribute to neutrophil extravasation into damaged tissue, including skeletal muscle. Regarding the function of neutrophils, exercise has both short- and long-term effects. Neutrophils respond to infection by adherence, chemotaxis, phagocytosis, oxidative burst, degranulation, and microbial killing. In general, moderate exercise boosts neutrophil functions, including chemotaxis, phagocytosis, and oxidative burst activity. Maximal exercise, by contrast, reduces these functions, with the exception of chemotaxis and degranulation which are not affected (32).

Repeated Dynamic Exercise and the Immune Response

Surprisingly, there have been few studies on the effects of repeated bouts of exercise on immune cells. The absence of experimental data is perplexing, given that many people, including athletes, engage in more than one exercise session on a single day or in a single week. (The direction of the effects on the various immune parameters has been inconsistent, owing to differences in exercise and recovery protocols, levels of training of the subjects, other experimental or methodological issues, and the outcome variability due to small sample sizes.)

One study evaluated a protocol of relevance for the untrained individual. Healthy untrained ($\dot{V}_{O_{2max}}$ 46 mL · kg^{-1} · min^{-1}) men performed repeated submaximal dynamic exercise on a cycle ergometer (65% $\dot{V}_{O_{2max}}$ for 1 h daily). This resulted in significant increases in the total number of blood leukocytes and in specific lymphocyte subpopulations (CD3$^+$, CD4$^+$, and NK cells) after the first but not after the third exercise trial (33).

Another study reflected the daily exercise and recovery regimen practiced by most elite endurance athletes, who typically have two or more exercise sessions per day. Rønsen and colleagues (34) investigated elite athletes ($\dot{V}_{O_{2max}}$ 69.1 mL · kg^{-1} · min^{-1}) and compared leukocyte counts and lymphocyte responsiveness during and after a second bout of high-intensity dynamic exercise on the same day with the response to a similar but single bout of exercise. All bouts consisted of 75 min at about 75% of maximal oxygen uptake on a cycle ergometer. The second bout of exercise in the second trial on the same day was associated with significantly increased concentrations of total leukocytes, neutrophils, lymphocytes, CD4$^+$, CD8$^+$, and CD56$^+$ NK cells. It also was associated with a decrease in the percentage of NK cells expressing the activation marker CD69 and the density of CD69 molecules following mitogen stimulation of CD56$^+$ cells. This increase in lymphocyte number was especially high if the recovery period was short (3 versus 6 h). The difference between the first and second bouts of exercise suggests a carryover effect in the immune system from a first to a second bout of exercise on the same day.

A likely biological mechanism for the pronounced leukocyte changes after repeated exercise sessions is exercise stress–mediated catecholamine release. Thus, in the elite athlete study, the plasma catecholamine levels increased significantly more during the second bout of exercise than during the first, even though the catecholamine levels were back to resting values before the second bout (35). Epinephrine, which is involved in the recruitment of lymphocytes to the blood, decreases the expression of cell adhesion molecules (such as CD62L and CD44$^+$) on leukocytes. The cortisol levels were also further increased in relation to the second bout of exercise. Dynamic-exercise–induced cortisol release could also be involved, since glucocorticoids down-regulate mRNA for lymphocyte function–associated antigen (LFA) 1 and CD2 expression in human peripheral blood mononuclear cells (36) and inhibit the expression in vitro of ICAM-1 cell adhesion molecules on leukocytes and endothelial E-selectin (37). Circulating cytokines IL-6 and IL-1 receptor antagonist (IL-1ra) have also been shown to be influenced by repeated exercise sessions in athletes, and increases may

be related to muscle glycogen depletion and limiting inflammatory damage.

Moderate Versus Intense Exercise

During both moderate and intense exercise, lymphocytes are mobilized to the blood compartment. However, dynamic exercise lasting more than 1 h of a relatively high intensity (more than 70% $\dot{V}_{O_{2max}}$) will induce a decrease in the circulating number of lymphocytes post exercise. Thus lymphocytes disappear from the circulation in the recovery period, but only if the exercise has been intense. As assessed in assays in vitro, an impairment of lymphocyte and NK cell function also follows heavy exercise. Thus, following intense long-duration exercise, the immune system is temporarily impaired. This period has also been called the open window. During the open window, bacteria and viruses can invade the host, and infections may be established more readily than when the immune system is not temporarily impaired. The concept of the open window is illustrated in Figure 23.4.

Exercise and Lymphocyte Proliferation

Following stimulation with antigen (e.g., virus) or mitogen (e.g., concanavalin A), immune cells that are in the quiescent (G0) phase of the cell cycle undergo activation. A commonly used method for evaluating the activation of lymphocytes is by the assessment of proliferative responses by measuring incorporation of [3H] thymidine in DNA fol-

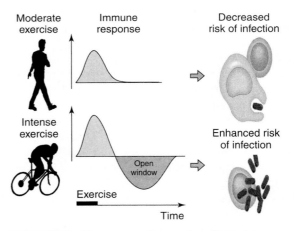

FIGURE 23.4 The open window model, which relates the intensity of exercise to risk of or protection from infection (and other clinical conditions). This increased or decreased risk presumably reflects intervening variables of immune system function. *(Reprinted with permission from Pedersen BK. Physical activity and the immune system—a stress model. Ugeskr Laeger 2000;162:2182.)*

lowing stimulation with an antigen or a mitogen. A mitogen is any substance that nonspecifically stimulates DNA synthesis and mitosis. Typical mitogens for lymphocytes are plant lectins, such as phytohemagglutinin and bacterial wall products such as lipopolysaccharide. These *in vitro* studies are performed either on a fixed number of BMNC or a fixed blood volume and will reflect the lymphocyte subpopulation composition. Thus, phytohemagglutinin and the mitogen concanavalin A stimulate primarily $CD4^+$ T cells. Several studies find a decline in the phytohemagglutinin and concanavalin A response during exercise and for up to several hours afterward (38). This is at least partly due to the increase in NK cells in the circulation and the relative decline of $CD4^+$ cells in assays *in vitro* (38,39). Furthermore, the shift in memory and naive cells and type 1 and type 2 cytokine–producing cells will also influence proliferation *in vitro*. In accordance, a recent study (40) found that 60 min of running at 95% of ventilatory threshold decreased mitogen-induced BMNC proliferation but had no effect on NK-depleted BMNC or BMNC again adjusted for $CD3^+$ percentage. In contrast, lymphocyte proliferation to B cell mitogens, pokeweed mitogen, and lipopolysaccharide, which stimulates monocytes, either increases or remains unchanged after exercise (41).

A few other representative findings and patterns are briefly described in this section. Heavy (80% $\dot{V}_{O_{2max}}$) intensity treadmill running, but not light intensity (50% $\dot{V}_{O_{2max}}$), is associated with a decrease in concanavalin A–stimulated lymphocyte proliferation immediately after exercise compared to baseline values (42). Short duration (<30 min) submaximal cycling at 50% peak work capacity significantly stimulated lymphocyte proliferation in young (26 ± 3 years) but not elderly (69 ± 5 years) subjects (43). The difference in proliferation responses between lymphocytes from young and older subjects may reflect a shift proportion of memory to naive lymphocytes, decreases in cyclin D2 (involved in the regulation of cell proliferation in association with cyclin-dependent kinases) and altered progression through the cell cycle (44), or a shift in the balance of type 1 and type 2 cytokine profiles (45).

Although studies that measure lymphocyte proliferation as determined by 3H-thymidine incorporation suggest changes in the cell cycle with exercise, further research is needed to pinpoint specific regulatory components.

Exercise and Lymphocyte Apoptosis

Heavy exercise and/or overtraining can impair the immune system, leading to immune suppression and loss of lymphocytes. One mechanism by which the loss of immune function with heavy exercise may occur is through apoptosis. Under normal circumstances, apoptosis, or programmed cell death, is tightly regulated and essential for normal immune system development and regulation (46). However, apoptosis can be induced by radiation, heat, hormonal triggering, anticancer drugs, and intense physical exercise stress. Apoptosis differs from necrosis in that apoptosis does not lead to an inflammatory response, whereas cell death through necrosis does. Apoptotic cells are rapidly endocytosed by neighboring healthy cells or phagocytized by macrophages or neutrophils that recognize a number of signals on the surface of injured cells. Eventually, irreversible DNA fragmentation and the formation of membrane-bound apoptotic bodies occur (47). The end result of apoptosis is cleavage of intracellular proteins essential for cell growth and survival.

Apoptosis occurs through two pathways: the intrinsic pathway and the extrinsic pathway. The intrinsic pathway is associated with changes in mitochondrial permeability and suicide signals originating from within the cell. Mitochondrial cytochrome *c* is released into the cytosol and becomes bound to caspase 9 (a cysteine protease) and other molecules to form a complex known as an apoptosome (48). In a cascade-like fashion, caspase 9 activates caspase 3, leading to proteolysis of downstream targets. Other mitochondrial activators can promote nuclear apoptosis, but in all cases a central mechanism leading to the activation of these proapoptotic proteins is the opening of the mitochondrial permeability transition pore and the resultant loss of mitochondrial membrane potential. The opening of this pore is regulated by members of the Bcl-2 family of intracellular proteins (for example, proapototic proteins such as Bax). Lymphocytes undergoing apoptosis are characterized by a number of intracellular changes, including the translocation of $NF_{-kappaB}$ (an inducible nuclear transcriptional activator), the exposure of phosphatidylserine at the cell membrane, and DNA fragmentation. Apoptosis also occurs through the activation of death receptors at the cell membrane. One of the best studied is that of Fas (CD95), which is expressed on the surface of target cells and which interacts with its ligand FasL, found on CTLs. This interaction of Fas-FasL leads to apoptosis of the target cell through caspase 8 and caspase 3 activation. Death receptor–mediated apoptosis can also occur through tumor necrosis factor (TNF) signaling following binding to TNF receptor, which is widely distributed in many cell types, including lymphocytes.

In summary, both the intrinsic and extrinsic pathways to apoptosis involve the sequential activation of caspase proteases resulting in the loss of cell viability. Unlike necrosis, the death of lymphocytes by apoptosis does not usually involve inflammation and activation of macrophages or inflammatory cytokines. Figure 23.5 illustrates the two pathways by which apoptosis can occur.

Maximal exercise influences a number of factors that trigger lymphocyte apoptosis. For example, increased GC secretion, growth factor withdrawal, catecholamine exposure, reactive oxygen species generation, and increased plasma

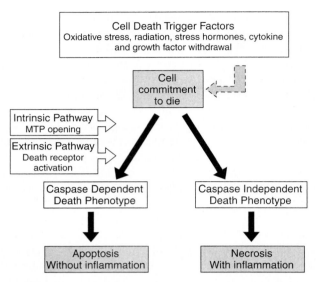

FIGURE 23.5 Apoptosis and necrosis pathways to cell death in response to physiological and pathophysiological stimuli. Apoptosis involves activation of the caspase enzyme cascade, triggered either through the intrinsic (mitochondrial) pathway or the extrinsic (death receptor) pathway leading to cell death. Necrosis does not involve caspase enzyme activation. *(Modified from Hoffman-Goetz L, Quadrilatero J, Patel H. Cellular life span. In Mooren FC, Voelker K, eds. Molecular and Cellular Exercise Physiology. Illinois: Human Kinetics, 2005: 29.)*

TNF-α are some of the signals that induce apoptosis in immune cells (46). These factors (especially GC, catecholamines, and reactive oxygen species) are notably elevated after strenuous, prolonged, or muscle-damaging exercise. Many studies have demonstrated that heavy exercise induces lymphocyte apoptosis in humans and animals. One of the earliest studies to address this was conducted by Concordet and Ferry (49), who found increased DNA fragmentation (using the TUNEL, or terminal deoxyribonucleotidyl transferase–mediated dUTP-digoxigenin nick end labeling assay) of thymic lymphocytes following two treadmill runs to exhaustion (separated by a 24-h rest) in rats. Thymocyte apoptosis could be blocked by administration of a GC receptor antagonist, RU-486 (mifepristone). (A precautionary note is that DNA fragmentation characterizes many kinds of cell death events, and the detection of DNA fragments may not be specific to apoptosis.) Increased oxygen consumption with exhaustive exercise leads to the generation of reactive oxygen species and lipid peroxidation of lymphocyte cell membranes. Dynamic exercise ($\dot{V}O_{2max}$ > 80%, 60 min) increases NF-$_{kappaB}$ activation in human peripheral blood lymphocytes (50), and this transient activation may be explained by oxidative stress and/or GC responses with exercise. Caspase 3 activity is greater in thymocytes after a single intensive bout of dynamic exercise (51) and annexin-V, a marker for phosphatidylserine externalization and early apoptosis, is increased in intraepithelial

intestinal T lymphocytes 24 h after exhaustive exercise (52). Overtraining and acute muscle-damaging exercise can also increase the expression of TNF-α (53), which could trigger lymphocyte apoptosis through the extrinsic pathway. Taken together, the human and animal studies suggest that heavy or maximal exercise induces apoptotic cell death in circulating and tissue lymphocytes through multiple pathways, including glucocorticoids, catecholamines, oxidative stress, and possibly TNF (Fig. 23.6). The loss of lymphocytes through apoptosis after intense exercise may contribute to the greater risk of infections during the open window (Fig. 23.4) and to immune function changes observed with repeated bouts of exercise and/or overtraining.

Lymphocyte Recirculation and Exercise

Lymphocyte recirculation ensures that the necessary subpopulations are distributed to appropriate extravascular sites when required. What follows is a brief overview of recirculation of lymphocytes with reference to exercise. For a complete description of the mechanisms of lymphocyte recirculation, consult a standard immunology textbook.

Lymphocytes continually move from the circulation and lymph to peripheral lymph nodes and spleen; lymphocytes also migrate to tissues that interface with the external environment, such as the skin and the mucosal epithelia of the gastrointestinal, pulmonary, and genitourinary tracts. This continual movement of lymphocytes increases the probability of antigenically committed lymphocytes contacting antigen. Extravasation and recirculation are linked to the expression of cell adhesion molecules on lymphocytes, on granulocytes, and on vascular endothelium. In the latter case, cell adhesion molecules are expressed in postcapillary venules of secondary lymphoid tissues known as high-

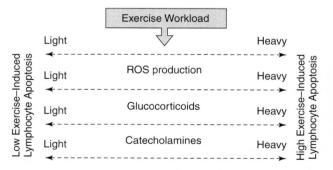

FIGURE 23.6 Exercise conditions, which trigger lymphocyte apoptosis above spontaneous levels. Reactive oxygen species (ROS), glucocorticoids (GC), and catecholamines released in response to high-intensity and/or long-duration exercise trigger apoptosis in lymphocytes. Below some intensity and duration threshold, exercise-induced apoptosis of lymphocytes will not occur because of absence of triggers.

endothelial venules. It has been estimated that more than 10,000 lymphocytes per second extravasate through high-endothelial venules of a single lymph node (5). High-endothelial venules express numerous leukocyte-specific cell adhesion molecules, including selectins, mucinlike adhesion molecules, and adhesion molecules of the Ig superfamily. Each cell adhesion molecule plays a role in white blood cell recirculation patterns: L-selectin (CD62L), found on all leukocytes, is involved in tethering and rolling, whereas the lymphocyte integrin molecule LFA-1 (CD11a/CD18) is involved in the adhesion and arrest of lymphocytes. ICAM-1 also participates in the movement of inflammatory cells, leukocyte effector functions, adhesion of antigen-presenting cells to T lymphocytes during antigen presentation, and signal transduction by activation of specific tyrosine kinases through phosphorylation with resultant transcription factor activation (54). Thus, in addition to enhancing leukocyte adhesion to vascular and mucosal endothelium, cell adhesion molecules contribute to the interactions between lymphocytes, antigen-presenting cells, and target cells.

Chemokines, small peptides with chemoattractant properties, also influence lymphocyte migration patterns. There are two patterns of chemokine expression. First, the homeostatic chemokines are constitutively expressed and are involved in regular lymphocyte recirculation. Second, the inflammatory chemokines are expressed only during specific inflammatory stimuli and are involved in recruitment of activated lymphocytes and inflammatory cells (55). The interaction of chemokines with specific receptors on lymphocytes initiates abrupt and extensive cytoskeletal changes. An important feature of lymphocyte recirculation is that memory lymphocytes (CD45RO$^+$) home selectively to the tissue in which antigen was first encountered, whereas naive CD45RA$^+$ lymphocytes (which haven't been exposed to antigen) extravasate nonpreferentially (5,6).

Exercise of various modalities affects the expression of cell adhesion molecules, the extent of which depends on the duration and intensity of the exercise and on which cell adhesion molecule is investigated (56). Generally, there is an increased expression on peripheral lymphocytes and neutrophils of CD62L and CD11a molecules, which may contribute to the transient exercise-associated leukocytosis. An increased expression of CD62L and CD11b on blood leukocytes occurs after both interval and eccentric exercise. In contrast, prolonged dynamic exercise does not influence macrophage or neutrophil adherence but may decrease soluble ICAM-1 levels many hours after completion of the exercise. The effect of dynamic exercise on the expression of the cell adhesion molecule CD103 (found on T lymphocytes in the gastrointestinal intestinal tract) has not been determined but would be important to characterize, since this compartment may serve as a reservoir for T cells. Among the potential mechanisms for the changes in the expression of adhesion molecules with dynamic exercise are (a) the action

of GC and catecholamines on marginated cell pools (57), (b) the selective apoptosis of leukocytes with a decreased expression of CD62L (58), and (c) the effects of oxidative products, such as endothelial-derived nitric oxide, which affect neutrophil adhesion (59).

Dynamic-Induced Cytokine Production

Cytokines are polypeptides originally discovered within the immune system. However, it appears that many cell types produce cytokines and that the biological roles of cytokines are beyond being immune regulatory. Recent data suggest that several cytokines have important metabolic functions and that they may either exert their effects locally or work in a hormonelike fashion. As described earlier, other cytokines, the chemokines, have a chemoattractant effect on blood leukocyte subpopulations and influence cell trafficking. Most studies on cytokines come from sepsis research. In sepsis models, the cytokine cascade consists of increased plasma levels (named in order) of TNF-α, IL-1β, IL-6, IL-1 receptor antagonist (IL-1ra), soluble TNF receptors (sTNF-R), IL-10, the chemokines IL-8 (chemoattractant for neutrophils), and macrophage inflammatory protein 1 (MIP-1) α and β (chemoattractant for lymphocytes). TNF-α and IL-1β are proinflammatory cytokines, whereas sTNF-R, IL-1ra and IL-10 have anti-inflammatory functions. Although IL-6 has been classified as both a proinflammatory and an anti-inflammatory cytokine, recent research suggests that circulating IL-6 is primarily anti-inflammatory (60). Infusion of IL-6 into humans will result in fever but does not cause shock or capillary leakage–like syndrome, as observed with the prototypical proinflammatory cytokines IL-1β and TNF-α. Unlike IL-1β and TNF-α, IL-6 does not up-regulate major inflammatory mediators, such as nitric oxide (61). Rather, IL-6 appears to be the primary inducer of hepatocyte-derived acute-phase proteins, many of which have anti-inflammatory properties. When infused into humans, IL-6 enhances the levels of the anti-inflammatory cytokines IL-1ra and IL-10.

Several cytokines can be detected in plasma during and after heavy or maximal exercise (62,63). Most studies report that exercise does not induce an increase in plasma levels of TNF-α except for a few studies demonstrating that prolonged heavy or maximal exercise, such as marathon running, results in an increase in the plasma concentration of TNF-α (64). Furthermore, most studies demonstrate that IL-1β does not increase in the blood, although a few studies have demonstrated relatively minor changes (63). The fact that the classical proinflammatory cytokines TNF-α and IL-1β do not increase or increase to only a minor degree is important to distinguish the cytokine cascade induced by exercise from the cytokine cascade in response to infections. Typically, the first cytokine that is present in the circulation following exercise is IL-6, which may increase 100-fold. The increase in IL-6 is followed by a marked increase in the concentration of IL-1ra and IL-10. The cytokine inhibitor sTNF receptor and the anti-inflammatory cytokine IL-10 furthermore increase. Also, the concentrations of the chemokines IL-8, MIP-1α and MIP-1β are elevated after a marathon race (65,66). Moreover, it has been demonstrated that endurance exercise induces systemic release of granulocyte colony–stimulating factor (G-CSF), macrophage CSF (M-CSF) and monocyte chemotactic protein 1 (MCP-1) (67). The early cytokine response to exercise is shown in Figure 23.7.

When BMNC are sampled during or following heavy or maximal exercise and stimulated *in vitro* to produce cytokines, cytokine production *in vitro* is impaired (68), not changed, or enhanced (69). These findings are likely to be explained by exercise-induced altered blood mononuclear cell composition.

IL-12 has dominated the field of cell-mediated immunity since its discovery more than 10 years ago, and it clearly plays an essential role in the development of Th1 cells under a variety of conditions. The role of IL-12 is not limited to initiating an immune response but may contribute to maintaining immunity. Thus, Th1 responses rapidly wane in the absence of IL-12, leading to a loss in protective immunity against intracellular pathogens. IL-12 production by NK cells is stimulated by several viruses (70), which again stimulate the production of IFN-γ. In response to exercise, circulating levels of IL-12 increase (63). The role of exercise-induced IL-12 has, however, not been identified.

Although TNF-α is normally not detected in plasma, it can be detected in urine 2 hours after exercise (63). IL-6 seems to be cleared by the hepatosplanchnic area (71) and in the urine as well. Additionally, it has been demonstrated that plasma concentrations of IL-4, G-CSF, granulocyte-macrophage CSF (GM-CSF), M-CSF, IL-8, and MCP-1 in-creased immediately after short-duration exercise and that the urine concentrations of these cytokines were high (63).

Initially it was thought that the cytokine response to exercise reflected a classic acute-phase response to muscle injury. Muscle damage occurs when the exercise emphasizes eccentric muscle contractions, such as in downhill running. However, a vast number of reports have demonstrated that this cytokine response occurs when the movements are performed by predominantly concentric muscle contractions of moderate intensity (72).

In relation to 1 h of heavy exercise involving eccentric muscle contractions, creatine kinase (CK) (an indicator of muscle membrane damage) was measured for 5 days in healthy young and elderly subjects. Despite a 100-fold increase in CK, plasma IL-6 was increased only a few fold immediately after the exercise, and then there was a second peak 4 hours into recovery. Plasma TNF hardly changed. The second IL-6 peak was tightly correlated to the CK level. Thus, IL-6 production in relation to muscle damage occurs later and is likely to reflect the invasion of monocytes into injured muscle.

Muscle Contraction–Induced Immune Regulation

For most of the last century, researchers have searched for a muscle contraction–induced factor that could mediate some of the exercise-induced changes in other organs, such as the liver and the adipose tissue. For lack of more precise knowledge, it has been called the work stimulus or the work factor (73). Today, we may prefer to use the term *exercise factor* to cover the effects of muscle contractions as such. It is clear that besides the nervous systems there are other signaling pathways from contracting muscles to other organs. Thus electrical stimulation of paralyzed muscles in spinal cord–injured patients induces many of the same physiological changes as in intact human beings (74). Recently, it has been demonstrated that exercise induces transcription of metabolic genes in exercising skeletal muscle (75), which shows that muscle contractions as such may directly influence metabolism. The finding that IL-6 gene transcription takes place locally in contracting skeletal muscle and that IL-6 is released to the blood in high amounts from an exercising limb (72) opens the possibility that exercise-induced immune changes are directly linked to a factor induced by muscle contractions.

A number of studies (76) have demonstrated that IL-6 mRNA in monocytes, the blood mononuclear cells responsible for the increase in plasma IL-6 during sepsis (77), did not increase as a result of exercise. Determining intracellular cytokine production, it was demonstrated that the number, percentage, and mean fluorescence intensity of monocytes staining positive for IL-6 either does not change

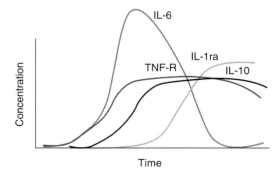

FIGURE 23.7 Early cytokine response to endurance exercise. IL-6, interleukin-6; TNF-R, soluble tumor necrosis factor receptor; IL-1ra, interleukin-1 receptor antagonist; IL-10, interleukin-10. *(Reprinted with permission from Pedersen BK. Physical activity and the immune system—a stress model. Ugeskr Laeger 2000; 162:2183.)*

during cycling exercise (78) or in fact decreases during prolonged running (79).

To test the possibility that working muscle produces IL-6, muscle biopsies were collected before and after dynamic exercise (80). IL-6 mRNA is present in small amounts in resting skeletal muscle but is enhanced up to 100-fold in contracting muscle, which indicates that exercise is responsible for the IL-6 gene-induction. This is also the case when concentric muscle contractions are responsible for the limb movements that occur with no muscle damage. Recently, it was shown that not only is the IL-6 gene activated in working muscle but that the IL-6 protein is released in large amounts from a contracting limb and markedly contributes to the exercise-induced increase in arterial plasma concentrations (81). Infusion of recombinant human IL-6 demonstrates that IL-6 enhances cortisol production with the same kinetic and to the same extent as during exercise (82). Furthermore, IL-6 induces neutrocytosis and late lymphopenia to the same magnitude and with the same kinetics as during dynamic exercise, which suggests that muscle-derived IL-6 may have a central role in exercise-induced leukocyte recirculation. In relation to highly exhaustive running exercise, large increases in muscle gene expression of IL-1β and IL-8 have been found as well as small increases in IL-10 and TNF-α (83). It is, however, not known whether these cytokines are also released into the circulation to play a role in exercise-induced immunomodulation.

Endocrine Regulation of Immune Function During Exercise

Exercise induces dramatic changes in the hormonal milieu. Acute, heavy muscular exercise increases the concentrations of a number of stress hormones in the blood, including epinephrine, norepinephrine, growth hormone, β-endorphins, and cortisol/corticosterone, whereas the concentration of insulin slightly decreases (84). This section discusses the evidence for exercise-induced changes in neuroimmune interactions, with emphasis on catecholamines and cortisol.

Catecholamines and Lymphocytes

During exercise epinephrine is released from the adrenal medulla and norepinephrine is released from the sympathetic nerve terminals. Arterial plasma concentrations of epinephrine and norepinephrine increase almost linearly with duration of dynamic exercise and exponentially with intensity, when it is expressed relative to the individual's maximal oxygen uptake (84). The expression of β-adrenoceptors on T, B, and NK cells, macrophages, and neutrophils in numerous species provide the molecular basis for these cells to be targets for catecholamine signaling (85). The numbers of adrenergic receptors on the individual lymphocyte subpop-

ulations may determine the degree to which the cells are mobilized in response to catecholamines. In accordance with this hypothesis, it has been shown that different subpopulations of BMNC have different numbers of β-adrenergic receptors (86). NK cells contain the highest number of β-adrenergic receptors, with CD4+ lymphocytes having the lowest number. B lymphocytes and CD8+ lymphocytes are intermediate between NK cells and CD4+ lymphocytes (87). Dynamic exercise up-regulates the β-adrenergic density, principally on NK cells. Interestingly, NK cells are more responsive to exercise and other stressors than any other subpopulation. CD4+ T cells are less sensitive, and CD8+ T cells and CD19+ B cells are intermediate (88). Thus, a correlation exists between numbers of β-adrenergic receptors on lymphocyte subpopulations and their responsiveness to exercise. Selective administration of epinephrine to obtain plasma concentrations comparable to those obtained during concentric cycling for 1 h at 75% $\dot{V}_{O_{2max}}$ mimicked the exercise-induced effect on BMNC subsets, NK cell activity, LAK cell activity, and the lymphocyte proliferation response (89). However, epinephrine infusion caused either a very small or no increase in neutrophil concentrations compared with that observed following exercise (90). Thus, epinephrine seems to contribute to the immediate recruitment of lymphocytes, in particular NK cells, to the blood during physical exercise.

Glucocorticoids and Lymphocytes

The plasma concentrations of GC increase in relation to exercise of long duration (91). Thus, short-term exercise does not increase the cortisol concentration in plasma, and only minor changes in the concentrations of plasma GC were described in relation to acute time-limited exercise stress of less than 1 h. However, exercise imposing significant psychological stress (for example, competition) would lead to elevated cortisol and corticosterone even if the exercise were of short duration. It is well documented that corticosteroids given intravenously to humans cause lymphocytopenia, monocytopenia, eosinopenia, and neutrophilia, which reach their maximum 4 h after administration (86). The increase in cortisol during exercise may be mediated in part by IL-6 (82). Linking exercise-induced lymphocyte changes to an effect of IL-6 on cortisol production is suggested by several studies demonstrating that carbohydrate loading during exercise attenuates both the exercise-induced increase in circulating IL-6 and the dynamic exercise effect on lymphocyte number and function (92).

To summarize, epinephrine and to a lesser extent norepinephrine contribute to the acute effects on circulating lymphocyte subpopulations. GC exerts its effects within about 2 h and contributes to the maintenance of lymphopenia and neutrocytosis after prolonged exercise. GC also may be responsible for the increase in apoptosis in tissue lymphocytes, such as in the thymus, observed after completion of heavy exercise of several hours. The effects of epinephrine, norepinephrine, and cortisol on circulating leukocyte numbers are shown in Figure 23.8.

Interactions Between Immune Function and Metabolism During Exercise

Alterations in metabolism and metabolic factors may contribute to dynamic-exercise–associated changes in immune function. Reductions in plasma glutamine concentrations due to muscular exercise have been hypothesized to influence lymphocyte function (93). However, although *in vitro* glutamine is an important fuel for lymphocytes, a number of glutamine supplementation studies have failed to demonstrate that glutamine can modulate exercise-induced immune changes (94).

Several studies have reported that carbohydrate ingestion attenuates elevations in plasma IL-6 during both running and cycling (92). As a consequence, carbohydrate diminishes the exercise-induced increase in cortisol and fluctuations in lymphocyte and neutrophil numbers. In addition, the increase in IL-6 mRNA, its nuclear transcriptional activity, and protein release from skeletal muscle are augmented when muscle glycogen availability is reduced (95,96). Furthermore, the increased expression of IL-6 was associated with increased glucose uptake during exercise. This suggests that IL-6 may at least in part be involved in mediating glucose uptake during exercise.

TNF-α and IL-6 are tightly linked, and TNF-α stimulates IL-6 production. On the other hand, both *in vitro* (97) and animal (98) studies have suggested that IL-6 may inhibit

TNF-α production. Recently it was demonstrated that both physical exercise and rhIL-6 infusion at physiological concentrations inhibit the production of TNF-α elicited by low-level endotoxemia in humans (99). Although it has been reported that both inflammatory and anti-inflammatory cytokines are present in the circulation after exercise, it appears that the net result of exercise involving concentric muscle contractions and not muscle damaging is a strong anti-inflammation. In support of a central role of IL-6 is that IL-6 infusion enhances plasma levels of IL-1ra and IL-10 and thereby markedly contributes to an anti-inflammatory response. Given that TNF-α induces insulin resistance (100) and that exercise that does not damage muscle inhibits TNF-α production, it is likely that exercise may also enhance insulin sensitivity via an induction of anti-inflammatory cytokines.

Exercise Training and the Immune Response

It has been hypothesized that moderate exercise training improves and strenuous or overtraining decreases a variety of immune functions on a tonic basis. This enhancement by moderate training and decrement by overtraining in immune function may be associated with greater protection from or risk of adverse exposures, such as bacterial or viral pathogens. This concept is presented as an open window (Fig. 23.4). However, the extent to which exercise training improves immune function in a clinically meaningful way has been difficult to establish. There have been few studies on exercise training and immune outcomes relative to the body of literature on acute exercise effects in various populations.

Immune Responses of Trained Individuals Sampled at Rest

Cross-sectional data consistently show little difference in the lymphocyte proliferative responses to a variety of mitogens between trained individuals and sedentary controls sampled at rest (101). Circulating NK cell numbers in highly trained athletes, sampled at rest, are generally quite similar to numbers found in nonathletes (102), although some reports indicate higher NK cell numbers (103). These differences are likely due to small sample sizes, the effects of various training regimens, and the time of NK cell measurement relative to training. Resting NK cell activity in male athletes (competitive cyclists, marathoners) also appears to be within the normal range compared with untrained individuals or even higher (102). Gender differences influence the functional responses, with significantly higher resting NK cell activity and T cell proliferative responses to mitogens reported in elite female rowers compared to nonathletes (104). The lack of

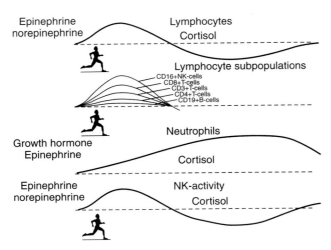

FIGURE 23.8 The important neuroendocrine mediators, which affect lymphocytes, neutrophils, and NK cells during exercise. *(Reprinted with permission from Pedersen BK. Physical activity and the immune system—a stress model. Ugeskr Laeger 2000;162: 2181.)*

consistency in results from cross-sectional training studies may be partly explained by factors that influence immune status, including nutrition, genetics, gender, and psychosocial factors.

Immune Responses of Individuals Undergoing Training

Longitudinal studies avoid many of these methodological issues but are expensive and are plagued by noncompliance and high dropout by participants. However, several studies have shown that the effect of strength training on T cell, NK cell, and cytokine responses in healthy individuals is quite modest (105). For example, 12 weeks of progressive resistance strength training had no significant effect on peripheral blood lymphocyte subset numbers or percentages, in vitro cytokine responses, lymphocyte proliferation responses, or delayed hypersensitivity responses in either young (22–30 years old) or elderly (65–80 years old) individuals (106). The exercise consisted of 80% one-repetition maximum, 8 repetitions per set, 3 sets per session twice weekly. The cytokine responses were IL-1β, TNF-α, IL-6, IL-2, and PGE2 production. The lymphocyte proliferation responses were two concentrations of phytohemagglutinin and concanavalin A. Although moderate resistance training has little effect on cytokine responses in healthy individuals, in individuals with preexisting cardiovascular disease, moderate combined dynamic and resistance exercises may reduce plasma-soluble TNF-α receptor 1 and TNF-α receptor 2 levels (107). The effect of resistance exercise training on salivary immunoglobulin A has also been studied. Using a combined resistance and endurance training program for 12 months, Akimoto and colleagues (108) reported an increase in concentration and secretion rate of surface membrane IGA for 45 healthy elderly individuals. Although this finding raises the possibility that mucosal immune functions may be more responsive to resistance exercise than cellular immune functions, because of the combined training program it is not possible to disassociate the separate effects of resistance from dynamic exercise.

Immune Responses to Overtraining

Dynamic exercise results in leukocytosis followed by leukopenia. These effects are transient, and the numerical effects when subjects are sampled at rest indicate normal values for most cell populations. However, during periods of heavy training and overtraining, including 7 months of swim training in elite swimmers (109), 10 days of interval training in military personnel (110), and 10 days of running at 200% of normal training volume (111), circulating leukocyte numbers, including NK cell numbers, tend to fall. The mechanisms for this decline may be related to migration of leukocytes out of the circulation consequent to changes in the expression of adhesion molecules or to cate-cholamine- and GC-mediated apoptosis of leukocyte changes in metabolism.

Animal Studies of Immune Function and Training

The effect of training on lymphocyte function as measured by proliferation to mitogen depends on the intensity. Light to moderate activity, such as walking or chair calisthenics, generally has little impact on immune parameters, or if there are changes, the associated variability is quite high (112). Animal studies consistently report that moderate endurance training enhances natural (NK and macrophage) immunity in vivo and in vitro compared with sedentary untrained controls (77). Differences between human and animal study findings are likely due to two factors: First, animal studies use genetically related individuals (e.g., highly inbred laboratory strains; congenic individuals differing at only one genetic locus). Second, the variability in the immune measure under study tends to be smaller than the variability observed in genetically unrelated individuals (either outbred animal strains or human subjects). Other factors, such as type and intensity of training, confounding by stress, differences in diet, and age, also may contribute to the differing results. Both high-intensity aerobic training and anaerobic training have been reported to decrease T-lymphocyte proliferation to mitogens, decrease NK cell activity to tumor targets, and reduce circulating lymphocyte numbers (113). These effects likely reflect metabolic factors, including the intracellular redox state of lymphocytes consequent to generation of reactive oxygen species and consumption of endogenous antioxidants (114).

Immune Responses to Exercise Across the Life Cycle

Little is known about the lymphocyte response to exercise in children. It seems, however, that the mobilization of lymphocytes to the blood compartment in response to exercise follows the same pattern in children as in adults (115). In children 8 to 17 years, swim training was associated with marginally lower baseline NK cell activity than that of untrained children sampled at rest (116). (This NK response in children is not unlike that observed in adults when NK cell activity is determined in trained subjects at rest.) It has further been demonstrated that elderly healthy people have a preserved ability to recruit T lymphocytes in response to acute physical stress (16). During aging, circulating levels of a number of cytokines increase. Thus, increased plasma levels of TNF-α (117,118), IL-6, IL-1ra (119) and sTNF-R (120) have been demonstrated in the elderly. In addition, aging is associated with increased levels of acute-phase proteins, such as CRP and serum amyloid A

(121) and with high neutrophil counts (122). Although levels of circulating cytokines and acute-phase proteins are only two to four times as high as levels in young subjects, low-grade inflammation is clearly associated with atherosclerosis, dementia, and diabetes in the elderly (119). Given that exercise, which accentuates concentric muscle contractions, may reduce inflammatory cytokines, it is most likely that some types of exercise in the elderly may contribute importantly to control chronic low-grade inflammation and associated diseases.

SUMMARY

Since the observations at the turn of the last century on leukocytosis after a marathon race, research in exercise immunology has increased exponentially. This chapter focuses on major immunological changes to acute endurance exercise, since these have been best documented. Given the scope of exercise immunology, some issues clearly could not be addressed (e.g., muscle injury and inflammation, exercise in the heat, gender effects, exercise and chronic diseases).

What is apparent, however, is that the field of exercise and the immune system has moved from descriptions of immune responses to studies on the underlying physiological, biochemical, and molecular biological processes causing these responses, reflecting the maturation of the science. It is now clear that the leukocytosis of exercise is due to changes in the expression of cell adhesion molecules and leukocyte trafficking, both of which reflect the hormonal and cytokine milieu during exercise. The mechanisms for the leucopenia of long-duration exercise are less clear, although evidence points to both apoptosis and changes in trafficking of cells. The role of cytokines released during exercise in coordinating the Th1 and Th2 responses of lymphocytes has implications for predominance of a cellular or humoral immune response and for inflammation or anti-inflammation. Muscle-derived IL-6 may have important metabolic regulatory effects well beyond the immune system. The strong anti-inflammatory effects of moderate exercise (especially those that emphasize concentric muscle contractions) are likely to be clinically important in terms of controlled low-grade inflammation and related disorders, such as atherosclerosis and insulin resistance.

A MILESTONE OF DISCOVERY

Are competitive athletes who overtrain really at risk for recurrent respiratory infections as a result of reduced mucosal immunity? A widespread belief held by athletes and by the exercising (and not exercising) public is that repeated fatiguing exercise makes an individual more susceptible to infection. Is this belief supported by empirical evidence? To what extent do immune changes with exercise affect risk of infection? An early observational report suggested that episodes of respiratory illness in children were related to participation in intense exercise resulting in acute fatigue (123). Later experiments with rats, rabbits, and guinea pigs in the 1920s tested whether fatiguing exercise increased mortality from bacterial infections (124,125). The results were equivocal, depending upon when the exposure took place. Thus, fatigue before exposure to bacterial challenge was associated with increased resistance, whereas fatigue after exposure was associated with decreased resistance. The use of revolving drums, which tumbled the animals rather than exercised them and which confounds stress with exercise, the lack of measures of either fatigue or exercise intensity, and the lack of immunological measures to mediate the increased or decreased resistance made interpretation of these early findings problematic.

Given the role of the mucosal immune system in protection from upper respiratory tract infections, Mackinnon and colleagues (24) were the first to systematically test whether exhaustive exercise affects the specific immunological components that provide barrier protection from pathogens at mucosal surfaces. Elite cyclists were exercised for 2 hours at 90% of anaerobic threshold (about 75% of each cyclist's maximum exercise

capacity), and serum, salivary, and nasal Ig titers were measured using modern techniques, including enzyme-linked immunosorbent assay (ELISA). Immediately after (and for 1 hour after) the exercise bout, salivary IgA concentrations (the key antibody in secretions) was significantly lower (9.5 ± 2.8 µg of Ig per mg protein) relative to levels before exercise (27.5 ± 6.9 µg of Ig per mg protein) and returned to baseline 24 hours after completion of the bout. In contrast to the salivary IgA and IgM, serum and nasal Ig concentrations were completely unaffected by the exercise bout. The importance of this study is threefold. First, this work (and many subsequent studies by other investigators) provided an immunological basis for the open window model, which relates intensity and duration of exercise to infection risk (see section on training and the immune response). Second, this study provided clear empirical insight into our assumptions about immune responses to exercise occurring in one compartment being mirrored in other tissue compartments, since saliva and serum Ig responses were quite different. Third, by sampling at multiple time points for up to 2 days after the exercise bout, Mackinnon and colleagues rigorously demonstrated that even with exhaustive exercise, the immune suppression is transitory and the immune system recovers quickly. The clinical and physiological meaning of transitory immune changes has been a consideration in the design of exercise immunology investigations ever since.

Mackinnon LT, Chick TW, van As A, Tomasi TB. The effect of exercise on secretory and natural immunity. Adv Exp Med Biol 1987;216A:869–876.

ACKNOWLEDGMENTS

Our research was supported by the Natural Sciences and Engineering Research Council of Canada and The Danish Research Council.

REFERENCES

1. Cannon WB. The Wisdom of the Body. New York: Norton, 1939.
2. Selye H. The Stress of Life. New York: McGraw-Hill, 1976.
3. Larrabee RC. Leucocytosis after violent exercise. J Med Res 1902;7:76–82.
4. Abbott AC, Gildersleeve N. The influence of muscular fatigue and of alcohol upon certain of the normal defences. Univ Penn Med Bull 1910;23:169–181.
5. Goldsby RA, Kindt TJ, Osborne BA, et al. Immunology. New York: Freeman, 2003.
6. Roitt IM, Delves PJ. Essential Immunology. Oxford: Blackwell Science, 2001.
7. Baldwin C. Constitutive host resistance. In Kreier JP, ed. Infection, Resistance, and Immunity. New York: Taylor & Francis, 2002;27–43.
8. Rehman J, Mills PJ, Carter SM, et al. Dynamic exercise leads to an increase in circulating ICAM-1: further evidence for adrenergic modulation of cell adhesion. Brain Behav Immun 1997;11:343–351.
9. Hickey MA, Taylor DW. The inducible defense system: the induction and development of the inducible defense. In Kreier JP, ed. Infection, Resistance, and Immunity. New York: Taylor & Francis, 2002;113–156.
10. Russell JH, Ley TJ. Lymphocyte-mediated cytotoxicity. Annu Rev Immunol 2002;20:323–370.
11. Mosmann TR, Li L, Sad S. Function of CD8 T-cell subsets secreting different cytokine patterns. Semin Immunol 1997;9:87–92.
12. McCarthy DA, Dale MM. The leucocytosis of exercise: a review and model. Sports Med 1988;6:333–363.
13. Pedersen BK. Exercise Immunology. Austin, TX: R. G. Landes, 1997.
14. Bell EB, Spartshott S, Bunce C. CD4+ T cell memory, CD45R subsets and the persistence of antigen: a unifying concept. Immunol Today 1998;19:60–64.
15. Gabriel H, Schmitt B, Urhausen A, et al. Increased CD45RA+CD45R0+ cells indicate activated T cells after endurance exercise. Med Sci Sports Exerc 1993;25:1352–1357.
16. Bruunsgaard H, Jensen MS, Schjerling P, et al. Exercise induces recruitment of lymphocytes with an activated phenotype and short telomere lengths in young and elderly humans. Life Sci 1999;65:2623–2633.
17. Steensberg A, Toft AD, Bruunsgaard H, et al. Strenuous exercise decreases the percentage of type 1 T cells in the circulation. J Appl Physiol 2001;91:1708–1712.
18. Welsh RM, Vargas-Cortes RM. Natural killer cells in viral infection. In Lewis CE, McGee JO, eds. The Natural Killer Cell. Oxford, UK: Oxford University, 1992;108–150.
19. O'Shea J, Ortaldo JR. The biology of natural killer cells: insights into the molecular basis of function. In Lewis CE, McGee JO, eds. The Natural Killer Cell. Oxford, UK: Oxford University, 1992;1–40.
20. Mackinnon LT. Exercise and natural killer cells: what is the relationship? Sports Med 1989;7:141–149.
21. Nielsen HB, Secher NH, Kappel M, et al. Lymphocyte, NK, and LAK cell responses to maximal exercise. Int J Sports Med 1996;17:60–65.
22. Liew, FY, Russell SM, Appleyard G, et al. Cross-protection in mice infected with influenza A virus by the respiratory route is correlated with local IgA antibody rather than serum antibody or cytotoxic T cell reactivity. Eur J Immunol 1984;14:350–356.
23. Tomasi TB, Trudeau FB, Czerwinski D, et al. Immune parameters in athletes before and after strenuous exercise. J Clin Immunol 1982;2:173–178.
24. Mackinnon LT, Chick TW, van As A, et al. The effect of exercise on secretory and natural immunity. Adv Exp Med Biol 1987;216A:869–876.
25. Tharp GD, Barnes MW. Reduction of saliva immunoglobulin levels by swim training. Eur J Appl Physiol 1990;60:61–64.
26. Steerenberg PA, van-Aspersen IA, van-Nieuw-Amerongen A, et al. Salivary levels of immunoglobulin A in triathletes. Eur J Oral Sci 1997;105:305–309.
27. McDowell SL, Hughes RA, Hughes RJ, et al. The effect of exhaustive exercise on salivary immunoglobulin A. J Sports Med Phys Fit 1992;32:412–415.
28. Tvede N, Heilmann C, Halkjaer Kristensen J, et al. Mechanisms of B-lymphocyte suppression induced by acute physical exercise. J Clin Lab Immunol 1989;30:169–173.
29. Bruunsgaard H, Hartkopp A, Mohr T, et al. In vivo cell mediated immunity and vaccination response following prolonged, intense exercise. Med Sci Sports Exerc 1997;29:1176–1181.
30. Kurokawa Y, Shinkai S, Torii J, et al. Exercise-induced changes in the expression of surface adhesion molecules on circulating granulocytes and lymphocytes subpopulations. Eur J Appl Physiol 1995;71:245–252.
31. Smith JA, Gray AB, Pyne DB, et al. Moderate exercise triggers both priming and activation of neutrophil subpopulations. Am J Physiol 1996;270:R838–R845.
32. Brines R, Hoffman-Goetz L, Pedersen BK. Can you exercise to make your immune system fitter? Immunol Today 1996;17:252–254.
33. Hoffman-Goetz L, Simpson JR, Cipp N, et al. Lymphocyte subset responses to repeated submaximal exercise in men. J Appl Physiol 1990;68:1069–1074.
34. Rønsen O, Haug E, Pedersen BK, et al. Increased neuroendocrine response to a repeated bout of endurance exercise. Med Sci Sports Exerc 2001;33:568–575.
35. Rønsen O, Pedersen BK, Oritsland TR, et al. Leukocyte counts and lymphocyte responsiveness associated with repeated bouts of strenuous endurance exercise. J Appl Physiol 2001;91:425–434.
36. Pipitone N, Sinha M, Theodoridis E, et al. The glucocorticoid inhibition of LFA-1 and CD2 expression by human mononuclear cells is reversed by IL-2, IL-7 and IL-15. Eur J Immunol 2001;31:2135–2142.
37. Cronstein BN, Kimmel SC, Levin RI, et al. A mechanism for the antiinflammatory effects of corticosteroids: the glu-

cocorticoid receptor regulates leukocyte adhesion to endothelial cells and expression of endothelial-leukocyte adhesion molecule 1 and intercellular adhesion molecule 1. Proc Natl Acad Sci USA 1992;89:9991–9995.

38. Fry RW, Morton AR, Crawford GP, et al. Cell numbers and in vitro responses of leukocytes and lymphocyte subpopulations following maximal exercise and interval training sessions of different intensities. Eur J Appl Physiol 1992;64:218–27.

39. Keast D, Cameron K, Morton AR. Exercise and the immune response. Sports Med 1988;5:248–267.

40. Green KJ, Rowbottom DG, Mackinnon LT. Exercise and T-lymphocyte function: a comparison of proliferation in PBMC and NK cell-depleted PBMC culture. J Appl Physiol 2002;92:2390–2395.

41. Field CJ, Gougeon R, Marliss EB. Circulating mononuclear cell numbers and function during intense exercise and recovery. J Appl Physiol 1991;71:1089–97.

42. Nieman DC, Miller AR, Henson DA, et al. Effect of high- versus moderate-intensity exercise on lymphocyte subpopulations and proliferative response. Int J Sports Med 1994;15:199–206.

43. Mazzeo RS, Rajkumar C, Rolland J, et al. Immune response to a single bout of exercise in young and elderly subjects. Mech Ageing Dev 1998;100:121–132.

44. Hale TJ, Richardson BC, Sweet LI, et al. Age-related changes in mature CD4+ T cells: cell cycle analysis. Cell Immunol 2002;220:51–62.

45. Sandmand M, Bruunsgaard H, Kemp K, et al. Is ageing associated with a shift in the balance between type 1 and type 2 cytokines in humans? Clin Exp Immunol 2002;127:107–114.

46. Phaneuf S, Leeuwenburgh C. Apoptosis and exercise. Med Sci Sports Exerc 2001;33:393–396.

47. Los M, Stroh C, Janicke RU, et al. Caspases: more than just killers? Trends Immunol 2001;22:31–34.

48. Ashe PC, Berry MD. Apoptotic signaling cascades. Prog Neuropsychopharmacol Biol Psychiatry 2003;27:199–214.

49. Concordet JP, Ferry A. Physiological programmed cell death in thymocytes is induced by physical stress (exercise). Am J Physiol 1993;265:C626–629.

50. Vider J, Laaksonen DE, Kilk A, et al. Physical exercise induces activation of NF-kappaB in human peripheral blood lymphocytes. Antioxid Redox Signal 2001;3:1131–1137.

51. Patel H, Hoffman-Goetz L. Effects of oestrogen and exercise on caspase-3 activity in primary and secondary lymphoid compartments in ovariectomized mice. Acta Physiol Scand 2002;176:177–184.

52. Hoffman-Goetz L, Quadrilatero J. Treadmill exercise in mice increases intestinal lymphocyte loss via apoptosis. Acta Physiol Scand 2003;279:289–297.

53. Steinacker JM, Lormes W, Reissnecker S, et al. New aspects of the hormone and cytokine response to training. Eur J Appl Physiol: 2003;91:382–391.

54. Hubbard AK, Rothlein R. Intercellular adhesion molecule-1 (ICAM-1) expression and cell signaling cascades. Free Radic Biol Med 2000;28:1379–1386.

55. Olson TS, Ley K. Chemokines and chemokine receptors in leukocyte trafficking. Am J Physiol 2002;283:R7–R28.

56. Shephard RJ. Adhesion molecules, catecholamines and leucocyte redistribution during and following exercise. Sports Med 2003;33:261–284.

57. Nakagawa M, Bondy GP, Waisman D, et al. The effect of glucocorticoids on the expression of L-selectin on polymorphonuclear leukocyte. Blood 1999;93:2730–2737.

58. Matsuba KT, van Eeden SF, Bicknell SG, et al. Apoptosis in circulating PMN: increased susceptibility in L-selectin-deficient PMN. Am J Physiol 1997;272:H2852–H2858.

59. Cuzzolin L, Lussignoli S, Crivellente F, et al. Influence of an acute exercise on neutrophil and platelet adhesion, nitric oxide plasma metabolites in inactive and active subjects. Int J Sports Med 2000;21:289–293.

60. Xing Z, Gauldie J, Cox G, et al. IL-6 is an antiinflammatory cytokine required for controlling local or systemic acute inflammatory responses. J Clin Invest 1998;101:311–320.

61. Barton BE. IL-6: insights into novel biological activities. Clin Immunol Immunopath 1997;85:16–20.

62. Ostrowski K, Rohde T, Asp S, et al. The cytokine balance and strenuous exercise: TNF-alpha, IL-2beta, IL-6, IL-1ra, sTNF-r1, sTNF-r2, and IL-10. J Physiol (Lond) 1999;515:287–291.

63. Suzuki K, Nakaji S, Yamada M, et al. Systemic inflammatory response to exhaustive exercise. Cytokine kinetics Exerc Immunol Rev 2002;8:6–48.

64. Pedersen BK, Steensberg A, Schjerling P. Muscle-derived interleukin-6: possible biological effects. J Physiol (Lond) 2001;536:329–337.

65. Niess AM, Sommer M, Schlotz E, et al. Expression of the inducible nitric oxide synthase (iNOS) in human leukocytes: responses to running exercise. Med Sci Sports Exerc 2000;32:1220–1225.

66. Ostrowski K, Rohde T, Asp S, et al. Chemokines are elevated in plasma after strenuous exercise in humans. Eur J Appl Physiol 2001;84:244–245.

67. Yamada M, Suzuki K, Kudo S, et al. Raised plasma G-CSF and IL-6 after exercise may play a role in neutrophil mobilization into the circulation. J Appl Physiol 2002;92:1789–1794.

68. Drenth JP, van Uum SH, van Deuren M, et al. Endurance run increases circulating IL-6 and IL-1ra but downregulates ex vivo TNF-alpha and IL-1beta production. J Appl Physiol 1995;79:1497–1503.

69. Haahr PM, Pedersen BK, Fomsgaard A, et al. Effect of physical exercise on in vitro production of interleukin 1, interleukin 6, tumor necrosis factor-alpha, interleukin 2 and interferon- gamma. Int J Sports Med 1991;12:223–7.

70. Scott P. IL-12: initiation cytokine for cell-mediated immunity. Science 1993;260:496–497.

71. Febbraio MA, Ott P, Nielsen HB, et al. Hepatosplanchnic clearance of interleukin-6 in humans during exercise. Am J Physiol 2003;285:E397–E402.

72. Febbraio MA, Pedersen BK. Muscle-derived interleukin-6: mechanisms for activation and possible biological roles. FASEB J 2002;16:1335–1347.

73. Winocour PH, Durrington PN, Bhatnagar D, et al. A cross-sectional evaluation of cardiovascular risk factors in coronary heart disease associated with type 1 (insulin-dependent) diabetes mellitus. Diabetes Res Clin Pract 1992;18:173–184.

74. Mohr T, Andersen JL, Biering-Sorensen F, et al. Long-term adaptation to electrically induced cycle training in severe spinal cord injured individuals. Spinal Cord 1997;35:1–16.

75. Pilegaard H, Ordway GA, Saltin B, et al. Transcriptional regulation of gene expression in human skeletal muscle during recovery from exercise. Am J Physiol 2000;279: E806–E814.

76. Ullum H, Haahr PM, Diamant M, et al. Bicycle exercise enhances plasma IL-6 but does not change IL-1alpha, IL-1beta, IL-6, or TNF-alpha pre-mRNA in BMNC. J Appl Physiol 1994;77:93–7.

77. Pedersen BK, Hoffman-Goetz L. Exercise and the immune system: regulation, integration and adaptation. Physiol Rev 2000;80:1055–1081.

78. Starkie RL, Angus DJ, Rolland J, et al. Effect of prolonged submaximal exercise and carbohydrate ingestion on monocyte intracellular cytokine production in humans. J Physiol (Lond) 2000;528:647–655.

79. Starkie RL, Rolland J, Angus DJ, et al. Circulating monocytes are not the source of elevations in plasma IL-6 and TNF-alpha levels after prolonged running. Am J Physiol 2001;280:C769–C774.

80. Ostrowski K, Rohde T, Zacho M, et al. Evidence that IL-6 is produced in skeletal muscle during prolonged running. J Physiol (Lond) 1998;508:949–953.

81. Steensberg A, van Hall G, Osada T, et al. Production of interleukin-6 in contracting human skeletal muscles can account for the exercise-induced increase in plasma interleukin-6. J Physiol (Lond) 2000;529Pt1:237–242.

82. Steensberg A, Fischer CP, Keller C, et al. IL-6 enhances plasma IL-1ra, IL-10, and cortisol in humans. Am J Physiol 2003;285:E433–E437.

83. Nieman DC, Davis JM, Henson DA, et al. Carbohydrate ingestion influences skeletal muscle cytokine mRNA and plasma cytokine levels after a 3–h run. J Appl Physiol 2003;94:1917–1925.

84. Kjaer M, Dela F. Endocrine responses to exercise. In Hoffman-Goetz L, ed. Exercise and Immune Function. Boca Raton, FL: CRC, 1996;1–20.

85. Madden K, Felten DL. Experimental basis for neural-immune interactions. Physiol Rev 1995;75:77–106.

86. Rabin BS, Moyna MN, Kusnecov A, et al. Neuroendocrine effects of immunity. In Hoffman-Goetz L, ed. Exercise and Immune Function. Boca Raton, FL: CRC, 1996; 21–38.

87. Maisel AS, Harris C, Rearden CA, et al. Beta-adrenergic receptors in lymphocyte subsets after exercise: alterations in normal individuals and patients with congestive heart failure. Circulation 1990;82:2003–2010.

88. Hoffman-Goetz L, Pedersen BK. Exercise and the immune system: a model of the stress response? Immunol Today 1994;15:382–7.

89. Kappel M, Tvede N, Galbo H, et al. Evidence that the effect of physical exercise on NK cell activity is mediated by epinephrine. J Appl Physiol 1991;70:2530–4.

90. Tvede N, Kappel M, Klarlund K, et al. Evidence that the effect of bicycle exercise on blood mononuclear cell proliferative responses and subsets is mediated by epinephrine. Int J Sports Med 1994;15:100–104.

91. Galbo H. Hormonal and metabolic adaptation to exercise. New York: Thieme Verlag, 1983.

92. Nehlsen-Canarella SL, Fagoaga OR, Nieman DC. Carbohydrate and the cytokine response to 2.5 hours of running. J Appl Physiol 1997;82:1662–1667.

93. Newsholme EA, Parry Billings M. Properties of glutamine release from muscle and its importance for the immune system. J Parenteral Enteral Nutr 1990;14:63S–67S.

94. Hiscock N, Pedersen BK. Exercise-induced immunodepression: plasma glutamine is not the link. J Appl Physiol 2002;93:813–822.

95. Keller C, Steensberg A, Pilegaard H, et al. Transcriptional activation of the IL-6 gene in human contracting skeletal muscle: influence of muscle glycogen content. FASEB J 2001;15:2748–2750.

96. Steensberg A, Febbraio MA, Osada T, et al. Interleukin-6 production in contracting human skeletal muscle is influenced by pre-exercise muscle glycogen content. J Physiol (Lond) 2001;537:633–639.

97. Fiers W. Tumor necrosis factor: characterization at the molecular, cellular and in vivo level. FEBS Lett 1991;285:199–212.

98. Matthys P, Mitera T, Heremans H, et al. Anti-gamma interferon and anti-interleukin-6 antibodies affect staphylococcal enterotoxin B-induced weight loss, hypoglycemia, and cytokine release in D-galactosamine-sensitized and unsensitized mice. Infect Immun 1995;63:1158–1164.

99. Starkie R, Ostrowski SR, Jauffred S, et al. Exercise and IL-6 infusion inhibit endotoxin-induced TNF-alpha production in humans. FASEB J 2003;17:884–886.

100. Hotamisligil GS, Shargill NS, Spiegelman BM. Adipose expression of tumor necrosis factor-alpha: direct role in obesity-linked insulin resistance. Science 1993;259: 87–91.

101. Nielsen HB, Pedersen BK. Lymphocyte proliferation in response to exercise. Eur J Appl Physiol 1997;75:375–379.

102. Nieman DC, Brendle D, Henson DA, et al. Immune function in athletes versus nonathletes. Int J Sports Med 1995;16:329–33.

103. Rhind SG, Shek PN, Shinkai S, et al. Differential expression of interleukin-2 receptor alpha and beta chains in relation to natural killer cell subsets and aerobic fitness. Int J Sports Med 1994;15:311–318.

104. Nieman DC, Nehlsen-Cannarella SL, Fagoaga OR, et al. Immune function in female elite rowers and non-athletes. Br J Sports Med 2000;34:181–187.

105. Woods JA, Lowder TW, Keylock KT. Can exercise training improve immune function in the aged? Ann N Y Acad Sci 2002;959:117–127.

106. Rall LC, Roubenoff R, Cannon JG, et al. Effects of progressive resistance training on immune response in aging and chronic inflammation. Med Sci Sports Exerc 1996;28: 1356–1365.

107. Conraads VM, Beckers P, Bosmans J, et al. Combined endurance/resistance training reduces plasma TNF-alpha receptor levels in patients with chronic heart failure and coronary artery disease. Eur Heart J 2002;23:1854–1860.

108. Akimoto Y, Kumai T, Akama E, et al. Effects of 12 months of exercise training on salivary secretory IgA levels in elderly subjects. Br J Sports Med 2003;37:76–79.

109. Gleeson M, McDonald WA, Cripps AW, et al. The effect on immunity of long-term intensive training in elite swimmers. Clin Exp Immunol 1995;102:210–216.

110. Fry RW, Grove JR, Morton AR, et al. Psychological and immunological correlates of acute overtraining. Br J Sport Med 1994;28:241–246.

111. Pizza FX, Flynn MG, Starling RD, et al. Run training vs cross training: influence of increased training on running economy, foot impact shock and run performance. Int J Sports Med 1995;16:180–184.

112. Woods JA, Ceddia MA, Wolters BW, et al. Effects of 6 months of moderate aerobic exercise training on immune function in the elderly. Mech Ageing Dev 1999;109: 1–19.

113. Mackinnon LT. Chronic exercise training effects on immune function. Med Sci Sports Exerc 2000;32: S369–S376.

114. Sen CK. Oxidants and antioxidants in exercise. J Appl Physiol 1995;79:675–686.

115. Perez CJ, Nemet D, Mills PJ, et al. Effects of laboratory versus field exercise on leukocyte subsets and cell adhesion molecule expression in children. Eur J Appl Physiol 2001; 86:34–39.

116. Boas SR, Joswiak ML, Nixon PA, et al. Effects of anaerobic exercise on the immune system in eight to seventeen year old trained and untrained boys. J Pediatr 1996;129: 846–855.

117. Dobbs RJ, Charlett A, Purkiss AG, et al. Association of circulating TNF-alpha and IL-6 with ageing and parkinsonism. Acta Neurol Scand 1999,100:34–41.

118. Paolisso G, Rizzo MR, Mazziotti G, et al. Advancing age and insulin resistance: role of plasma tumor necrosis factor-alpha. Am J Physiol 1998;275:E294–E299.

119. Bruunsgaard H, Pedersen M, Pedersen BK. Ageing and proinflammatory cytokines. Curr Opinion Hematol 2001;8:131–136.

120. Bruunsgaard H, Andersen-Ranberg K, Jeune B, et al. A high plasma concentration of TNFalpha is associated with dementia in centenarians. J Gerontol 1999;54A:357–364.

121. Ballou SP, Lozanski FB, Hodder S, et al. Quantitative and qualitative alterations of acute-phase proteins in healthy elderly persons. Age Ageing 1996;25:224–230.

122. Bruunsgaard H, Pedersen AN, Schroll M, et al. Impaired production of proinflammatory cytokines in response to lipopolysaccharide (LPS) stimulation in elderly humans. Clin Exp Immunol 1999;118:235–241.

123. Cowles WN. Fatigue as a contributory cause of pneumonia. Boston Med Surg 1918;179:555.

124. Nicholls EE, Spaeth RA. The relation between fatigue and the susceptibility of guinea pigs to infections of type I pneumococcus. Am J Hygiene 1922;2:527–535.

125. Oppenheim H, Spaeth RA. The relation between fatigue and the susceptibility of rats towards a toxin and an infection. Am J Hygiene 1922;2:51–66.

CHAPTER 24

The Body Fluid and Hemopoietic Systems

GARY W. MACK

Introduction

Within the human body optimal cellular function is maintained as long as the internal environment maintains the proper concentration of nutrients (i.e., oxygen and glucose), ions (i.e., sodium and potassium), and other essential constituents (i.e., amino acids). The constancy of the body fluid bathing each cell or what Claude Barnard called the *milieu interieu* is determined by interaction of several sophisticated physiological control systems that act to attain homeostasis. Regulatory mechanisms involved in fluid homeostasis include the kidney, which ultimately determines the rates of water and electrolyte output, and numerous extrarenal reflexes that modify rates of fluid and salt intake and adjust fluid distribution between various fluid compartments within the body. During exercise fluid homeostasis is challenged in several ways. There is a redistribution of body water consisting of fluid shifts between the vascular compartment and interstitial fluid (ISF) compartment and water movement between the extracellular fluid (ECF) and intracellular fluid (ICF) compartments. During prolonged exercise the loss of body water to thermoregulatory sweating provides another impetus for body water redistribution. The redistribution of body water evokes reflexes that act to restore the constancy of the *milieu interieu*. Because the level of circulating blood volume must be protected to ensure adequate circulatory control and stability during exercise, the body also evokes reflexes that act to limit the magnitude of fluid loss from the vascular compartment. Finally, dynamic exercise training can alter the absolute size of various fluid compartments and redistribution of fluid during exercise-induced dehydration. Specifically, exercise-induced hypervolemia (blood volume expansion) is considered a hallmark adaptation of dynamic exercise (endurance) training. It is clear that the increase in blood volume provides an individual with a physiological and thereby performance advantage during exercise. This chapter addresses the general characteristics of the body fluid compartments, their distribution at rest and during exercise, the impact of exercise on homeostatic control of body fluid balance, and adaptations of the fluid compartments to exercise training. Since blood volume is composed of plasma and RBC volumes, the regulation of RBC volume and its influence on exercise performance will be discussed.

Body Fluid Compartments

Most total body water (TBW) resides within the cells, or ICF space, while about one-third is found in the space surrounding the cells, or ECF space (1). Water moves passively via osmosis, along with the solutes, across boundary layers. The composition of the ICF is determined by the permeability and transport characteristic of the cell membrane;

however, total osmolality of the ICF and ECF spaces are similar (about 286 mOsm · kg water^{-1}). The ECF is mixed throughout the body in a two-stage process. First, it is rapidly transported and distributed via circulating plasma. Second, it is mixed between the plasma and fluid outside the vascular compartment, or ISF space, by diffusion and bulk transport across the capillary wall. A change in water content of any of the body's fluid compartments will result in redistribution of body water and an alteration of the solute concentration in all of the compartments.

With use of deuterium, TBW can be estimated from a measured dilution space with a relative precision of 1.5%, or about 0.6 L. Other dilution tracers, such as ethanol, are a viable alternative, but ethanol dilution underestimates TBW by 5–10%, and the methodology has slightly less precision (2.6%) (2). Bioelectrical impedance analysis can also be used to predict TBW; however, these measurements should be made with some caution. Single-frequency (50-kHz series) bioelectrical impedance instruments should be able to predict absolute TBW in a population of normal, healthy individuals as long as the ratio of extracellular to intracellular fluid compartment size is within a physiological range. However, these instruments are not accurate if drugs or disease significantly alters the ratio of ICF to ECF. Also, single-frequency units cannot detect small changes in TBW. A multifrequency bioelectrical impedance instrument using a 0–∞kHz parallel Cole-Cole model will better predict small changes in TBW (3).

For the sedentary individual TBW averages approximately 60% of body weight, or about 600 mL · kg body weight^{-1} (Fig. 24.1). The literature indicates that TBW varies with the age, sex, weight, and lean body mass (1). However, when TBW is expressed as a function of fat-free mass (about 780 ± 7 mL · kg FFM^{-1}), it is similar across a wide age range (20–90 years old), which suggests that differences in body composition contribute to most of the reported variability in TBW (4,5). The distribution of TBW between the various fluid compartments is illustrated in Figure 24.1. Heterogeneity within the extracellular compartments and the inherent limitations of dilution methodology prevent precise identification of the other fluid compartment sizes. Therefore, the values for the distribution of TBW presented in Figure 24.1 should be viewed as approximate.

The ICF compartment accounts for 55% of the water content (about 50% for females and 60% for males), while the ECF compartment accounts for the remaining 45% (50% for females and 40% for males) of TBW. Within the ECF compartment fluid is distributed between the intravascular and extravascular fluid space. In the classical description, the ECF is distributed between the plasma, which contains 7.5% of the TBW, and the ISF compartment, which holds about 20% of the TBW. However, portions of the ISF fluid space, identified by its inability to rapidly equilibrate with conventional tracer molecules, are found in dense connective tissue and bone and account for 7.5 and 7.5% of TBW, respectively (1). In addition, the activity of secretory cells produces a fluid that is not a simple ultrafiltrate of plasma but is still considered a portion of the ISF compartment. This fluid space, identified as the transcellular fluid compartment, accounts for 2.5% of TBW. This distribution of TBW is illustrated in Figure 24.1.

In general, for a 70-kg man the ECF volume averages 260 mL · kg body weight^{-1}, or 43% of TBW, and is determined primarily by the total body sodium content. ICF volume averages 340 mL · kg body weight^{-1}, or about 55% of TBW. Plasma volume (PV) is about 17% of the ECF space and averages 40 mL · kg body weight^{-1}, while RBC volume (RCV) averages 31 mL · kg body weight^{-1}. The result is that blood volume averages about 71 mL · kg body weight^{-1} in sedentary adults. Figure 24.2 illustrates the relationship between vascular compartment size and body weight.

Table 24.1 summarizes the fluid compartment sizes and includes the norms published by the International Commission on Radiological Protection (6). Compartment sizes for sedentary and exercise-trained individuals reported in Table 24.1 represent average values reported in the literature. Deviation of these numbers from the expected norms will reflect both individual variability and measurement errors associated with the various tracers used to estimate TBW, ECF, PV, and RCV.

Dynamic exercise training, specifically for endurance, causes an increase in most fluid compartments (Table 24.1). Limited data on the measurement of TBW, ICF, and ECF compartment sizes in endurance-trained athletes make comparison with sedentary individuals for these fluid spaces somewhat speculative; however, the data in Table 24.1 provide a reasonable view of the available literature.

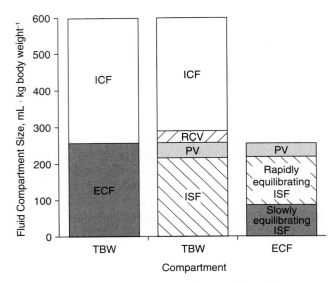

FIGURE 24.1 Distribution of total body water (TBW) between various fluid compartments. ICF, intracellular fluid; ECF, extracellular fluid; RCV, red cell volume; PV, plasma volume ISF, interstitial fluid.

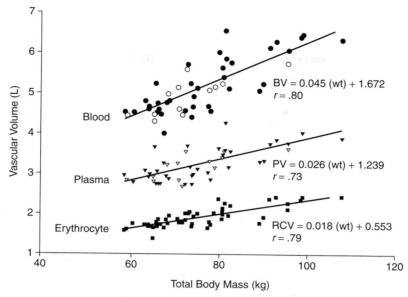

FIGURE 24.2 The relationships between erythrocyte, plasma, and blood volumes and total body mass in healthy young men. *(Reprinted with permission from Sawka MN, Young AJ, Pandolf KB, Dennis RC, Valeri CR. Erythrocyte, plasma, and blood volume of healthy young men. Med Sci Sports Exerc 1992;24:451.)*

Because TBW expressed per kilogram of fat-free mass is fairly constant over one's lifespan, it is possible that the differences in TBW (expressed in milliliters per kilogram of body weight) between trained athletes and untrained individuals will disappear when the data are normalized to fat-free mass (7).

Sufficient data have been published to establish that endurance-trained athletes demonstrate considerable blood volume expansion (Table 24.1). A cross-sectional look at the available data indicates that PV, RCV, and blood volume are about 30% larger in endurance-trained athletes than in sedentary individuals. In sedentary individuals PV averages about 45 mL $\cdot$ kg body weight^{-1}, or approximately 18% of the ECF compartment size. In endurance-trained athletes PV averages 58 mL $\cdot$ kg^{-1}, or about 23% of the ECF space. Based upon data collected from cross-sectional analysis of endurance-trained athletes and sedentary individuals, the increase in blood volume with endurance training is shared by an increase in PV and RCV. In longitudinal training studies lasting 3 to 21 days, the increase in blood volume is limited to only 10 to 15%. In addition, the increase in PV is usually greater than the increase in RCV (noticeable hemodilution). Figure 24.3 illustrates the time course of the change in vascular compartments during endurance training. A high blood volume, even in individuals with no history of exercise training, is associated with a high $\dot{V}O_{2max}$ (8).

TABLE 24.1	Body fluid compartment size in sedentary individuals and trained athletes						
Category	TBW mL $\cdot$ kg^{-1}	ICF mL $\cdot$ kg^{-1}	ECF mL $\cdot$ kg^{-1}	ISF mL $\cdot$ kg^{-1}	PV mL $\cdot$ kg^{-1}	RCV mL $\cdot$ kg^{-1}	BV mL $\cdot$ kg^{-1}
NORMS	600	340	260	220	40	31	71
Sedentary	627	366	246	201	45	31	76
Trained Athlete	671	424	247	189	58	42	100
Relative Increase	Δ%	Δ%	Δ%	Δ%	Δ%	Δ%	Δ%
Cross-Sectional	7	16	—	−6	29	35	32
Training Studies					11	8	9

TBW, total body water; ICF, intracellular fluid space; ECF, extracellular fluid space; ISF, interstitial fluid space; PV, plasma volume; RCV, red cell volume; BV, total blood volume. Absolute volumes are expressed as mL per kg body weight and relative changes are expressed as a change in volume as a percent of the appropriate control. The values for TBW, ICF, ECF, and ISF volumes for sedentary and trained athletes represent mean values calculated from limited data available in the literature (5, 25, 26). The values for PV, RCV, AND blood volume volumes represent the average of reported values in the literature (8, 40, 48, 49, 64). The clinical database (NORMS) represents values for the standard man reported by the International Commission on Radiological Protection in 1975.

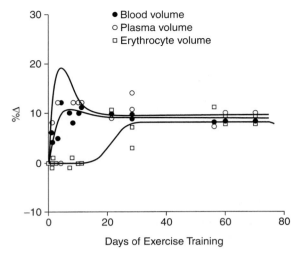

FIGURE 24.3 Estimated time course of changes in plasma volume (PV), erythrocyte volume, and total blood volume with endurance exercise training. During the early phases of training increases in plasma volume account for most of the increase in total blood volume. After 8 weeks of training the contribution of plasma volume and erythrocyte volume to the increase in TBV are about equal. *(Reprinted with permission from Sawka MN, Convertino VA, Eichner ER, et al. Blood volume: importance and adaptations to exercise training, environmental stresses, and trauma/sickness. Med Sci Sports Exerc 2000;32:333.)*

Water Balance and Dynamic Exercise

Water homeostasis and osmoregulation are critical for the survival of all organisms. Water and salt balance are maintained by behavioral and physiological reflexes that act to control ingestive behaviors (water intake, sodium appetite) and water and electrolyte loses. Exercise affects water and electrolyte homeostasis in several ways. First, exercise causes a fluid shift out of the vascular compartment, initiating reflex responses that act to defend PV and thereby blood volume during exercise. Second, prolonged thermoregulatory sweating during dynamic exercise leads to a loss of water and electrolytes, hence to exercise-induced dehydration and the initiation of osmoregulatory reflexes. Control of urinary excretion of water through osmoregulatory control of arginine vasopressin (AVP) secretion will help limit the magnitude of water loss by the kidney during exercise. The restoration of water deficits following exercise-induced dehydration is controlled by the sensation of thirst and ingestive behaviors that regulate fluid intake. Maintenance of water and electrolyte homeostasis under any set of conditions (during exercise or during recovery from dehydration) reflects the balance between ingestive behaviors that restore lost water and electrolytes and water and electrolyte retention by renal mechanisms. This section examines these three aspects of dynamic exercise and fluid balance.

Water Distribution at Rest

The steady-state volumes for each fluid compartment are listed in Table 24.1. They reflect the effect of net water movement under resting conditions. At rest and during exercise water is continually exchanged between the fluid compartments. The forces guiding theses water fluxes are osmotic and hydrostatic. Osmosis is the primary mechanism by which water exchange occurs between the ICF and ISF compartments. The osmotic gradient for water exchange is determined by the concentration gradient of osmotically active substances. The concentration of osmotically active substances, or osmolality (expressed as milliosmoles per kilogram of water), is determined by the total solute concentration. Electrolytes contribute predominantly to the transmembrane osmotic gradient. However, as the result of active transport and metabolic processes, the cell contains high concentrations of amino acids, nucleotides, and small organic molecules that are impermeable to the plasma membrane. These molecules are charged, and their counter ions (Donnan effect) contribute to the total osmolality of the intracellular compartment. van't Hoft's law defines the relationship between solute concentration and osmotic pressure:

$$\pi = [\text{solute}] \cdot R \cdot T$$

where π = osmotic pressure in millimeters of mercury; R = universal gas constant; T = absolute temperature.

Intracellular osmolality is controlled by adjusting the rate of transport of solute into (to prevent dehydration) or out of (to prevent overhydration) the cell to regulate cell volume.

Transcapillary Exchange of Fluid

The distribution of fluid between the intravascular compartment and the ISF space is governed by parameters outlined by Starling in 1896 and experimentally verified by Landis in 1927. Transcapillary fluid movement follows the difference in hydrostatic pressure and osmotic pressure across the capillary and is described in the following equation (Starling-Landis equation [9]):

$$J_v / S = Lp \left(PRES_{cap} - PRES_{ISF} \right) + \sigma_d \left(\pi_{cap} - \pi_{ISF} \right)$$

where J_v = solvent (water) flux across the capillary per unit surface area (S); Lp = hydraulic conductivity (permeability); S = capillary surface area; PRES = hydrostatic pressure in millimeters of mercury; cap = capillary; ISF = interstitial fluid; σ_d = osmotic reflection coefficient; π = colloid osmotic pressure in millimeters of mercury.

Classically substituting global values for hydrostatic and colloid osmotic pressures in plasma and tissue ISF solves this equation. Standard values for the parameters of the Starling-Landis equation under resting conditions are listed in Table 24.2.

At the arteriolar end of the capillary the net hydrostatic pressure gradient trying to force fluid out of the capillary

TABLE 24.2	Approximate Starling forces in resting skeletal muscle							
Capillary	$PRES_{cap}$	$PRES_{ISF}$	$\Delta PRES$	π_{cap}	π_{ISF}	$\Delta\pi$	Net	
Arteriolar	+32	−2	+34	+25	+5	−20	+14	filtration
Venular	+10	−2	+12	+25	+5	−20	−8	reabsorption

Hydrostatic and colloid osmotic pressures are given in mm Hg. $PRES_{cap}$, capillary hydrostatic pressure; $PRES_{ISF}$, interstitial fluid hydrostatic pressure; $\Delta PRES$, hydrostatic pressure gradient; π_{cap}, capillary colloid osmotic pressure; π_{ISF}, interstitial fluid colloid osmotic pressure, $\Delta\pi$, colloid osmotic pressure gradient; Net, sum of $\Delta PRES$ and $\Delta\pi$ (9, 12).

($\Delta PRES$ = 34 mm Hg) exceeds the net colloid osmotic pressure gradient that is pulling fluid into the vascular compartment ($\Delta\pi = -20$ mm Hg). Therefore, fluid filters out of the vascular compartment. At the venular end of the capillary the net colloid osmotic pressure gradient pulling fluid into the capillary ($\Delta\pi = -20$ mm Hg) exceeds the net hydrostatic pressure gradient forcing fluid out of the capillary ($\Delta PRES$ = 12 mm Hg). In these conditions fluid moves back into the vascular compartment (reabsorption). Normally, the amount of fluid filtered only slightly exceeds the volume of fluid reabsorbed. The remaining fluid is returned to the vascular compartment via the lymphatic capillaries.

Transcapillary Exchange of Macromolecules

Transcapillary exchange of macromolecules is described by a set of equations derived by Kedem and Ksatchchalsky (10):

$$J_s/S = J_v/S \left(1 - \sigma_d\right) \cdot [solute]_{mean} + P_d \cdot \left([solute]_{cap} - [solute]_{ISF}\right)$$

where J_s/S = solute flux per unit area and P_d = diffusional permeability.

This equation describes the important parameters that govern microvascular exchange across a homoporous membrane in a global sense but does not directly address the exact relationship of structure to function of microvascular transport. Recent advances in microvascular exchange have significantly improved our understanding of this process and should be reviewed by all students interested in the study of fluid balance (11,12). Rippe and Haraldsson (12) described a two-pore theory of capillary permeability in which capillary barrier characteristics can be described in terms of pore (channel) size and number. In this model the pathways for macromolecule transport through microvascular walls of continuous capillaries (i.e., those found in skeletal muscle) are depicted as water-filled pores (or channels) of fixed diameter (small pores with a radius of about 40 Å and large pores with a radius of 250–200 Å). The spaces between adjacent endothelial cells (interendothelial clefts or slits) are the most likely candidates for these small pores. The large pores are thought to represent either interendothelial clefts that are wider than the typical small pore or large-radius (300–700 Å) transcellular channels. In general, the solute transport across most capillary beds can be described

by the presence of small pores that restrict proteins and few non–size-selective large pores. The number and type of pores per unit of area can account for differences in Lp between various vascular beds. The two-pore concept is the simplest model to account for most but not all of the transport characteristics of capillary macromolecule exchange and fluid flux. More recently, Michel and Curry (11) described a fiber matrix model of capillary permeability. Here the pore size is not determined by the tight junction size (interendothelial clefts) but by the characteristics of a molecular filter (fiber matrix) associated with the endothelial cell glycocalyx. This surface glycocalyx acts as a primary molecular sieve and diffusion barrier for plasma proteins. In the fiber matrix model the Starling forces that determine fluid exchange are the hydrostatic and oncotic pressure gradients across the glycocalyx or fenestral diaphragm rather than the typical global gradients in hydrostatic and oncotic pressure between plasma and tissue. This view of transcapillary exchange leads to two dramatic changes in our view of Starling forces. First, local Starling forces are heterogeneous across the length of the capillary. Second, the local protein and tissue pressure just behind the glycocalyx or fenestral diaphragm determine the hydrostatic and oncotic pressure gradients for fluid and solute movement rather than some global tissue pressure or protein concentration. These concepts help to explain large spatial variations in local water flux across the surface glycocalyx. Both models provide a better understanding of the biophysics of capillary exchange.

Fluid Shifts and Dynamic Exercise

In contracting muscles fluid exchange between the vascular compartment and the interstitial space are controlled by the prevailing Starling forces across microvascular beds and the osmotic gradients between ICF and ECF spaces. In human research rapid changes in ECF or ICF spaces are difficult to measure. However, rapid fluid shifts into or out of the vascular compartment can be estimated reliably and accurately. One of the first observations associated with the effect of exercise on hematological variables was the observation of an increase in the volume of packed RBCs (hematocrit, Hct). The increase in Hct was associated with a shift of protein-free fluid out of the vascular compartment into the tissue ISF space. It is now recognized that this PV shift in response to exercise can be estimated by measuring changes in Hct and hemoglobin using the following equation (13):

$$\%\Delta PV = 100 \times \left[\frac{Hb_{CON}}{Hb_t} \times \frac{(1 - Hct_t \times 100)}{(1 - Hct_{CON} \times 100)} \right] - 100$$

where $\%\Delta PV$ = percent change in PV; Hb = hemoglobin concentration in grams per deciliter; Hct_t = hematocrit, or fraction of packed RBCs, at time t after the control sample; HCT_{CON} = control blood sample.

This equation describes the change in PV relative to a control condition. This calculation is only as accurate as the precision of the control condition. The simple act of changing posture from supine to standing is associated with significant hemoconcentration: the upright posture moves fluid out of the vascular space, with maximal hemoconcentration occurring some 40–60 minutes later. This posture-dependent hemoconcentration may or may not mask the impact of exercise on the PV shift. For example, in the upright posture on a cycle ergometer the PV shift during dynamic exercise of 70% of $\dot{V}O_{2max}$ averages about −17% if the exercise is preceded by a 10- to 15-min control period. On the other hand, the PV shift during dynamic exercise is negligible if the control period lasts 60 min or longer. There is no absolute answer as to how long one must wait in a given posture before body fluid reaches equilibrium. If one controls for posture and time spent in the posture before exercise, then reasonable comparisons between control and experimental groups can be made. However, a 60-min postural control period provides an excellent starting point for any experiment designed to measure accurate changes in PV using the Dill-Costill equation. Contraction of the spleen occurs during exercise in humans; however, release of red blood cells (RBCs) by the spleen into the circulation has little impact on circulating erythrocyte volume or peripheral hematocrit. This means that contraction of the spleen does not influence estimates of PV shifts using the Dill-Costill equation.

Fluid Shifts During Mild Dynamic Exercise

Early research has clearly shown that PV shifts during exercise interact with posture. For this reason this discussion focuses primarily on upright cycle ergometer exercise when describing the general phenomenon of fluid shifts during exercise. During upright dynamic cycle ergometer exercise the PV shift out of the vascular compartment is proportional to relative exercise intensity ($\%\dot{V}O_{2max}$) (14–16). At maximal aerobic power ($\dot{V}O_{2max}$) a fluid volume equal to 20 to 25% of the initial PV will move out of the vascular compartment during the first 5–15 minutes of exercise. The plasma composition of electrolytes is unaltered by the fluid shift at exercise intensities lower than 40% $\dot{V}O_{2max}$, indicating that the fluid that leaves the vascular compartment is isotonic with plasma. At the onset of muscle contraction $PRES_{cap}$ rises rapidly and is sustained at this elevated level for the duration

of the exercise (17). The rise in $PRES_{cap}$ during exercise is proportional to the rise in mean arterial blood pressure. This is an interesting observation because normally $PRES_{cap}$ is autoregulated so that it changes very little over a wide range of arterial blood pressures. However, during exercise this autoregulation is lost. The coupling of $PRES_{cap}$ to mean arterial pressure during exercise is most likely related to the large increase in blood flow to active skeletal muscle as a result of metabolic hyperemia and functional sympatholysis. At the onset of exercise the rise in $PRES_{cap}$ promotes a rapid efflux of isotonic fluid from the vascular compartment.

Fluid Shifts During Moderate to Heavy Dynamic Exercise

At higher exercise intensities hypotonic fluid is shifted out of the vascular compartment, causing plasma osmolality to increase. In addition, increased activity of skeletal muscles results in local intracellular and interstitial hyperosmolality. During heavy dynamic exercise skeletal muscle ICF lactate concentration can increase from 5 to more than 29 mmol · L^{-1}, and extracellular lactate can increase from 1.3 to more than 13 mmol · L^{-1} (18). These increases in lactate concentration create a favorable osmotic gradient for water into the ICF space of the active skeletal muscle cell. During heavy exercise the increase in skeletal muscle ECF space is about 10 times greater than the increase in ICF space. Lag times in the rate of equilibrium between the ISF and vascular compartment indicate that a rapid increase in interstitial osmolality could also contribute to the movement of water out of the vascular compartment.

During heavy exercise plasma osmolality will increase by 15 mOsm · kg water^{-1}. According to van't Hoff's law, this equates to an osmotic gradient of 200 mm Hg. The increase in plasma osmolality during exercise acts to limit excessive reductions in PV and thereby helps to maintain circulating blood volume. An interesting observation is that during graded exercise the rise in plasma sodium concentration is proportional to the rise in plasma lactate (19). The stoichiometry of the increase in lactate and sodium in the plasma during exercise suggests that the negatively charged lactate ion restricts Na^+ efflux from the vascular compartment, as its accompanying H^+ is buffered by the carbonic anhydrase reaction. This coupling of Na^+ with the lactate will act to limit fluid efflux from the plasma compartment and aid in maintaining circulating blood volume and cardiovascular stability. Figure 24.4 illustrates the general relationship between relative exercise intensity, plasma osmolality, and PV during upright cycle ergometer exercise.

Starling Equilibrium During Prolonged Dynamic Exercise

As exercise continues, the rate of fluid efflux from the plasma declines, and a new Starling equilibrium is established as a result of several adjustments. First, increased blood flow to

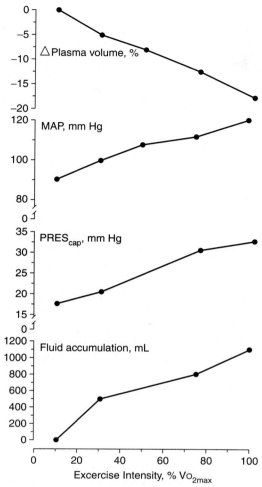

FIGURE 24.4 Impact of relative exercise intensity on plasma volume, plasma osmolality, capillary pressure, and tissue fluid accumulation during upright cycle ergometer exercise.

The magnitude of the fluid accumulation in active skeletal muscle immediately following exercise has been measured. During upright cycle ergometer exercise the total volume of fluid accumulating in active skeletal muscle averages about 18, 30, and 45 mL per kilogram of active muscle during light, moderate, and heavy exercise, respectively (22). For a 70-kg human these represent absolute volume accumulations of about 500, 800, and 1100 mL following light, moderate, and heavy exercise, respectively. During heavy exercise the net reduction in PV averages about 600 mL, or 20% of the initial PV (23). To compensate for the large fluid accumulation in active skeletal muscle during exercise, the vascular compartment must simultaneously absorb fluid from inactive tissue to minimize the reduction in PV (24). Again, the driving forces for this fluid absorption are the Starling forces. Increased sympathetic nerve signals sent to inactive tissues during exercise will result in vasoconstriction. Arteriolar vasoconstriction will cause a reduction in $PRES_{cap}$, causing the ΔPress gradient to favor absorption of fluid into the vascular compartment. During heavy exercise plasma osmolality (Posm) and plasma protein concentration (i.e., π_{cap}) will increase. Thus, both a decrease in hydrostatic pressure gradient and an increase in the osmotic pressure gradient contribute to fluid absorption into the vascular compartment from inactive tissues (i.e., noncontracting muscle, skin, intestines). Without the absorption of water from inactive tissues the fall in PV during exercise would likely limit cardiovascular and exercise performance.

Modulation of Fluid Shifts During Dynamic Exercise

While Starling forces are the primary regulators of fluid exchange during exercise, several factors modulate fluid shifts. The extensive list of variables that are thought to impact PV regulation during exercise includes such things as hormones, exercise mode (e.g., cycle, treadmill, swimming), posture, exercise intensity, muscle mass (arm versus leg exercise), gender, phase of menstrual cycle, hydration status, and fitness level. The following section focuses on only a few important factors that act as modulators of fluid shifts during exercise.

Atrial natriuretic peptide directly alters capillary permeability to water and albumin. Also, it indirectly alters capillary permeability by increasing the hydrostatic pressure gradient for fluid efflux by changing the ratio of capillary resistance before and after exercise (arteriolar dilation leads to an increase in $PRES_{cap}$). During upright exercise (treadmill walking) the plasma concentration of atrial natriuretic peptide is increased in proportion to exercise intensity. If the identical treadmill exercise (i.e., identical energy cost) is performed in water (up to xiphoid process) we see a greater release of atrial natriuretic peptide and a larger plasma fluid shift out of the vascular space (25). These observations provide

the active skeletal muscle and a slight rise in local tissue hydrostatic pressure ($PRES_{ISF}$) wash out local ISF solute (20). The rise in ISF hydrostatic pressure is a function of the pressure–volume relationship (or compliance) of the ISF compartment. The rise in capillary filtration and an increase in muscle pump activity will also lead to an increase in lymph flow. The increase in lymph flow serves a dual purpose. First, the increased filtration and lymph flow will flush lymph proteins into the vascular compartment, causing a small decline in π_{ISF} (21). Second, the increase in lymph flow will cause an influx of lymphatic protein into the vascular space and thus increase π_{cap}. In addition, as hypotonic fluid leaves the vascular compartment, there is an accompanying rise in plasma oncotic pressure. This rise in plasma oncotic pressure will oppose the hydrostatic pressure gradient. These adjustments in Starling forces act to limit fluid efflux from the vascular compartment and maintain circulating blood volume.

evidence of the role of atrial natriuretic peptide in the modulation of the PV shift during dynamic exercise.

Exercise mode affects fluid shifts during exercise. Arm-cranking exercise produces a larger PV shift than does leg exercise at the same $\dot{V}O_{2max}$ (16). The greater PV shift during arm exercise is proportional to the larger mean arterial pressure and thereby the greater increase in the critical Starling force, $PRES_{cap}$. At similar absolute exercise intensity (i.e., same $\dot{V}O_{2max}$), swimming and upright cycling produce the same shift in PV out of the vascular compartment (26). Body fluid status prior to exercise will also affect fluid shifts during exercise. During light treadmill exercise in air, hemodilution occurs in euhydrated subjects but hemoconcentration occurs in hypohydrated (-5% of body weight) subjects (27).

As one examines the literature it is difficult to derive a simple description of fluid shifts during exercise. What is clear is that the maximal degree of PV shift during exercise is limited to about 20%. Therefore, regardless of which factor dominates—exercise or gravity—the fluid shift out of the vascular compartment is limited and balanced by a rise in $PRES_{ISF}$, Posm, and π_{cap}.

Exercise-induced Dehydration

As exercise continues, body water is lost to thermoregulatory sweating and insensible water loss. Body temperatures (core and skin) and ambient conditions determine thermoregulatory sweating during exercise. Maximal whole-body sweat loss during dry heat exposure in man has been reported to be 1.5–2.0 kg · h^{-1}, but some researchers have reported values as high as 3.0–4.0 kg · h^{-1} during heavy exercise in the heat (27,28). However, local sweat rates at different sites on the body surface vary considerably. In man, water loss from the respiratory system (insensible water loss) contributes an additional 0.12 kg · h^{-1} of water loss during heavy exercise. Thus, a 70-kg adult could lose on the order of 2.5% of water content per hour of heavy exercise in the heat. Most of that water loss is due to sweating. Offsetting sensible and insensible water loss is the gain of water from metabolism and release of water bound to glycogen. Exercising at an oxygen cost of 42 mL of oxygen per minute per kilogram of body weight will result in the production of about 122 g water per hour. As glycogen is metabolized, the water complexed with this molecule (about 2.7 g water per gram of glycogen) is released. Burning 100 g glycogen per hour could liberate 0.3–0.4 L of water per hour into the TBW pool. During exercise-induced dehydration you can observe a drop in body weight (loss of sweat and respiratory water) but maintain TBW (gain of body water from metabolism and release from glycogen).

Sweat is a hypotonic fluid with an average [Na$^+$] and [K$^+$] of 56.4 (range 30.6–105.7) and 9.6 (range 6.9–11.5) mEq · L^{-1}, respectively (20). Assuming an average sweat concentration of 55 mEq Na$^+$ per liter, we can estimate that a 70-kg adult will lose about 96 mEq Na$^+$ per hour, or about

3.3% of total exchangeable Na$^+$ per hour. Thus, the loss of water due to sweating is accompanied by a concomitant loss of electrolytes. Previous discussions make it clear that both ECF and ICF compartments share the exercise-induced water and electrolyte deficits. It is also clear that the body's ability to mobilize water from the extravascular to the intravascular space during exercise will aid in maintenance of circulating blood volume, an important step in optimal regulation of both arterial blood pressure and temperature regulation.

Water and Electrolyte Losses During Light Dynamic Exercise

During light dynamic exercise in the heat (body weight decrease of 2.0 to 6.0 kg), the water losses are equally distributed between the ECF and ICF spaces (28). Within the ECF compartment, water loss from the plasma averages approximately 20% of the ECF volume loss. This is what you would expect, since at rest prior to dehydration plasma water accounts for about 20% of the ECF volume. Since extracellular Na$^+$ content determines the size of the ECF compartment, it is easy to see why the loss of Na$^+$ from the body closely predicts the decrease in ECF space. During dehydration the [Na$^+$] in sweat determines the amount of free water loss from the body via the sweat gland (analogous to free water loss by the kidney) and the subsequent increase in Posm (29). The rise in Posm contributes to the osmotic gradient between the ICF and ECF compartments in inactive tissue and determines the amount of water mobilized into the vascular compartment by osmosis. The mobilization of fluid from the ICF into the ECF space prevents excessive reductions in PV and circulating blood volume and provides cardiovascular stability during dehydration. The mobilization of fluid from the ICF to ECF space cannot prevent the decline in PV, as the reduction in PV during dehydration is generally proportional to the reduction in TBW. However, the magnitude of the reduction in PV during dehydration can be attenuated. Maintenance of circulating blood volume during exercise-induced dehydration is a function of the body's ability to mobilize fluid from the ICF space, which itself is linked to the sodium concentration in sweat (29). Thus, dilute sweat allows conservation of the PV during dehydration, primarily because of the greater movement of water from the intracellular fluid compartment. Sweat [Na$^+$] is generally relatively low in heat-acclimated individuals and trained athletes, which indicates an improved ability to maintain circulating blood volume during exercise-induced dehydration.

Osmoregulatory Responses to Exercise-induced Dehydration

Exercise-induced dehydration results in hyperosmolality and hypovolemia. Physiological compensation for the reduction in the size and tonicity of the cellular and extracellular fluid compartment involves modification of water and sodium losses by the kidney through the action of water- and sodium-retaining hormones and through modulation of efferent renal sympathetic nerve activity. Two prominent responses to exercise-induced dehydration are the release of AVP and the increase in plasma renin activity.

During exercise plasma levels of AVP increase in a linear fashion once Posm exceeds some threshold level. At rest that threshold is about 280 to 285 mOsm · kg water^{-1} (30,31). During exercise this threshold increases in proportion to the exercise intensity (19). The threshold plasma osmolality that elicits the increase in AVP also depends on the size of the intravascular compartment, such that during dehydration both the increase in Posm and the reduction in PV contribute to the increase in AVP and result in a high AVP level at any given osmotic drive. Several other factors contribute to the release of AVP: an elevation in body temperature, muscle receptor activation, and elevated plasma levels of angiotensin II. Convertino and associates (32) showed that during heat stress, elevated body temperature increased plasma AVP from 1.2 to 5.5 pg · mL^{-1} while plasma osmolality increased only 2 to 4 mOsmol. The increase in AVP per unit change in plasma osmolality seen during passive heat stress was twice as high as predicted from the linear relationship between Posm and AVP during hypertonic saline infusion. Thus, an increase in body temperature provides an additional stimulus for AVP release during dynamic exercise.

Following exercise-induced dehydration, human urine osmolality has been found to be in the order of 1000–1400 mOsm · kg water^{-1}, which is greater than that seen during infusions of large doses of AVP. Thus, the maximal concentrating ability of the kidney following exercise-induced dehydration is not entirely dependent on the action of elevated AVP. In response to a decrease in PV during dehydration, renin release from the juxtaglomerular cells will be increased in response to a reduction in sodium load to the macula densa (i.e., reduced glomerular filtration rate), reduced arterial blood pressure in afferent arterioles, increased renal sympathetic nerve activity, or increased levels of circulating catecholamines. The activation of the renin–angiotensin–aldosterone axis will enhance renal sodium reabsorption during prolonged exercise in the heat.

Rehydration Following Exercise

Following exercise-induced dehydration, water balance is restored by the integration of behavioral and physiological reflexes that act to control ingestive behaviors (water intake) and urinary excretion (water loss). Control of urinary excretion through osmoregulatory control of AVP secretion limits water loss by the kidney. However, this control system has no ability to restore lost water. Therefore, the restoration of body fluid balance after dehydration induced by exercise (or any other stress) ultimately depends on reflexes that regulate fluid intake. Unfortunately, the pattern of rehydration in humans displays a distinct delay in the restoration of water bal-

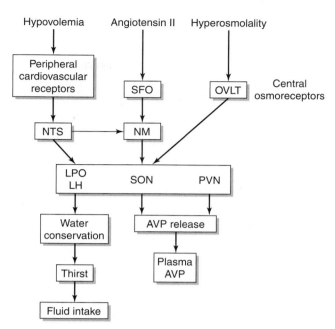

FIGURE 24.5 Central nervous system integration of input (osmotic, volume, and angiotensin II) for control of thirst and arginine vasopressin (AVP) secretion. SFO, subfornical organ; OVLT, organum vasculosum laminae terminalis; NTS, nucleus of the solitary tract; NM, nucleus medians; LPO, lateral preoptic hypothalamus; LH, lateral hypothalamus; SON, supraoptic nucleus; PVN, paraventricular nucleus.

ance despite unlimited access to water, a problem called involuntary dehydration (33). Such a delay is not seen in all animal species. In fact, the dehydrated dog will drink exactly the required volume of water to restore fluid balance within a 5-min period (34). However, humans (and other species) are considered to be slow hydrators. The next section describes the physiological and behavior control systems that contribute to the restoration of body fluid balance following dehydration and tries to explain the physiological nature of involuntary dehydration.

Dipsogenic[1] Signals

A primary dipsogenic signal driving thirst or drinking behavior following dehydration is an increase in Posm. The sensation of thirst and AVP secretion are under similar yet distinct physiological control (Fig. 24.5). Both are initiated by osmoreceptors in the circumventricular organs of the anterior third ventricle (35) that respond to changes in plasma osmolality and by sodium sensors in the anterior wall of the third ventricle that respond to changes in cerebrospinal and brain extracellular sodium concentration. Thirst and AVP secretion are controlled so that above a certain osmotic threshold (about 280 mOsm · kg water^{-1}) there is a linear relationship

---

[1]From the term dipsas, after a serpent whose bite was fabled to produce a raging thirst.

between the increase in Posm and the increase in [AVP] plasma or thirst (30). In addition, animal studies provide evidence for the existence of peripheral osmoreceptors, possibly in the hepatic portal system. Rapid dilution of hepatic portal blood could account for some of the rapid adjustments in thirst and AVP secretion during the early phase of rehydration (0–60 minutes). However, this hypothesis requires further support, particularly from human studies. The supraventricular and supraoptic nuclei of the hypothalamus also have a high expression of water channels, or aquaporin 4, which leads to the hypothesis that aquaporin 4 channels may participate in osmoregulation. Further research is also necessary to identify and characterize the role of these water channels in osmoregulation.

Thirst and AVP secretion also occur in response to a reduction in extracellular fluid volume. The sensory pathway for this reflex is thought to involve an increase in plasma angiotensin II acting on circumventricular organs and neural signals from mechanoreceptors in the great vessels and atrium of the heart (low-pressure baroreceptors) (35). The sensory information with regard to plasma tonicity and extracellular fluid volume influence the supraoptic and paraventricular nuclei within the hypothalamus and modulate the synthesis and release of AVP. This same sensory information also subserves thirst sensation. Following dehydration, fluid intake is determined in large part by the magnitude of the increase in Posm and decrease in PV. Removal of the volume-dependent dipsogenic signal in dehydrated individuals, by having the person either lie supine or assume the head-out water immersion position, will markedly reduce thirst ratings and attenuate the total volume of fluid ingested. In dehydrated humans rehydration during head-out water immersion results in only 40% of the fluid intake of rehydration occurring in air (36).

The neural pathways involved in the consciousness of thirst have only recently been identified. The combination of positron emission tomography and magnetic resonant imaging has demonstrated that the sensory input from osmoreceptors feed into higher brain regions, the anterior cingulate region, and specific sites in the middle temporal gyrus and periaqueductal gray area (37). Activation of these brain regions occurs in proportion to the increase in plasma sodium concentration during hypertonic saline infusion. Specific sites within the anterior cingulate region (Brodmann's areas 32, 24, and 31) remain active after a dry mouth is rinsed with water but disappear rapidly following drinking. These latter brain regions may play an important role in the consciousness of thirst (37).

Preabsorptive Signals

Afferent signals originating from the oropharyngeal region influence thirst and AVP secretion. The sensation of a dry mouth provides an important drive for thirst and the initiation of drinking. The sensation of dry mouth (38) is known to rise in proportion to Posm and is closely correlated with an individual's perceived rating of thirst. However, a dry mouth is not a principle physiological signal that drives fluid intake following dehydration. Rather it is a perceived sensation that can act to initiate drinking, regardless of the body fluid status.

Sensory pathways associated with the oropharyngeal region and the stomach also act to signal termination of thirst and can modulate osmotic and volume-dependent dipsogenic signals. For example, rinsing a dry mouth with water will transiently reduce thirst ratings despite the persistence of a strong osmotic and/or volume-dependent dipsogenic signal. Rinsing the mouth with water does not appear to significantly impact AVP secretion. The act of swallowing water produces a steep and sudden inhibition of [AVP] and thirst. This inhibition cannot be attributed to the dilution of plasma or a reduction in osmoreceptor activity, because it occurs before any substantive changes in Posm can be detected. This rapid response cannot be explained by the possible presence of hepatic osmoreceptors because the rapid reduction in thirst occurs after ingestion of isotonic saline. The rapid inhibition of thirst and AVP secretion appear to be a response to oropharyngeal stimulation as dehydrated subjects swallow water (but not food).

The oropharyngeal region also participates in the restoration of fluid balance by monitoring the rate and/or volume of ingested fluid via a process called oropharyngeal metering. Oropharyngeal metering plays a dominant role in determining total fluid replacement in species that rapidly rehydrate, such as the dog (34). Despite the slower recovery of fluid balance in humans, oropharyngeal metering also provides important sensory information (38). Dehydrated humans allowed to drink *ad libitum* but with all of the ingested fluid rapidly removed from the stomach via a nasogastric tube drink only 15% more fluid than when the fluid is allowed to be absorbed. Despite the presence of a marked and persistent elevation in Posm and reduction in PV, fluid intake increased only 15%. These data support the hypothesis that in humans, the act of swallowing and oropharyngeal metering provide an integrated signal proportional to the cumulative volume of ingested fluid that acts to limit the overall rate of fluid ingestion (38). Finally, gastric distention can also provide sensory input to signal termination of fluid intake. However, the importance of gastric distention in the early termination of drinking in humans has not been clearly established.

To summarize, oropharyngeal stimulation contributes to drinking behavior in two general ways. First, it provides a signal for initiation of drinking via an impact on thirst drive, through the sensation of dryness in the oropharyngeal region. Second, it provides a signal to terminate drinking via two mechanisms: (*a*) by a reflex inhibition of osmotically stimulated thirst and AVP secretion and (*b*) by oropharyngeal metering.

The hedonic (pleasurable) properties of the ingested fluid can also have a profound impact on the rate and volume of ingested fluid. Specific properties of the ingested fluid, such as flavor and temperature, affect consumption. During exercise in the heat, water intake is markedly reduced if the drinking water temperature is increased to 40°C (39). With persistent dehydration the impact of temperature becomes less as the dipsogenic drive (osmotic and volume) override the hedonic properties. Following exercise-induced dehydration, maximal rates of rehydration have been seen with water at 15°C. Flavoring a rehydration fluid will also increase drinking, and this effect is independent of fluid temperature (39). Hedonic preferences, such as temperature and flavor, are culturally influenced; that is, the preferred water temperature or flavor may vary considerably from group to group.

Involuntary Dehydration

Several observation about human rehydration provide the background for understanding involuntary dehydration. First, the increase in Posm and reduction in PV as a result of exercise-induced dehydration are proportional to the magnitude of water loss. Second, the overall volume of fluid ingested during rehydration is proportional to the level of dehydration (33). Third, the rate of fluid intake during the first few minutes of rehydration is proportional to the peak thirst rating (28). Fourth, the total volume of fluid ingested within a 3-h rehydration period (without food) will constitute only about 60–70% of the fluid lost during dehydration. These generalizations can be applied to many situations; however, it is clear that magnitude of involuntary dehydration may be manipulated by other factors, such as aging. To explain this lack of full rehydration in humans one must look at the time-dependent responses of the principle dipsogenic signals.

In human studies the rates of fluid intake during the early phase of rehydration (0–60 min) appears independent of small differences in the volume or osmosis-dependent dipsogenic factors (40). Thus, the primary dipsogenic drives are directing drinking, and the preabsorptive factors, such as oropharyngeal metering and gut distension, are providing inputs that act to limit drinking during this period. During this early phase of rehydration one can manipulate the primary dipsogenic drives and cause marked changes in drinking. For example, when the volume-dependent dipsogenic drive is eliminated in dehydrated individuals (with either a supine posture or immersion in water up to the neck before the onset of drinking), fluid intake is reduced by 40–50% (36). With the person upright, reflexes that want to restore ECF volume and Posm to normal levels drive the act of drinking.

As drinking continues (60–180 min), fluid balance and cation balance are linked. That is, an individual who ingests pure water will replace sufficient fluid to return the ECF space (i.e., Posm) to its original isotonic level (Fig. 24.6). However, while this behavior will control Posm, the loss of

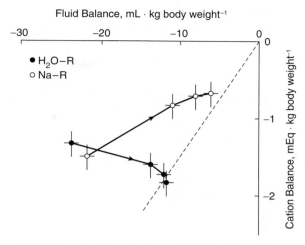

FIGURE 24.6 Relationship between fluid balance and electrolyte (cation) balance during ad libitum rehydration with water (H$_2$O-R) or 0.04% NaCl (Na-R). The broken line represents a theoretical isotonic line. *(Modified with permission from Nose H, Mack GW, Shi XR, et al. Role of osmolality and plasma volume during rehydration in humans. J Appl Physiol 1988;65:329.)*

electrolytes during sweating results in an absolute reduction in ECF volume. In other words, the degree of rehydration in each fluid compartment is determined by the ability to restore the ions lost from each compartment during exercise-induced dehydration.

In summary, during recovery from moderate whole-body dehydration, the delay in rehydration is caused both by the electrolyte deficit in the intracellular and extracellular spaces and by the removal of a volume-dependent dipsogenic drive as a result of the retention of ingested fluid in the vascular space.

Exercise-Induced Hypervolemia

PV expansion is a well-described consequence of upright endurance exercise training (41–43). Overall, the literature is almost universally supportive of PV expansion being a hallmark of endurance exercise training. A few researchers have been unable to document changes in PV with endurance training. There is no clear reason that these studies failed to induce hypervolemia. However, short-term exercise training in an environment without full gravitational forces (i.e., supine exercise or exercise in water) does not produce any remarkable hypervolemia. On the other hand, endurance-trained swimmers have a larger blood volume than sedentary controls but not as large as that of endurance-trained runners. It may be that in the absence of gravity, the time course and magnitude of the blood volume adaptation to training are delayed and/or attenuated. To allow some level of generalization, the next section focuses on exercise-induced hypervolemia in response to upright cycle ergometer exercise training and discusses its time course and mechanisms.

Mechanisms of Exercise-Induced Hypervolemia

Within 24 h after a high-intensity intermittent upright exercise bout, PV expands (42). This essentially isotonic hypervolemia occurs in the context of increased intravascular total protein content, approximately 85% of which is in the form of albumin (42). Convertino and associates (41) demonstrated a progressive expansion of plasma albumin content during the first 3 days of an endurance training protocol. Gillen and associates (42,44) have shown that albumin content expands by 1 h after exercise to the level it maintains for the next 48 h.

Exercise-Induced Hypervolemia: Role of Plasma Proteins

The immediate increase in PV 24 h following heavy exercise may be accomplished by two possible mechanisms: (*a*) a net decrease in filtration forces or (*b*) a net increase in absorptive forces acting across and along the capillary membranes. An elevation of albumin content after exercise would cause expansion of the intravascular fluid compartment at the expense of the extravascular fluid compartment through the latter mechanism because of an increase in plasma oncotic pressure. Since each gram of added albumin will bind approximately 18 mL of water, it is not surprising that the fluid volume associated with a 10% increase in albumin content (15 g) corresponds well to the measured PV expansion that Gillen and associates described 24 h after heavy exercise (42,44). Therefore, plasma albumin content expansion facilitates PV expansion through albumin's colloid osmotic properties (41,42). The rapid increase in intravascular albumin content cannot be explained by changes in albumin metabolism (synthesis or degradation) or in albumin vascular permeability but must be ascribed primarily to redistribution of albumin stores from the interstitial to the intravascular compartment. However, the simple act of increasing intravascular albumin content cannot explain the PV expansion at 24–48 h, because direct infusion of 12 g of albumin into the vascular compartment of man is entirely lost within 24 h (45).

Several mechanisms promote the increase and/or maintenance of this extra protein in the intravascular space and the retention of isotonic fluid. First, a rapid accumulation of albumin in the intravascular space occurs as a result of increased translocation of albumin (protein) from the interstitial compartment to the vascular compartment. Second, the rate of albumin escape from the vascular compartment is reduced (46). Finally, an increase in hepatic albumin synthesis rate can contribute to a long-term increase

in plasma albumin content and the maintenance of the expanded PV.

Rapid translocation of fluid and protein into the vascular compartment is critical to the restoration and maintenance of PV immediately following exercise. This phase of fluid balance following exercise is due to simple reabsorption of isotonic fluid from the interstitium, a process regulated primarily by changes in local Starling forces across the capillary wall. Exercise stimulates lymph flow as much as 10-fold, promoting translocation of protein from the interstitial to the intravascular compartment. The rapid rise in plasma albumin content following exercise must be explained by such a mechanism. Under conditions of increased lymphatic outflow pressure (i.e., supine posture), lymph flow and albumin return to the vascular compartment are limited. That is to say, in the supine posture elevated central blood pressure will act to increase lymphatic outflow pressure and thereby limit lymphatic albumin delivery to the vascular compartment.

Exercise-Induced Hypervolemia: Starling Forces

In previously active skeletal muscle, the colloid osmotic pressure difference (ISF versus plasma) is similar before and after exercise and does not contribute to retention of fluid in the vascular space. However, a reduction in the transcapillary hydrostatic pressure gradient in skeletal muscle following exercise because of a slight increase in $PRES_{ISF}$ favors the movement of fluid into the vascular space following exercise. The increase in $PRES_{ISF}$ should also promote increased lymphatic flow and the return of fluid and protein to the vascular space. Over a longer time the increased skeletal muscle lymph flow will lead to oncotic buffering within the interstitial space, producing a small reduction in π_{ISF}. In inactive tissues (i.e., subcutaneous tissue) the transcapillary colloid osmotic pressure difference is increased to favor fluid movement back into the vascular space, primarily as a result of an increase in π_{plasma}.

The transcapillary clearance of albumin in previously active skeletal muscle declines 24 h following exercise (46). In addition, the whole-body transcapillary escape rate of albumin (measured by the rate of washout from the vascular compartment of labeled albumin) also decreases following dynamic exercise (46). Overall, the net accumulation of albumin in the vascular compartment is the result of a translocation of albumin from the interstitial to the vascular compartment and increased retention of the translocated protein.

Changes in albumin metabolism occur too slowly to contribute to the rapid changes in plasma albumin content within the first few hours following exercise. At rest the fractional synthetic rate of albumin is about 5% per day, and 24 h following heavy exercise a small but significant increase in fractional synthetic rate to 6–7% per day occurs (47,48).

This increase in albumin synthesis rate is insufficient to account for the elevation of albumin content during the first 6 hours post exercise rate but can fully account for the increase in albumin content by 24 h of recovery. In recent research by Nagashima and associates (47) the effect of heavy exercise on PV expansion, plasma albumin content, and albumin fractional synthetic rate were negated when the subject was supine during the exercise and recovery period. That is, the rapid expansion of PV was prevented when subjects were supine. These observations indicate that the mechanism of exercise-induced hypervolemia is posture specific, and the upright posture provides an important stimulus for an increase in plasma albumin content and PV following heavy exercise.

Exercise-Induced Hypervolemia: Water and Salt Retention

Plasma volume expansion during dynamic exercise training is isotonic (49), indicating that increased sodium and water retention by the kidney contributes to this volume expansion. Plasma aldosterone and plasma renin activity are elevated following moderate to heavy dynamic exercise and should mediate an increase renal sodium retention from the distal tubules (41,50). Following a single bout of heavy exercise, reduced sodium and water excretion by the kidney occurs within 24 h (50). The heavy dynamic exercise bout increased sodium reabsorption in the proximal and distal tubules. The increased sodium reabsorption in the proximal tubule is most likely mediated by a reduction in renal blood flow. In addition, baroreflex-mediated reductions in fluid-regulating hormones are delayed and attenuated following heavy dynamic exercise. Thus, plasma renin activity, aldosterone, and vasopressin levels remain at control levels despite a 10–12% elevation in PV following heavy dynamic exercise. These renal mechanisms complement the role of albumin in the expansion of PV immediately following heavy dynamic exercise. However, renal adaptation lags the increase in plasma albumin content. Therefore, within the first 24–48 h after heavy dynamic exercise PV expansion occurs at the expense of the ISF space. With chronic dynamic exercise training the ECF space expands, and the increase in PV is eventually matched by an appropriate expansion of the ECF space. The time course of these adaptations during dynamic exercise training has not been fully identified. However, during heat acclimation an expansion of the ECF space has been noted by the eighth day of acclimatization (51).

In summary, the process of exercise-induced hypervolemia can be described on the basis of acute and long-term adjustments. The acute adjustment, within the first 24–48 hours, involves selective expansion of PV, primarily due to an increase in intravascular albumin content (42,44). On the long-term basis the size of the intravascular compartment does not appear to be disproportionately larger than the increase in extracellular volume (49). Taken together, these data suggest that the overall adjustments in fluid compartment sizes take considerable time and that selective expansion of PV has precedence in this procedure. During the acute phase, the increase in plasma albumin content occurs within 1–2 h of exercise and is subsequently maintained (42,44,52). Another mechanism is the attenuation of volume regulating reflexes (44,52). This latter mechanism is characterized by an attenuated cardiopulmonary baroreflex control of peripheral vascular tone 2 h after exercise (44) and the maintenance of fluid-regulating hormones such as renin and aldosterone (15,52,53). In combination these mechanisms appear to play a role in exercise-induced hypervolemia by allowing the increase in fluid volume and albumin content to remain for extended periods. The increase in PV 24 h post exercise is closely related to the increase in plasma albumin content, and the increased albumin synthesis rate contributes to the rise in plasma albumin content.

Regulation of Red Cell Mass and Exercise

The major function of RBCs (erythrocytes) is to transport the oxygen-carrying molecule hemoglobin from the lungs to the tissues. However, these same RBCs also provide a large amount of the buffering capacity of the blood. RBCs contain a large quantity of the enzyme carbonic anhydrase to catalyze the reaction between carbon dioxide and water. Thus, the RBC promotes the transport of large quantities of carbon dioxide, in the form of bicarbonate ion, from the tissue to the lungs. In addition, the hemoglobin molecule itself is an excellent acid-base buffer. The average concentration of RBCs per milliliter of blood is 5.2 million for men and about 4.7 million for women. These numbers equate to Hct (the percentage of blood that is cells) of 45 and 41 for men and women, respectively. The RBC concentrates hemoglobin to a level of 34 g $\cdot$ dL^{-1} of ICF. As such, the average hemoglobin concentration in whole blood averages 16 g $\cdot$ dL^{-1} blood in men and 14 g $\cdot$ dL^{-1} in women.

Regulation of Erythropoiesis

In adults circulating RBCs are produced exclusively by the bone marrow from pluripotential hemopoietic stem cells. These cells reproduce to create differentiated cells (committed stem cells named colony-forming units) that are destined to become one of several circulating blood cells (e.g., erythrocytes, lymphocytes, monocytes). Multiple proteins called growth inducers and differentiation inducers control this process of growth and differentiation. The formation of these inducers is controlled by factors outside the bone marrow.

Role of Erythropoietin

The principal factor that stimulates RBC production in bone marrow is a circulating hormone called erythropoietin (EPO) (166–amino acid residues linked to three carbohydrate chains, 34 KD glycoprotein) (54). In adults about 90% of the EPO is formed in the kidneys, either in the proximal tubular cells or in the peritubular capillary endothelial cells. Liver hepatocytes account for the remaining 10% of circulating EPO. EPO binds to its receptors on the membranes of the committed erythroid progenitor cells (colony-forming-unit erythrocytes) in the bone marrow to increase erythropoiesis by stimulating both proliferation and maturation of colony-forming-unit erythrocytes. EPO levels in resting individuals at sea level average about 15 mU EPO · mL^{-1} plasma (95% confidence limits: 10 to 30 mU EPO · mL^{-1} plasma) (54,55). The principle stimulus for EPO production by the kidney is low oxygen tension in the tissue. The balance of oxygen delivery and oxygen consumption of the renal tissue determines the oxygen tension in the renal tissue. General hypoxemia in the absence of EPO will not stimulate RBC production.

Hormones That Modulate Erythropoiesis

Several hormones modulate EPO release by modifying the balance between oxygen delivery and oxygen consumption of the renal tissue or modulate the effect of EPO on the erythroid progenitor cells. Thyroxin increases the rate of EPO production by increasing the rate of oxygen use by renal tissue. Angiotensin II impacts EPO production by reducing oxygen delivery to renal tissue via a reduction in renal blood flow and by increasing renal oxygen consumption by stimulating sodium reabsorption in the proximal tubules. Androgenic steroids do not impact oxygen tension in the renal tissue but rather act directly on renal cells to augment production of EPO to a given hypoxic stimulus and by direct stimulation of erythroid precursor cells to stimulate maturation (56).

Dynamic Exercise and Erythropoiesis: Role of EPO

The oxygen-dependent feedback regulation of EPO production is widely accepted (55). Anemia or hypoxemia signals the renal oxygen sensors and EPO-producing cells to increase EPO production. Increased EPO stimulates bone marrow erythropoiesis and an increase in RBC mass. The increase in RBC mass and improved oxygen delivery to the tissues reduce the hypoxic drive for EPO release. This feedback loop explains the typical response of EPO following acute exposure to altitude (hypobaric hypoxia) (see Chapter 27). For example, during a sojourn to 4350 m plasma EPO levels increase to 120 mU EPO · mL^{-1} by day 3 (55). New RBCs appear in the circulation within 5 to 7 days, improving oxygen saturation of the blood, and EPO levels begin to return

toward baseline. A major question is whether the increased RBC mass associated with exercise training is linked to EPO and this same feedback control loop, or is it related to some other nonrenal factor?

Oxygen desaturation during exercise seems to be a likely candidate for stimulating EPO production during exercise. However, for arterial desaturation to occur at sea level, two requirements must be met: (*a*) Exercise intensities must be near $\dot{V}O_{2max}$. (*b*) The athletes must be highly trained. Acute continuous exposure (5–60 minutes) to normobaric hypoxia (10.5% FiO_2) does not induce a rise in plasma EPO levels (55). On the other hand, short bursts of supramaximal exercise performed at an altitude of 1000–2000 m will result in exercise-induced hypoxemia ($SaO_2 < 91\%$) and an increase in plasma EPO levels (55). These observations indicate that there may be an exercise factor other than simple hypoxemia that also contributes to the EPO response. The problem is that most exercise studies have not seen a measurable change in plasma EPO levels. For example, Schmidt and associates (59) did not see an increase in plasma EPO following 60 min of moderate exercise (60% $\dot{V}O_{2max}$) or following a maximal exercise test. Klausen (55) failed to alter plasma EPO following 60 min of cycle ergometer exercise at 85–90% of heart rate max ($SaO_2 > 95\%$). Any small increase in plasma EPO level (about 3 U EPO · L^{-1}) following exercise would easily fall within the normal diurnal variation observed for plasma EPO. Use of a bioassay to estimate EPO activity finds that the rate of iron incorporation into bone marrow cell cultures is increased following exercise (60). In this case the plasma containing EPO is used to stimulate erythropoietic activity in a cell culture and is thought to indicate EPO activity of the serum. However, the serum post exercise also contains all of the other hormones released during exercise. One interpretation of these finding is that despite the relatively small increase in EPO following exercise, the serum is able to enhance erythropoietic activity in bone marrow cells.

Dynamic Exercise and Erythropoiesis: Role of Circulating Hormones

GH release during exercise may also contribute to EPO-mediated erythropoiesis. The increase in plasma GH during exercise depends on exercise intensity and duration. During graded exercise the threshold intensity required to induce an increase in plasma GH is similar to that required to increase plasma catecholamine and blood lactate (61). At lower intensities of exercise the duration of the bout must exceed about 15 min before a detectable rise in plasma GH can be seen. So given an adequate exercise stimulus, a rise in plasma GH following exercise is expected. It is known that administration of pharmacological doses of GH to adults (and children) results in an increase in total blood volume (57). More important, GH receptors are known to be located in bone marrow (58). Studies examining the mechanism of action of GH *in vitro,* based upon work with isolated erythroid progenitor cells from humans, indicate that the effects of GH on erythropoiesis are mediated by IGF-I. Based upon the available evidence, it is likely that release of GH during exercise will contribute to erythropoiesis.

Dynamic Exercise and Red Cell Turnover

The impact of exercise on the erythrocyte life span will influence the time course and magnitude of blood volume expansion during training. During endurance training erythrocyte turnover increases (62). Endurance training is associated with an increase in reticulocytosis (increase in number of immature RBCs) and increase in erythrocyte destruction. Increased erythrocyte turnover dictates that trained athletes will have younger erythrocytes than sedentary individuals. Younger erythrocytes demonstrate a rightward shift in their oxyhemoglobin dissociation curve, explaining in part the observed rightward shift in the oxyhemoglobin dissociation curve of blood from endurance-trained athletes (63,64). Mean erythrocyte lifespan in male endurance athletes averages just less than 70 days compared to the 120-day average for sedentary individuals.

Several pathways contribute to accelerated erythrocyte loss during exercise training. They include gastrointestinal bleeding, dietary iron deficiency, insufficient erythropoiesis, and intravascular hemolysis (65). Of these pathways intravascular hemolysis has received the most attention as clinically relevant. Exercise-induced hemolysis has been implicated in the development of sports anemia and suboptimal iron status in the endurance trained. Exercise-induced erythrocyte destruction may occur from several distinct mechanisms, including mechanical trauma (usually associated with foot strike or compression of erythrocytes within small blood vessels during muscle contraction), elevated body temperature, dehydration, hemoconcentration, and oxidative stress. Exercise-induced oxidative stress may contribute to erythrocyte destruction, and this pathway may be modulated by antioxidant treatment. However, endurance training will enhance activity of antioxidant enzymes and improve coupling of the electron transport chain. As such, the role of exercise-induced oxidative stress in the destruction of RBCs will be diminished significantly with exercise training. In general, circulatory trauma to RBCs during exercise appears to be the primary contributor to exercise-induced hemolysis. During running the mechanical trauma of the foot strike is considered to be the major contributor to exercise-induced hemolysis (65).

To summarize, an increase in RBC mass with exercise training appears to occur sometime after the first 2 weeks of training (Fig. 24.5). The timing of the increase in RBC mass with exercise training is similar to that seen during exposure to short-term intermittent hypobaric hypoxia. In both cases the hematological response is a slight rise in EPO levels following exercise or hypobaric hypoxia. Repeated for 3–4 wk, the result is an increase in RBC mass. Because the intensity of exercise during most training sessions would be insufficient to evoke clear hypoxemia, the rise in erythropoietic activity of the plasma must result from a combination of relative renal hypoxemia coupled with the impact of exercise on the hypophysoadrenal, hypophysogonadal, growth hormone, and renin–angiotensin axes. The impact of exercise on the erythropoietic activity of the plasma is not simply the increase in EPO levels.

Red Cell Expansion and $\dot{V}O_{2max}$

Changes in RBC mass influence aerobic capacity through two important pathways. Changes in hemoglobin concentration ([Hb]) will affect aerobic capacity by altering the maximal oxygen transport capacity of blood, while changes in total blood volume will affect aerobic capacity by altering cardiac output (43,66). Reductions in hemoglobin concentration in humans via acute and chronic isovolemic anemia cause a reduction in maximal aerobic capacity but not always a reduction in maximal cardiac output. The removal of 900 mL of blood by phlebotomy results in an 11% reduction in [Hb], which rapidly begins to recover 2 wk after phlebotomy but requires a total of 5–6 wk for [Hb] to return to control levels (66). The time course of recovery is slightly longer in trained runners (67).

The removed blood can be stored frozen indefinitely. Autologous infusion of the stored RBCs, or blood doping, produces an abnormally high [Hb]. Twenty-four hours following infusion of RBCs stored in this manner, a process also referred to as induced erythrocythemia, there is an 8% increase in [Hb]. More important, this elevation in [Hb] is maintained for a week after an autologous infusion of RBCs (66). Hemoglobin concentration will gradually return toward baseline levels in a somewhat linear manner over the next 12–15 wk. Using this type of autologous blood transfusion technique, Buick and associates (67) demonstrated significant increases in [Hb] (9%), maximal aerobic capacity (5%), and run time to exhaustion post infusion (34%). Greater improvements are seem with larger volumes of blood transfused (1350 mL blood); however, this also results in an excessive rise in Hct (66).

Integration of Physiological Control Systems

Osmotic Control of AVP Secretion With Dynamic Exercise Training

AVP secretion and thirst are governed by sensory information related to both plasma osmolality and blood volume

(35). Osmotic regulation of thirst and AVP secretion are characterized by a threshold level of plasma osmolality (about 282 mOsm · kg⁻¹) above which thirst or AVP rises in proportion to the increase in plasma osmolality. According to animal studies, the stimulus-response curve for Posm and AVP shifts upward during hypovolemia and downward with hypervolemia. Because training is accompanied by hypervolemia, one might expect some alteration in the osmotic control plasma AVP (or thirst) in endurance-trained athletes. However, an increase in blood volume in endurance-trained athletes is also accompanied by an attenuation of low-pressure baroreceptor function (68). Figure 24.7 shows the effect of hypertonic saline infusion (to stimulate thirst and AVP secretion) during normovolemia, hypovolemia, and hypervolemia in groups of sedentary and endurance-trained subjects.

Iso-osmotic hypovolemia was achieved by administering diuretic pills for 3 days prior to testing, and iso-osmotic hypervolemia was induced by infusion of isotonic saline equal to 2% of body weight 30 min prior to hypertonic saline infusion. Osmoregulatory control of thirst is increased during hypovolemia but unchanged during hypervolemia in sedentary individuals. These observations confirm the role of low-pressure baroreceptors in modulating osmotically stimulated AVP secretion in healthy adults (36). In contrast, osmotically stimulated thirst was not significantly modulated by changes in PV in endurance-trained individuals. Do these data indicate an alteration in osmotically stimulated AVP secretion in endurance-trained individuals? This cannot be directly addressed by the present data, because as hypertonic saline is infused into an individual, the rise in Posm is also accompanied by a rise in PV. Isovolumetric plots of AVP versus Posm are necessary to answer this question correctly. At present such data are not available.

Osmotic Inhibition of Thermoregulatory Function

Progressive dehydration during exercise produces a decrease in PV, an increase in plasma osmolality, and an increase in heat storage. The higher heat storage is a result of a reduced ability to dissipate heat. Figure 24.8 illustrates that hypohydration results in a lower sweat rate at a given body core temperature. This decrement in sweat rate is proportional to the level of hypohydration. The mechanism responsible for mediating the reduction in sweat rate during hypohydration is not fully understood. However, it is clear that plasma hypovolemia and plasma hyperosmolality act independently to reduce evaporative water loss. This is illustrated by the data of Sawka and associates (69), which showed a rightward shift of the sweat rate–esophageal temperature relationship in humans following graded hypohydration.

A reduction in the rate of evaporative water loss following thermally induced dehydration has been demonstrated in several animal species. In humans, hypertonic saline infusion during exercise results in a reduced sweat rate at any given body core temperature. These results, in combination with observations of altered thermoregulatory function following dehydration in man and other species, are consistent with neurophysiological data demonstrating the modulating influence of osmotic stimuli on thermosensitive neurons in the hypothalamic thermoregulatory center. These data support the hypothesis that modulation of sweating during heat stress may be accomplished by modifying neural information in the thermoregulatory control centers in the hypothalamus, either through the central effects of osmolality or release of central neural transmitters. A study by Takamata and associates (70) provides an interesting look at this interaction. In these experiments, thermoregulatory sweating was established in humans (by heating the lower legs to

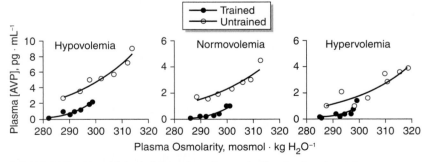

FIGURE 24.7 Unpublished observation of osmotically stimulated arginine vasopressin release in sedentary (n = 5) and endurance-trained (n = 4) subjects in hypovolemic, normovolemic, and hypervolemic conditions. Isoosmotic hypovolemia was induced by diuretic treatment, and the isoosmotic hypervolemia was caused by an acute infusion of isotonic saline. Osmotic regulation of AVP secretion is attenuated in trained group. Hypervolemia did not alter osmotic regulation of AVP secretion for either group. Hypovolemia did not markedly alter osmotic regulation of AVP secretion in trained group.

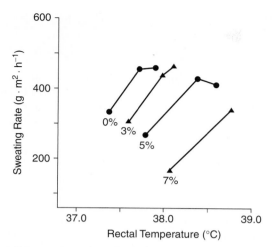

FIGURE 24.8 Effect of hypohydration on thermo-regulatory sweating in humans. Hypohydration attenuates thermoregulatory sweating in a dose-dependent manner. *(Modified with permission from Sawka MN, Young AJ, Francesconi RP, et al. Thermo-regulatory and blood responses during exercise at graded hypohydration levels. J Appl Physiol 1985; 59:1397.)*

43°C) with the subjects in a iso-osmotic or hyperosmotic state. In the hyperosmotic state thermoregulatory sweating was attenuated. The subject was then allowed to ingest a single bolus of water (4.3 mL · kg body weight^{-1}). Ingestion of the water caused a rapid reduction in thirst rating and plasma AVP levels. In addition, there was a marked transient increase in local sweat rate. These data demonstrated the vital and dynamic interaction between osmoregulatory and thermoregulatory systems in humans. Figure 24.9 provides a schematic summery of these interactions.

SUMMARY

Maintaining constancy of the volume, composition, and distribution of fluids within the body is a fundamental problem facing all animal species. With multiple sensory inputs the integrative function of the central nervous system provides the necessary regulatory stability. Exercise simply adds to the already burdensome sensory information that the central nervous system must filter and integrate. This chapter presents a variety of specific interactions between homeostatic control systems and their role in body fluid balance during exercise (or exercise-induced dehydration). It also reviews the adaptations of the body fluid system with endurance training and their ability to improve physiological function. The well-defined expansion of blood volume is a perfect example. This adaptation within the fluid-regulating system stabilizes cardiovascular function during exercise, especially in the heat. Another example is the improved sodium retention by sweat glands following exercise training or heat acclimatization that results in a lower sweat sodium concentration. This adaptation also provides for an enhanced ability to maintain circulating blood volume in the face of a TBW deficit. It should become apparent that exercise-induced adaptations in the fluid regulatory system are focused on providing support for the cardiovascular system during the next exercise session.

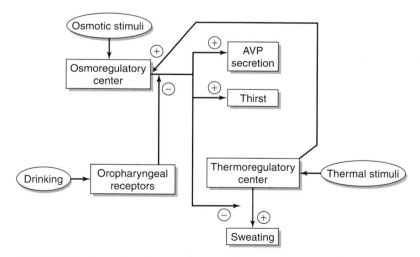

FIGURE 24.9 Interaction between osmoregulatory control of thirst and arginine vasopressin (AVP) secretion and thermoregulatory control of sweating and oropharyngeal stimulation during drinking. Oropharyngeal stimulation during drinking attenuates the osmotic inhibition input into the thermoregulatory center as well as osmotically stimulated thirst and AVP secretion. Increased body temperature also modulates osmotically stimulated AVP secretion and thirst.

A MILESTONE OF DISCOVERY

Following thermal or exercise-induced dehydration, what causes the long delay in rehydration, or involuntary dehydration, in humans? Since 1947 the phenomenon of delayed rehydration puzzled researchers. Earlier studies provided important background information emphasizing that two factors unique to human dehydration contributed to involuntary dehydration: Na^+ loss in sweat and the upright posture. It was following a series animal studies examining involuntary rehydration in rodents (71) that Hiroshi Nose proposed a unique approach to the study of involuntary dehydration in humans. Nose and associates (29,40,72) designed an eloquent experiment that allowed them to quantify the changes in body fluid compartments during dehydration and monitor the distribution and fate of ingested water during rehydration. Nose and associates (29,40,72) proposed that a high retention of ingested fluids in the vascular space during rehydration would rapidly dilute plasma constituents and restore PV, thereby accounting for the rapid removal of osmotic and volume-dependent dipsogenic drives. Nose and associates (29) carefully documented the shift in body fluid compartments following dehydration, demonstrating that the body's ability to maintain circulating blood volume during dehydration induced by dynamic exercise in the heat is a function of the body's ability to mobilize fluid from the intracellular fluid space, which itself is linked to the sodium concentration in sweat. This observation provided insight into the benefit of producing a more dilute sweat during heat adaptation—to enhance the individual's ability to maintain circulating blood volume during exercise in the heat. During *ad libitum* drinking with pure water, individuals replaced only 68% of the water lost during dehydration over a 3-hour observation period. However, a disproportionate amount of the ingested water was retained in the vascular compartment, restoring 78% of the PV deficit following dehydration. This restoration of PV was sufficient to diminish volume-dependent dipsogenic stimulation. The selective retention of water in the vascular compartment also caused a rapid decline in plasma osmolality, thereby rapidly removing the osmotic-dependent dipsogenic drive. The most critical finding of this work was that when dehydrated subjects drank water *ad libitum* while ingesting sodium chloride capsules (equivalent to a 0.45% NaCl solution) they restored significantly more of their lost body water (40). This experiment demonstrated that the recovery of fluid balance during rehydration was linked to the recovery of cation balance (Fig. 24.6). An important aspect of their experimental design was that fluid recovery was followed for 3 hours, or well beyond the time frame of earlier researchers. This is important, since the difference in fluid balance only occurs about 2 hours after rehydration. This work provided a well-defined experimental approach to the study of fluid balance in humans. This series of experiments unraveled some of the mysteries behind involuntary dehydration in humans. Overall, the research showed that during recovery from moderate (2.3% body weight loss) whole-body dehydration, a delay in rehydration is caused by the electrolyte deficit from the intracellular and extracellular spaces and the rapid removal of a volume-dependent dipsogenic drive due to the selective retention of ingested fluid in the vascular space.

Nose H, Mack GW, Shi X, Nadel ER. Role of osmolality and plasma volume during rehydration in humans. J Appl Physiol 1988;65: 325–331.

ACKNOWLEDGMENTS

My research interest in body fluid balance and exercise is supported by grants from the Heart, Lung, and Blood Institute of the National Institutes of Health (HL-39818 & HL-20634) and performed at the John B. Pierce Laboratory and Yale University School of Medicine in New Haven.

REFERENCES

1. Edelman IS, Leibman J. Anatomy of body water and electrolytes. Am J Med 1959;27:256–277.
2. Norberg A, Sandhagen B, Bratteby LE, et al. Do ethanol and deuterium oxide distribute into the same water space in healthy volunteers? Alcohol Clin Exp Res 2001;25:1423–1430.
3. Gudivaka R, Schoeller DA, Kushner RF, et al. Single- and multifrequency models for bioelectrical impedance analysis of body water compartments. J Appl Physiol 1999;87: 1087–1096.
4. Lesser GT, Markofsky J. Body water compartments with human aging using fat-free mass as the reference standard. Am J Physiol 1979;236:R215–R220.
5. Visser M, Gallagher D, Deurenberg P, et al. Density of fat-free body mass: relationship with race, age, and level of body fatness. Am J Physiol 1997;272:E781–E787.
6. International Commission on Radiological Protection. Report of the Task Group on Reference Man. Elmsford, NY: Pergamon, 1975.
7. Shimamoto H, Komiya S. Comparison of body water turnover in endurance runners and age-matched sedentary men. J Physiol Anthropol Appl Human Sci 2003;22:311–315.
8. Convertino VA. Blood volume: its adaptation to endurance training. Med Sci Sports Exerc 1991;23:1338–1348.
9. Landis EM, Pappenheimer JR. Exchange of substances through the capillary walls. In Hamilton WF, Dow P, eds. Handbook of Physiology. Washington: American Physiological Society, 1963;961–1034.
10. Kedem O, Katchalsky A. Thermodynamic analysis of the permeability of biological membranes to non-electrolytes. Biochim Biophys Acta 1958;27:229–246.
11. Michel CC, Curry FE. Microvascular permeability. Physiol Rev 1999;79:703–761.

12. Rippe B. Haraldsson B. Transport of macromolecules across microvascular walls: the two-pore theory. Physiol Rev 1994; 74:163–219.

13. Dill DB, Costill DL. Calculation of percentage changes in volumes of blood, plasma, and red cells in dehydration. J Appl Physiol 1974;37:247–248.

14. Convertino VA, Keil LC, Bernauer EM, et al. Plasma volume, osmolality, vasopressin, and renin activity during graded exercise in man. J Appl Physiol 19;8150:123–128.

15. Convertino VA, Keil LC, Greenleaf JE. Plasma volume, renin, and vasopressin responses to graded exercise after training. J Appl Physiol 1983;54:508–514.

16. Miles DS, Sawka MN, Glaser RM, et al. Plasma volume shifts during progressive arm and leg exercise. J Appl Physiol 1983; 54:491–495.

17. Bjornberg J. Forces involved in transcapillary fluid movement in exercising cat skeletal muscle. Acta Physiol Scand 1990; 140:221–236.

18. Saltin B, Sjogaard G, Gaffney FA, et al. Potassium, lactate, and water fluxes in human quadriceps muscle during static contractions. Circ Res 1981;48:18–24.

19. Nose H, Takamata A, Mack GW, et al. Water and electrolyte balance in the vascular space during graded exercise in humans. J Appl Physiol 1991;70:2757–2762.

20. Mohesinin V, Gonzalez RR. Tissue pressure and plasma oncotic pressure during exercise. J Appl Physiol 1984;56: 102–108.

21. Aukland K, Reed RK. Interstitial-lymphatic mechanisms in the control of extracellular fluid volume. Physiol Rev 1993; 73:1–78.

22. Jacobsson S, Kjellmer I. Accumulation of fluid in exercising skeletal muscle. Acta Physiol Scand 1964;60:286–292.

23. Sawka MN, Francesconi RP, Pimental NA, et al. Hydration and vascular fluid shifts during exercise in the heat. J Appl Physiol 1984;56:91–96.

24. Lundvall J, Mellander S, Westling H, et al. Fluid transfer between blood and tissues during exercise. Acta Physiol Scand 1972;85:258–269.

25. Nagashima K, Nose H, Yoshida T, et al. Relationship between atrial natriuretic peptide and plasma volume during graded exercise with water immersion. J Appl Physiol 1995;78: 217–224.

26. McMurray RG. Plasma volume changes during submaximal swimming. Eur J Appl Physiol 1983;51:347–356.

27. Sawka MN, Pandolf KB. Effects of body water loss on physiological function and exercise performance. In Gilsolfi CV, Lamb CV, Lamb DR, eds. Fluid Homeostasis During Exercise. Carmel, IN: Benchmark, 1990;1–38.

28. Mack GW, Nadel ER. Body fluid balance during heat stress in humans. In Blatteis CM, Fregly CM, Fregly MJ, eds. Handbook of Physiology: Environmental Physiology. New York: Oxford University, 1996;187–214.

29. Nose H, Mack GW, Shi XR, et al. Shift in body fluid compartments after dehydration in humans. J Appl Physiol 1988;65:318–324.

30. Baylis PH. Osmoregulation and control of vasopressin secretion in healthy humans. Am J Physiol 1987;253:R671–R678.

31. Thompson CJ, Burd JM, Baylis PH. Plasma osmolality of thirst onset is similar to the threshold for vasopressin release in man. Clin Sci 1985;69:39P.

32. Convertino VA, Greenleaf JE, Bernauer EM. Role of thermal and exercise factors in the mechanism of hypervolemia. J Appl Physiol 1980;48:657–664.

33. Greenleaf JE, Sargent F. Voluntary dehydration in man. J Appl Physiol 1965;20:719–724.

34. Thrasher TN, Keil, Ramsay DJ. Drinking, oropharyngeal signals, and inhibition of vasopressin secretion in dogs. LC Am J Physiol 1987;253:R509–R515.

35. Johnson AK. Brain mechanisms in the control of body fluid homeostasis. In Gisolfi CV, Lamb DR, eds. Perspectives in Exercise Science and Sports Medicine. Carmel, IN: Benchmark, 1990;347–424.

36. Sagawa S, Miki K, Tajima F, et al. Effect of dehydration on thirst and drinking during immersion in men. J Appl Physiol 1992;72:128–134.

37. Denton D, Shade R, Zamarippa F, et al. Neuroimaging of genesis and satiation of thirst and an interoceptor-driven theory of origins of primary consciousness. Proc Natl Acad Sci USA 1999;96:5304–5309.

38. Figaro MK, Mack GM. Regulation of fluid intake in dehydrated humans: role of oropharyngeal stimulation. Am J Physiol 1997;272:R1740–R1746.

39. Hubbard RW, Maller O, Sawka MN, et al. Voluntary dehydration and alliesthesia for water. J Appl Physiol 1984;57: 868–875.

40. Nose H, Mack GW, Shi XR, et al. Role of osmolality and plasma volume during rehydration in humans. J Appl Physiol 1988;65:325–331.

41. Convertino VA, Brock PJ, Keil LC, et al. Exercise training-induced hypervolemia: role of plasma albumin, renin, and vasopressin. J Appl Physiol 1980;48:665–669.

42. Gillen CM, Lee R, Mack GW, et al. Plasma volume expansion in humans after a single intense exercise protocol. J Appl Physiol 1991;71:1914–1920.

43. Sawka MN, Convertino VA, Eichner ER, et al. Blood volume: importance and adaptations to exercise training, environmental stresses, and trauma/sickness. Med Sci Sports Exerc 2000;32:332–348.

44. Gillen CM, Nishiyasu T, Langhans G, et al. Cardiovascular and renal function during exercise-induced blood volume expansion in men. J Appl Physiol 1994;76:2602–2610.

45. Haskell A, Gillen CM, Mack GW, et al. Albumin infusion in humans does not model exercise induced hypervolaemia after 24 hours. Acta Physiol Scand 1998;164:277–284.

46. Haskell A, Nadel ER, Stachenfeld NS, et al. Transcapillary escape rate of albumin in humans during exercise-induced hypervolemia. J Appl Physiol 1997;83:407–413.

47. Nagashima K, Cline GW, Mack GW, et al. Intense exercise stimulates albumin synthesis in the upright posture. J Appl Physiol 2000;88:41–46.

48. Yang RC, Mack GW, Wolfe RR, et al. Albumin synthesis after intense intermittent exercise in human subjects. J Appl Physiol 1998;84:584–592.

49. Maw GJ, MacKenzie IL, Comer DA, et al. Whole-body hyperhydration in endurance-trained males determined using radionuclide dilution. Med Sci Sports Exerc 1996;28:1038–1044.

50. Nagashima K, Wu J, Kavouras SA, et al. Increased renal tubular sodium reabsorption during exercise-induced hypervolemia in humans. J Appl Physiol 2001;91:1229–1236.

51. Patterson MJ, Stocks JM, Taylor NA. Sustained and generalised extracellular fluid expansion following heat acclimation. J Physiol (Lond) J Physiol 2004;559(Pt 1): 327–334.

52. Nagashima K, Mack GW, Haskell A, et al. Mechanism for the posture-specific plasma volume increase after a single intense exercise protocol. J Appl Physiol 1999;86: 867–873.

53. Convertino VA, Mack GW, Nadel ER. Elevated central venous pressure: a consequence of exercise training-induced hypervolemia? Am J Physiol 1991;260:R273–R277.

54. Kendall RG. Erythropoietin. Clin Lab Haematol 2001;23: 71–80.

55. Klausen T. The feed-back regulation of erythropoietin production in healthy humans. Dan Med Bull 1998;45: 345–353.

56. Fried W, Morley C. Effects of androgenic steroids on erythropoiesis. Steroids 1985;46:799–826.

57. Christ ER, Cummings MH, Westwood NB, et al. The importance of growth hormone in the regulation of erythropoiesis, red cell mass, and plasma volume in adults with growth hormone deficiency. J Clin Endocrinol Metab 82:2985–2990, 1997.

58. Dardenne M, Mello-Coelho V, Gagnerault MC, et al. Growth hormone receptors and immunocompetent cells. Ann NY Acad Sci 1998;840:510–517.

59. Schmidt W, Eckardt KU, Hilgendorf A, et al. Effects of maximal and submaximal exercise under normoxic and hypoxic conditions on serum erythropoietin level. Int J Sports Med 1991;12:457–461.

60. De Paoli Vitali E, Guglielmini C, Casoni I, et al. Serum erythropoietin in cross-country skiers. Int J Sports Med 1988; 9:99–101.

61. Chwalbinska-Moneta J, Krysztofiak F, Ziemba A, et al. Threshold increases in plasma growth hormone in relation to plasma catecholamine and blood lactate concentrations during progressive exercise in endurance-trained athletes. Eur J Appl Physiol 1996;73:117–120.

62. Smith JA. Exercise, training and red blood cell turnover. Sports Med 1995;19:9–31.

63. Schmidt W, Maassen N, Trost F, et al. Training induced effects on blood volume, erythrocyte turnover and haemoglobin oxygen binding properties. Eur J Appl Physiol 1988;57: 490–498.

64. Weight LM, D Alexander, T Elliot, et al. Erythropoietic adaptations to endurance training. Eur J Appl Physiol 1992;64:444–448.

65. Telford RD, Sly GJ, Hahn AG, et al. Footstrike is the major cause of hemolysis during running. J Appl Physiol 2003;94: 38–42.

66. Gledhill N, Warburton D, Jamnik V. Haemoglobin, blood volume, cardiac function, and aerobic power. Can J Appl Physiol 1999;24:54–65.

67. Buick FJ, Gledhill N, Froese AB, et al. Effect of induced erythrocythemia on aerobic work capacity. J Appl Physiol 1980;48:636–642.

68. Mack GW, Thompson CA, Doerr DF, et al. Diminished baroreflex control of forearm vascular resistance following training. Med Sci Sports Exerc 1991;23:1367–1374.

69. Sawka MN, Young AJ, Francesconi RP, et al. Thermoregulatory and blood responses during exercise at graded hypohydration levels. J Appl Physiol 1985;59:1394–1401.

70. Takamata A, Mack GW, Gillen CM, et al. Osmoregulatory modulation of thermal sweating in humans: reflex effects of drinking. Am J Physiol 1995;268:R414–R422.

71. Nose H, Yawata T, Morimoto T. Osmotic factors in restitution from thermal dehydration in rats. Am J Physiol 1985;249:R166–R171.

72. Nose H, Mack GW, Shi XR, et al. Involvement of sodium retention hormones during rehydration in humans. J Appl Physiol 1988;65:332–336.

CHAPTER 25

The Renal System

Edward J. Zambraski

Introduction

The kidneys play an essential role in the maintenance of total-body homeostasis. By varying the amount and chemical composition of the urine, the renal system can regulate total-body water, extracellular volume and tonicity, plasma electrolyte levels, and plasma pH. The kidneys can also produce and release into the circulation a large number of compounds, such as angiotensin II (Ang II), prostaglandins (PG), norepinephrine (NE), erythropoietin, and nitric oxide (NO), that can affect circulatory function (blood pressure and flow), metabolism, thermoregulation, and red blood cell production. All of these responses are designed or intended either to maintain or to restore homeostasis. The fact that acute exercise extremely perturbs homeostasis therefore predicts that the renal response to exercise will be fundamental and essential, in terms of our ability to do continued work. It follows that there should be a large amount of interest in and research on renal function and exercise, whereas in fact this has not been the case. Historically, there has been very little mechanistic work on the kidney and exercise. The exercise studies of the 1930s and 1940s provided only a general description of the renal excretory and hemodynamic response to exercise. After a hiatus, it was not until the 1970s to 1990s that interest in this topic increased and more mechanistic studies began to appear. Since then there has been in increased interest in the renal response to exercise and to the

factors that control this response. This chapter describes the renal response to exercise, the mechanisms involved, and the relative importance of the renal response to acute and chronic exercise.

Extrinsic Control of Kidney Function During Exercise

To understand kidney function during exercise one must be aware of the fundamental factors that control renal function. The three major controls are neural (autonomic nervous system), endocrine, and hemodynamic (blood pressure). During exercise the kidneys are essentially targeted by these factors. The neural input to the kidney is largely sympathetic-adrenergic (NE releasing), with essentially no functional parasympathetic innervation. Renal sympathetic nerve activity (RSNA) has the potential to directly affect renal hemodynamics (renal blood flow, or RBF; glomerular filtration rate, or GFR), salt and water excretion, and the renal release of compounds such as renin, PG, and NE. The adrenoreceptors involved in the renal response include the α_1-receptor for renal vasoconstriction and augmented tubular sodium reabsorption and the β_1-receptor for renin release. Endocrine and/or chemical control of renal function, via compounds such as antidiuretic hormone (ADH), aldosterone, atrial natriuretic peptide, and NO, influence GFR and RBF and the renal handling of sodium and water. Last, since renal excretory function is totally dependent upon filtration (i.e., adequate GFR) and GFR is directly dependent upon blood pressure, changes in systemic blood pressure will markedly alter renal function. Consequently, the renal response to exercise is totally dependent upon these three foci of control. Also, the greater the change in the control (e.g., increase in RSNA or endocrine level), the larger will be the magnitude of the renal response.

Techniques to Assess Kidney Function with Exercise

To understand the renal response to exercise, one must understand the techniques or tools, and their inherent limitations, available to study renal function. Table 25.1 lists all of the techniques that have been used to assess renal function with exercise, both in animals and man. Until the 1980s and 1990s the only techniques used in humans were urine collections and clearance methods. Only in the past 2 decades have more sophisticated techniques been used, both in man and animals, to provide new, more mechanistic information.

Renal Hemodynamics and Exercise

Renal hemodynamics include RBF (or renal plasma flow), GFR, the intrarenal distribution of RBF (i.e., cortex vs. medulla), and the filtration fraction (the fraction of renal plasma flow that is filtered). Table 25.2 illustrates the changes in renal hemodynamics in response to progressive steady-state exercise at three relative exercise intensities.

Renal Blood Flow

As measured by clearance techniques, renal plasma flow (both kidneys) is approximately 800 mL $\cdot$ min^{-1} at rest. When corrected for hematocrit, RBF is approximately 1300 mL $\cdot$ min^{-1}. With exercise at increasingly high intensities, RBF decreases in a linear fashion. The decline in RBF with exercise is somewhat greater if the subjects are exercising in the heat

and/or dehydrated (1). At heavy or near maximal exercise intensities the absolute decrease in RBF is approximately 300 mL $\cdot$ min^{-1}. The decrease in RBF is due to active vasoconstriction of the renal blood vessels, and it is generally assumed that two strong renal vasoconstrictor mechanisms, increased RSNA and increased Ang II, are responsible for this reduction in RBF. Changes in directly measured RSNA in an exercising animal are shown in Figure 25.1. Indirect findings have implicated an important role for the increased RSNA; however, no existing data support the concept that Ang II causes active renal vasoconstriction with dynamic exercise.

The change in RBF with exercise is almost exclusively described not in an absolute fashion but rather as a percent of cardiac output. At rest, RBF represents approximately 20% of cardiac output, whereas during maximal exercise this declines to 3–5% of cardiac output. This approach gives a false impression that the magnitude of change in RBF during exercise is large. What many fail to consider is that cardiac output is going from 5 to 25 to 30 L $\cdot$ min^{-1} with heavy exercise; consequently, 3% of this larger amount is not very different from 20% of only 5 L $\cdot$ min^{-1}. The widely held belief that renal vasoconstriction during exercise is important because it redistributes a large quantity of blood from the kidneys to support active skeletal muscle is misleading (2). Relative to a cardiac output increase of 20 to 25 L $\cdot$ min^{-1} seen with exercise, the 300-mL decline in RBF is negligible.

The importance of renal vasoconstriction during exercise relates to the change in total peripheral resistance. The intense renal vasoconstriction offsets the vasodilation seen in active skeletal muscle, thereby preventing total peripheral resistance from falling dramatically. Thus, this renal response helps to maintain blood pressure (2).

Glomerular Filtration Rate

Glomerular filtration is essential for kidney function. Water and various chemical compounds must be filtered, or translocated from the circulation to the renal tubule, if they are to be excreted. GFR is determined by the Starling forces at the glomerular capillary, as is the case for all capillaries. One unique factor in the kidney is that the glomerular capillary hydrostatic pressure, the major force favoring filtration, is

TABLE 25.1	Techniques Used to Study Renal Function During Exercise in Conscious Humans and Animal Models	
Humans		**Animals**
Single urine sample		Urine collections, clearance methods
Timed urine collection		Doppler, electromagnetic flow probes—RBF
Clearance methodology—GFR, RPF		Radioactive microspheres
Pharmacological interventions		Pharmacological interventions
Radiographic, NMR imaging		Surgical renal denervation
NE spillover estimates of RSNA		Renal vein cannulation, blood sampling
		Directly measured renal nerve activity

RPF, renal plasma flow.

TABLE 25.2	Changes in Renal Hemodynamics and Excretory Function With Graded Exercise			
	Resting	25% $\dot{V}O_{2max}$	40% $\dot{V}O_{2max}$	>80% $\dot{V}O_{2max}$
RBF, mL · min⁻¹	1330.0	1250.0	1100.00	990
GFR, mL · min⁻¹	120.0	135.0	110.00	>80
UV, mL · min⁻¹	1.0	1.2	0.75	0.30–0.50
U Na V, % resting	100.0	125.0	60.00	20–50

Values represent workloads as expressed as a percent of $\dot{V}O_{2max}$.
UV, urine volume; U Na V, sodium excretion.
Data adapted from Freund BJ, Shizuru EM, Hashiro GM, et al. Hormonal, electrolyte, and renal responses to exercise are intensity dependent. J Appl Physiol 1991;70:900–906.

usually high enough that filtration always occurs, unlike the situation in muscle capillaries, where filtration or absorption may occur. Filtration depends on two variables: the net filtration pressure and permeability characteristics of the capillary membrane.

At rest, GFR is approximately 120 mL · min⁻¹ (3). As shown in Table 25.2, with light exercise GFR is either increased or maintained, but it falls with moderate to heavy exercise (4). It has been hypothesized but never proven that

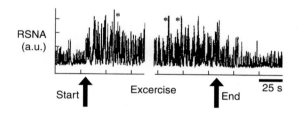

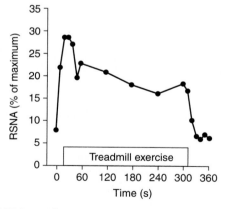

FIGURE 25.1 With acute exercise there is a rapid increase in RSNA. *Top.* An actual renal nerve recording obtained from chronically instrumented rabbits at rest, during treadmill exercise, and with recovery. *Bottom.* The quantitative changes in RSNA expressed as a percent of resting values. Note the rapidity with which the RSNA response turns on with exercise and diminishes with the end of exercise. *(Data courtesy of Dr. K. O'Hagan, Department of Physiology, Midwestern University, Downers Grove, IL.)*

the rise in GFR with light exercise may due to increased atrial natriuretic peptide (4). With increased exercise intensity there is more active renal preglomerular vasoconstriction, the effects of atrial natriuretic peptide are overridden, and GFR falls. The mechanisms responsible for the decline in GFR are the same as those described for the control of RBF. As mentioned earlier, GFR is also determined by the membrane permeability. Glomerular membrane permeability can differentially influence the movement of small molecules, such as water and electrolytes, versus larger molecules, like plasma protein. Several compounds that increase during exercise may decrease glomerular capillary surface area and/or permeability to facilitate a decrease in GFR. These include ADH, Ang II, endothelin, thromboxane A2, and NE. There is also the concomitant release of PGI₂, NO, and atrial natriuretic peptide, which increase glomerular capillary surface area and permeability. Whether glomerular capillary surface area and/or permeability is actually altered during exercise and influencing water translocation across the glomerular capillary and contributing to the fall in GFR is unknown. As discussed later in the chapter, glomerular permeability to larger molecules, such as albumin, is increased during acute dynamic exercise.

Site of Renal Vasoconstriction

The renal vasculature is densely innervated with sympathetic nerves. This innervation goes to both preglomerular and postglomerular vessels (5). Since these vessels are in series, constriction at either site will decrease RBF. In contrast, selective constriction of the preglomerular afferent arteriole will decrease glomerular capillary pressure and cause a fall in GFR, while constriction of the postglomerular efferent arteriole will have just the opposite effect. The fact that during moderate to heavy exercise RBF and GFR decline in parallel suggests that most renal vasoconstriction during exercise occurs at the preglomerular afferent arteriole.

Filtration Fraction and Exercise

The filtration fraction is the fraction of renal plasma flow that is filtered (i.e., GFR/renal plasma flow). This value at rest is normally approximately 20%. With exercise, if GFR and renal plasma flow fell similarly, the filtration fraction would remain constant. The fact that GFR is unchanged or slightly increased with light exercise and decreases to a lesser extent with moderate to heavy exercise, as compared to renal plasma flow, means that the filtration fraction actually increases with the intensity and duration of exercise. The mechanism may involve elevated postglomerular constriction. One possible mediator of this response may be Ang II, since it has been shown to act preferentially at the postglomerular vessels and to increase proportionally with exercise intensity (6). This possibility has not been confirmed or tested.

Distribution of Renal Blood Flow

It is known that of the total RBF received by the kidneys, more than 90% perfuses the cortex, with the remaining 10% going to the medulla through the special medullary circulation known as the vasa recta. Small plastic spheres with radioactive labels have been used to measure the distribution of blood flow within the kidney in various animal models. It has been shown that the distribution of intrarenal blood flow does not change with exercise (i.e., the decline in RBF is proportional across the cortex and medulla (7). This finding, although negative, is important because if exercise increased medullary blood flow, it would have the potential to wash out the high concentrations of sodium and urea in the medullary interstitium. The resultant loss of the high medullary tonicity would dramatically impair the ability of ADH to produce concentrated urine (discussed later).

Renal Handling of Sodium During Exercise

Sodium is one of the most important ions because it determines extracellular tonicity. Since the body must keep extracellular tonicity constant, if extracellular sodium changes, more or less water will have to be added to that compartment to restore tonicity to normal. Thus extracellular sodium content determines extracellular volume; this includes plasma volume. Under resting conditions, the amount of sodium in the body is determined by the amount of sodium ingested (dietary intake) versus sodium lost in the urine. At rest, various control factors regulate renal tubular sodium reabsorption to maintain sodium balance at zero (i.e., intake equals loss). During exercise, especially when there is a thermal challenge, excessive sodium is lost via sweating. This decrease may result in a net loss of total body sodium (i.e., negative sodium balance). Conceptually, during exercise the role of the kidney would be to decrease urinary sodium loss to offset sodium lost in the sweat and thereby maintain or restore sodium balance.

One of the primary controls over sodium excretion is GFR. If sodium (and/or water) is not filtered into the renal tubule, it cannot be excreted. The decrease in GFR with exercise is one of the fundamental responses to minimize urine sodium loss or to conserve sodium.

Absolute Changes in Sodium Excretion With Exercise

As shown in Table 25.2, sodium excretion declines with increases in exercise intensity. Studies have shown a very tight inverse linear relationship with sodium excretion and exercise intensity (percent $\dot{V}_{O_{2max}}$) (4). With maximal exercise, sodium excretion can be as low as 10–20% of the resting value. While the decline in GFR contributes to this antinatriuretic affect, it is also known that the magnitude of the reduction in sodium excretion with moderate to heavy exercise cannot be fully accounted for by the decrease in GFR or filtered sodium load (8). This means an increase in renal tubular sodium reabsorption must be occurring.

Mechanisms of Control

There are multiple redundant controls over renal tubular sodium reabsorption. Increased RSNA, Ang II, and aldosterone all directly stimulate tubular sodium reabsorption, and all of these factors increase with exercise. It is widely stated that during exercise an increase in aldosterone and/or Ang II is responsible for the renal conservation of sodium. Unfortunately, no data support this belief. In fact, in both animal and human studies pharmacological interventions to block Ang II or aldosterone have shown that these maneuvers do not alter the renal handling of sodium during exercise; sodium ion conservation is unaffected (9,10). The control factor that is probably responsible for the augmented sodium reabsorption during exercise is the increase in RSNA (11). Definitive experiments to prove this assertion, even in animal models, are difficult to design and have not been undertaken.

Importance of Renal Sodium Conservation

The amount of sodium in the urine at rest is relatively small, approximately 130 mEq · L^{-1}. With steady-state heavy exercise, both in laboratory and field experiments, sodium excretion decreases by approximately 50–75%. While this percent change appears impressive, when one calculates the absolute amount of sodium conserved (approximately 5 mEq · h^{-1}) and compares this with the amount lost in sweat (>30 mEq · h^{-1}), it is noted that the kidneys are able to conserve only about 10% of the total sodium that was lost. This demonstrates that the renal antinatriuretic response during exercise is inadequate and that if dietary sodium intake is not supplemented, large deficits in total body sodium will occur. As indicated, this will compromise extracellular and plasma volume.

An essential role of the kidneys in this regard is the restoration of normal body sodium content during the hours to days following long-term strenuous exercise. The control factors operating in this setting are elevated aldosterone and Ang II (6).

Renal Handling of Water During Exercise

The excretion of water is necessary, as it is the solvent required to remove dissolved electrolytes, acids, and metabolic wastes. Normal urine volume, or excretion of water, is approximately 1.0 mL · min^{-1} at rest. As shown in Table 25.2, urine volume goes down to 0.3–0.5 mL · min^{-1} with maximal exercise.

The renal handling of water, especially in the context of an exercise stress, is largely misunderstood. Various factors should be clarified. First, the major control over the excretion of water is GFR. As was indicated for sodium, if water is not filtered, it cannot be excreted. Second, of the huge amount of water normally filtered (GFR 120 mL · min^{-1}), 60–80% is reabsorbed or returned to the circulatory compartment via iso-osmotic reabsorption. This means that for every reabsorbed molecule of solute, such as sodium, chloride, or calcium, the resultant osmotic pressure is responsible for the reabsorption of a molecule of water. Since one is removing an equal amount of solute and solvent, the osmolarity of the fluid in the renal tubule does not change; hence the term *iso-osmotic*. This process has two important implications. First, if mechanisms are activated to increase the reabsorption of sodium and other solutes, this will cause an increase in water reabsorption. Second, if all water reabsorption were accomplished solely by iso-osmotic reabsorption, the resultant osmolarity of urine would have to be similar to that of plasma (approximately 300 mOsm · L^{-1}). Since urine osmolarity varies from approximately 700 to 800 mOsm · L^{-1} in a well-hydrated person at rest to 1200 mOsm · L^{-1} in someone who is exercising at maximum intensity and likely dehydrated, another mechanism for water reabsorption must exist.

The ability to concentrate urine, or make a urine that is more concentrated than plasma, is derived from the affect of ADH. ADH increases the permeability of the collecting duct such that the high osmotic pressure of the medullary interstitium is allowed to extract water from the renal tubule. The higher the ADH, the greater the urine osmolarity and the lower the urine volume. If ADH is suppressed, a voluminous amount of urine with a low osmolarity will be excreted. Even if ADH is decreased, dilute urine can be produced only if an adequate amount of water is delivered to the distal tubule. With a decrease in GFR and augmented iso-osmotic reabsorption of water early in the renal tubule, minimal free water will be present in the collecting duct. In this situation a decrease in ADH will not result in excretion of a high volume of dilute urine (discussed next).

Renal Excretion of Water During Exercise

As shown in Table 25.2, with moderate to heavy dynamic exercise urine volume will decrease by 50–70%. The primary mechanisms are a decrease in GFR and an increase in iso-osmotic reabsorption of water. All of the factors discussed with respect to increasing sodium reabsorption during exercise will also cause a proportional increase in water reabsorption. In addition, elevation of ADH will increase urine osmolarity and decrease volume.

Antidiuretic Hormone

ADH, also known as arginine vasopressin, is released from the posterior pituitary gland. One of the major factors stimulating the release of ADH is increased tonicity sensed by osmoreceptors in the brain. If tonicity is elevated, ADH is released, urine volume is reduced, and the return of this water to the circulation will restore normal tonicity. ADH release is also stimulated by a wide variety of other factors, such as stress, anesthesia, and exercise. With acute exercise, plasma levels of ADH do not increase appreciably until one performs moderate to heavy exercise (1). Resting ADH levels of 3–5 pg · mL^{-1} may increase 10-fold with exercise of maximum intensity (12).

ADH acts selectively on the cells of the renal tubule collecting duct. It promotes the formation of microtubules within the cytoplasm of these cells, which increases the ability of water to move through these cells. The driving force for this water movement is the high tonicity of the medullary interstitium.

Importance of Renal Water Conservation During Exercise

As discussed for sodium, there is a widespread impression that the renal response to exercise is very important in terms of the conservation of water to offset fluid lost via sweating. As shown in Table 25.2, urine flow rate is approximately 1.0 mL · min^{-1}. With heavy exercise the excretion of water decreases to 0.3–0.5 mL · min^{-1}. If these values were to remain constant for 1 h, the kidneys would be conserving only 30–36 mL · h^{-1}. These amounts are dwarfed by the amount of fluid lost in the sweat, which can be well above 1,000 mL · h^{-1}. Since the kidneys are not excreting a large amount of water at rest, the antidiuretic effect seen with exercise is inconsequential. A key point, however, is that the renal conservation of water (and sodium) will persist for hours or days following exercise to restore total body water and electrolyte levels (6).

Renal Acid Excretion and Metabolism During Exercise

At rest one excretes slightly acidic urine. With exercise urine pH drops further, to 4.0–5.0. This is due to several mechanisms, including active secretion of hydrogen ions, excretion of fixed acids, and increased reabsorption of water resulting in concentrated urine.

The renal handling of lactic acid may vary with exercise. With exercise lactic acid excretion increases. Lactic acid is freely filterable at the glomerular capillary, and it is also reabsorbed along the renal tubule. The excretion of lactic acid appears to involve a plasma threshold of 5–6 mmol $\cdot$ L^{-1} (13). Above this concentration, the maximal ability of the tubules to reabsorb lactic acid is exceeded and excretion increases. Nevertheless, the amount of lactic acid removed by excretion, relative to the total amount produced with heavy exercise, is estimated to be less than 2% (13).

It has been shown that the renal arterial-venous difference in lactic acid concentration is positive. That is, the kidneys remove lactic acid from the circulation during exercise, but the amount is not believed to be large. Lactic acid removed by the kidney could be used directly for energy or for gluconeogenesis. As observed by Krebs and Yoshida, lactate-derived gluconeogenesis in the kidney increased by approximately 50% immediately after exercise (14).

Water Intoxication

In both competitive and recreational athletics, there are increased reports of water intoxication. This occurs when an exercising individual is consuming pure water in amounts that far exceed water being lost via sweating (15). This causes a fluid imbalance (overhydration), expanded plasma volume, and lowered plasma electrolyte concentrations. Central nervous system and/or cardiac problems may ensue. An important issue is why the kidneys do not respond to this situation by excreting this excess water and thus preventing this condition. It has been suggested that this may reflect an abnormality in renal function (15). This is simply not correct; renal function is normal, but control factors and conditions prevent excretion of the excess water.

As indicated earlier, during exercise various control factors are activated to promote sodium and water reabsorption. The ability of these controls, when activated during acute exercise, is dramatic in terms of minimizing the excretion of sodium and water. For example, it was shown that if a subject drank 200 mL of water every 20 min and had resultant urine flow rates of 10–12 mL $\cdot$ min^{-1}, urine flow rates after exercise fell to 2–3 mL $\cdot$ min^{-1}, even if the subject continued to drink the fluids (3). In these subjects and in those who are becoming water intoxicated, ADH levels will be markedly suppressed. As mentioned earlier, during exercise, if free water being delivered to the distal tubule is limited, a reduction of ADH will have no effect, since there will be a very limited volume of water to be excreted due to the decrease in ADH.

Exercise Proteinuria

Exercise proteinuria is defined as an increase in urine protein concentration either during or following exercise. Normally, because of the size and electrical charge of protein molecules, only a small amount of protein is filtered through the glomerular capillary membrane. Of the amount that is filtered, a large fraction (>90%) is reabsorbed by the renal tubule cells. Conceptually, exercise proteinuria could result from either an increase in the filtration of protein or decreased reabsorption or both. In fact, studies have shown that both pathways are involved, with the major contributing mechanism being an increase in glomerular membrane permeability to protein (13). With acute exercise there is an increase in the permeability to albumin due to the loss of the negative charge characteristics of the glomerular membrane (3). The anionic quality of the glomerular membrane normally prevents negatively charged plasma proteins from passing through it. In a diseased kidney the glomerular membrane allows protein to pass through it; hence proteinuria is observed. It is important not to confuse exercise proteinuria with disease-induced proteinuria. Exercise proteinuria is a benign, reversible process. Within 24–48 h after exercise the proteinuria is resolved (3). Quantitatively, the amount of protein in the urine is proportional to both intensity and duration of exercise. Historically, the common belief was that the intense renal vasoconstriction associated with exercise was responsible for exercise proteinuria (3). While this mechanism may contribute to the proteinuria, studies have shown that renal PG are involved. If exercising subjects are given a drug to block the renal production of PG, the exercise proteinuria is markedly reduced in the absence of any renal hemodynamic changes (16).

Renal Endocrine Release During Exercise

The importance of the kidney in the maintenance or restoration of fluid–electrolyte homeostasis is commonly accepted. Less well recognized is the fact that the kidneys also release into the circulation several endocrines, or compounds with widespread effects that are important components of the integrated response to exercise. Several of these compounds are discussed next.

Renin–Angiotensin

Renin is released from the juxtaglomerular cells in the kidney. Renin release is proportional to exercise intensity. Resting plasma renin values of 1–3 ng $\cdot$ mL $\cdot$ h^{-1} are significantly increased, to levels of 10–12 ng · mL · h^{-1}, when exercise intensity exceeds 80% $\dot{V}O_{2max}$ (12). Renin acts upon angiotensinogen to form the decapeptide angiotensin I. Angiotensin I is converted to the octapeptide Ang II by an angiotensin-converting enzyme. Ang II is an extremely important biologically active compound. In brief, Ang II is a potent vasoconstrictor that affects systemic blood pressure, alters thirst, is a growth factor for various types of tissues, and promotes sodium reabsorption (5). Numerous mechanisms are capable of causing an increase in renin release. The major mechanism for renin release during exercise involves the increase in RSNA and the stimulation of β$_1$-adrenoreceptors (17).

Renal Prostaglandins

The kidney has a very high capacity to produce PG, which consist of a group of related compounds with diverse properties, the major ones being PGE$_2$ and PGI$_2$. PGE$_2$ and PGI$_2$ are vasodilators, and they inhibit sodium transport (18).

PG also have a wide array of other effects, including an important role in mediating the inflammatory process (e.g., musculoskeletal injury). Compounds designed to inhibit the synthesis of PG are the nonsteroidal anti-inflammatory drugs (NSAIDs). Examples include widely used drugs such as ibuprofen (Advil, Nuprin), indomethacin (Indocin), and meclofenamate (Meclofan). The major biochemical effect of aspirin is also to inhibit PG synthesis (18).

Exercise has the capacity to increase renal PG synthesis; with exercise there is an increase in PGE$_2$ and PGI$_2$ in both urine and renal venous blood (19). Since these PG are vasodilators and natriuretic, an important issue is this: would the use of NSAIDs during acute exercise and the resultant reduction in renal PG alter the renal hemodynamic or excretory response, or even cause acute renal failure? Fortunately, studies examining the effects of renal PG synthesis inhibition, using NSAIDs or aspirin, have not shown deleterious changes in renal function during exercise in normal subjects tested under controlled laboratory conditions (16,19). It is known that PG control over renal function increases when a person is dehydrated, is in a negative sodium balance, and/or has very high levels of RSNA. The term *renal PG dependent* has been used to describe the fact that under such conditions the use of a NSAID will predictably cause renal vasoconstriction and sodium retention (18). Such conditions would be likely during a long-term endurance event, such as the marathon, especially with concomitant heat stress. There are anecdotal suggestions that NSAIDs may cause kidney problems during events such as the marathon. These combined conditions of sodium deprivation, dehydration, heat stress, and long-term exercise have been replicated in the laboratory to determine whether NSAIDs have a deleterious effect on kidney function in these extreme physiological circumstances. When ibuprofen is administered, there is an exaggerated renal vasoconstrictor response; however, there were no reports of overt renal failure or salt and water retention (20).

Norepinephrine

During exercise of various intensities in animals and humans there is an increase in total body peripheral sympathetic nerve activity. However, the sympathetic outflow is not uniform in all organs, as the kidneys receive a disproportionately elevated amount of sympathetic nerve activity. Studies in animals have directly measured sympathetic nerve traffic over the renal nerves during exercise as shown in Figure 25.1 (21,22).

Also, investigations in humans measuring NE spillover from the kidneys with exercise confirm that RSNA is markedly increased with exercise (23). The increase is proportional to the exercise intensity. The effect of this large increase in RSNA with exercise, along with the fact that the kidneys are so densely innervated with sympathetic adrenergic nerves, is that a large amount of NE spills over from the synaptic spaces and enters the circulation through the renal vein. It has been estimated that at rest renal spillover of NE accounts for about 20% of the plasma circulating NE. In contrast, the adrenal gland contribution to circulating NE at rest is less than 5% (24). With exercise the marked increase in RSNA will increase the renal contribution to circulating NE, which in turn will have widespread systemic affects on cardiovascular function and metabolism.

Nitric Oxide

NO is produced from the endothelium from L-arginine by NO synthase. NO is a vasodilator, and it is believed to be responsible for setting the vascular tone and control of local blood flow. Acting as a vasodilator, NO contributes to muscle blood vessel dilation in response to dynamic exercise (25). Within the kidney there is potential for interaction among three control factors: RSNA, endothelin, and NO. Acting as a vasodilator, if NO synthesis was increased with acute dynamic exercise, this could attenuate the renal vasoconstrictor effects of increased RSNA and/or increased endothelin. Such an effect could assist in preventing renal failure during exercise (discussed later). Alternatively, if NO synthesis decreased during acute exercise, this change could be mediating the decrease in RBF.

In animal studies in which NO production is pharmacologically blocked, decreases in RBF with acute dynamic exercise are not changed (26). Other studies suggest that renal NO synthesis may be selectively reduced during exercise, perhaps as a result of an increase in endothelin (25). This reduction in NO could partially mediate the decrease in RBF (i.e., decreased vasodilatory NO may increase renal vascular resistance). One way to study the role of NO in various physiological processes is to administer a false analogue of L-arginine (e.g., L-NAME). This can be done in human subjects. One problem with trying to elucidate NO control of renal function during exercise using inhibitors such as L-NAME is that other systemic affects, such as an increase in blood pressure, will alter renal function.

Injury or Acute Renal Failure Induced by Exercise

With exercise the kidneys are stressed. Renal oxygen consumption, which is proportional to the amount of sodium being reabsorbed, is increased. At the same time RBF, or oxygen delivery, is being compromised. At rest the renal arteriovenous difference in oxygen is very small (i.e., oxygen extraction is minimal) when compared to that of muscle. Oxygen extraction will increase with exercise to meet metabolic demand. It has never been shown that heavy exercise damages the kidney or the renal tubule cells in terms of an inadequate amount of oxygen. However, there have been concerns about individuals who are not only exercising but also severely dehydrated, such as wrestlers attempting to lose weight. Studies have shown that the urine of wrestlers contains extremely high amounts of potassium and leucine amino peptidase (27). It has been suggested but never proved that the release of these compounds may be due to or reflect renal tubule cell damage or death as a result of the combined effects of exercise and dehydration (11). What is needed in this regard is identification and validation of novel biomarkers of renal damage that can be measured in the urine.

Acute renal failure (ARF) is defined as a sudden decrease in renal function associated with a significant decline in GFR. Factors that result in a decrease in renal perfusion, or RBF, such as increased RSNA, increased Ang II, hypovolemia, and hypotension, could all contribute to ARF. Rhabdomyolysis, the breakdown of muscle tissue, could also cause ARF. Heavy exercise, especially combined with dehydration, heat stress, and the sympathetic responses created by intense competition, could cause ARF. For that reason, it is surprising that exercise-induced ARF is relatively rare (11). Despite thousands of people participating in marathons and other long-term endurance events, only isolated cases of ARF have been reported. It has been hypothesized that some yet-unidentified factor or factors vasodilate the kidney during exercise and thus protect against ARF (11). One additional protective mechanism may be changes in RSNA seen with exercise training (discussed in the next section).

Changes in Kidney Function with Exercise Training

As indicated earlier, changes in kidney function are largely dictated by neural and endocrine controls activated by exercise. Changes in renal function with training, therefore, would be anticipated if training altered the magnitude of a change in a particular control factor.

In general, at rest there are no substantial measurable changes either in renal hemodynamics or excretory function as a consequence of training. This finding is consistent with the fact that training does not appear to change resting levels of ADH, atrial natriuretic peptide, aldosterone or renin–Ang II (12). With exercise, the renal response (i.e., vasoconstriction, sodium reabsorption) is proportional to the relative workload. Therefore, at the same absolute workload some of the renal responses of the trained subject will be dampened compared with those of the untrained subject because the trained person is working at a lower relative workload.

While it may be difficult to measure changes in kidney excretory function as a consequence of dynamic exercise training, another way to view or assess any adaptations of the kidneys is to focus on sodium balance. If there is a steady-state change in a person's extracellular or plasma volume, two things should be occurring. First, a person who is in a steady state must be in sodium balance. More important, if plasma volume changes, extracellular sodium content often also changes. The primary way this can occur is with a change in renal function. For example, an expansion of plasma volume can be achieved if the renal excretion of sodium initially decreases, allowing extracellular sodium to rise, with excretion subsequently finding a new steady state and reestablishing sodium balance. In other words, a maintained expansion of plasma volume often occurs with a change in the control of sodium excretion by the kidneys. It is well known that with dynamic exercise training, plasma volume is expanded (2). This adaptation associated with training is often mediated or controlled by a change in renal function; however, a redistribution of extracellular fluid to the plasma can also contribute via elevated circulating protein increasing plasma oncotic pressure.

Changes in RSNA With Dynamic Exercise Training

One major change with training is an alteration in RSNA. Studies using NE spillover calculations and catheterization across the kidney in humans have been able to estimate RSNA both at rest and with exercise. In 1991 in a landmark study RSNA was measured in human subjects before and after a 4-wk training program (Milestone of Discovery) (28). In these subjects dynamic exercise training caused arterial NE levels to decrease by 21%. As shown in Figure 25.2, total body NE spillover also fell by 24%. More important, the changes in RSNA were dramatic, as the decreased RSNA accounted for 70% of the decrease in whole-body NE spillover. In contrast, cardiac NE spillover, or sympathetic activity, was not altered by training, which suggests that exercise training had a selective affect on decreasing RSNA.

The decrease in RSNA with training essentially means that certain renal parameters influenced by the renal nerves (e.g., RBF, GFR, sodium reabsorption, renin release) are probably altered by training. These changes are undoubtedly

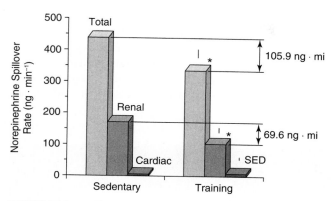

FIGURE 25.2 With exercise training total peripheral sympathetic nerve activity at rest decreases. This can be measured using calculated total NE spillover. With 1 month of exercise training in humans, total NE spillover was decreased by approximately 25%. RSNA or renal NE spillover was also markedly decreased. The decrease in RSNA was responsible for approximately 70% of the change in total NE spillover. Cardiac sympathetic activity was unchanged with training. This shows that with training a selective decrease in RSNA is responsible for most of the decrease in total sympathetic activity. This training adaptation could help protect the kidneys against acute renal failure. *(Modified from Meridith IT, Friberg P, Jennings GL, et al. Exercise training lowers resting renal but not cardiac sympathetic activity in humans. Hypertension 1991;18:579.)*

very subtle, and with the techniques available, they simply cannot be accurately measured.

Chapter 9 well documents that in a trained individual the peripheral sympathetic response is reduced with a given exercise challenge, as reflected with notable decreases in plasma catecholamine concentrations. Recent animal studies (21,29) in which renal neurograms directly measured RSNA during exercise indicate that dynamic exercise training will reduce RSNA in response to acute exercise.

That exercise training conditions decrease RSNA at rest and during exercise has important ramifications, because RSNA controls renal tubular sodium reabsorption; that is, increased RSNA increases reabsorption or decreases excretion. A decrease in RSNA therefore could alter total-body sodium balance. With a decrease in RSNA the directional change would be a reduction in total body sodium and water. This response would be advantageous for an individual with hypertension, congestive heart failure, or other condition in which sodium retention is problematic.

Earlier the issue of ARF with exercise was discussed. A reduction of RSNA with exercise training results in attenuation of renal vasoconstriction during exercise. This adaptation could be the most important protective mechanism responsible for the low incidence of exercise-induced ARF. It also means that an untrained person may be more likely to develop ARF if he or she attempts to do long-term strenuous exercise than is a trained person who has this adaptation in the RSNA response.

The mechanisms responsible for the decrease in RSNA with training have not been identified. Organs such as the heart and kidneys have an extensive complex of afferent nerves that provide information to the central nervous system. In general, increases in renal or cardiac afferent activity have a tonic inhibitory affect on sympathetic outflow (5). Very recent studies suggest that an increase in cardiac afferent nerve activity observed with exercise training was responsible for measured reductions in RSNA seen with acute exercise (21). To date, the possible involvement of the renal afferent nerves in this response has not been examined.

Aging, Exercise, and Renal Function

Age-related changes in renal function at rest have been well characterized. There is a decrease in RBF and GFR, decreased ability to excrete sodium, and a decline in renal concentrating ability. The most dramatic of these changes is the decrease in GFR, which is approximately 10% per decade starting at 30 years of age.

In contrast, the renal response to exercise in young versus old subjects has been assessed in a very limited number of studies. Experiments on exercise proteinuria suggest that in older subjects, the exercise proteinuric response to the same absolute workload is increased (13). In addition, it has been shown that the RBF response (i.e., vasoconstriction) to exercise is reduced in older subjects (30). This change may be important for thermoregulation, in that less blood will be available for heat transfer to the skin. At present there is not enough information to know whether any of these age-related changes in renal function with exercise are gender specific.

The importance of RSNA in controlling renal function is emphasized throughout this chapter. As one ages, circulating plasma NE increases, and this increase in total body peripheral sympathetic activity is believed to be due to an increase in muscle sympathetic nerve activity. RSNA does not appear to increase with aging (23). In addition, it does not appear that the increase in RSNA stimulated by exercise is changed by aging (31). One difference, however, is that the renal clearance of NE at rest is decreased in older subjects. This change contributes to higher levels of circulating NE. Whether the renal clearance of NE during exercise is also decreased with aging is unknown.

SUMMARY

The renal response to exercise is complex, involving hemodynamic changes, alterations in tubular function, and the release of a wide array of compounds into the circulation. The inaccessibility of the kidneys renders it extremely difficult to examine inherent kidney function in the exercise setting. The importance of the renal response to acute dynamic exercise is not, as most believe, conservation of sodium and water, but rather intense renal vasoconstriction to help maintain blood pressure and the release of large amounts of NE into the circulation. The importance of the exercise-induced increase in renal NO synthesis remains to be determined. One of the fundamental changes seen with

exercise training is a decrease in RSNA, both at rest and during exercise. Changes in this control factor may be the crucial element in preventing exercise-associated ARF. The resultant potential changes in renal function with a training-induced decrease in RSNA, while having little affect on exercise performance, may also have widespread clinical benefits.

A MILESTONE OF DISCOVERY

Before the 1990s it was well known that regular endurance exercise, or training, lowers circulating plasma NE. This change reflects a general decrease in peripheral sympathetic nerve activity (SNA). Also known was that SNA was not uniform or global. The amount of SNA to various sites or organs varies markedly, and the kidneys were believed to receive a disproportionately high amount of SNA. A research group from Australia headed by Murray D. Esler refined the technique of measuring NE spillover in human subjects to estimate SNA. In addition, by placing both arterial and venous catheters across different organs, such as the heart, kidneys, or liver, they could actually measure the amount of SNA going to each of these areas. This research group's influence on the exercise physiology research community began in 1991, when they examined the effects of exercise training on total-body, renal, and cardiac NE spillover. Normal but sedentary men were exercise-trained on a bicycle for 1 month. The program involved training only three times per week, 40 min for each session, at an intensity of 60–70% of their maximal capacity. With this "minimal" train-

ing regimen plasma NE concentration and total-body NE spillover fell by 20–24%. More important, renal NE spillover, which reflects RSNA, fell by 41%. Of this decrease in total-body NE spillover, two-thirds was attributable to a selective decrease in RSNA. In contrast, as shown in Figure 25.2, cardiac NE spillover did not change. Blood pressure was also significantly reduced by training. This study showed that the decrease in total SNA seen with regular exercise is primarily due to a change in RSNA. Also, since RSNA is a major control factor over various aspects of renal function, the potential clinical implications of this decline in RSNA are extensive. In addition, the demonstration that this spillover technique could be used in conjunction with exercise and training has led to several other studies using this technique to assess RSNA in various exercise settings.

Meredith IT, Friberg P, Jennings GL, et al. Exercise training lowers resting renal but not cardiac sympathetic activity in humans. Hypertension 1991;18:575–582.

REFERENCES

1. Radigan L, Robinson S. Effects of environmental heat stress and exercise on renal blood flow and filtration rate. J Appl Physiol 1949;2:185–191.
2. Rowell LB. Human cardiovascular adjustments to exercise and thermal stress. Physiol Rev 1974;54:75–159.
3. Poortmans JR. Exercise and renal function. Sports Med 1984;1:25–153.
4. Freund BJ, Shizuru EM, Hashiro GM, et al. Hormonal, electrolyte, and renal responses to exercise are intensity dependent. J Appl Physiol 1991;70:900–906.
5. Dibona GF, Kopp UC. Neural control of renal function. Physiol Rev 1997;77:75–197.
6. Wade CE, Dressendorfer RH, O'Brien JC, et al. Renal function, aldosterone, and vasopressin excretion following repeated long-distance running. J Appl Physiol 1981;50:709–712.
7. Sanders M, Rasmussen S, Cooper D, et al. Renal and intrarenal blood flow distribution in swine during severe exercise. J Appl Physiol 1976;40:932–935.
8. Castenfors J. Renal function during prolonged exercise. Ann NY Acad Sci 1977;301:151–159.
9. Wade C, Ramee S, Hunt M, et al. Hormonal and renal responses to converting enzyme inhibition during maximal exercise. J Appl Physiol 1987;63:1796–1800.
10. Zambraski EJ. Renal regulation of fluid homeostasis during exercise. In Gisolfi C, Lamb D, eds. Fluid Homeostasis During Exercise. Carmel, IN: Benchmark, 1990;247–280.
11. Zambraski EJ. The kidney and body fluid balance during exercise. In Buskirk E, Puhl S, eds. Body Fluid Balance. Exercise and Sports. New York: CRC, 1996;75–95.
12. Wade C. Hormonal control of body fluid volume. In Buskirk E, Puhl S, eds. Body Fluid Balance. Exercise and Sports. New York: CRC, 1996;53–73.
13. Poortmans JR, Vanderstraeten J. Kidney function during exercise in healthy and diseased humans: an update. Sports Med 1994;18:419–437.
14. Krebs HA, Yoshida T. Muscular exercise and gluconeogenesis. Biochem Z 1963;338:241–244.
15. Noakes TD, Goodman N, Rayner BL, et al. Water intoxication: a possible complication during endurance exercise. Med Sci Sports Exerc 1985;17:370–375.
16. Mittleman KD, Zambraski EJ. Exercise-induced proteinuria is attenuated by indomethacin. Med Sci Sport Exerc 1992;24:1069–1074.
17. Zambraski EJ, Tucker MS, Lakas CS, et al. Mechanisms of renin release in exercising dogs. Am J Physiol 1984;246:E71–E78.
18. Vane JR, Bakhle YS, Botting RM. Cyclooxygenases 1 and 2. Annu Rev Pharmacol Tox 1998;38:97–120.

19. Zambraski EJ, Dodelson R, Guidotti SM, et al. Renal prostaglandin E2 and F2 alpha synthesis during exercise: effects of indomethacin and sulindac. Med Sci Sports Exerc 1986;18:678–684.

20. Farquhar WB, Morgan AL, Zambraski EJ, et al. Effects of acetaminophen and ibuprofen on renal function in the stressed kidney. J Appl Physiol 1999;86:598–604.

21. DiCarlo SE, Stahl LK, Bishop VS. Daily exercise attenuates the sympathetic nerve response to exercise by enhancing cardiac afferents. Am J Physiol 1997;273:H1606–H1610.

22. O'Hagan KP, Alberts JA. Uterine artery blood flow and renal sympathetic nerve activity during exercise in rabbit pregnancy. Am J Physiol 2003;285:R1135–R1144.

23. Mazzeo RS, Rajkumar C, Jennings G, et al. Norepinephrine spillover at rest and during submaximal exercise in young and old subjects. J Appl Physiol 1997;82:1869–1874.

24. Esler MG, Jennings P, Korner P, et al. Measurement of total and organ-specific norepinephrine kinetics in humans. Am J Physiol 1984;247:E21–E28.

25. Miyauchi T, Maeda S, Iemitsu M, et al. Exercise causes a tissue specific change of NO production in kidney and lung. J Appl Physiol 2003;94:60–68.

26. Shen W, Lundborg M, Wang J, et al. Role of EDRF in the regulation of regional blood flow and vascular resistance at rest and during exercise. J Appl Physiol 1994;77:165–172.

27. Zambraski EJ, Foster DT, Gross PM, et al. Iowa Wrestling Study: Weight loss and urinary profiles of collegiate wrestlers. Med Sci Sports 1976;8:05–108.

28. Meridith IT, Friberg P, Jennings GL, et al. Exercise training lowers resting renal but not cardiac sympathetic activity in humans. Hypertension 1991;18:575–582.

29. Negrao CE, Irigoyen MC, Moreira ED, et al. Effect of exercise training on RSNA, baroreflex control, and blood pressure responsiveness. Am J Physiol 1993;265:R365–R370.

30. Kenney WL, Ho C. Age alters regional distribution of blood flow during moderate-intensity exercise. J Appl Physiol 1995;79:1112–1119.

31. Esler MD, Turner AG, Kaye DM, et al. Aging effects on human sympathetic neuronal function. Am J Physiol 1995;268:R278–R285

The Effects of Exercise in Altered Environments

CHAPTER 26

Physiological Systems and Their Responses to Conditions of Heat and Cold

MICHAEL N. SAWKA AND ANDREW J. YOUNG

Introduction

Individuals exercise and work in a wide range of environmental conditions (temperature, humidity, sun, wind, rain, other water). Depending upon the environmental conditions, metabolic rate, and clothing, exercise can accentuate either heat gain or heat loss, causing body temperature to rise or fall. Humans normally regulate body (core) temperatures near 37°C, and fluctuations within the narrow range of 35° to 41°C can degrade exercise performance. Fluctuations outside that range can be lethal (1). Therefore, heat or cold stress can have profound effects on exercise capability as well as morbidity and mortality.

In this chapter the term *exercise* refers to dynamic exercise, and *training* refers to repeated days of exercise in a specific modality. Throughout this chapter, *stress* refers to environmental exercise conditions tending to influence the body's heat content and *strain* refers to physiological consequences of stress. The magnitude of stress and the resulting strain depends upon the complex interaction of environmental factors (e.g., ambient conditions, clothing), the individual's biological characteristics (e.g., acclimatization status, body size) and exercise task (e.g., metabolic rate, duration). Acclimatization refers to adaptations to both natural (acclimatization) and artificial (acclimation) environmental conditions.

This chapter examines the effects of both heat stress and cold stress on physiological responses and exercise capabil-ities. Human thermoregulation during exercise is addressed, but more detailed reviews on human thermoregulation during environmental stress can be found elsewhere (2–4). This chapter includes information on pathogenesis of exertional heat illness and exertional hypothermia, since exercise can increase morbidity and mortality from thermal injury. Other chapters emphasize acute and chronic (training) exercise, whereas in this chapter the focus is on acute and chronic (acclimatization) environmental exposure, although the effects of exercise training on physiological responses during thermal (heat or cold) stress are discussed.

Thermal Balance and Control

Biophysics of Heat Exchange and Balance

Figure 26.1 schematically shows energy (heat) transfers of an exercising athlete. Muscular contraction produces metabolic heat that is transferred from the active muscle to blood and the body core. Since skeletal muscle contraction is about 20% efficient, about 80% of expended energy is released as heat and must be dissipated from the body to avoid heat storage and increasing body temperature. Physiological adjustments redirect blood flow from the body core to periphery, thereby facilitating heat transfer from within the body to the skin, where it can be dissipated into the environment. Heat exchange between skin and the environment is governed

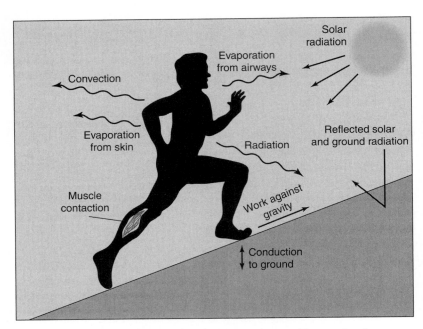

FIGURE 26.1   Avenues of energy (heat) exchange for an athlete performing exercise in air.

by biophysical properties dictated by surrounding air or water temperature; air humidity; air or water motion; solar, sky, and ground radiation; and clothing (5). The biophysical avenues of this heat exchange are conduction, convection, radiation, and evaporation. The nonevaporative (conduction, convection, and radiation) avenues are often collectively called dry heat exchange.

Conduction is heat transfer between two solid objects in direct contact, and convection is heat exchange between a surface and a fluid, including air or water. Heat exchange by conduction or convection occurs as long as there is a temperature gradient between the body surface and contacting object or surrounding fluid. When a person is standing, walking, or running and wearing shoes, heat exchange by conduction is minimal, because the thermal gradients between the body and contacted solids are usually small. Convective heat exchange is facilitated if the surrounding fluid is moving (e.g., wind, water circulation), relative to the body surface. In air environments, convective heat transfer can be significantly increased by wind if clothing does not create a barrier, and for swimmers convective heat loss can be very large, even when the difference between body surface and surrounding fluid temperature is small, since water's heat capacity is much greater than that of air: its convective heat transfer coefficient is about 25 times that of air (3). Heat loss by convection to air or water occurs when the air or water temperature is below body temperature; conversely, heat gain by convection from air or water occurs when the temperature exceeds that of the body.

Heat loss by radiation occurs when surrounding sun, sky, ground, or other large natural or manmade objects have lower surface temperatures than the body, and heat gain by radiation occurs when surrounding objects have higher surface temperatures than body surface temperature. Radiative heat exchange is independent of air temperature or motion. Accordingly, temperature combinations of the sky, ground, and surrounding objects may result in body heat gain due to radiation, even though the air temperature is below that of the body. For example, on a very sunny day a mountaineer on a snowy surface may gain a significant amount of heat despite low air temperature, and heat loss from exposed skin is greater under a clear night sky than in daylight, even when ambient air temperatures are the same.

Evaporative heat loss occurs with the phase change when liquid turns to water vapor. For humans, physiological vectors of evaporative heat loss are associated with breathing and perspiration. When water secreted onto the skin via sweat glands or rained or splashed onto the skin evaporates, or water from respiratory passages evaporates, the kinetic energy of the motion of the water molecule, latent heat of evaporation, eliminates heat from the body. Evaporative cooling accounts for almost all heat loss during exercise at ambient temperatures equal to or above skin temperatures.

Body temperature reflects the balance between internal heat production and body heat transfer to the environment. The energy balance equation describes these relationships between the body and environment:

$$S = M - (\pm W) \pm (R + C) \pm K - E$$

where S = rate of body heat storage; M = rate of metabolic energy (heat) production; W = mechanical work of either concentric (positive) or eccentric (negative) exercise; R + C =

rate of radiant and convective energy exchanges; K = rate of conduction (important only during direct contact with an object, such as clothing, or a substance, such as water); and E = rate of evaporative loss. The sum of these, heat storage, represents heat gain if positive or heat loss if negative. Body temperature increases when S is positive, decreases when S is negative, and remains constant when S equals zero (5).

Physiological Thermoregulation

Humans regulate core temperature through two collaborative processes: behavioral and physiological temperature regulation (2). Behavioral temperature regulation operates through conscious alterations in behavior that influence heat storage. It includes things like modifying activity levels, changing clothes, and seeking shade or shelter. Physiological temperature regulation operates through responses that are independent of conscious voluntary behavior. It includes control of: (a) rate of metabolic heat production (e.g., shivering), (b) body heat distribution via the blood from the core to the skin (e.g., cutaneous vasodilation and constriction), and (c) sweating. Persons often choose to ignore effective behavioral thermoregulation strategies because of their motivation to win or complete a task.

The function of the human thermoregulatory system is shown schematically in Figure 26.2 (2). This scheme presumes that thermal receptors in the core and skin send information about their temperature to some central integrator. Any deviation between the controlled variable (body temperature) and a reference variable (e.g., set-point temperature)

constitutes a load error that generates a thermal command signal to control sweating, vasodilation, vasoconstriction, and shivering. The notion of such a thermal command signal is supported by two observations: (a) Core temperature (70–90%) and skin temperature (10–30%) provide similar influence on the control of both sweating and skin blood flow responses. (b) The threshold temperatures for both sweating and skin blood flow are simultaneously shifted by a similar magnitude, by factors such as biological rhythms, endogenous pyrogens, and heat acclimatization. It is useful to think of such similar and simultaneous shifts in various thermoregulatory thresholds as representing (or as being the result of) a shift in thermoregulatory set point (6). In contrast, dynamic exercise can increase the threshold temperature for skin blood flow but not alter the threshold for sweating, so this would not be interpreted as a change in set-point temperature (7).

A disturbance in the regulated variable, core temperature, elicits graded heat loss or heat gain responses. Peripheral (skin) and central (brain, spinal column, large vessels) thermal receptors provide afferent input into hypothalamic thermoregulatory centers (8), where this information is processed, producing a load error and proportionate thermoregulatory command signal to initiate responses to regain and maintain heat balance. In addition, very small changes in hypothalamus (anterior preoptic area) temperature elicits changes in the thermoregulatory effector responses, as this area contains many neurons that increase their firing rate in response either to warming or to cooling. The magnitudes of changes in heat loss (e.g., sweating, skin blood flow), heat

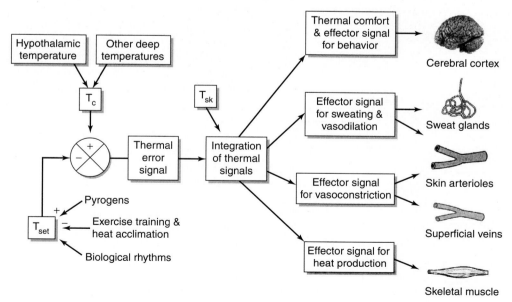

FIGURE 26.2 Human thermoregulation. *(Adapted from Sawka MN, Wenger CB, Pandolf KB. Thermoregulatory responses to acute exercise heat stress and heat acclimation. In Fregly MJ, Blatteis CM, eds. Handbook of Physiology: Section 4. Environmental Physiology. New York: Oxford University, 1996;160.)*

conservation (e.g., vasoconstriction) or production (e.g., shivering) are proportional to the displacement of the regulated variable (core temperature) from the thermoregulatory set-point temperature. The set-point temperature serves as a reference (analogous to a thermostat setting) in the control of all of the thermoregulatory responses (9). There is controversy as to whether a set point truly exists, and there are alternative theories (10).

Exercise and fever can both increase core temperature, but acute exercise does not involve a set-point increase, whereas fever does (6). Figure 26.3 shows schematically the difference in thermoregulatory control between fever and exercise hyperthermia (11). Metabolic heat production increases immediately with the initiation of exercise, causing heat storage and thus a load error (−e) or difference between set-point temperature and the elevated core temperature. The set-point temperature is unchanged, and therefore heat-dissipating responses are elicited as core temperature increases until heat loss responses sufficient to match heat production are achieved and a new thermal balance is established. When exercise stops, heat loss exceeds heat production, so core temperature falls back toward the set point. This diminishes the signal (load error) eliciting the heat dissipation responses, and they decline to baseline levels as the thermal balance conditions prevailing before exercise are reestablished. Therefore, the primary event elevating core temperature during exercise is increased metabolic heat production.

In fever, the primary event is an elevation of set-point temperature, which initially causes a negative load error (11). Heat-dissipating responses are inhibited and/or heat production is stimulated until core temperature increases enough to correct the load error and reestablish thermal balance at a new set-point temperature in which heat production and heat loss are near their values before the fever. The inhibition of heat dissipation and/or stimulation of heat production acts independently as a result of the person's thermal state and environmental temperature. When the fever abates (set point returns to normal), the heat-dissipating responses are increased and/or heat production is reduced until normal thermal balance is reestablished. If individuals perform exercise while having a fever, their exercise hyperthermia is imposed above the fever temperature.

In summary, when changes in metabolic heat production or environmental temperature upsets the thermal balance between heat dissipation and heat production, heat will be stored or lost from the body, and temperatures in the core or skin or both will change. Those temperature changes will be detected by the thermal receptors. In response to information from these receptors, the thermoregulatory controller in the central nervous system will call for responses that alter heat loss and/or production. Unless the thermal stress exceeds the capacity of the thermoregulatory system, these responses will continue until they are sufficient to restore heat balance and prevent further change in body temperatures.

Core Temperature

Fundamental to the experimental study of human temperature regulation is the measurement of body core temperature. Core temperature is measured either to provide an estimate of the core temperature input to thermoregulatory control or to estimate average internal temperature to compute changes in heat storage in the core (2). Brain (i.e., hypothalamic) temperature during exercise is probably similar to blood temperature; however, recent evidence suggests that it could be slightly higher (12). There is no one true core temperature because temperature varies among sites deep inside the body. The temperature within a given deep body region depends upon (*a*) the local metabolic rate of the surrounding tissues, (*b*) the source and magnitude of local blood flow, and (*c*) the temperature gradients between contiguous body regions. Considerable temperature gradients exist between and within orifices, body cavities, and blood vessels. For resting humans, internal organs and viscera within the body core produce about 70% of the metabolic heat. During dynamic exercise, however, skeletal muscles produce up to about 90% of the metabolic heat. Because metabolic heat sources change during exercise as compared to rest, temperature changes measured in one body region during exercise may be disproportionate to changes measured in other body regions. For example, during rest in a comfortable environment, skeletal muscle temperature is lower than core temperature, but during exercise, the temperature within active skeletal muscle often exceeds core temperature (temperature within inactive skeletal muscle usually does not increase). Blood perfusing active skeletal muscles is warmed, and the blood carries that heat to

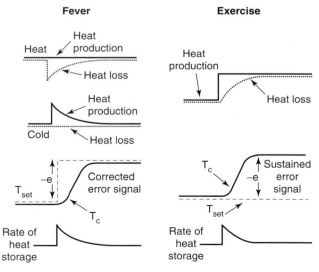

FIGURE 26.3 Differences between the elevation of core temperature in fever and during exercise. (*Adapted from Stitt JT. Fever versus hyperthermia. Fed Proc 1979;38:41, 42.*)

other body regions, and consequently, core temperature is elevated.

Core temperature during exercise is often measured at the esophagus, rectum, mouth, tympanum, and auditory meatus (2). Measurement methods employed for each of these sites and the advantages and disadvantages of each are summarized in Table 26.1. In brief, most thermal physiologists consider esophageal temperature to be the most accurate and reliable noninvasive index of core temperature for humans, followed in preference by rectal temperature and gastrointestinal tract temperature measured using ingestible temperature sensor pills. The pills are ideally suited for ambulatory monitoring outside of laboratories. Tympanic and auditory meatus temperatures are widely used, but all are influenced to some degree by head and face skin temperatures and ambient temperature and sensitive to inaccuracies related to proper placement of the sensor. Rectal and gastrointestinal tract temperatures are often slightly higher and slower to respond than esophageal temperature.

Heat Stress

Core Temperature Response to Exercise

Figure 26.4 illustrates the core (rectal and esophageal) temperature responses to two exercise bouts interspersed by a brief rest period (13). During exercise and recovery both measures of core temperature show similar patterns but with somewhat different kinetics and absolute values (rectal temperature slower to respond and slightly higher). Heat production increases almost immediately at the onset of exercise, so that during the early stages of exercise, rate of heat production exceeds rate of dissipation, and the undissipated heat is stored, primarily in the core, causing core temperature to rise. As core temperature rises, heat-dissipating reflexes are elicited, and the rate of heat storage decreases, so that core temperature rises more slowly. Eventually, as exercise continues, heat dissipation increases sufficiently to balance heat production, and essentially steady-state values are achieved. When exercise is discontinued, core temperature returns toward baseline levels, and with subsequent exercise the process is repeated.

The heat exchange components to achieve steady-state core temperature are dependent upon the environmental conditions; however, exercise type (arm vs. leg) can influence regional body heat exchange (14). Figure 26.5 illustrates the whole-body heat exchanges that might be expected during exercise (650-W metabolic rate) in a broad range of ambient temperatures (5–36°C, dry-bulb temperatures with low humidity) (15). The difference between metabolic rate and total heat loss represents the energy used for mechanical work (and heat storage or heat debt, if none steady-state). Total heat loss, and therefore heat storage and elevation of core temperature, are essentially the same in all environments. The relative contribution of dry and evaporative heat exchange to the total heat loss, however, varies with the environment. As the ambient temperature increases, the gradient for dry heat exchange diminishes and evaporative heat exchange becomes more important. When ambient temperature approaches or exceeds skin temperature, evaporative heat exchange will account for virtually all heat loss.

Heat stress can be divided into compensated heat stress (CHS) and uncompensated heat stress (UCHS). CHS and UCHS are primarily determined by biophysical factors (environment, clothing, metabolic rate) and are modestly affected by biological status (heat acclimatization and hydration status). CHS exists when heat loss occurs at a rate in balance with heat production, so that a steady-state core temperature can be achieved at a sustainable level for a requisite activity. CHS occurs in most situations. UCHS occurs when the individual's evaporative cooling requirements exceed the environment's evaporative cooling capacity. During UCHS, an individual cannot achieve steady-state core temperature, and core temperature rises until exhaustion occurs at physiological limits. Examples of UCHS include performing intense exercise in oppressive heat and wearing a football uniform while exercising in hot weather (16).

During CHS and dynamic exercise, the magnitude of the steady-state core temperature elevation is largely independent of the environment and is proportional to the metabolic rate. This idea, that steady-state core temperature elevation during exercise is independent of the CHS environment, may be inconsistent with the personal experience of some individuals. This is because there are biophysical limits to heat exchange between the environment and the

TABLE 26.1	Core Temperature Measurements	
Site	Advantage	Disadvantage
Esophageal	Accurate, rapid response	Uncomfortable, affected by swallowing
Rectal	Accurate, easy to measure	Slow response, cultural objections
Auditory canal, tympanic membrane	Easy to measure	Inaccurate (biased by skin and ambient temperature), uncomfortable
Oral	Easy to measure	Inaccurate (affected by mouth breathing)
Pill	Accurate, easy to measure	Pill movement from stomach and location influence measurement

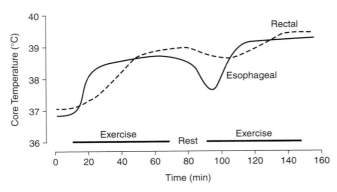

FIGURE 26.4 Core temperature (rectal and esophageal) responses to two exercise bouts separated by a brief rest period. *(Reprinted from Sawka MN, Wenger CB. Physiological responses to acute exercise heat stress. In KB Pandolf, Sawka MN, Gonzalez RR, eds. Human Performance Physiology and Environmental Medicine at Terrestrial Extremes. Indianapolis: Cooper, 1988;110.)*

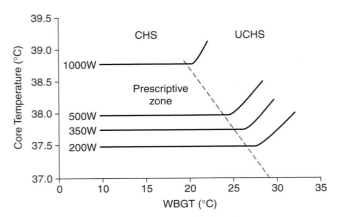

FIGURE 26.6 Possible core temperature (steady-state) responses during exercise at four metabolic rates during compensable (CHS) and uncompensable (UCHS) heat stress. *(Adapted from Lind AR. A physiological criterion for setting thermal environmental limits for everyday work. J Appl Physiol 1963;18:53.)*

performer, and core temperature may have to be elevated further to facilitate heat exchange. Actually, the magnitude of core temperature increase during exercise is independent of the environment only within a range of CHS conditions, or the "prescriptive zone" (17). Outside the prescriptive zone within CHS, a steady-state core temperature will be achieved, but it is elevated. Figure 26.6 provides an illustration of the steady-state core temperature elevation for a lightly clothed person that might be expected at several metabolic rates and wet-bulb globe temperature (WBGT) conditions in low humidity (17). The 200-, 350-, and 500-W metabolic rates approximate very light, moderate, and hard-intensity dynamic exercise for occupational tasks, respectively. For many individuals, the upper limit for sustained exercise corresponds to a metabolic rate of about 1000 W. The prescriptive zone narrows as metabolic rate increases.

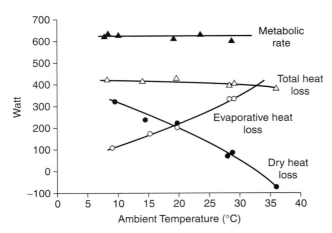

FIGURE 26.5 Heat exchange during exercise in a broad range of environmental temperatures with low humidity. *(From Nielsen M. Die Regulation der Körpertemperatur bei Muskelarbeit. Scand Arch Physiol 1938;9:216.)*

During CHS the core temperature increases in proportion to the metabolic rate during exercise (17,18). The greater the metabolic rate, the higher the steady-state core temperature during exercise. This relationship between metabolic rate and core temperature holds true for a given person but not always for comparisons between people. The use of relative intensity (percent of maximal oxygen uptake) rather than absolute metabolic rate (absolute intensity) reduces the variability between subjects for the core temperature elevation during exercise in CHS.

Acute Exercise Heat Stress

Sweating and Evaporative Cooling

For humans, unlike most animals, respiratory evaporative cooling is small compared to total skin evaporative cooling. Human skin provides the advantage over respiratory tract by virtue of a greater surface area directly exposed to ambient conditions for evaporation. Thermoregulatory sweating can begin within a few minutes after starting muscular exercise. The onset time of thermoregulatory sweating can vary and is influenced by skin temperature, acclimatization status, hydration status, and nonthermal stimuli (19).

The increase in thermoregulatory sweating closely parallels the increase in body temperature. As the sweating rate increases, first sweat glands are recruited and then sweat secretion per gland increases. Therefore, the sweat secretion for a given region of skin is dependent upon both the density of sweat glands and secretion per gland (20). In addition, different body regions of skin have different sweating responses (threshold and/or sensitivity) for a given core temperature. For a given core temperature, the back and chest have the highest sweating rates, while the limbs have relatively high sweating rates only after a substantial elevation in core temperature (21).

The eccrine glands secrete sweat onto the skin, which causes evaporative cooling by conversion of sweat from liquid to water vapor. The evaporation rate is dependent upon the gradient between the skin and water vapor pressure and the coefficient of evaporative heat transfer; and the wider the water vapor gradient, the greater the rate of evaporation for a given mass transfer coefficient (5). When 1 g of sweat is vaporized at 30°C, 2.43 kJ of heat energy becomes kinetic energy (latent heat of evaporation). The following calculations provide the minimal sweat requirements for persons performing exercise at 600-W metabolic rate in severe heat, in which only evaporative cooling is possible. If the activity is 20% efficient, the remaining 80% of metabolic energy produced is converted to heat in the body, so that 480 W (0.48 kJ · s^{-1}, or 28.8 kJ · min^{-1}) must be dissipated to avoid heat storage. The specific heat of body tissue (amount of energy required for 1 g of tissue to increase temperature by 1°C) approximates 3.5 kJ · °C^{-1}, so a 70-kg man has a heat capacity of 245 kJ · °C^{-1}. If this person performed exercise in a hot environment that enabled only evaporative heat loss and did not sweat, body temperature would increase by approximately 1.0°C every 8.5 min (245 kJ per °C, 28.8 kJ · min^{-1}). Since the latent heat of evaporation is 2.43 kJ · g^{-1}, this person would need to evaporate approximately 12 g of sweat (28.8 kJ · min^{-1}/2.43 kJ · g^{-1}) per minute, or 0.72 L · h^{-1}. Sweating, however, is not 100% efficient, because secreted sweat can drip from the body and not be evaporated. Therefore, higher sweat secretions than calculated may actually be needed to satisfy demands for cooling.

Skin Blood Flow and Dry Heat Loss

Blood transfers heat by convection from the deep body tissues to the skin. When core and skin temperatures are low enough that sweating does not occur, raising skin blood flow brings skin temperature nearer to blood temperature, and lowering skin blood flow brings skin temperature nearer to ambient temperature. Thus, the body can control dry heat loss by varying skin blood flow and thereby skin temperature. When sweating occurs, the tendency of skin blood flow to warm the skin is approximately balanced by the tendency of sweat evaporation to cool the skin. Therefore, after sweating has begun, skin blood flow serves primarily to deliver to the skin the heat that is being removed by sweat evaporation. Skin blood flow and sweating thus work in tandem to dissipate heat.

Skin circulation is affected by temperature in two ways: local skin temperature affects the vascular smooth muscle directly, and temperatures of the core and of the skin elsewhere on the body affect skin blood flow by reflexes operating through the sympathetic nervous system. Blood flow in much of the human skin is under dual vasomotor control (22). In the palm of the hand, sole of the foot, lips, ears, and nose, adrenergic vasoconstrictor fibers are probably the predominant vasomotor innervation, and the vasodilation that occurs in these regions during heat exposure is largely the result of withdrawing vasoconstrictor activity. Over most of the skin area, there is minimal vasoconstrictor activity at skin temperatures of about 39°C and above (23), and vasodilation during heat exposure depends on intact sympathetic innervation. This vasodilation depends on the action of neural signals and as such is sometimes referred to as active vasodilation. Both active vasoconstriction and active vasodilation play a major part in controlling skin blood flow of the arm, thigh, and calf. However, active vasodilation is primarily responsible for controlling skin blood flow on the torso. The mechanism or mechanisms responsible for active cutaneous vasodilation are not fully understood. It is known that active cutaneous vasodilation is usually closely associated with sweating. Whether this link is due to a cotransmitter or linkage to sudomotor neural activity is unresolved, but possible vasoactive substances include vasoactive intestinal peptide, calcitonin gene–related peptide, substance P, and nitric oxide (22).

Skin blood flow requirements to achieve heat dissipation needs change with the skin (ambient conditions and sweat evaporation) and core temperatures. Table 26.2 provides calculations for minimal skin blood flow requirements at several core and skin temperature levels. These estimates assume that blood entering and leaving the cutaneous vasculature is equal to core and skin temperatures, respectively (24). If the exercise-mediated heat production is 10 kcal · min^{-1} (about 698 W of heat production so requires a metabolic rate of 872 W [about 2.5 L oxygen uptake] with 80% of energy converted to heat) and core temperature is 38°C, the minimal skin blood flow requirement will be about 5 L · min^{-1} if skin temperature is 36°C but will decrease to 2.5 L · min^{-1} if skin temperature decreases to 34°C. This clearly demonstrates the advantage of improved evaporative cooling (lowering skin temperature) on reducing cardiovascular requirements for skin blood flow.

TABLE 26.2	Skin Blood Flow Requirements for Several Core and Skin Temperatures During Exercise Heat Stress			
Heat Production	Core Temperature	Skin Temperature	Core-to-Skin Gradient	Skin Blood Flow
10	38	36	2	5.0
10	38	34	4	2.5
10	39	36	3	3.3

Heat production in kilocalories per minute; temperatures in degrees Celsius; blood flow in liters per minute.
SKBF = 1/SH · HP/Tc − Tsk. SKBF = skin blood flow; SH = specific heat of blood ~1 Kcal per °C per liter of blood; HP = heat production.

During exercise under environmental conditions that do not allow skin cooling, the body can employ a different approach to reduce skin blood flow requirements, one of which is to tolerate an additional elevation in core temperature. If skin temperature remains at 36°C, a core temperature elevation by 1°C increases the core-to-skin temperature gradient and minimal skin blood flow requirement from 5.0 to 3.3 L · minute⁻¹ (Table 26.2). This explains the advantage of an elevated core temperature outside the prescriptive zone during CHS (Fig. 26.6). Therefore, accentuated core temperature elevations during exercise should not always be interpreted as an undesirable outcome; they may reflect a strategy to reduce cardiovascular strain to sustain thermal balance and exercise performance.

Cardiovascular Effects

During exercise heat stress, maintaining high skin blood flow can impose a substantial burden on the cardiovascular system (24). Skin blood flow can approach 8 L · min⁻¹ for an average adult during heat stress. High skin blood flow is associated with reduced right atrial pressure and filling (24). This reduction in cardiac filling occurs because the cutaneous venous bed is large and compliant and dilates during heat stress. For these reasons, the venous bed of the skin—especially below heart level—tends to become engorged with blood at the expense of central blood volume as skin blood flow increases. Sweat secretion can result in a net body water loss, thereby reducing blood volume. Therefore, heat stress can reduce cardiac filling both through pooling of blood in the skin and through reduced blood volume. To compensation for reduced cardiac filling during rest and exercise, cardiac contractility increases to maintain stroke volume because of elevated sympathetic activity and parasympathetic withdrawal and perhaps temperature effects on the cardiac pacemaker cells. In addition, whole-body heating in resting subjects can reduce carotid baroreflex control of blood pressure and vagal baroreflex regulation of heart rate, which might contribute to orthostatic intolerance during heat stress (25,26).

During exercise in the heat, the primary cardiovascular challenge is to increase cardiac output sufficiently to support both high skin blood flow for heat dissipation and high muscle blood flow for metabolism. Exercise heat stress increases skin blood flow and usually sustains muscle blood flow relative to temperate conditions; however, reduced muscle blood flow has been observed during maximal exercise with heat stress (27). Figure 26.7 provides an analysis of cardiac output and distribution during rest and dynamic exercise in temperate and hot climates (24). This figure depicts cardiac output as being elevated during mild and perhaps moderate exercise in the heat compared to similar exercise in temperate conditions. During high- and maximal-intensity exercise in the heat, cardiac output can be below levels observed during similar exercise in temperate conditions. The lower cardiac output during maximal exercise results from an inability to maintain stroke volume because of skin blood flow and pooling (28).

Brain, spinal cord, and coronary blood flow are believed to be unaffected by exercise heat stress. However, as a result of increased sympathetic activity and thermal receptor stimulation, visceral (splanchnic, renal) blood flow is reduced by both exercise and heat stress. The visceral blood flow reductions are graded to the intensity of exercise, and the effects of exercise and heat seem to be additive (24). The mechanisms responsible for changes in this splanchnic blood flow are probably quite complex (29). Reduced visceral blood flow allows a corresponding diversion of cardiac output to skin and

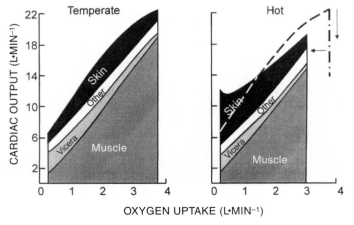

FIGURE 26.7 Comparison of cardiac output responses to exercise performed at various metabolic rates in temperate and heat stress conditions. *(From Rowell LB. Human circulation: regulation during physical stress. New York: Oxford University Press, 1986:385.)*

exercising muscle and helps support blood pressure. Also, secondary to reduced visceral blood flow, a substantial volume of blood can be mobilized from the compliant splanchnic beds to help maintain cardiac filling during exercise heat stress. If these compensatory responses are insufficient, skin and muscle blood flow may be compromised. Although Figure 26.7 indicates that muscle blood flow decreases during severe exercise heat stress, this is controversial and probably occurs only with a combination of maximal exercise or severe heat strain and dehydration (27,30).

Metabolism

The relationship between tissue temperature and metabolic processes is described by a temperature quotient (Q_{10}), which is the increase in a reaction that occurs as a function of a positive 10°C temperature change. Positive thermal dependence occurs when Q_{10} is greater than 1.0. Most mechanical (contraction velocity, power output) and chemical (enzymatic) reactions of skeletal muscle display thermal dependence on the order of 2.0–3.0.

Acute heat stress increases the metabolic rate to perform submaximal exercise, possibly because the rate of adenosine triphosphate (ATP) utilization to develop a given muscle tension is increased as muscle temperature increases (31). Aerobic metabolism and muscle total adenine pool may decrease, while oxygen debt, blood and muscle lactate accumulation, skeletal muscle glycogen utilization, and inosine 5-monophosphate concentration may all increase during exercise with higher muscle temperatures (31,32). The increased glycogen utilization is probably mediated by elevated epinephrine and muscle hyperthermia. In addition, lactate uptake and oxidation by the liver and probably nonexercising muscle are impaired during exercise heat stress. Elevated muscle temperature does not appear to alter oxidative adaptations or mitochondrial biogenesis (33,34).

Heat acclimatization usually lowers total metabolic rate during exercise because of reductions in aerobic and anaerobic components, but this effect is probably too small to reduce heat storage (31). On the other hand, changes in substrate metabolism induced by heat acclimatization may help to improve endurance. Blood and muscle lactate accumulation and muscle glycogen depletion during exercise are often reduced following heat acclimatization. The fact that these metabolic effects of heat acclimatization are observed during exercise in both temperate and hot environments suggests that chronic heat exposure may result in metabolic adaptations that are independent of thermoregulatory and cardiovascular alterations (31,32).

Exercise Performance Limitations

Performance Effects

Heat strain will degrade dynamic exercise performance and increase variability between athletes. High maximal aerobic power enables performance of tasks that require sustained high metabolic rates; therefore, a lower maximal aerobic power often translates to reduced exercise performance. Most investigators find that maximal aerobic power is lower in hot than in temperate climates. For example, maximal aerobic power was 0.25 L · min^{-1} (7%) lower at 49°C than at 21°C in one study, and the state of heat acclimatization did not alter the magnitude of the maximal aerobic power decrement (35).

What physiological mechanisms might be responsible for such a reduction in maximal aerobic power? Heat stress, by dilating the cutaneous vascular beds, might divert some cardiac output from skeletal muscle to skin, leaving less blood flow to support the metabolism of exercising skeletal muscle (27). In addition, dilation of the cutaneous vascular bed may increase cutaneous blood volume at the expense of central blood volume, reducing venous return and maximal cardiac output. For example, Rowell and associates (28) reported that during intense (73% of maximal aerobic power) exercise in the heat, cardiac output can be reduced by 1.2 L · min^{-1} below control levels. Such a reduction in cardiac output during heat exposure could account for a 0.25 L · min^{-1} decrement in maximal aerobic power, assuming each liter of blood delivers 0.2 L of oxygen (1.34 mL O_2 · g Hb^{-1} × 15 g Hb · 100 mL^{-1} of blood).

Submaximal exercise performance is also reduced by heat stress. For example, marathon performance declines by about 1 min for each 1°C increase in air temperature beyond 8 –15°C (36). Figure 26.8 presents time to fatigue during cycle ergometer exercise performed at four ambient temperatures (37). Subjects exercised 45% longer at an air temperature of 11°C compared with 31°C and had less cardiovascular strain. Core temperature at exhaustion was inversely related to air temperature but ranged narrowly from

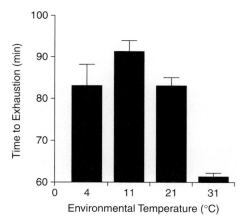

FIGURE 26.8 Exercise endurance time at a given metabolic rate in cold (4°C), cool (11°C), temperate (21°C) and warm (31°C) ambient temperatures. *(Adapted from Galloway SD, Maughan RJ. Effects of ambient temperature on the capacity to perform prolonged cycle exercise in man. Med Sci Sports Ex 1997;29:1242.)*

about 39–40°C despite large differences in exercise duration. Likewise, time to fatigue in a cool (10°C) environment even after completing a muscle glycogen–reducing regimen is even markedly longer (>30 min) than time to fatigue for glycogen-loaded subjects in a hot (30°C) environment (38). Finally, muscle heating does not have a consistent effect on maximal voluntary contraction (MVC) and will generally reduce muscle endurance at a given percentage of MVC.

Heat Strain Mechanisms of Exhaustion

Table 26.3 presents physiological mechanisms that can reduce exercise performance in the heat. These mechanisms include increased thermal and cardiovascular strain, diminished central nervous system drive for exercise, accelerated glycogen depletion with increased metabolite accumulation, and perhaps increased discomfort. The exact mechanism or mechanisms are unknown but probably depend upon the specific heat stress, exercise task, and biomedical state of the individual. For example, the increased glycogen depletion would be critical to reducing performance only if the individual could minimize the adverse consequences of elevated cardiovascular strain.

Core temperature provides the most reliable physiological index to predict the incidence of exhaustion from heat strain (39). However, as discussed earlier, the skin temperature associated with a given core temperature can greatly modify the physiological strain. Figure 26.9 illustrates some relationships between core temperature and incidence of exhaustion from heat strain for heat-acclimated persons exercising in uncompensable (most likely very hot skin) and compensable (most likely cool skin) heat stress (40). During uncompensable heat stress, exhaustion is rarely associated with a core temperature below 38°C, and exhaustion will almost always occur before a core temperature of 40°C (39). Remember, a skin temperature above 35°C, as seen during uncompensable heat stress, will be associated with greater cardiovascular strain for a given core temperature (41) and therefore result in earlier exhaustion. If skin is relatively cool, higher core temperatures can be better sustained during exercise.

Some elite athletes can tolerate core temperatures above 40°C and continue to exercise. It is unknown whether their tolerance to high core temperatures results from extensive heat acclimatization, training practices, natural selection, or a combination of these factors. Regardless, for a given athlete the exercise heat stress condition and how the high core temperature with skin temperature is achieved contribute to this variability. For example, skin temperature that starts low and rises throughout exercise will allow a higher core temperature than if skin temperature is constantly hot. For many hot weather conditions, the expected incidence of exhaustion will probably fall somewhere between the two extremes in Figure 26.9.

The role of cardiovascular strain on reducing exercise performance has been discussed earlier. Another possible mechanism is that hyperthermia itself might be an impetus for a central nervous system–mediated diminished drive to exercise (42). There is growing evidence in both humans and animals of a role for serotonin contributing to the genesis of fatigue from exercise hyperthermia. The effects of serotonin in the nervous system may be excitatory or inhibitory, depending largely on the brain region and the receptor involved, but general agreement is that acute serotonin accumulation produces an overall feeling of sleepiness and lethargy. Peripheral measurements of prolactin concentrations have been used as a biomarker for brain serotonergic activity and may increase with core temperature elevations above 38°C (43). Therefore, heat strain may elevate brain serotonin levels and reduce the desire to continue exercise. Consistent with this hypothesis, exercise in the heat can induce changes in electroencephalographic activity from the frontal cortex that are consistent with changes seen with drowsiness (44).

The first convincing demonstration that the central nervous system may mediate reduced exercise performance in the heat was provided by Lars Nybo and Bodil Nielsen of Denmark (42) (Milestone of Discovery). These experiments demonstrated that exercise hyperthermia (40°C) markedly reduces voluntary force-generating capacity during a prolonged MVC in both active (leg) and inactive (forearm) muscles when compared to that measured at a core temperature of 38°C. However, electrical stimulation of these hyperthermic muscles restored total force generation to that of the lower-temperature trial. These data strongly suggest a central

TABLE 26.3	Physiological Mechanisms Contributing to Reduced Exercise Performance During Heat Stress	
Mechanism	**Causes**	**Consequence**
Cardiovascular strain	High skin blood flow Compliant skin Dehydration	Inability to maintain required cardiac output and blood pressure
Central fatigue	High brain temperature	Reduced neural drive to exercise
Thermal discomfort	Hot and wet skin High heart rate	Reduced desire to exercise
Muscle glycogen depletion	High muscle temperature High sympathetic activity	Insufficient carbohydrate substrate

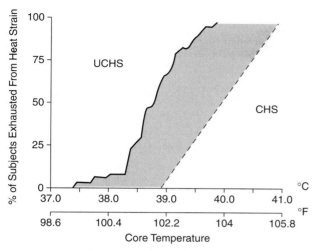

FIGURE 26.9 Relationship between core temperature and incidence of exhaustion from heat strain during exercise in compensable heat stress (CHS) and uncompensable heat stress (UCHS). *(Adapted from Sawka MN, Young AJ. Physical exercise in hot and cold climates. In: Garrett WE, Kirkendall DT, eds. Exercise and Sports Science. Philadelphia: Lippinocott Williams & Wilkins, 2000:389.)*

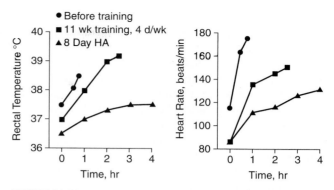

FIGURE 26.10 Core temperature and heart rate responses during standardized exercise heat stress when untrained and not acclimatized to heat, after 11 weeks of physical training and after 8 days of heat acclimatization. *(Adapted from Cohen, JS, Gisolfi CV. Effects of interval training on work-heat tolerance of young women. Med Sci Sports Exerc 1982;14:46–52.)*

nervous system component contributing to the reduced exercise performance of individuals exercising in hyperthermic conditions.

Psychological strain is probably an important factor determining an individual's desire to continue exercise in the heat. Thermal discomfort is influenced by factors including skin temperature and wetness (10), while rated perceived exertion is influenced by both of these factors as well as heart rate. It is doubtful that high core temperature alone can be sensed, but high brain temperature might induce neurochemical changes that modify perception of strain. During exercise in the heat, skin temperature, wetness, and heart rate will increase. Athletes' individual tolerance to such perceptual cues will most likely influence their exercise capabilities.

Exercise Training and Heat Acclimatization
Dynamic Exercise Training

Dynamic exercise training in a temperate climate with emphasis on improved aerobic performance can reduce physiological strain and improve exercise capabilities in the heat, but such exercise training programs alone cannot replace the benefits of heat acclimatization (45,46). Figure 26.10 depicts an exercise training program with heat acclimatization on reducing physiological strain and improving endurance during exercise heat stress (47). After completing an initial (pretraining) exercise heat test (4 h at about 35% maximal aerobic power in hot, dry conditions) the subjects completed the training program (1 h a day, 4 times per wk for 11 wk in temperate conditions), then again completed the exercise heat test. Finally, subjects completed a heat acclimatization

program (35% maximal aerobic power, 4 h per day for 8 days) then again completed the exercise heat test. The exercise training reduces physiological strain and improves endurance, but these improvements are modest compared to those obtained by heat acclimatization.

Dynamic exercise training in temperate climates can improve heat loss responses during exercise heat stress, but not to the same magnitude as is induced by heat acclimatization (45,46). Figure 26.11 illustrates the impact of exercise training and heat acclimatization on improving sweating responses. Local sweating responses during exercise heat stress were measured on untrained and not acclimatized subjects, after 10 days of exercise training (70–80% maximal aerobic power in temperate conditions), and after 10 days

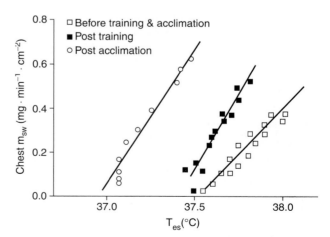

FIGURE 26.11 Local sweating responses during standardized exercise heat stress when untrained and unacclimatized to heat, after completing a physical training program, and after completing a heat acclimatization program. *(From Roberts MF, Wenger CB, Stolwijk JAJ, et al. Skin blood flow and sweating changes following exercise training and heat acclimation. J Appl Physiol 1977;43:135.)*

of heat acclimatization (1 hour at 50% maximal aerobic power in hot, wet conditions) (48). Exercise training increased the slope of the sweating response, but heat acclimatization markedly reduced threshold temperature to initiate sweating as soon as core temperature started to rise. The net effect of heat acclimatization is a substantially increased sweating rate for a given core temperature during exercise. The skin blood flow responses change in a similar manner to sweating after exercise training and heat acclimatization. Clearly, exercise training can improve heat loss responses; however, these improvements are modest compared to those obtained by heat acclimatization.

For exercise training to improve thermoregulation and exercise capabilities in the heat, the training sessions must produce a substantial elevation of core temperature and sweating rate (45). To achieve optimal improvement in thermoregulation with aerobic exercise training in temperate climates, the intensity should be at least 50% of maximal aerobic power with a minimal duration of 1 wk and for perhaps as long as 8 wk (45).

Heat Acclimatization

Heat acclimatization induces biological adjustments that reduce the negative effects of heat stress. Heat acclimatization develops through repeated heat exposures that are sufficiently stressful to elevate both core and skin temperatures and provoke perfuse sweating. The biological adjustments are mediated by integrated changes in thermoregulatory control, fluid balance, and cardiovascular responses. In addition to these systemic adaptations, emerging research information demonstrates that cellular adaptations occur (49).

The magnitude of biological adaptations induced by heat acclimatization depends largely on the intensity, duration, frequency, and number of heat exposures. Exercise in the heat is the most effective method for developing heat acclimatization; however, even resting in the heat results in limited acclimatization. Usually, about 7–10 days of heat exposure is needed to induce heat acclimatization. Optimal heat acclima-tization requires a minimum daily heat exposure of about 2 h (can be broken into two 1-h exposures) combined with dynamic exercise that requires cardiovascular endurance rather than resistance training for development of muscular strength. Individuals in training should gradually increase the exercise intensity or duration each day of heat acclimatization.

During the initial exercise heat exposure, physiological strain is high, as manifested by elevated core temperature and heart rate. The physiological strain induced by the same exercise heat stress decreases each day of acclimatization. Most of the improvements in heart rate, skin and core temperatures, and sweat rate are achieved through daily exercise in a hot climate during the first week of exposure. The heart rate reduction develops most rapidly in 4–5 days. After 7 days, the reduction in heart rate is virtually complete. The thermoregulatory benefits from heat acclimatization are generally thought to be complete after 10–14 days of exposure (46). However, improvements in physiological tolerance may take longer (39).

Heat acclimatization is transient and gradually disappears if not maintained by continued repeated heat exposure (45,46). The benefits of heat acclimatization will be retained for about 1 week and then decay, with about 75% lost by about 3 wk once heat exposure ends. A day or two of intervening cool weather will not interfere with acclimatization to hot weather. The heart rate improvement, which develops more rapidly during acclimatization, is also lost more rapidly than thermoregulatory responses.

Table 26.4 provides a brief description of the actions of heat acclimatization. Heat acclimatization improves thermal comfort and submaximal aerobic exercise capabilities. These benefits of heat acclimatization are achieved by improved sweating and skin blood flow responses, better fluid balance and cardiovascular stability, and a lowered metabolic rate (2). Heat acclimatization is specific to the climate (desert or jungle) and physical activity level. However, heat acclimatization to a desert or jungle climate can markedly improve exercise capabilities in the other hot climate.

TABLE 26.4	Actions of Heat Acclimatization	
Thermal Comfort Improved	**Exercise Performance Improved**
Core temperature reduced	*Cardiovascular stability improved*
Sweating improved	Heart rate lowered
Earlier onset	**Stroke volume increased**
Higher rate	Blood pressure better defended
Redistribution (*jungle*)	Myocardial compliance improved
Hidromeiosis resistance (*jungle*)	Fluid balance improved
	Thirst improved
Skin blood flow improved	Electrolyte loss (sweat, urine) reduced
Earlier onset	Total body water increased
Higher rate (*jungle*)	**Plasma (blood) volume increased,** better defended
Metabolic rate lowered	Acquired thermal tolerance improved

Heat acclimatization does not improve maximal exercise performance. For example, heat stress–mediated reductions in maximal aerobic power are not abated by heat acclimatization (35). In addition, heat acclimatization probably does not alter the maximal core temperature a person can tolerate during exercise during CHS (50,51). There is some evidence, however, that persons who live and physically train over many weeks in the heat may be able to tolerate higher maximal core temperatures during UCHS (39).

The effect of heat acclimatization on submaximal exercise performance can be quite dramatic, such that acclimatized subjects can easily complete tasks in the heat that earlier were difficult or impossible (Fig. 26.10). Heat acclimatization mediates improved submaximal exercise performance by reducing body temperature and physiological strain (Fig. 26.10). The three classical signs of heat acclimatization are lower heart rate and core temperature and higher sweat rate during exercise heat stress. Skin temperatures are often lower after heat acclimatization, and thus dry heat loss is less (or if the environment is warmer than the skin, dry heat gain is greater). To compensate for the changes in dry heat exchange, an increase in evaporative heat loss is necessary to achieve heat balance.

After acclimatization, sweating starts earlier and at a lower core temperature; that is, the core temperature threshold for sweating is decreased (Fig. 26.11). The sweat glands also become resistant to hidromeiosis and fatigue, so that higher sweat rates can be sustained. Sweating rate is often increased by the second day of heat acclimatization. Earlier and greater sweating improves evaporative cooling (if the climate allows evaporation) and reduces body heat storage and skin temperature. Lower skin temperatures decrease the cutaneous blood flow required for heat balance (because of greater core-to-skin temperature gradient) and reduce cutaneous venous compliance, so that blood volume is redistributed from the peripheral to the central circulation. All of these factors reduce cardiovascular strain and enhance exercise heat performance.

The effects of heat acclimatization on cardiac output responses to exercise heat stress are not clearcut. Some studies report little change in cardiac output, while most find an increase in cardiac output during submaximal exercise performed after heat acclimatization as compared to before it. Heart rate is much higher and stroke volume is lower (than in temperate conditions) during exercise heat stress on the first day of heat acclimatization. Thereafter, heart rate begins to decrease as early as the second day. These changes are rapid at first but continue more slowly for about a week. Probably numerous mechanisms participate, and their relative contributions will vary, both over the course of the program and also among subjects (2). These mechanisms include (a) improved skin cooling and redistribution of blood volume, (b) plasma volume expansion, (c) increased venous tone from cutaneous and noncutaneous beds, and (d) reduced core temperature. In addition, myocardial changes from heat acclimatization include increased compliance and isoenzyme transition, reducing the myocardial energy cost (52).

Fluid balance improvements from heat acclimatization include better matching of thirst to body water needs, increased total body water, and increased blood volume (53,54). Most but not all studies report that heat acclimatization increases total body water (54). The magnitude of increase often approximates 2.0 L, or about 5% of total body water. This increase is well within the measurement resolution for total body water and thus appears to be a real physiological phenomenon. The division of the total body water increase between intracellular fluid and extracellular fluid varies: studies have reported that extracellular fluid accounts for greater, equal, and smaller amounts of the percentage increase compared to intracellular fluid after heat acclimatization (54). Measures of extracellular fluid have relatively high variability, and therefore trends for such small changes are difficult to interpret. The extent to which intracellular fluid increases is unclear, because typically it is calculated as the difference between total body water and extracellular fluid, and thus measurement variability inherent in both these techniques is compounded in the calculation of intracellular fluid. If total body water and extracellular fluid increase after heat acclimatization, then expansion of plasma volume might be expected.

Plasma volume expansion is usually but not always present after repeated heat exposure and heat acclimatization (55). Erythrocyte volume does not appear to be altered by heat acclimatization. Heat acclimatization studies report that plasma volume expansion generally ranges from about 5% to about 30%, and the magnitude of increase somewhat depends on (a) whether the person is at rest or performing exercise, (b) the day of heat acclimatization, and (c) the hydration state when measurements are made. Plasma volume expansion seems to be greatest during upright exercise on about the fifth day of heat acclimatization in fully hydrated persons who are living in the heat.

The mechanisms responsible for this hypervolemia are unclear, but they include an increase in extracellular fluid mediated by retention of crystalloids (primarily sodium chloride) and perhaps an increase in plasma volume selectively mediated by the oncotic effect of increased volume of intravascular protein (no change in content) (54). The increase in total body water can be explained in part by increased aldosterone secretion and/or renal sensitivity to a given plasma concentration. An unacclimatized person may secrete sweat with a sodium concentration of 60 mEq $\cdot$ L^{-1} or higher and if sweating profusely, can lose large amounts of sodium. With acclimatization, the sweat glands conserve sodium by secreting sweat with a sodium concentration as low as 10 mEq $\cdot$ L^{-1}. This salt-conserving effect of acclimatization depends on the hormone aldosterone, which is secreted in response to exercise and heat exposure as well as to sodium depletion. The conservation of salt also helps to maintain the number of osmoles in the extracellular fluid and thus to maintain or increase extracellular fluid volume.

Acquired Thermal Tolerance and Molecular Changes

Individuals who are repeatedly exposed to the hyperthermia of exercise can become more resistant to exertional heat injury and stroke. The repeated heating of body tissues results in acquired thermal tolerance, cellular changes resulting from severe nonlethal heat exposure that allow the organism to survive a subsequent otherwise lethal heat exposure (1,56). Acquired thermal tolerance and heat acclimatization are complementary, as acclimatization reduces heat strain and thermal tolerance increases survivability in a given heat load. For example, rodents with fully developed thermal tolerance can survive 60% more heat load than what would have been initially lethal (57).

Acquired thermal tolerance is associated with heat shock proteins (HSP) binding to denatured or nascent cellular polypeptides and providing protection and accelerating repair from heat stress, ischemia, monocyte toxicity, and ultraviolet radiation in cultured cells and animals. These HSP are grouped into families by molecular mass (56). Each has a variety of cellular locations and functions that include processing of stress-denatured proteins, management of protein fragments, maintenance of structural proteins, and chaperone of proteins across cell membranes. For example, HSP 27 (sometimes referred to as sHSP), resides in the cytosol and nucleus and has antiapoptotic and microfilament stabilization functions. The HSP 70 family (HSP 72, 73, 75, 78) resides in the cytosol and nucleus (HSP 72 and 73), endoplasmic reticulum (HSP 78), and mitochondria (HSP 75) and has molecular chaperone (HSP 73,75, 78), cytoprotection (HSP 72) and antiapoptotic (HSP 73) functions.

The HSP responses increase within several hours of the stress and last for several days after the exposure. After the initial heat exposure, mRNA levels peak within an hour, and subsequent HSP synthesis depends upon both severity of heat stress and cumulative heat stress (57). Both heat exposure and high-intensity dynamic exercise elicit HSP synthesis; however, the combination of dynamic exercise and heat exposure elicits a greater HSP response than either stressor independently (58). In addition, HSP responses vary with specific tissue, as brain and liver demonstrate greater responses than skeletal muscle. The cellular mechanisms mediating thermal tolerance are not fully understood, but it seems probable that the stress kinase pathways (59) and other cellular systems contribute (60,61).

Fluid and Electrolyte Imbalances

Water balance represents the net difference between water intake and loss. During exercise in the heat, water losses primarily occur from respiration and sweating. Renal water losses will be minimal and respiratory water losses will usually be approximately offset by metabolic water production (62). Therefore, sweat losses determine most of a person's water needs. Also, since sweat contains electrolytes (primarily sodium and chloride), prolonged periods of high sweat losses can lead to electrolyte deficits.

A person's sweating rate depends on the climatic conditions, clothing, and exercise intensity. Persons in desert and tropical climates often have sweating rates of 0.3–1.0 L $\cdot$ h^{-1} while performing occupational activities. Competitive marathon runners' sweating rates average about 0.8 L $\cdot$ h^{-1} (range 0.7–1.4 L $\cdot$ h^{-1}) and about 1.2 L $\cdot$ h^{-1} (range 0.9–2.8 L $\cdot$ h^{-1}) in cool to temperate and warm to hot weather, respectively (63). Active individuals, however, have high sweating rates only for several hours per day, and the remainder of time, when more sedentary, they have lower sweating rates. For competitive athletes training in temperate and hot weather, daily fluid requirements may range from 3–5 L and 4–10 L, respectively (62).

Dehydration

Persons dehydrate (sustain a body water deficit) during exercise because of unavailability of fluid or a mismatch between thirst and body water requirements. In these instances, the person starts the exercise task with normal total body water and dehydrates over time. This scenario is common for most athletic and occupational settings; however, sometimes the person starts exercise with a body water deficit. For example, in several sports (e.g., boxing, power lifting, wrestling) athletes purposefully dehydrate to compete in lower weight classes. Also, persons medicated with diuretics may be dehydrated prior to exercise. Dehydration from water deficit without excessive sodium chloride loss is the most commonly seen type during relatively short-term exercise in the heat if a normal diet is consumed. If the person has a large sodium chloride deficit, the extracellular fluid volume will contract and cause salt depletion dehydration. If the sodium chloride deficit is combined with excessive water consumption, hyponatremia, or water intoxication, can more easily occur (64).

Regardless of the approach used to induce dehydration, there is great similarity in altered physiological function and performance consequences. Dehydration can decrease dynamic exercise performance, including maximal aerobic power (54). Dehydration by more than 2% of body weight degrades endurance exercise, especially in heat (65). The magnitude of the performance decrement is variable and probably depends on the individual, the environment, and the exercise mode. However, for a given person and event, the greater the dehydration level (after achieving the threshold for performance degradation), the greater the performance decrement. Dehydration probably does not alter muscle strength but sometimes has been reported to reduce anaerobic performance (66). In addition, dehydration of more than 2% often adversely influences cognitive function in the heat; however, this area requires more research (62).

Physiological factors that contribute to dehydration-mediated performance decrements include increased hyperthermia, increased cardiovascular strain, altered metabolic function, and perhaps altered central nervous system function. Though each factor is unique, evidence suggests that they interact to contribute in concert, rather than in isolation, to degrading exercise performance. The relative contribution of each factor may differ depending on the endurance event, environmental conditions, and athlete prowess, but elevated hyperthermia probably acts to accentuate the performance decrement (65).

Dehydration increases core temperature responses during exercise in temperate and hot climates (54). A body water deficit of as little as 2% of body weight can elevate core temperature during exercise. As the magnitude of water deficit increases, there is a concomitant graded elevation of core temperature during exercise in the heat. The magnitude of core temperature elevation approximates 0.2°C for every percent body weight lost, and it is influenced by the environment. The hotter the environment and greater the evaporative heat loss requirement, probably the greater the core temperature elevation. Dehydration not only elevates core temperature; it negates the core temperature advantages conferred by high aerobic fitness and heat acclimatization. In addition, dehydration lowers the core temperature that can be tolerated before exhaustion from heat strain during uncompensable heat stress.

When a person is dehydrated, the elevated core temperature responses during exercise result from reduced heat dissipation. Both sweating and skin blood flow are reduced for a given core temperature during dehydration (54). For both thermoregulatory effector responses (sweat secretion and active cutaneous vasodilation), threshold temperature (body temperature at initiation of heat loss response) is increased and sensitivity (increase in heat loss for a given increase in body temperature) is reduced during dehydration. For thermoregulatory sweating, the increased threshold temperature and reduced sensitivity are proportional to the level of dehydration. Therefore, the degraded sweating response represents an attempt to conserve body water losses. Whole-body sweating is usually either reduced or unchanged during exercise at a given metabolic rate in the heat. However, even when dehydration is associated with no change in whole-body sweating rate, core temperature is usually elevated, so that whole-body sweating rate for a given core temperature is lower when dehydrated.

Both the singular and combined effects of plasma hyperosmolality and hypovolemia mediate the reduced heat loss response during exercise heat stress (67). Plasma hyperosmolality with no change in blood volume can increase core temperature by reducing heat loss during rest or exercise in the heat. In addition, reestablishment of blood volume that is still hyperosmotic does not alter the core temperature elevation compared to responses to dehydration during prolonged exercise in the heat. Plasma volume reductions with no change in osmolality can increase core temperature and impair heat loss during exercise in the heat (67).

Dehydration increases cardiovascular strain during dynamic exercise in temperate and hot climates (54). During submaximal dynamic exercise with little heat strain, dehydration elicits an increase in heart rate and decrease in stroke volume but usually no change in cardiac output relative to euhydration levels. Heat stress and dehydration, however, have additive effects on cardiovascular strain. If evaporative cooling is reduced, the skin temperature will be elevated, which increases compliance (superficial cutaneous veins) and acts to transfer blood from central to peripheral circulation. This transfer of blood volume, combined with the hypovolemia, acts to reduce cardiac filling and stroke volume, making it more difficult to sustain sufficient cardiac output to support muscle metabolism. The inability to sustain sufficient cardiac output provides a cardiovascular limitation to exercise in the heat. During submaximal dynamic exercise with moderate or severe heat strain, dehydration (3–4% body weight) leads to a decrease in cardiac output. The dehydration-mediated cardiac output reduction (below euhydration levels) during heat stress is greater during high-intensity (65% maximal aerobic power) than low-intensity (25% maximal aerobic power) exercise. In addition, severe water deficit (7% body weight) in the absence of heat strain can reduce cardiac output during submaximal exercise.

During severe exercise heat stress when dehydration mediates a reduction in cardiac output, the skeletal muscle blood flow can also be decreased (30). Despite having decreased muscle blood flow, substrate delivery and lactate removal are not impaired by dehydration. However, dehydration can reduce free fatty acid uptake and increase muscle glycogen utilization and muscle lactate production during intense exercise. The dehydration-associated increase in muscle glycogen utilization during exercise is probably mediated by elevated catecholamine levels.

Dehydration might reduce exercise performance through mechanisms mediated by the central nervous system. As discussed earlier, dehydration elevates body temperature, and there is evidence that hyperthermia might diminish the drive to exercise and reduce exercise tolerance time.

Hypervolemia and Hyperhydration

Hypervolemia, or blood volume expansion, can improve thermoregulation and exercise performance in the heat if the erythrocyte volume alone or erythrocyte volume and plasma volume together are expanded (54,68). Plasma volume expansion alone does not provide a thermoregulatory benefit, but it does reduce cardiovascular strain (54). Studies that only expanded erythrocyte volume have demonstrated small thermoregulatory benefits, but when both erythrocyte volume and plasma volume were expanded, more substantial benefits were observed. The former experiments were on unacclimatized subjects, and the latter experiments were on heat-acclimatized subjects, so it is unclear whether accentuated thermoregulatory benefits resulted from simultaneous expansion of both vascular volumes or the subjects' acclimatization state (68).

Hyperhydration, or above-normal body water, has been suggested to improve, above euhydration levels, thermoregulation and exercise heat performance (54). The concept that hyperhydration might be beneficial for exercise performance arose from the recognition of the adverse consequences of dehydration. It was theorized that an increase in body water might reduce cardiovascular and thermal strain of exercise by expanding blood volume and reducing blood tonicity, thereby improving exercise performance. In some studies that have evaluated hyperhydration effects on thermoregulation in the heat, smaller core temperature elevations during exercise were observed with hyperhydration, but those studies generally have confounding factors in experimental procedures. Studies that were carefully controlled for these confounding factors have not observed any thermoregulatory advantages with either water hyperhydration or glycerol hyperhydration during exercise heat stress (54).

Hyponatremia

Symptomatic hyponatremia (serum sodium concentration of 125–130 mEq $\cdot$ L^{-1}) has been observed during prolonged marathon and ultramarathon competition, military training, and recreational activities (64). Symptomatic hyponatremia is very rare, and hospitalizations occur at a rate of less than 1 per 100,000 person years for U.S. Army soldiers (69). The severity of symptoms is probably related to the serum sodium concentration and the rapidity with which it develops. If hyponatremia develops over many hours, there may be less brain swelling and less adverse symptoms than when changes are rapid. Hyponatremia usually develops because a person drinks excessively large quantities of hypotonic fluids for many hours. However, other factors, such as excessive sodium losses, nausea (which increases vasopressin

levels), and heat or exercise stress (which reduce renal blood flow and urine output), can contribute when excessively large volumes of fluids are consumed. For a person to become hyponatremic, total body water usually must be markedly increased, and excessive intake of hypotonic fluids and/or significant sodium loss must occur (64).

Table 26.5 presents the predicted serum sodium response to prolonged exercise (90-km ultramarathon foot race) for two individuals of low and average body mass, with three sweat sodium concentrations, who replace their sweat losses with sodium-free fluid (64). For the example, it is assumed that total body water is 63% of body mass and that water distributes within the extracellular fluid and intracellular fluid until osmotic equilibrium is reached. This analysis illustrates that sweat sodium losses are an important contributor to the reduction of serum sodium when water or a sodium-free solution is used to replace sweat lost during exercise. In the example provided, if a 70-kg man had sweat sodium concentrations of 25, 50, and 75 mEq $\cdot$ L^{-1} and drank sufficient sodium-free water to replace all of the 8.6 L of sweat loss, serum sodium would be expected to decline about 5, 10, and 15 mEq $\cdot$ L^{-1}. However, to lower the serum sodium to the average value reported for individuals with symptomatic hyponatremia (121 mEq $\cdot$ L^{-1}), the 70-kg man would still have to accrue a fluid excess of 5.1, 3.3, and 1.6 L at the low, moderate, and high sweat sodium concentrations, respectively. Example calculation for a 70-kg person with low sweat sodium: x / 44 L TBW × 135 mEq $\cdot$ L^{-1} / 121 mEq $\cdot$ L^{-1} = 49.1 L; then 49.1–44 = 5.1 L.

This analysis also illustrates that smaller individuals with similar sweat sodium concentrations will develop symptoms in the presence of less fluid excess to dilute serum sodium than larger persons. Therefore, if a group of people are drinking at the same rate (as may happen if they follow drinking schedules that are not adjusted for body mass), the individuals with smaller body mass will dilute their extra-

TABLE 26.5	Predicted Serum Sodium Values to Prolonged Exercise[a]					
Body mass, kg		50			70	
Total body water, L		31.5			44	
extracellular fluid, L		12.5			17.5	
Serum [Na$^+$], mEq $\cdot$ L^{-1}		140			140	
extracellular fluid Na$^+$, mEq		1750			2450	
Running velocity, km $\cdot$ h^{-1}		10			10	
Sweat loss, liters		6.1			8.6	
Calculations of serum sodium dilution if water intake is equal to sweat loss						
Sweat [Na$^+$], mEq $\cdot$ L^{-1}	25	50	75	25	50	75
Na$^+$ loss, mEq	153	305	458	215	430	645
Δ TBW osmol $\cdot$ L^{-1}	4.9	9.7	14.5	4.9	9.8	14.7
Serum [Na$^+$], mEq $\cdot$ L^{-1}	135.1	130.3	125.5	135.1	130.2	125.3
Fluid excess to dilute serum Na$^+$ to 121 mEq $\cdot$ L^{-1}	3.7	2.4	1.2	5.1	3.3	1.6

[a]90-km ultramarathon foot race for two body masses, when body mass is preserved by ingestion of sodium-free water.

cellular sodium levels more quickly and further than those with larger body mass. On the other hand, to produce the magnitude of sodium dilution observed in symptomatic hyponatremia cases, persons who are larger than 70 kg either would have to substantially overdrink relative to sweating rate or would have to have an abnormally high sweat sodium concentration.

Environmental Heat Stress

Sports and occupational medicine communities commonly use WBGT to quantify environmental heat stress and set limits on exercise in planned strategies designed to minimize the risk of serious exertional heat illness. WBGT is an empirical index of climatic heat stress: outdoor WBGT = 0.7 natural wet bulb + 0.2 black globe + 0.1 dry bulb. Indoor WBGT = 0.7 natural wet bulb + 0.3 black globe. (Natural wet bulb is a stationary wet-bulb thermometer exposed to the sun and prevailing wind. The black globe thermometer consists of a 6-inch hollow copper sphere painted flat black on the outside, containing a thermometer with its bulb at the center of the sphere.) High WBGT values can be achieved either through high air (dry bulb) temperature and solar load, as reflected in black-globe temperature, or through high humidity, as reflected in high wet-bulb temperature. However, WBGT underestimates heat stress risk for humid conditions, so different guidance tables should be used in low-, moderate-, and high-humidity climates. Table 26.6 provides the relative risk of excessive hyperthermia and possibly serious exertional heat illness for an individual exercising in the heat or an athlete competing in running events while lightly clothed and sustaining a high metabolic rate (70).

Exertional Heat Illness

Serious exertional heat illnesses occupy a continuum of increasing severity of heat exhaustion, heat injury, and heat stroke (69). Heat exhaustion is defined as a mild to moderate illness characterized by inability to sustain cardiac output with moderate (>38.5°C) to high (>40°C) body temperature resulting from strenuous exercise and environmental heat exposure. Exertional heat injury is defined as a moderate to severe illness characterized by organ (e.g., liver, renal) and tissue (e.g., gut, muscle) injury with high body temperature resulting from strenuous exercise and environmental heat exposure. Exertional heat stroke is defined as a severe illness characterized by central nervous system dysfunction, organ (e.g., liver, renal), and tissue (e.g., gut, muscle) injury with high body temperatures resulting from strenuous exercise and environmental heat exposure.

Risk factors for serious exertional heat illness include lack of heat acclimatization, low physical fitness, dehydration and high body fat or mass, and certain medications (Table 26.7). However, serious exertional heat illness can occur in low-risk persons who are practicing sound heat mitigation procedures. Exertional heat injury and stroke often occur under conditions the victim has been exposed to many times before or while others are concurrently being exposed to the same condition without incident. This suggests that these victims were inherently more vulnerable that day and/or some unique event triggered the heat injury.

Many victims of exertional heat stroke were sick the previous day. Exertional heat stroke often occurs during the initial hours of exercise heat stress and may not occur during the hottest part of the day. These facts suggest that on that day, the victim began the exercise already heat stress compromised. Fever and inflammatory responses from muscle injury may adversely influence thermoregulation and may help mediate subsequent exertional heat injury or stroke. Gastrointestinal problems will induce dehydration and increase the risk of serious exertional heat illness or may indicate previous heat injury (e.g., gut ischemia causing endotoxin leakage). Evidence suggests that some cases of exertional heat injury or stroke might be explained by an association between susceptibility to malignant hyperthermia and exertional heat stroke.

Recent research shows that exertional heat injury (unlike heat shock *in vitro*), produces a broad spectrum of

TABLE 26.6	Risk of Hyperthermia and Possible Exertional Heat Illness for a Typical Marathon Racer[a]			
Risk of Hyperthermia	Color Code (flag)	WBGT, °C (°F) RH, 100%	WBGT, °C (°F) RH, 75%	WBGT, °C (°F) RH, 50%
Excessive	Black	>28	>29	>33
High	Red	24–28 (73–82)	26–29 (77–85)	28–33 (82–92)
Moderate	Amber	18–23 (65–72)	20–25 (68–76)	24–27 (75–81)
Low	Green	<18 (<65)	<20 (<68)	<24 (<75)
Low (some risk of hypothermia)	White	<10 (<50)	<10 (<50)	<10 (<50)

[a]Based on wet-bulb globe temperature (WBGT) and relative humidity (RH).

TABLE 26.7	Drugs Implicated in Intolerance to Heat Stress
Drug or Drug Class	**Proposed Mechanism of Action**
Anticholinergics (Atropine)	Impaired sweating
Antihistamines	Impaired sweating
Glutethimide (Doriden)	Impaired sweating
Phenothiazines (antipsychotic drugs, e.g., chlorpromazine [Thorazine], trifluoperazine [Stelazine], perphenazine [Trilafon])	Impaired sweating, (possibly) disturbed hypothalamic temperature regulation
Tricyclic antidepressants, e.g., imipramine, amitriptyline	Impaired sweating, increased motor activity and heat production
Amphetamines, cocaine	Increased psychomotor activity, activated vascular endothelium
Ergogenic stimulants, e.g., ephedrine, ephedra	Increased heat production
Lithium	Nephrogenic diabetes insipidus and water loss
Diuretics	Salt depletion and dehydration
β-Blockers, e.g., propranolol, atenolol	Reduced skin blood flow, reduced blood pressure
Ethanol	Diuresis, possible effects on intestinal permeability

gene expression changes, including interferon-induced sequences (61). Elevated levels of circulating interferon-γ are reported in victims of classic heat stroke, and it can increase cellular mortality by apoptosis after heat shock. A prior incident of cellular heat shock or some other unknown event might mediate expression of interferon genes and subsequently elevated circulating interferon-γ levels. Expression of this or another cytokine might contribute to the pathogenesis of exertional heat injury (71).

Figure 26.12 provides a diagram of the possible progression of heat strain to exertional heat injury and/or stroke (71). The hyperthermia and cardiovascular responses to exercise heat stress can result in reduced perfusion of the intestine and other body tissues, resulting in ischemia and excessively high tissue temperatures (heat shock, >41°C). The magnitude and duration of the heat shock will influence whether the cell responds by adaptation (acquired thermal tolerance), injury, or death (apoptotic or necrotic) (56,59). This can result in a variety of systemic coagulation and inflammatory responses (71). It is suspected that the inflammatory response is primed (e.g., leukocytosis, expression of inflammatory cytokines) so that a subsequent exposure to severe exercise heat induces an accentuated acute-phase response. This exaggerated acute-phase response could mediate fever (in addition to exercise hyperthermia) and/or enhance likelihood of tissue injury and cellular death.

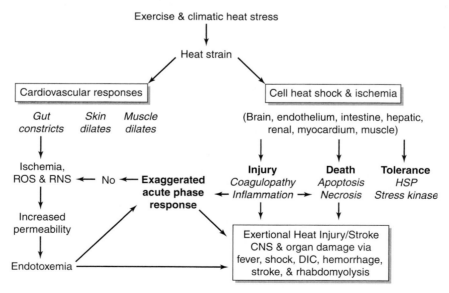

FIGURE 26.12 Possible pathogenesis for progression of exercise heat strain to exertional heat injury and stroke. (*Adapted from Bouchama A, Knochel P. Heat stroke. N Engl J Med 2002;346:1982.*)

The severity of heat injury is often not apparent on presentation. Individuals performing or competing in strenuous activities in hot weather who exhibit signs and symptoms of serious exertional heat illness (e.g., unsteady gait; sweaty, flushed skin; dizziness; headache; tachycardia; paresthesias; weakness; nausea; cramps) should be immediately evaluated for mental status, core (rectal) temperature, and vital signs. Poor or worsening mental status (ataxia, confusion) is a true medical emergency, and these individuals need rapid intervention and evacuation to a medical treatment facility.

Regardless of the pathogenesis, serious exertional heat illness poses a risk to healthy persons who are active in warm weather. Guidelines for the prevention and treatment of serious exertional heat illness can be readily obtained (http://usariem.army.mil/HeatInjury.htm and http://www.naspem.org/pos_stmts/) and should be followed.

All persons suspected of having exertional heat injury or stroke must have early initiation of cooling in the field. Delay in cooling probably is the single most important factor leading to death or residual serious disability. The patient should lie down, and as much clothing should be removed as is practical. Body cooling should be initiated and continued until core temperature is less than 38.5°C by the most practical means as quickly as possible. Immersion in cool or iced water with skin massage is the most rapid method, but ice sheets and ice packs can be effective.

Cold Stress

Environmental Cold Stress

The principal determinants of cold stress during outdoor events in cold weather are air temperature and wind speed. Most body heat loss during cold exposure occurs via conductive and convective mechanisms, so when ambient temperature is colder than body temperature, the thermal gradient favors body heat loss, and wind exacerbates heat loss by facilitating convection at the body (5). Wind chill charts and tables have been constructed to depict, for every combination of air temperature and wind speed, a corresponding temperature in calm air (i.e., no wind) that is calculated to produce the same theoretical heat flow through bare skin, and this value is the equivalent chill temperature for the temperature and wind combination (72). The effect of increasing wind speed with decreasing air temperature on equivalent chill temperature is illustrated in Figure 26.13.

Although widely reported and broadly accepted as an overall cold stress index, wind chill temperatures really only estimate the danger of cooling the exposed flesh of sedentary persons. Wind chill effects are greatly reduced by wearing windproof clothing and/or engaging in strenuous exercise. Further, wind chill provides no meaningful estimate of the risk of hypothermia. Thus, wind chill tables probably somewhat exaggerate the risk of cold injury during endurance competition, and events in which participants are properly dressed

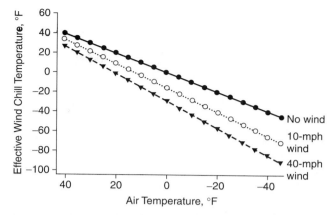

FIGURE 26.13 Effects of increasing wind speed with decreasing air temperature on equivalent chill temperature (ECT). Prepared from wind chill index values extracted from the National Weather Service Wind Chill Chart. *(Data from National Weather Service. Wind chill temperature index. Office of Climate, Water, and Weather Services, NOAA, National Weather Service, 2001 http://www.nws.noaa.gov/om/windchill/index.shtml)*

and maintain high metabolic rates need not be canceled because of the wind chill alone. Lacking a better tool, equivalent chill temperature is useful for guiding decisions regarding the need to cancel outdoor activities, but, as with the WBGT, the limitations to this approach should be appreciated. Prudence does warrant increased safety surveillance of competitors when equivalent chill temperatures fall below −30°C, since injured or fatigued athletes may be unable to sustain high metabolic rates and skin temperatures that protect them from wind chill.

As described at the beginning of this chapter, water has a much higher thermal capacity than air, and the heat transfer coefficient in water is 25 times greater than in air (3). Therefore, heat conduction away from the body is greater during exposure to a given cold air temperature when skin and clothing are wet (e.g., from rain) than when the skin is dry. With an air temperature of 5°C, heat loss in wet clothes may be double that in dry ones (73). Even so, heat loss predictions (74) indicate that core temperature of an average-sized individual performing high-intensity endurance exercise (metabolic rate of 600 W) in an air temperature of 5°C and continuous rain will not fall below 35°C for at least 7 h, and experimental observations tend to confirm those predictions (75). The enhancement of conductive heat loss is much more pronounced during full or partial immersion. During exercise in water, skin heat conductance can be 70 times greater than comparable exercise in air at the same temperature; thus, swimmers can lose considerable body heat even in relatively mild water temperatures. However, as will be explained later, anthropomorphic factors, exercise type and intensity, metabolic rate, aerobic capacity, and water temperature all interact in a complex manner to determine net thermal balance during immersion in cold water, so individuals vary considerably with respect to the water temperature they can tolerate without a dangerous decline in core temperature during exercise.

Safe limits for allowable duration of recreation involving immersion in different water temperatures can be predicted using thermoregulatory models (76) or estimated according to actual observations of survival times following accidental immersion (77), the latter being the less conservative approach. Figure 26.14 illustrates both approaches to establishing water temperature safety limits for aquatic events. However, in both cases, expected time to death due to hypothermia or drowning due to the inability to maintain consciousness or sustain useful physical activity is used to define the limits, and this approach may be too liberal for athletic competition.

Physiological Responses to Cold

Acute Cold Exposure

Humans exhibit peripheral vasoconstriction upon exposure to cold. The resulting decrease in peripheral blood flow reduces convective heat transfer between the body's core and shell (skin, subcutaneous fat, and skeletal muscle), effectively increasing insulation by the body's shell. Since heat is lost from the exposed body surface faster than it is replaced, skin temperature declines. During whole-body exposure to cold, the vasoconstrictor response extends beyond the fingers and spreads throughout the entire body's peripheral shell. Vasoconstriction begins when skin temperature falls below about 35°C and becomes maximal when skin temperature is about 31°C or less (78). Thus, the vasoconstrictor response to cold exposure helps retard heat loss and defend core temperature but at the expense of a decline in temperature of peripheral tissue.

The vasoconstriction-induced blood flow reduction and fall in skin temperature probably contribute to the causation of peripheral cold injuries. Cold-induced vasoconstriction has pronounced effects in the hands and fingers, making them particularly susceptible to cold injury and loss of manual dexterity (79). In these areas, another vasomotor response, cold-induced vasodilation, modulates the effects of vasoconstriction. Periodic fluctuations of skin temperature follow the initial decline during cold exposure, resulting from transient increases in blood flow to the cooled finger. A similar cold-induced vasodilation in the forearm appears to reflect vasodilation of muscle as well as cutaneous vasculature (80). Originally thought to be a local effect of cooling, evidence suggests that a central nervous system mechanism medicates cold-induced vasodilation (81).

Cold exposure also elicits increased metabolic heat production in humans, which can help offset heat loss. In humans, cold-induced thermogenesis is attributable to skeletal muscle contractile activity. Humans initiate this thermogenesis by voluntarily modifying behavior, that is, increasing physical activity (e.g., exercise, increased fidgeting) or by shivering. While certain animals increase metabolic heat production by noncontracting tissue in response to cold exposure, that is, nonshivering thermogenesis, adult humans lack this mechanism.

Shivering, which consists of involuntary repeated rhythmic muscle contractions during which most of the metabolic energy expended is liberated as heat and little external work is performed, may start immediately or after several minutes of cold exposure. It usually begins in torso muscles, then spreads to the limbs (82). The intensity and extent of shivering vary according to the severity of cold stress. As shivering intensity increases and more muscles are recruited to shiver, whole-body metabolic rate increases, typically reaching about 200 to 250 W during resting exposure to cold air but often exceeding 350 W during resting immersion in cold water. Maximal shivering is difficult to quantify, but the highest metabolic rate reported in the literature to date appears to be 763 W, recorded during immersion in 12°C water, and this corresponded to 46% of that test subject's maximal aerobic power (83).

Patterns of Human Cold Acclimatization

Athletes exposed to cold weather can acclimatize, but the specifics of the physiological adjustments are modest and depend on the severity of the exposures. Cold acclimatization in persons repeatedly or chronically exposed to cold manifests in three patterns of thermoregulatory adjustments: habituation, metabolic acclimatization, and insulative acclimatization. Figure 26.15 summarizes the characteristic features of each pattern (4).

The most commonly observed acclimatization pattern is habituation. With habituation, physiological responses to cold become less pronounced than before acclimatization,

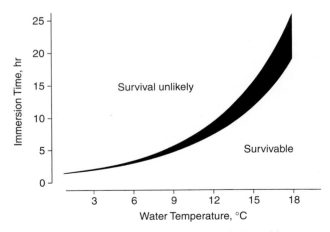

FIGURE 26.14 Approximate survival times during cold water immersion. *(From Pandolf KB, Young AJ. Assessment of environmental extremes and competitive strategies. In Shephard RJ, Astrand PO, eds. Endurance in sport. Oxford: Blackwell Science, 2000;292.)*

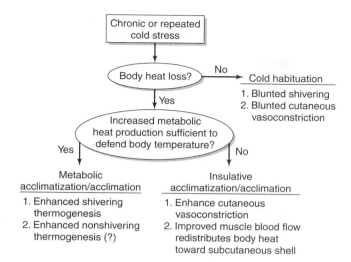

FIGURE 26.15 Theoretical flow chart to explain how humans develop different patterns of cold acclimatization. *(From Young AJ. Homeostatic responses to prolonged cold exposure: human cold acclimatization. In MJ Fregly, CM Blatteis, eds. Handbook of Physiology: Section 4: Environmental Physiology. New York: Oxford University, 1996;435.)*

and blunting of both shivering and cold-induced vasoconstriction are the hallmarks of habituation (4). Sometimes, but not always, cold-habituated persons with blunted shivering and vasoconstrictor responses to cold also exhibit a more pronounced decline in core temperature during cold exposure than nonacclimatized persons, a pattern called hypothermic habituation. Findings from different cold acclimatization studies viewed collectively (see Young [4] for a detailed review) suggest that the distinction between studies observing hypothermic habituation and those in which habituation of shivering and vasoconstriction occurred without effect on core temperature responses to cold probably reflect differences in experimental protocols rather than physiological mechanisms.

The second distinct pattern of acclimatization induced by chronic cold exposure is characterized by a more pronounced thermogenic response to cold, hence is termed metabolic acclimatization (4). Studies in which subjects appeared to demonstrate development of an enhanced thermogenic response to cold exposure seem to have observed subjects chronically (months to lifetime) exposed to relatively mild whole-body cold that was tolerated without producing hypothermia (4). Enhanced thermogenic responses to cold could arise either through an exaggerated shivering response or through development of nonshivering thermogenesis. Experimental evidence purporting to document the existence of both thermogenic adjustments has been reported (for review see Young [4]), but a critical analysis of those reports suggests little support for the development of a nonshivering thermogenic response in humans.

The third major pattern of cold acclimatization, referred to as insulative cold acclimatization, is characterized by enhanced heat conservation mechanisms (4). With insulative acclimatization, cold exposure elicits a more rapid and more pronounced decline in skin temperature and lower thermal conductance at the skin than in the unacclimatized state. The response is mediated by a pronounced vasoconstrictor response to cold, possibly due to enhanced sympathetic nervous response to cold. In addition, some data suggest that insulative cold acclimatization may also involve development of enhanced circulatory countercurrent heat exchange mechanisms to limit convective heat loss, as evidenced by the observation that before wet suits came into common usage, Korean diving women immersed in cool water exhibited less forearm heat loss than control subjects, despite the fact that concomitant forearm blood flow remained higher in the diving women. After wet suit use became widespread, Korean diving women no longer exhibited any thermoregulatory adjustments compared to control subjects, which suggests that the previous differences truly reflected adjustments to frequent exposure to cold while diving (for review see Young [4]).

The nature of the cold exposure may determine the pattern of acclimatization. In a suggested theoretical model the key determinant for cold acclimatization is the degree to which cold exposure results in body heat loss (4), and some recently reported experimental data support that concept (84). This model, illustrated in Figure 26.15, postulates that brief, intermittent cold exposures in which limited areas of the body surface are cooled and whole-body heat losses are negligible produces habituation. By contrast, repeated cold exposures prolonged and/or severe enough to preclude increased metabolic heat production from balancing body heat loss (i.e., deep body temperature declines), will induce insulative acclimatization. That model also postulates that an enhanced thermogenic capability will develop when repeated and prolonged cold exposures produce significant body heat loss, but increased body heat production can be sustained sufficiently to prevent significant core temperature declines. An alternative to that model's explanation for development of different patterns of cold acclimatization is that the metabolic, hypothermic habituative, and insulative patterns do not represent different types of cold acclimatization but are actually different stages in the development of complete cold acclimatization. Thus, initially humans respond to whole-body cold exposure by shivering, which becomes more pronounced over time; eventually, however, shivering disappears and is replaced by insulative adaptations to help limit body heat loss.

Compared to the effects of heat acclimatization, physiological adjustments to chronic cold exposure are less pronounced, slower to develop, and less practical in terms of relieving thermal strain, defending normal body temperature, and preventing thermal injury. Therefore, researchers have directed less attention to these physiological adjustments than to effects of heat acclimatization. Nonetheless, physiologists need to appreciate these adjustments, as they may be sufficient to influence physiological responses observed during exercise and/or exposure to environmental stress, particularly under controlled experimental conditions.

Individual Factors Modifying Responses to Cold

Anthropometric Characteristics

Most variability between individuals in their thermoregulatory responses and capability to maintain normal body temperature during cold exposure is attributable to anthropometric differences. Large individuals lose more body heat in the cold than smaller individuals because they have larger body surface area, but this effect is somewhat mitigated, since a large body mass favors maintenance of a constant temperature by virtue of a greater heat content than a small body mass. In general, persons with a large ratio of surface area to mass have greater declines in body temperature during cold exposure than those with a smaller ratio (3,5).

All body tissues provide thermal resistance to heat conduction (i.e., insulation) from within the body. In resting individuals, unperfused muscle tissue provides a significant contribution to the body's total insulation. However, that contribution declines during exercise or other physical activity because increased blood flow through muscles facilitates convective heat transfer from core to the body's shell. The thermal resistivity of fat is greater than that of other tissues (3), and as illustrated in Figure 26.16, subcutaneous fat provides significant insulation against heat loss in the cold. Consequently, fat persons have smaller body temperature changes and shiver less during cold exposure than lean persons (3).

Gender-associated differences in thermoregulatory responses and ability to maintain normal thermal balance during cold exposure appear almost entirely attributable to anthropometric characteristics (3). For example, in men and women having equivalent total body mass, surface areas are similar, but the women's greater fat content enhances insulation. However, in women and men of equivalent subcutaneous fat thickness, the women have a greater surface area but smaller total body mass (and lower total body heat content) than men. Thus, while insulation is equivalent, total heat loss would be greater in the women because they have a larger surface area for convective heat flux, and body temperature would tend to fall more rapidly for any given thermal gradient unless shivering thermogenesis compensated with a more pronounced increment than in the men. This compensation may be possible when heat flux is low (mild cold conditions), but women's smaller lean body mass limits their maximal capacity for thermogenic response; therefore, a more rapid core temperature decline might occur under severely cold conditions than in men of comparable body mass (85,86).

Aerobic Fitness and Training

Overall, exercise training and aerobic fitness appear to have only minor influences on thermoregulatory responses to cold. Most cross-sectional comparisons of aerobically fit and less fit persons find no relationship between maximal aerobic power and temperature regulation in cold, and in studies purportedly demonstrating a relationship, differences in thermoregulation appear more likely attributable to anthropometric differences between the aerobically fit and less fit subjects than to an effect of maximal aerobic power *per se* (87). Longitudinal studies have shown interval training to have no measurable effects on thermoregulatory response to cold (88), and while endurance training was shown to improve cutaneous vasoconstrictor response during cold water immersion, that effect had little impact on core temperature changes during cold exposure (34). The effects of resistance training programs on thermoregulatory responses to cold have not been documented, but it seems likely that any such effects would be primarily attributable to training-related changes in body composition. The primary thermoregulatory advantage provided by the increased strength and aerobic power resulting from exercise training is that the fitter individual can sustain voluntary activity at higher intensity and thus higher rates of metabolic heat production for longer periods than less fit persons during cold exposure.

Clothing

A wide variety of athletic clothing is available to provide protection during exercise and recreational activity in cold conditions. Detailed consideration of the biophysics and heat transfer properties of cold-weather athletic clothing is considered elsewhere (89) and is beyond the scope of this text. However, it should be intuitively obvious that the amount of clothing insulation required to maintain comfort and insulate against excessive body heat loss during cold-weather activity

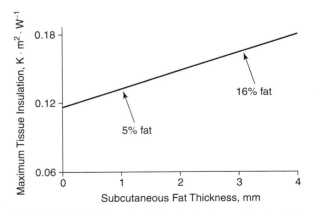

FIGURE 26.16 Tissue insulation during immersion in cold water as a function of subcutaneous fat thickness. *(Adapted from Hong SK. Pattern of cold adaptation in women divers of Korea (Ama). Fed Proc 1973;32:1618.)*

will depend on combined effects of two opposing factors: thermal gradient for heat loss (i.e., ambient temperature) and rate of metabolic heat production (i.e., exercise intensity). Increasing clothing insulation will be required as ambient temperature decreases, while decreasing clothing insulation will be required as metabolic rate increases. Heat production during high-intensity exercise can be sufficient to prevent a fall in deep body temperature without the need for heavy clothing even when air temperature is extremely low, but athletes dressed optimally during events may be inadequately protected from cold before starting or when exercise ceases because of fatigue, injury, or completion of the event. Thus, modern cold-weather athletic clothing incorporates design features enabling adjustable insulation, such as ventilating openings and clothing layering. Further, since much of the insulation provided by cold-weather clothing is achieved by trapping stagnant air layers within the clothing or against the skin, the clothing must also provide a barrier against moisture and wind, which degrade insulation by disrupting trapped air layers. Also, even during activity of sufficiently high intensity that metabolic heat production completely obviates heavy cold-weather clothing to protect against hypothermia, exposed skin of the fingers, nose, and ears may be susceptible to freezing injuries, and clothing to protect those regions from surface cooling should be worn when wind chill conditions are extreme. Finally, since the insulation provided by cold-weather clothing adds to insulation provided by body fat and other tissues, clothing requirements will vary among individuals, depending on anthropometric factors discussed earlier.

Exercise in the Cold

Oxygen Uptake and Systemic Oxygen Transport

As the noted environmental physiologist Dave Bass once observed (90), "man in the cold is not necessarily a cold man." Thus, whether physiological responses to exercise are altered by cold environment depends on whether the interactive effects of environment, clothing, anthropometric factors, and exercise intensity are such that cold stress elicits additional physiological strain beyond that associated with the same exercise under temperate conditions.

If cold stress is severe enough to cause a significant decline in core or muscle temperature, maximal aerobic power can be reduced, compared to that measured at normal core and muscle temperatures (91). The mechanism for this effect is not definitively demonstrated, but it probably reflects an effect of low tissue temperature on contractile function of heart (91) and/or skeletal (92) muscle. An impairment of myocardial contractility could limit maximal cardiac output, thus accounting for the reduced maximal aerobic power. Further, impairment of skeletal muscle contractile function associated with muscle cooling could reduce maximal aerobic power by simply limiting demand for oxygen transport. However, there must be a threshold temperature for this effect,

as exposure to cold conditions that lower core temperature 0.5°C or less have no significant effect on maximal aerobic power and associated responses (93).

Whether cold exposure influences oxygen uptake during steady-state submaximal exercise depends on whether exercise thermogenesis is sufficient to balance the rate of body heat loss to the ambient environment and maintain core and skin temperatures warm enough that shivering does not develop. During exercise at intensities too low for metabolic heat production to balance heat loss to the cold environment and prevent shivering, oxygen uptake will be higher than in warm conditions, with the increased oxygen uptake representing the added oxygen requirement for metabolism in the shivering muscles. With increasing exercise intensity, metabolic heat production rises and core and skin temperatures are maintained warmer. Therefore, the afferent stimulus for shivering declines along with the shivering-associated component of total oxygen uptake during exercise until eventually exercise metabolism becomes high enough to prevent shivering, and the steady-state oxygen uptake at that intensity and higher is the same in cold and warm conditions.

Figure 26.17 illustrates conceptually the influence of exercise intensity on steady-state submaximal oxygen uptake during exercise (94). The precise effect of exercise intensity on the shivering component of total oxygen uptake during exercise and the specific intensity at which metabolic heat production is sufficient to prevent shivering will depend on the severity of cold stress, clothing insulation, and anthropometric factors influencing body heat flux.

Cold exposure can also affect cardiovascular responses to submaximal exercise. When shivering occurs during exercise in the cold, cardiac output is elevated relative to the cardiac output elicited by that same exercise intensity in temperate conditions. However, the increment in cardiac output simply reflects the requirement for increased systemic oxygen transport to sustain shivering, so cardiac output for any given oxygen uptake level remains unchanged (95,96).

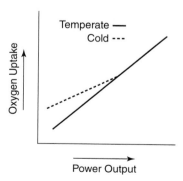

FIGURE 26.17 Steady-state oxygen uptake response during submaximal exercise at given power output in temperate and cold conditions. *(From Young AJ, Sawka MN, Pandolf KB. Physiology of cold exposure. In Marriott BM, Carlson SJ, eds. Nutritional needs in cold and in high-altitude environments. Washington: National Academy, 1996, 137.)*

Nevertheless, shivering during exercise could somewhat increase cardiovascular strain for a given submaximal exercise bout over the strain of that same bout without shivering. Cold exposure can also alter the way that a given cardiac output is achieved (95,96). During exercise in cold air or cold water, bradycardia and increased stroke volume are observed for a given cardiac output and oxygen uptake level compared to exercise at the same oxygen uptake in temperate conditions (95,96). Whether a baroreflex, a change in the inotropic state of the heart (cold-induced increase in plasma norepinephrine), or the effects of increased central blood volume resulting from peripheral vasoconstriction accounts for the bradycardia and stroke volume increase seen during exercise during cold exposure await definitive experimental determination (95,96).

Muscle Energy Metabolism

Cold exposure may also affect muscle energy metabolism during exercise. If shivering occurs during exercise, higher blood lactate concentrations may be attained in cold than in temperate conditions, but when oxygen uptake is the same (i.e., no shivering), blood lactate accumulation during exercise in cold and temperate conditions is the same (31). Muscle glycogen depletion has been observed to be more pronounced during low-intensity (e.g. below 25% maximal oxygen uptake) exercise in cold, when oxygen uptake levels were elevated compared to an exercise bout similar in intensity and duration performed under temperate conditions, but differences are not seen when bouts of higher-intensity exercise are compared (31). Earlier interpretations of that observation were that added energy requirements of shivering increased glycogen breakdown during exercise and that shivering preferentially metabolized muscle glycogen as an energy source. However, recent findings show instead that shivering, like low-intensity exercise, relies on lipid as the predominant metabolic substrate, but blood glucose, muscle glycogen, and even protein are metabolized as well (97). The accelerated muscle glycogen utilization previously observed during low-intensity exercise in cold conditions might result from increased motor unit recruitment to compensate for impaired force generation induced by muscle cooling. However, cold exposure would probably have to be extreme or entail prolonged immersion in cold water to induce a sufficiently pronounced decline in muscle temperature to impair force generation during sustained dynamic exercise (92).

Body Fluid Balance

Cold exposure is thought to influence both physiological and behavioral mechanisms affecting body fluid balance during exercise. For one thing, fluid intake can become inadequate during cold exposure. Thirst sensation may be blunted in cold persons, and cold environments often present practical constraints on voluntary drinking (frozen drinking supplies, desire to avoid urinating outdoors in the cold). Cold exposure is also thought to exacerbate fluid losses, but the extent that these effects are operational during exercise is unclear.

Perhaps the most widely recognized effect of exposure to cold air or immersion in cold water is an increased urine flow rate, or cold-induced diuresis, but controversy still exists regarding its precise mechanism. Experimental findings appear to rule out hormonal mechanisms and suggest that the increased systemic and renal blood pressure associated with cold-induced vasoconstriction may increase filtration and decrease reabsorption of water and solute by the kidney (98). However, whatever the mechanism or mechanisms, exercise counteracts or blocks them, because cold-induced diuresis is prevented by even moderate exercise during cold exposure (98).

Breathing cold air has also been suggested to exacerbate respiratory water loss during exercise, since cold air has lower water content than warmer air, and it is assumed that each inspired breath warms to body temperature and becomes 100% saturated with water as it passes through the respiratory passages (98). However, that assumption may not be valid. Experimental observations (99) illustrate that cold inspired air (−12°C) does not warm to the same temperature as warmer air (23°C), and in fact, less rather than more water was lost in the exhaled cold air. The difference in temperature between ambient and inspired air temperature becomes even greater when ventilation rate increases, as during exercise (99). Therefore, respiratory water losses are probably no more important for fluid balance during exercise in the cold than in warm conditions, and the most significant avenue of fluid loss during exercise in cold is the same as in warm conditions—sweating.

Even in cold environments, metabolic heat production can exceed heat loss, with the resulting heat storage causing hyperthermia and initiating thermoregulatory sweating. The problem is that clothing insulation needed for warmth and comfort in cold environments is much higher during rest and light activity than during strenuous activity (5). Therefore, if one begins exercising vigorously while wearing clothing selected for sedentary activities in the cold, sweating and the resultant drinking requirements can increase substantially. If those increased drinking requirements go unmet, dehydration will ensue, just as with exercise in the heat, with possibly similar adverse physiological and performance consequences (100) as discussed earlier in this chapter. Otherwise, there is little evidence that cold exposure has any unique impact on regulation (101).

Exercise Performance Limitations

As discussed earlier, cold exposure can reduce maximal aerobic power and increase metabolic and cardiovascular strain during submaximal exercise, both of which would be predicted to limit or impair exercise performance to some extent. However, as described, both of those effects appear to be mediated by significant body heat loss and cooling of deep body and skeletal muscle. Thus, how exercise influences the ability to maintain thermal balance in the cold is probably the key factor determining whether cold exposure is associated with performance decrements. In addition, certain patho-physiological responses elicited by cold exposure can degrade performance by impairing an individual's ability to exercise.

Exercise and Thermal Balance

As described earlier, exercise elicits both thermogenesis and an increased peripheral blood flow (skin and muscles), which facilitates body heat loss by enhancing convective heat transfer from the central core to peripheral shell, and both responses increase concomitantly as exercise intensity increases. During exposure to cold air, the thermogenic response during exercise is sufficiently pronounced that the increased metabolic heat production usually matches or exceeds any exercise-related facilitation of heat loss, and exercise performance would not be affected by inability to maintain thermal balance (3). In contrast, because the higher convective heat transfer coefficient is so much greater during water immersion than in air, the exercise-associated increase in heat loss during exercise in water can be so large that metabolic heat production during even intense exercise is insufficient to maintain thermal balance (3).

Exercise affects thermal balance during cold exposure in two other ways. Arms have a greater ratio of surface area to mass and thinner subcutaneous fat than legs, so exercise-induced increments in muscle and skin blood flow to the limb tend to increase convective heat transfer more during arm than leg exercise (14). As a result, metabolic heat production is less effective for sustaining thermal balance during arm than leg exercise at a similar intensity (3). In addition, limb movement disrupts the stationary boundary layer of air or water that develops at the skin surface in a still environment, and the loss of that insulation further favors increased convective heat loss from the body surface. Experimental observations confirm that these effects have a measurable influence on thermal balance during exercise in cold water (102). The practical implications of those effects for performance in the cold remains to be fully explored, but they may have implications for design of cold-weather athletic clothing.

Hiker's Hypothermia: Exertional Fatigue and Thermoregulation in the Cold

Strenuous exercise can lead to exertional fatigue, and when strenuous exercise and high levels of energy expenditure are sustained for long periods, people have difficulty maintaining sufficiently high energy intake to offset expenditure. Fatigue due to exertion, sleep restriction, and underfeeding impairs an individual's ability to maintain thermal balance in the cold (103), and an anecdotal association between exertional fatigue and susceptibility to hypothermia has also been reported (104). This syndrome has been referred to as

hiker's hypothermia. The simplest explanation proposed is that prolonged exercise produces fatigue, so the exercise intensity and rate of metabolic heat production that can be sustained decline, and if ambient conditions are sufficiently cold, negative thermal balance and declining core temperature ensue. When underfeeding is a factor, effects probably result from development of hypoglycemia, since acute hypoglycemia impairs shivering through a central nervous system–mediated effect. Also, declining peripheral carbohydrate stores probably contribute to an inability to sustain exercise or activity and the associated exercise-induced thermogenesis in the cold. Recent studies also indicate that shivering and peripheral vasoconstriction may themselves be directly impaired following strenuous exercise (75,105), repeated or prolonged cold exposure (106), or both. Irrespective of mechanism, when strenuous exercise produces fatigue, either acute or chronic, ability to maintain thermal balance appears to be degraded, and that in turn can further limit performance.

Cold-Induced Bronchospasm

For the most part, inhaling cold air during exercise has negligible effects. Upper airway temperatures, which normally remain unchanged during exercise under temperate conditions, can decrease substantially when extremely cold air is breathed during strenuous exercise, but temperatures of the lower respiratory tract and deep body temperatures are unaffected (107). Pulmonary function during exercise in healthy athletes is usually unaffected by breathing cold air, but allergy-prone athletes frequently have bronchospasm (108). The triggering mechanism for bronchospasm in susceptible persons remains unresolved, but it may be related to thermally induced leakage in the lung's microcirculation with subsequent edema (99). Persons who have bronchospasm when breathing cold air during heavy exercise exhibit a reduced forced expiratory volume (108), which can limit maximal ventilation, thus maximal performance. Further, even healthy persons can have an increase in respiratory passage secretions and decreased mucociliary clearance when breathing very cold air during exercise, and any associated airway congestion may impair pulmonary mechanics and ventilation during exercise, also impairing performance (109).

SUMMARY

Body temperature is regulated by two distinct control systems, behavioral and physiological. Behavioral thermoregulation involves the conscious, willed use of whatever means are available to minimize thermal discomfort. Physiological thermoregulation employs unconscious responses that are controlled by the autonomic nervous system in proportion to the core and skin temperatures. The physiological responses modifying body heat loss are increased skin blood flow and sweating, and those modifying heat conservation are vasoconstriction and shivering.

A MILESTONE OF DISCOVERY

Does central fatigue contribute to reduced exercise performance associated with hyperthermia? Human tissues retain their function and tolerate temperatures above 40°C without injury, but irrevocable damage can result beyond tissue temperatures above 42°C (1,110). Therefore, an inability or unwillingness to exercise beyond destructive internal body temperatures may be a type of protection against catastrophic hyperthermia. Animal research has shown that exercise performance can sometimes decrease when hypothalamic temperature exceeds 42°C (independent of body temperature), suggesting that very high brain temperatures can mediate protective thermoregulatory behavior (111). However, such high brain temperatures would not normally be expected in exercising humans.

Prior to the study of Nybo and Nielson (42) there was no conclusive evidence that central fatigue contributes to reductions in exercise performance in the heat for humans. These investigators had 14 subjects exercise at 60% of $\dot{V}O_{2max}$ for 1 hour in a hot (40°C) and temperate (18°C) climate. Immediately after that exercise bout, subjects performed 2 minutes of sustained MVC of handgrip and knee extension with electrical stimulation (EL) periodically applied to the nervus femoralis. EL superimposed during the MVC generated the maximal total force (MVC + EL) and maximal voluntary activation percentage (MVC / MVC + EL). Core temperature increased to 40°C (exhaustion after 50 minutes of exercise) and 38°C (completed 1 hour of exercise) in the hot and temperate climates, respectively. Knee extension MVC force was initially unaffected by prior exercise, but after 5 seconds the decline in MVC force was greater after the hyperthermia than after the temperate trials. Total maximal force was similar, so the voluntary activation percentage was lower after exercise in hot (54%) than temperate (82%) conditions. Two subjects were passively heated to 39°C and demonstrated the same pattern of voluntary force decline during sustained maximal handgrip contractions. The experiments showed that hyperthermia significantly reduced force-generating capacity during a sustained MVC in both active (leg) and inactive (forearm) muscles compared to that measured at a lower core temperature. However, the capacity of the skeletal muscles was not altered by hyperthermia when EL was applied.

The study provides strong support for the idea that central fatigue may contribute to reduced capabilities for dynamic exercise in hot weather. It is unclear whether brain or other tissue temperature (or feedback inhibition from hot muscles) might have been influenced by the hyperthermia to send signals affecting motor activity. The mechanism for attenuated neuromuscular activity at a higher body temperature remains unresolved but may possibly be linked to the neurotransmitter serotonin within the brain, as discussed in the chapter.

Nybo L, Nielsen B. Hyperthermia and central fatigue during prolonged exercise. J Appl Physiol 2001;91:1055–1060.

Climatic heat stress and exercise interact synergistically and may push physiological systems to their limits. Heat stress reduces an athlete's ability to exercise. Physiological mechanisms contributing to this reduced performance include cardiovascular, central nervous system, and metabolic perturbations. Heat acclimatization provides many physiological adaptations that enable sustained exercise and protection from heat injury. Athletes routinely have high sweating rates during exercise heat stress that can lead to dehydration and adversely influence exercise performance.

In the cold, heat balance and requirements for shivering depend on the severity of climatic cold stress, effectiveness of vasoconstriction, and intensity and mode of exercise. Cold-induced vasoconstriction decreases blood flow to peripheral tissues, allowing them to cool and making them susceptible to cold injury. Cooling of peripheral tissues can degrade finger dexterity and impair skeletal muscle contractile function, while reduced core temperature can degrade the ability to achieve maximal metabolic rates and submaximal endurance performance. Body composition is the most important physiological determinant of thermoregulatory tolerance to cold exposure. The clothing requirement for warmth and comfort is much higher during rest and light activity than during strenuous activity, and overinsulation can cause heat stress that elicits sweating, wet clothing, and dehydration. Each of those factors can have undesirable affects on athletic performance and susceptibility to cold injury.

ACKNOWLEDGMENTS

The views, opinions, and findings in this report are those of the authors and should not be construed as an official Department of the Army position or decision unless so designated by other official documentation. Approved for public release; distribution unlimited.

REFERENCES

1. Katschinski DM. On heat and cells and proteins. NIPS 2004;19:11–15.
2. Sawka MN, Wenger CB, Pandolf KB. Thermoregulatory responses to acute exercise heat stress and heat acclimation. In Fregly MJ, Blatteis CM, eds. Handbook of Physiology, section 4: Environmental Physiology. New York: Oxford University, 1996;157–185.
3. Toner MM, Mcardle WD. Human thermoregulatory responses to acute cold stress with special reference to water immersion. In Fregly MJ, Blatteis CM, eds. Handbook of Physiology, Section 4: Environmental Physiology. New York: Oxford University, 1996;379–418.

4. Young AJ. Homeostatic responses to prolonged cold exposure: human cold acclimatization. In Fregly MJ, Blatteis CM, eds. Handbook of Physiology, Section 4: Environmental Physiology. New York: Oxford University, 1996;419–438.

5. Gagge AP, Gonzalez RR. Mechanisms of heat exchange: biophysics and physiology. In Fregly MJ, Blatteis CM, eds. Handbook of Physiology, Section 4: Environmental Physiology. New York: Oxford University, 1996;45–84.

6. Gisolfi CV, Wenger CB. Temperature regulation during exercise: old concepts, new ideas. Exerc Sport Sci Rev 1984;12:339–372.

7. Johnson JM, Park MK. Effect of upright exercise on threshold for cutaneous vasodilation and sweating. J Appl Physiol 1981;50:814–818.

8. Boulant JA. Hypothalamic neurons regulating body temperature. In Fregly MJ, Blatteis CM, eds. Handbook of Physiology, Section 4: Environmental Physiology. New York: Oxford University, 1996;105–125.

9. Cooper KE. Some historical perspectives on thermoregulation. J Appl Physiol 2002;92:1717–1724.

10. Hensel HT. Neural processes in thermoregulation. Physiol Rev 1973;53:948–1017.

11. Stitt JT. Fever versus hyperthermia. Fed Proc 1979;8:39–43.

12. Nybo L, Secher NH, Nielsen B. Inadequate heat release from the human brain during prolonged exercise with hyperthermia. J Physiol 2002;545:697–704.

13. Sawka MN, Wenger CB. Physiological responses to acute exercise heat stress. In Pandolf KB, Sawka MN, Gonzalez RR, eds. Human Performance Physiology and Environmental Medicine at Terrestrial Extremes. Indianapolis: Cooper, 1988;97–151.

14. Sawka MN. Physiology of upper body exercise. Exerc Sport Sci Rev 1986;14:175–211.

15. Nielsen M. Die Regulation der Körpertemperatur bei Muskelarbeit. Scand Arch Physiol 1938;9:193–230.

16. Mccullough EA, Kenney WL. Thermal insulation and evaporative resistance of football uniforms. Med Sci Sports Exerc 2003;35:832–837.

17. Lind AR. A physiological criterion for setting thermal environmental limits for everyday work. J Appl Physiol 1963;18:51–56.

18. Nielsen B, Nielsen M. Body temperature during work at different environmental temperatures. Acta Physiol Scand 1962;56:120–129.

19. Shibasaki M, Kondo N, Crandall CG. Non-thermoregulatory modulation of sweating. Exerc Sports Sci Rev 2003;1:34–39.

20. Sato K. The mechanism of eccrine sweat secretion. In Gisolf CV, Lamb DR, Nadel ER, eds. Exercise, Heat, and Thermoregulation. Dubuque, IA: Brown & Benchmark, 1993;85–117.

21. Nadel ER, Mitchell JW, Saltin B, et al. Peripheral modifications to the central drive for sweating. J Appl Physiol 1971;31:828–833.

22. Johnson JM, Proppe DW. Cardiovascular adjustments to heat stress. In Fregley MJ, Blatteis CM, eds. Handbook of Physiology, Section 4: Environmental Physiology. New York: Oxford University, 1996;215–243.

23. Taylor WF, Johnson JM, O'Leary DS, et al. Modification of the cutaneous vascular response to exercise by local skin temperature. J Appl Physiol 1984;7:1878–1884.

24. Rowell LB. Human Circulation: Regulation During Physical Stress. New York: Oxford University, 1986.

25. Crandall CG. Carotid baroreflex responsiveness in heat-stressed humans. Am J Physiol 2000;279:H1955–H1962.

26. Crandall CG, Zhang R, Levine BD. Effects of whole body heating on dynamic baroreflex regulation of heart rate in humans. Am J Physiol 2000;279:H2486–H2492.

27. Gonzalez-Alonso J, Calbet JA. Reductions in systemic and skeletal muscle blood flow and oxygen delivery limit maximal aerobic capacity in humans. Circulation 2003;107:824–830.

28. Rowell LB, Marx HJ, Bruce RA, et al. Reductions in cardiac output, central blood volume, and stroke volume with thermal stress in normal men during exercise. J Clin Invest 1966;45:1801–1816.

29. Massett MP, Lewis SJ, Bates JN, et al. Effect of heating on vascular reactivity in rat mesenteric arteries. J Appl Physiol 1998;85:701–708.

30. Gonzalez-Alonso J, Calbet JA, Nielsen B. Muscle blood flow is reduced with dehydration during prolonged exercise in humans. J Physiol (Lond) 1999;513:895–905.

31. Young AJ. Energy substrate utilization during exercise in extreme environments. Exerc Sport Sci Rev 1990;18:65–117.

32. Febbraio MA. Does muscle function and metabolism affect exercise performance in the heat? Exerc Sport Sci Rev 2000;28:171–176.

33. Mitchell CR, Harris MB, Cordaro AR, et al. Effect of body temperature during exercise on skeletal muscle cytochrome c oxidase content. J Appl Physiol 2002;93:526–530.

34. Young AJ, Sawka MN, Levine L, et al. Metabolic and thermal adaptations from endurance training in hot or cold water. J Appl Physiol 1995;8:793–801.

35. Sawka MN, Young AJ, Cadarette BS, et al. Influence of heat stress and acclimation on maximal aerobic power. Eur J Appl Physiol 1985;53:294–298.

36. Zhang S, Guanglin M, Yanwen W, et al. Study of the relationships between weather conditions and the marathon race, and the meteorotrophic effects on distance runners. Int J Biometeor 1992;6:63–68.

37. Galloway SD, Maughan RJ. Effects of ambient temperature on the capacity to perform prolonged cycle exercise in man. Med Sci Sports Ex 1997;29:1240–1249.

38. Pitsiladis Y, Maughan JR. The effects of exercise and diet manipulation on the capacity to perform prolonged exercise in the heat and in the cold in trained humans. J Physiol (Lond) 1999;517:919–930.

39. Sawka MN, Latzka WA, Montain SJ, et al. Physiological tolerance to uncompensable heat: intermittent exercise, field vs laboratory. Med Sci Sports Exerc 2001;33:422–430.

40. Sawka MN, Young AJ. Physical exercise in hot and cold climates. In Garrett WE, Kirkendall DT, eds. Exercise and Sport Science. Philadelphia: Lippincott Williams & Wilkins, 2000;385–400.

41. Cheuvront SN, Kolka MA, Cadarette BS, et al. Efficacy of intermittent, regional microclimate cooling. J Appl Physiol 2003;94:1841–1848.

42. Nybo L, Nielsen B. Hyperthermia and central fatigue during prolonged exercise in humans. J Appl Physiol 2001;91:1055–1060.

43. Radomski MW, Cross M, Buguet A. Exercise-induced hyperthermia and hormonal responses to exercise. Can J Physiol Pharmacol 1998;76:547–552.

44. Nielsen B, Hyldig T, Bidstrup F, et al. Brain activity and fatigue during prolonged exercise in the heat. Eur J Physiol 2001;442:41–48.

45. Armstrong LE, Pandolf KB. Physical training, cardiorespiratory physical fitness and exercise heat tolerance. In Pandolf KB, Sawka MN, Gonzalez RR, eds. Human Performance Physiology and Environmental Medicine at Terrestrial Extremes. Indianapolis: Benchmark, 1988;199–226.

46. Wenger CB. Human heat acclimatization. In Pandolf KB, Sawka MN, Gonzalez RR, eds. Human Performance Physiology and Environmental Medicine at Terrestrial Extremes. Indianapolis: Benchmark, 1988;153–197.

47. Cohen JS, Gisolfi CV. Effects of interval training on work-heat tolerance of young women. Med Sci Sports Exerc 1982;14:46–52.

48. Roberts MF, Wenger CB, Stolwijk JAJ, et al. Skin blood flow and sweating changes following exercise training and heat acclimation. J Appl Physiol 1977;43:133–137.

49. Horowitz M. Matching the heart to heat-induced circulatory load: heat acclimation responses. NIPS 2003;18:215–221.

50. Nielsen B, Hales JRS, Strange S, et al. Human circulatory and thermoregulatory adaptations with heat acclimation and exercise in a hot, dry environment. J Physiol (Lond) 1993;460:467–485.

51. Nielsen B, Strange S, Christensen NJ, et al. Acute and adaptive responses in humans to exercise in a warm, humid environment. Pflüger's Arch 1997;434:49–56.

52. Horowitz M. Do cellular heat acclimation responses modulate central thermoregulatory activity? NIPS 1998;13:218–225.

53. Mack GW, Nadel ER. Body fluid balance during heat stress in humans. In Fregly MJ, Blatteis CM, eds. Environmental Physiology. New York: Oxford University, 1996;187–214.

54. Sawka MN, Coyle EF. Influence of body water and blood volume on thermoregulation and exercise performance in the heat. Exerc Sport Sci Rev 1999;27:167–218.

55. Sawka MN, Convertino VA, Eichner ER, et al. Blood volume: importance and adaptations to exercise training, environmental stresses, and trauma/sickness. Med Sci Sports Exerc 2000;32:332–348.

56. Kregel KC. Heat shock proteins: modifying factors in physiological stress responses and acquired thermotolerance. J Appl Physiol 2002;92:1–10.

57. Maloyan A, Palmon A, Horowitz M. Heat acclimation increases the basal HSP72 level and alters its production dynamics during heat stress. Am J Physiol 1999;276:R1506–R1515.

58. Skidmore R, Gutierrez JA, Guerriero V, et al. HSP70 induction during exercise and heat stress in rats: role of internal temperature. Am J Physiol 1995;68:R92–R97.

59. Gabai VL, Sherman MY. Interplay between molecular chaperones and signaling pathways in survival of heat shock. J Appl Physiol 2002;92:1743–1748.

60. Sonna LA, Fujita J, Gaffin SL, et al. Effects of heat and cold stress on mammalian gene expression. J Appl Physiol 2002;2:1725–1742.

61. Sonna LA, Wenger CB, Flinn S, et al. Exertional heat injury and gene expression changes: A DNA microarray analysis study. J Appl Physiol 2005;73–185.

62. Institute of Medicine. Water. In Dietary Reference Intakes: Water, Potassium, Sodium, Chloride, and Sulfate. Washington: National Academies, 2005;73–185.

63. Cheuvront SN, Haymes EM. Thermoregulation and marathon running: biological and environmental influences. Sports Med 2001;31:743–762.

64. Montain SJ, Sawka MN, Wenger CB. Hyponatremia associated with exercise: risk factors and pathogenesis. Exerc Sport Sci Rev 2001;29:113–117.

65. Cheuvront SN, Carter R, Sawka MN. Fluid balance and endurance exercise performance. Curr Sports Med Rep 2003;2:202–208.

66. Sawka MN, Pandolf KB. Effects of body water loss on physiological function and exercise performance. In Gisolfi CV, Lamb DR, eds. Perspectives in Exercise Science and Sports Medicine, Volume 3: Fluid Homeostasis During Exercise. Carmel, IN: Benchmark, 1990;1–38.

67. Sawka MN. Physiological consequences of hydration: exercise performance and thermoregulation. Med Sci Sports Exerc 1992;24:657–670.

68. Sawka MN, Young AJ. Acute polycythemia and human performance during exercise and exposure to extreme environments. Exerc Sport Sci Rev 1989;17:265–293.

69. Departments of Army and Air Force. Heat stress control and heat casualty management. Technical Bulletin Medical 507 / Air Force Pamphlet 48–152 (I): 2003.

70. Gonzalez RR. Biophysics of heat exchange and clothing: applications to sports physiology. Med Exerc Nutr Health 1995;4:290–305.

71. Bouchama A, Knochel P. Heat stroke. N Engl J Med 2002;346:1978–1988.

72. National Weather Service. Windchill temperature index. Washington: Office of Climate, Water, and Weather Services, 2001.

73. Kaufman WC, Bothe DJ. Wind chill reconsidered, Siple revisited. Aviat Space Environ Med 1986;57:23–26.

74. Stolwijk JAJ, Hardy JD. Control of body temperature. In Lee DHK, Falk HL, Murphy SD, Geiger SR, eds. Handbook of Physiology, Section 9: Reactions to Environmental Agents. Bethesda: American Physiological Society, 1977;45–68.

75. Castellani JW, Young AJ, Degroot DW, et al. Thermoregulation during cold exposure after several days of exhaustive exercise. J Appl Physiol 2001;90:939–946.

76. Tikuisis P. Prediction of survival time at sea based on observed body cooling values. Aviat Space Environ Med 1997;8:441–448.

77. Molnar GW. Survival of hypothermia by men immersed in the ocean. JAMA 1946;131:1046–1050.

78. Veicsteinas A, Ferretti G, Rennie DW. Superficial shell insulation in resting and exercising men in cold water. J Appl Physiol 1982;2:1557–1564.

79. Brajkovic D, Ducharme MB, Frim J. Influence of localized auxiliary heating on hand comfort during cold exposure. J Appl Physiol 1998;85:2054–2065.

80. Ducharme MB, Vanhelder WP, Radomski MW. Cyclic intramuscular temperature fluctuations in the human forearm during cold-water immersion. Eur J Appl Physiol 1991;63:188–193.

81. Lindblad LE, Ekenvall L, Klingstedt C. Neural regulation of vascular tone and cold induced vasoconstriction in human finger skin. J. Autonom Nerv Syst 1990;30:169–174.

82. Bell DG, Tikuisis P, Jacobs I. Relative intensity of muscular contraction during shivering. J Appl Physiol 1992;72:2336–2342.

83. Golden FS, Hampton IF, Hervery GR, et al. Shivering intensity in humans during immersion in cold water. J Physiol (Lond) 1979;277: 48.

84. O'Brien C, Young AJ, Lee DT, et al. Role of core temperature as a stimulus for cold acclimation during repeated immersion in 20°C water. J Appl Physiol 2000;89:242–250.

85. Mcardle WD, Magel JR, Spina RJ, et al. Thermal adjustment to cold-water exposure in exercising men and women. J Appl Physiol 1984;56:1572–1577.

86. Mcardle WD, Magel JR, Spina RJ, et al. Thermal adjustments to cold-water exposure in resting men and women. J Appl Physiol 1984;56:1565–1571.

87. Bittel JHM, Nonott-Varly C, Livecchi-Gonnot GH, et al. Physical fitness and thermoregulatory reactions in a cold environment in men. J Appl Physiol 1988;65:1984–1989.

88. Savourey G, Bittel J. Thermoregulatory changes in the cold induced by physical training in humans. Eur J Appl Physiol Occup Physiol 1998;78:379–384.

89. Gonzalez RR. Biophysical and physiological integration of proper clothing for exercise. Exerc Sport Sci Rev 1987;15:261–295.

90. Bass DE. Metabolic and energy balances in men in a cold environment. In Horvath SM, ed. Cold injury. Montpelier, VT: Josiah Macy Foundation, 1960;317–338.

91. Bergh U, Ekblom B. Physical performance and peak aerobic power at different body temperatures. J Appl Physiol 1979;46:885–889.

92. Bergh U, Ekblom B. Influence of muscle temperature on maximal muscle strength and power output in human skeletal muscles. Acta Physiol Scand 1979;107:33–37.

93. Schmidt V, Brück K. Effect of a precooling maneuver on body temperature and exercise performance. J Appl Physiol 1981;50:772–778.

94. Young AJ, Sawka MN, Pandolf KB. Physiology of cold exposure. In Marriott BM, Carlson SJ, eds. Nutritional Needs in Cold and in High-altitude Environments. Washington: National Academy, 1996;127–147.

95. Mcardle WD, Magel JR, Lesmes GR, et al. Metabolic and cardiovascular adjustment to work in air and water at 18, 25 and 33. J Appl Physiol 1976;40:85–90.

96. Pendergast DR. The effects of body cooling on oxygen transport during exercise. Med Sci Sports Exerc 1988;20:S171–S176.

97. Haman F, Peronnet F, Kenny GP, et al. Effect of cold exposure on fuel utilization in humans: plasma glucose, muscle glycogen, and lipids. J Appl Physiol 2002;93:77–84.

98. Freund BJ, Young AJ. Environmental influences body fluid balance during exercise: cold exposure. In Buskirk ER, Puhl SM, eds. Body Fluid Balance: Exercise and Sport. New York: CRC, 1996;159–181.

99. Mcfadden ER, Nelson JA, Skowronski ME, et al. Thermally induced asthma and airway drying. Am J Resp Critical Care Med 1999;160:221–226.

100. Lennquist S, Granberg PO, Wedin B. Fluid balance and physical work capacity in humans exposed to cold. Arch Environ Health 1974;29:241–249.

101. O'Brien C, Young AJ, Sawka MN. Hypohydration and thermoregulation in cold air. J Appl Physiol 1998;84:185–189.

102. Toner MM, Sawka MN, Pandolf KB. Thermal responses during arm and leg and combined arm-leg exercise in water. J Appl Physiol 1984;6:1355–1360.

103. Young AJ, Castellani JW, O'Brien C, et al. Exertional fatigue, sleep loss, and negative energy balance increase susceptibility to hypothermia. J Appl Physiol 1998;85:1210–1217.

104. Pugh LGCE. Cold stress and muscular exercise, with special reference to accidental hypothermia. BMJ 1967;2:333–337.

105. Castellani JW, Young AJ, Kain JE, et al. Thermoregulation during cold exposure: effects of prior exercise. J Appl Physiol 1999;87:247–252.

106. Castellani JW, Young AJ, Sawka MN, et al. Human thermoregulatory responses during serial cold-water immersions. J Appl Physiol 1998;85:204–209.

107. Jaeger JJ, Deal EC, Roberts DE, et al. Cold air inhalation and esophageal temperature in exercising humans. Med Sci Sports Exerc 1980;12:365–369.

108. Helenius IJ, Tikkanen HO, Haahtela T. Exercise-induced bronchospasm at low temperatures in elite runners. Thorax 1996;51:628–629.

109. Giesbrecht GG. The respiratory system in a cold environment. Aviat Space Environ Med 1995;66:890–902.

110. Bynum GD, Pandolf KB, Schuette WH, et al. Induced hyperthermia in sedated humans and the concept of critical thermal maximum. Am J Physiol 1978;235:R228–R236.

111. Caputa M, Feistkorn G, Jessen C. Effect of brain and trunk temperatures on exercise performance in goats. Pflüger's Arch 2001;406:184–189.

Physiological Systems and Their Responses to Conditions of Hypoxia

ROBERT S. MAZZEO AND CHARLES S. FULCO

Introduction

Hypoxia, or decreased availability of oxygen in inspired air, will affect the millions of individuals who are exposed to high-altitude environments on an intermittent or regular basis during recreational (e.g., skiing, climbing, mountaineering, sightseeing) or business pursuits. Depending on the elevation, many unacclimatized individuals have difficulty during the first hours to days of exposure, particularly during periods of intense physical exercise. With more prolonged residence at high altitude, specific adaptations of nearly all physiological systems are called upon to promote improved oxygen exchange, transport, and utilization. When the added stress of exercise is imposed during hypoxia, it is essential that the responses of the physiological systems be appropriately orchestrated to maintain oxygen delivery and utilization. Additionally, in recent years the use of hypoxia as part of a physical training regimen to improve athletic performance has proliferated throughout the world. High-altitude camps enable athletes to train using either ambient air or supplemental oxygen while living at altitude. Also, commercially available devices such as hypoxic tents and rooms allow athletes to sleep or to train under moderate- to high-elevation equivalents while continuing to live at a lower elevation.

This chapter describes the physiological and metabolic responses associated with exposure to high altitude during both rest and exercise. Adaptations associated with acclimatization to altitude are also addressed. As numerous scientific studies have been conducted at the summit of Pikes Peak, Colorado (4300 m), this altitude is frequently referenced throughout the chapter.

Basic Concepts and Overview

Hypoxia is defined as an oxygen deficiency caused by a reduction in the partial pressure of oxygen (P_{O_2}) in ambient air because of a decrease in either the ambient barometric pressure (P_B) or the oxygen concentration of the inspired gas. The reduction in P_B, or hypobaria, occurs as one ascends above sea level. According to Boyle's law, the volume of a gas is inversely proportional to its pressure. As the P_B decreases with increasing elevation, the volume of any given gas will increase. The significance of this observation directly relates to the partial pressures of the gases (oxygen, nitrogen, and carbon dioxide) that make up most of the ambient air. With the expanding volume of ambient air at altitude, the partial pressure of each gas declines in proportion to the decline in ambient P_B. In other words, as the elevation increases, the P_{O_2} (as well as the pressure of the other gases) decreases, resulting in less oxygen per liter of air (Table 27.1). Thus, exposure to altitude reduces the P_{O_2} presented to the lungs, which leads to less oxygen diffusing into the arterial circulation for utilization by tissues throughout the body.

TABLE 27.1	Ambient Gas Pressures	
Gas (mm Hg)	Sea Level	4300 m
Carbon dioxide	0.3	0.2
Oxygen	159	96
Nitrogen	601	364
Total	760	460

As per Boyle's law, the volume of a gas is inversely proportional to it pressure at constant temperature. Thus, a given volume of gas at sea level (760 mm Hg) will expand at altitude as the ambient barometric pressure decreases (e.g., Pikes Peak, 460 mm Hg). This reduces oxygen per liter of air at altitude. However, the relative percentages of all the gases remain the same.

Alternatively, hypoxia can be induced by lowering the oxygen concentration of the inspired gas mixture. The hypoxic stimulus of the two methods is considered identical as long as the product of P_B and percent oxygen is identical between methods. For example, to produce the same hypoxic simulation at sea level ($P_B = 760$ mm Hg) as at the summit of Pikes Peak (4300 m; $P_B = 460$ mm Hg and 20.93% oxygen), a gas containing 12.67% oxygen should be utilized ($460 \cdot 20.93\% = 760 \cdot 12.67\%$). The fact that the two methods provide an equivalent hypoxia stimulus has important implications. It means that the two methods can be used interchangeably or in some combination for a desired outcome and for a variety of purposes.

Adjustments in a number of physiological systems occur in response to the disruption of homeostasis imposed by the stress of hypoxia (Fig. 27.1). The respiratory response is an increase in both rate and volume in an attempt to get more oxygen into the lungs. The oxyhemoglobin dissociation curve initially shifts to the left as a result of respiratory alkalosis allowing more oxygen to become bound to Hb at the level of the lungs. Heart rate, and thus cardiac output, increase to compensate for the reduced oxygen content of blood so that similar amounts of oxygen are transported to tissues. Additionally, to improve oxygen-carrying capacity, there is a reduction in plasma volume and an increase in red blood cell (RBC) volume. Unloading of oxygen at the tissue is also facilitated, as is oxygen diffusion from blood into cells. Muscle energetics are also altered to reflect a limitation in oxygen availability and to maintain adenosine triphosphate (ATP) production. Many of these adjustments are regulated in part by activation of key components of the neuroendocrine system. Specifically, the autonomic nervous system and the adrenal glands play a major role. These concepts are discussed in more detail in later sections.

The extent to which altitude exposure disrupts homeostasis and the degree of the physiological and metabolic responses are determined by the level of hypoxia. Generally, at low altitudes (0–1499 m, or 0–4918 ft, 760–635 mm Hg) resting arterial oxygen saturation (SaO_2) is well maintained and represents minimal stress on the body. At moderate altitudes (1500–2999 m, or 4921–9840 ft, 635–525 mm Hg) individuals will experience slight decreases in resting SaO_2 (95–92%) as the ambient PO_2 can range from 130 to 110 mm Hg (compared to 159 mm Hg at sea level) (Fig. 27.2). As one ascends to higher altitudes (3000–5000 m, or 9841–16,405 ft, 525–405 mm Hg), ambient PO_2 will decrease to 110 to 85 mm Hg, with resting SaO_2 ranging from 91% to less than 80%. Thus, the decrease in resting SaO_2 is proportional to the elevation. During exercise at altitude, SaO_2 falls below resting values, with the additional decline proportional to both elevation and exercise intensity. Exercise-induced reduction in SaO_2 at altitude is discussed in the next sections.

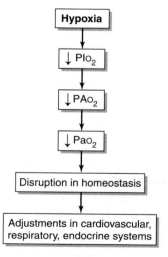

FIGURE 27.1 Exposure to hypoxia directly results in a reduction in arterial oxygen pressure (PaO_2). This disruption in homeostasis triggers neuroendocrine responses that help regulate important adjustments in key systems, such as the cardiovascular, respiratory, and endocrine systems.

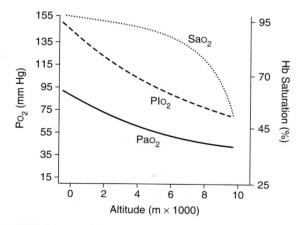

FIGURE 27.2 Alterations in Hb saturation (SaO_2), inspired oxygen pressure (PIO_2) and arterial oxygen pressure (PaO_2) as a function of increasing altitude. Values for SaO_2 and PaO_2 are for resting acclimatized individuals.

Gas Exchange, Delivery, and Extraction

The transport of oxygen from the atmosphere to the cells of various tissues starts with pulmonary ventilation, in which gas molecules are actively transferred from the ambient air to the alveoli. Then there is pulmonary gas exchange, in which oxygen diffuses from the alveoli into capillary blood and combines with Hb. The oxygenated Hb is transported to the tissues, where it diffuses out of the systemic capillaries and into the cells and their centers of respiration, the mitochondria.

Ventilation

Peripheral chemoreceptors in the aortic arch and carotid arteries are sensitive to reductions in the partial pressure of arterial oxygen (PaO_2). As PaO_2 falls during ascent, the chemoreceptors are stimulated, and within seconds ventilation increases. Then, over the ensuing hours to days at altitude, ventilation increases progressively to a sustained higher level whose magnitude depends on the elevation. The hypoxic ventilatory response results in an increase in the partial pressure of alveolar oxygen (PAO_2), which in turn increases PaO_2 and SaO_2 throughout the same period. The induced hyperventilation also causes more carbon dioxide than normal to be exhaled, resulting in below normal levels of $PACO_2$ and $PaCO_2$ and a rise in arterial pH. One of the physiological outcomes of the resulting alkalosis includes the opposition and limitation of the rise in ventilation over the first few days relative to what it would be without the inhibitory effects. Thereafter, the inhibitory influence of low PCO_2 on ventilation is overridden by the hypoxic ventilatory drive. The term *ventilatory acclimatization* is often used to describe the interrelated and time dependent changes in ventilation, PAO_2, PaO_2, $PACO_2$, pH, and SaO_2 that occur over the first weeks of residence at a given elevation (1). Presented in Table 27.2 are the resting ventilatory, pH and SaO_2 responses representing a typical successful ventilatory acclimatization of a sea level resident exposed to an elevation of 4300 m for 2 wk.

Exercise at sea level stimulates ventilation for reasons that are described in detail in other chapters in this textbook. Ventilation at rest and during exercise at a given power output is generally higher at altitude than at sea level (Fig. 27.3).

However, the difference between resting and exercise ventilation widens in proportion to an increase in elevation. This observation suggests that there is a synergistic rather than a simple additive relationship between exercise and hypoxia that may be related to changes in carotid chemoreceptor responsiveness (2). Interestingly, maximal exercise ventilation will be similar, even at extreme elevations.

Alveolar–Arterial Oxygen Pressure Gradient

The pressure gradient between PAO_2 and the partial pressure in pulmonary capillary blood and the diffusion capacity of the lung for oxygen determine the rate of oxygen uptake by Hb during its transit through lung capillaries (about 0.75 s during rest) (see Chapter 11). The higher the PAO_2 and the wider the pressure gradient, the more rapid will be the diffusion of oxygen. At sea level, the pressure gradient is 65 mm Hg (PAO_2 is 105 mm Hg and entering capillary blood is 40 mm Hg). In approximately 0.25 s at sea level, the rise in SaO_2 is complete ($\geq 96\%$) before Hb leaves the lung capillary. Even with a reduction in RBC transit time through the pulmonary capillaries, as would occur with an increase in cardiac output ($\dot{Q}$) during exercise, the end capillary PO_2 for most individuals will be nearly equal to PAO_2 (1).

During initial exposure to 4300 m the oxygen pressure gradient is reduced to about 30 mm Hg ($PAO_2 = 50$ mm Hg—entering capillary blood of 20 mm Hg), which ultimately reduces the rate of rise in PO_2 to its lower equilibrium, resulting in a SaO_2 of about 80% at rest during capillary transit time. During dynamic exercise, the increase reduces Hb transit time (i.e., increases RBC speed through pulmonary capillaries) to a level that may be insufficient to allow equilibrium between PAO_2 and capillary PO_2, hence result in a further reduction in SaO_2. The resultant widening of the PAO_2–PaO_2 gradient (and reduced SaO_2) at altitude indicates that oxygen uptake during moderate to heavy exercise is at least in part diffusion limited by the lowered PAO_2 (1,3).

The adequacy with which gas exchange occurs is also dependent upon the distribution of the ratio of alveolar ventilation to blood perfusion ($\dot{V}_A/\dot{Q}$) throughout the lung. At rest, not all alveoli are ventilated equally, nor is blood flow through the alveolar capillary the same for each alveolus. Therefore, $\dot{V}_A$ and alveolar capillary blood flow are usually

TABLE 27.2	Typical Resting Responses for PAO_2, $PACO_2$, Ventilation, pH, and SaO_2 for a Sea-Level Resident Exposed to an Elevation of 4300 m for 2 Weeks				
	Sea Level	Day 1	Day 7	Day 14
PAO_2 (mm Hg)	100	47	52	56
$PACO_2$ (mm Hg)	39	35	31	28
Ventilation (L·min⁻¹)	8	9	11	12
pH	7.40	7.46	7.50	7.45
SaO_2 (%)	97	80	86	88

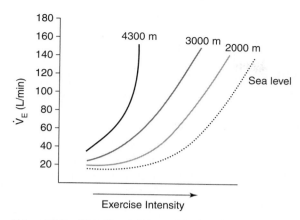

Figure 27.3 The effect of increasing altitude on ventilation during graded-intensity exercise.

not distributed uniformly. The upper lobes are ventilated more but perfused less than the lower lobes. At altitudes above 2500 m, the increase in $\dot{V}_A$ is matched by an increase in pulmonary perfusion in poorly perfused areas of the lung, such as the apices, likely because of hypoxia-induced pulmonary vasoconstriction. The net effect is an enlarged surface area for gas exchange. Both a diffusion limitation and a $\dot{V}_A/\dot{Q}$ mismatch contribute to the widening of the PAO_2–PaO_2 gradient during exercise at altitude, but the contribution of a diffusion limitation becomes proportionally greater with increasing exercise intensity and elevation (3).

Transportation of Oxygen

As described in Chapter 11, oxygen diffuses into the pulmonary capillary, where the blood carries it to the tissues. Most oxygen is transported in a loose, reversible chemical combination with Hb and not in a dissolved state (<1%). The sigmoid shape of the oxyhemoglobin dissociation curve describes the relationship between the PaO_2 and the completeness with which Hb is saturated with oxygen (i.e., SaO_2). The curve has potential for shifting position relative to a given PO_2 to provide a means to match oxygen exchange capabilities of the lung with that of the tissues. Changes in PCO_2, pH, temperature, and 2,3 diphosphoglycerate (2,3 DPG) affect the position of the curve and thereby alter the relationship of PaO_2 and SaO_2. The position of the curve is influenced by the strength of each of the factors relative to the others. During initial altitude exposure under resting conditions, hyperventilatory alkalosis causes a leftward shift in the oxyhemoglobin dissociation curve (increasing oxyhemoglobin affinity) so that the rate of oxygen loading into the lungs is increased. After a few hours at elevations up to about 4500 m, the curve progressively shifts to the right (decreasing oxyhemoglobin affinity) owing to an increase in 2,3-DPG and then to gradual renal compensation (i.e., increased bicarbonate excretion) to correct the respiratory alkalosis throughout the next couple of weeks (1). At first, it would seem that a right-ward shift would be advantageous, since oxygen release to the tissues would be enhanced. However, an increase in 2, 3-DPG also makes it more difficult for oxygen to combine with Hb in the lungs. At elevations less than 3500 m, there appears to be a net advantage of the rightward shift; at progressively higher altitudes, the relative inability of Hb to combine with oxygen at the lungs may outweigh the advantage provided to the tissues.

Systemic oxygen transport is the product of oxygen content of arterial blood (CaO_2) and $\dot{Q}$. Arterial oxygen content is determined by the product of Hb concentration [Hb], SaO_2, and a constant (1.35 mL · oxygen^{-1} · g Hb^{-1}). Initial exposure to hypoxia causes CaO_2 to be reduced in direct proportion to the reduction in SaO_2. But because of compensatory increases in muscle blood flow and $\dot{Q}$, oxygen transport to the active muscles is maintained similarly for any fixed submaximal power output at altitude as at sea level. Thus, a higher $\dot{Q}$ at altitude than at sea level maintains a similar level of oxygen transport to the tissues. The increase in $\dot{Q}$ is achieved by an increase in heart rate that is evident within the first hour of hypoxia (Fig. 27.4), a result of stimulation of the cardiac β-adrenergic receptors by the cardiac sympathetic nerves and circulating epinephrine.

Within hours to weeks, there is a continued reduction in plasma volume (Fig. 27.5) that is linked to the degree of hypocapnia and alkalosis secondary to the magnitude of hypoxic stress (4). Although the exact mechanism for the reduction in plasma volume at altitude remains unclear, contributing factors include increased urinary, respiratory, and transcutaneous fluid losses and loss of plasma protein content (5). For elevations greater than about 2000 m, there is a significant decrease in plasma volume that is proportional to the elevation. At altitudes of 2300, 3000, 4300, and 5400 m, plasma volume decreases on average by approximately 5, 10, 18, and 28%, respectively (5), resulting in increases in hematocrit and [Hb] (Fig. 27.5). Because of the

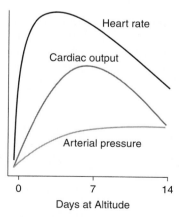

FIGURE 27.4 Cardiovascular adjustments in response to acute and chronic exposure to high altitude. These responses are observed at rest and during submaximal exercise at a given power output.

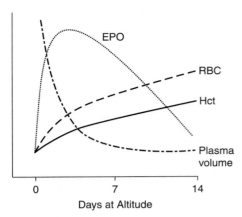

FIGURE 27.5 Effect of altitude on plasma volume over time. A reduction in plasma volume can occur quickly upon exposure to high altitude. This will increase oxygen-carrying capacity of blood by concentrating existing red blood cells (RBC), thereby increasing hematocrit. The hypoxia also stimulates the synthesis and release of erythropoietin (EPO) from the kidneys, which results in a true increase in RBC volume during more prolonged altitude acclimatization.

hemoconcentration and an increase in SaO_2 (due to ventilatory acclimatization), CaO_2 is restored to near sea level values after a week or two of residence at a given altitude. Over the same period, for a given exercise power output, $\dot{Q}$ is reduced from initial exposure because of a decrease in stroke volume due to reduced venous filling and to a decrease in heart rate linked to attenuation in cardiac responsiveness to β-adrenergic stimulation (6) and/or an increase in vagal tone (7). For all exercise intensities, systemic oxygen transport to active muscles is maintained by the restored CaO_2 despite reduced $\dot{Q}$.

Additionally, as a direct result of the hypoxia stimulus, the production of erythropoietin (EPO), a hormone produced primarily by the kidneys to promote synthesis of new RBCs, will increase within the first day of exposure to altitude. EPO will accelerate RBC production in the bone marrow that can persist for weeks with continued residence at altitude (Fig. 27.5). The time course and magnitude of change for a true increase in RBC volume is not clear, although it appears to be one of the slowest adjustments that occurs with acclimatization (5). The EPO response varies greatly among individuals exposed to a given altitude, as does RBC production to a given level of EPO response (8). Nevertheless, for the first few weeks of exposure to altitudes of less than approximately 4000 m, there is likely no measurable true increase in RBC volume. One exception may relate to highly conditioned subjects who lived for 4 wk at 2500 m and trained intensely either at that altitude or a lower altitude (1250 m) (9). In that study (9), RBC volume increased by 9%. After a several weeks at higher elevations, a true ex-

pansion of RBC volume does appear to occur, but the magnitude of change is not well defined (5).

Tissue Oxygenation and Oxygen Extraction

As described in Chapter 14, oxygen travels from the peripheral capillaries through the interstitial fluid and finally into the cell and mitochondria. Once oxygenated blood enters the capillary bed of the tissue, it is the affinity of Hb for oxygen and the capillary-to-cell PO_2 gradient that affects the unloading of oxygen. The increased temperature, acidity, and other local factors associated with exercising muscle also shift the oxyhemoglobin dissociation curve to the right and reduce the affinity of Hb for oxygen to favor the release of oxygen into muscle tissue. Oxygen extraction from the circulation for a given rate of oxygen delivery is further promoted because of the lower tissue intracellular PO_2 at altitude. Tissue oxygen extraction (as indicated by a widening of the arterial-venous oxygen difference) at the same power output is significantly greater during dynamic exercise after about a week at altitude when compared to sea level (1). Thus, at a given submaximal power output at high altitude, muscle oxygen uptake is defended in part by increasing tissue oxygen extraction (Milestone of Discovery).

A number of skeletal muscle changes often associated with altitude acclimatization produce a favorable effect on the rate of oxygen utilization and aerobic energy production. These include increases in capillary density, myoglobin concentration, mitochondrial number, and oxidative enzyme activity (10). However, numerous confounding factors also associated with long-term altitude exposure, such as differing levels of physical activity and caloric intake, reduced muscle mass compared to sea level, and differences in the fitness of the individuals studied, have made it difficult to determine definitively whether skeletal muscle adaptations occur as a result of altitude exposure *per se* (10).

Metabolism and Energetics

Ascent to altitude increases basal metabolic rate above sea level values (11). The increase in basal metabolic rate is apparent after just 1 day at altitude and can persist for days to weeks of altitude residence (11). Further, the total energy requirement that maintains stable body weight and composition at altitude remains elevated for weeks during residence at high elevations (12). Thus, the increase in the energy requirement associated with exposure to altitude must be coupled with an equal increase in energy intake to avoid a negative energy balance and remain weight stable. However, cachexia (weight loss) is a commonly reported consequence during the initial weeks of altitude exposure. This weight loss exceeds what would be expected from loss of total body water normally associated with acclimatization to altitude. The extra weight loss most likely results from a combination of the increase in total energy requirement coupled with loss of appetite and lower energy intake (11). While a number of mechanisms have been suggested to play a role in the suppression of appetite at altitude (e.g., leptin, insulin, cytokines), exact causes of this phenomenon remain to be elucidated.

The implications of the occurrence of a negative energy balance at altitude may account for early reports suggesting a shift toward fat metabolism during the acclimatization period. These assumptions were primarily based on the observations that the rate of muscle glycogen degradation was lower and circulating free fatty acid levels were higher during exercise after altitude acclimatization than during acute altitude exposure (13). However, more recent data reporting subjects who were in energy balance and thus weight stable indicate a greater reliance on carbohydrate than fat with altitude exposure (14–16). With use of isotopic tracer infusions, it has been demonstrated that upon arrival to altitude (4300 m) there is a higher dependence on blood glucose as a substrate both at rest and during steady-state submaximal exercise than at sea level (14). This reliance on blood glucose as a substrate source for muscle persisted after acclimatization (21 days) (Fig. 27.6). These observations were later reaffirmed when it was found that acclimatization to altitude resulted in a decreased reliance on fat as a substrate source with a concomitant increase in the use of glucose (17). It was suggested that this adaptation would be oxygen efficient, since glucose yields more energy per liter of oxygen than do fats and proteins. From a mechanistic standpoint, hypoxia can promote glucose uptake via translocation of glucose transporters to the cell surface of the plasma membrane independently of insulin or skeletal muscle contraction.

A particular phenomenon that has interested high-altitude and exercise physiologists alike is known as the lactate para-

dox. Upon arrival to altitude, exercise elicits a significantly greater blood lactate response than the same absolute power output at sea level. This finding alone is not surprising, as the same absolute power output performed at altitude represents a greater relative stress. As a result, it elicits hormonal and metabolic changes that in turn promote increased glycogenolysis and elevated glycolytic flux (Table 27.3). The traditional concept has been that in the presence of reduced arterial oxygen levels at altitude, a Pasteur-like effect could contribute to an elevation of glycolysis and thereby lactate production. After acclimatization, at the identical power output (both absolute and relative) as that of acute altitude exposure, blood lactate is significantly lower (Fig. 27.7A). The paradox is that this occurs despite the finding that whole-body and working muscle oxygen uptake do not differ as a function of duration at altitude. Thus, the lower lactate concentration with acclimatization cannot be explained by improved oxygen delivery and utilization by exercising muscle. Further, despite the presence of hypoxia, blood lactate at maximal exercise is lower than at sea level (1).

A number of explanations have been postulated to explain the lactate paradox. One involves the hormonal regulation of muscle glycogenolysis via increased epinephrine stimulation of β-adrenergic receptors that would increase glycolytic flux and result in an increase in lactate production. As described later, the adrenal medullary secretion of epinephrine is elevated with acute exposure to hypoxia but subsides during acclimatization. It has been shown that with [3-^{13}C] isotopic lactate infusions, significant temporal correlations exist (r = .95) between arterial epinephrine levels (Fig. 27.7B) and the rate of lactate appearance both at rest and during steady-state exercise at sea level and during acute and chronic altitude exposures (18). A follow-up study utilizing β-adrenergic blockade clearly indicated that epinephrine has a critical role in lactate production at altitude, although it could not entirely account for the lactate response observed with acclimatization (17).

Other factors that may contribute to the lactate paradox include intracellular calcium concentration and its regulation and the control of glycolysis by ATP and adenosine diphosphate (ADP). Because excitation-contraction coupling in muscle involves alterations in calcium flux, it is likely that calcium plays a role in stimulating glycogenolysis (e.g., via stimulation of phosphorylase kinase) during muscular contraction independently of epinephrine. This line of reasoning agrees with the finding of a transient increase in muscle lactate production during exercise at 4300 m (19) and may at least partially explain why lactate concentration always increases during exercise, even after acclimatization, when epinephrine levels are greatly reduced. However, whether the reliance on or sensitivity to calcium is altered with acute or chronic altitude exposure is unknown. It has been suggested that a tighter coupling between oxidative phosphorylation and glycolytic flux may explain the lower lactate level with acclimatization at altitude (20). A higher ratio of ATP

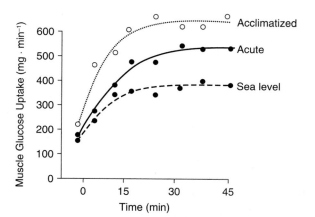

FIGURE 27.6 Muscle glucose uptake during 45 minutes of submaximal cycle exercise at 100 watts at sea level, on day 1 of exposure to 4300 m (acute) and on day 21 at 4300 m (acclimatized). *(Reprinted with permission from Brooks GA, Wolfel EE, Groves BM, et al. Muscle accounts for glucose disposal but not blood lactate appearance during exercise after acclimatization to 4,300 m. J Appl Physiol 1992;72:2439.)*

TABLE 27.3	Absolute and Relative Oxygen Uptake When Cycling at Power Output of 100 W at Sea Level and at 4300 m		
	Sea Level	4300 m Acute Exposure	4300 m Chronic Exposure
Power output (W)	100	100	100
Oxygen uptake (L · min⁻¹)	1.5	1.5	1.5
% Maximal oxygen uptake	50	70	70

to ADP after acclimatization than during acute exposure would, via allosteric regulation, result in a lower glycolytic flux and consequently reduced lactate production. Further research is necessary to determine whether this potential mechanism contributes to the lactate paradox.

Hormonal and Autonomic Adjustments to Exercise During Hypoxia

Sympathetic Nervous System and Catecholamines

As stated earlier, exposure to high altitude is an environmental stressor with many physiological consequences. The necessary adaptations to high altitude are further complicated by the added stress of dynamic exercise. In response to the disturbance in resting homeostasis, a number of regulatory systems are called upon in an attempt to preserve oxygen delivery to essential tissues. Principal among these are the central nervous system, which is capable of making very rapid adjustments to large segments of the body, and the endocrine system, which can have a more global and farther-reaching effect but requires more time to respond. Specifically, the sym-

pathetic nervous system and the adrenal glands play a critical role in helping an individual respond to the stress of hypoxia.

Catecholamines, both as neurotransmitters and as hormones, have very powerful regulatory properties that exert control over a number of critical physiological and metabolic functions central to the ability to sustain oxygen availability (see Chapter 9). Included among these responses are their capacity to affect cardiac function, regulation of blood flow and pressure, and substrate mobilization and utilization. These responses are specific to the target tissue involved and to the type of adrenergic receptor (e.g., α or β) to which the catecholamines interact. The extent of these responses depends on a number of factors, including the degree of hypoxia, time at altitude, and elapsed time between altitude exposures. When all facets of the neuroendocrine system are performing in harmony, the ability to coordinate and regulate key physiological functions under the perturbations imposed by hypoxia is quite remarkable.

Hypoxemia directly stimulates the adrenal medulla. Within 4 h of arrival at altitude, plasma concentrations of epinephrine in a person at rest are significantly higher than at sea level. This response persists during submaximal exercise, yielding epinephrine levels that are significantly greater than those for the same absolute exercise power output at sea level

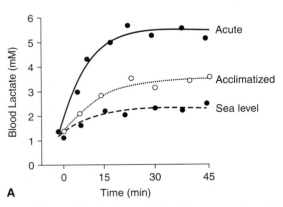

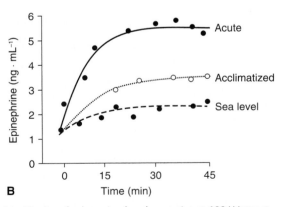

FIGURE 27.7 **A.** The change in blood lactate concentration during 45 min of submaximal cycle exercise at 100 Watts at sea level on day 1 of exposure to 4300 m (acute) and on day 21 at 4300 m (acclimatized). Since $\dot{V}O_{2max}$ did not change from day 1 to day 21 at altitude, subjects exercised at the same absolute and relative exercise intensities on both days. Thus, a change in exercise intensity could not account for the fall in blood lactate associated with acclimatization. **B.** The plasma epinephrine response during conditions identical to those in part A. Note the similarities in response at sea level and at altitude for lactate and epinephrine (correlation coefficient = .95). (*Modified from Mazzeo RS, Bender PR, Brooks GA, et al. Arterial catecholamine responses during exercise with acute and chronic high-altitude exposure. Am J Physiol 1991;261:E421–E422.*)

(Fig. 27.7B). The two explanations for this exaggerated epinephrine response to submaximal exercise during acute altitude exposure are a direct effect of hypoxemia on adrenal medullary epinephrine release and a greater relative exercise intensity at altitude than at sea level (Table 27.3 and the section "Submaximal Exercise Performance"). As consistently demonstrated at sea level, the relative intensity plays a critical role in determining the magnitude of sympathoadrenal responses elicited during exercise (see Chapter 9).

As SaO_2 increases during acclimatization, an inverse relationship between SaO_2 and plasma epinephrine concentration becomes apparent. Thus, during acute hypoxia, in which SaO_2 is at its lowest levels, plasma epinephrine concentration is observed to be at its highest. As arterial oxygenation improves with acclimatization, SaO_2 increases and epinephrine levels decline toward sea level values.

The epinephrine response to acute high-altitude exposure is primarily mediated via the β-adrenergic receptors and is designed to immediately improve oxygen delivery to tissues. For example, epinephrine increases heart rate and contractility (i.e., positive chronotropic and inotropic effects) to increase cardiac output and causes vasodilation in blood vessels of skeletal muscle to improve peripheral oxygen transfer. Further, epinephrine activates both muscle and liver glycogenolysis, thereby enhancing carbohydrate utilization. As stated earlier, this likely plays a role in the lactate paradox. Additionally, the increase in β-adrenergic stimulation contributes to the elevation in metabolic rate associated with acute high-altitude exposure.

The resting plasma norepinephrine response to hypoxia (which is a marker of whole-body sympathetic nervous system activity) is different from that observed for epinephrine. When compared to sea level values, resting plasma norepinephrine levels generally do not change significantly with acute hypoxia (21). A lack of an increase in plasma norepinephrine levels does not necessarily indicate that increases in regional sympathetic nerve activity are not occurring, however. While breathing 8–12% oxygen or during acute hypobaric hypoxia simulating 4000–6000 m, resting muscle sympathetic nerve activity has been reported to increase despite plasma norepinephrine remaining unchanged. An elevation in sympathetic nervous system also is confirmed: with no measurable change in plasma norepinephrine levels, within 4 h after arrival to 4300 m measurements of net norepinephrine release from resting legs are greater than values measured at sea level (22).

Dynamic exercise at the same absolute power output during acute hypoxia results in higher plasma norepinephrine levels and sympathetic nervous system activity than at sea level. It appears that this norepinephrine response during acute hypoxia is primarily dependent upon the relative exercise intensity. Thus, if subjects exercise at a similar percentage of maximal oxygen uptake under both environmental conditions, the norepinephrine response is not significantly different between sea level and acute hypoxia.

Sympathetic nervous system activity at rest and in response to exercise at the same power output steadily increases during the first week of altitude residence and remains elevated for quite some time (1–2 months). While the mechanisms responsible for this consistent and robust response are unknown, the physiological consequences are becoming more apparent. Persistent elevations in sympathetic nervous system activity and circulating norepinephrine levels after chronic exposure to high altitude contribute to the rise in systemic vascular resistance, mean arterial blood pressure, elevation in metabolic rate, altered substrate selection, and impaired immune function (21, 23–25).

Parasympathetic Nervous System

An increase in heart rate observed at rest and during exercise can be due to an increase in sympathetic nervous system activity, a decrease in parasympathetic nervous system activity, or both. At sea level and during the first week of altitude exposure, atropine blockage of parasympathetic activity results in similar increases in heart rate at rest and during submaximal exercise. This finding is consistent with the postulate that parasympathetic activity is the same during acute altitude exposure as at sea level. Over a prolonged exposure to altitude (2–3 wk), resting heart rate and submaximal heart rates for a given power output progressively fall. This response is associated with a decline in adrenergic receptor responsiveness in the heart (i.e., down-regulation of β-receptors of the heart). Whether it is also associated with an increase in parasympathetic nervous system activity has not been definitively determined.

During maximal exercise at sea level, the administration of atropine does not increase heart rate, which indicates that parasympathetic activity is completely withdrawn (7). In contrast, administration of atropine during maximal exercise after 5 days of exposure to an altitude of 4300 m significantly increases heart rate (7). This finding clearly shows that parasympathetic activity contributes to the reduction in maximal heart rate from sea level to altitude. With more prolonged exposure to altitudes greater than about 4000 m, maximal heart rate continues to decline, which suggests that parasympathetic activity also may progressively increase with continued exposure (1). However, no studies have determined whether parasympathetic activity during maximal exercise varies as a function of altitude exposure duration. More studies are necessary to assess the role of the parasympathetic nervous system during both acute and chronic altitude exposure. Additionally, the effect of hypoxia on altering muscarinic receptor function and characteristics should be addressed.

Insulin

Fasting insulin levels at altitude are generally similar to those found at sea level. However, the response to a high carbohydrate meal in acute hypoxia suggests a reduction in insulin sensitivity compared to sea level (18). This alteration in insulin sensitivity appears to be transient, since insulin sensitivity returns toward sea level values with altitude acclimatization. In fact, after 9 days at 4300 m, insulin sensitivity was found to increase in response to a high carbohydrate meal compared to sea level (18). These findings likely contribute to the observation of greater oxidation of carbohydrates and in particular blood glucose during acclimatization to altitude. Insulin levels decline gradually during submaximal exercise during both acute and chronic altitude exposure in a manner similar to that observed at sea level. With chronic altitude exposure, submaximal insulin levels are not different from those observed at sea level; however, glucose turnover for the same absolute power output is elevated at altitude (19). These observations are consistent with the concept of enhanced insulin sensitivity associated with acclimatization to altitude.

Cortisol and Glucagon

Surprisingly, despite the stress associated with exposure to hypoxia, cortisol levels generally remain unchanged or only transiently elevated at rest when compared to sea level. Furthermore, the increase in cortisol levels during an acute bout of exercise is more closely related to the relative exercise intensity than to the hypoxia *per se*. Similarly, glucagon levels at rest and during exercise are not appreciably different from those found at sea level.

Immune Function at Altitude

Given the stress imposed by altitude exposure and the associated changes in the sympathoadrenal system, which can independently influence immune function and responsiveness, it is not surprising that recent evidence suggests that both acute and chronic exposure can alter immune function. Blood lymphocyte level and natural killer cell activity increase under conditions of acute hypoxia, with a potentiated response when exercise is added (26). Potential mechanisms include both neural and hormonal interactions with immune function. The alterations in lymphocyte and natural killer cell activity appear to be transient, since levels do not differ from sea level after 4 wk of hypoxic exposure (27).

Recently, alterations in interleukin-6 (IL-6) responses to altitude exposure have been reported (27). IL-6 is an important cytokine involved in a number of biological processes, including the regulation of the immune inflammatory reaction to various stressors. Thus, circulating IL-6 is elevated when homeostasis is disrupted, such as during high-intensity exercise or acute and chronic altitude exposures (27). Resting IL-6 levels increase immediately upon arrival to altitude and remain elevated throughout the duration of stay at 4300 m (3–4 wk). Thus, the elevation in IL-6 persists while individuals are becoming acclimatized to high altitude. Recent evidence suggests that both α- and β-adrenergic mechanisms contribute to the acute and chronic changes in IL-6 levels at altitude (23).

While the physiological significance of the IL-6 response to hypoxia is not well understood, a number of possibilities have been suggested. It is generally believed that the function of IL-6 during acute hypoxia is not to mediate inflammation or acute-phase protein response, since serum values of IL-1β, IL-1ra, TNFα, and C-reactive protein remain unchanged (28). One possible explanation relates to the ability of IL-6 to promote angiogenesis. IL-6 expression is elevated in tissues that undergo active angiogenesis and may play a role via induction of vascular endothelial growth factor (28). The benefit of forming new blood vessels during extended periods of hypoxia (and reduced SaO_2) are obvious and have been reported in both animal and human studies. Additionally, IL-6 can modulate production of EPO, as the addition of IL-6 to hypoxic human hepatoma cells results in a dose-dependent stimulation of hypoxia-induced EPO production by as much as 81% (28). The associated increases in RBC volume and oxygen-carrying capacity are well-documented markers of adaptation to high altitude.

Gender Differences

There have only been a few studies examining the effect of acute hypoxia on women and even fewer investigations related to chronic adaptations. Despite the lack of studies, there is evidence to suggest that in some variables, women adapt to hypoxia slightly differently than men. Early investigations suggested that women may not increase their hematocrit as fast and to the same extent as men (7). This is true particularly for women who come to altitude with inadequate or borderline iron stores. Iron supplementation prior to and during their stay at altitude will increase hematocrit similarly to men. Thus, it is recommended that prior to coming to altitude, women (and men) should ensure that they have adequate iron stores. This is true especially for athletes who plan on training or competing at high elevations (8).

Another possible gender difference is observed on examination of substrate utilization during the acclimatization period. As stated previously, men demonstrate a greater reliance on carbohydrates as a fuel source for muscle after they have acclimatized to altitude than with the same exercise performed at sea level. However, for women, it has been shown that whole-body carbohydrate utilization was lower at rest and during exercise after 10 days of acclimatization to 4300 m than with the same relative exercise intensity performed at sea level (29). The mechanism for this gender difference is unknown, although differences in substrate utilization between men and women also have been reported at sea level. Factors related to differences in adiposity and fat distribution coupled with the known effects of estrogen and progesterone on fat and carbohydrate metabolism have been suggested as possible mechanisms. No effect of menstrual cycle phase has been found with respect to substrate utilization while at altitude (29).

Exercise Performance at Altitude

Maximal Oxygen Uptake

Maximal oxygen uptake ($\dot{V}O_{2max}$) is the product of the total quantity of blood transported to tissues (i.e., $\dot{Q}$) and the difference in CaO_2 and venous ($C\bar{v}O_2$) blood (i.e., atrial-venous oxygen difference). Adjustments in any of the processes involved in oxygen transport or utilization therefore affect $\dot{V}O_{2max}$. During ascent to altitude, there is a progressive decrease in P_B, with resultant declines in PIO_2, PAO_2, and PaO_2. With initial exposure to altitudes up to approximately 4300 m, the reduced $\dot{V}O_{2max}$ is primarily due to a reduced CaO_2 secondary to the decline in PaO_2, while maximal $\dot{Q}$, [Hb], and $C\bar{v}O_2$ are not meaningfully changed from values obtained at sea level. With initial exposure to higher elevations, reductions in $\dot{V}O_{2max}$ are greater than would be expected only from a reduced CaO_2; a recent study conducted at 5300 m equivalent (i.e., breathing 10.5% oxygen at sea level) implicates significant reductions in $\dot{Q}$ and leg blood flow (30). Regardless of the elevation, $\dot{V}O_{2max}$ must necessarily decline during initial exposures to altitude, since maximal $\dot{Q}$ cannot increase to levels greater than those at sea level to compensate for the reduced CaO_2 to maintain maximal oxygen transport.

Within 2–3 wk of residence at 4300 m, CaO_2 will be restored to near sea level values as a result of hemoconcentration and an increase in SaO_2 (due to ventilatory acclimatization). However, within days of exposure maximal $\dot{Q}$ falls to below sea level values. A reduction in maximal stroke volume is the primary factor responsible for the reduction in maximal $\dot{Q}$ at elevations up to approximately 4000 m. At higher elevations, maximal heart rate will also decline with acclimatization, at least in part because of an increase in vagal tone (7). Thus, the potential advantage of a restored CaO_2 is largely negated by the reduction in maximal $\dot{Q}$, and at least at higher elevations, a preferential redistribution of $\dot{Q}$ to nonexercising tissues (31). Restoration of CaO_2 after 2–10 wk of altitude acclimatization does not improve $\dot{V}O_{2max}$ at altitude as much as might be expected from the large improvement in systemic oxygen transport unless aerobic fitness also improves as a result of augmented exercise training. Whether $\dot{V}O_{2max}$ significantly improves with altitude acclimatization has been debated for decades. While many research studies indicate that $\dot{V}O_{2max}$ may be improved at altitude as a result of altitude acclimatization (32), very few well-controlled research studies have actually observed a significant improvement (9).

The solid line in Figure 27.8 illustrates the curvilinear relationship of the measured percentage decline in $\dot{V}O_{2max}$ (expressed as milliliters per kilogram per minute) with increasing actual (mountain laboratories) or simulated (hypobaric chambers or breathing hypoxic gas mixtures) elevations. For ex-

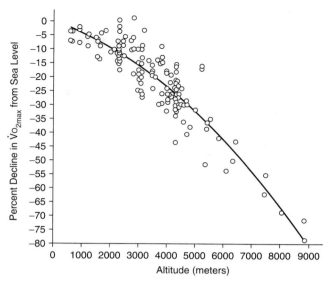

FIGURE 27.8   Change in $\dot{V}O_{2max}$ with change in altitude. Each of the 146 points (circles) represents the average $\dot{V}O_{2max}$ decrement of a group of test subjects participating in one of 67 research studies conducted at actual or simulated altitudes from 580 to 8848 m. Multiple data points were included from a study if more than one elevation, group of test subjects, or exposure was used. Since each data point is a mean value of many intrastudy individual determinations of $\dot{V}O_{2max}$, the drawn regression line represents thousands of $\dot{V}O_{2max}$ test values and therefore can be considered to provide a true approximation of the expected average decrement at each elevation. (*Fulco CS, Rock PB, Cymerman A. Maximal and submaximal exercise performance at altitude. Aviat Space Environ Med 1998;69:794. The figure is printed with permission.*)

ample, on average, $\dot{V}O_{2max}$ declines by about 9, 14, 24, and 32% at 2000, 3000, 4000, and 5000 m, respectively. Note the wide range in percent $\dot{V}O_{2max}$ decline at nearly all elevations. A decrement in $\dot{V}O_{2max}$ that is much less than expected at elevations exceeding approximately 2000 m generally indicates that sedentary subjects participated in a training program at altitude that was more severe than what they were accustomed to at sea level. In other words, it was augmented exercise training *per se* and not the combination of exercise training and altitude exposure that improved $\dot{V}O_{2max}$. Other often-cited potential sources of variation include factors such as aerobic fitness level before exposure, gender, residence at altitude or level of acclimatization prior to a study, amount of exercise-induced arterial hypoxemia, heredity, hypoxic tolerance, lactate threshold, amount of lean body mass, motivation, age, hypoxic ventilatory response, presence of altitude sickness, duration of exposure, inappropriate exercise testing mode for subject population or type of training, and amount of altitude-induced muscle wasting (8,33,34).

One of the biggest contributors to the variation in the decline in $\dot{V}O_{2max}$ at altitude is aerobic fitness level before exposure. To illustrate this point, Figure 27.9 was redrawn from data presented in Figure 27.8 but including only the results of studies of highly conditioned and less well conditioned individuals up to 4300 m. In addition, to minimize possible confounding effects of altitude acclimatization and/or improved aerobic fitness due to training while at altitude, data collected beyond the first 3 days of altitude exposure were excluded.

Figure 27.9 clearly indicates that the much of the variability in $\dot{V}O_{2max}$ at altitudes up to about 4500 m is associated with fitness level before exposure. For example, at approximately 3000 m, the mean decline in $\dot{V}O_{2max}$ for highly conditioned individuals can be expected to be about 22%, whereas for less well conditioned individuals the decline will be about 13%. Although the data presented in Figure 27.9 were dichotomized to compare widely differing fitness levels, the amount of decline in $\dot{V}O_{2max}$ at a given elevation appears to exist on a continuum (35). The difference in $\dot{V}O_{2max}$ between highly conditioned and less well conditioned individuals has been associated with a widened PAO_2–PaO_2 gradient attributed to either greater capillary diffusion limitation or ventilation–perfusion mismatch (3, 36).

It has also been determined that a decrease in $\dot{V}O_{2max}$ is detectable at elevations as low as 580 m, and the minimal altitude may be even lower for highly conditioned individuals. During residence at elevations exceeding about 5000 m, the more rapid decline in $\dot{V}O_{2max}$ may be linked to a failure of $\dot{Q}$ to approach sea level values, preferential redistribution of

$\dot{Q}$ to tissues that are not exercising, reduced blood flow, reduction in muscle mass, or metabolic deterioration often associated with long-term extreme altitude exposures (31,37,38). Finally, when men and women are matched on aerobic fitness level, there generally is no gender difference in $\dot{V}O_{2max}$ decline, nor is there a difference in $\dot{V}O_{2max}$ decline between follicular and luteal menstrual cycle phases (33).

Submaximal Exercise Performance

Although $\dot{V}O_{2max}$ is measured during maximal effort of a relatively brief duration, the decrease in $\dot{V}O_{2max}$ at altitude is also reflected in more prolonged exercise bouts at power outputs less than that required to elicit $\dot{V}O_{2max}$. The metabolic cost for a particular exercise task performed in a steady state at a specified absolute power output is similar at sea level and altitude. But because of the progressive reduction in $\dot{V}O_{2max}$ with increasing elevation, a fixed power output represents progressively greater relative exercise intensity (i.e., a higher percentage of $\dot{V}O_{2max}$) as the elevation increases (Table 27.3). The greater relative stress during exercise at a fixed power output requiring an identical oxygen uptake will shorten time to exhaustion at altitude. Similarly, for activities in which a fixed distance or amount of work must be performed (e.g., 10-km race), completion time will be extended. During initial altitude exposure, ratings of perceived exertion, and various physiological responses associated with exercising at higher submaximal exercise intensities, such as blood lactate and heart rate, also will be higher. After 2–4 wk of altitude acclimatization, exercise at the same submaximal power output will result in lower values for ratings of perceived exertion, blood lactate, and heart rate and will demonstrate enhanced endurance performance compared to initial exposure (39).

It is difficult to predict exactly how much submaximal exercise performance will be impaired at a given elevation or how much variability exists from one individual to another. Unlike the objectivity of the $\dot{V}O_{2max}$ plateau, which indicates high motivation and ensures maximal short-term effort, there are no similar criteria for ensuring all-out effort during many submaximal physical activities or work-related tasks. Moreover, test-retest variability for some commonly used performance testing paradigms is very large, even at sea level under identical experimental conditions (40).

In an effort to minimize such sources of variability, performance results were obtained from 11 studies that used the same male and female athletes ranked nationally or higher, primarily during competitions at sea level and then at altitude (33). Using a homogeneous group of people who are presumed to be healthy and highly motivated and who are performing all-out in precisely timed running or swimming events for which they are trained allows the effects of altitude exposure *per se* on exercise performance to be quantitated. To minimize confounding factors, such as acute mountain sickness and lack of familiarity with the altitude environ-

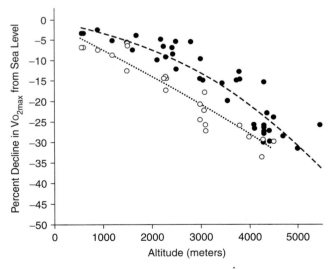

FIGURE 27.9 The effect of physical fitness on $\dot{V}O_{2max}$ decrement at altitude. Highly conditioned individuals (baseline $\dot{V}O_{2max}$ > 63 mL · kg^{-1} · min^{-1}, white circles and dotted line) generally have a greater decrement in $\dot{V}O_{2max}$ than less well conditioned individuals ($\dot{V}O_{2max}$ < 51 mL · kg^{-1} · min^{-1}, black circles and broken line) at elevations up to 4300 m. *(Fulco CS, Rock PB, Cymerman A. Maximal and submaximal exercise performance at altitude. Aviat Space Environ Med 1998;69:794. The figure is reprinted with permission.)*

ment, only the performances of athletes who had lived and trained at altitude for more than 10 days or more were used. Figure 27.10 illustrates the performance decrements as functions of event duration and elevations up to 4300 m.

Much information can be gathered from the data illustrated in Figure 27.10. Athletic events lasting less than 2 min at sea level were not adversely affected by increasing elevation. In general, for events lasting more than 2 minutes at sea level, the longer the event, the greater was its impairment at a given elevation. In addition, the higher the elevation, the greater were the impairments for long events. Data illustrated in Figure 27.10 can also be used to estimate the approximate elevation where measurable performance impairments might consistently be detected. For example, impaired performance during an event lasting 2–5 min at sea level might not be detected until the elevation exceeds approximately 1600 m; for an event lasting 20–30 min at sea level, the impairment might occur at a somewhat lower elevation (about 800 m).

Although Figure 27.10 was derived using highly trained athletes who were participating in competitive athletic events, it could also be used as a guide to estimate hypoxia-induced impairments for less fit individuals participating in other physical activities and work-related tasks of similar durations at similar elevations. Regardless of fitness level, the principle is the same: endurance exercise tasks take longer and have to be performed at a lower metabolic rate at altitude than at sea level.

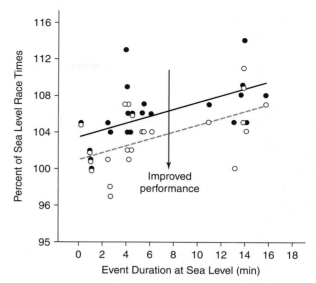

FIGURE 27.11   Effect of altitude acclimatization (2240–2800 m) on athletic events lasting up to 16 min. Data are from athletes whose race times were recorded in the conduct of their primary event at the beginning (<5 days, black circles and solid line) and end (>10 days, white circles and broken line) of their altitude exposure. *(Fulco CS, Rock PB, Cymerman A. Maximal and submaximal exercise performance at altitude. Aviat Space Environ Med 1998;69:793–801. The figure is reprinted with permission.)*

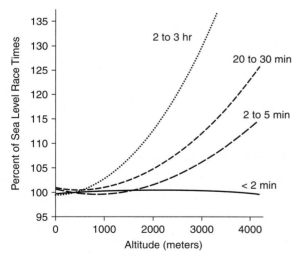

FIGURE 27.10   Physical performance decrements as a function of event duration and elevations up to 4300 m. Data are from athletes who lived and trained at altitude for more than 10 days. Each regression line illustrates how performances changed at altitude for sea level events that lasted less than 2 minutes, 2–5 min, 20–30 min, and 2–3 h. *(Fulco CS, Rock PB, Cymerman A. Maximal and submaximal exercise performance at altitude. Aviat Space Environ Med 1998;69:793–801. The figure is reprinted with permission.)*

The endurance performance decrements illustrated in Figure 27.10 were attenuated relative to the decrements that occurred earlier in the exposure. In other words, the amount of acclimatization that took place during more than 10 days at altitude significantly improved exercise performance. Figure 27.11 illustrates the effects of altitude acclimatization (2240–2800 m) on athletic events lasting up to 16 min. Data are from six of the studies used for Figure 27.10 (33). The illustrated data points are for the same individuals and events but for two different altitude durations (<5 days and >10 days). On average, event performance improved by approximately 2–3% in the relatively short time as a result of altitude acclimatization *per se*. Because of their high aerobic fitness levels and a relatively short interval between evaluation and reevaluation, the improvement in athletic performance at altitude was not likely due to altered aerobic fitness or increased training. Not surprisingly, there was wide variation in improvement between individuals (8).

Improvements in endurance performance at altitude occur not only in highly aerobically fit athletes (e.g., $\dot{V}O_{2max} >$ 63 mL · kg^{-1} · min^{-1} at sea level) who maintain intense training while at low to moderate altitudes but also for less aerobically fit individuals (e.g., $\dot{V}O_{2max} <$ 51 mL · kg^{-1} · min^{-1}1 at sea level) who reside at higher elevations and undergo no additional physical training. For example, endurance time to exhaustion at a given power output while residing at 4300 m improved by 45% on day 10 (39) and by 59% on day 16 (41) compared to day 2 for individuals with $\dot{V}O_{2max}$ of approximately 49 mL · kg^{-1} · min^{-1} at sea level. The dramatic improvements in endurance performance were not likely related to augmented systemic or peripheral oxygen transport, because steady-state $\dot{V}O_2$ was identical on both days. (If steady-state $\dot{V}O_2$ did increase, it would suggest that the enhanced performances were associated with alleviation of active muscle hypoxia.) One possibility (5) relates to the restored CaO_2 resulting from hemoconcentration and ventilatory adaptation that allowed a given $\dot{V}O_2$ to be achieved with a lower $\dot{Q}$, thereby reducing cardiac work. In addition, a reduced $\dot{Q}$ would allow more peripheral diffusion time and perhaps more oxygen extraction for a given power output. Such changes would improve exercise tolerance during whole-body dynamic exercise. Collectively, the results from both athletic events and laboratory research studies clearly indicate that endurance performance improves with residence for a few weeks at altitude for both trained and untrained individuals independently of changes in $\dot{V}O_{2max}$ or training volume.

The reduced air resistance due to the lower air density may also benefit exercise performance in some athletic events at altitude. At 2300 m, the 24% reduction in air density will increase the shot put, hammer throw, javelin, and discus distances by 6 cm, 53 cm, 69 cm, and 162 cm, respectively (42). For running very short distances, in which there is a small aerobic component but high velocity, the advantage of reduced air resistance can result in faster times at altitude than at sea level (43) (Fig. 27.10). Similarly, for events such as speed skating and track cycling, in which velocity is much greater than in running, the reduced air resistance allows a greatly improved performance compared to sea level, even though $\dot{V}O_{2max}$ may be significantly reduced. In fact, a theoretical model suggests that 4000 m would be the optimal elevation for breaking the 1-h unaccompanied cycle race (44) despite an approximately 25% decline in $\dot{V}O_{2max}$. At higher elevations, cycling performance would be impaired by the further reduction in $\dot{V}O_{2max}$ and would more than offset the improving aerodynamic benefit.

Muscle Strength and Power

Muscle strength and maximal muscle power, determined by the force generated during a single brief (1–5 s) maximal muscle contraction (static or dynamic) are generally not adversely affected by acute or chronic altitude exposure (45,46) as long as muscle mass is maintained (47). There is some indication that the first 20 min of hypoxia exposure (equivalent to about 4000–4500 m) may alter the recruitment pattern of the monosynaptic Hoffman (H) reflex and of the direct motor (M) excitation of α-motor fibers (48). However, with longer exposures to altitudes exceeding 4500 m, α-motor neuron excitability, nerve and muscle conduction velocity, and neuromuscular transmission are similar relative to sea level baseline values (49). Anaerobic performance of 20–30 s or less is generally not adversely affected (50).

Improving Athletic Performance at Sea Level

Overview

If the training stimulus at sea level lacks sufficient intensity, duration, frequency, and specificity to affect the appropriate muscle groups and fibers and the energy system, exercise performance will either not improve or deteriorate. Weeks to months of aerobic exercise training enhances both the delivery of oxygen to the exercising muscles and the utilization of oxygen by the muscles and will typically result in improvements in $\dot{V}O_{2max}$ and endurance performance. Reversible changes include increases in blood volume, stroke volume, cardiac output, capillary density, mitochondria, and oxidative enzymes. Moreover, for a given power output, there will be an increase in fat utilization and decreases in heart rate, plasma epinephrine, norepinephrine, lactate and H^+ accumulation, muscle glycogen utilization, and perceived exertion. The magnitude of improvement and physiological change are inversely related to the initial level of aerobic fitness (51).

Many of the changes associated with altitude acclimatization are similar to changes induced by exercise training *per se*. For example, for a given power output after altitude acclimatization compared to initial exposure, there is enhanced blood oxygen carrying capacity; reductions in heart rate, muscle glycogen utilization, lactate accumulation, and perceived exertion; and increased endurance (19,39). Increases in EPO, reticulocytes, RBC volume, capillary density (via reduced muscle fiber size), skeletal muscle buffer capacity, and mitochondrial oxidative enzyme activities have also been observed (5,10). Many athletes and coaches supplement aerobic exercise training programs with an altitude or hypoxia component to improve athletic performance at altitude and sea level. Unfortunately, the interaction of the severity, duration, and frequency of the altitude and hypoxia stimuli that will optimize performance for a given individual are not well defined, and results of many studies have been inconclusive or contradictory (8).

Training While Living at Altitude

Many early studies (1960s and early 1970s) reported that training while living at altitude improved $\dot{V}O_{2max}$ or endurance performance upon return to sea level. However, many of these studies did not include a control group of individuals of similar aerobic fitness who trained at sea level in a similar manner to those who trained at altitude (32). Lack of a sea level control group makes it impossible to determine whether the improvement in performance was due to training or to altitude exposure. Even when sea level control groups were added for comparison in studies conducted in more recent years, results conflicted. Many studies supported a beneficial effect of training and living at altitude for eventual competitions at altitude. However, there is less justification for using such a strategy to improve sea level performance. Most studies having a control group indicated that there was no additional benefit of living and training at altitude for sea level $\dot{V}O_{2max}$ or endurance performance (32,52).

The reason the collective results suggest there may be little to be gained from training while living at altitude for sea level performance relates to alterations in one or more of the training stimuli or strategies, or a reduced blood volume. Ironically, the higher the elevation to optimize the potential beneficial effects associated with altitude acclimatization, such as increases in EPO concentration and RBC volume, the greater the disruption of the training stimulus, which reduces the likelihood of a beneficial effect. If the power output used during altitude training was to be equivalent to that at sea level, the training intensity would be increased (i.e., higher percent $\dot{V}O_{2max}$), training duration shortened, and recovery times lengthened. If the higher-altitude training intensity was to be maintained, there existed an increased possibility that the athlete would train too hard or in an unaccustomed manner (e.g., more intervals, less base training). In contrast, if power output was reduced to maintain equivalent relative exercise intensity (i.e., same percent $\dot{V}O_{2max}$) at altitude as at sea level, the task would take longer, and pacing strategies (e.g., length of the final kick) would be affected. Moreover, there may actually be a detraining effect related to a reduced oxygen turnover and substrate flux through the mitochondrial enzyme systems that lead to a down-regulation of muscle function (52). The practical implication for a highly conditioned and competitive athlete is that training at altitude would be conducted at a reduced sea level race pace, with related reductions in $\dot{V}O_2$, heart rate, and lactate levels (9). Moreover, living at altitude for up to a few weeks is associated with a reduced blood volume and cardiac output, which is opposite to the hematological changes usually observed at sea level when highly conditioned athletes are compared to sedentary individuals or after completion of a prolonged, intense endurance training program. Thus, on balance, living and training at altitude would not seem to be the optimal training strategy for endurance athletes competing in sea level events.

Training but Not Living in Hypoxic Conditions

Living at sea level (or normal ambient P_B) but resting or training under hypoxic conditions (e.g., hypoxic gas breathing) is another strategy used by many highly aerobically fit athletes to improve sea level performance. Typically athletes will rest and/or train in hypoxia (e.g., 2300–6400 m equivalent) for up to 2–5 h per day, 3–5 days per wk, for weeks to months. The principle is that the interaction of training and hypoxic exposure will be more beneficial than training only at sea level. The primary goal is to improve skeletal muscle oxygen transfer by intensifying physical effort. Rarely have studies reported increases in RBC volume, Hb levels, and hematocrit during the experimental periods, despite some studies showing an increase in blood EPO during initial hypoxic exposure. Absolute exercise intensity or power

output is usually reduced during training to a degree proportional to the level of hypoxia for reasons already mentioned. Lack of hematological changes and/or reduced exercise intensity stimuli may be why performance results have been inconclusive. Some studies indicate that performance at sea level after hypoxic training are greater than what would be expected with equivalent training at sea level; others show no performance benefit. If a significant improvement in sea level performance resulting from training in hypoxia is reported, it generally is related to anaerobic power and capacity. Improvements in $\dot{V}O_{2max}$ and endurance are sometimes reported but generally only when assessed under hypoxic conditions. Typically, sea level $\dot{V}O_{2max}$ and endurance performance are not improved with hypoxic training relative to a control group training similarly but under sea level conditions.

Living High, Training Low

In recent years, a live high, train low (LHTL) approach has emerged that allows some of the potentially beneficial changes associated with altitude acclimatization to be combined with maintained power output and race pace strategies. In the landmark study using this approach, Levine and Stray-Gundersen (9) had 39 competitive male and female runners first train together under supervision at sea level for 6 wk before randomly assigning each subject to one of three groups matched by gender, training history, and 5000-m time trial performance. Then, for the next 4 wk, one group lived high, at 2500 m (>20 h per day), and trained low, at 1250 m (LHTL group). Another group lived and trained at 2500 m (LHTH group), and the third group lived and trained at 150 m (LLTL group). Before, during, and for 3 wk after the LHTL, LHTH, or LLTL intervention, numerous field and laboratory performance and blood measures were periodically obtained. There were no significant differences among groups in training distances or duration or for any of the groups over time. At sea level, after the intervention phase, the LHTL and the LHTH groups had increases in $\dot{V}O_{2max}$ (about 5%), RBC volume (about 9%), and Hb (about 10%); but only the LHTL group had improved 5000-m time trial performance, with the improvement persisting for 3 wk after the LHTL intervention. There were no performance changes for the LLTL control group. The authors concluded that because LHTL resulted in an improvement in sea level 5000-m running performance that was not observed in the LHTH and LLTL groups, the mechanism was related to the combination of an increased blood oxygen carrying capacity and $\dot{V}O_{2max}$ along with high-intensity interval training equivalent to sea level training velocities and oxygen flux.

In the context of similarly designed follow-up studies by the same group, these findings have also been confirmed: (a) The LHTL approach improves performance for athletes of differing levels of aerobic fitness (53). (b) Performance varies widely in response to altitude training regardless of the type of altitude intervention used. (c) Subjects (responders) having the greatest initial and sustained increase in

EPO leading to an increased RBC volume had most improvements in $\dot{V}O_{2max}$ and 5000-m run times; this was in contrast to nonresponders, who had a lesser EPO response, no change in RBC volume, and no improvement in $\dot{V}O_{2max}$ or 5,000-m run time (8). (d) Iron-deficient athletes are unable to increase RBC volume during altitude acclimatization, so iron supplementation is advised. (e) Speed maintenance during high-intensity intervals while training is essential for competitive performance at sea level and for the maintenance of muscle fiber size, myoglobin concentration, and muscle buffer capacity. The research group also determined that the level of hypoxia required for sustained increased release of EPO over a 24-h period for most individuals is equivalent to 2100–2500 m (20).

Despite consistent growing evidence that the LHTL paradigm is the most beneficial altitude-training method for improving sea level performance in competitive endurance athletes, it may be impractical or inconvenient for many groups to use it as it was originally implemented by Levine and Stray-Gundersen (9). In their paradigm (9), LHTL athletes lived more than 20 h per day at 2500 m and were driven to 1250 m to participate in high-intensity training daily for 28 days. To simulate the LHTL experience, some research groups have used alternative approaches that include hypoxic sleeping units or apartments to live high and continue normal training near sea level. Others have used supplemental oxygen to train low while living at altitude. All alternative LHTL approaches should yield equivalent physiological and performance-enhancing stimuli relative to the original LHTL paradigm. However, results of most of the recent studies using the alternative LHTL approaches are equivocal. Closer inspection of all of the results to date seem to indicate clearly that to yield similar physiological adaptations that will improve sea level performance, none of the experimental design factors of the alternative LHTL approaches may deviate greatly from the original LHTL paradigm. That is, significant beneficial changes will not likely occur if: (a) The living high elevation is less than about 2100 m. (b) The hypoxic exposure is less than about 16 h per day. (c) The duration of exposure is less than about 20 days. (d) High-intensity training is not maintained at lower elevations. It is unknown to what extent, if any, changing one factor (e.g., elevation) can offset a change in another factor (e.g., hours of exposure per day).

A **MILESTONE** OF DISCOVERY

In the fall of 1985, a team of investigators began what is now known as Operation Everest II. This multifaceted project, which had been in preparation for approximately 5 years, was conducted in the hypobaric chamber in Natick, Massachusetts, under the direction of the U.S. Army Research Institute of Environmental Medicine. This investigation resulted in more than 40 published works that have significantly added to our understanding of adaptations made by the body in response to exposure to extreme high altitude. The study by John Sutton and his associates specifically examined the role of oxygen transport during exercise under such conditions. As ambient oxygen pressure decreases with increasing altitude, it was a primary purpose of this study to examine how well oxygen transport is maintained under such extreme conditions, particularly when the added demand of exercise is placed upon the body. Further, the extent to which the various links in the oxygen transport chain or cascade could respond and function was of primary interest. Nine subjects began the investigations and a total of six subjects completed all phases of the experiment. A simulated ascent to the summit of Mount Everest (8848 m) was accomplished by gradual decompression over time, with a total of 40 days being spent inside the chamber. Subjects were studied at rest and while cycling on a bicycle ergometer to maximal capacity, with each workload lasting 5–8 min. The main finding was that oxygen transport at extreme altitude was defended primarily by the first (pulmonary ventilation) and last (diffusion from capillary and mitochondrial utilization) links in the oxygen transport chain. Table 27.4 shows data for the highest exercise power output achieved, which was common to all altitudes (PIO_2) studied.

The observation of a progressive increase in both resting and exercise ventilation indicated maintenance of the hypoxic ventilatory control at these extreme altitudes. Further, the results suggested that despite severe hypoxemia, there was no depression of ventilatory drive or respiratory muscle fatigue.

The next link in the chain, diffusion of oxygen from alveoli to capillary blood, while diffusion-limited at altitude, was found to contribute only marginally to the reduction in PaO_2. The finding that at high altitude cardiac output for a given workload was similar to that found at sea level led the authors to conclude that cardiac output defends oxygen transport only at the higher exercise workloads. This was further supported by the observation that tissue oxygen extraction, indicated by decrements in $P\bar{V}O_2$, during the initial workloads was significantly greater at altitude than at sea level. Thus, at a given submaximal power output at high altitude, muscle $\dot{V}O_2$ is defended by increasing tissue oxygen extraction in preference to increasing cardiac output. Only at the higher workloads, when oxygen extraction becomes limited, are there adjustments in cardiac output. The time and effort required for such a multifaceted study, the number of subjects and investigators involved, and the voluminous amount of data collected and analyzed under such finely controlled conditions makes Operation Everest II truly a remarkable achievement in high-altitude physiology.

Sutton JR, Reeves JT, Wagner PD, et al. Operation Everest II: oxygen transport during exercise at extreme simulated altitude. J Appl Physiol 1988;64:1309–1321.

TABLE 27.4	Data Collected at Power Output of 120 W During Operation Everest II				
Elevation	PIo$_2$ (mm Hg)	V̇E (L · min⁻¹)	Pao$_2$ (Torr)	Q̇ (L · min⁻¹)	Pvo$_2$ (Torr)
Sea level	150	47.7 ± 3.5	99.7 ± 5.8	16.5 ± 2.4	26.0 ± 2.0
4527 m	80	71.8 ± 6.8	42.2 ± 2.7		
6100 m	63	92.4 ± 12.7	33.8 ± 2.9	14.6 ± 1.7	15.4 ± 1.7
7620 m	49	161.8 ± 18.0	33.1 ± 1.2	15.9 ± 0.6	14.4 ± 1.4
8848 m	43	183.5 ± 34.0	27.6 ± 0.6	16.1 ± 0.1	13.8 ± 0.6

PIo$_2$, inspired Po$_2$; V̇E, minute ventilation (BTPS); Pao$_2$, arterial Po$_2$; Q̇, cardiac output; Pvo$_2$, mixed venous P o$_2$; Values are means + or − SD. For sea level and 4572 m, n = 8; for 6100 m, n = 6; for 7620 and 8848 m, n = 3.

SUMMARY

During ascent to high elevations, a decrease in atmospheric pressure reduces the oxygen gradient between lung and target tissues. Depending on the elevation, many unacclimatized individuals have difficulty during the first few hours to days of exposure. Changes in numerous ventilatory, hemodynamic, hematological, neural, hormonal, metabolic, acid-base, and body water processes are initiated almost immediately to counteract the hypoxia. In general, there is a wide range in the rate and magnitude of each change that characterizes physiological stability at a given elevation. Moreover, the magnitude of the early physiological adjustments of each process and the subsequent rate of acclimatization at a given elevation are related to factors such as rate of ascent, amount of physical exertion, and individual variability.

It has often been observed that many of the physiological changes that occur with altitude acclimatization parallel those that occur after a period of endurance exercise training at sea level. For example, for a given submaximal power output, heart rate and blood lactate decline and endurance performance improves during altitude acclimatization and during augmented physical conditioning. For such reasons, athletes and coaches have used numerous strategies and combinations of hypoxia and altitude supplementation during a period of exercise training to induce an additive or potentiating effect on athletic performance at sea level. In recent years, the living high and training low approach, which combines some of the advantageous changes of acclimatization (e.g., an increase in RBC volume) with an undiminished exercise intensity stimulus, has been accumulating scientific and popular support as the most beneficial altitude and training paradigm for improving endurance performance at sea level.

REFERENCES

1. Young AJ, Reeves JL. Human adaptation to high terrestrial altitude. In Lounsbury DE, Bellamy RF, Zajtchuk R, eds. Medical aspects of harsh environments. Washington, DC: Office of the Surgeon General, Borden Institute, 2002, 647–691.
2. Dempsey JA, Forster HV, Birnbaum ML, et al. Control of exercise hyperpnea under varying durations of exposure to moderate hypoxia. Respir Physiol 1972;16:213–231.
3. Wagner PD, Sutton JR, Reeves JT, et al. Operation Everest II: pulmonary gas exchange during a simulated ascent of Mt. Everest. J Appl Physiol 1987;63:2348–2359.
4. Grover RF, Reeves JT, Maher JT, et al. Maintained stroke volume but impaired arterial oxygenation in man at high altitude with supplemental CO$_2$. Circ Res 1976;38:391–396.
5. Sawka MN, Convertino VA, Eichner ER, et al. Blood volume: importance and adaptations to exercise training, environmental stresses, and trauma/sickness. Med Sci Sports Exerc 2000;32:332–348.
6. Maher JT, Denniston JC, Wolfe DL, et al. Mechanism of the attenuated cardiac response to beta-adrenergic stimulation in chronic hypoxia. J Appl Physiol 1978;44:647–651.
7. Hartley LH, Vogel JA, Cruz JC. Reduction of maximal exercise heart rate at altitude and its reversal with atropine. J Appl Physiol 1974;36:362–365.
8. Chapman RF, Stray-Gundersen J, Levine BD. Individual variation in response to altitude training. J Appl Physiol 1998;85:1448–1456.
9. Levine BD, Stray-Gundersen J. "Living high–training low": effect of moderate-altitude acclimatization with low-altitude training on performance. J Appl Physiol 1997;83:102–112.
10. Mathieu-Costello O. Muscle adaptation to altitude: Tissue capillarity and capacity for aerobic metabolism. High Altitude Medicine Biology 2001;2:413–425.
11. Butterfield GE, Gates J, Fleming S, et al. Increased energy intake minimizes weight loss in men at high altitude. J Appl Physiol 1992;72:1741–1748.
12. Mawson JT, Braun B, Rock PB, et al. Women at altitude: energy requirement at 4300 m. J Appl Physiol 2000;88:272–281.
13. Young AJ, Evans WJ, Cymerman A, et al. Sparing effect of chronic high-altitude exposure on muscle glycogen utilization. J Appl Physiol 1982;52:857–862.
14. Brooks GA, Butterfield GE, Wolfe RR, et al. Increased dependence on blood glucose after acclimatization to 4,300 m. J Appl Physiol 1991;70:919–927.
15. Brooks GA, Wolfel EE, Groves BM, et al. Muscle accounts for glucose disposal but not blood lactate appearance during exercise after acclimatization to 4,300 m. J Appl Physiol 1992;72:2435–2445.
16. Roberts AC, Butterfield GE, Cymerman A, et al. Acclimatization to 4,300-m altitude decreases reliance on fat as a substrate. J Appl Physiol 1996;81:1762–1771.

17. Roberts AC, Reeves JT, Butterfield GE, et al. Altitude and β-blockade augment glucose utilization during submaximal exercise. J Appl Physiol 1996;80:605–615.

18. Braun B, Rock PB, Zamudio S, et al. Women at altitude: short-term exposure to hypoxia and/or α1-adrenergic blockade reduces insulin sensitivity. J Appl Physiol 2001;91:623–631.

19. Brooks GA, Butterfield GE, Wolfe RR, et al. Decreased reliance on lactate during exercise after acclimatization to 4,300 m. J Appl Physiol 1991;71:333–341.

20. Ge RL, S Witkowski, Y Zhang, et al. Determinants of erythropoietin release in response to short-term hypobaric hypoxia. J Appl Physiol 2002;92:2361–2367.

21. Mazzeo RS, Bender PR, Brooks GA, et al. Arterial catecholamine responses during exercise with acute and chronic high-altitude exposure. Am J Physiol 1991;261:E419–E424.

22. Mazzeo RS, Brooks GA, Butterfield GE, et al. Acclimatization to high altitude increases muscle sympathetic activity both at rest and during exercise. Am J Physiol 1995;269:R201–R207.

23. Mazzeo RS, Donovan D, Fleshner M, et al. Interleukin-6 response to exercise and high-altitude exposure: influence of α-adrenergic blockade. J Appl Physiol 2001;91:2143–2149.

24. Mazzeo RS, Dubay A, Kirsch JS, et al. Catecholamine response to exercise and high-altitude exposure: influence of α-adrenergic blockade. Metabolism 2003;52:1471–1477.

25. Wolfel EE, Selland MA, Mazzeo RS, et al. Systemic hypertension at 4,300 m is related to sympathoadrenal activity. J Appl Physiol 1994;76:1643–1650.

26. Klokker M, Kjaer M, Secher NH, et al. Natural killer cell response to exercise in humans: effect of hypoxia and epidural anesthesia. J Appl Physiol 1995;78:709–716.

27. Meehan R, Duncan U, Neale L, et al. Operation Everest II: alterations in the immune system at high altitudes. J Clin Immunol 2004;8:397–406.

28. Pedersen BK, Steensberg A. Exercise and hypoxia: effects on leukocytes and interleukin-6—shared mechanisms? Med Sci Sports Exerc 2002;34:2004–2012.

29. Braun B, Mawson JT, Muza SR, et al. Women at altitude: carbohydrate utilization during exercise at 4300 m. J Appl Physiol 2000;88:246–256.

30. Calbet JAL, Boushel R, Radegran G, et al. Determinants of maximal oxygen uptake in severe acute hypoxia. Am J Physiol 2003;284:R291–R303.

31. Calbet JA, Boushel R, Radegran G, et al. Why is VO2max after altitude acclimatization still reduced despite normalization of arterial oxygen content? Am J Physiol 2003;284:R304–R316.

32. Fulco CS, Rock PB, Cymerman A. Improving athletic performance: is altitude residence or altitude training helpful? Aviat Space Environ Med 2000;71:162–171.

33. Fulco CS, Rock PB, Cymerman A. Maximal and submaximal exercise performance at altitude. Aviat Space Environ Med 1998;69:793–801.

34. Robergs RA, Quintana R, Parker DL, et al. Multiple variables explain the variability in the decrement in VO2max during acute hypobaric hypoxia. Med Sci Sports Exerc 1998;30:869–879.

35. Young AJ, Cymerman A, Burse RL. The influence of cardiorespiratory fitness on the decrement in maximal aerobic power at high altitude. Eur J Appl Physiol 1985;54:12–15.

36. Gore CJ, Hahn AG, Scroop GS, et al. Increased arterial desaturation in trained cyclists during maximal exercise at 580 m altitude. J Appl Physiol 1996;80:2204–2210.

37. Boutellier U, Marconi C, di Prampero PE, et al. Effects of chronic hypoxia on maximal performance. Bull Europ Physiopath Resp 1982;18:39–44.

38. Rose MS, Houston CS, Fulco CS, et al. Operation Everest. II: nutrition and body composition. J Appl Physiol 1988;65:2545–2551.

39. Maher JT, Jones LG, Hartley LH. Effects of high-altitude exposure on submaximal endurance capacity of men. J Appl Physiol 1974;37:895–898.

40. Jeukendrup A, Saris WHM, Brouns F, et al. A new validated endurance performance test. Med Sci Sports Exerc 1996;28:266–270.

41. Horstman D, Weiskoff R, Jackson RE. Work capacity during 3-wk sojourn at 4,300 m: effects of relative polycythemia. J Appl Physiol 1980;49:311–318.

42. Dickinson ER, Piddington MJ, Brain T. Project Olympics. Schweizerische Zeitschrift Fur Sportmedizin 1966;14:305–308.

43. Arsec LM. Effects of altitude on the energetics of human best performances in 100 m running. Eur J Appl Physiol 2002;87:78–84.

44. Capelli C, di Prampero PE. Effects of altitude on top speeds during 1 h unaccompanied cycling. Eur J Appl Physiol 1995;71:469–471.

45. Fulco CS, Cymerman A, Muza SR, et al. Adductor pollicis muscle fatigue during acute and chronic altitude exposure and return to sea level. J Appl Physiol 1994;77:179–183.

46. Fulco CS, Lewis SF, Frykman P, et al. Muscle fatigue and exhaustion during dynamic leg exercise in normoxia and hypobaric hypoxia. J Appl Physiol 1996;81:1891–1900.

47. Kayser B, Narici M, Milesi S, et al. Body composition and maximum alactic anaerobic performance during a one month stay at high altitude. Int J Sports Med 1993;14:244–247.

48. Willer JC, Miserocchi G, Gautier H. Hypoxia and monosynaptic reflexes in humans. J Appl Physiol 1987;63:639–645.

49. Garner SH, JR Sutton, RL Burse, et al. Operation Everest II: neuromuscular performance under conditions of extreme simulated altitude. J Appl Physiol 1990;68:1167–1172.

50. Coudert J. Anaerobic performance at altitude. Int J Sports Med 13 Suppl 1992;1:S82–S85.

51. Blomqvist GC, Saltin B. Cardiovascular adaptations to physical training. Ann Rev Physiol 1983;45:169–189.

52. Levine BD. Intermittent hypoxic training: fact and fancy. High Alt Med Biol 2002;3:177–193.

53. Stray-Gundersen J, Chapman RF, Levine BD. "Living high-training low" altitude training improves sea level performance in male and female elite runners. J Appl Physiol 2001;91:1113–1120.

Physiological Systems and Their Responses To Conditions of Hyperbaria

John R. Claybaugh, Keizo Shiraki, and Robert Elsner

Introduction

When humans enter a hyperbaric environment, the purpose is typically to exercise or work. Such work includes the age-old occupations of breath-hold diving, helmet diving, and diving with self-contained breathing apparatus (SCUBA). In addition, underwater tunnel construction and deep saturation diving are often done in dry pressurized-gas environments. The work force in these occupations is relatively small. For instance, there are approximately 20,000 commercial breath-hold divers. Also, the Association of Diving Contractors International estimates that there are 4200 commercial divers in the United States. Most are helmet divers, some use SCUBA, and approximately 600 are engaged in saturation diving. Worldwide, there are an estimated 13,000 to 15,000 commercial divers. These figures do not include professions that may use diving as part of their job, for example policemen, firemen, military workers, commercial fishermen, and scientific divers. In addition, the Professional Association of Diving Instructors estimates that 854,000 SCUBA divers are certified each year worldwide. Thus, a labor force and a large recreational population are exposed to hyperbaric work and exercise, justifying consideration of the unique problems associated with this environment.

The units of pressure used to describe the high-pressure environments are unfortunately not consistent. Pressures are given in units of pounds per square inch, bar, atmospheres, atmospheres absolute, torr, and pascals (Table 28.1), and the depth is usually given in fsw (feet sea water) or msw (meters sea water). In this text we will express pressures in atmospheres absolute (atm abs), sometimes abbreviated ATA in the older literature. The term *absolute* indicates that the atmospheric pressure at sea level is included in the value. For instance, for every 33-fsw increase in depth, there is an additional 1 atm of pressure in the environment. Thus, at a depth of 66 fsw, the absolute pressure is 2 atm plus 1 atm at the surface if the surface is assumed to be sea level.

The hyperbaric environment poses many obstacles that must be overcome before human habitation is possible. The most elementary is that the underwater environment lacks gaseous oxygen and requires that lung-breathing animals hold their breath. If longer stays under water are required, oxygen from compressed gas is used. When depths are greater than approximately 180 fsw (55 msw), the partial pressure of nitrogen is more than six times that of sea level, and then has a narcotic effect. At greater depths helium is used instead of nitrogen in the compressed-gas mixture. Additionally, the high partial pressures of oxygen become poisonous because of the induction of free radicals with depths as little as 33 fsw. Therefore, at depths of several atmospheres a reduced percentage of oxygen is used in the gas breathed, but it is usually maintained at about twice the sea level partial pressure of oxygen, 0.4–0.5 atm abs. Thus, the mixture of gas is a factor to be considered.

TABLE 28.1	Pressure Unit Equivalents of 1 atm
1.01325 bar	760 torr
101.325 kPa	33.08 fsw
14.6959 psi	10.13 msw

atm, atmosphere; kPa, kilopascal; psi, pounds per square inch; torr, Torricelli unit (mm Hg); fsw, feet sea water; msw, meters sea water. The unit of pressure defined by the International System of Unit (SI) is the pascal ($Pa = N \cdot m^{-2}$), often the preferred unit of pressure in current publications.

Other factors to be considered when the body is under water include the state of weightlessness, which causes blood to be displaced from the legs to the thorax. This causes an increase in preload to the heart and affects certain exercise responses. Additionally, the partial pressures of all gases become higher in the body tissues at high pressure, and the risk of bubble formation upon decompression, similar to opening a bottle of champagne, can be influenced by exercise. Thus slow decompression, long enough to allow for the gases to be exhaled from the body without the formation of bubbles in the tissues, must occur.

When divers descend to greater and greater depths, the amount of time that the diver can spend at depth becomes shorter relative to the amount of time required for safe decompression. Therefore, with dives of several hundred feet, the body is allowed to come to equilibrium with gases in the environment. In this way, extended bottom times can be achieved with a constant amount of decompression time necessary for safe decompression. Such dives are called saturation dives, and human performance has been studied at great pressures equivalent to more than 2000 fsw (1) (Milestone of Discovery). The advantage of saturation dives is that saturation allows work at depth for several days. The divers can remain at pressure in a dry chamber on a surface vessel for sleep and rest. Complications of the dry high-pressure environment, including changes in insensible water loss and hormonal control of water balance, also become a factor affected by exercise.

Therefore, the definition of hyperbaric environment compatible with human habitation changes with increasing depth and with the state of immersion or dryness. This means that the response to exercise is likely to change as a function of depth or immersion, not only because of the depth *per se* but because of the necessary change in other characteristics of the environment necessary to support human life, such as gas mixture and density.

Exercise During Submersion

Three important physiological disturbances occur with exercise during submersion. First, we must hold our breath or breathe from a pressurized source, since there is no gaseous source of oxygen. These two modes of underwater diving cause distinct differences in the physiological responses to dynamic exercise and are considered separately. Second, the hydrostatic gradient in air causes a certain proportion of blood to be in sequestered in the legs, but submersion removes the gradient. This shifts blood from the legs to the thorax. The third disturbance involves the physiological adjustments that must take place for a person to tolerate the challenges to thermal regulation. Exercise or work in water usually takes place in a cooler setting than thermal neutral, and the impact of heat loss and its interaction with exercise are important.

Exercise During Breath Holding

Cessation of respiration, represented by simple breath holding, fundamentally contradicts what seems natural and supports life. It deprives the organism of oxygen and of the facility for dumping carbon dioxide. It is the beginning step toward asphyxia, that is, the threatening combination of tissue hypoxia, hypercapnia, and acidosis, the triad that disrupts physiological integrations and ultimately leads to reversal of life-sustaining functions. Human breath-holding dive performances appear trivial when matched with those of aquatic mammals. We do not breath-hold comfortably, as seals and whales routinely do in their facile underwater excursions. Nevertheless, breath-hold skin dives are our most immediate and simplest means of acquaintance with submersion for work or pleasure.

Marine Mammals: A Model of Breath-Hold Diving

Just as asphyxia applies to cessation of respiration by the whole animal, ischemia refers to reduction or occlusion of blood flow within an organ or tissue. Resistance to asphyxia varies with species, and tolerance of ischemia varies from tissue to tissue. Some seal and whale species can tolerate breath-holding apnea longer than an hour; most of us struggle to breath-hold for 1 min. We lose consciousness when our brain is deprived of blood circulation for longer than a few seconds, but we can tolerate limb ischemia by a tourniquet for 30 min or more.

The superior breath-holding capacities of seals, especially the phocid or "true" seals, depend upon several physiological characteristics that support their diving habit. Seals' adaptive mechanisms are not, strictly speaking, unique to them; rather, they exploit fundamental mammalian functions and regulations and expand them quantitatively. Their combined adaptations result in some impressive dive depths and durations. Harbor seals, *Phoca vitulina*, common on both U.S. coasts, can dive to 200 m and remain submerged for 25 min; Antarctic Weddell seals, *Leptonychotes weddelli*, 700 m, more than 1 h; northern elephant seals, *Mirounga angustirostris*, can dive to 1500 m.

The marine mammal's advantage for underwater life is accounted for by several specializations, among them enhanced oxygen supply in high blood volume and enriched hemoglobin concentration and some physical features, such as collapsible lungs that may prevent inert gas bubble formation upon decompression, or the bends, in these species. However, the seals display other mechanisms of oxygen conservation during a dive, such as a reduction and redistribution of circulation heralded by bradycardia, the marked slowing of heart rate that is characteristic of most dives but less noticeable in breath-holding terrestrial animals. The redirected circulation favors continued blood flow to the most vulnerable and obligatory aerobic organs, brain and heart, at the expense of organs having greater anaerobic facility, for example, kidney, gut, and skin. Additional advantages that the seal has in its underwater excursions are those of high tolerance for low oxygen and low pH, well beyond human limits (2). For instance, harbor seals and Weddell seals reach arterial P_{O_2} levels of 10 torr and pH values of 6.8 and recover without incident.

The seal's muscle perfusion is partially reduced during dives, and that tissue depends on richly oxygenated myoglobin content. As a consequence of these various reductions in circulatory perfusion, overall metabolism declines, and body temperature falls slightly in the longest dives. Ultimately, metabolic resources are exhausted, and the seal's superior mechanisms for dealing with problems of acid-base balance and cerebral tolerance of hypoxia further extend diving time (2,3). The responses are variable in timing and intensity; brief dives, for example, sometimes show relatively little effect, whereas longer submersions are supported by more profound reactions. The result is metabolic conservation and lowering of energetic demands during apneic dives in support of extending the underwater episode. Therefore, this metabolic conservation can be adjusted to some extent by behavioral alterations of swimming activity.

Human Breath-Hold Diving

Most of us relate enjoyably to recreational breath-hold diving as a sport. Throughout long human history, however, such diving has been an important occupation in the harvest of food and employment in industry, as in pearl culture and underwater operations. These activities continue today in several locations: Japan, Korea, Indonesia, and Oceania and to a lesser extent in other littoral regions of the world. This work employs 16,000 men and women in Japan and 3000 women in Korea. The Japanese ama divers are active during the summer, and Korean divers work throughout the year. Diving activity patterns vary depending on local custom and harvesting conditions. Invertebrates such as abalone and sea snails are an important part of the products foraged from the sea floor.

Japanese and Korean breath-hold divers traditionally worked in considerable cold, but modern divers are better protected by a wet suit. This relief from severe cold exposure permits the full expression of diving capabilities without the need for frequent rewarming interruptions. Dive range from 5 to 20 m, and durations seldom exceed 1 min. Some divers average 100 dives during a 5-h workday (4).

HUMAN DIVE RESPONSES Human breath-holding capabilities pale by comparison with those of the marine diving specialists, seals and whales. Still, some traces of their responses are demonstrable in humans. Most human subjects show bradycardia and reductions of peripheral circulation during submersion, even when only the face is immersed. A seal, for example, immediately upon immersion will reduce its heart rate to 5–30% of its rate before the dive, but the human diver usually undergoes a slow decline in heart rate over 30 s to about 70% of the value before the dive. These effects are consistently more responsive to water immersion than to breath-holding in air, whether the immersion involves the whole body or the face alone. Over the past half-century, roughly 1000 subjects have been studied in various apneic diving experiments in differing conditions (2,5). Of these, nearly all have had slowing of the heart rate, usually of considerably less magnitude than that of diving seals. However, a few human subjects have shown remarkably slow cardiac rates, less than 20 beats per minute. Limb blood flow was reduced in subjects in whom it was measured. Despite these reactions suggesting physiological possibilities that might extend the usable dive duration, the overall savings in oxygen demand for humans is small. Still, an oxygen-saving response to face immersion can be demonstrated in human subjects during dynamic exercise. Andersson and associates (6) reported, for instance, that the reduction in arterial oxygen saturation resulting from a breath-hold for 30 s in air while exercising at 100 W was 6.8%, but with a breath-hold during face immersion and exercising at a similar rate, the decrement in oxygen saturation was only 5.2%. Accompanying these responses were corresponding reductions in heart rate of 21–3%, and the blood pressure increases were augmented by 34–42%.

Incidentally, far beyond the routine of usual human dive activities, depth and duration records resulting from bizarre competitions stand at 130 m and 6 min! Prior hyperventilation, especially on oxygen, makes possible considerably longer dives. Such practices are not common in normal breath-hold diving excursions, however. Hyperventilation before breath holding can lower circulating carbon dioxide levels to such an extent that subsequent stimulation for ventilation is suppressed. Thus, a diver can use up available oxygen in the circulation with no sensation of a need to break the breath hold and can lose consciousness, a sequence of events termed shallow water blackout (5).

CONTRADICTIONS OF BREATH HOLDING AND DYNAMIC EXERCISE Apneic diving is usually accompanied by swimming. In several respects the reactions to breath holding are antithetical to those of exercise, working in direct opposition to each other. The demands for increased oxygen consumption during exercise and oxygen conservation during apneic diving are in fundamental conflict. Increased cardiovascular responses of exercise, that is, tachycardia and elevated muscle blood flow, act directly against the requirements of sustained apneic dives. It is the resolution of this conflict that defines the practical range of underwater activities for seal and skin diver alike. Seal dive times are shortened when accompanied by vigorous swimming, and humans are similarly affected by underwater exercise. Several investigations have been undertaken for the specific purpose of examining this issue.

The results of studies in which breath-hold dives and dynamic exercise are combined have shown, somewhat surprisingly, that reduced heart rate is the prevailing cardiac response, usually overriding the tachycardia of exercise. In fact, some examples of profound human bradycardia have been observed in apneic diving or simple face immersion by inexperienced subjects while performing moderate exercise (2,7,8). As an example, Figure 28.1 shows the data of Strømme and associates (8) and demonstrates that over a range of exercise intensities heart rate was greatly decreased during breath-hold swimming compared with free swimming. The mechanisms by which this modification of the cardiac response to exercise is produced have not been completely resolved. However, there is evidence that a moderate decline

in alveolar P_{O_2}, such as occurs early during immersion in which breath holding is combined with exercise can, via chemoreceptor activation, interact with airway stimulation or tactile stimuli from face immersion to augment the bradycardia. The resulting combined effect is greater than either one alone. Experimental verification of this heightened dive response has been derived from both human and animal (dogs and seals) studies (9).

An exception to the general reactions of untrained human breath-hold divers has been observed in highly experienced professional Japanese and Korean ama divers. In contrast to the responses of relatively untrained human subjects, further activation of diving bradycardia in ama divers is suppressed by exercise, and they have moderately higher heart rates during underwater exercise than during resting immersion (10). Explanation of these diverse results is not readily discernible. The ama divers may, through long underwater experience with apneic exercise, have become readapted for sustained circulatory support of exercising muscle, thus maintaining higher cardiovascular integrity than that of untrained dive subjects.

Effects of Submersion on Cardiorespiratory Responses to Dynamic Exercise

Whether in a breath-hold dive or using SCUBA, the body becomes weightless in the water. This results in a shift of the blood from the legs into the thoracic cavity. Intuitively this suggests that an increased preload probably exists and therefore results in alterations of exercise-induced cardiorespiratory responses. For instance, when measured with the subject in the resting seated position during water immersion to the suprasternal notch, right atrial pressure increased 10.7 mm Hg, pulmonary arterial pressure increased 9.9 mm Hg, and the cardiac index and stroke index both increased over 70% compared with similar measurements taken in the dry environment (11). Mean arterial pressure was not affected by immersion.

Christie and associates (11) performed these measurements in the same subjects at similar percentages of $\dot{V}_{O_{2max}}$ in both dry and immersed conditions and noted that these determinations remained at a similar absolute difference despite increasing during exercise. They remained significantly elevated during immersion exercise compared with dry land conditions. In this study heart rate was similar at lower workloads performed during immersion compared to air, but at higher workloads and maximal exercise heart rate was lower during immersion. Despite the reduced maximal heart rate during immersion, a similar $\dot{V}_{O_{2max}}$ was achieved in the two conditions of exercise. Similar results were reported more than 20 years earlier for cycling exercise while completely submerged and breathing on SCUBA. Accordingly, bradycardia seems to occur only at heavy workloads but is accompanied by modest or no differences in $\dot{V}_{O_2}$ at heavy or maximal work loads. Despite reductions in maximal heart

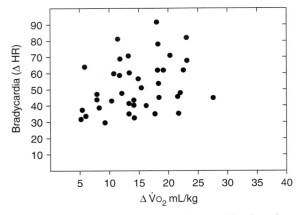

FIGURE 28.1 Comparison between degree of bradycardia during apneic face immersion while swimming and metabolic intensity of work performed. Bradycardia (ΔHR) is the difference between heart rate during steady-state swimming and heart rate after 20 s of swimming with apneic face immersion. Δ $\dot{V}_{O_2}$ is the difference between resting metabolic rate and metabolic rate during the steady state of swimming, expressed in milliliters of oxygen per kilogram of body weight per minute. Each black dot designates one subject. *(Modified with permission from Strømme SB, Kerem D, Elsner R. Diving bradycardia during rest and exercise and its relation to physical fitness. J Appl Physiol 1970;28:619.)*

rate by approximately 10 beats per minute and ventilatory volume ($\dot{V}E$) by 15 L · min^{-1} compared to the air environment, $\dot{V}O_{2max}$ remains similar during exercise while submerged and breathing by SCUBA or during exercise performed during head-out immersion as tested by cycle exercise (12). The ability to deliver adequate supplies of oxygen to reach $\dot{V}O_{2max}$ despite reduced heart rate and reduced $\dot{V}E$ is apparently achieved by the increased cardiac output owing to the increased stoke volume. However, this reduction in heart rate during immersed exercise occurs only at high workloads, unlike breath-hold diving discussed earlier, in which relative heart rate is reduced by 30 or more beats per minute, even at lower work loads (8).

At greater depths, equivalent to 1600 fsw (13), $\dot{V}E$ is greatly reduced, to about 50% relative to sea level control values, and sensations of breathlessness seem to limit performance of work at high oxygen consumption levels. For instance, three divers able to work with a $\dot{V}O_2$ of more than 3 L · min^{-1} on a bicycle while submersed at 1 atm abs were able to work only at a $\dot{V}O_2$ of 1.9 L · min^{-1} at 1600 fsw (13). This inability to perform work at high $\dot{V}O_2$ requirements is apparently a consequence of the state of submersion and breathing through a mouthpiece, because similar exercise performed in the dry gas environment at similar pressures does not cause great reductions in $\dot{V}O_{2max}$ (1).

Interactions of Water Submersion and Exercise on Thermal Balance

Heat conduction from the human body is about 25 times faster in water than air, and the heat capacity of water, the product of density and specific heat, exceeds that of air by approximately 3500 times. Because of these physical characteristics, human thermoregulatory mechanisms are incapable of preventing a decrease in internal body heat during prolonged cold-water exposure without additional insulation.

Divers protect themselves against cold by wearing thick underwear covered by a dry suit or a closed-cell foam rubber wet suit. Dry suits usually provide satisfactory thermal protection for most cold-water diving, but they often limit the diver's mobility. Most contemporary divers engaged in either breath-hold or SCUBA diving are protected from cold-water stress by wearing a wet suit. However, as the closed-cell foam is compressed when hydrostatic pressure increases, it loses thickness, resulting in a loss of protective value of the wet suits against cold (14).

Effects of Water Submersion on Thermal Balance

Body temperature represents a balance between rates of metabolic heat production and heat dissipation. Heat loss in humans occurs mainly through the skin and partly through the respiratory tract. The range of ambient temperature in air between 28 and 31°C is considered as the zone of vasomotor regulation of body temperature in an unclothed human, and this range is termed thermoneutral. In water, the range of the thermoneutral zone is approximately 33–35°C, much narrower than that in air. Tissue conductance is a term used to describe the delivery of heat from the core to surface, and the reciprocal of conductance is defined as tissue insulation. The lowest value of the zone of vasomotor regulation is called the critical temperature and in water is termed critical water temperature. Below these values, core temperature cannot be maintained in the normal range without increasing metabolic heat production by shivering. However, the shivering markedly increases the convective heat loss in water because of body movements, leading to increases in conductance and total heat loss. The faster body heat loss in water is the dominant thermal problem for divers, and in fact it determines the duration of dive exposure.

The primary pathways of heat transfer from the body surface to the surrounding water are convection and conduction. The combined heat transfer coefficient for convection and conduction varies from 38 kcal · (m^2 · h· °C)$^{-1}$ in still water to an average of 55 kcal · (m^2 · h · °C)$^{-1}$ in stirred water. Shivering in still water raises the heat transfer coefficient considerably. According to Rapp (15), the conductive heat transfer coefficient is about 9 kcal · (m^2 · h · °C)$^{-1}$ regardless of the degree of stirring, whereas the convective heat transfer coefficient increases from 81 kcal · (m^2 · h · °C)$^{-1}$ in still water to 344 kcal · (m^2 · h · °C)$^{-1}$ at a swimming speed of 0.5 m · s^{-1}. These values are 100–200 times those in air (1–2 kcal · [m^2 · h · °C]$^{-1}$). Despite such marked differences in the convective heat transfer coefficient between air and water, the heat loss in water has been estimated to be only about two to five times that in air at the same temperature. This indicates that heat loss in water is largely determined by core-to-skin tissue insulation.

The range of neutral water temperature for a resting unprotected man is 33–35°C, varying inversely with the thickness of subcutaneous fat (16). The critical water temperature for humans is 29–33°C, which is also inversely dependent upon the thickness of subcutaneous fat (17). Because water temperature of typical dives is lower than this neutral temperature range, divers are often exposed to cold-water stress.

Effects of Dynamic Exercise on Thermal Balance During Submersion

When the cold-water stress is moderate (water temperature 25–32°C), it is possible to maintain reasonable thermal equilibrium by increasing heat production with exercise.

For instance, humans can maintain their normal body temperature in water of 32°C when they are engaged in continuous underwater work that doubles their resting oxygen consumption (2-MET exercise); and a 3-MET exercise keeps body temperature normal in water temperature at 26°C (18). However, when the water temperature falls below 24°C, heat loss becomes so great that it is virtually impossible to maintain thermal balance by increases in the metabolic rate unless wearing protective clothing. Thus, the core temperature of humans immersed in water is determined by several physical and physiological factors, including water temperature, intensity and type of exercise, subcutaneous fat thickness, ratio of surface area to mass, and duration of immersion (19).

Effects of Exercise Intensity on Maintenance of Body Temperature in Cold Water Submersion

Exercise accelerates the rate of heat loss from the body compared with that seen during rest in cold water. However, this does not necessarily reduce the core temperature. The intensity of exercise influences the core temperature response to cold water immersion; in fact, the performance of heavy exercise during immersion in water of 17–24°C can lessen the rate of fall of core temperature as compared with that observed during static immersion. The type of exercise also plays a role in determining core temperature response to cold-water immersion. For instance, leg exercise is more effective than whole-body exercise in maintaining the core body temperature in water of 18°C (20).

The exercise intensity required to keep core body temperature within physiological range in water has been investigated over a range of exercise intensities and water temperatures. Sagawa and associates (18) conducted experiments in male subjects in which 30 min of rest in water of different temperatures was followed by a series of graded leg exercises of 2–4 MET for 30 mins. Four water temperatures were used: (a) 2°C below critical water temperature (29°C), (b) critical water temperature (31°C), (c) thermoneutrality (34°C), and (d) 2°C above thermoneutrality (36°C). The top panel of Figure 28.2 illustrates typical effects of leg exercise on the esophageal temperature at critical water temperature (31°C). During rest in water, esophageal temperature gradually decreased. During 30 min of exercise, however, esophageal temperature increased to a higher level than recorded following 30 min of rest in water, and the rise in core temperature depended on the exercise intensity.

The time course of cumulative heat storage is shown in the bottom panel of Figure 28.2, which reveals changes in body heat content during rest and exercise at different intensities in water of various temperatures. During 30 min of rest in thermoneutral water, cumulative heat storage re-

mained near zero, whereas it increased in water above thermoneutrality and decreased in water below thermoneutrality. Leg exercise increased cumulative heat storage in proportion to the intensity at all water temperatures, indicating that heat production during underwater exercise exceeded heat loss into the water at these temperatures. Following 30-min resting in water at critical temperature (31°C), negative heat storage occurs, but 30 min of work intensity at 4 MET returned the heat storage to the initial level. In contrast, heat storage did not return to the initial level (0 heat storage) even during the 4-MET exercise at 2°C below critical water temperature. Thus, leg exercise is effective in maintaining core temperature during cold-water exposure, and the effectiveness increases with increasing intensity of exercise. In practice, an exercise intensity more than 200 kcal · m² · h⁻¹ (about 4 MET) cannot be long continued in water, but this level of exercise intensity, as determined from several related exercise studies (18), could maintain body temperature in water at a temperature of about 25°C. Therefore, 25°C approaches the lowest water temperature in which an average unprotected person can continue to perform dynamic exercise without lowering core temperature, and this water temperature can be defined as *crucial water temperature*. Below this value body temperature continues to decrease even with continued exercise at an intensity of approximately 4 MET.

Tissue Insulation and Muscle Mass

Classically, a close inverse relationship has been observed between the fall in core temperature and the skinfold thickness of subjects during immersion (19). However, Veicsteinas and associates (21) have suggested that during rest in cold water, the muscle acts in series with fat and skin to provide tissue insulation. Furthermore, the vasoconstricted muscle provides the major tissue insulation in the resting state. During swimming or severe shivering, the variable insulation of muscle will be lost because of increased blood perfusion through exercising muscle, leaving only the fixed insulation of the subcutaneous fat and skin. It thus appears that during static cold water immersion one might expect the fall in core temperature of subjects to be more closely related to body weight (or muscle mass) than to subcutaneous fat thickness. On the other hand, during dynamic cold water immersion, the variable insulation of muscle is reduced and the role of subcutaneous fat becomes a more important factor in tissue insulation (21).

The results of limb exercise studies suggest that the arms are a significant source of heat loss during whole-body exercise in cold water (18,20), and most swimming strokes require a high level of energy expenditure by the arms. Even at similar work levels, the arms, because of their smaller muscle mass, will receive higher blood flows per

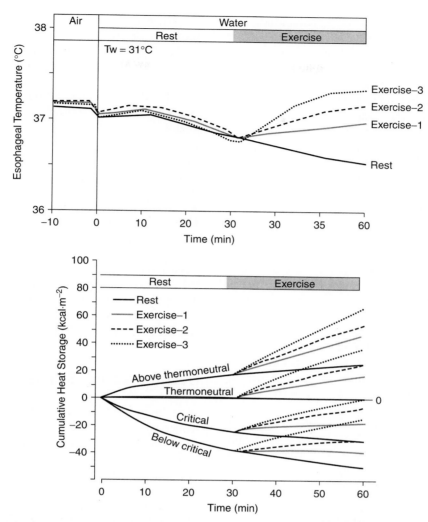

FIGURE 28.2 Changes in esophageal temperature and cumulative heat storage during underwater exercise at various work intensities. *Top*. Typical time changes in core (esophageal) temperature at different work levels during immersion in water of critical temperature (31°C). Exercise 1, 2, and 3 refer to exercise intensity at 2, 3, and 4 MET, respectively. (Adapted from Shiraki K, Claybaugh JR. Effect of diving and hyperbaria on response to exercise. Exerc Sport Sci Rev 1995;23:464, with permission of Lippincott Williams and Wilkins.) *Bottom*. Average time course of cumulative heat storage during rest and the three different exercises in water of above thermoneutral (36°C), thermoneutral (34°C), critical (31°C), and below critical (29°C) temperatures. (Adapted with permission from Sagawa S, Shiraki K, Yousef MK, et al. Water temperature and intensity of exercise in maintenance of thermal equilibrium. J Appl Physiol 1988;65: 2416.)

unit of weight than the legs. This will result in more circulatory delivery of heat to the arms. In other words, the ability of the arms to retain heat is less than that of the legs because the arms have approximately twice the ratio of surface area to mass of the legs, and the conductive pathway from the core to the surface of the limbs is shorter in the arms than in the legs.

Regional Heat Loss During Dynamic Exercise in Water

There are regional differences in tissue insulation during underwater exercise (18). Specifically, insulation is less in the trunk than the limbs in water of cooler than critical temperature (29°C). This is probably because of a longer conduction pathway in the limbs, an enhanced countercurrent heat exchange in the limbs, and/or the predominance of shivering in the trunk. On the other hand, during immersion in water of neutral (34°C) or warmer (36°C) temperature, limb insulation decreases more than that of the trunk, probably because of an attenuated countercurrent heat exchange in the limbs. The results indicate that when water temperature is lower than thermoneutral (<34°C) but above critical temperature, leg exercise facilitates heat loss from the limbs by releasing vasoconstrictor tone in skin vessels. By contrast, dynamic exercise in water warmer than thermoneutral (36°C) causes trunk vasodilation and facilitates heat loss to the water. Exercise in water cooler than thermoneutrality does not increase heat loss from the trunk as exercise intensity increases. If this observation applies to other dynamic immersions, we may expect that exercise-generated heat is preserved more efficiently in the trunk than the limbs and that the trunk keeps its maximum insulation during muscular exertion as well as at rest in cold water. Tissue insulation in the limbs, on the other hand, is high during rest but decreases as the intensity of leg exercise increases. These findings suggest that the most effective protection against heat loss during underwater exercise may be attained by preventing or minimizing heat loss from the limbs. Thus, dynamic exercise in cold water with thermal protection on the limbs would help to preserve body heat.

In conclusion, several factors determine whether exercise during cold water immersion will accelerate or retard the fall in core temperature. These factors include water temperature, water agitation, fitness (muscle mass) and fatness (subcutaneous fat thickness) of the person, type of clothing worn, and the intensity and type of dynamic exercise.

Thermal Balance in Wet-Suited Divers and Effects of Pressure

The insulation of neoprene wet-suits is provided by trapped air. Therefore, the volume of the trapped air, and thus suit insulation, will be inversely proportional to the depth of immersion (hydrostatic pressure). The apparent suit insulation is reduced by approximately 45% at 2 atm abs (10 m sea water) and 52% at 2.5 (15 m) atm abs as compared with the 1 atm abs (sea level) value (14). When the reciprocal relation of depth to insulation is extended to high pressure, suit insulation at 31 atm abs (300 m) during a saturation dive, for instance, would be almost negligible. Fortunately, however, this is not the case in a prolonged helium-oxygen saturation dive, because the wet suit regains its original thickness in 24 h by diffusion of environmental gas into the neoprene. In a typical SCUBA dive, suit insulation decreases curvilinearly as the diving depth increases, and the diver loses heat even in moderately cold water (14).

Park and associates (14) observed changes in the critical water temperature in subjects wearing wet suits at 2 and 2.5 atm abs in comparison with 1 atm abs, with the average critical water temperature of wet-suited subjects being 22,

26, and 28°C at 1, 2, and 2.5 atm abs, respectively. The reduction in wet suit insulation at pressure is exactly compensated for by increasing critical water temperature, such that the suit heat loss remained similar at different pressures, resulting in a similar degree of skin cooling when measured at critical water temperature. Consequently, the vasomotor control for transfer of internal heat loss at critical water temperature is identical at all pressures. These data indicate that the increase in the critical water temperature of wet-suited subjects at high pressure is most likely a simple consequence of changes in suit insulation and not alterations in physiological mechanisms controlling body heat conservation. The available data on critical water temperature at depth are limited to a maximum pressure of 2.5 atm abs.

Another potentially critical problem associated with dives is related to heat loss from the respiratory tract. A diver engaged in heavy exercise and breathing cold gas (7°C) at 3 atm abs loses heat through the respiratory system, which represents 65% of metabolic heat production (22). The respiratory heat loss of a diver in cold water at depth can lead to a severe negative heat balance unless the breathing gas is heated.

Decompression Sickness

Work in the hyperbaric environment is not restricted to activities while immersed. Early applications of hyperbaric work began with the development of the first caisson in 1788 (23). The caisson was originally devised as a bell, open at the bottom, with air supplied to the top. This allowed workers to remove silt and clay from river bottoms until bedrock could be located for the positioning of bridge piers. The Eads Bridge over the Mississippi River in St. Louis, Missouri, completed in 1874, was the first major caisson project in the United States. The depth of the caisson work was 112 ft, and decompression sickness was yet to be defined. Of 352 workers employed, 13 died and 30 others were seriously injured. Similar incidences in the construction of the Brooklyn Bridge led to the use of the word *bends* or *bent* because of the bent-over posture that caisson workers developed from the effects of decompression sickness. Since this time, with the advent of more sophisticated underwater breathing support to free-swimming workers, decompression sickness is reported in most forms of hyperbaric work. The neurological damage resulting from decompression is likely to be a result of gas bubble formation in the brain and spinal tissues.

General Concepts Regarding Bubble Formation Upon Decompression

Formation of gas bubbles during decompression depends on two major factors (24). The first is a requirement for supersaturation of a gas in a fluid, such that the pressure of the gas in the fluid plus the vapor pressure of the gas exceeds the atmospheric pressure. It is possible for supersaturation to occur without bubble formation. Other factors, therefore, contribute to the process of bubble formation, and an important second factor is the presence of preexisting gas nuclei in solution because of surface tension. As decompression proceeds and supersaturation becomes greater, bubbles from the gas nuclei form. Thus, theoretical approaches to prevention of bubble formation include limiting the supersaturation by slow decompression rates and by reducing the number of gas nuclei. For example, prior compression removes gas nuclei and therefore reduces bubble formation upon decompression. The latter has been demonstrated in several demonstrations *in vitro* and animal experiments (24).

Caisson work, also used in tunnel construction, continues today with improvements in safety owing to scheduled decompressions allowing more time for gas elimination from the body and the use of oxygen during decompression. Sometimes oxygen is substituted for nitrogen because it can be eliminated from the body by metabolism to carbon dioxide. This metabolism converts the relatively insoluble oxygen into carbon dioxide that is 21 times more soluble and therefore less likely to come out of solution to form bubbles. The inert nitrogen can be eliminated only by diffusion down a concentration gradient, and therefore it is a slower process than the elimination of oxygen (24). With these added precautions in more recent projects, the reported rate of decompression illness is about 1.5%, based on the number affected seriously enough to report for treatment. The greatest practical pressures that are used in compressed air work are about 4.4 atm abs (445 kPa), about the depth of the Eads Bridge piers, because slightly beyond this pressure mixed gases become necessary and the cost is prohibitive.

Exercise and Decompression Sickness

Generally held concepts of exercise and bubble formation resulting from decompression involve the understanding that exercise while at depth would increase blood flow and consequently nitrogen uptake. With more nitrogen in the body, the time required to unload the additional nitrogen would be greater. Studies have shown, for instance, that more nitrogen is eliminated from a person at sea level after a dive in which exercise was performed at depth than a dive without exercise (25). This observation is in agreement with the finding that more bubbles are detected when subjects exercise during or immediately following completion of decompression, and the intravascular bubbles impede the elimination of inert gases. Summarization of prior reports generally led to the conclusion that dynamic exercise performed either prior to or during exposure to pressure increased the risk of decompression sickness (24).

Such impressions led to conclusions that otherwise unexplainable cases of decompression sickness might have been due to heavy exercise performed prior to an incident. On the other hand, more recent reports have indicated that when arm or leg exercise was performed at a moderate intensity, approximately 50% of each subject's arm or leg aerobic capacity, during decompression Doppler-detected gas emboli were reduced by more than 50% at all body sites monitored (26). Doppler-detected gas emboli in the venous circulation, venous gas emboli, can be detected in subjects lacking symptoms of decompression sickness. Furthermore, these circulating gas emboli are not thought to be the cause of decompression sickness, which is most likely caused by the formation of bubbles in the tissues. Thus there is no direct correlation between the detection of venous gas emboli and decompression sickness, but high incidence rates of venous gas emboli are associated with a significant probability of developing decompression sickness (26). The potential beneficial effects of dynamic exercise during decompression are similarly thought to be a result of increased blood flow but in this case cause increased gas elimination. So the timing of exercise performed at depth and the intensity of the exercise become critical factors as to whether the effects are harmful or beneficial.

Recently a new theory involving exercise and decompression sickness has been proposed by a research group in Norway (27,28). Studies conducted in rats have shown that prevention of bubble formation and death from decompression could be achieved by exercise 20 h prior to a dive to 7 atm abs. This beneficial effect did not occur if the exercise was done too close to the dive time, within 10 h, or too much in advance of the dive time, for example 48 h (28). These authors proposed a mechanism whereby exercise-induced suppression of bubble formation is related to nitric oxide production, which may reduce the number of gas nuclei. They showed earlier that nitric oxide inhibition exacerbated the decompression sickness occurrence in this animal model (29). They then demonstrated that administration of a nitric oxide–releasing agent reduced bubble formation (28). However, this could be demonstrated when the nitric oxide was given just 30 min prior to hyperbaric exposure. Thus, the timing of the responses between exercise and nitric oxide administration were quite different, suggesting that the mechanism of the exercise response may not be resolved.

Perhaps most interesting is their subsequent report that dynamic exercise performed in human subjects 24 h before a dive to 2.8 atm abs reduced venous gas emboli by 78% (27). The exercise involved treadmill running at 90% of maximum heart rate for 3 minfollowed by running at 50% of maximum heart rate for 2 min. This series was repeated eight times. It is not clear why dynamic exercise, performed only within a window of time near 24 h prior to the dive, can produce the effect if the mechanism is linked to a nitric oxide–dependent reduction in bubble nuclei. Whether the exercise-dependent reduction of bubble formation operates through the formation of nitric oxide, as the authors hypothesize, or through another mechanism, these studies provide new avenues for ameliorating the formation of bubbles upon decompression in humans. Further standardization and study of the contribution of this effect is necessary before it can be widely used as a predictable safeguard to decompression sickness.

Breath-Hold Divers and Decompression Sickness

There is a persisting question regarding the possibility that breath-hold divers might under some circumstances be susceptible to the bends. There is little information on this concern, but the most direct evidence comes from a self-imposed experiment by a Danish submarine officer to test the potential for inert gas accumulation precipitated by an enforced severe bout of frequent and deep breath-hold diving. He performed 60 apneic dives to 20 m during a 5-h period, allowing only brief surface intervals. At the conclusion of the diving bout he had incipient decompression symptoms. He promptly recovered after being placed in a recompression chamber, which verified that he had indeed had decompression sickness (30). The extreme circumstances of this experiment are noteworthy, and it seems clear that ordinarily benign apneic diving is unlikely to impose a hazard of inert gas sequestration.

Exercise in the Dry Hyperbaric Environment

When humans enter increased atmospheric pressure in the air, approximately 80% nitrogen and 20% oxygen, several factors with a bearing on exercise performance immediately change. First, and of longstanding interest, the density of the air increases. At 33 fsw (2 atm abs), the gas is twice as dense as at sea level. With increasing gas density the resistance to breathing increases and the work involved in breathing increases. Second, the partial pressure of oxygen increases. Studies conducted nearly eight decades ago by Hill and associates (31) demonstrated that breathing 50% oxygen could increase $\dot{V}_{O_{2max}}$. One might expect, therefore, that the increased partial pressure of oxygen at hyperbaria could also result in an increased $\dot{V}_{O_{2max}}$. Third, heart rate decreases (32,33).

Effects of Compressed Gas Environments on Cardiorespiratory Responses to Exercise

Many studies have shown that increasing environmental gas pressure greatly reduces the maximum voluntary ventilation.

This is evident even at pressures of 3 atm abs, approximately 66 fsw. Of particular importance was the demonstration that altering the density of the gas could duplicate the changes in maximum voluntary ventilation observed at high pressure. Maio and Farhi (34) were able to demonstrate sequentially greater decrements in maximum voluntary ventilation with increasing gas density by replacing the nitrogen in air with helium or sulfur hexafluoride to achieve breathing gas densities that were approximately one-third and four times the density of air, respectively.

The increase in breathing resistance caused by the increased gas density also contributes to a predictable decrease in maximum $\dot{V}_E$. Fagraeus (35) studied maximal exercise in subjects in compressed air environments ranging from 1 to 6 atm abs (Fig. 28.3).

With increasing pressures, $\dot{V}_{E_{max}}$ decreases, but $\dot{V}_{O_{2max}}$ was not greatly affected. It can be seen in the figure that $\dot{V}_{O_{2max}}$ was actually enhanced at 1.4 atm abs compared to 1 atm abs in the air. This confirms the observation that at least in some instances, a small increase in $\dot{V}_{O_{2max}}$ can be achieved by breathing higher concentrations of oxygen (Table 28.2). At higher pressures of air, however, these workers and others reported no increase in $\dot{V}_{O_{2max}}$. Thus, it can be seen from Figure 28.3 that reductions in $\dot{V}_{E_{max}}$ by more than 40% could still be accompanied by only modestly reduced $\dot{V}_{O_{2max}}$ values. Also, it can be seen that the reduction in ventilation is accompanied by a significant increase in Pa_{CO_2}. This decrease in $\dot{V}_E$ associated with exercise is evident not only during maximum efforts (Table 28.2) but is uniformly reported at submaximal workloads and at pressures ranging from 2 atm abs to 66 atm abs.

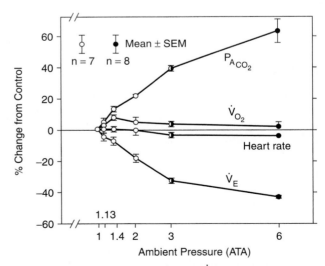

FIGURE 28.3 Alveolar carbon dioxide, $\dot{V}_{O_2}$, heart rate, and expiratory volume ($\dot{V}_E$) responses to maximal exercise at different pressures in a dry compressed-air environment. *(Modified with permission from Fagraeus L. Cardiorespiratory and metabolic functions during exercise in the hyperbaric environment. Acta Physiol Scand 1974;Supp414:20.)*

TABLE 28.2	Exercise-Induced Changes in Heart Rate, Expiratory Volume, and Oxygen Consumption at Maximal Exercise Intensities in Dry Pressurized Environments of Various Gas Mixtures and Densities					
Total Pressure ATA	P_{O_2} (ATA)	Density (g·L⁻¹)	ΔHR_{max} (%)	$\Delta \dot{V}_{E\,max}$ (%)	$\Delta \dot{V}_{O_2\,max}$ (%)	Reference
1.4 (air)	0.28	1.5	↔	↓ 7	↑11	35
3 (air)	0.60	3.3	↓ 3	↓33	↔	35
3 (He-O_2)	0.60	1.08	↓<3	↓14	↑13	35
6 (air)	1.20	7.2	↓ 5	↓46	↔	35
18.6 (He-O_2)	0.30	3.8	↓ 4	↓26	↑ 3	41
18.6 (He-O_2)	0.21	2.8	↓ 4	↓21	↔	41
31 (He-O_2)	0.40	7.3	↓ 9	↓45	↓13	37
37 (He-N_2-O_2)	0.50	9.2	↓ 7	↓41	↓10	38
47–66 (He-N_2-O_2)	0.50	12.3–17.1	↓ 4	↓16	↓13	31

ΔHR_{max}, change in heart rate; $\Delta \dot{V}_{E\,max}$, change in expiratory volume; $\Delta \dot{V}_{O_2\,max}$, change in oxygen consumption.

The reduction in $\dot{V}_E$ is a consequence not only of increased gas density and airway resistance; also, increased pressure and gas density have been shown to reduce the ventilatory drive in response to the increased carbon dioxide (36,37). The slowing of the incremental increase in respiration in response to increased carbon dioxide produced by rebreathing expired carbon dioxide while maintaining inspired oxygen constant was determined by Lambertsen and associates (36). They tested rebreathing at increasing gas densities up to the equivalent of 5000 fsw in the helium-oxygen environment, 25 times the density at sea level. This was accomplished by substituting neon as the inert gas in a chamber pressurized to 1200 fsw. Through these experiments it was observed that maximum voluntary ventilation decreased rather steeply up to gas densities equivalent to about 2000 fsw in a helium-oxygen environment and then leveled off at a decrement of about 60%. On the other hand, the $\dot{V}_E$ at about 80% $\dot{V}_{O_2\,max}$ steadily decreased, reaching an 80% decrement at the gas densities equivalent to 5000 fsw in the helium-oxygen environment. Thus, a "predicted work load maximum" could be constructed in which maximum voluntary ventilation equals $\dot{V}_E$ at maximum $\dot{V}_{O_2}$. In their experiments on two subjects, this point would be reached at 5000 fsw in the helium-oxygen environment. These two subjects were able to exercise for 4 min of a scheduled 6-min bout before voluntarily stopping. The Pa_{CO_2} was approximately 60 mm Hg and not considered limiting; instead it was believed that $\dot{V}_E$ had been reduced to maximum voluntary ventilation and the oxygen demand could not be met.

Surprisingly, even at these extreme environmental gas densities, subjects were able to exercise at 80% of their sea level maximums with no report of dyspnea. Although no studies have been performed at such extreme depths, maximum exercise has been performed at 37.5 atm abs, slightly greater than 1200 fsw, with no evidence of dyspnea despite a 30% reduction in $\dot{V}_E$, and nearly sea level values for $\dot{V}_{O_2\,max}$ were achieved (38). Similarly, Salzano and associates (1) re-

ported dyspnea as a "rare occurrence" at nearly maximum workloads performed by subjects at over 2000 fsw. Thus, predictive experiments and direct observations indicate that relatively similar levels of exertion can be performed at hyperbaria with no negative respiratory consequences. This interpretation must be considered with caution, however, because as mentioned earlier in this chapter, others have observed, at moderate workloads at 1600 fsw, dyspnea that severely limited exercise performance in upright subjects during submersion (13). These and similar reports suggest an effect of submersion and/or a need to optimize the equilibration pressure of the breathing apparatus, an issue that remains unresolved.

Effects of Compressed Gas Environments on Water Balance and Hormonal Responses to Dynamic Exercise

The increased gas density at hyperbaria also decreases insensible water loss that is not accompanied by a decrease in water intake. Thus, the accumulation of free water must be voided in the urine. This appears to be accomplished by a chronic reduction in circulating arginine vasopressin (AVP), which is accompanied by the production of about an additional 200–500 mL of relatively dilute urine per day (32). This new set point for the homeostatic regulation of fluid and electrolytes would be expected to alter the hormonal and renal responses to exercise. This possibility has been investigated in only one study (38). At sea level, maximal dynamic exercise is invariably accompanied by several-fold increases in levels of AVP, atrial natriuretic peptide, renin, and aldosterone (39). In addition, for reasons that are unclear, urine osmolality decreases during exercise despite the increase in plasma AVP concentration and plasma osmolality. In contrast, the AVP and atrial natriuretic peptide responses to maximal dynamic exercise are greatly blunted, while the renin and aldosterone responses are unaffected in the hyperbaric environment at 37 atm abs (38). Despite the greatly reduced rise in plasma AVP, maximal and submaximal exercise were associated with increases in urine osmolality and a decrease in urine flow in hyperbaria. An explanation of the blunted AVP response is not readily apparent. It seems likely that the decreased insensible water loss associated with the hyperbaric environment may result in a slight state of hyperhydration. This could lead to small reductions in plasma osmolality that may contribute to the significant lowering of the resting plasma AVP. However, a state of hyperhydration would not be expected to blunt the ANF response. Such a response is more expected with dehydration, which is in better agreement with increased hematocrit and decreased plasma volume observed in other studies (32). Thus, the blunted AVP response to dynamic exercise at hyperbaria is probably a result of other factors in addition to plasma osmolality.

Hyperbaric Bradycardia

We have mentioned reduced heart rate during exercise associated with breath holding, with face immersion, and with head-out immersion. Apparently by different mechanisms, the dry hyperbaric environment is also accompanied by a slight decrease in heart rate (22,33). Consequently, when exercise is performed at hyperbaria, the heart rate at any given workload and at all pressures studied is reduced relative to 1 atm abs values (Fig. 28.4).

However, as noted earlier, the effects on oxygen consumption and the ability to perform work do not appear to be greatly affected. There appear to be several reasons for the so-called hyperbaric bradycardia. Most obvious is the increase in oxygen concentration. That is, breathing increased concentrations of oxygen will reduce heart rate by a combination of vasoconstriction, increased vagal tone, and decreased sympathetic activity via baroreceptor and chemoreceptor input (32,33). Experimental data support such responses in hyperbaria. For instance, significantly reduced basal plasma norepinephrine, 15%, and muscle sympathetic nerve activity, 60%, have been shown when comparing human subjects at 3 atm abs in compressed air to subjects at 1 atm abs. Additionally, the baroreceptor stimulation of these measurements, as assessed by lower body negative pressure applications, were blunted in the hyperbaric environment (40). However, when oxygen concentration is held constant by breathing 100% oxygen at 1 atm abs and breathing normal air at 4.5 atm abs, Fagraeus (35) observed greater bradycardia at pressure. Also, if normoxia is maintained between 1 atm abs and 18.6 atm abs, maximal exercise at hyperband is accompanied by 4% bradycardia (41). Thus, hyperoxia is not the only factor causing the bradycardia. Another factor that can be shown to reduce the heart rate response to exercise, independent of oxygen, is an increase in the partial pressure of nitrogen. However, hyperbaric bradycardia is also observed in a helium-oxygen hyperbaric environment with nitrogen essentially absent. So unidentified factors other than hyperoxia and increased nitrogen reduce heart rate in the hyperbaric environment.

SUMMARY

Exercise in the hyperbaric environment is never a unifactorial effect of high pressure on the human physiological response to dynamic exercise. In fact, that single effect, if any exists, is difficult to identify and perhaps meaningless, since it is invariably commingled with other more profound factors, such as breath holding, immersion, cold exposure, and gas density. For the most part, these effects on exercise have been shown to be unaffected by different ambient pressures. For instance, we have discussed evidence for increasing ambient pressure up to 2.5 atm abs with no effects on critical temperature and duplication of ventilatory effects of hyperbaria by changing gas density with no changes in atmospheric pressure. Finally, when physical barriers are minimized, man is able to perform at near maximal intensities even at pressures of 66 atm abs or depths greater than 2000 fsw. This performance most likely does not represent a limit of pressure tolerance but rather a limit resulting from practicality and need in the face of technological development of robots and deep, highly manageable submarines.

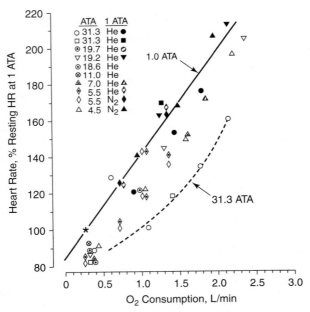

FIGURE 28.4 Heart rate during submaximal exercise in hyperbaric environments. *(The data for this figure are based on multiple sources cited in original publication. Redrawn with permission from Lin YC, Shida KK. Brief review: mechanisms of hyperbaric bradycardia. Chinese J Physiol 1988;31:5.)*

A MILESTONE OF DISCOVERY

In the late 1970s it was not clear whether man could safely perform strenuous work at extreme pressures. Predictive studies had shown that moderate work up to 80% of $\dot{V}O_{2max}$ at sea level could be performed with no severe dyspnea in dry hyperbaric environments at gas densities equivalent to 5000 fsw in a helium-oxygen environment. Thus it was concluded that breathing limitations posed no significant barrier to the performance of fairly intense exercise at gas densities 22 times that at sea level. However, when moderate work was performed during submersion at 1600 fsw, severe dyspnea was encountered. This raised the question whether gas density was the single limiting feature in breathing during exercise at extreme hyperbaria or there was an effect of high pressure in addition to gas density. Alternatively, the disparate results could have been attributable to the submersed state.

At the same time, others had explored the utility of adding some nitrogen (5 to 10% of total gases) to the helium-oxygen gas mixture, a mixture called trimix, as a means of reducing high-pressure nervous syndrome associated with compression to depths over 1000 fsw. Trimix provided a means of safely placing divers at a greater depth, up to 2250 fsw, but at the same time increased gas density and therefore raised additional questions regarding the use of trimix on exercise performance at high pressure.

As shown in Figure 28.5, through a series of dry saturation dives, Salzano and associates (1) studied exercise-induced changes in cardiorespiratory measurements at work rates of rest, 360, 720, 1080, and 1440 (kpm · minute^{-1}) at gas densities of 1.1 g · L^{-1} (air with 50% oxygen), 10.1 g · L^{-1} (trimix with 5% nitrogen at 47 atm abs), 12.3 g · L^{-1} (trimix with 10% nitrogen at 47 atm abs), and 17.1 g · L^{-1} (trimix with 10% nitrogen at 66 atm abs).

A work rate of 1080 kpm · minute^{-1} produced oxygen consumption of 75 to 92% of sea level maximum for four individuals. The fifth subject was able to perform work at 1440 kpm · minute^{-1} at approximately 80% of sea level $\dot{V}O_{2max}$ at 66 atm abs.

Two decades later these experiments represent the most extreme environmental pressures where exercise responses have been studied in man. They demonstrated that work performed at

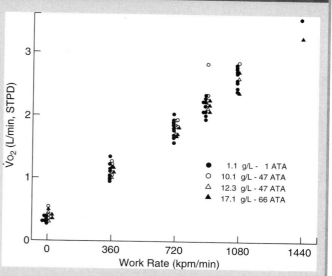

FIGURE 28.5 Cardiorespiratory responses to exercise at 47 and 66 ATA by five subjects at different work rates and gas densities. Each symbol represents one exercise session among five subjects. *(Redrawn with permission from Salzano JV, Comporesi EM, Stolp BW, et al. Physiological responses to exercise at 47 and 66 ATA. J Appl Physiol 1984;57:1060.)*

360 kpm · minute^{-1} at approximately three to four times resting $\dot{V}O_2$ results in physiological responses essentially the same as at sea level. Also, greater work loads could be achieved, with most individuals able to perform work at about 80% of their sea level $\dot{V}O_{2max}$ at pressures of 47 atm abs, and one subject at 66 atm abs.

Salzano JV, Camporesi EM, Stolp BW, Moon RE. Physiological responses to exercise at 47 and 66 ATA. J Appl Physiol 1984;57:1055–1068.

ACKNOWLEDGMENT

The views expressed in this manuscript are those of the authors and do not reflect the official policy or position of the Department of the Army, Department of Defense, or the United States government.

REFERENCES

1. Salzano JV, Comporesi EM, Stolp BW, et al. Physiological responses to exercise at 47 and 66 ATA. J Appl Physiol 1984;57:1055–1068.

2. Elsner R, Gooden B. Diving and asphyxia: a comparative study of animals and man. Monographs of the Physiological Society no. 40. Cambridge: Cambridge University, 1983;168–189.

3. Elsner R. Living in water: solutions to physiological problems. In Reynolds JE, Rommel SA, eds. Biology of Marine Mammals. Washington: Smithsonian Institution, 1999;73–116.

4. Mohri M, Torii R, Nagaya K, et al. Diving patterns of ama divers of Hegura Island, Japan. Undersea Biomed Res 1995;22:137–143.

5. Lin YC, Hong SK. Hyperbaria: breath-hold diving. In Fregly MJ, Blatteis CM, eds. Handbook of Physiology, Section 4: Environmental Physiology, vol II. New York: Oxford University, 1996;979–995.

6. Andersson JP, Linér MH, Runow E, et al. Diving response and arterial oxygen saturation during apnea and exercise in breath-hold divers. J Appl Physiol 2002;93:882–886.

7. Butler PJ, Woakes AJ. Heart rate of humans during underwater swimming with and without breath-hold. Respir Physiol 1987;69:387–399.

8. Strømme SB, Kerem D, Elsner R. Diving bradycardia during rest and exercise and its relation to physical fitness. J Appl Physiol 1970;28:614–621.

9. Daly M, Angell-James JE, Elsner R. Role of carotid body chemoreceptors and their reflex interactions in bradycardia and cardiac arrest. Lancet 1979;1:764–767.

10. Shiraki K, Elsner R, Sagawa S, et al. Heart rate of Japanese male ama divers during breath-hold dives: diving bradycardia or exercise tachycardia? Undersea Hyperbaric Med 2002;29:59–62.

11. Christie JL, Sheldahl LM, Tristani FE, et al. Cardiovascular regulation during head-out water immersion exercise. J Appl Physiol 1990;69:657–664.

12. Dressendorfer RH, Morlock JF, Baker DG, et al. Effects of head-out water immersion on cardiorespiratory responses to maximal cycling exercise. Undersea Biomed Res 1976;3:177–187.

13. Spaur WH, Raymond LW, Knott MM, et al. Dyspnea in divers at 49.5 atm abs; mechanical, not chemical in origin. Undersea Biomed Res 1977;4:183–198.

14. Park YH, Iwamoto J, Tajima F, et al. Effect of pressure on thermal insulation in humans wearing wet suits. J Appl Physiol 1988;64:1916–1922.

15. Rapp GM. Convection coefficients of man in a forensic area of thermal physiology: heat transfer in underwater exercise. J Physiol (Paris) 1971;63:392–396.

16. Craig Jr AB, Dvorak M. Thermal regulation during water immersion. J Appl Physiol 1966;21:1577–1585.

17. Rennie DW. Thermal insulation of Korean diving women and non-divers in water. In Rahn H, Yokoyama T, eds. Physiology of Breath-Hold Diving and the Ama of Japan. Washington: National Academy of Science National Research Council, 1965;315–324.

18. Sagawa S, Shiraki K, Yousef MK, et al. Water temperature and intensity of exercise in maintenance of thermal equilibrium. J Appl Physiol 1988;65:2413–2419.

19. Craig AB Jr, Dvorak M. Thermal regulation of man exercising during water immersion. J Appl Physiol 1968;25:28–35.

20. Toner MM, Sawka MN, Pandolf KB. Thermal responses during arm and leg and combined arm-leg exercise in water. J Appl Physiol 1984;56:1355–1360.

21. Veicsteinas A, Ferretti G, Rennie DW. Superficial shell insulation in resting and exercising men in cold water. J Appl Physiol 1982;52:1557–1564.

22. Shiraki K, Claybaugh JR. Effects of diving and hyperbaria on responses to exercise. Exerc Sport Sci Rev 1995;23:459–485.

23. Kindwall EP. Compressed air work. In Bennett PB, Elliott DH, eds. The physiology and Medicine of Diving. 4th ed. Philadelphia: Saunders, 1993;1–18.

24. Vann RD, Thalmann ED. Decompression physiology and practice. In Bennett PB, Elliott DH, eds. The Physiology and Medicine of Diving. 4th ed. Philadelphia: Saunders, 1993;376–432.

25. Dick APK, Vann RD, Mebane GY, et al. Decompression induced nitrogen elimination. Undersea Biomed Res 1984;11:369–380.

26. Jankowski LW, Nishi RY, Eaton DJ, et al. Exercise during decompression reduces the amount of venous gas emboli. Undersea Hyperbaric Med 1997;24:59–65.

27. Dujić Z, Duplančić D, Marinović-Terzić I, et al. Aerobic exercise before diving reduces venous gas bubble formation in humans. J Physiol (Lond) 2004;555:637–642.

28. Wisløff U, Richardson RS, Brubakk AO. NOS inhibition increases bubble formation and reduces survival in sedentary but not exercised rats. J Physiol (Lond) 2003;546:577–582.

29. Wisløff U, Richardson RS, Brubakk AO. Exercise and nitric oxide prevent bubble formation: a novel approach to the prevention of decompression sickness? J Physiol (Lond) 2004;555:825–829.

30. Paulev P. Decompression sickness following repeated breath-hold dives. J Appl Physiol 1965;20:1028–1031.

31. Hill AV, Long CNH, Lupton H. Muscular exercise, lactic acid, and the supply and utilization of oxygen. Parts VII and VIII. Proc R Soc Edinburgh Section B: Biology 1;92497:155–176.

32. Hong SK, Bennett PB, Shiraki K, et al. Mixed-gas saturation diving, part V: the hyperbaric environment. In Blatteis CM, Fregley MJ, eds. Handbook of Physiology, Section 4: Adaptation to the Environment. New York: Oxford University, 1995;1023–1045.

33. Lin YC, Shida KK. Brief review: mechanisms of hyperbaric bradycardia. Chin J Physiol 1988;31:1–22.

34. Maio DA, Fahri LE. Effect of gas density on mechanics of breathing. J Appl Physiol 1967;23:687–693.

35. Fagraeus L. Cardiorespiratory and metabolic functions during exercise in the hyperbaric environment. Acta Physiol Scand 1974;Supp414:5–40.

36. Lambertsen CJ, Gelfand R, Peterson R, et al. Human tolerance to He, Ne, and N2 at respiratory gas densities equivalent to He-O₂ breathing at 1200, 2000, 3000, 4000 and 5000 feet of sea water (predictive studies III). Aviat Space Environ Med 1977;48:843–855.

37. Ohta Y, Arita H, Nakayama H, et al. Cardiopulmonary functions and maximal aerobic power during a 14-day saturation dive at 31 ATA (Seadragon IV). In Bachrach AJ, Matzen MM, eds. Underwater Physiology VII: Proceedings of the VII Symposium on Underwater Physiology. Bethesda, MD: Undersea Medical Society, 1981;209–221.

38. Claybaugh JR, Freund BJ, Luther G, et al. Renal and hormonal responses to exercise in man at 46 and 37 atmospheres absolute pressure. Aviat Space Environ Med 1997;68:1038–1045.

39. Freund BJ, Shizuru EM, Hashiro GM, et al. The hormonal, electrolyte, and renal responses to exercise are intensity dependent. J Appl Physiol 1991;70:900–906.

40. Yamauchi K, Tsutsui Y, Endo Y, et al. Sympathetic nervous and hemodynamic responses to lower body negative pressure in hyperbaria in men. Am J Physiol 2002;282:R38–R45.

41. Dressendorfer RH, Hong SK, Morlock JF, et al. Hana Kai II: a 17–day dry saturation dive at 18.6 ATA. V. Maximal oxygen uptake. Undersea Biomed Res 1977;4:283–296.

CHAPTER 29

Physiological Systems and Their Responses to Conditions of Microgravity and Bed Rest

SUZANNE M. SCHNEIDER AND VICTOR A. CONVERTINO

Introduction

When Columbus sought funding to explore a new route to the Orient, critics predicted that his ships would sink, his men would die of scurvy or other hideous diseases, or he would sail off the end of the Earth. Prior to April 12, 1961, similar catastrophes were predicted for human space flight. The rocket would explode on takeoff, the astronauts would die of weightlessness, or they would burn up during reentry. Happily for Yuri Gagarin, the first human to fly in space, the critics were wrong. We now know that the human body adapts and functions quite well during extended space flight. However, we must wait for further data to understand the consequences of very long exposures to flight (during interplanetary travel) on physiological functions when crew members return to normal terrestrial activities. In the process of unraveling the mechanisms by which physiological systems respond to changes in gravity, new insights are being discovered about how the human body responds to environmental and disease stressors. The techniques and procedures (countermeasures) developed to ease the transition between space flight and normal gravity may prove useful for ameliorating adverse consequences of aging or chronic illness. For example, during space flight the decrease in bone mass is similar in many ways to the osteoporosis of aging; and the loss of muscle mass is similar to that in immobilized patients. As examined in this chapter, one of the most effective countermeasures for preventing space flight–induced deconditioning is exercise training.

Microgravity and Weightlessness

The term *microgravity* describes a condition in which gravitational forces acting on the long axis of the body are minimized. It is a technical (physics) definition that applies to low gravitational forces in space. Brief periods of microgravity are experienced on Earth during free fall, such as during some amusement park rides. There are several methods to simulate microgravity. For example, during bed rest (BR) subjects are confined to a horizontal or head-down tilt position, which minimizes the effects of gravity on the body. These subjects are in a condition of simulated microgravity.

During space flight, astronauts often are said to be weightless, but this is technically not correct. According to Newton's law of gravitation, every particle in the universe attracts every other particle with a force that is directly proportional to the product of their masses and inversely proportional to the square of the distance between them (1). For a human standing on Earth, gravity therefore depends on the product of the person's mass, the Earth's mass, and distance from the center of the Earth. During orbital space flight the distance between the astronaut and the center of the Earth is about 5% greater than when the astronaut is standing on the Earth, and the mass of the Earth and the astronaut are relatively constant. Thus, orbital space flight is associated with only a minor decrease in gravity (2). Instead, weightlessness during orbital space flight is caused by the fact that the spacecraft is in free fall. The spacecraft circles the Earth at a rate such that the craft's centrifugal force counterbalances the force of gravity, so that a scale used for weighing and the weight to be measured (the astronaut) are accelerating at the same rate. The crew member therefore seems weightless, even in the presence of gravity.

Weightlessness is a term that refers to what the crew perceives during space flight, and it is one of the major factors contributing to the total syndrome of space flight deconditioning. During BR, the simulated microgravity is a major factor contributing to the total syndrome of BR deconditioning. These two types of deconditioning have many similar physiological changes, but the other unique stressors associated with space flight or with BR must also be considered when comparing data from these two conditions.

Space Flight

During space flight, an astronaut is exposed to a variety of environmental and psychological stressors (3). A potent environmental stressor felt immediately upon insertion into orbit is microgravity, which unloads body tissues and redistributes body fluids. Also, during orbital flight external light and dark cycles occur every 90 min, disrupting normal pituitary–hypothalamic regulation. Ultraviolet radiation is nearly abolished, which decreases vitamin D production. Ionizing radiation exposure is elevated, posing potential health hazards. Microflora in the air and water proliferate in the enclosed spacecraft while immune responses may be compromised. And carbon dioxide levels inside the craft are chronically elevated to about 0.4% during nominal crew activity, with peaks of 1–3% during intense exercise and while other crews visit. Stress levels may be high in the diverse crew members exposed to relatively confined living quarters, high noise levels, and altered sleep and eating patterns. The crew members are required to exercise vigorously during long flights, often more intensely than they did before flight. Therefore, it is a misconception to view space flight as a condition of reduced activity (hypodynamia). Taken together, the physiological changes that occur in response to all of these stressors are referred to as space flight deconditioning. Astronauts are deconditioned in relation to how they could perform upon return to a 1g environment, but during space flight, they adapt appropriately and can function normally.

Free Fall and Parabolic Flight

Free fall occurs when a person plunges downward at the rate of acceleration due to gravity (980 cm · s^{-2}). This can happen in a falling elevator, after release from a drop tower, in some amusement park rides, or in a diving aircraft. Astronauts undergo short-term weightlessness when training in a special plane that flies parabolic arcs (3). During this ma-

neuver the airplane dives to gain speed, then pulls up at a 45° angle into the first arm of the parabolic arc, producing hypergravity (1.8 g). The pilot then powers back the engines, allowing the plane to glide over the top of the arc to begin a controlled 45° nose-down free-fall dive. The passengers inside the plane immediately go into free fall (weightlessness). As the plane reaches the bottom of its parabola, the passengers again are subjected to 1.8 g. The average duration of weightlessness during this technique is 20 to 25 s. If you watch the movie *Apollo 13* closely, the actors actually are weightless, as scenes from this movie were filmed during parabolic flight. During parabolic flight, the brief exposures to microgravity interspersed with exposures of hypergravity make interpretation of physiological responses challenging and often unique to the parabolic flight condition.

Simulated Microgravity

Microgravity can be simulated by changing the angle of the person relative to the gravitational vector or by unweighting all or portions of the body. Unweighting can be done by immersion in water, by suspension, or by immobilization of limbs.

Bed Rest

The most common model used to simulate the physiological effects of microgravity on Earth in humans is prolonged BR. A subject is placed in a horizontal or slightly head-down tilt position for the duration of a study that can last for hours or for longer than a year. The physiological responses to BR depend upon the duration and the angle of head-down tilt. The earlier BR studies were performed with subjects in a horizontal position. Then, in the mid 1970s, Kakurin and coworkers demonstrated that an antiorthostatic head-down tilt position of 4–16° induces body fluid and cardiovascular responses to tilting or exercise that more closely match changes accompanying space flight (4). Since then, because responses to 6° head-down tilt most closely approximate those during space flight deconditioning, this angle is used most frequently to study cardiovascular responses to microgravity (3). It is unclear whether this 6° head-down tilt angle offers greater validity than use of horizontal BR in the study of other physiological systems, such as bone remodeling.

Physiological systems respond to BR with differing rates of deconditioning. Decrease in muscle mass and loss of strength become apparent after approximately 2 wk of BR (5), while the decrease in bone mineral density requires about 12 wk to be detected by standard dual-energy absorptiometry imaging (6). A decrease in cardiac mass is measurable after approximately 6 wk of BR without exercise (7). Impairment in exercise responses are evident after only a few days of BR, but maximal exercise capacity may not decline for a few weeks, and it depends on the initial fitness level of the subject (5). Thus, it is important to consider the most appropriate BR protocol when designing a study to simulate the effects of space flight.

Immersion

Immersion is another model to simulate microgravity. American astronauts prepare to perform extravehicular activity (EVA) by training in the Neutral Buoyancy Laboratory, a large pool at the Johnson Space Center. This laboratory has a 6.2 million-gallon pool containing a mockup of the space station on the bottom. Astronauts don their EVA suits and are slowly lowered into the pool. As they stand completely submerged on a platform, weights are added to their suit until they reach neutral buoyancy. Astronauts report that the sensations of working underwater are similar to those of working in space. This model of microgravity has obvious limitations for performing experimental investigations. The friction of the water causes resistance to fast movements, but this is not a problem during EVA because the pressurized EVA suit limits the speed of their limb movements.

Unconfined water immersion (without a space suit) is also used to simulate microgravity. Subjects are immersed in a small pool of usually thermoneutral (34.5°C) water either with their head just above water or submerged while breathing through a snorkel. A major difficulty of such studies is the high rate of heat transfer between the subject and the surrounding water, requiring that body temperature be closely monitored. This model is used to simulate responses of body fluids and electrolytes during the first few days of microgravity. During immersion, the water pressure against the surface of the body causes a central fluid redistribution from legs to thorax, resulting in body fluid and cardiovascular responses that occur more rapidly and may be more pronounced than those during space flight or with other microgravity simulation models (3).

To avoid problems during immersion associated with heat exchange and from prolonged exposure of the skin to the immersion fluid, some investigators enclose the subjects in a waterproof material. This dry immersion method was first used during the 1960s and is still used occasionally by Russian investigators (3). Physiological responses are similar to those during wet water immersion; study duration can be weeks.

Suspension and Immobilization

Musculoskeletal unloading can be produced by suspending subjects above the ground with springs or by supporting them from below with air jets (air-bearing floors). Such methods create regions of tissue compression that can be tolerated for only short periods. Limb immobilization or casting has been used to study regional changes in muscle. A limb is casted at a fixed angle, and the reported changes in muscle generally are greater and occur faster than those reported during BR or space flight. Fixing the limb may not replicate the conditions of space flight, during which astronauts move their limbs freely (8).

There are two methods of unilateral lower limb suspension to unweight a limb and simulate microgravity. In one method a support strap is used to suspend one limb while the other limb is used for mobilization via crutches. In the second method a high platform shoe is fitted on one foot while the subject walks with crutches, allowing the unloaded leg to hang freely. The strap method produces muscle changes similar to those with casting, possibly because of the limited ability to move the limb. The platform shoe method produces muscle responses similar to those reported in astronauts during flight and similar to those of subjects during BR (8).

In summary, space flight exposes astronauts to extreme environmental conditions imposed by a variety of stressors that result in pronounced deconditioning upon return to Earth. To study the mechanisms of the physiological responses to space flight and to develop countermeasures to prevent deconditioning, microgravity simulations are often used. The most frequently used simulation is BR; however, one must use caution when extrapolating BR results to flight, since BR does not involve many of the stressors of living and working in space.

Effects of Microgravity on Human Physiological Systems

Exposure to microgravity could affect human tissues through several mechanisms. First, the reduction in apparent body mass unloads the postural or supportive tissues, resulting in atrophy of these tissues. Second, microgravity causes body fluids to redistribute caudally, such that hydrostatic forces equilibrate throughout the body, increase perfusion in upper body regions, and decrease perfusion in lower body regions. A result of the increased upper body fluid volume is a reduction in total blood volume. The concomitant changes in regional intravascular pressures must be counterbalanced by modifications in vascular permeability and tissue oncotic pressures to reestablish homeostatic body fluid exchange. Microgravity engenders much smaller fluctuations in vascular pressures than naturally occur during change in posture in terrestrial gravity. Without such pressure fluctuations the baroreceptors and other reflexes that regulate blood pressure lose responsiveness and are less able to maintain blood pressure upon return to 1g or during positive acceleration (9). Third, the effects of increased stress and altered light and dark cycles may result in alterations of the hypothalamic–pituitary–adrenal axis or the sympathetic–adrenal medullary axis, resulting in marked changes in hormonal, neural, and immune functions.

Cardiovascular System

Exposure to microgravity initiates alterations in the body's homeostasis that can lead to profound effects on the capacity of the body to maintain orthostatic (fainting) tolerance and to perform physical exercise. Data from both space flight and BR experiments demonstrate an early reduction in blood volume due to contraction of the plasma followed by a more gradual stabilization between 30–60 days of exposure (Fig. 29.1). Results from BR experiments indicate that the rapid reduction in plasma volume occurs within 24–72 h and is a result of diuresis and natriuresis induced by the headward fluid shifts. There is also a more gradual decrease of red blood cell volume. Loss of circulating blood volume probably contributes directly to the limitation of cardiac filling, as evidenced by reduction in echocardiographic end-diastolic and stroke volumes (5,10–14).

In addition to reduced circulating vascular volume, there is evidence that cardiovascular structures alter during adaptation to microgravity and its simulations. Echocardiographic measurements demonstrated lower resting heart volume in subjects after exposure to BR (13,14) and space flight (10). Subsequent magnetic resonance imaging (MRI) measurements of cardiac muscle mass before and after exposure to space flight and BR have revealed that in addition to reduced filling, cardiac atrophy may lead to a smaller myocardial mass in both humans and animals (7,12). It is possible that less cardiac muscle could contribute to reduced myocardial contractility and stroke volume following adaptation to microgravity. Contrary to data on myocardial atrophy in space, recent evidence from ground-based and flight experiments on animals suggests that cardiac atrophy may not occur in microgravity but that reports of atrophic effects on the myocardium may simply reflect the negative caloric balance and body mass routinely observed in astronauts during space flight (15). Despite the controversy of evidence for cardiac atrophy, measures of myocardial function curves, ejection fractions, and arterial pulse wave velocities all suggest that there is little effect of exposure to microgravity on cardiac contractility (5,11–13).

Alterations in cardiac mechanical factors have also been associated with exposure to microgravity. The observation that stroke volume remained higher at any given filling pressure after confinement to BR for less than 2 wk (11) suggested that cardiac compliance was increased in the early stage of exposure. Elevated cardiac compliance (the change in intraventricular pressure for a given change in cardiac filling) may be a mechanism to defend stroke volume in the presence of hypovolemia and reduced cardiac filling pressure. However, as the duration of confinement to BR exceeds 2 wk, myocardial compliance and cardiac filling are reduced (7).

Increased venous compliance of the lower extremities has also been reported during exposure to space flight and BR (5,11,12). Greater compliance of capacitance vessels can compound the effect of hypovolemia on venous return and stroke volume by providing a greater capacity to pool blood under the same hydrostatic pressure. A positive correlation between the magnitudes of reduction in size of the muscle compartment and elevated calf compliance has been reported in BR subjects. This relationship supports the premise that increased venous compliance may be influenced by a loss of tissue mass that normally provides structural support for the veins. When the muscle compartment is reduced, compliance increases (5); when the muscle compartment loss is attenuated with routine muscular activity during BR, the compliance changes are eliminated (5).

Exposure to space flight and BR is also associated with alterations of autonomically mediated baroreflex mechanisms that control cardiovascular functions. Data from both space flight and BR experiments have provided evidence for reduced cardiac vagal nerve activity, increased heart rate response with aortic baroreceptor stimulation, elevated sympathetic nerve activity and circulating catecholamines, and greater cardiac β-adrenergic receptor reactivity (12). These alterations in autonomic function alone or in combination could explain, at least in part, the tachycardia and compromised orthostatic performance following exposure to space flight and BR. However, there is no evidence that these autonomic adaptations are associated with compromised exercise performance.

Exposure to microgravity causes alterations in the structure and function of vascular smooth muscle. Elevated peripheral vascular resistance (12) after exposure to space flight or BR reflects a reflex compensatory response to the reduction in stroke volume and cardiac output. Since maximal vasoconstriction is finite, elevated resting vasoconstriction reflects a reduction in vasoconstrictive reserve and lowers the capacity to buffer alterations in blood pressure. Increased vascular β-adrenoreceptor (vasodilatory) sensitivity has been reported after BR (12). In the presence of elevated sympathetic nerve traffic, increased vasodilatory adrenergic receptor reactivity could limit vasoconstrictive capacity. An alternate explanation for attenuated vasoconstriction post-BR or flight is that the vasoconstrictor response is impaired, due to reduced release or end-organ sensitivity to norepinephrine (16,17). There is also consistent and compelling evidence from animal experiments that vascular smooth muscle contraction is reduced

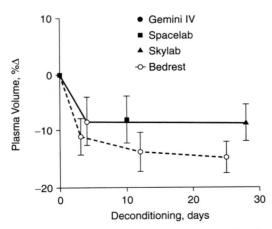

FIGURE 29.1 Time courses of percent change (%Δ) in plasma volume during space flights (*closed symbols, solid line*) and bed rest (*open circles, broken line*). (*Adapted from Convertino VA. Exercise and adaptation to microgravity environments. In Fregly MJ, Blatteis CM, eds. Handbook of Physiology. Section 4: Environmental Physiology. III. The Gravitational Environment. New York: Oxford University, 1996;824.*)

during exposure to low gravity and is associated with altered morphology, atrophy, and lower vasoreactivity (18).

Pulmonary System

Gravity profoundly influences the lung. In a 1g environment gravity helps determine the shape of the lungs, the distribution of ventilation and blood flow, alveolar size, intrapleural pressure, chest mechanics, and gas exchange. Therefore, it is predicted that pulmonary function will be altered greatly during microgravity, although the direction of change is uncertain because some alterations may impair pulmonary function while others may be beneficial. Prisk and coworkers (19,20) argue that the effects of "true microgravity," such as space flight or parabolic flight, differ from the effects caused by simulated microgravity, such as BR. For this reason, space flight and BR responses will be discussed separately.

LUNG FUNCTION DURING SPACE FLIGHT   Prisk (19) extensively reviewed the effects of space flight on pulmonary function, and many of his findings are summarized in Table 29.1. Lung volumes decrease upon entry to microgravity in part because of the headward fluid shifts. Both vital capacity and forced vital capacity decreased during the first 24 h compared to a preflight standing control and then returned to preflight levels by 72 h and remained there for the remainder of the 9-day flight. The initial decrease in lung volumes was attributed to the rapid increase in intrathoracic blood volume and the later recovery to a gradual reduction in thoracic blood volume as plasma volume decreased. A 10% decrease in functional residual capacity also occurred immediately as a result of an upward movement of the diaphragm and abdominal contents and an outward movement of the rib cage with gravitational unloading. Residual volume decreased compared to preflight standing and was attributed to more uniform closure of airways in dependent lung regions so that less air was trapped in the bottom of the lungs during expiration. Airway resistance, assessed by measurement of peak expiratory flow, decreased early in flight but recovered after 9 days. Prisk (19) suggested that this airway response was due to measurement difficulties and requires further verification.

The most surprising finding from the SLS-1 and SLS-2 space flight missions (9 and 14 days, respectively) was that the normal ventilation ($\dot{V}_A$) and perfusion ($\dot{Q}$) gradients in the lung, although improved, still persisted during weightlessness. This remaining nongravitational inhomogeneity of ventilation and perfusion was unexpected, and the cause remains unclear. An improvement in the $\dot{V}_A/\dot{Q}$ matching would be expected to enhance gas exchange and possibly increase arterial P_{O_2} and lower arterial P_{CO_2}. Instead, arterial oxygen pressure fell, as estimated from arterialized capillary blood samples obtained during long-duration Soviet Mir missions. Arterial desaturation has yet to be confirmed with direct arterial measurements.

Another unexpected finding from the 16-day Neurolab mission (19) was that the ventilatory response to hypoxia was reduced during space flight. This altered hypoxic drive was attributed to an increase in arterial pressure at the carotid bodies, which may decrease the sensitivity of these chemoreceptor organs. In contrast, the ventilatory response to hypercapnia was reported to be unchanged during flight (19).

Resting oxygen consumption and carbon dioxide production were unchanged during the SLS-1 and SLS-2 missions (19). Tidal volume was smaller and breathing frequency was faster but not fast enough to compensate totally because ventilation was reduced by about 7% compared to preflight values. Alveolar ventilation was maintained, however, because of a reduction in physiological dead space.

A particular concern during space flight is that aerosol deposition in the lungs will be impaired. Gravity plays an important role in causing potentially toxic inhaled particles to be deposited and cleared in the airways before reaching the alveoli; but there have been no studies of aerosol deposition during space flight. However, during parabolic flight there is an almost linear positive relationship between gravity level and the amount of particle deposition (19).

LUNG FUNCTION DURING BED REST   During space flight the changes in mechanical forces on the lungs—caused by removal of gravity from the surface of the lungs, chest, and abdominal walls—is greater than those during BR. True microgravity causes the rib cage to expand slightly, creating more negative intrapleural pressure. A decrease in central venous pressure at the heart has been measured during space flight despite an increase in intrathoracic blood volume (19). These mechanical influences are not replicated during BR, during which body tissues continue to be compressed by gravity. Unlike during space flight, central venous pressure increases transiently upon assumption of a supine or head-down position (9). Although the changes in lung volumes, pulmonary blood flow, $\dot{V}_A/\dot{Q}$ matching, gas diffusion, and physiological dead space are in the same direction as during space flight (9), they are not as pronounced. In agreement with space flight data, pulmonary tissue volume does not increase during exposure to BR despite the increase in thoracic blood volume and central venous pressure. This resistance to formation of pulmonary edema is explained by the ample compliance of the pulmonary circulation (19).

As the BR continues and central blood volume returns toward levels before BR, lung volumes also return toward values before BR (9); BR differs from space flight in this respect. During BR the lung volumes and diffusing capacity recover toward a supine position value before BR, while during space flight these values return toward a preflight standing position value. Prisk and associates (20) attributed this difference to the differing mechanical influences on the lung, chest, and abdominal wall. Peak expiratory flow rate is unaffected even during prolonged BR, which has been interpreted as evidence against respiratory muscle deconditioning during

TABLE 29.1	Respiratory Changes During 1 to 17 Days of Space Flight	
Physiological Response	**Flights**	**Changes**
Pulmonary blood flow		
Total pulmonary blood flow (cardiac output)	SLS1, SLS2, D2	Initial 35% increase, then reduction to about 25% above preflight upright
Diffusing capacity (carbon monoxide)	SLS1	25% increase
Pulmonary capillary blood volume		25% increase
Diffusing capacity of alveolar membrane	SLS1	25% increase
Pulmonary tissue volume		No change at 24 h, 20–25% decrease after 9 d
Pulmonary blood flow distribution	SLS1	More uniform but some inequality remained
Pulmonary ventilation		
Respiration frequency	SLS1, SLS2	9% increase
Tidal volume	SLS1, SLS2	15% decrease
Alveolar ventilation	SLS1, SLS2	Unchanged
Total ventilation	SLS1, SLS2	7% decrease
Ventilatory distribution	SLS1, SLS2, D2	More uniform but some inequality remained
Maximal peak expiratory flow	SLS1	Decreased ≤12.5% early in flight then returned to normal by 4th day
Gas Exchange		
Oxygen uptake	SLS1, SLS2	Unchanged
CO_2 output	SLS1, SLS2	Unchanged
End-tidal P_{O_2}	SLS1	Unchanged
End-tidal P_{CO_2}	SLS1	Small increase when CO_2 concentration in spacecraft increased
$\dot{V}_A/\dot{Q}$ matching	SLS1, SLS2	Increase but still some mismatching remains
Lung Volumes		
Vital capacity	SLS1	5% decrease at 24 h, return to control values by 72 h
Function residual capacity	SLS1	15% decrease
Residual lung volume	SLS1	18% decrease
Closing volume (argon bolus)	SLS1	Unchanged
Control of Breathing		
Hypoxic response	Neurolab, LMS	50% reduction
Hypercapnic response	Neurolab, LMS	No change

Data are summarized from Prisk GK. Microgravity and the lung. J Appl Physiol 2000;89:385–396. Flight durations were SLS1, 9 days; SLS2, 14 days; D2, 10 days; Neurolab, 16 days; and LMS, 17 days.

microgravity (21). In agreement with space flight data, some authors have reported arterial desaturation during prolonged BR, which they attributed to pulmonary circulatory stasis or to a reduced threshold for airway closure (9). Unlike during space flight, carbon dioxide sensitivity was reduced after 120 days of BR (9). Changes in breathing mechanics during BR are similar to those reported during space flight: an increase in breathing frequency and a decrease in tidal volume, although ventilation was unchanged (9).

Muscular System

Exposure to space flight and BR causes unloading and relative disuse atrophy of skeletal muscles, especially those of the lower extremities. The magnitude of the resulting decrease in limb size is similar in individuals exposed to flight and BR and has been used as an indication of muscle atrophy (Fig. 29.2). Muscle biopsies taken from subjects before and after exposure to both flight and BR revealed significant muscle atrophy, as evidenced by reduction in cross-sectional areas of slow-twitch (type I) and fast-twitch (type II) muscle fibers of the vastus lateralis (22,23). The relative reduction in muscle fiber cross-sectional area was approximately 50 to 60% greater in larger fast-twitch than smaller slow-twitch fibers. Muscle atrophy was also accompanied by a reduced ratio of capillaries to fiber in both slow- and fast-twitch fibers after exposure to BR and flight (22,23). Various ultrastructural abnormalities—such as disorganized myofibrils, cellular edema, irregular Z-bodies, and fiber necrosis (disrupted fiber membranes), as indicated by disrupted sarcolemma, abnormal mitochondria, disrupted striation patterns, and mitochondria in the intercellular spaces—have been observed from electron microscopic analyses of muscle biopsy samples obtained from humans confined to BR (22).

In addition to changes in muscle morphology, exposure to microgravity has been associated with histochemical alterations. Although there were no significant changes in activities of glycolytic enzymes (e.g., ATPase, α-glycerophosphate

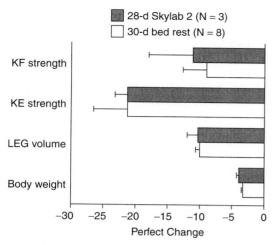

FIGURE 29.2   Percent change in strength of knee flexors (KF), knee extensors (KE), leg volume, and body weight following 30 days of bed rest compared to 28 days of space flight (*Skylab 2*). Values are mean ± SE. (*Adapted from Convertino VA. Neuromuscular aspects in development of exercise countermeasures. Physiologist 1991;34(Suppl):S125–S128.*)

dehydrogenase, lactate dehydrogenase, phosphofructokinase) in soleus and/or vastus lateralis muscles following BR or flight, the activities of enzymes associated with aerobic metabolic pathways (succinate dehydrogenase, citrate synthase, β-hydroxyacyl–coenzyme A dehydrogenase) were reduced in both slow- and fast-twitch muscle fibers (22,23). These data indicate that in addition to compromised capability to generate force, the effect of prolonged muscle unloading and reduced energy requirements associated with exposure to microgravity may reduce the capacity for oxygen delivery to and utilization by muscle fiber cells.

Skeletal System

Bone mass and bone mineral density (BMD) decrease during exposure to microgravity, and this loss of bone tissue is one of the critical issues to resolve before planetary exploration can be pursued. Factors that influence bone remodeling include gravitational forces, dynamic mechanical forces during movement, nutrition, hormonal changes, and biochemical effects produced during mineral and acid-base imbalances. Age, gender, and ethnicity also have important effects on bone homeostasis. Bone loss begins immediately upon unloading, particularly during BR, and is evidenced by a rapid and sustained increase in calcium excretion. The increased blood and urinary calcium concentrations increase the risk of cardiac arrhythmias and kidney stones (3).

The qualitative changes in bone are similar after BR and flight and to those reported in patients with disuse osteoporosis (21). For this reason, gravitational unloading and reduced dynamic mechanical forces are believed to be primary stimuli for bone changes in microgravity. During 4- to 14-month space flights, whole-body BMD decreased at approximately 0.6% per month (6), faster than during BR despite the fact that the crew members were exercising 1–2 h · day^{-1} but the BR subjects were not. It is unclear from these results whether the space flight subjects would have lost bone at an even greater rate without the exercise countermeasures or whether the in-flight exercise was ineffective in preventing bone loss.

Decreases in BMD during BR and flight are not uniform; 95% of the changes occur from weight-bearing regions of the body, including the hip, spine, and legs (6). Fortunately, these changes appear to be reversible upon exposure to gravity. Smith and coworkers (25) predict that the rate of bone loss during flight and recovery is linear but that it takes approximately 2.5 times longer to regain bone than to lose it. However, the rate of recovery varies greatly among individuals and among different regions of the body (26).

The decline in bone mass with BR and flight is attributed primarily to mechanical factors, such as gravitational unloading, and a lack of dynamic forces on bones during walking. However, during space flight the nongravitational effects may account for the faster rate of bone loss than during BR. Changes in secretion of calcium-regulating hormones, such as parathyroid hormone, vitamin D, and calcitonin, have been reported during flight (27), while other hormonal changes, such as reduced growth hormone and increased cortisol, may contribute to the bone loss but are not observed consistently during space flight (3). Nutritional factors, including reduced energy and calcium intake, impaired absorption of calcium from the gastrointestinal tract, and possible effects related to the high-sodium diet, may also contribute to the bone loss (27).

Bone calcium (Table 29.2) is lost at rates of up to 140 mg · day^{-1} during flight (25); countermeasures including exercise, increased calcium intake, reduced sodium intake, vitamin D supplementation, and exposure to ultraviolet light have proved ineffective for preventing these bone losses (24). Bisphosphonate administration (alendronate) appears to be a promising countermeasure to reduce bone loss (26). However, data from BR have shown that pharmacological treatment alone does not prevent all bone loss, but treatment with two of the early bisphosphonates (etidronate and clodronate) was most effective when combined with exercise (26).

Intensive research is being conducted to discover the mechanisms by which unloading (deconditioning) causes bone loss. Bone mass turnover is determined by net balance between resorption and formation. Bone resorption, as indicated by the urinary markers hydroxyproline and urinary collagen crosslinks, increases within the first few days of BR and flight (2,25). Kinetic tracer data indicated a 50% increase in bone resorption during long flights (25). On the other hand, findings regarding the changes in bone formation conflict. Biochemical markers, including osteocalcin and bone-specific alkaline phosphatase, are unchanged or slightly decreased

TABLE 29.2 Calcium and Bone During Bed Rest and Space Flight

Bed Rest

Time	Change	Reference[a]
2 d	Urinary calcium increased Resorption markers increased	Baecker et al., 2003
7 d	Resorption markers increased Formation markers increased or no change	Leukin et al, 1993
10 d	Hydroxyproline increased Urinary calcium increased Serum calcium, phosphate increased Vitamin D decreased	Van der Wiel, 1991
20 d	Formation markers no change Resorption markers increased Cytokines transiently increased	Fukuoka et al., 1994
3 mo	BMD in spine and hip decreased Urinary, serum calcium increased Serum calcium increased PTH, vitamin D decreased Formation markers no change Resorption markers increased	Zerwekh et al., 1998

Space Flight

Change	Time	Reference[b]
Ionized calcium increased Serum 1,25 vitamin D decreased Formation markers decreased Resorption markers increased	21 d	Turner, 2000
BMD decrease in flight and no return in 5 yr	28–48 d	Turner (2)
Urinary calcium increased during flight	28–84 d	Turner, 2000
Urinary collagen breakdown markers increased	28–84 d	Turner (2)
Resorption markers increased Formation markers no change	51 d	Turner, 2000
Urinary calcium increased during flight	60 d	Turner, 2000
Formation markers decreased Resorption markers no change	1, 6 mo	Collet et al., 1997

Reference	Duration	Findings	Reference
LeBlanc et al., 2002	4 mo	BMD decreased in lower body; BMD no change in upper body; Resorption markers increased; Formation markers no change; PTH, vitamin D decreased	
	4–14.5 mo	BMD decreased in lower body; BMD no change in upper body	LeBlanc et al., 2000
	3 mo	Calcium intake and absorption decreased; Urinary calcium increased; Resorption markers increased; Formation markers increased	Smith et al., 1999
	180 d	Serum PTH decrease (Turner, 2000); Formation markers decreased; Resorption markers increased	
Donaldson et al., 1970	210 to 252 d	Urinary calcium, sustained increase; Fecal calcium increased; Sweat calcium not increased; Whole-body calcium loss 4.2%; Phosphorus balance similar to calcium; Os Calcis, 25–45% loss in mass in central region	
	30–438 d	Serum calcium increased; PTH increased; Calcitonin decreased	Turner, 2000
	115 d	Intestinal calcium absorption decreased; GI and kidney calcium excretion increased	Turner, 2000

[a]Bed rest references
Baecker N, Tomic A, Mika C, et al. Bone resorption is induced on the second day of bed rest: results of a controlled crossover trial. J Appl Physiol 2003;95:977–982. Lueken SA, Arnaud SB, Taylor AK, Baylink DJ. Changes in markers of bone formation and resorption in a bed rest model of weightlessness. J Bone Miner Res 1993;8(12):1433–1438. Van der Wiel HE. Biochemical parameters of bone turnover during ten days of bed rest and subsequent mobilization. Bone Miner 1991;13:123–129. Fukuoka H, Kiriyama M, Nishimura Y, et al. Metabolic turnover of bone and peripheral monocyte release of cytokines during short-term bed rest. Acta Physiol Scand Suppl. 1994;616:37–41. Zerwekh JE, Ruml LA, Gottschalk F, Pak CY. The effects of twelve weeks of bed rest on bone histology, biochemical markers of bone turnover, and calcium homeostasis in eleven normal subjects. J Bone Miner Res 1998;13(10):1594–1601. LeBlanc AD, Driscoll TB, Shackelford LC, et al. Alendronate as an effective countermeasure to disuse induced bone loss. J Musculoskelet Neuronal Interact 2002;2(4):335–343. Donaldson CL, Hulley SB, Vogel JM, et al. Effect of prolonged bed rest on bone mineral. Metabolism 1970;19(12):1071–1084.
[b]Space flight references
Turner RT. Physiology of a microgravity environment invited review: what do we know about the effects of space flight on bone? J Appl Physiol 2000;89:840–847.
Collet PH et al. Bone 1997;20:547–551. Effects of 1- and 6-month spaceflight and bone mass and biochemistry in two humans.
LeBlanc A, Schneider V, Shackelford L, et al. Bone mineral and lean tissue loss after long duration space flight. J Musculoskeletal Neuronal Interact 2000;1(2):157–160.
Smith SM, Wastney ME, Morukov BV, et al. Calcium metabolism before, during, and after a 3-mo space flight: kinetic and biochemical changes. Am J Physiol 1999;277:R1–R10.

during BR (26) and during flight (25,27). Following both flight and BR, bone formation markers increase promptly well above the preflight values (25). Thus, it appears that bone loss in microgravity is due to increased bone resorption compounded by a slowly developing decrease in bone formation. Animal data suggest that decreased bone blood perfusion of lower body regions during microgravity simulations may alter nutrient delivery and vascular wall shear forces to stimulate endothelial cytokine activity that results in regional bone loss (28).

Immune Function

There is strong evidence that humans who fly in space flight have compromised immune function; see Sonnenfeld (26) for a recent overview of results from human and animal studies during flight. During the Apollo missions, 15 of 29 astronauts reported bacterial or viral infections either during flight or within the first week after landing. During the infamous *Apollo 13* mission, the travails of one of the crew members was further compounded because he had a severe urinary tract infection. Most human space flight studies have examined the effects of flight on cell-mediated immunity. Blood samples drawn from astronauts and cosmonauts after the *Apollo-Soyuz* test project, Skylab, and space shuttle flights revealed inhibition of mitogen-induced formation of leukocytes. After a combined Soviet and Hungarian flight, cosmonauts had a severe decrease in ability of leucocytes to produce interferon-α and interferon-β. Compared to ground-based controls, crew members immediately after flight have an altered leukocyte subset distribution and interferon production and reduced natural killer cell activity. Delayed hypersensitivity responses to skin tests were inhibited after short- and long-term space flights, and reactivation of latent viruses (e.g., Epstein-Barr) may occur, possibly in response to the elevated catecholamine levels.

The causes of these changes in immune function are uncertain. During space flight, it could be a direct effect of microgravity, or it could related to the confined environment, increased stress, exposure to radiation, nutrition, sleep deprivation, or other as yet undefined factors. The concern is that changes in immune function might make the crew more susceptible to bacterial or viral infections, to tissue radiation damage, and to future development of tumors and cancers.

Alterations in immune responses also have been reported following BR (30). Many of the responses are similar to those reported during flight, such as decreased interleukin (IL) 2 production and increased IL-1 production by monocytes, which may be involved in promoting bone mineral loss. Other flight changes, such as alteration in leukocyte subsets, have not been consistently observed in humans during BR (31).

In summary, microgravity has profound effects on human tissues, resulting in physiological responses often seen during aging or detraining or associated with inactivity-related diseases. The long-term effects of such changes have been minimal following space flight or BR studies thus far, possibly related to the limited duration of the microgravity or simulated microgravity exposures. For a long-term mission to Mars, estimated to require at least 3 years in continuous microgravity, the most significant concerns regard the health consequences of bone loss and the effects of radiation. As is discussed later in the chapter, it is hoped that exercise countermeasures may help to prevent the bone changes and possibly improve immune function to minimize radiation effects.

Changes in Aerobic and Anaerobic Exercise Responses During and After Space Flight or Bed Rest

Many of the adaptive responses to microgravity discussed earlier can have significant impact during aerobic and anaerobic exercise. A loss of aerobic capacity during space flight could impair the ability to perform in an emergency. Deconditioning in a bedridden patient could compound the effects of illness; for example, the changes in fluids and electrolytes associated with BR (9) may complicate the management of arrhythmias in a cardiac patient.

Cardiorespiratory Responses

In microgravity the circulatory and respiratory responses with exertion are impaired before any significant change in maximal exercise capacity occurs. For example, after only 5 days of BR the heart rate and respiratory exchange ratio were elevated during submaximal cycle exercise, yet the peak oxygen uptake ($\dot{V}O_{2pk}$) was maintained (32). This finding raises questions about results from BR or flight when a change in aerobic capacity is assumed because of changes observed in submaximal exercise responses.

Cardiorespiratory Responses During Exposure to Weightlessness

A basic cardiorespiratory response to exercise during BR and flight is impaired cardiac filling (33). Cardiac output was measured (using the single-breath carbon dioxide rebreathing method) several times during the 9- and 15-day SLS-1 and SLS-2 shuttle missions. At rest the cardiac output was similar to preflight supine levels, with slightly larger stroke volume and slightly lower heart rate. During exercise at 30 and 60% of preflight $\dot{V}O_{2pk}$, the in-flight heart rate increased more rapidly than before the flight, while stroke volume decreased with increased exercise intensity. As a result of this unusual decreased stroke volume, the increase in cardiac output was attenuated significantly from preflight levels, such that the slope of the cardiac output (L $\cdot$ min^{-1}) to $\dot{V}O_2$ (L $\cdot$ min^{-1}) relationship was only 3.5 compared to the normal value of 6.0. The blood pressure response at rest and during exercise was similar to that of the supine subject before the flight. The reason for the attenuated cardiac output response to exercise in microgravity is unclear. Shykoff and coworkers (33) suggested that it may be due to lower cardiac output requirements in flight, as the peripheral muscle tissues may have better perfusion and be better able to extract oxygen from the circulating blood. Because of the reduced red cell mass and generally attenuated perfusion in the lower extremities during flight, this explanation seems unlikely. Alternatively, a reduction in circulating blood volume due to sequestration of blood in the pulmonary circulation could limit the ability to increase cardiac output.

During a 237-day Russian space flight, cosmonauts exercising at 125 and 175 W also had lower stroke volume, cardiac output, and end-diastolic volume than before the flight. Also, end-systolic volumes were smaller and ejection fractions were larger than before the flight, which suggests that reduction in cardiac contractility could not account for the reduced cardiac output (5). Perhonen and associates (7) evaluated cardiac function before and after 2, 6, and 12 wk of BR and after flight and noted significant cardiac muscle atrophy between 2 and 6 wk of BR and a 12% reduction in cardiac mass after only 10 days of flight. The authors cautioned, however, that a reduction in cardiac mass does not necessarily indicate impairment in cardiac contractile function, as spinal cord–injured patients have a much smaller heart but normal systolic function. Instead, an important clinical outcome of cardiac atrophy is decline in diastolic function caused by a leftward shift in the end-diastolic pressure–volume curve resulting in a reduced left ventricular end-diastolic volume for any given filling pressure, which would result in a smaller stroke volume. Thus, cardiac atrophy during flight may contribute to the inability to maintain stroke volume, which could impair both exercise and orthostatic responses.

Cardiorespiratory Responses After Weightlessness

Cardiorespiratory responses are further compromised following flight, even in crew members whose aerobic capacity was maintained or increased during flight (3,34). Sitting submaximal cycle exercise tests were performed during Skylab flights at 25, 50, and 75% of preflight $\dot{V}_{O_{2pk}}$. When this test was performed on landing day, cardiac output was 30% lower and stroke volume was 50% lower than before the flight; heart rate and total peripheral resistance were elevated, while arterial blood pressure was similar to those before the flight. A profound reduction in cardiac output and stroke volume during exercise post flight also was reported following Russian flights of 30, 63, and 96 days (5), when accompanying systolic blood pressure was elevated and diastolic blood pressure was similar to those before the flight (unchanged during exercise).

Interpretation of exercise responses post flight depends on the position of the subject during testing. Cardiorespiratory changes in exercise post flight are more pronounced with the subject sitting than supine. For example, on landing day following the *Skylab 4* mission, three crew members exercised at approximately 25% of their preflight $\dot{V}_{O_{2pk}}$ both sitting and supine. During supine exercise the cardiac output was maintained despite a decrease in stroke volume; during sitting exercise the cardiac output fell and was accompanied by an accentuated increase in heart rate and a decrease in stroke volume (35). Similar changes in cardiorespiratory responses to exercise and effects of posture have been reported following BR (5).

Oxygen Uptake and Mechanical Efficiency

Oxygen uptake ($\dot{V}_{O_2}$) at the same absolute power output on a cycle ergometer is consistently lower during flight and BR than baseline $\dot{V}_{O_2}$ values measured before such exposures (5,11,36) and is greater with dynamic exercise during recovery from flight and BR (5). Thus the lower submaximal $\dot{V}_{O_2}$ at equal power outputs might be explained by increased mechanical efficiency in flight. Alternatively, the lower inflight $\dot{V}_{O_2}$ might involve a change in the time constant for the $\dot{V}_O$ to reach a steady state. If the rate change of $\dot{V}_{O_2}$ during the transient phase of exercise were lengthened during flight or BR, then the $\dot{V}_{O_2}$ measured at 3–5 min of exercise may not have reached steady state, and it would be lower than preexposure levels without a change in mechanical efficiency. This idea is supported by the measurement of a slower $\dot{V}_{O_2}$ kinetics during the transient phase of exercise after BR with a greater recovery of oxygen uptake (Fig. 29.3). These attenuated changes in $\dot{V}_{O_2}$ kinetics during the tran-

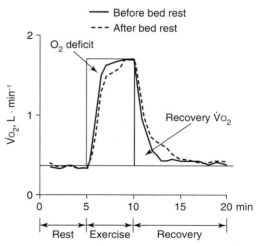

FIGURE 29.3 Oxygen uptake ($\dot{V}_{O_2}$) kinetics during constant-load exercise (115 W) before (*solid line*) and after (*broken line*) bed rest. *(Modified from Convertino VA. Exercise and adaptation to microgravity environments. In Fregly MJ, Blatteis CM, eds. Handbook of Physiology. Section 4: Environmental Physiology. III. The Gravitational Environment. New York: Oxford University, 1996;818.)*

sient periods at the beginning and completion of exercise following deconditioning may reflect a greater requirement for anaerobic metabolism to provide for adequate energy demand, and the findings are further supported by higher blood lactate and ventilation and respiratory exchange ratios following BR (5).

When exercise metabolism reaches steady state during post-BR cycle ergometry, the energy requirement is equal to the pre-BR level (5), which suggests that mechanical efficiency does not change. These BR results have been verified during flight in that a predicted $\dot{V}O_2$ of 2.25 L · min⁻¹ during in-flight exercise at 160 W on a cycle ergometer was virtually equal to the measured $\dot{V}O_2$ of 2.31 L · min⁻¹ (approximately 20% mechanical efficiency, the same as that generally reported on the ground). Since the basal metabolic rate is similar prior to and during exposure to BR or flight, the gross efficiency of performing exercise on a mechanically stabilized device (cycle ergometer) appears to be unaltered during flight.

The energy cost of locomotion in flight may be much higher when the body cannot be stabilized by postural muscles as in terrestrial gravity. This hypothesis is supported by comparisons of the average power output and metabolic cost of exercise on a cycle ergometer with those on a treadmill during flight. The energy expenditure during treadmill exercise, using a system of bungee cords to stabilize a subject, was 7.4 kcal · min⁻¹ during flight compared to 5.7 kcal · min⁻¹ when the same treadmill exercise was performed on Earth (5). Thus, the predicted mechanical efficiency of 20% on Earth was reduced to 15% in flight. These findings demonstrate the importance of gravity stabilization of the body when measuring mechanical efficiency during in-flight exercise in weightlessness.

Maximal Oxygen Uptake

Maximum aerobic capacity, whether expressed as $\dot{V}O_{2max}$ or $\dot{V}O_{2pk}$ (subjects exercise to voluntary exhaustion without attaining a plateau of the oxygen consumption–work level curve), is reduced by 5–35% in individuals exposed to BR or flight, and the magnitude of this loss is dependent upon the duration of the exposure (Fig. 29.4). Since $\dot{V}O_{2max}$ is regarded as a very good single indicator of maximal endurance and aerobic physical fitness, measurement of reduction in $\dot{V}O_{2max}$ during BR or flight should provide a good assessment of the magnitude of the deconditioning process on the cardiorespiratory and other physiological systems. The Fick equation expresses the relationship between oxygen uptake (oxygen utilized by the total body), A-$\dot{V}O_{2diff}$ (difference between arterial and venous oxygen concentrations resulting from the amount of oxygen extracted by working muscles) and cardiac output (heart rate times stroke volume): $\dot{V}O_2$ = heart rate × stroke volume × A-$\dot{V}O_{2diff}$. Thus mechanisms that underlie reduction in $\dot{V}O_{2max}$ during adaptation to deconditioning can be assessed and elucidated by evaluating changes

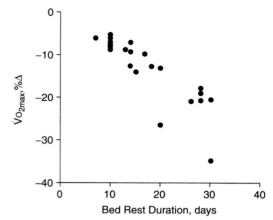

FIGURE 29.4 Regression of duration of bed rest and percent change (%Δ) in $\dot{V}O_{2max}$. Compilation of data from 19 independent investigations. The linear regression of best fit is %Δ$\dot{V}O_{2max}$ = –0.85 [days] + 1.4; r = .73. (*Modified from Convertino VA. Exercise and adaptation to microgravity environments. In Fregly MJ, Blatteis CM, eds. Handbook of Physiology. Section 4: Environmental Physiology. III. The Gravitational Environment. New York: Oxford University, 1996;819.*)

in factors that influence the control of heart rate, stroke volume, and oxygen delivery.

After exposure to BR or space flight, the rate of increase in heart rate is similar at the same oxygen uptake, including that at $\dot{V}O_{2max}$ (Fig. 29.5). The mechanisms of elevated exercise heart rate after BR represent a combination of several probable factors, including increased sympathetic nerve ac-

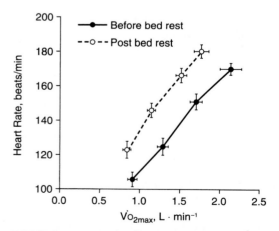

FIGURE 29.5 Mean (±SE) relationship between $\dot{V}O_2$ and heart rate before and post (*open circles, broken line*) 10 days of bed rest in 12 healthy middle-aged men. (*Modified from Hung J, Goldwater D, Convertino VA, et al. Mechanisms for decreased exercise capacity following bed rest in normal middle-aged men. Am J Cardiol 1983;51:344–348.*)

tivity at maximal levels as evidenced by higher plasma nor-epinephrine concentrations (11). In addition, the heart rate response to a 0.02 μg · kg · min⁻¹ steady-state dose of isoproterenol is increased significantly after BR (11), which suggests that cardiac β-adrenergic receptor sensitivity may be increased. Therefore, increased sympathetic nerve activity and sensitivity of cardiac adrenergic receptors can partly explain the elevated maximal heart rate after deconditioning.

Despite increased heart rate, cardiac output during submaximal and maximal exercise is decreased following exposure to BR and flight deconditioning (5,11,13,36). Thus, the reduction in maximal cardiac output is accounted for entirely by reduced stroke volume. Absence of change in A-$\dot{V}O_{2diff}$ suggested that the primary mechanism for reduction in $\dot{V}O_{2max}$ following deconditioning was a severely compromised stroke volume.

Lower resting heart volume (measured echocardiographically) after deconditioning advanced the possibility that reduced stroke volume during exercise reflects decreased ventricular performance resulting from myocardial atrophy (7,14). To test this hypothesis, cardiac output and stroke volume were measured during exercise in subjects before and

after BR using radionuclide imaging (13). A 17% reduction in $\dot{V}O_{2max}$ was due solely to a 23% reduction in cardiac output and 28% decrease in stroke volume, with little change in the A-$\dot{V}O_{2diff}$. Despite a significant reduction in the exercise stroke volume after BR, the ejection fraction actually increased at rest and during exercise (Fig. 29.6, left panels). This reduction in stroke volume and increased ejection fraction at baseline rest and during exercise has been substantiated during flight (Fig. 29.6, right panels). Together, the reduced stroke volume in the presence of higher ejection fraction suggests that ventricular performance is maintained and that functional myocardial deterioration is not significant after exposure to weightlessness.

In the absence of evidence of any significant loss of myocardial function, the reduced cardiac output with increased ejection fraction and heart rate during exercise after deconditioning points to reductions in venous return and cardiac filling, which probably constitute the primary mechanism by which maximal stroke volume is decreased. Reduced myocardial compliance and increased peripheral venous pooling (compliance) could limit cardiac filling. However, a rapid decrease in maximal stroke volume and $\dot{V}O_{2max}$ occurs during

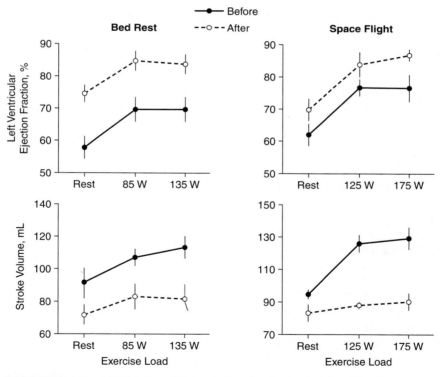

FIGURE 29.6 Mean (±SE) left ventricular ejection fraction (*top*) and stroke volume (*bottom*) during rest and graded exercise before and after bed rest (*left*) and space flight (*right*). (*Adapted from bed rest data in Hung J, Goldwater D, Convertino VA, et al. Mechanisms for decreased exercise capacity following bed rest in normal middle-aged men. Am J Cardiol 1983;51:344–348. Space flight data from Convertino VA. Exercise and adaptation to microgravity environments. In Fregly MJ, Blatteis CM, eds. Handbook of Physiology. Section 4: Environmental Physiology. III. The Gravitational Environment. New York: Oxford University, 1996;827,828.*)

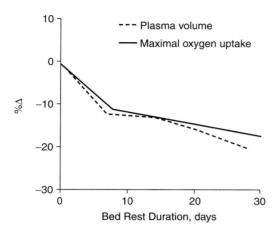

FIGURE 29.7 Average time course of percent change (%Δ) in plasma volume and maximal oxygen uptake from five male subjects during bed rest. *(Modified from Convertino VA. Cardiovascular consequences of bed rest: effects on maximal oxygen uptake. Med Sci Sports Exerc 1997;29:191–196.)*

the initial period of weightlessness (Fig. 29.7), when cardiac compliance may be unchanged or even increased (11).

Since limited cardiac filling cannot be explained by compromised myocardial mechanics during the initial 2 or more weeks of BR (11), a primary factor associated with reduced stroke volume during maximal exercise is lower circulating blood (plasma) volume. This hypothesis is supported by the close relationship between the magnitude of changes in blood volume and in $\dot{V}O_{2max}$ (5,11). The time course of relative reduction in $\dot{V}O_{2max}$ shows a steep decline within the first few days of BR followed by a more gradual reduction thereafter, which is similar to the time course of hypovolemia (Fig. 29.7). Cross-sectional comparison of data from 12 independent investigations demonstrated a high correlation ($r = .85$) between percent change in plasma volume and $\dot{V}O_{2max}$ (Fig. 29.8). This relationship suggests that reduction in plasma volume contributes significantly (approximately 70% of the variability) to the limitation of maximal stroke volume, cardiac output, and $\dot{V}O_2$ following flight deconditioning. The effect of lower circulating blood volume on venous return and cardiac filling may be compounded by the increased venous pooling (compliance) in the lower extremities, which is supported by the observations that the reductions in maximal stroke volume and $\dot{V}O_{2max}$ after BR are greater during exercise in the sitting position than in the supine position (5,11,13).

Peripheral mechanisms of oxygen delivery and utilization may also contribute to lower $\dot{V}O_{2max}$ during extended space flight. Oxygen utilization by exercising muscle appears to be lower during BR, as evidenced by greater accumulation of blood lactate at the same work rate as before BR (5,14). Lower muscle oxygen utilization is consistent with reduced oxidative enzyme activities and compromised capacity for

oxygen delivery because of less capillary density, lower maximal conductance, and decreased red blood cell volume. Although changes in the peripheral mechanisms associated with restricted delivery to and utilization of oxygen by skeletal muscle could contribute to lower $\dot{V}O_{2max}$ after BR, this mechanism was not apparent when based on calculation of maximal A-$\dot{V}O_{2diff}$ (13,14). It is probable that the reduction of cardiac output is such an overwhelming limiting factor that the input from peripheral mechanisms is relatively insignificant. However, if blood volume and cardiac filling are not fully limiting, then the influence of peripheral mechanisms for limiting $\dot{V}O_{2max}$ may become more important.

In summary, the deconditioning effects of bed BR or space flight on $\dot{V}O_{2max}$ can be accounted for by alterations in several central (cardiac) and peripheral mechanisms (Fig. 29.9). An increased maximal heart rate is associated with elevations in sympathetic activity (norepinephrine release) at maximal exercise and increased cardiac β-adrenergic reactivity. These adrenergic responses following deconditioning could also increase cardiac contractility, which would increase ejection fraction during exercise, even with reductions in stroke volume and cardiac filling. Despite elevated maximal heart rate and probably cardiac contractility, maximal cardiac output is reduced dramatically from the significant decrease in stroke volume. Since cardiac contractility is probably enhanced, the lowered stroke volume must be due primarily to reduced cardiac filling associated with lower blood volume. Increased compliance of leg veins may also limit venous return, especially after return to the upright posture. Although A-$\dot{V}O_{2diff}$ has been reported to be unaltered following BR and flight, reductions in oxidative enzymes, capillaries, and maximal blood flow in skeletal muscle could limit oxygen delivery and utilization. The ultimate consequence of

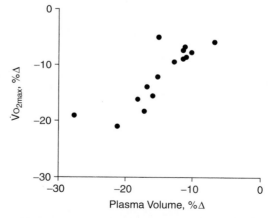

FIGURE 29.8 Regression of percent change (%Δ) in $\dot{V}O_{2max}$ on %Δ in plasma volume after bed rest. Data from 12 investigations. The linear regression equation is %Δ$\dot{V}O_{2max}$ = + 0.82 [%Δ PV] +0.3; $r = .84$. *(Modified from Convertino VA. Cardiovascular consequences of bed rest: effects on maximal oxygen uptake. Med Sci Sports Exerc 1997;29:191–196.)*

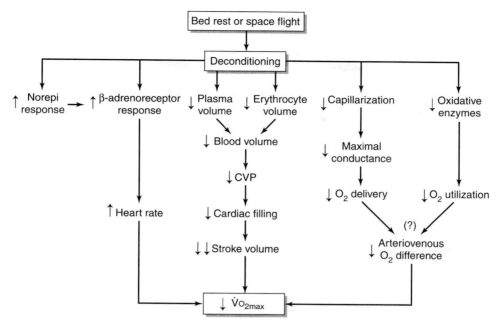

FIGURE 29.9 Summary of factors influencing maximal oxygen uptake during bed rest.

alterations in cardiac and vascular functions resulting from deconditioning is reduction in aerobic power.

Exercise Endurance

Both space flight and BR experiments designed to determine the effects of deconditioning on exercise endurance are limited. Increased heart rate and reduced stroke volume were associated with decreased endurance in two crew members, as evidenced by their inability to complete a 5-minute standardized exercise test at relatively low work intensity on the 24th day of a 96-day flight aboard the Soviet *Salyut 6* space station (5). Results from numerous BR investigations have provided quantitative evidence of reduced endurance after BR by demonstrating that less time was required to reach volitional exhaustion during graded exercise (5). However, information about the ability of the crew to complete prolonged submaximal work tasks following flight is limited, since all experiments employed exercise durations of no more than 5–10 min.

Thermoregulation

Both resting and exercise body temperatures are altered during BR and space flight. Basal temperatures were unchanged after 14- and 30-day BR but were decreased by 0.05–0.07°C after 56 days of horizontal BR (9). Body temperature circadian rhythm is blunted during BR and flight, with increases in the minimum night temperature (0.22°C) and decreases in the maximal daily temperature (0.20°C). Thermal sensations are altered; subjects feel cooler than normal, especially in the legs.

During dynamic exercise after BR or flight the ability to dissipate body heat is impaired, resulting in a faster rise in core temperature for a given absolute level of work. Skin blood flow is reduced at rest, possibly because of enhanced sympathetic vasoconstriction, and during exercise the sensitivity of the active vasodilatory response is impaired. Crandall and associates (37) postulated that the reduced skin blood flow during exercise may be due not only to enhanced sympathetic vasoconstriction but also to vascular remodeling, which reduces maximal blood flow, and to a reduced vascular responsiveness or release of nitric oxide. The sweating response also is impaired following BR or flight. Although 14 days of BR did not alter the sensitivity of the sweat glands to exogenously applied acetylcholine and did not affect the number of active sweat glands, the maximal sweat output per gland was reduced, possibly because of sweat gland atrophy (37). Dynamic exercise training (90 min · day^{-1} at 75% of pre-BR HR$_{max}$) during 14 days of BR prevented these exercise-induced changes in skin blood flow and sweating.

Age and Gender

Limited sample size, particularly with female astronauts, and a relatively homogeneous age group have limited evaluation of age and gender factors on the exercise response to weightlessness to the use of BR data. Because of significant differences in baseline $\dot{V}O_{2max}$ between men and women and young and middle-aged subjects, the relative (percent) changes in $\dot{V}O_{2max}$ resulting from exposure to similar durations of BR were similar; $\dot{V}O_{2max}$, measured during supine cycle ergometry, decreased by 9% in young men, 10% in young women, 8% in middle-aged men, and 8% in middle-aged women (5). The corresponding changes in maximal power output and maximal exercise duration, both indices of functional exercise capacity, were also similar among the age and gender groups. Despite significant differences in the absolute $\dot{V}O_{2max}$ between men and women of varying ages, the percent changes in $\dot{V}O_{2max}$ are equal across age and gender. However, the slope of the regression line between initial $\dot{V}O_{2max}$ and post-BR change in $\dot{V}O_{2max}$ was significantly steeper in the younger subjects than in the older subjects (38), which suggests that the rate of absolute reduction in aerobic power is greater in younger subjects. The attenuated reduction in absolute $\dot{V}O_{2max}$ for older subjects must be partly explained by aging; however, middle-aged persons appear to have the same relative ability as younger subjects to reduce their aerobic power with adaptation to BR.

Level of Physical Fitness

An active (fit) individual with a large $\dot{V}O_{2max}$ reserve has greater potential to lose that reserve during space flight or BR than does a more sedentary individual with smaller $\dot{V}O_{2max}$ reserve (14). This idea is supported by early descriptive reports of a 22% reduction in $\dot{V}O_{2max}$ following BR in a subject with an initial $\dot{V}O_{2max}$ of $4.15\ L \cdot min^{-1}$ compared to a 13% reduction observed in a subject with initial $\dot{V}O_{2max}$ of $3.54\ L \cdot min^{-1}$ (5). Also, two subjects with greater aerobic capacity showed greater relative loss of their $\dot{V}O_{2max}$ than three less fit subjects after 20 days of BR (14). In a more systematic approach, changes in $\dot{V}O_{2max}$ before and after BR in 10 moderately fit subjects ($\dot{V}O_{2max} = 48.5 \pm 1.9\ mL \cdot kg^{-1} \cdot min^{-1}$) compared to those in 10 less fit subjects ($\dot{V}O_{2max} = 38 \pm 1.8\ mL \cdot kg^{-1} \cdot min^{-1}$) revealed that the percent reduction in blood volume and $\dot{V}O_{2max}$ was nearly threefold greater in the moderately fit subjects than in the less fit group (5). Although some analyses have not supported this relationship, general findings are consistent with the hypothesis that the relative magnitude of reduction in aerobic capacity during deconditioning is associated with the initial $\dot{V}O_{2max}$ reserve and that levels of physical conditioning may influence the results.

Changes in Muscle Strength and Endurance Following Bed Rest and Space Flight

As discussed previously, weightlessness results in changes not only in muscle mass but also in biochemical properties of skeletal muscles. Lean body mass, muscle volume, and postural muscle cross-sectional areas decrease after approximately 2 wk of BR or after a few days of flight (5). Both type 1 and type 2 muscle fibers become smaller, capillarity density decreases, and enzymatic properties and myosin isoforms adapt, creating a smaller, faster, more anaerobic phenotype (8).

Muscular Strength

Standard clinical methods have been used to assess muscle strength following space flight; those most frequently used were isokinetic because of perceived greater safety for the crew

(Table 29.3). However, strength tests during flight have been performed rarely and only when special hardware was flown. Change in strength occurs in two phases during flight: an initial rapid decline in which the decrease post flight was much greater than predicted by the change in muscle volume and a later, slower decline in strength. In BR and flight studies, this initial decrease in strength (attributed to neuromotor changes) was followed by a more gradual decrease in strength that was more closely related to the decreased muscle mass. However, the changes in strength following flight are highly variable among crew members and do not correlate positively with flight length. This variability may be related to a protective effect provided by in-flight exercise countermeasures, although this has never been verified. In general, strength changes are greater in lower body muscle groups than in upper body groups and in extensor than in flexor muscles (Table 29.3). Few flight follow-up data are available to describe changes in the force or torque–velocity relationship of muscles. From the biochemical changes in muscle favoring a greater expression of fast-twitch myosin isoforms and increased glycolytic enzymes, one might expect that strength would be better maintained at faster contraction velocities. This hypothesis was supported by space flight findings in which after 175 days of flight the greatest losses in ankle plantar flexor strength occurred at the highest angular velocities (8).

Results generated from BR experiments have consistently substantiated that the strength in both small-muscle (arm, forearm, hand) and large-muscle (trunk, thigh, leg) groups is decreased. Analysis of cross-sectional data reveals that the relative reduction in strength of muscle groups does not substantially decrease until after 7–14 days of BR and is dependent on the specific muscle group and duration of rest (Fig. 29.10). Linear regression of cross-sectional changes in maximal muscle force development over 120 days of BR suggests decreases in strength in all muscle groups at a rate of 0.4% per day. Mean reductions in handgrip (−8%) and arm (−6%) strengths are only about one-third as great as the strength losses in the trunk (−22%) and leg (−20%) muscle groups during periods of 1–120 days. The greater use of arms than legs in flight and the possibility that arm muscles that generate smaller forces, hence are less affected by unloading than the antigravity muscles of the lower extremities, which use larger forces in terrestrial gravity, could account for the smaller strength loss after BR in muscles of the upper compared to the lower extremities.

After 2–4 wk of BR, the average decrease in angle-specific peak torque across multiple speeds of concentric muscle action is approximately 20% for knee extensors and 10% for knee flexors of the dominant leg (Fig. 29.2). These decreases in muscle strength are associated with average body weight losses of about 3% and average leg volume reduction of about 10%. These changes in body weight, leg volume, and muscle function following BR compare favorably with the average changes in body weights, leg volumes, and concentric peak torque development in the same muscle groups exposed

TABLE 29.3	Muscle Changes Following Space Flight		
Variable	Flight Length	Changes	Reference[a]
Muscle volume (MRI)	17 d	Largest changes in calf, back muscles, 12 and 10%	LeBlanc A et al., 2000
Muscle volume (MRI)	112–196 d	Largest changes in calf, back muscles, 24 and 20%	LeBlanc A et al., 2000
Isokinetic strength 5 d post flight	Skylab 2, 28 d, 30-min cycle exercise	10% decrease in arm flexor extensor isokinetic strength 25% decrease in leg extensors, 5% decrease in leg flexors	Rummel JA et al., 1975
Isokinetic strength 5 d post flight	Skylab 3, 56 d, 60-min cycle, some resistive arm exercise	Minimal change in arm strength 18% decrease in leg flexors, 25% decrease in leg extensors	Rummel JA et al., 1975
Isokinetic strength 5 d post flight	Skylab 4, 84 d, 90-min cycle, some resistive arm exercise, passive treadmill plate	No change in arm flexors; 15% decrease in arm extensors 5% decreases in leg flexors, extensors	Rummel JA et al., 1975
Isokinetic strength, landing day	Shuttle 5–13-d flights, minimal in-flight aerobic exercise	No change biceps, triceps, deltoids, tibialis anterior, gastrocnemius, soleus Back, 23% concentric, 14% eccentric Abdomen 10% concentric, 8% eccentric Quads, 12% concentric, 7% eccentric Hamstrings, no sign changes	Greenisen MC et al., 1999
Isokinetic strength, 5–7 d post flight	ISS missions, 129–145 d 2 h · d⁻¹ in-flight countermeasures	Knee extension, 26% decrease Knee flexion, 29% decrease	Lee SMC et al., 2003
Isokinetic endurance, 5–7 d post flight	ISS missions, 129–145d 2 h · d⁻¹ in-flight countermeasures	Knee extension, 19% decrease Knee flexion, 24% decrease	Lee SMC et al., 2003
Isometric strength	17-d LSM mission, frequent strength measurements	No change in calf muscle strength	Trappe SW et al., 2001
Isometric strength	Mir missions, 180 d	Triceps surae group, 42% decrease	Koryak Y, 2001
Isometric force, endurance	180 d	Plantar flexor force decreased 20–48% Force decrease not correlated with decreases in muscle volume Shortened endurance due to reduced metabolic efficiency	Zange J et al., 1996

(continued)

611

TABLE 29.3   Muscle Changes Following Space Flight (*Continued*)

Variable	Flight Length	Changes	Reference[a]
Peak tetanic force	Mir missions, 180 d	Triceps surae group, 25% decrease	Koryak Y, 2001
Maximal explosive power	30 d	Reduced 30%	Di Prampero PE, Antonutto G, 1997
Maximal explosive power	180 d	Reduced 55%	Antonutto G. et al., 1999
Myosin isoforms	11 d	Reduced proportion of vastus lateralis fibers expressing only slow myosin heavy chain	Zhou MY et al., 1995
Fiber size, capillarity, ATPase, GPD	5 and 11 d	6–8% fewer slow fibers 16–32% decrease fiber cross-sectional area ATPase activity increased in type 2 (fast) fibers GPD activity in type 1 fibers increased 80% 24% decrease capillarity	Edgerton VR et al., 1995.
Skinned myofiber velocity of shortening	17 d	Increased force and velocity of shortening of slow fibers	Widrick JJ et al., 1999

[a]References

LeBlanc A, Lin C, Shackelford L, et al. Muscle volume, MRI relaxation times (T2), and body composition after spaceflight. J Appl Physiol 2000;89:2158–2164.

Rummel JA et al. Exercise and long duration space flight through 84 days. J Am Med Womens Assoc 1975;30:175–187.

Greenisen MC et al. Functional performance evaluation. In: NASA/SP-199-534 1999;3-1–3-8.

Lee SMC et al. Isokinetic strength and endurance after international space station (ISS) missions. Med Sci Sport Exerc 2003;35:S262.

Trappe SW, Trappe TA, Lee GA, et al. Comparison of a space shuttle flight (STS-78) and bed rest on human muscle function. J Appl Physiol. 2001;91:57–64.

Koryak YU. Electrically evoked and voluntary properties of the human triceps surae muscle: effects of long-term spaceflights. Acta Physiol Pharmacol Bulg 2001;26(1–2):21–27.

Zange J et al. Changes in calf muscle performance energy metabolism, and muscle volume caused by long term stay on space station MIR. Proc. 6th Eur Symp on Life Sciences Res in Space. ESA SP-390, 287–290, 1996.

di Prampero PE, Antonutto G. Cycling in space to simulate gravity. Int J Sports Med 1997;18(Suppl 4):S324–S326.

Antonutto G, Capelli C, Girardis M, et al. Effects of microgravity on maximal power of lower limbs during very short efforts in humans. J Appl Physiol 1999;86:85–92.

Zhou MY, Klitgaard H, Saltin B, et al. Myosin heavy chain isoforms of human muscle after short-term spaceflight. J Appl Physiol. 1995;78:1740–1744.

Edgerton VR, Zhou MY, Ohira Y, et al. Human fiber size and enzymatic properties after 5 and 11 days of spaceflight. J Appl Physiol 1995;78:1733–1739.

Widrick JJ, Knuth ST, Norenberg KM, et al. Effect of a 17 day spaceflight on contractile properties of human soleus muscle fibres. J Physiol 1999;516(Pt 3):915–930.

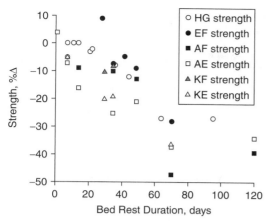

FIGURE 29.10 Regression of percent change (%Δ) in strength of handgrip (HG), elbow flexors (EF), ankle flexors (AF), ankle extensors (AE), knee flexors (KF), and knee extensors (KE) on duration of bed rest. Compilation of data from 17 independent investigations. *(Adapted from Convertino VA. Exercise and adaptation to microgravity environments. In Fregly MJ, Blatteis CM, eds. Handbook of Physiology. Section 4: Environmental Physiology. III. The Gravitational Environment. New York: Oxford University, 1996;823.)*

to similar durations of flight (Fig. 29.2). The general conclusion is that weightlessness reduces strength approximately twice as much in extensor as in flexor muscles.

Change in the torque–velocity relationship of BR subjects *in vivo* demonstrated a reduction in force development across all speeds of limb movement during concentric muscle contractions. Strength loss occurred with eccentric as well as concentric muscle actions, and the reduction of angle-specific peak torque was not significantly influenced by the type or speed of muscle action.

Muscular Endurance

Muscle endurance has been assessed after short and long space flights by measuring the total isokinetic work performed during multiple contractions. Following short shuttle flights, the total work during knee flexion and extension was reduced on landing day but had returned to baseline within 7 days (30). Following 129- to 145-day space station missions, knee extensor and flexor endurance (21 contractions at $180° \cdot s^{-1}$) were reduced by 19% (extension) and by 24% (flexion) 7 days after landing and had not recovered to preflight levels by 20 days of recovery (40).

Data regarding fatigability characteristics of muscle groups in humans following BR are limited. Right-leg plantar flexor exercise (60 contractions per minute with a target force of 588 N) was performed by seven supine men before and after 16 days of BR during which the lower limb was made ischemic by inflation of a pneumatic cuff just above the knee. After BR

the time to fatigue (inability to maintain cadence and/or force for >5 s) during ischemic plantar flexion exercise was decreased by 18% (41). Upper body muscular strength and endurance are especially important for crew members who perform EVA. During an EVA the crew member must move against the pressurized space suit to move and to perform work. These activities involve mostly upper body exertions at approximately 26–32% of the crew member's upper body maximal oxygen uptake (42). Normally this would not be a problem, except that this work must be continued for 5–8 h, during which time the crew member has limited access to fluids and may become dehydrated by up to 2.6% of body weight. During BR simulations without exercise countermeasures, arm strength decreased by 10–20% (42). This decrease in strength also would reduce upper body endurance and thus compromise the EVA timeline and possibly even the success of the EVA.

Neuromotor Function

The decrease in strength following flight is often much greater than would be expected from the corresponding decreases in muscle mass. For example, peak isometric force of the legs was reduced by 17%, while the corresponding muscle mass was reduced by only 11% in 14 cosmonauts after 90–180 days of flight (8). EMG activity from the contracting muscles was reduced by 39%. The authors concluded that their results were due to impairment of neuromotor function from either an effect on the intrinsic characteristics of the motor units or a change in their recruitment pattern.

Maximal Explosive Power

In a space flight emergency, maximal explosive power may be critical for survival. Antonutto and coworkers (43) measured maximal explosive power (single maximal contractions with both legs) with a dynamometer after as long as 180 days of flight. The maximal explosive power was reduced by 30% after 1 month and by 50% after 6 months of flight. Since these reductions in maximal explosive power were much larger than the concomitant decrease in muscle mass of 6–0%, these results support the hypothesis of deterioration in motor control and coordination after flight.

In summary, loss of muscle mass, strength, and endurance frequently are observed following microgravity exposure, although the changes are not a simple function of duration of exposure. The greatest changes occur in muscle groups involved in postural control or locomotion. The initial rapid decline in strength is most likely caused by changes in neuromotor function. The continuing decline in strength and changes in endurance are related to the muscle atrophy and biochemical changes (a more glycolytic, fast-twitch phenotype). Although microgravity is the primary stimulus for deconditioning, changes in nutrition and endocrine and immune functions may compound the unloading effects.

Exercise Countermeasures

A prescription containing both dynamic (aerobic) and resistive exercise would be expected to prevent most of the deconditioning effects of microgravity described earlier. Dynamic exercise should be effective in preventing the cardiorespiratory changes, while resistive exercise should help to maintain muscle function. In addition, heavy dynamic and resistive exercise may prevent the decreases in bone mass and BMD.

Exercise to Maintain Exercise Tolerance Post Flight

Following BR or flight, deconditioning of the cardiorespiratory system is evident from the reductions in orthostatic tolerance and exercise capacity (i.e., decreased $\dot{V}O_{2max}$). Specific exercise prescriptions performed during flight or BR may provide therapeutic benefit by helping to preserve cardiac function, cardiovascular reflexes, skeletal muscle mass, oxidative capacity of muscle fibers, neuromotor coordination, and body fluid homeostasis (5). Few studies have been performed during space flight to determine the most effective exercise prescription. In the Skylab program, as the duration of each mission increased from 28 to 56 to 84 days, in-flight exercise was increased from 30 to 60 to 90 min $\cdot$ day^{-1}, respectively. Submaximal cycle exercise tests were performed before flight, every 5–6 days during flight, and 2 days post flight. While the in-flight exercise responses were maintained, exercise response post flight significantly decreased, including decreased cardiac output, stroke volume, and oxygen pulse and elevated heart rate and ventilation. The decrement post flight did not worsen with increasing flight duration, which led the investigators to conclude that the in-flight exercise was useful to shorten the recovery period post flight (3,35).

The effect of in-flight dynamic exercise during shuttle missions to improve exercise responses post flight was evaluated for the 30 shuttle crew members who performed varying levels of in-flight exercise (39). Exercise responses post flight were evaluated by measuring the change in heart rate during a graded cycle exercise test. Even moderate volumes of in-flight dynamic exercise (cycle or treadmill exercise performed three times per week for more than 20 minutes per session) reduced the exercise heart rate response following flight. As maximal exercise testing is not allowed within the first 5–7 days following space station missions, it may never be possible to directly assess the effect of countermeasures on exercise capacity following long space flight.

BR findings, however, do strongly support a positive effect of dynamic exercise to prevent the deconditioning effects of simulated microgravity. Numerous studies have demonstrated that various modes of dynamic exercise performed daily with intensities from 20 to 100% of $\dot{V}O_{2max}$ for 15–60 min reduced the average reduction in $\dot{V}O_{2max}$ to only 4%, compared to 13% when no exercise training was performed (5). These observations indicate the importance of regular physical exercise for maintenance of $\dot{V}O_{2max}$ during prolonged exposure to BR.

Exercise to Prevent Orthostatic Intolerance

Although dynamic exercise training with a high aerobic component has proved successful in maintaining $\dot{V}O_{2max}$ when performed during BR (44,45) and space flight (35), it has failed to protect against orthostatic intolerance after BR (5,12,46). Few studies have been performed during flight to determine the most effective exercise prescription for orthostatic intolerance post space flight. However, there is evidence that a single bout of maximal dynamic exercise within 24 h of the end of BR can increase or restore blood volume, stroke volume, sympathetic nerve activity, vascular α-receptor reactivity, and various baroreflex functions associated with control of heart rate and vascular peripheral resistance (5,12,47). Orthostatic hypotension and intolerance also were ameliorated by a single bout of maximal dynamic exercise in individuals restrained for extended periods to wheelchairs or to BR (5,12,47). To test the hypothesis that a single bout of maximal exercise would improve orthostatic function after space flight, four shuttle crew members performed maximal cycle exercise within 24–48 h of landing, and cardiovascular responses to the operational 10-min stand test were examined before and after flight. Four control crew members from the same flights did not perform the exercise countermeasure. Although the post-flight heart rate and blood pressure responses to standing were similar for both groups, cardiac stroke volume (by echocardiography) was better maintained in the exercisers (48). In the BR studies, a smaller reduction in stroke volume was found in the subjects who had the smallest decrement in orthostatic tolerance (5,12). However, to validate the effectiveness of this maximal exercise countermeasure, a more provocative orthostatic test or longer flights are required to evaluate improvements in orthostatic tolerance.

Submaximal dynamic exercise performed frequently during short flights may improve orthostatic responses post flight (49). Heart rate and blood pressure response to standing were evaluated for the same 30 shuttle crew members described previously, who were categorized as high-, medium-, or low-volume exercisers. The medium- and high-volume exercisers had significantly smaller increases in heart rate and decreases in pulse pressure during the stand test. These results suggest that even moderate amounts of in-flight dynamic exercise may reduce orthostatic stress after short flights. Again, however, more provocative tests must be performed to validate an effect to protect orthostatic tolerance.

Exercise to Prevent Muscle Deconditioning

During the 17-day LMS space shuttle mission a torque velocity isokinetic dynamometer was used to assess changes in muscle properties in four crew members. However, since strength tests were performed frequently during the mission, no significant changes in isometric calf strength, force velocity characteristics, or muscle fiber composition or size were found post flight (7). Thus, infrequent maximal resistive contractions appear to preserve muscle function during space flight. Exercise training performed on a passive treadmill by four crew members during shuttle missions resulted in a 12% increase in post-flight isokinetic calf extensor eccentric strength compared to a 13% reduction in a control group who did not exercise (39).

Results from muscle biopsies obtained from subjects before and after exposure to BR argue that resistive exercise, in addition to dynamic exercise, will be necessary to counteract the muscle atrophy and dysfunction during exposure and adaptation to extended weightlessness. Application of regular axial-load resistance to the musculoskeletal system of the arms, legs, and torso using various resistance exercise devices ameliorates many expected reductions in muscle size and strength associated with exposure to BR (5,50). The effects of exercise training employed during BR corroborate flight results in that the 0.4–0.6% daily reductions in muscle strength during BR are virtually eliminated with regular performance of resistive exercise (50). Perhaps more significant is the probability that preservation or restoration of muscle structure and function during weightlessness will require restoration of muscle actions and forces that occur in the normal 1g environment. Nearly all muscle actions in flight or BR require fiber shortening (concentric actions), whereas fiber lengthening (eccentric actions) is virtually eliminated in both environments because of negation of effects of gravity. Since eccentric muscle actions are involved as a regular part of our daily ambulatory activities on Earth, an efficient exercise countermeasure designed to ameliorate muscle atrophy during flight and BR should include eccentric in addition to concentric contractions.

Exercise to Prevent Bone Deconditioning

Bone loss during space flight was first suspected from radiographic changes in Gemini and Apollo crew men post flight. Bone loss (photon absorptiometry) was observed following Skylab flights, despite the progressive increase in dynamic exercise volume during the three missions (3). Cosmonauts and astronauts performed approximately 2 h $\cdot$ day^{-1} of heavy treadmill (footward loading of approximately 50% body weight), cycle and resistive expander exercises during Mir flights. Yet all crew members had decreases in BMD in lower extremities that directly correlated with flight length (6). This continuing loss of bone mass during space flight, even with the various exercise training regimens being used, will persist until more effective countermeasures (exercise, drugs, or hormones) are developed.

Early BR studies of 5–36 weeks' duration evaluated the effectiveness of various exercise training programs to prevent the increase in calcium excretion (51). Countermeasures included a resistance pulley system (Exer-Genie) used for 80 min $\cdot$ day^{-1}, a static body longitudinal compression de-

vice applied for 4 h $\cdot$ day^{-1} at a force of 80% body weight, and impact loading with longitudinal compression of 80% body weight. However, these countermeasures failed to attenuate the negative calcium balance after 12 or 17 wk of BR. During 120 days of BR (52), 1 hour of heavy exercise (with isokinetic cycle and isokinetic devices and bungee expanders), applied three of every four BR days, maintained bone formation but did not prevent resorption. Ingested diphosphonates reduced bone resorption and bone formation. Exercise plus diphosphonates also decreased resorption, but exercise alone did not prevent reduction in bone formation. In a following 360-day BR study (53), 1 h $\cdot$ day^{-1} of dynamic exercise (horizontal treadmill, cycling) during the first 120 days of BR did not prevent the negative calcium balance, which was similar to that of the controls, who did not exercise. During the second 120 days, when the dynamic exercise training regimen was increased to two 60-min exercise sessions per day, bone resorption was reduced, thus improving calcium balance significantly, by 52%. When exercise was combined with bisphosphonate administration (900 mg daily), the calcium balance was normalized throughout BR. Thus, from these early Russian BR studies it appeared that very vigorous and prolonged exercise training could reduce but not prevent bone loss. In a recent 30-day BR study, 30 min $\cdot$ day^{-1} of treadmill exercise (6 of 7 days per week) within a lower-body negative pressure (LBNP) chamber (which provides a ground reaction force of 1–1.2 times body weight) significantly reduced the increase in bone resorption markers as seen in the subjects who did not exercise (54). Thus, heavy-impact dynamic exercise training, heavy-intensity resistive exercise training, or both may help to maintain bone integrity during simulated microgravity.

In summary, exercise countermeasures are used extensively (approximately 2 h $\cdot$ day^{-1}) during current space station missions. Dynamic (aerobic) exercises are intended to minimize cardiorespiratory changes to weightlessness, as assessed by responses to exercise and orthostatic challenges post flight. The continuing decrements in responses post flight suggest that further improvements in these countermeasures are necessary. To date, the implementation of resistive exercise during flight has been severely limited; thus exercise has not been effective in preventing musculoskeletal responses to space flight.

Exercise to Prevent Decompression Sickness During Extravehicular Activity

A lesser-known role for exercise during space flight is for prevention of decompression sickness. Decompression sickness is a risk during EVA because the pressure surrounding the astronaut decreases from 14.7 psi (normal ambient pressure in the spacecraft) to 4.3 psi, the pressure in the U.S. EVA suit. With a sudden reduction in ambient pressure, nitrogen from the blood desaturates and forms bubbles in the tissues that move to the circulation and block blood flow. To prevent decompression sickness during weightlessness, the shuttle is decompressed to 10.2 psi for 12 h before EVA. The EVA crew members then breathe with 100% oxygen for 1 h to reduce their tissue nitrogen before donning their EVA suit. Without the 10.2-psi cabin decompression, crew members would have to breathe oxygen for 4 h prior to an EVA. On the international space station (ISS), however, it is impractical to decompress the entire space station, and so the crew members use exercise to accelerate nitrogen elimination (55). The ISS crew members perform 10 min of moderate arm and leg exercise during a 2-h oxygen-breathing period before the EVA to increase tissue perfusion and retard nitrogen bubble formation during their EVA.

Repeated Exposure to Bed Rest and Space Flight

Although over 100 crew members have flown more than once in space, there has been no systematic evaluation comparing the physiological effects of repeated space flight. Is there an adaptation to space flight, such that having flown once, physiological changes during repeated missions will be attenuated? Or do the detrimental effects accumulate with repeated space flight? Is the interval (recovery) between flights important? Cardiorespiratory responses to exercise appear to recover within 30 days and have no lasting effect. Cosmonaut V. V. Ryumin performed a 185-day flight only 6 months after landing from a 175-day flight. His pre-flight aerobic capacity was nearly identical before both missions, suggesting full recovery (5). Bone decrements, on the other hand, may be additive, since full recovery often takes several years. LeBlanc and coworkers (6) found that the rate of bone loss in three cosmonauts who flew twice was similar, suggesting no protective effect on their second flight. The best protection against bone loss may be to select crew members who have the greatest bone mineral density or to screen for those who resist bone loss during flight. Perhaps a countermeasure for long space missions will be to select those with genetic profiles that indicate resistance to bone demineralization.

SUMMARY

1. Astronauts during space flight and patients on BR undergo profound physiological changes.
2. Some immediate effects of space flight or BR occur in the cardiovascular system in response to the headward redistribution of body fluids. Within hours of assuming a horizontal or head-down position, plasma volume is reduced and orthostatic and exercise responses are impaired.
3. With continued exposure to space flight or BR, changes in baroreceptor function, cardiac function, venous tone, and vascular reactivity further impair blood pressure regulation and the ability to maintain stroke volume and cardiac output during subsequent orthostatic or exercise stresses.
4. Pulmonary function is susceptible to the effects of gravity. During space flight and BR the lung volumes decrease in relation to changes in thoracic blood volume; residual volume decreases in response to upward movement of the abdominal contents; and the ventilation–perfusion inhomogeneity is improved yet still persists. Pulmonary responses to space flight are generally in the same direction but larger than those to BR.
5. Muscle mass is reduced during space flight and BR. Initially muscle strength declines faster than muscle mass. Maximal explosive power also is reduced to a much greater extent than the decline in muscle mass, suggesting impairment in neuromotor function. Morphological and biochemical changes include smaller muscle fibers with faster velocity of shortening and greater reliance on glycolytic metabolism. These changes reduce strength and endurance.
6. Bone content and bone mineral density decrease gradually during space flight and BR as a result of a rapid increase in bone resorption and possibly a more gradual decrease in bone formation. The recovery of bone mass and density varies for different body regions and often requires several months, sometimes years.
7. Aerobic capacity decreases during space flight and BR, primarily because of inability to maintain stroke volume, hence maximal cardiac output. Reduced muscle capillarity and decreased activity of muscle oxidative enzymes also impair cardiorespiratory endurance.
8. Current exercise training countermeasures, consisting primarily of treadmill and cycle dynamic exercises and low-intensity resistive exercise, are capable of attenuating the decline in aerobic capacity during flight. However post flight, especially during upright exercise, cardiac filling is impaired and aerobic capacity is reduced for several weeks.
9. High-intensity resistance exercise training performed only two or three times a week during BR is effective for preventing muscular deconditioning. The use of resistive exercise during space flight to improve muscle or bone responses has not been systematically tested.
10. There is no evidence of additional detrimental effects from repeated space flight or BR exposures.
11. Exercise training treatments and procedures developed to prevent space flight or BR-induced deconditioning have been used for treatment of many Earth-based conditions, such as disuse osteoporosis, orthostatic hypotension, muscle diseases associated with sarcopenia, sedentary disease syndrome, and aging.

A MILESTONE OF DISCOVERY

Although the debilitating effects of BR confinement on physical performance have been well recognized and described for decades in the clinical literature, the physiology underlying the reduction in $\dot{V}_{O_{2max}}$ and working capacity was not understood. In a landmark investigation of the effects of BR and recovery on responses to exercise, Saltin and coworkers demonstrated an average reduction in treadmill $\dot{V}_{O_{2max}}$ of 26% in five young male subjects (aged 19–21 yr) after they were confined for 21 days in bed. Specific hemodynamic and pulmonary function measurements performed during baseline rest and exercise provided the first evidence for the mechanisms of reduction in $\dot{V}_{O_{2max}}$ following exposure to BR. The magnitude of the decrease in $\dot{V}_{O_{2max}}$ was equal to the average 26% reduction in maximal cardiac output from 20.0 L · min^{-1} before to 14.8 L · min^{-1} after BR. A slight compensatory elevation in maximal heart rate after BR failed to compensate for the average reduction in stroke volume from 104 to 74 mL. Absence of a significant change in pulmonary function or arterial-venous oxygen difference indicated that the primary cause for the reduction in $\dot{V}_{O_{2max}}$ during BR was severely compromised stroke volume (a central cardiac effect) rather than decrements in gas exchange or in peripheral oxygen delivery or utilization. New insights into the adaptation process during exposure to weightlessness were provided by comparisons of responses during both upright and supine exercise, as well as measurements of heart volume, blood volume, and various blood biochemical parameters at rest and during exercise. It is clear that over more than four decades results from this study have stimulated numerous investigations designed to test new hypotheses that described effects of deconditioning on structural and functional relationships of cardiac and skeletal muscles, blood pressure regulation, and metabolic and hemodynamic responses during exercise and their clinical implications.

Although the subject sample was small, Saltin and associates introduced the premise that persons with a large $\dot{V}_{O_{2max}}$ (physiological) reserve have a greater absolute loss of that reserve during deconditioning than more sedentary individuals with smaller $\dot{V}_{O_{2max}}$ reserve. They found that the two subjects with the highest $\dot{V}_{O_{2max}}$ before BR (average = 4.48 L · min^{-1}) showed greater absolute loss of their $\dot{V}_{O_{2max}}$ (average = −1.01 L · min^{-1}) than three less fit subjects (average $\dot{V}_{O_{2max}}$ = 2.52 L · min^{-1} before BR) with an average absolute reduction of $\dot{V}_{O_{2max}}$ of 0.75 L · min^{-1}. Some subsequent data have provided support for this hypothesis in several physiological systems.

Data from this study are often cited as evidence favoring the use of exercise training for enhancing recovery from the deleterious effects of deconditioning on exercise performance following BR. In the three sedentary subjects $\dot{V}_{O_{2max}}$ was restored within 10–14 days of recovery from BR and continued to increase by 36% above baseline levels at 60 days of recovery. However, the two habitually active subjects required 30 to 40 days of physical activity to restore $\dot{V}_{O_{2max}}$ to baseline levels. These results emphasize the importance of regular exercise in the rehabilitation of BR patients, particularly in relatively fit individuals.

In an interesting 30-yr follow-up investigation, McGuire and associates (56) studied these same five subjects to assess their maximal aerobic capacity. On average, their $\dot{V}_{O_{2max}}$ had decreased by 11%. Their body weight had increased 25%, entirely because of a 100% change in body fat and little change in fat-free mass. Maximal heart rate declined by 6% while maximal stroke volume increased by 16%, resulting in no significant change in maximal cardiac output. The entire decline in $\dot{V}_{O_{2max}}$ could be accounted for by a 15% decrease in the maximal arterial-venous oxygen difference. Thus, 3 weeks of BR when these men were 20 years of age had a more profound effect on their physical work capacity than 30 years of aging.

Saltin B, Blomqvist G, Mitchell JH, et al. Response to exercise after bed rest and after training. Circulation 1968;38(suppl 7):1–78.

REFERENCES

1. McArdle WD, Katch KI, Katch VL. Microgravity: the last frontier. In Exercise Physiology. Baltimore: Lippincott Williams & Wilkins, 2001;678–748.

2. Turner RT. Physiology of a microgravity environment invited review: what do we know about the effects of space flight on bone? J Appl Physiol 2000;89:840–847.

3. Nicogossian AE, Huntoon CL, Pool SL. Space Physiology and Medicine. Philadelphia: Lea & Febiger, 1994.

4. Kakurin LI, Lobachik I, Mikhailov VM, Senkevich YA. Antiorthostatic hypokinesia as a method of weightlessness simulation. Aviat Space Environ Med 1976;47:1083–1086.

5. Convertino VA. Exercise and adaptation to microgravity environments. In Fregly MJ, Blatteis CM, eds. Handbook of Physiology: Section 4. Environmental Physiology. III. The Gravitational Environment. New York: Oxford University, 1996;815–843.

6. LeBlanc A, Schneider V, Shackelford L, et al. Bone mineral and lean tissue loss after long duration space flight. J Musculoskel Neuron Interact 2000;1:157–160.

7. Perhonen MA, Franco F, Lane LD, et al. Cardiac atrophy after bed rest and space flight. J Appl Physiol 2001;91:645–653.

8. Adams GR, Caiozzo VJ, Baldwin KM. Invited review: skeletal muscle unweighting: space flight and ground based models. J Appl Physiol 2003;95:2185–2201.

9. Fortney SM, Schneider VS, Greenleaf JE. The physiology of bed rest. In Fregly MJ, Blatteis CM, eds. Handbook of Physiology. Section 4: Environmental Physiology. III. The Gravitational Environment. New York: Oxford University, 1996;889–939.

10. Bungo MW, Johnson PC Jr. Cardiovascular examinations and observations of deconditioning during the space shuttle orbital flight test program. Aviat Space Environ Med 1983;54:1001–1004.

11. Convertino VA. Cardiovascular consequences of bed rest: effects on maximal oxygen uptake. Med Sci Sports Exerc 1997;29:191–196.

12. Convertino VA. Mechanisms of microgravity-induced orthostatic intolerance and implications of effective countermeasures: overview and future directions. J Grav Physiol 2002;9:1–12.

13. Hung J, Goldwater D, Convertino VA, et al. Mechanisms for decreased exercise capacity following bed rest in normal middle-aged men. Am J Cardiol 1983;51:344–348.

14. Saltin B, Blomqvist G, Mitchell JH, et al. Response to exercise after bed rest and after training. Circulation 1968;38(suppl7):1–78.

15. Ray CA, Vasques M, Miller TA, et al. Effect of short-term and long-term hindlimb unloading on rat cardiac mass and function. J Appl Physiol 2001;91:1207–1213.

16. Buckley JC, Lane LD, Levine BD, et al. Orthostatic intolerance after spaceflight. J Appl Physiol 1996;81:7–18

17. Fritsch-Yelle JM, Whitson PA, Bondar RL, Brown TE. Subnormal norephinephrine release relates to presyncope in astronauts after spaceflight. J Appl Physiol 1996;81: 2134–2141.

18. Delp MD, Colleran PN, Wilkerson MK, et al. Structural and functional remodeling of skeletal muscle microvasculature is induced by simulated microgravity. Am J Physiol 2000;H1866–H1873.

19. Prisk GK. Physiology of a microgravity environment invited review: microgravity and the lung. J Appl Physiol 2000;89:385–396.

20. Prisk GK, Fine JM, Elliott AR, et al. Effect of 6° head-down tilt on cardiopulmonary function: comparison with microgravity. Aviat Space Environ Med 2002;73:8–16.

21. Montmerle S, Spaak J, Linnarsson D. Lung function during and after prolonged head-down bed rest. J Appl Physiol 2002;92:75–83.

22. Convertino VA. Neuromuscular aspects in development of exercise countermeasures. Physiologist 1991;34(Suppl):S125–S128.

23. Edgerton VR, Zhou MY, Ohira Y, et al. Human fiber size and enzymatic properties after 5 and 11 days of space flight. J Appl Physiol 1995;78:1733–1739.

24. Vico L, Collet P, Guignandon A, et al. Effects of long-term microgravity exposure on cancellous and cortical weight-bearing bones of cosmonauts. Lancet 2000;355:1607–1611.

25. Smith SM, Wastney ME, Morukov BV, et al. Calcium metabolism before, during, and after a 3–mo space flight: kinetic and biochemical changes. Am J Physiol 1999;277:R1–R10.

26. LeBlanc AD, Driscol TB, Shackelford LC, et al. Alendronate as an effective countermeasure to disuse induced bone loss. J Musculoskel Neuron Interact 2002;2:335–343.

27. Smith SM, Heer M. Calcium and bone metabolism during space flight. Nutrition 2002;18:849–852.

28. Colleran PN, Wilkerson MK, Bloomfield SA, et al. Alterations in skeletal muscle perfusion with simulated microgravity: a possible mechanism for bone remodeling. J Appl Physiol 2000;89:1046–1054.

29. Sonnenfeld G. The immune system in space and microgravity. Med Sci Sports Exerc 2002;34:2021–2027.

30. Sonnenfeld G. Space flight, microgravity, stress, and immune responses. Adv Space Res 1999;23:1945–1953.

31. Schmitt DA, Schaffar L, Taylor GR, et al. Use of bed rest and head-down tilt to simulate space flight-induced immune system changes. J Interferon Cytokine Res 1996;16:151–157.

32. Lee SMC, Bennett BS, Hargens AR, et al. Upright exercise or supine lower body negative pressure exercise maintains exercise responses after bed rest. Med Sci Sport Exerc 1997; 29:892–900.

33. Shykoff BE, Farhi LE, Olszowka AJ, et al. Cardiovascular response to submaximal exercise in sustained microgravity. J Appl Physiol 1996;81:26–32.

34. Sawin CF, Rummel JA, Michel EL. Instrumented personal exercise during long-duration space flights. Aviat Space Environ Med 1975;46:394–400.

35. Michel EL, Rummel JA, Sawin CF, et al. Results of medical experiment M171—metabolic activity. In Biomedical results from Skylab, NASA SP-377. Washington: 1977; 372–387.

36. Levine BD, Lane LD, Watenpaugh DE, et al. Maximal exercise performance after adaptation to microgravity. J Appl Physiol 1996;81:686–694.

37. Crandall CG, Shibasaki M, Wilson TE, et al. Prolonged head-down tilt exposure reduces maximal cutaneous vasodilator and sweating capacity in humans. J Appl Physiol 2003;94:2330–2336.

38. Convertino VA, Goldwater DJ, Sandler H. Bedrest-induced peak VO_2 reduction associated with age, gender and aerobic capacity. Aviat Space Environ Med 1986;57:17–22.

39. Greenisen MC, Hayes JC, Siconolfi SF, et al. Functional performance evaluation. In Extended duration orbiter medical project final report. NASA SP-1999–534. Houston: 1999; 3-1-3.17.

40. Lee SMC, Loehr JA, Guilliams ME, et al. Isokinetic strength and endurance after international space station (ISS) missions. Med Sci Sport Exerc 2003;35:S262 (Abstract).

41. Engelke KA, Convertino VA. Restoration of peak vascular conductance after simulated microgravity by maximal exercise. Clin Physiol 1998;18:544–553.

42. Cowell SA, Stocks JM, Evans DG, et al. The exercise and environmental physiology of extravehicular activity. Aviat Space Environ Med 2002;73:54–67.

43. Antonutto G, Capelli C, Girardis M, et al. Effects of microgravity on maximal power of lower limbs during very short efforts in humans. J Appl Physiol 1999;86:85–92.

44. Greenleaf JE. Deconditioning and reconditioning. Boca Raton, FL: CRC, 2004.

45. Greenleaf JE, Bernauer EM, Ertl AC, et al. Work capacity during 30–days of bed rest with isotonic and isokinetic exercise training. J Appl Physiol 1989;67:1820–1826.

46. Greenleaf JE, Wade CE, Leftheriotis G. Orthostatic responses following 30–day bed rest deconditioning with isotonic and isokinetic exercise training. Aviat Space Environ Med 1989;60:537–542.

47. Engelke KA, Doerr DF, Crandall CG, et al. Application of acute maximal exercise to protect orthostatic tolerance after simulated microgravity. Am J Physiol 1996;271: R837–R847.

48. Moore AD, Lee SMC, Charles JB, et al. Maximal exercise as a countermeasure to orthostatic intolerance after space flight. Med Sci Sport Exerc 2001;33:75–80.

49. Lee SMC, Moore AD, Fritsch-Yelle JM, et al. Inflight exercise affects stand test responses after space flight. Med Sci Sport Exerc 1999;31:1755–1762.

50. Convertino VA. Exercise as a countermeasure for physiological adaptation to prolonged space flight. Med Sci Sports Exerc 1996;28:999–1014.

51. Schneider VS, McDonald J. Skeletal calcium homeostasis and countermeasures to prevent disuse osteoporosis. Calcif Tissue Int 1984;36:S151–S154.

52. Vico L, Chappard D, Alexandre C, et al. Effects of a 120 day period of bed-rest on bone mass and bone cell activities in man: attempts at countermeasure. Bone Min 1987;2:383–394.

53. Grigoriev AI, Morukov BV, Oganov VS, et al. Effect of exercise and bisphosphonate on mineral balance and bone density during 360 day antiorthostatic hypokinesia. J Bone Min Res 1992;7:Suppl2, S449–S455.

54. Smith SM, Davis-Street JE, Fesperman JV, et al. Evaluation of treadmill exercise in a lower body negative pressure chamber as a countermeasure for weightlessness-induced bone loss: a bed rest study with identical twins. J Bone Min Res 2003;18:2223–2230.

55. Webb JT, Fischer MD, Heaps CL, et al. Exercise-enhanced preoxygenation increases protection from decompression sickness. Aviat Space Environ Med 1996;67:618–624.

56. McGuire DK, Levine BD, Williamson JW, et al. A 30–year follow-up of the Dallas Bedrest and Training Study: II. Effect of age on cardiovascular adaptation to exercise training. Circulation 2001;104:1358–1366.

Genomics in the Future
of Exercise Physiology

CHAPTER 30

Exercise Genomics and Proteomics

FRANK W. BOOTH AND P. DARRELL NEUFER

Introduction

The concept of a gene as a functional unit of hereditary information was first proposed in the mid nineteenth century by Gregor Mendel. In the early 1900s, scientists surmised that genes were located in chromosomes. However, despite the new field of genetics providing increasingly detailed knowledge of inheritance and development over the next several decades, the prevailing wisdom was that genes were simple substances required to support the structure of cells and that only proteins were structurally complex enough to carry genetic information. The discovery of the double-helix structure of DNA by James Watson and Francis Crick in 1953 definitively transformed this way of thinking by providing a new concept of how genetic information could be encoded in the structure of nucleic acids and transmitted from one generation to the next. Soon it became evident that each protein within the cell is encoded for by a single gene and that variations in the sequence of a gene can alter the amino acid sequence of the resulting protein, sometimes with profound physiological and clinical consequences.

The purpose of this chapter is to introduce genomics, proteomics, and bioinformatics and their application to exercise physiology. Genomics is a rapidly evolving discipline; therefore, much of this chapter offers perspectives for future research for the aspiring student. To serve as a foundation, the terms and methods of genomics research are introduced, followed by a comprehensive discussion of the principles of homeostasis (the driving force upon which all cells respond and adapt) in the context of physical activity or inactivity (exercise or lack of exercise). Particular emphasis is placed on the potential application of genomic and proteomic approaches and technologies to decipher the mechanisms responsible for diseases linked to chronic physical inactivity and for the cellular and molecular basis for the prevention and treatment of these diseases by increased physical activity. Finally, methods and concepts to form hypotheses for functions of genes altered by physical activity or inactivity and how they might integrate to orchestrate the new phenotype are given. As this is the final chapter in the text, particular effort has been placed on attempting to provide insight to what the future may hold for research in physical activity or inactivity and exercise physiology. The tides of technology will undoubtedly shift the research sands in ways that we can not foresee; however, it is the unknown that we look forward to the most.

Genomics: Terms and Definitions

Genomics is traditionally defined as the study of the genetic material (genome) of an organism; that is, all of the DNA in the chromosomes of an organism. The year 2000 is an approximate demarcation in genomics research between the twentieth century, when genomics was largely confined to geneticists working to identify and sequence one or a few genes at a time, and the twenty-first century, when scientists from nearly every discipline have the opportunity to examine the function and interaction of all genes within cells, tissues, and organ systems. This transition can be attributed in large part to the recent sequencing of the entire genome (all of the nucleotide sequences, including structural genes, regulatory sequences, and noncoding DNA segments) for several species (e.g., human, mouse, *Caenorhabditis elegans,* yeast) and to the tremendous advances in biotechnology, that is, the methods of science.

Functional, Physiological, and Environmental Genomics

This transition has also spawned a number of new terms, including functional genomics, physiological genomics, and environmental genomics, to name a few. Genomics is obviously common to all three terms, reflecting an evolution in its connotation. In other words, genomics now addresses questions such as these: What are the proteins encoded for by every gene in the genome? How do variations in gene sequence (polymorphisms) affect gene expression and function? What is the genetic basis for diversity within species and among different species? What genes are expressed in specific cell types, and how does global gene expression in those cell types change under different conditions, such as physical activity? Although still evolving, functional genomics generally is the study of the function of all gene products within a cell. Physiological genomics addresses the functional interaction among gene products within a larger setting (tissue, organ, or whole body) to maintain homeostasis. Environmental genomics is the study of the ways influences outside of the cell, tissue, organ, or whole body (e.g., physical activity or inactivity, diet, oxygen content, toxins) affect the regulation of gene expression. It also addresses how such regulation is influenced by polymorphisms among individuals (e.g., susceptibility to obesity because of variations in specific genes in the environmental context of sedentary behavior or a high-fat diet).

Application of Genomics to Exercise: Exercise Genomics

How does exercise physiology fit into the genomics era? It is recognized that athleticism is at least in part inherited. However, it also became appreciated in the latter half of the twentieth century that exercise training improves physical performance through changes in gene expression. Thus, it is now clear that elite athletes not only are born but must also train to optimize the expression of an undefined subpopulation of genes that predispose to superior physical performance (application of exercise to genomics). Indeed, numerous investigators proved that training changes protein levels within cells by altering both their concentration (milligrams per unit of cell) and content (milligrams of tissue) in a manner that improves the functional capacity of muscle as well as the whole

body (1). The challenge for exercise physiologists in the twenty-first century is not only to identify all genes that are responsive to exercise but to decipher the mechanisms by which those genes are regulated, the functional impact of the proteins that are encoded by those genes, how such protein interactions form the basis for the cellular adaptations generated by exercise training, and how such adaptations among all affected organs integrate to improve whole-body function and health.

Application of Genomics to the Sedentary Diseases

In the last decade of the twentieth century, it was firmly established that lack of daily dynamic exercise in otherwise healthy individuals significantly increases the risk of developing chronic health disorders. The application of genomics research to study diseases caused by sedentary living represents a clear challenge for the twenty-first century exercise scientists. For example, the ability of an individual to perform increased maximal aerobic work is linked to a reduced prevalence of chronic disease. This raises the obvious and important question: what are the genes shared by maximal aerobic performance and the prevention of chronic health disorders? Thus, in the transition between centuries, exercise genomics has grown from the study of a small number of elite athletes to an application of science (application of genomics to the sedentary diseases) targeting a public health need for nearly all persons in sedentary cultures. An additional challenge for the exercise physiologist in the twenty-first century will be to decipher the mechanisms by which physical inactivity alters the expression of disease susceptibility genes until ultimately a biological threshold is passed to cause overt clinical disease.

Methods of Genomics and Proteomics Research

Many important hypotheses to understand the scientific basis of physical activity can now be tested, thanks to rapid technological advances, with the challenge to apply them to exercise research. To discuss future uses of genomics in physical activity research, techniques of genomics are presented, followed by a discussion of some concepts that may be employed to decipher the functions for the thousands of changes in gene expression that are likely occurring with physical activity. This will be followed by a section on proteomics. It is assumed that the reader is familiar with basic molecular biology techniques (e.g., DNA sequencing, Northern blotting, reverse transcriptase polymerase chain reaction). The intent in the following section is to present newly developed techniques of global analyses. This section is divided into tools for human research and animal investigations.

Human Research

DNA and Genes

The amino acid sequence of every protein in the body largely determines the location, 3-dimensional structure, and ultimately, therefore, the function of that protein. Because the amino acid sequence is derived from the gene that encodes for that protein, it is not hard to imagine that specific variations in DNA sequence (insertions, deletions, or single-nucleotide polymorphisms [SNPs, pronounced *snips*]) may alter the amino acid sequence in a way that affects the function of the protein. In fact, it is this natural variation in gene sequence that accounts for the uniqueness of all humans. As one might expect, the frequency of SNPs varies considerably across all genes, depending on the functional impact of the particular variation and the evolutionary pressure to conserve critical sequences.

SINGLE-NUCLEOTIDE POLYMORPHISMS   Most complex diseases, such as cancer and diabetes, do not arise from a defect in a single gene (e.g., cystic fibrosis is a single gene defect); rather, they arise from the influence of a host of environmental factors on multiple genes interacting over the course of many years. The susceptibility to such complex diseases is thought to reside within each individual's polymorphic profile. One strategy being employed by geneticists is to identify the frequency and locations of all SNPs, under the assumption that specific SNPs will be associated with specific diseases. Of particular interest and importance is to determine which of these polymorphisms double as SNPs responsive to physical activity or inactivity.

However, the hunt for genetic markers of disease susceptibility thus far has been an extremely daunting task. SNPs occur as frequently as one in every 1000 bases, which means that huge numbers of SNPs must be analyzed in large populations before links between DNA and disease can be truly correlated. An alternative to the genome-wide search is to employ a selective strategy in which the search for disease-associated SNPs is restricted to previously suspected regions of a chromosome associated with a disease. For example, such a strategy recently proved successful in identifying, in a 66,000-nucleotide stretch of chromosome 2, three SNPs associated with a heightened susceptibility to diabetes in a population of Mexican Americans (2). It is anticipated that restricting searches to the promoter regions, protein coding segments (exons) and 3′ untranslated regions of candidate genes, thereby eliminating intron sequence from the analysis, may prove to be a more efficient and fruitful strategy for identifying meaningful SNPs.

DNA–PROTEIN INTERACTIONS   A recently developed technique, chromatin immunoprecipitation (ChIP), permits global analysis of the interaction of a particular protein with DNA. In ChIP assay, protein and DNA interactions are first cross-linked in a muscle or nuclear homogenate. The specific protein is then immunoprecipitated by antibody, and the DNA fragments are amplified by polymerase chain reaction (PCR) and sequenced to determine whether proteins bind to the specific DNA region of interest. An advantage of this method is that it can be used to determine chromatin regulation at both local and global levels. Local effects refer to regulation of single genes: ChIP can be used to determine whether a specific transcription factor is binding to a specific gene regulatory region. ChIP assays can also be used to determine global effects on gene expression involving alterations in the properties of enormous chromosome domains (termed epigenetic action). While genetic information is encoded by DNA sequences, epigenetic information is encoded by differential methylation of DNA on cytosines (primarily in CpG dinucleotides), by proteins that associate with DNA and their covalent modifications, and by the chromatin structures that these form within the nucleus. DNA-associated proteins include histones—which may be modified covalently by acetylation, methylation, phosphorylation, and/or ubiquitination—methyl CpG–binding proteins, and others (3). For example, activation of muscle-specific genes by members of the myocyte enhancer factor 2 (MEF2) and MyoD families of transcription factors has recently been shown to be coupled to histone acetylation and is inhibited by class II histone deacetylases 4 and 5, which interact with MEF2 (4).

ADVANTAGES AND LIMITATIONS   Some advantages of identifying disease and activity SNPs will be that predisposition to disease can be more accurately predicted on an individual basis and primary preventive prescriptions made (individualized medicine). Some of the potential limitations to analyzing SNPs are as follows: (*a*) The data are initially associative, not causal. (*b*) Very large populations are required to obtain statistical confidence. (*c*) Because of multiple SNPs whose prevalence varies within each person, discerning the interaction between disease-susceptible genes and disease- or inactivity-predisposing genes will likely prove to be very challenging in terms of developing a quantitative predication of inactivity-related disease risk.

RNA

Messenger RNA (mRNA) for analysis of changes in pretranslational regulation produced by exercise in human studies can be obtained from skeletal muscle or adipose tissue biopsies, myonuclei isolated from the biopsies, and tissue sections. As opposed to DNA, which is the same in different cell types, mRNA expression varies by cell type and experimental treatment.

MICROARRAY ANALYSIS   Simultaneous analysis of all mRNAs in a given cell type or tissue is now possible. Complementary DNA (cDNA) or oligonucleotide microarrays can be used to measure the expression patterns of thousands of genes in parallel, generating clues to gene function. The cDNA microarray technique uses discrete DNA sequences that have been arrayed onto a glass slide and then interrogated with fluorescently labeled cDNA probes that were reverse-transcribed from an mRNA population. Oligonucleotide arrays from Affymetrix, a microarray manufacturer, have 11–20 separate short oligonucleotides from the same gene arrayed on a glass plate. Each of the oligonucleotides is paired with its identical cDNA sequence, which has a single base mismatch to serve as a control. Both techniques do result in false-positive differences (a gene whose expression is indicated as different when it is not different) between two experimental groups if the sample sizes are small and if either improper statistics or no statistics are employed. Oligonucleotide microarrays, while allowing the simultaneous analysis of thousands of mRNAs, require larger sample sizes to maximize the number of significant differences while minimizing the percentage of false positives. While array analysis is expensive, its power is its unbiased identification of previously unknown changes in mRNA and the ability to group mRNAs with similar patterns of change in expression to discover functional classes of genes (5). Bioinformatics, which is obligatory for analysis of function, is discussed later.

Although microarray analysis offers a comprehensive snapshot of mRNA expression under a given experimental condition, there is not always a direct relationship between the concentration of an mRNA and its encoded protein. Differential rates of mRNA translation into protein, protein assembly, and variations in specific rates of protein degradation influence the predictive power of mRNA expression to protein expression profiles. The correlation coefficients between changes in mRNA and protein in yeast are not high. Microarrays have been applied to isolated polysomes to determine differential expression of mRNAs attached to ribosomes. While microarrays are not quantitative, they provide an unbiased global database from which unique insights and new hypotheses can be generated based on the identification of specific genes of interest that would otherwise remain indefinitely unknown. As such, microarrays should be viewed as an initiator of new information for undreamed hypotheses (6).

REAL-TIME POLYMERASE CHAIN REACTION Because many microarray analyses use small sample size and/or do not employ rigorous statistical evaluations, differentially expressed mRNAs identified for further study require confirmation with an independent measurement, usually real-time PCR. Real-time PCR technology combines rapid thermocycling with real-time fluorescent probe detection of amplified target mRNAs or nucleic acids with high sensitivity. Once analysis of a given mRNA is established for real-time PCR, the potential is present for high throughput analysis. However, each mRNA change of interest must be normalized to an mRNA that is unaffected by the experimental treatment to account for potential differences in the initial total mRNA concentration across samples. Finding an mRNA or riboso-

mal RNA (rRNA) for real-time PCR analysis that is not changed in a comparison of two physical activity levels can be very difficult, as exercise often produces global changes in mRNA expression. For example, the quantity of almost every house-keeping gene and rRNA in the soleus muscle of rats was recently found to be altered by 10 days of hindlimb immobilization (7). Even mRNAs not found to be statistically significant with microarray analysis became statistically different when they were reanalyzed by the more sensitive real-time PCR method. Thus, how to normalize mRNA expression data continues to represent a challenge for experimental researchers.

Proteomics

Proteomics is the study of global protein expression. There are estimated to be approximately 30,000 genes in humans, rats, and mice, and no protein profiling techniques can approach the capability of microarrays to qualitatively profile the expression of more than 25,000 genes. For example, two-dimensional (2D) gels separate known and unknown proteins by charge and then molecular weight. However, a single 2D gel detects only about 1000 proteins, which means multiple gels have to be run to approach a true global determination of all proteins expressed in a given cell or tissue. A factor further compounding the magnitude of the global detection of proteins is that each protein is likely to be modified by phosphorylation, acetylation, acylation, glycosylation, and/or myristoylation, with an unknown percentage of these modifications changing the bioactivity of the modified protein. Thus, the number of proteins with different bioreactivities exceeds 30,000 and is likely greater than 200,000; that is, each protein has multiple bioreactivities. As different levels of daily physical activity are associated with adaptive alterations in protein levels, knowledge of the tens of thousands of proteins and their modified forms will be required to decipher the precise mode by which the human body functions in its daily life. The following section highlights some of the latest proteomic biotechnologies being developed and used.

2D FLUORESCENCE DIFFERENCE GEL ELECTROPHORESIS Similar to conventional 2D electrophoresis, 2D fluorescence difference in-gel electrophoresis (DIGE) resolves and separates proteins initially by charge (i.e., isoelectric point) followed by molecular weight in the second dimension. However, with DIGE, mass- and charge- matched fluorescent dyes (Cy3 and Cy5) are used to label two different protein samples (with either Cy3 or Cy5) prior to electrophoresis of both samples on the same gels. (Standard 2D electrophoresis would run the control and treatment samples on different gels and compare the intensity of a stained protein spot between the gels.) In addition, an internal standard can be created by pooling aliquots from all control and experimental protein samples into a single tube and labeling with a third dye (Cy2). The internal standard is run with each gel in the experiment, permitting quantification of each separated protein relative to the amount of the same protein in the internal standard. After electrophoresis, the gel is scanned for fluorescence of each of the three dyes. The images are then overlaid to identify differentially expressed proteins between the control and experimental sample relative to the internal standard. Because DIGE is based on fluorescence, detection is over a large dynamic range (10^4), allowing a wide range of protein quantifications. Changes in protein content from as little as 1.3-fold to more than 100-fold between control and experimental samples may be detected. Spots of interest may then be excised for further analysis (e.g., trypsin digestion followed by mass spectroscopy) and possible identification by comparison with existing peptide databases.

MASS SPECTROMETRY Mass spectrometry is often used to identify a protein that is differentially expressed between two experimental groups on a 2D gel. In standard mass spectrometry, molecules are ionized and accelerated through a vacuum by an electric field. The particles are then separated according to their ratio of mass to charge by either deflection in a magnetic field or by measurement of their time of flight to the detector. The multiple types of mass spectrometry allow not only identification of a protein but also modifications to the protein, such as glycosylation and phosphorylation.

ADVANTAGES AND LIMITATIONS An overriding advantage of proteomics is that proteins are the unit of biological action in a cell. As physical activity likely alters the expression of thousands of proteins, categorization of these changes is necessary to decipher the signals that react to and counterbalance disturbances to homeostasis during exercise and the signals that lead to long-term adaptations with training to improve function during physical activity. Proteomics will continue to progress to the forefront of biomedical research as existing techniques are improved and new techniques are developed.

Bioinformatics

Genomics- and proteomics-based research presents an enormous challenge in terms of the sheer volume of raw data that must be managed. Thousands and thousands of data points (each corresponding to a single SNP, mRNA, or protein) are obtained with each sample. Each experiment in turn requires multiple samples or subjects to obtain sufficient statistical power to determine with some confidence that a given finding is truly relevant. Adding to the complexity is the fact that the locations, functions, and activities of proteins are continually subject to allosteric interactions, covalent modifications, and binding to other proteins. Thus, deciphering all of the molecular, cellular, and physiological events responsible for the improvements in physical performance and health that

accompany exercise or the decrements associated with the development of overt clinical disorders in response to physical inactivity, is a daunting task. It is not unreasonable to estimate that up to 200,000 individual gene expression or protein changes will occur in all tissues with physical activity or inactivity, which must be catalogued, interpreted, and integrated to explain normal and pathological functions of the human body. For the first time in history, biologists face the realization that the ability to interpret and integrate their own data may be beyond their ability to remember the facts. Although still evolving, bioinformatics is the only discipline providing hope for this monumental task.

The role of bioinformatics extends beyond the management and analysis of the reams of data generated by genomics- and proteomics-based techniques; bioinformatics is also a tool to transform biological knowledge to alter the ways researchers frame the questions that shape research projects and the design of experiments. For example, researchers working on cardiovascular disease can now run a computer search of the more than 5 million known human SNPs. With this information they can test their control groups for SNPs to screen out those who might have unidentified disease, thus removing one source of uncertainty from their experiment. It has been predicted that in the near future new services and software products will permit the expertise of a professional bioinformatician to be downloaded onto a desktop computer.

Another example of the impact that bioinformatics is likely to have in the near future comes from consideration of the signaling pathways regulating glucose transport in skeletal muscle. The activation of glucose transport by contractile activity occurs through a signaling mechanism independent of that activated by insulin. Recently, while investigating the regulation of fatty acid metabolism in skeletal muscle during exercise, researchers discovered a new exercise signaling pathway (adenosine monophosphate [AMP] kinase) for contraction-induced glucose into skeletal muscle (8). However, subsequent research revealed that expression in mouse muscle of a dominant inhibitory mutant of AMP kinase only partially reduced contraction-stimulated glucose uptake, suggesting that AMP kinase transmits only a portion of the signal by which muscle contraction increases glucose uptake (9). In other words, other signaling factors and pathways must exist for the exercise-induced uptake of glucose into skeletal muscle. In the future, when signaling pathways or factor databases are established, it will be possible for researchers to use bioinformatics software to predict likely components missing from their data, providing logical targets for their next experiments. In fact, bioinformatic databases and software will likely be created for specific areas of biology (e.g., insulin-responsive signaling mechanisms, contractile activity–induced signaling mechanisms). For example, it is predicted that many as yet unknown signaling pathways provide a survival advantage during physical activity, particularly when food intake is low, since physical activity was required for food acquisition during evolution (10). Thus, it is likely that bioinformatics tools will be required to make a conceptual model of physical activity to integrate the predicted 200,000 pieces of information.

The necessity for bioinformatics is reinforced by a recent review article in which the authors wrote that the biggest challenge for exercise physiologists in the forthcoming years will be to link signaling cascades to defined metabolic responses and specific changes in gene expression that occur during and after exercise (11). Computers will allow storing and sorting of the details of enormous cross-talk, feedback regulation, and transient activation occurring during and after exercise.

Animal Research

This section is subdivided into two parts: techniques and physical activity interpretations of genetically modified animals.

Historical Perspective

As early as the 1960s the principal technique to identify new hormones was to remove a tissue (e.g., the thyroid gland) from an animal, observe the phenotype, grind up the gland, and inject it into the animal to see if the initial phenotype could be rescued. If the phenotype was rescued, the proteins were isolated from the ground-up gland, and then each individual isolated protein was injected alone until a specific biochemical (e.g., thyroxine) restored the original phenotype. The rescue identified the chemical (hormone) responsible for the phenotype. These principles can be applied to understanding gene manipulation methods that identify genes responsible phenotypical adaptations in response to physical activity.

Transgenic technologies originated in the early 1980s with the development of pronuclear microinjection, in which the gene of interest is directly injected into the pronuclei of fertilized eggs and the functional outcome is observed. By the late 1980s to early 1990s, a major breakthrough for altering gene expression was forged. With use of homologous recombination, it was discovered that DNA could be exchanged between the host genome and a transgene (a new gene transferred into the host genome); that is, a transgene could be inserted into a precise location in the mouse genome (12).

This finding afforded scientists with the ability to replace, or knock out, a specific endogenous gene with a replacement DNA sequence of their design (Fig. 30.1). It also enabled researchers to insert extra copies of a gene or insert genes with special promoters to cause overexpression of a gene. The result of transgenic technologies is that genetically modified animals can be created and studied to reveal the functions of genes and gene-related diseases (13). The introduction of transgenic and knockout mice into biology provided powerful techniques to study the function of individual genes. The major purpose of this section is to explain the many

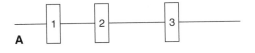

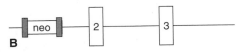

FIGURE 30.1 Homologous recombination. **A.** An endogenous gene with 3 exons (*rectangles 1, 2, and 3*) that can make protein A. The line between the rectangles represents introns. **B.** A new gene constructed from gene A so that a neomycin (*neo*) coding sequence replaces a part of the promoter A and exon 1, inactivating the coding sequence of gene A, so that no protein A would be made if gene B were to replace gene A in an egg by homologous recombination.

advantages of genetic modulation technologies in living animals and their great potential for advancing the understanding of exercise science. Another important aspect of this section is to introduce an appreciation of the potential limitations of genetically modified animals to the study of exercise adaptations. This section presents first techniques and then examples of interpretations of exercise responses from genetically modified animals.

The Knockout Animal

Knockout is jargon for generation of a mutant animal in which the function of a particular gene has been eliminated by the insertion of a replacement DNA sequence. Normally, the replacement sequence causes a portion of the original gene to be lost, and thus the original gene fails to function normally. Phenotypes of the knockout mice are compared with those of wild-type mice (with all their genes intact), allowing researchers to deduce the function of the knocked-out gene (analogous to a loss-of-function study in which removal of a gland is used to prove that the gland produces the missing hormone). For example, if a gene necessary for muscle hypertrophy was knocked out, the knockout animal might no longer be capable of muscle growth with training. One advantage of a knockout model is that it might show a loss-of-function phenotype; that is, the animal loses a function or ability to adapt. Another advantage is that the gene disruption is made in the germ line, so that subsequent generations will carry the same genetic composition. Because some gene knockout models faithfully mimic the phenotype of human diseases, those mice can be used as model systems for the study of human diseases. For example, apoprotein E (ApoE) knockouts develop cardiovascular disease and are being used to study the development of atherosclerosis and potential treatments for cardiovascular disease (14). Knockout mice can also be used to test specific hypotheses about exercise. For example, hippocampal neurogenesis is increased within 3 weeks when mice are housed in cages with running wheels (15). Activation of *N*-methyl D-aspartate (NMDA) receptors is thought to be involved in neurogenesis; therefore, the hypothesis was made that NMDA receptor signals may be involved in exercise-induced neurogenesis. To test this hypothesis, knockout mice lacking the NMDA receptor-ε_1 subunit gene were housed in cages with running wheels. No increases in hippocampal neurogenesis and brain-derived neurotrophic factor occurred in the knockout mice, whereas wild-type mice with the intact NMDA receptor gene showed marked increases in brain-derived neurotrophic factor production and neurogenesis. These findings led to the suggestion that hippocampal neurogenesis in mice induced by voluntary running is likely mediated, at least in part, via NMDA receptor signaling (16).

Disadvantages of the knockout animal include that they sometimes show surprisingly little phenotypic change, often because there are alternative or redundant genes or mechanisms that compensate for the deficient gene during development and maturation of the animal. Thus, the lack of a phenotypic change with exercise would not allow for a definitive conclusion on whether the disrupted gene is necessary for the phenotype or function. Another disadvantage of traditional knockout models is that some genes are necessary for normal development. In this situation, the mice often die *in utero* or shortly after birth as a result of developmental defects. Even if the animal survives, some genetically modified models have somewhat different phenotypes from their human counterparts, limiting their utility as models of human disease. Another limitation is that it may be impossible to delineate whether the observed phenotype is the result of a deficiency during development, adolescence, or adulthood. The latter shortcoming with the traditional knockouts can be overcome with a new technology known as conditional knockout or tissue-specific gene targeting (reviewed later in the chapter).

The Overexpression Animal

Transgenic animals are often designed to overexpress a gene so that its protein product is overproduced, yielding a gain-of-function phenotype. This technique is also employed for misexpressing a mutated nonfunctional copy (known as negative because the overexpression of a catalytically inactive protein overwhelms the amount of endogenous protein) in the animal. In some instances, it is desirable to restrict expression of the target gene to a specific tissue. For example, selection of a skeletal muscle–specific promoter restricts expression to skeletal muscle myofibers as opposed to other tissues or cell types in skeletal muscle, such as fibroblasts and smooth muscle cells. This strategy was recently employed to generate transgenic mice overexpressing hexokinase II by using a construct consisting of the muscle creatine kinase promoter fused to the human hexokinase II cDNA (17,18). These mice were generated to examine whether hexokinase II,

which catalyzes the first step (phosphorylation) in the metabolism of glucose once it enters the cell, plays a role in determining the rate of glucose uptake in muscle. Under basal conditions, glucose uptake into muscle did not differ between wild-type mice and those overexpressing hexokinase II. However, in response to both hyperinsulinemia and exercise, mice overexpressing hexokinase II had a significantly greater rate of glucose uptake into muscle than their wild-type litter mates, providing evidence that hexokinase II–mediated phosphorylation of glucose may be an important determinant of the overall rate of glucose uptake in skeletal muscle during exercise.

Another potentially useful strategy is to select a promoter that contains one or more binding sites for a specific transcription factor of interest and place this promoter in front of a reporter gene. When the transcription factor is present and active, the reporter gene will be expressed. This strategy was recently used to examine the molecular pathways involved in the control of exercise-responsive genes (A Milestone of Discovery).

Disadvantages of gene overexpression include that the transgenic technique results in the transgene randomly inserting into the genome, with an unknown integration site, and possibly affecting the expression of a second unknown gene. Another limitation inherent to this technique is that the copy number of inserted genes is variable: 1 to 100 copies of the transgene could be inserted. The variable copy number can lead to inconsistent phenotypical characteristics (expression pattern and level of expression). Thus, to verify the phenotype in transgenic animals, the development of several independent transgenic lines is required.

Conditional Knockouts

The purpose of conditional knockouts, in contrast to traditional knockouts, is to delete a gene in a specific organ, tissue type, or cell type at a specific time determined by the investigator. This technique can be used to knock out portions of genes, entire genes, or even promoter regions of genes. The creation of a conditional knockout is typically executed through a mechanism of site-specific recombination. The most widely used method is the Cre-loxP recombinase system. The second most popular system is the Flp-FRT system. Both Cre and Flp are site-specific recombinases, that is, enzymes that act to trade DNA segments by recognizing specific DNA sequences. Recombinases act like molecular scissors (targeting their actions to the specific DNA recognition sites of loxP or FRT) to cut out designated regions of DNA flanked on both sides by loxP or FRT and replace the region with a new DNA fragment. These systems are referred to as binary systems because they require the interaction of two components, the recombinase and the splice sites.

In practice, a researcher might design a transgenic mouse with a tissue-specific promoter that drives the Cre recombinase gene. Next the investigator would create a second transgenic animal that contains loxP sites around the region of DNA (typically in introns [noncoding sequences surrounding a regulatory exon) to be spliced out. These two transgenic animals are mated to produce progeny with tissue-specific knockout of a specific gene. Because Cre will be expressed only in the tissue or cells where the promoter is activated to transcribe Cre, the targeted gene will be knocked out only in the specified tissue or cells. Thus, the mouse will express its wild-type phenotype until induction of the tissue-specific promoter, at which time the Cre protein will be expressed and its recombinase activity will delete the gene segment between its recombinase recognition sites. This approach makes it possible to circumvent the problem of embryonic lethality, if an appropriate promoter was chosen to be activated only in the adult animal, not during embryogenesis. Both recombination systems offer exquisite specificity for testing gene function. Thus, the advantage of a tissue-specific conditional knockout is that it allows the scientist to study a gene's mechanism of action in a specific tissue (without the complications of observing the side effects of the gene deficiency in other surrounding tissues) and by choice of promoter. Tissue-specific conditional knockouts also give a higher level of specificity and control over whole-body knockouts, but they do not allow the investigator to turn the gene on again once the gene has been excised from the genome. In one effective conditional knockout experiment, inactivation of the myostatin gene in striated muscle by the Cre-lox system has recently been shown to result in generalized muscular hypertrophy (19). Although these findings were similar to that observed with constitutive myostatin knockout mice, the conditional knockout system eliminated the possibility of mitigating developmental influences in the general knockout mice by using a muscle-specific promoter only expressed in differentiated skeletal muscle, leading the researchers to suggest the hypothesis that a myostatin antagonist could be used to treat muscle wasting and to promote muscle growth in humans and animals.

Inducible Transgenic Systems

In an ideal research design, an exercise investigator would have control over a genetic switch that could be flipped to activate or to silence a transgene. Additionally, the transgene would have a high level of gene expression when on and no expression when off. The switch would be a chemical that is foreign to the animals and that would not interfere with or be affected by other cellular components. Most of the qualities of the ideal genetic switch have been achieved through the use of conditional (tissue specific) or inducible transgenic systems (20). Conditional or inducible systems allow gene manipulation not only in a specific organ, tissue type, or cell type as for the conditional knockout but also at a stage of development or life selected by the investigator. The tetracycline system allows for the control of target gene expression in eukaryotic systems via the application of the antibiotic tetracy-

cline or a tetracycline analogue, such as doxycycline, to study gain of function or loss of function for any given gene. Use of this kind of technology allows tissue-specific gene expression to be turned on or off by a drug (tetracycline) not normally present in the body. Additionally, because these systems are inducible, genes critical for development can express normally through development, then later in adolescence or adulthood be manipulated by the addition or subtraction of the drug. Because the amount of transgene expression is roughly proportional to the amount of drug, the investigator may be able to titrate the levels of target gene expression. The biggest advantage of these techniques is that they can overcome the limitation of a gene alteration being present throughout the life of the animal. Thus the gene can be turned on in a mature animal just prior to or during the exercise training and compared to an animal whose gene is kept off during the exercise training. This advantage of temporal control of gene expression offers the researcher exquisite control for analyzing the functional significance of a gene with exercise. When tetracycline systems were introduced, they were leaky, such that it was nearly impossible to completely silence the expression of the transgene. Since then researchers have redesigned the promoters to achieve nearly complete silencing. While in general gene expression is barely detectable or undetectable in the noninduced state, transcription is usually stimulated to levels of more than 10^5-fold above background in the induced state.

Future Genetically Modified Animal Models

Current transgenic technologies permit the generation of double knockouts, that is, a single mouse with two genes functionally eliminated. It is anticipated that future technological developments may permit the researcher to selectively activate or deactivate the expression of multiple genes in a given tissue or animal to allow for a more comprehensive study of signaling pathways and regulatory mechanisms. Since exercise alters multiple signaling pathways simultaneously, an ideal future model would be to block multiple signaling events instantaneously at the start of an exercise bout.

Gene Transfer Techniques

NAKED DNA INJECTIONS Gene transfer into skeletal muscle by the direct injection of naked plasmid DNA results in sustained gene expression in a small percentage of muscle fibers. Detection of the exogenous gene product is facilitated by incorporation of a reporter gene that encodes for a fluorescent or otherwise easily detected protein (e.g., luciferase). This strategy was recently used to characterize the effects of mutations of the skeletal α-actin promoter (driving a reporter gene) in a plasmid injected into a mechanically overloaded muscle (21). Deletional mutations identified a hypertrophy-responsive region, which was later confirmed by site-specific mutations of suspected promoter elements within the responsive region. The hypertrophy response was blocked by a plasmid expressing a mutated serum response element 1 (SRE1) DNA regulatory region, suggesting that in this overload model, SRE1 is a hypertrophy-responsive element on the skeletal α-actin promoter. A limitation of gene transfer of plasmids is the highly variable level of promoter expression among animals. Although this limitation can be lessened by coinjection with and normalization to a second non–exercise-sensitive promoter driving a second reporter gene, exercise can often alter the expression of the putative non–exercise-responsive promoter. Naked plasmid gene transfer has not been shown to very successful in tissues other than skeletal muscle.

ELECTROPORATION The temporary application of an electric field to skeletal muscle can increase the uptake of injected DNA by 100-fold or more, enhancing both the quantity and consistency of expression from the exogenous gene. Although the mechanism of electroporation is not entirely clear, the electric field is thought to cause temporary formation of pores across the sarcolemma, allowing the normally impermeable DNA to gain access to the cytoplasm (22). Despite the fact that nearly 99% of injected DNA is lost or degraded within 24 h, a portion does wind up in the nucleus, where it remains viable and expresses for up to 2–3 months. A certain degree of muscle damage and the presence of an inflammatory infiltrate have also been reported with the electroporation technique, and the altered gene expression of the damage and inflammation must be separated from the exercise-induced change in gene expression.

VIRAL INJECTIONS Adenoviral (AV) infection of adult skeletal muscle is unsuccessful because the virus fails to diffuse. However, adeno-associated viral (AAV) infection transfer of genes into adult muscle has been shown to be successful. This strategy has been used to rescue aged mouse skeletal muscle from sarcopenia with a single injection of an AAV expressing insulinlike growth factor I (IGF-I) into skeletal muscle (23). The advantage of injection into skeletal muscle with AAV over plasmids is that 80% of the muscle fibers may be infected with AAV, whereas only 1–2% may take up and express a plasmid. Both AAV and plasmid methods have minimal or no immune response, providing an advantage over AV. A lentivirus vector has just been reported as a tool for gene transfer and expression in mature muscle fibers.

Interpretations of Chronic Exercise Responses in Genetically Modified Animals

As challenging as or more challenging than the production of the transgenic animal will be the skill to interpret the results from a perspective of the exercise literature while integrating vast amounts of information from multiple organs and disciplines. A definitive cause-and-effect relationship for the function of a gene altered by physical activity or inactivity will normally require a sequence of gene modification ex-

periments likely published as separate venues (Table 30.1). The next example illustrates this approach. In 1998, it was reported that overexpression of calcineurin in the mouse heart induced cardiac hypertrophy, providing evidence that calcineurin participates in signal transduction leading to cardiac hypertrophy (24). In Table 30.1, overexpression of a gene to obtain an exercise phenotype is designated as step 1 in a process of determining cause and effect for exercise.

However, little was known about whether calcineurin actually participated in the signaling of exercise-induced hypertrophy, as most studies had used animals with pathological hypertrophy to study calcineurin signaling. The breakthrough came in 2000, when it was found that calcineurin was activated by 150% in the enlarged hearts of rats that had run 2.4 km each night for 10 wk as compared to caged controls (25). This illustrates step 2 of Table 30.1, in which it is determined whether physiological exercise increases the protein concentration or activity to a similar degree as found in the transgenic animal in step 1. While treatment with the calcineurin antagonist drug cyclosporin A completely inhibited the development of left ventricular hypertrophy in a subgroup of the voluntarily running rats, a controversy existed over whether cyclosporin could or could not block pathological hypertrophic responses in hearts of animal models of pressure overload or genetic cardiomyopathy. A different experimental approach would be necessary to resolve this controversy. In 2001, the forced overexpression of the calcineurin-inhibitory protein myocyte-enriched calcineurin-interacting protein-1 (hMCIP1) in hearts of transgenic mice was found to attenuate 57% of the hypertrophic response from voluntary running (step 3 in Table 30.1) (26). Thus, only after step 3 did it become possible to claim a cause-and-effect role for calcineurin in the hypertrophic response of the myocardium triggered by exercise as performed by mice in voluntary running wheels.

TABLE 30.1	Experimental Steps to Establish the Function of a Gene Altered by Physical Activity or Inactivity
Step 1	Overexpress a gene (Sedentary transgenic animal or tissue culture) ↓
Step 2	Exercise-train animal or human ↓
	Does protein or activity change? (Protein level in transgenic of step 1 equal or unequal to value in step 2?)
Step 3	Block expression of gene in exercising animal ↓
	Limit exercise phenotype in exercise-trained nontransgenic animal?

A suggested protocol for determination of a more definitive cause-and-effect function for a protein in exercise experiments.

Use of the Concept of Physiological Exercise and Models Showing the Limits of Adaptation With Nonphysiological Models

While electrical stimulation of skeletal muscle $24 \text{ h} \cdot \text{day}^{-1}$ induces a number of adaptive responses similar to dynamic exercise training (27), it is clear that the changes evoked by chronic stimulation exceed those induced by any other form of increased contractile activity. In effect, the chronic stimulation model provides information as to the limits of muscle adaptation. Unfortunately, results from this model are often translated as occurring in humans at levels of exercise less than that of chronic stimulation. For example, many contend that sedentary humans switch from type II to I fibers with dynamic training, as in the nonphysiological model of chronic stimulation of muscle for $24 \text{ h} \cdot \text{day}^{-1}$. Unfortunately, the published literature does not support this contention. Sedentary humans and animals do not increase their type I percentage with endurance exercise training. On the other hand, humans and animals do switch from type I to II fibers when sedentary populations undergo hindlimb unloading, hindlimb immobilization, or spinal isolation, and upon retraining, they switch back toward the percentage level found in sedentary populations (28). Thus, a future challenge will be to differentiate between physiological exercise and models providing information as to the limits of muscle adaptation when interpreting results from transgenic animals.

Summary

This section of the chapter delineates multiple approaches to manipulation of gene expression in animals prior to exercise testing. The challenge will be to interpret the exercise results. The best-guess interpretation on the functional outcome of a single modified gene in a sea of at least 200,000 other exercise-induced changes in multiple tissues of genetically modified animals will require a strong working knowledge of the literature.

Principles of Homeostasis: The Foundation for Exercise Genomics and Proteomics

An understanding of principles of homeostasis provides a foundation necessary for future genomics- and proteomics-based research efforts to identify the essential mechanisms mediating the effect of physical inactivity on the etiology of chronic disease as well as the ability of regular physical activity to prevent disease.

Definitions of Homeostasis: Pre-Genomic Era

Homeostasis is classically defined as the ability to maintain relative constancy or uniformity in the internal environment in the face of significant changes in the external environment. This definition can be applied in many contexts. For example, cells are surrounded by membranes that allow nutrients, ions, gases, and so on to move in and out passively or selectively while maintaining their own internal consistency or milieu, a property known as cell homeostasis. Physiologists also define homeostasis as the ability of the whole body or organism to maintain constancy under varying environmental conditions outside of the body. In this context, various organs contribute to maintaining whole-body homeostasis; for example, the lungs facilitate the exchange of carbon dioxide for oxygen in the blood to maintain arterial blood P_{CO_2} within a narrow range of 40 mm Hg in the resting healthy individual; the cardiovascular system delivers oxygen to the peripheral tissues to keep skeletal muscle P_{O_2} within a range of 6–10 mm Hg at rest; the gastrointestinal system assists in maintaining blood Ca^{++} within a narrow range by absorbing Ca^{++} under the control of the parathyroid glands; and the kidneys remove metabolic byproducts and help to maintain ion and fluid balance.

Definition of Homeostasis: The Era of the Genome

With the complete genome sequencing of an ever-growing list of species, basic science is evolving rapidly in terms of the complexity level at which researchers view cellular, organ, and whole-body physiology. Recognizing that every gene contains information required for the product of that gene (protein) to function (e.g., localization, enzymatic activity, binding properties) begins to give one a sense of how the baseline or genetic set point of each cell is determined by the collective functions and interactions of all proteins that are expressed within that cell type, some of whose expression contributes to homeostasis. Cells of course are not isolated entities but reside within an aqueous environment of extracellular fluid and blood, as well as neighboring cells that may secrete autocrine or paracrine factors. In other words, two cells that are the same type (e.g., two hepatocytes) may differ slightly in their gene expression profile, depending on their surrounding environment (i.e., fluid milieu, proximity to other cell types). It is the context of this surrounding environment that establishes the homeostatic set point of a given cell; that is, the adjustment of the genetic set point according to the surrounding environment. Other environmental influences, such as exercise, can challenge the maintenance of cellular homeostasis, as described in the next section.

Homeostasis in Skeletal Muscle

The external environment for cells in skeletal muscle is a composite derived from the various cell types that occupy the tissue: skeletal myofibers, satellite cells, neurons, vascular endothelial and smooth muscle cells, fibroblasts, and various immune cells. Homeostasis within a resting myofiber is a balance among competing systems, such as substrate flux through the various metabolic pathways, ion distribution across the plasma membrane, calcium sequestration in the sarcoplasmic reticulum, and contractile protein cycling (to name but a few). An analogy to homeostasis is the set point of the body's thermostat, which defends against changes in core body temperature (set point) in response to both internal and external environmental challenges. Collectively, it is the relative set points among all the dynamic systems of the cell that define the resting homeostatic state of the myofiber. In the face of changes to the environment outside and inside of the cell (e.g., oxygen concentration, ion concentration, substrate delivery), cellular systems react to ensure that homeostasis—be it metabolic, electrochemical, or physical—is maintained during the initial perturbation.

Not all myofibers are defined by the same homeostatic set point. Skeletal muscle fibers are broadly divided into two categories, slow and fast fibers, based on their speed of contraction, although a continuum exists between the two extremes.[1] The homeostatic level of high-energy phosphates (adenosine triphosphate [ATP]) is almost twice as great in fast fibers as in slow fibers. Muscle fiber types also differ in their calcium-handling properties, glycolytic and oxidative capacities, mitochondrial content, and capillary density. For example, the homeostatic level of resting free Ca^{++} is twice as high in slow as in fast fibers. The variation in homeostatic regulation among fiber types is relevant, as each muscle fiber, and likely each myonuclear domain, has to provide slightly different global gene expression patterns to maintain different (local) homeostatic levels at rest. Future research will likely reveal that the molecular mechanisms to defend disruptions from homeostasis in exercising muscle also vary among myonuclei within a single fiber and among different muscle fiber types.

Contribution of Other Organ Systems to Homeostasis in Skeletal Muscle

At rest, most energy is used to support other organs—heart, lung, liver, kidney, gastrointestinal system, and brain. The cardiovascular and gastrointestinal systems, lung, and liver

all contribute to maintaining homeostasis in skeletal muscle by providing for the exchange of oxygen and metabolic substrates for carbon dioxide and metabolic byproducts. In fact, one could argue that skeletal muscle is a rather selfish tissue, relying on other organs to maintain its own homeostasis while offering little in return. During exercise, muscle's reliance on other organ systems obviously intensifies. Under most conditions of exercise, the priority of other organ systems is to provide the support necessary for skeletal muscle to maintain contractile activity (e.g., increased cardiac output to allow increased muscle blood flow, enhanced respiratory minute volume to permit maintenance of a constant arterial P_{O_2}). However, as the exercise continues, particularly under adverse conditions such as a hot environment, the needs of these other organ systems begin to increase in priority, limiting their support to skeletal muscle and therefore the ability to continue exercise. Competition for blood volume between exercising muscle and skin to dispose of the metabolic byproduct heat, particularly in a hot environment and the competing need for glucose between exercising muscle and brain are two prime examples of times when the requirements of contracting muscle may be overridden in favor of homeostatic needs elsewhere in the body.

Contribution of Skeletal Muscle to Other Organs and Whole-body Homeostasis

Does skeletal muscle contribute to whole body homeostasis, and if so, how? Cardiac muscle makes an obvious contribution by pumping blood to other organs, but the contribution of skeletal muscle to whole-body homeostasis is less obvious. After all, skeletal muscle does not secrete ions, nutrients, or hormones that are required by any other organ to maintain homeostasis. In a very real sense, skeletal muscle does provide the means to gather the nutrients other organs need; if our ancestors couldn't move, they couldn't hunt or harvest or for that matter escape from being hunted. Much less apparent (and perhaps less appreciated) is the importance of skeletal muscle to whole-body metabolic homeostasis.

Simply put, skeletal muscle is a major consumer of energy. It constitutes about 40% of total body weight and accounts for 20–25% of basal metabolic rate. When carbohydrate intake is insufficient (prolonged physical activity, fasting, malnutrition, cachexia), defending blood glucose concentration, the major source of energy for the brain, becomes the metabolic priority for the body. Under such conditions, glucose utilization must be conserved by peripheral tissues. Skeletal muscle, which normally relies heavily on blood glucose, shifts to alternative fuel sources (i.e., free fatty acids and proteins). This conservation of glucose, coupled with the activation of glucose production by the liver in response to numerous counterregulatory hormones (e.g., glucagon, epinephrine, cortisol), ensures that the brain continues to be supplied with a sufficient amount of glucose. As these conditions persist, skeletal muscle also becomes the major source of

---

[1]Other classification systems of muscle fibers are based on myosin heavy chain isoform expression (MHC I and MHC IIA, IIX), color (red and white), or metabolic characteristics (oxidative and glycolytic). Human skeletal muscle contains three types of fibers: MHC type I (slow, red, oxidative), MHC IIA (fast, red, oxidative), and MHC IIX (fast, white, glycolytic). A small number of hybrid fibers (e.g., I/IIA, IIA/IIX) are also present.

amino acids (released via protein breakdown), many of which serve as gluconeogenic precursors for the liver.

This example serves as a representative illustration for a future challenge in genomic and proteomic profiling: to integrate multiple changing gene expression profiles in various organs to determine organ integration in whole-body stresses such as physical exercise. A future research endeavor will thus be to put together the changes in global gene expression communicating signals among individual organs to integrate a reduction in homeostatic disruptions.

In times of plenty, skeletal muscle's contribution to metabolic homeostasis can go awry with devastating consequences. In healthy, physically fit individuals, skeletal muscle is responsible for about 80% of the clearance of both glucose and lipids from the blood after a meal. However, when a chronic positive caloric imbalance exists in the body (particularly associated with high-fat diets), skeletal muscle can begin to lose its ability to clear glucose from the circulation, a condition known as insulin resistance. If insulin resistance persists for years, the pancreas in some individuals may no longer be able to produce enough insulin to maintain hyperinsulinemia to compensate for the insulin resistance in skeletal muscle. Consequently, blood glucose concentration remains elevated after as well as between meals—the clinical transition to type II diabetes.

Although the mechanism of insulin resistance in skeletal muscle is not fully understood, it is clear that a chronic disturbance to metabolic homeostasis in the form of a chronic positive caloric balance generated by excess intake and/or inadequate expenditure is a major underlying factor. This should make it readily apparent that the level of daily physical activity, and thus the level of energy consumed by skeletal muscle to support the activity, is a major determinant of energy balance, that is, metabolic homeostasis on a day-to-day basis. Thus, when considered in the context of obesity and type II diabetes, two disease states classified as epidemics in the United States, the contribution of skeletal muscle to glucose homeostasis and overall energy balance is profound and yet often underappreciated. Therefore, a major future research need not only for exercise physiology but for medicine will be to understand the mechanisms of physical inactivity–induced chronic health disorders. Usage of genomics, proteomics, and bioinformatics will be required to identify which genes in skeletal muscle orchestrate the pathologies of insulin resistance and of those genes which are metabolic signals between all involved organs or tissues when insufficient physical activity produces metabolic dysfunctions from a chronic positive caloric imbalance.

Principles of Cellular Homeostasis

The maintenance of cellular homeostasis is a dynamic process, as to optimize survival the cell has to retain the ability to adapt to changes in its external environment. Thus, proteins that control these adjustments must be able to increase or

decrease, which means they have to be continuously turning over, replacing the old with the new. (If a protein had no turnover, it would likely have no synthesis or degradation processes to call upon when an adaptive change in protein level was required to adjust to a new external environment.) The concentration of any protein at any given time thus reflects the balance between its rate of synthesis and rate of degradation. As long as these rates remain equal, the concentration of the protein will remain the same. This is known as the steady-state concentration. The next sections provide a series of examples to illustrate how specific changes in protein synthesis and degradation lead to a change in the steady-state level of proteins. Because the proteome represents the future of research in exercise physiology as well as all biomedical research, an understanding of the principles that govern protein turnover in all cells is required.

Protein Turnover: Kinetics of Normal Cellular Life

Imagine that you turned off the synthesis of a particular protein in a cell but degradation remained unchanged. By following the decrease in concentration of that protein in the cell over time, you could determine its fractional rate of degradation or turnover rate. By plotting time on the X-axis and protein concentration on the Y-axis, you would discover that the turnover rate is not a linear but a curvilinear or exponential decay (Fig. 30.2A). This is known as a first-order relationship and is given by Equation 30.1:

$$\text{Turnover Rate} = \frac{d[\text{protein}]}{dt} = k\,[\text{protein}]$$

[Equation 30.1]

where k = the fractional degradation rate constant expressed as reciprocal units of time (i.e., fraction or percentage degraded per minute or per day). This is called a first-order reaction because the degradation or turnover rate also depends on the concentration of the protein to the first power. In other words, the turnover rate is a certain percentage of the concentration of the protein at any given time. This means that as the protein concentration decreases exponentially over time, less and less protein is available to be degraded, which in turn means that the absolute turnover rate (i.e., the absolute amount of protein degraded per unit of time) also decreases exponentially.

The integrated form of Equation 30.1, which is more useful for making calculations, is

$$\log \frac{[A_o]}{[A_t]} = \frac{kt}{2.303}$$ [Equation 30.2]

where $[A_o]$ is the initial concentration of protein A at time zero and $[A_t]$ is the concentration at any time t. To allow for comparison among proteins when synthesis is artificially set to zero, the loss of protein can be set to 50% ($[A_o]/[A_t] = 2$). Solving for t gives the half-life ($t_{1/2} = 0.693 \cdot k^{-1}$) of the protein, the time required for half of the protein concentration

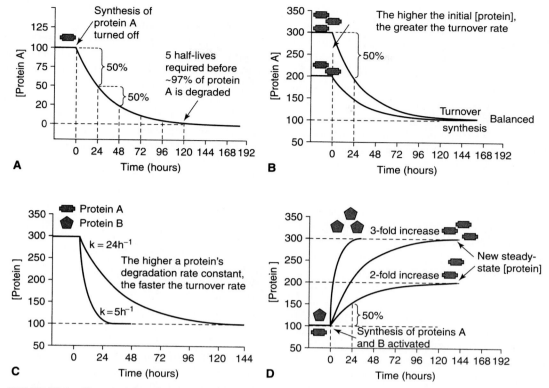

FIGURE 30.2 The principles of protein turnover in cells. See text for details.

to be degraded. Under these conditions, fractional turnover rate is synonymous with half-life. In the example shown in Figure 30.2A, protein A has a half-life of 24 h; thus 50% of the decrease in protein A concentration occurs during the first 24 h another 50% loss (of the remaining protein concentration) occurs during the following 24 h, and so on such that a total of 5 half-lives, or 5 days, are required before about 97% of the initial protein is degraded.

Now we move our example to the context of the cell. As mentioned, the concentration of a particular protein at any given time reflects the balance between its rate of synthesis and rate of degradation. When homeostasis is disturbed within a cell, the rate of synthesis and/or degradation of a target protein may be adjusted to allow an adaptive change in the protein level to minimize either acute or chronic disruptions in homeostasis. For purposes of discussion, we assume that the fractional degradation rate constant remains unchanged and that control for change in protein level is exerted only by changing the rate of synthesis. In the example shown in Figure 30.2B, the stimulus to the cell requires that the concentration of protein A be lowered from 200 to 100 (milligrams per muscle weight). Protein synthesis rate will be reduced to the level required to generate the new desired concentration (in this case halved), resulting in a loss in the concentration of protein A that follows a pattern identical to that shown in Figure 30.2A, requiring about 5 days (5 half-lives) before the degradation rate of protein A equals the syn-

thesis rate and the new steady-state concentration of protein A is established. What if the initial concentration of protein A is 300 instead of 200 mg per muscle weight? How long will it take to reduce protein A to the same baseline concentration of 100 mg per muscle weight, again assuming that the fractional degradation rate constant (k) is unchanged? As depicted in Figure 30.2B, the answer is the same, about 5 days. Protein synthesis rate will again be reduced to the level required to generate a concentration of 100 mg per muscle weight. Because the fractional turnover rate of protein is directly proportional to protein concentration (see Equation 30.1), the higher protein concentration will result in a greater absolute amount (milligrams) of protein being degraded per day. Thus, when the synthesis of a given protein is abruptly changed to a new rate, the time required to achieve the new steady-state concentration is independent of the initial protein concentration and solely a function of the fractional degradation rate constant, or half-life, of the protein.

Thus far we have considered protein A, with a characteristic half-life of 24 h. Fractional turnover rate, as you might imagine, varies considerably among proteins and is typically given as percent per day, for example 50% per day for a protein with a half-life of 24 h. For proteins with a much shorter half-life, the time required to reach a new steady-state concentration will be much less. Figure 30.2C compares the fractional turnover rate of protein A, with a half-life of 24 h, and protein B, with a half-life of 5 h.

Adjusting the concentration of both proteins from an initial concentration of 300 to a new steady-state concentration of 100 mg protein per muscle weight will require a total of 25 h (5 half-lives) for protein B as compared with 5 days (5 half-lives) for protein A. This example illustrates the concept that the time required to achieve a new steady-state concentration is solely a function of the fractional degradation rate constant, or half-life, of each individual protein.

There are three take-home points to this section. First, the absolute turnover rate of a protein is a product of the fractional degradation rate constant (percent per given time period) for that specific protein and the concentration (milligrams of protein per whole muscle or other tissue) of the protein at any given time. Second, regardless of the initial concentration of a particular protein, a change in the synthesis rate (with no change in the fractional degradation rate constant) will require 5 half-lives before the concentration of that protein reaches about 97% of its new steady-state concentration. The new concentration simply represents the balance between the new rate of synthesis (expressed as milligrams of protein synthesized per day per whole muscle) and the absolute rate of degradation (milligrams of protein degraded per day per whole muscle). Third, the higher the fractional degradation rate constant (i.e., the shorter the half-life), the less total time required for the protein to assume its new steady-state concentration (5 half-lives).

The Rate of Adaptive Increase in Protein Concentration Is Also a Function of Protein Turnover

Up to this point we have considered only the dynamics governing a decrease in protein concentration. What if the disturbance to cell homeostasis requires an increase in protein concentration? It turns out the same principles apply. Remember that anytime there is an increase in protein concentration, there is more protein available for degradation. In this example, let us assume that the stimulus doubles the protein concentration by doubling the protein synthesis rate (milligrams of protein synthesized per day) while keeping the protein degradation rate unchanged (percent per day). Thus, the doubling in protein synthesis is partially offset by an increase in the milligrams of protein degraded per day (determined by constant percent degraded per day multiplied by progressively increasing protein concentration in milligrams of protein per whole muscle). Returning to protein A, with a half-life of 24 h, a plot of the concentration of protein A versus time in response to an inducing stimulus shows that 50% of the adaptive change in protein concentration occurs during the first half-life, 50% of the remaining adaptive increase occurs in the second half-life, and so on, resulting in a nonlinear or exponential rate of increase in protein concentration. (Fig. 30.2D). As with protein degradation, the overall time required for protein A to adjust from its initial concentration to the new steady-state concentration requires about 5 half-lives, or 5 days, irrespective of the

level of activation of protein synthesis or magnitude of the final increase in protein concentration (twofold vs. threefold in Figure 30.2D). Again, the new steady-state concentration simply reflects the point at which the elevated amount of protein synthesized per day is balanced by the increased amount of protein degraded per day. In effect, the set point for homeostasis within the cell, at least with respect to protein A, has been reset in the context of the new environmental conditions. As long as these conditions persist, the concentration of protein A will remain stable at its new higher level.

It should also be clear from Figure 30.2D that the time required to reach the new steady-state concentration depends entirely on the half-life of the protein. Protein B, for example, with a half-life of only 5 h, will reach its new steady-state level in 25 h. This is because the fractional turnover rate is much faster, effectively allowing adjustments in concentration to occur at a much greater rate. At this point, you may be thinking that if protein A and protein B have the same initial concentration (e.g., 100 mg per muscle weight), how can the concentration of protein B, with the higher fractional turnover rate constant, increase faster than the concentration of protein A, with the lower fractional turnover rate constant? The key to thinking about this question is to recognize that even though protein A and protein B have the same initial concentrations, the initial synthesis rate of protein B is five times that of protein A because the half-life of protein B (5 h) is about one-fifth of the half-life of protein A (24 h). Thus, to triple the concentration of both protein A and protein B, the absolute increase in synthesis (milligrams of protein synthesized per day) of protein B will have to be five times greater than for protein A; that is, the relative rates of protein synthesis will have to be tripled for both A and B. Under these conditions, protein B will reach its new steady-state concentration much sooner than protein A (Fig. 30.2D).

What if the intensity of the stimulus to increase protein A is far greater, sufficient to induce a 10-fold increase in protein A concentration? How long will it take to generate the full response? The answer should be evident from the discussion of protein B; the half-life of protein A has not changed, so it will still require about 5 days to achieve the new steady-state concentration. The increase in protein A concentration (milligrams of protein A per whole muscle) will be 10 times greater, but the total time required for the adaptive response will remain the same.

Points of Cellular Control Regulating Protein Expression

Exactly how do cells adjust the concentration of specific proteins? In response to a stimulus, components of both protein synthesis (e.g., mRNA concentration, translation initiation, and processing, assembly), and protein degradation (e.g., ubiquitination) are subject to regulation, usually in a coordinated manner. Of course, genetic information ultimately flows from DNA (via transcription) to mRNA (via translation) to protein. The steady-state level of expression of a given gene product (protein) therefore reflects a series of synthetic and degradative processes and is ultimately determined by the kinetics of the rate-limiting step. Although it is difficult to determine in living animals, the rate-limiting step likely varies considerably among proteins and may shift from one step to another in response to a given stimulus. For example, proteins that are constitutively expressed in skeletal muscle (e.g., contractile proteins, many metabolic enzymes) tend to be fairly stable (i.e., long half-lives) and are backed by relatively steady rates of transcription, such that adjustments in protein concentration may be fine-tuned by altering protein translation or stability and altered on a larger scale by changes in mRNA.

In contrast, for proteins that fluctuate or are expressed as needed (e.g., stress proteins, certain transcription factors), the rate of synthesis for the final product (protein) often is primarily a function of the concentration of the corresponding mRNA. Similar to proteins, the concentration of a given mRNA in a cell is a function of its rate of synthesis (transcription) and fractional degradation rate (mRNA turnover). In addition, all mRNAs have a characteristic turnover rate, or half-life. Thus, the principles governing protein turnover also apply to the control of mRNA turnover. In fact, the half-life of most mRNAs is typically much shorter than the half-life of the corresponding proteins, which means that adjustments in mRNA concentration in response to a given stimulus occur much faster. This also implies that although regulation may be exerted at multiple steps, the rate-limiting step for altering the expression of many acutely regulated proteins likely resides at the level of transcription of the corresponding gene. Knowledge of the degree and time course of change in protein level can be used as one criterion to form hypotheses for functions of gene expression altered by physical activity or inactivity, as discussed later.

Principles Governing the Adaptive Response to Altered Physical Activity

The principles of protein turnover discussed in the preceding sections are based upon the responses of a cell in the face of a constant change in the environment that evokes a challenge to homeostasis. In other words, the stimulus imparted on the cell is the same throughout the adaptive period. But what if the disturbance to homeostasis in a cell is not constant? Exercise training, for example, is an intermittent stimulus that induces only temporary disruptions to homeostasis; yet when performed daily for several weeks, it is a stimulus that evokes clear adaptations. The next section discusses the kinetic principles governing the cellular responses to intermittent stimuli, such as repeated exercise bouts.

Dynamic Exercise Transiently Activates Transcription of Select Metabolic Genes

The increasing use of molecular biology approaches in the late 1980s revealed that dynamic-training–induced increases in mitochondrial proteins (such as the cytochromes of electron transport and Krebs cycle enzymes) were preceded by increases in corresponding mRNAs. This suggested that at least a portion of the adaptive response to training is mediated at the pretranslational level (i.e., transcription and/or mRNA stability). Indeed, over the past decade, a number of studies have provided direct evidence that contractile activity activates transcription of select metabolic genes. Importantly, these regulatory events were found to be acute and transient, occurring primarily during the recovery period after exercise. The implication of studies showing changes in gene transcription and mRNA within hours of a change in contractile activity is that the training adaptations generated by exercise training stem from the cumulative effects of the acute transient responses to each individual exercise bout. As illustrated in the next section, the factor determining whether a particular exercise-responsive protein accumulates during the course of a training program is determined solely by the half-life of that protein.

Kinetics of the Acute Adaptive Response to Exercise

Figures 30.3 to 30.5 present an analogy to help conceptualize how the dynamics governing changes in gene expression in response to an acute bout of exercise ultimately provide

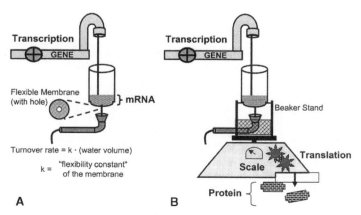

FIGURE 30.3 The flow of genetic information from a gene to mRNA (**A**) to protein (**B**). See text for details.

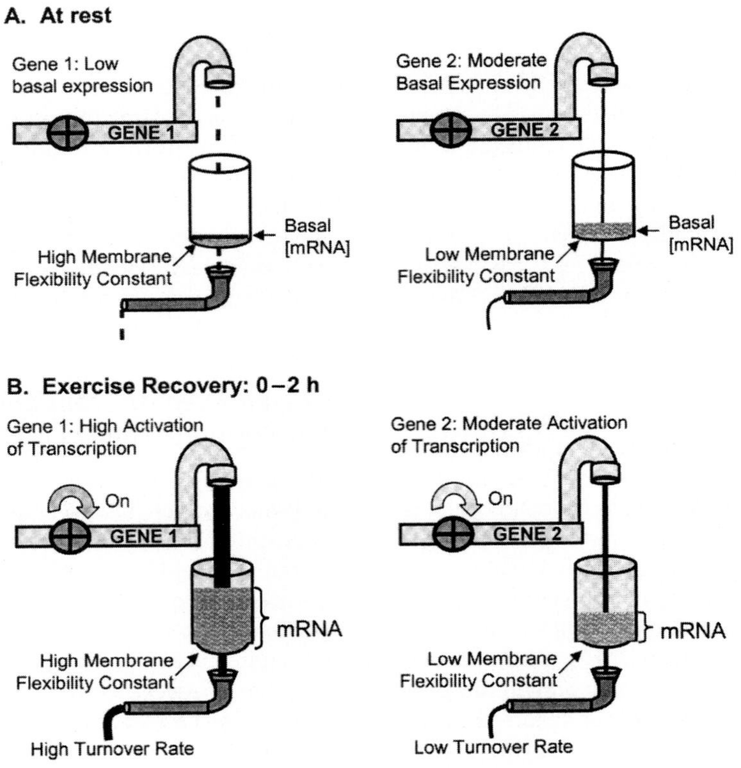
A. At rest
Gene 1: Low basal expression
GENE 1
Basal [mRNA]
High Membrane Flexibility Constant
Gene 2: Moderate Basal Expression
GENE 2
Basal [mRNA]
Low Membrane Flexibility Constant
B. Exercise Recovery: 0–2 h
Gene 1: High Activation of Transcription
On
GENE 1
mRNA
High Membrane Flexibility Constant
High Turnover Rate
Gene 2: Moderate Activation of Transcription
On
GENE 2
mRNA
Low Membrane Flexibility Constant
Low Turnover Rate

FIGURE 30.4 The dynamics governing changes in gene expression for two different genes in response to an acute bout of exercise. **A.** Regulation at rest. **B.** The 2-hour period immediately after exercise. See text for details.

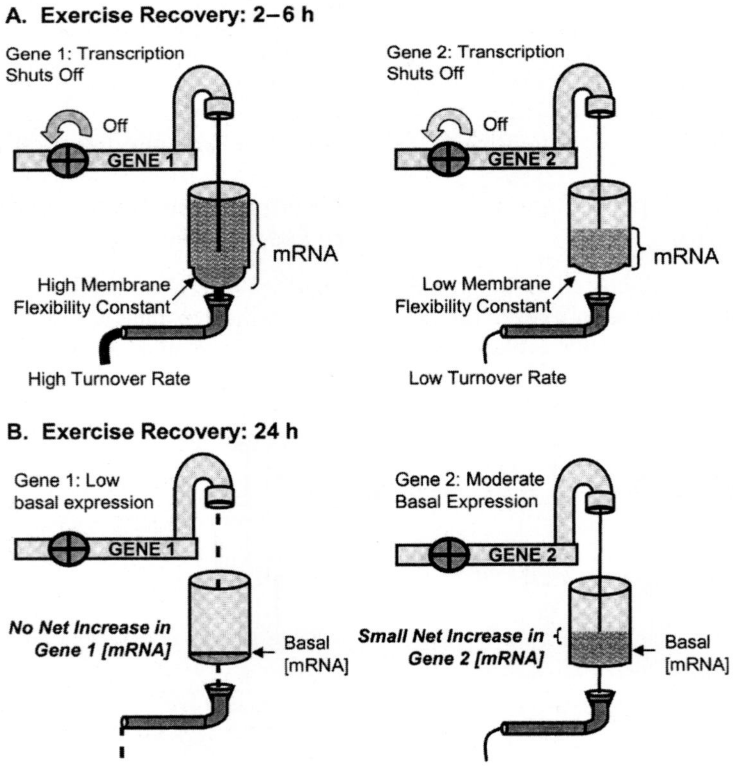
A. Exercise Recovery: 2–6 h
Gene 1: Transcription Shuts Off
Off
GENE 1
mRNA
High Membrane Flexibility Constant
High Turnover Rate
Gene 2: Transcription Shuts Off
Off
GENE 2
mRNA
Low Membrane Flexibility Constant
Low Turnover Rate
B. Exercise Recovery: 24 h
Gene 1: Low basal expression
GENE 1
No Net Increase in Gene 1 [mRNA]
Basal [mRNA]
Gene 2: Moderate Basal Expression
GENE 2
Small Net Increase in Gene 2 [mRNA]
Basal [mRNA]

FIGURE 30.5 The dynamics governing changes in gene expression for two different genes in response to an acute bout of exercise. **A.** Regulation at 2–6 hours. **B.** Regulation 24 h after exercise. See text for details.

the underlying basis for the adaptations to endurance training. In this analogy (Fig. 30.3A), transcriptional activity of a gene is depicted by the rate of water flow out of a faucet, the regulation of which is controlled by an on-off valve.

The water collects in a glass beaker, the volume of which represents the concentration of mRNA at any given time. To account for the turnover of mRNA, the bottom of the beaker is constructed with a flexible rubber membrane with a small hole in the middle, allowing water to drain from the beaker. Because the membrane is flexible, the hole in the membrane expands in direct proportion to the rise in the volume of water in the beaker, increasing the volume of water loss as a constant fraction of the total water volume (representing the fractional degradation rate constant). Different beakers possess membranes with different flexibility constants, representing the different degradation rate constants among mRNAs. Thus the fractional turnover rate of the water (mRNA) is a function of the membrane flexibility constant (mRNA fractional degradation rate constant) and the amount of water in the beaker (mRNA concentration), similar to Equation 30.1, which describes protein turnover.

To complete the analogy, the beaker is placed on a balance. The balance is mechanically linked to a machine that makes building blocks representing new proteins. The balance is designed to activate the building block machine (translation and protein synthesis) in direct portion to the weight of the beaker. For the sake of simplicity, mRNA stability, translation, and protein turnover are not subject to regulation in the analogy. Thus, the level of water (mRNA) in the beaker will determine the rate of building block production (protein synthesis).

Let us consider the response to exercise of two genes (Fig. 30.4A). Gene 1 encodes for a specialized protein (e.g., a transcription factor) that is needed by the cell only under certain conditions. Expression of gene 1 in the basal state is very low. The basal water flow from this faucet (transcriptional activity) is low, the membrane flexibility constant (mRNA fractional degradation rate constant) is high, and as a result, the basal level of water in the beaker (mRNA concentration) is low. Gene 2 encodes for a protein that is required for normal day-to-day function in the cell (e.g., a mitochondrial enzyme). It possesses a modest level of basal water flow from the faucet, a moderate membrane flexibility constant, and as a result, a modest basal level of water in the beaker. This stable level of water in the beaker produces a constant rate of building block synthesis (gene 2 encoded protein).

In response to a single bout of exercise, the faucet valve (mRNA transcription) for gene 1 is completely turned on (Fig. 30.4B). During the initial 2 h or so of recovery, water accumulates quickly in the beaker, followed by a rapid rise in the rate of gene 1 building block (protein). (Note: For the sake of simplicity, this example assumes a constant proportion between the concentration of a given mRNA and its translation into protein, which is often not held upon transition from rest to exercise.) The valve for gene 2 is also turned on, but not

nearly to the same extent, producing a relatively small increase in water flow from the faucet and a small rise in the water level in the beaker. The inherently high membrane flexibility constant of gene 1 also results in a much greater rate of water loss (mRNA fractional turnover) from the beaker.

Nevertheless, as the flow of water from each faucet (transcription) slows during the next several hours of recovery (about 2–6 h), the total accumulation of water in the beaker (mRNA concentration) for gene 1 still far exceeds that of gene 2 (Fig. 30.5A). However, within 24 hours after exercise, the level of water in the beaker for gene 1 has returned to its initial low basal level, while the level of water in the beaker for gene 2, because of the much slower rate of water loss for gene 2, remains slightly higher than basal (Fig. 30.5B). Thus, for gene 2 there has been a small net accumulation of water in the beaker (mRNA concentration) 1 day post exercise. When this scenario is repeated day after day, the level of water for gene 2 gradually accumulates with each transient response to exercise, eventually producing a net twofold to threefold increase in water (mRNA) level, or training adaptation. Presumably, the gradual or net cumulative increase in the water level (mRNA concentration) of gene 2 translates into a corresponding overall increase in the rate of synthesis for its protein and accumulation of building block 2 (protein). In contrast, despite the dramatic transient activation of water flow for gene 1 occurring in response to each exercise bout, the rate of water loss from the gene 1 beaker post exercise prevents any net mRNA accumulation from one day to the next, and thus no cumulative training adaptation occurs.

There are a two key points to take away from this analogy. First, the magnitude of increase in a specific mRNA or protein to an acute stimulus, such as exercise, depends largely on the degree of activation of the rate-limiting process (i.e., activation of transcription in the analogy), while the duration of increase depends primarily on the fractional degradation rate constants (half-lives) of the specific mRNAs and proteins involved. Second, for an mRNA or protein to undergo a cumulative increase in concentration in response to repeated bouts of exercise, as with exercise training, the half-life of the mRNA or protein must be long enough to result in a net increase between each exercise bout. Although it is not depicted specifically, the rate-limiting step in the synthetic process for a given gene may reside at steps other than transcription (e.g., posttranscriptional processing, mRNA stability, translation, assembly), may vary with the type of stimulus, and/or may shift during the course of the adaptive period. Regardless of the site of control, the disturbance to homeostasis during any training program is intermittent and therefore governed by standard kinetic principles.

Implications Regarding the Kinetic Principles Governing Exercise and Exercise Training

EXERCISE: A TRANSIENT DISTURBANCE TO HOMEOSTASIS
Although predominantly theoretical, it seems reasonable to assume that the acute molecular responses to exercise in

muscle are triggered by the relative stress imparted on the cell—the disturbance to homeostasis and the cell's effort to reestablish homeostasis. The time required for the various systems in myofibrils to recover and to return can vary on the order of minutes (ion balance) to several days or more (protein synthesis for damage repair). Thus, it is apparent that the cellular and molecular responses to exercise can extend well beyond the period of contractile activity, which implies that the signaling mechanisms within muscle may not simply reflect the residual effects of the exercise bout but rather are sensitive to specific disturbances in homeostasis independent of how they are evoked. In other words, until that disturbance is resolved, the specific regulatory mechanism will remain activated in an attempt to restore that portion of cell homeostasis. A perfect example of this concept is the regulation of glucose uptake during recovery from exercise. Despite the absence of contractile activity or insulin (two known activators of glucose uptake), glucose uptake has been shown to remain elevated in muscle during the initial 30-min recovery period after exercise (29). Moreover, insulin sensitivity (the amount of glucose taken up for a given amount of insulin) is also enhanced and remains elevated in a previously exercising muscle until muscle glycogen content is fully restored. Although the mechanisms are not well understood, it is reasonable to suggest that signaling mechanisms sensitive to muscle glycogen content, rather than contractile activity itself, may remain activated to ensure that glucose continues to enter the cell until substrate reserves are replenished.

THE ACUTE RESPONSES TO EXERCISE LIKELY DEPEND ON THE RELATIVE INTENSITY, DURATION, AND MODE OF EXERCISE

The magnitude of increase in the mitochondrial protein cytochrome c in response to a 12-wk endurance training program has been found to be directly related to the intensity and duration of exercise (30,31). Although data at the molecular level are limited, the conjecture can be made that the acute activation of gene expression is also directly related to intensity, duration, and mode of exercise (32). Clearly, the impact of a given exercise bout will depend on the relative stress perceived by a particular cellular system. For example, one might expect that genes involved in defense against reactive oxygen species would be induced to a greater degree during high-intensity exercise, particularly in fibers with low antioxidant defenses and high susceptibility to oxidative stress. Likewise, growth-promoting resistance exercise would be expected to elicit a much different set of genes from those induced by endurance exercise. Identifying the full complement of genes that respond under different intensities, durations, and modes of exercise is a challenge for future research in exercise physiology. Furthermore, identifying the polymorphisms that account for the wide variation in adaptive response to the same exercise stimulus among humans and animals also represents a particularly challenging but important area for future research.

TRAINING PRODUCES A RELATIVELY STEADY-STATE CHANGE IN PROTEIN CONCENTRATION

As exercise training continues over the course of several weeks, the products of those genes, such as cytochrome c, with a sufficiently long enough half-life will continue to gradually accumulate (33). If a progressive training program is used (gradual increases in training intensity) and protein concentration is measured at the same time each week, the change in protein concentration may appear to be linear and fairly slow. However, if the daily exercise stimulus follows the pattern of a square wave (same intensity used each day), the change in protein concentration will be exponential. After several weeks of training, the acute increase in synthesis in response to each exercise bout will be balanced by an increased absolute degradation rate. In addition, as the adaptations to training continue, a progressive resetting of the homeostatic set point occurs such that the disruption to homeostasis in response to each exercise bout is lessened. Unless the training intensity is increased, no further net increase in protein concentration will occur, and the protein will level off at a new higher relative steady-state. However, maintenance of the trained state is dependent upon regular intervals of exercise. Thus, in a sense, the concentrations of proteins adapting to a stimulus that is intermittent are in a constant state of flux.

THE CUMULATIVE INCREASES IN GENE EXPRESSION LIKELY DEPEND ON THE FREQUENCY OF TRAINING

As with the intensity and duration of exercise, it is well established that frequency of exercise during a training program directly influences the rate at which mitochondrial protein concentration increases. Again, although information at the molecular level is limited, it is reasonable to assume that the level of acute increase in protein or mRNA is inversely related to the time between exercise bouts. In other words, the shorter the period between exercise bouts, the more protein or mRNA will remain from the adaptive response to the previous bout and the faster the accumulation will be during training. For example, 2 h of dynamic exercise 2 or 6 days each week increased cytochrome c protein concentration 30% and 85% after 14 wk (34). Furthermore, it is also likely that with shorter intervals between exercise bouts, the expression of a greater number of genes will be elevated and thus accumulate with successive bouts of exercise. However, if a minimal rest period is not obtained, some components, such as contractile proteins, decrease in quantity, as in the continuous chronic stimulation of skeletal muscle.

SOME TRAINING ADAPTATIONS ARE RAPIDLY LOST WITH THE CESSATION OF TRAINING

It is painfully obvious to anyone who has undergone a period of detraining that training adaptations disappear rapidly, and recovery to the trained state requires a disproportionately longer time than detraining. This, of course, is due to the first-order nature of protein turnover as discussed earlier; that is, 50% of the loss of a protein occurs in one half-life (which for this example was the duration of the detraining), while 5 half-lives are required to regain the total protein lost once training resumes.

Historically, in many studies the effects of an endurance training program were assessed 48–96 h after the last training session to avoid the acute effects of the last exercise bout and to obtain the "true training" effect. While this strategy may be fine for proteins with relatively long half-lives (>1 wk; e.g., citrate synthase and succinate dehydrogenase have an estimated half-life of 12 days), it will significantly underestimate the training effect for proteins with shorter half-lives (<2–3 days). Moreover, some regulatory proteins with half-lives on the order of less than 1 day (e.g. transcription factors) may return to their resting concentration less than 24–48 h post exercise.

Although it is difficult to directly measure the degradation rates of specific proteins in living animals, it is generally agreed from indirect estimates that protein degradation rates increase as a result of enhancements in skeletal muscle usage. The higher the protein degradation rate becomes, the shorter is its protein half-life; that is, the more rapid the turnover rate. Thus, it is likely that protein turnover may actually be faster in exercise-trained muscle.

Application of Theoretical Concepts to Predict Functions of Proteins Whose Activities Are Altered by Exercise

The application of transcript profiling techniques will undoubtedly lead to the identification of novel proteins that change with physical activity or inactivity. One enlightening way to approach the interpretation of changes in gene expression with alterations in physical activity or inactivity may be to question the existence of a gene. For example, do activity-induced changes in the levels of some proteins reflect evolutionary selection of those genes for a particular survival function? Should the assignment of function for genes whose expression changes during physical training be based upon the philosophy that the gene usurped an exercise function from a gene selected by evolution to perform a function other than exercise? Or is it possible that exercise research in the new millennium is unmasking, in an otherwise sedentary population, the function of genes that evolved to support physical activity as a means of survival? With the advent of genomics, proteomics, and bioinformatics, some of the following concepts (Table 30.2) may be used to form hypotheses to test for functions of identified changes in protein levels with physical activity or inactivity.

Application of Various Time Courses or Patterns of Changes in Gene Expression to Identify Potential Functions for Genes Altered by Physical Activity

The pattern of change in the expression of a gene can provide clues to the function of that gene. If the response pattern shows an abrupt spike or repression, it will be designated as

TABLE 30.2	Concepts Allowing Generation of Potential Functions of Proteins or mRNAs Changing as a Result of Physical Activity or Inactivity
Pattern of change with physical activity or inactivity	
Homeostasis	
Phenotype of elite physical performer	
Environment–gene interaction	
Physical activity–gene interaction	
Thrifty genotype or gene hypothesis	
Chronic diseases	
Bioinformatics	
Search through multiple databases containing protein functions	
Chromosomal position	

an acute response as described in the next two examples. In example 1, the interleukin-6 (IL-6) gene is markedly activated in muscle during the latter stages of long-term exercise (3–4 h) but then shuts off immediately upon cessation of exercise (35). Such a pattern suggests a potential function downstream in an exercise sensor pathway communicating that exercise is ongoing. A second transient pattern is exemplified by the uncoupling protein 3 (UCP3) gene, a gene that encodes for a mitochondrial protein whose expression increases dramatically during the first several hours after exercise but then returns to resting levels within 24 h after exercise (32,36). A pattern of this type suggests that UCP3 may be needed for a specific function during recovery from exercise, although exactly what that function is has yet to be determined. Abrupt changes in mRNA per protein are possible only for gene products with very short half-lives. Because many regulatory proteins and rate-limiting enzymes have short half-lives to allow for speedy adjustments in control mechanisms, it is reasonable to hypothesize that proteins with similar transient expression patterns may perform similar functions. Many of these types of proteins are also normally not expressed at appreciable levels under resting conditions, as they may fulfill a specific need of the cell that under normal conditions is not required or even is potentially detrimental.

However, if the pattern is a gradual change over days to weeks, different potential functions may be proposed. The protein may have a role in reducing an exercise-induced disruption in homeostasis rather than a role as the regulator of other protein expression. The level of the mRNA or protein is often relatively high in the sedentary subject and requires multiple exercise bouts to generate a measurable increase in the mRNA or protein level. Proteins in this category have a relatively long half-life (e.g., days). One substance falling into this category is cytochrome *c*. The half life of cytochrome *c* protein is 7 days in rat skeletal muscle undergoing training or detraining, and it thus takes several days of daily exercise before a significant increase in its concentration can be detected.

Application of the Concept of Homeostasis to Identify Potential Functions for Genes Altered by Physical Activity

If at least one function of a gene and its pattern of change in response to a change in physical activity are known, an educated guess can be made as to whether the protein could play a role in homeostasis. (Concepts of homeostasis were presented earlier in the chapter.) If the directional change in the protein with exercise training is such as to invite a prediction that the exercise-induced disruption of homeostasis would be attenuated, it is feasible to hypothesize that the adaptive change in protein level may minimize the disturbance to homeostasis in response to exercise. An example of an adaptation that was eventually shown to minimize homeostatic disruption is the doubling of mitochondrial density, using cytochrome c protein concentration as an index, with endurance training. The hypothesis was that muscle with twice as many mitochondria but consuming the same oxygen as other muscle would have only half the flux through each electron transport chain, implying that adenosine diphosphate (ADP) concentration would increase only half as much. The hypothesis was later proved; that is, the disruption of the homeostatic level of ADP is less in the muscle with twice as much mitochondrial density at the same workload (37).

Homeostasis is classically defined as maintaining a constant level of a chemical. However, some functions of the body involve cycling and are considered normal. For example, the cycling of biochemical and hormonal events associated with the menstrual cycle can be considered as homeostatic cycling. Another example of homeostatic cycling is the hormonal response to ingestion of food, which includes a transient pulse in blood insulin and subsequent effects of insulin receptor signaling, all of which are a normal response to the ingestion of food, ingestion being periodical, not constant. Therefore, homeostatic cycling includes the physiological cycling of biochemicals such as insulin and glucose in normal human functions. Consequently, it is reasonable to propose that biochemical cycling associated with the exercise–recovery cycle is a normal function. During the most recent tens of thousands of years, the final selection of the current 30,000 human genes was made. As the survival of a gene pool involves the cycling of such fundamental life processes as reproduction, food consumption, the physical labor related to food gathering, and defense against the environment, they may be designated as homeostatic cycling processes. The absence of cycling (amenorrhea, starvation, or immobility) are surmised to be associated with selection for extinction. Therefore, it is speculated that the proper fluctuation of biochemicals supporting the exercise–recovery cycle were likely selected during evolution and are still present today, when exercise is performed. Thus, exercise–recovery cycles are an example of homeostatic cycling. In the presence of chronic physical inactivity, however, the normal homeostatic cycling of biochemicals stalls, leading to chronic metabolic dysfunctions that underlie chronic health conditions. Thus, if proteins that cycle in tandem with exercise and recovery do not cycle in physical inactivity, the hypothesis can be made that they could play some role in metabolic diseases. Observation of a protein whose concentration cycles with exercise and rest in the healthy but which published data indicate does not cycle in a disease state provides a hypothesis that the protein may be a candidate for affecting health. For example, GLUT4 cycles to the sarcolemma with increased insulin after a meal or with exercise and from the sarcolemma 12 h after the last meal or in physical inactivity. However, GLUT4 does not cycle in type 2 diabetes and remains at its intracellular site. Exercising diabetic patients increase sarcolemmal GLUT4 concentration, which leads to the hypothesis that GLUT4 protein has dual exercise functions, that is, a role post exercise to replenish muscle glycogen and in the primary prevention of type 2 diabetes.

Application of Elite Physical Performance to Identify Potential Functions for Genes Altered by Physical Activity

In the 1960s most of the applications of exercise physiology were directed toward understanding how to improve the physical performance of world-class athletes. One example is the use of muscle biopsies from world-class athletes. Cyclists were shown to have an 80% higher mitochondrial density in legs than arms, while canoeists had the opposite, having 36% higher mitochondria in their arms. Distance runners had a very high percentage of type I fibers compared to the average population, while sprinters had a high percentage of type II fiber. In his book *A Scientific Approach to Distance Running*, David Costill wrote that athletes having less than 60% type I fibers in their gastrocnemius muscle stood little chance of achieving success in national or international distance running competition (38). Thus, associating world-class performance with phenotype differences allowed functions to be deduced, that is, higher mitochondrial density and type I fiber percentage being related to athletic events. The identification of the functions of novel genes is allowing new experiments to determine whether these genes have a role in elite performance. One example is the myostatin gene, which was identified in 1997. Knockout of the myostatin gene in mice doubled skeletal muscle mass and created excited speculation that variations in sequence or expression might explain differences in human muscle mass (39). Although two common polymorphisms were subsequently identified in the myostatin gene, neither was found to be related to the change in muscle mass in response to strength training in either whites or African Americans (39). In addition, no significant correlations were observed between myostatin expression and any muscle strength or volume measure.

Application of the Concept of Environmental Gene Interaction to Identify Potential Functions for Genes Altered by Physical Activity or Inactivity

Gene expression (defined by the concentration of specific proteins) is not constant throughout the lifespan. While some genes have programmed changes in expression (development), and others are regulated by biological clocks (menstrual cycle or sleep), a major factor eliciting altered gene expression is the environment. The term *environment* refers to milieu within and surrounding the cell. Environment can alter the periodicity of the menstrual cycle. For example, the menstrual cycle can be overridden by chronic excessive physical exercise due to a negative caloric imbalance producing an alteration in the hypothalamic–pituitary–gonadal axis, which is responsible for the menstrual disorders. Another example of an environmental factor is resistance training that increases skeletal muscle size and strength. Thus, physical activity or inactivity is an environmental perturbation on gene expression.

Application of Physical Activity–Gene Interaction to Understand Protein Function

The concept of interaction between physical activity and genes received strong support at the biochemical level in 1967, when John Holloszy reported increases in mitochondrial protein and enzyme activities in the skeletal muscles of rats that had been forced to run on treadmills while their cage mates remained sedentary (40). As detailed in Chapter 21, Holloszy showed that expression of mitochondrial proteins was malleable by the level of habitual physical activity. Thus, he applied known information about exercise to explain an observed interaction between physical activity and a gene.

Another example of interaction between physical activity and genes comes from recent research on the effects of exercise on cognitive ability. As discussed earlier in the chapter, providing mice with voluntary running wheels is associated with improved hippocampal neurogenesis and cognitive function (15). Epidemiological data show that women who are 65 years or older have a 50% reduction in cognitive impairment, Alzheimer disease, and dementia of any type if they engage three or more times per week in exercise at an intensity greater than walking (41). Therefore, a future research endeavor will be to define further the interactions between removal of running activity and changed gene expression that allow a biologically significant threshold to be passed wherein overt clinical cognitive dysfunction occurs.

Application of the Thrifty Genotype Hypothesis to Identify Potential Functions for Genes Altered by Physical Activity or Inactivity

Thrifty Gene Hypothesis

In 1962 Neel proposed a hypothesis that a " 'thrifty' genotype would be exceptionally efficient in the intake and/or utilization of food" (42). Most published interpretations of Neel's 1962 hypothesis emphasize that humans who could most efficiently store foods as fat were most likely to survive a famine because of their larger stores of fat at the start of the famine than those without thrifty fat storage. The common deduction made since 1962 is that individuals with gene pools having polymorphisms to allow a more efficient storage of fat were more likely to survive via natural selection than those who could not as efficiently store fat. Less often mentioned in the current interpretations of the original thrifty genotype hypothesis is the other part of Neel's original definition, that is, the role of exceptional efficiency in the utilization of stored fat during a famine. Simply stated, individuals with polymorphisms that could conserve the limited body stores of carbohydrate and triglycerides longer during physical activity would have a survival advantage. Per O. Åstrand in 1986 wrote that because food was not continuously available for 99% of human existence, physical activity had to have been obligatory for survival (43). Likely humans and animals had to endure periods when food was not available (famine). Thus, the selection of polymorphisms is surmised to have occurred during thousands of years of feast-and-famine cycles when the environmental component of physical activity was required for food procurement during starvation (10). Humans without an ability to undertake physical activity or without polymorphisms that relatively efficiently conserve glycogen in the search for food were likely to be selected for extinction because food acquisition during evolution was not from grocery stores or restaurants. Such logic, if valid, supports the hypothesis that a subpopulation of the human genotype was selected to support physical activity during food shortage. Interaction between the environment and genes was likely a fundamental determinant in the conjectured selection of the thrifty genotype that was more efficient in the usage of carbohydrate and fat during physical activity. Therefore, the thrifty genotype is an example of a hypothesis that can be addressed by future exercise physiologists when studying the functions of polymorphisms identified by genomic scans.

Extension of Thrifty Genotype to Include Thrifty Genes to Understand Protein Functions During Exercise

It is interesting to consider that during evolution, specific genes, in addition to polymorphisms, were selected to maximize the efficiency of physical activity required for survival, particularly during periods of starvation, and the efficiency of energy restoration during feeding. To address this concept further, the next sections provide examples of candidate thrifty genes in the context of the regulation of fuel metabolism during physical activity.

GLUCOSE HOMEOSTASIS DURING PHYSICAL ACTIVITY AS AN EVOLUTIONARY FORCE FOR THE SELECTION OF THRIFTY GENES

The energy required to support life is derived from the

metabolism of carbohydrate, fat, and proteins. In the absence of food intake, existing stores of fat and protein can supply the needed energy for several weeks. Carbohydrate reserves (i.e., muscle and liver glycogen), however, are extremely limited and will be depleted within about 24 h. This presents a serious challenge to intermediary metabolism because the brain relies almost exclusively on blood glucose to support its energy needs: free fatty acids bound to albumin cannot cross the blood-brain barrier. Fortunately, metabolic catastrophe is avoided under such conditions because of the liver's ability to activate endogenous synthesis of both glucose (gluconeogenesis) and ketone bodies, an alternative fuel that can cross into and be metabolized by the brain. In fact, most hormonal control exerted over intermediary metabolism is targeted to the regulation of blood glucose to ensure that hypoglycemia does not occur during prolonged periods with limited or no carbohydrate intake.

Prolonged physical activity also represents a significant challenge to intermediary metabolism and specifically to glucose homeostasis. Although skeletal muscle, unlike the brain, can utilize carbohydrate, fatty acids, and amino acids to meet the energy demands of contractile activity, it is well established that as muscle glycogen concentration approaches zero during exercise, work cannot be continued at the same intensity. That is, fatigue occurs if the same exercise power is continued. Obviously, the challenge to both glucose homeostasis and exercise endurance is exacerbated if physical activity is performed under conditions of limited fuel intake. The thrifty gene hypothesis postulates that genes (and polymorphisms within, i.e., the original thrifty genotype hypothesis) that could most efficiently conserve muscle glycogen during work would be more likely to be conserved during evolution. In other words, being unable to perform the level of physical activity necessary for survival (hunting, gathering) because of an unfavorable metabolic gene profile would be incompatible with survival.

To illustrate how insight into functions for genes identified as being altered by physical activity may be gained when viewed in the context of both cellular homeostasis and evolutionary selection (e.g., thrifty gene hypothesis), consider a recently discovered "exercise-responsive" gene known as pyruvate dehydrogenase kinase 4 (PDK4). PDK4 is expressed primarily in skeletal and cardiac muscle, where it catalyzes the phosphorylation of the E1 component of pyruvate dehydrogenase (PDH) enzyme complex, inhibiting the conversion of pyruvate to acetyl-coenzyme A and thus preventing the entry of glycolytic products into the mitochondria for oxidation (44). The PDH complex is a pivotal step in metabolism because (a) the decarboxylation of pyruvate represents the irreversible loss of a major three-carbon gluconeogenic precursor and (b) skeletal muscle, because of its large percentage of the total body mass, accounts for nearly 20–25% of the resting energy expenditure in young adults. PDK4 mRNA is nearly undetectable in muscle under normal resting conditions when carbohydrate reserves are plentiful.

However, transcription of the PDK4 gene to PDK4 mRNA increases dramatically during the late stages of prolonged low-intensity exercise (32,36). This induction of PDK4 mRNA is consistent with the steady decline in oxidation of carbohydrates that occurs in muscle during such exercise. Thus, PDK4 induction may be an important mechanism for reducing the rate of both glucose and muscle glycogen utilization during prolonged activity as a means of delaying hypoglycemia, glycogen depletion, and therefore fatigue.

If PDK4 is to qualify as a candidate thrifty gene, then regulation of the gene must be consistent in response to other metabolic challenges. Indeed, both starvation and streptozotocin-induced diabetes also elicit marked increases in PDK4 expression in skeletal muscle (45). In each of these metabolic states (prolonged exercise, fasting, diabetes), there is a real or at least a perceived deficit in carbohydrate availability in the form of either low blood glucose or low muscle glycogen concentration. Consistent with this view is the finding that activation of the PDK4 gene is significantly enhanced when exercise is initiated with low muscle glycogen concentration (46), presumably reflecting the need to conserve glucose and/or glycogen utilization much earlier during exercise than in the fed state. In the big picture, these findings collectively raise the possibility that PDK4 may have been selected as a gene for induction in skeletal muscle during feast-and-famine cycles to minimize carbohydrate utilization during periods of starvation when physical activity was required to maintain survival. In other words, fatigue precipitated by an inability to conserve adequate carbohydrates when reserves are limited would be incompatible with survival.

ENERGY HOMEOSTASIS DURING PHYSICAL ACTIVITY AS AN EVOLUTIONARY FORCE FOR THE SELECTION OF THRIFTY GENES

Another candidate for a thrifty gene that would more efficiently utilize stored energy for physical activity is myosin heavy chain (MHC) I protein. More than two decades ago, it was found that muscles with a preponderance of MHC type I fibers use less than half the energy to perform the same contractile work as expended by muscles with a preponderance of MHC type II fibers (47). Thus, MHC I uses fuels more efficiently, fitting Neel's definition of thrifty.

The preceding are examples of how expanding the context in which exercise research findings regarding the regulation of a particular gene are viewed allows for further insight into the function of that gene product. One of the primary adaptations to dynamic exercise training is a reduced utilization of carbohydrate stores by the working muscle at a given absolute exercise intensity. A future research interrogation using genomics or proteomics could include a search for genes selected to permit a more efficient usage of substrate, that is, conservation of muscle glycogen and body glucose during exercise after endurance training. The conjecture is that genes involved in conserving muscle glycogen during physical activity can be called thrifty genes.

Application of Chronic Disease to Drive an Identification of Potential Functions for Genes Altered by Physical Activity or Inactivity

Type 2 diabetes is associated with defective post-receptor insulin signaling. It has been known for a century that exercise improves glucose uptake into skeletal muscle of diabetic patients, so an early hypothesis was that exercise increased insulin signaling. The studies to test the hypothesis found that contractile activity surprisingly did not increase proximal insulin signaling. As a result, investigators were forced to look for candidates other than insulin-signaling proteins to determine which proteins were involved in the exercise-induced increase in glucose uptake by skeletal muscle. Attention soon focused on an energy-sensing protein known as AMP kinase (mentioned earlier in the chapter). It was found that (*a*) exercise increased AMP kinase activity, (*b*) increasing AMP kinase activity by administering a drug also activated glucose transport in muscle of resting animals, and (*c*) expression of a dysfunctional form of AMP kinase in transgenic mice at least partially attenuated the activation of glucose transport in muscle. Thus, these studies proved that AMP kinase is at least one of the signaling proteins required for the exercise-induced increase in glucose uptake by skeletal muscle.

In a second example, an apparent association between increased physical activity levels and decreased coronary heart disease was published in the early 1950s. Later investigations showed that exercise training increased coronary blood flow transport capacity, but not as a result of an enhanced structural capacity of blood vessels. Rather they showed that blood vessels from trained animals and humans had better vasodilation, allowing more blood flow, than sedentary subjects. Since earlier literature indicated that nitric oxide produced vasodilation, researchers used the nitric oxide studies to pose the hypotheses leading to the findings that exercise training increased endothelial nitric oxide synthase mRNA and protein in vascular endothelial cells in the heart.

Concluding Comments to the Section on the Application of Theoretical Concepts to Predict Functions of Proteins Whose Activities Are Altered by Exercise

Hypotheses in genomics research must be stated with a clear understanding of the principles that guide not only the immediate homeostasis of the cells, tissues, and whole organism but also the factors that allow for the selection and reinforcement of the genes in the human genome during evolution. A future genomic research endeavor in exercise physiology will be to prove the postulate that some of the molecular adaptations to physical training consist of genes permitted to invoke their ancient functions during physical activity or training by sedentary humans or animals. Thousands of genes change expression during physical activity or inactivity.

Exercise-induced genes can be used as a query for the discovery of why some of the 30,000 genes in the human genome survived selection and are still present. The inclusion of the concept of thrifty genes in physical activity adaptations may provide an additional approach to delineate the true function for genes whose expression is altered by physical activity or inactivity. If the truth is that some genes that compose the human genome were selected for their survival functions to support physical activity, then basic science demands that the original role of this subset of genes must be understood to fully understand the human genome. After all, discerning the correct function of a gene leads to a true understanding of the essence of life.

The Role of Exercise in Future Genomic Research

Individualized Medicine for the Prediction of Disease

Grand Challenge II-3 of the Human Genome Project is to develop genome-based approaches to prediction of disease susceptibility. The discovery of variants that affect risk of disease could be used in individualized preventive medicine, including diet, exercise, lifestyle, and pharmaceutical intervention, to maximize the likelihood of staying well. Individualization of an exercise prescription for prevention of disease (primary, secondary, and tertiary) must include the recognition from the Heritage study that the same training program that resulted in a change of less than 0.2 L in maximal oxygen uptake for 5 of 47 subjects also found that 12 subjects gained 0.2–0.4 L of oxygen per minute, 16 gained 0.4–0.6 L of oxygen per minute, 4 gained 0.6–0.8 L of oxygen per minute, and 11 gained 0.8–1.0 L of oxygen per minute (48). However since progressively large increases in maximal oxygen uptake with training have yet to be shown to be associated with step increases in bone hippocampal neurogenesis (decreased dementia), bone density (osteoporosis), and other health benefits, it is erroneous to conclude prematurely that those whose genes predict minimal increase in maximal oxygen uptake with training should not train because they would receive no health benefit.

It is also clear that inheritance plays a major role in predisposing to prevalence of a specific disease and furthermore that physical inactivity determines whether expression of these inherited genes surpasses a biological threshold for the overt occurrence of this disease (a concept called gene–environmental interaction). Figure 30.6 illustrates gene–physical inactivity interaction in determining the risk of type 2 diabetes.

Population medicine describes the prescription of the same amount of physical activity to everyone. For example, the current prescription is a minimum of 30 min of moderate physical activity per day to provide a minimal health ben-

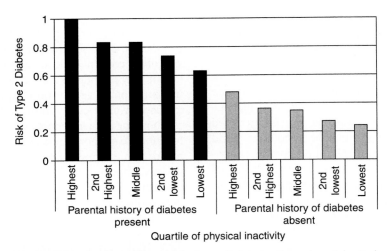

FIGURE 30.6 Predisposition to risk of type 2 diabetes depends on inherited genes (deduced from greater prevalence with parental history of type 2 diabetes) and on environmental interaction with genes predisposing to type 2 diabetes. This figure shows the quartile of physical inactivity instead of physical activity on the X-axis as the cause of type 2 because exercise does not cause type 2 diabetes, whereas physical inactivity does. The risk of type 2 diabetes increases 59% and 100% from the lowest to the highest quartile of physical inactivity in siblings with and without, respectively, a parental history of type 2 diabetes. Subjects were 70,102 women aged 46–72 and were free from diagnosed diabetes, cardiovascular disease, and cancer at the start of the 6-yr study. *(Modified with permission from Hu F et al. Walking compared with vigorous physical activity and risk of type 2 diabetes in women: a prospective study. JAMA 1999;282:1433–1439.)*

efit (U.S. Surgeon General) or 60 minutes of physical activity per day to prevent weight gain on the average U.S. caloric intake (U.S. Institute of Medicine). However, a shortcoming of population medicine for physical activity is that not all individuals respond identically to physical training. For example, a rare proportion of individuals, nonresponders, do not increase maximal oxygen consumption with aerobic training. These nonresponders may not obtain a health benefit from daily physical activity; it is unknown whether the genes responsible for the failure to increase maximal oxygen consumption in response to training are same genes that interact with disease-predisposing genes to produce overt clinical chronic health conditions. Individualized medicine describes the determination of gene polymorphisms for a given individual and then prescription of treatment based upon the identified cocktail of disease-susceptible and physical inactivity polymorphisms present in the individual's genome.

Population studies aiming to locate polymorphisms related to physical inactivity causing chronic health conditions in the United States are ongoing. In the Heritage Family Study the aim is to use genome-wide scans, including targeted dense SNP mapping and skeletal muscle gene expression studies with serial analysis of gene expression, to search for genes and mutations. The aim is to document the con-

tribution of cardiovascular and metabolic responses to endurance training and of genetic factors to the concomitant risk of cardiovascular disease and type 2 diabetes risk factors among nearly 1000 individuals. A second population study aims to characterize environmental effects on 87 biological and positional candidate genes for genotyping in a population-based sample of 11,000 subjects. The study addresses dietary measures, obesity, measures of physical activity, smoking, and in women, menopause status and hormone use. The outcome of these studies could provide a foundation of polymorphisms for future personalized physical activity prescriptions by physicians to primarily prevent chronic health conditions (individualized medicine for physical activity). The success of such studies will depend on of large populations of subjects. Within 100 years, it is possible that healthy patients may be provided with access to gene chips predicting susceptibility to future diseases based upon the polymorphisms in their genome, including genes susceptible to physical inactivity. The goal will be to provide a personalized preventive lifestyle prescription designed to prevent the interaction of physical inactivity genes (by including a personalized physical activity plan) with existing disease susceptibility genes, such that the threshold for development of overt clinical disease is not crossed. Although the hypothesis is as yet unproved, it is anticipated that an individualized, genomics-based preventive approach to medicine will result in an improved, economically beneficial health care system.

Designation of Control Group Based Upon Genomics

If it is believed to be true that (*a*) hunter-gatherers were more physically active in their acquisition of food than members of sedentary cultures and (*b*) some genes exist in the human genome because they were selected to support physical activity, then the control group based upon the human genome must be the physically active group. It is speculated that few sedentary humans in hunter-gatherer societies had their gene pool selected for the human genome (the lack of physical activity would not permit food gathering and thus an early death is presumed). Thus, physical activity was the norm for nearly all of the population during nearly all of human existence on Earth. The deduction is that the control group would have consisted of physically active individuals throughout evolution until sometime in the 1900s. Sedentary individuals, by their rareness (<1% of the population), could not be considered as a representative control group for most of the population during more than 99% of human existence on Earth. Thus, a future challenge is to designate physically active individuals as the control group for genomic studies whose purpose is to understand the function of genes.

In the early 1900s, the average person included in the control group was more physically active in their daily routine compared to the average person in the late 1900s. The exercise group in the early 1900s consisted of the same cohort and was called the treatment group. The initial terminology has been retained; that is, the less physically active group is still designated as the control group. However, the control group has switched from physically active individuals (walking for transportation, manual labor on the farm, in housekeeping, and employment) in 1900 to physically inactive or sedentary (driving cars for short distances, automatic washing machines and sweepers, robotic machines) in 2000. In other words, the levels of physical activity in experimental groups are as follows: A trained group of physically active individuals in the early 1900s was more active than in the physically active control group in the 1900s. Controls in the 1900s were about as active as the exercise-trained group of physically active individuals in 2000, who are more active than the sedentary control group in 2000. Between 1900 and 2000, the control group designation has been retained for the group not undergoing the experimental exercise treatment, but the control group went from being physically active in 1900 to sedentary in 2000. Thus, in the future, physically active individuals have to be designated as the control group, since their activity levels are closer to those of the control group in the early 1900s and to the hunter-gatherer than are the sedentary majority in the United States in 2003.

The pioneering studies of Jeremy N. Morris and Ralph S. Paffenbarger Jr., published in the 1970s, were awarded the 1996 Olympic Prize for studies showing that exercise protects against heart disease. Their Olympic Prize indicated that their research findings had changed the practice of medicine, inspired the fitness revolution, and stimulated additional studies that have contributed enormously to insight into the relationship between physical activity and a reduction in the incidence of coronary heart disease. Morris's early studies showed that bus drivers, whose occupation was sedentary, had more clinical heart disease than conductors, who continuously walked through a London bus with an upper and lower floor. It is now well established that sedentary populations have 40% higher prevalence of coronary heart disease and stroke than do middle-aged women who walk a minimum of 30 min · day^{-1}. It is dogma in medicine that the healthy individuals are the control group and the sick patients are the treatment group. The exercise literature calls healthier physically active individuals the treatment group and the sicker sedentary subjects the controls. Thus exercise physiologists are one of a few, if not the only, medical group who designate the sicker population as the controls for experimental purposes. This assignment has led to the perception by some scientists in disciplines other than exercise that exercise as the treatment group is not normal and that sedentary is physiologically the norm. Thus, in the future physically active individuals have to be designated as the control group.

A negative byproduct of the misdesignation of the proper physical activity level for the control group is the misconception by some that the cellular and molecular mechanisms underlying exercise adaptations explain with 100% fidelity the cause of inactivity-related diseases. However, this experimental approach is flawed, because exercise does not cause obesity or type 2 diabetes. In order to understand the mechanistic etiology of inactivity-related diseases, physical inactivity must be the research focus. A similar tenet of medicine is that understanding the molecular mechanisms of diseases provides the scientific basis for therapy and prevention. Again, the only way to decipher the mechanisms of disease prevention is to study the process itself as it is evoked by increased physical activity, diet, and so on. It is therefore anticipated that future research will investigate the molecular mechanisms of the sicker physically inactive population, because physical inactivity, not activity, causes genes to misexpress proteins, producing the metabolic dysfunctions that result in overt clinical disease if continued long enough.

Drug Development

Remarkable development of pharmaceutical agents is predicted to occur with the sequencing of the human genome. Multiple references to an "exercise pill" have appeared in news reports. However laudable is the idea of a pill to replace all physical activity, the term exercise pill is a misnomer for the following reasons. A true full-exercise pill would produce at least the following effects:

- Physiological cardiac hypertrophy
- Bradycardia
- Enhanced nitric oxide synthase in vascular endothelial cells
- Lower systolic blood pressure
- Decreased arterial stiffness
- Less prevalence of stroke
- Cardioprotective effect
- Higher blood levels of high-density lipoprotein
- Improved cognitive function
- Lower incidence of depression
- Better immune function
- Less C-reactive protein
- Skeletal muscle hypertrophy and prevention of physical frailty
- Increased skeletal muscle mitochondria and capacity to oxide fatty acids
- Increased whole-body insulin sensitivity
- Reduction in colon and breast cancers
- Increased bone density
- Normal body mass index

Any single pill that incorporates one or two of the aforementioned benefits is accurately scientifically termed a "small-part exercise pill." The public and medical profession would be misled into missing all of the health benefits from exercise if they were induced to give up physical activity for such a pill, which would miss most of the health benefits of exercise. Nonetheless, such pills will be of great benefit to those unable to exercise (e.g., physically challenged). However, developers of drugs have a responsibility for their proper usage.

Summary: Future Research Questions That Can Be Addressed With Genomics and Proteomic Methods

The purpose of the chapter is to provide a link to the future. Only time will determine whether all suggestions, concepts, and predictions become reality. However, one fact seems indisputable: compared to the exercise physiology graduate student in the 1960s, similar students in the first decade of 2000 have immensely more significant research questions and methods. We encourage students to use genomic concepts and methodology to address mechanistic issues in all of the systems being addressed in this textbook using sample questions provided below (not meant to be all inclusive).

- What are the mechanisms by which mechanical loading hypertrophies human skeletal muscle?

- Why is mechanical loading in microgravity less effective for stimulating hypertrophy of skeletal muscle than in full gravity?
- What are the differential gene expressions between exercise-induced physiological cardiac hypertrophy and cardiac pathophysiology?
- Should exercise-induced hypertrophic heart rather than the atrophied sedentary heart be the norm for clinical medicine?
- What are the mechanisms by which bone loading during physical activity reduces the risk of osteoporosis?
- What are the underlying mechanisms for the loss of muscle fibers and motor units with aging? Which is lost first? Do muscle fibers cause the loss of nerves, or does motor neuron loss initiate the loss of muscle fibers?
- What are the mechanisms causing aged skeletal muscle to exhibit defective muscle regrowth following atrophy?
- By what mechanisms does physical inactivity increase the risk of most site-specific cancers, such as breast, colon, lung, rectal, and pancreatic cancer?
- By what mechanisms does physical activity maintain somatic cells in a nonimmortalized condition?
- How is blood flow regulated through the microcirculation during exercise?
- By what mechanisms does moderate exercise enhance the immune system?
- What are the mechanisms that moderate exercise uses to suppress local inflammation, such as in walls of arterial blood vessels?
- How does muscle inactivity cause insulin resistance?
- By what mechanisms does muscle inactivity initiate prediabetes?
- What additional signaling mechanisms to AMP kinase activate glucose transport in response to contractile activity?
- What is the connection between physical inactivity, mitochondrial dysfunction, and insulin resistance?
- How many ways does skeletal muscle communicate with other organs and tissues?
- Is skeletal muscle an endocrine organ?
- How is the metabolic state of the working skeletal muscle communicated to the brain? Does it use type III or IV sensory neurons?
- What are the mechanisms by which physical activity improves learning, memory, and cognitive function?
- By what mechanisms does physical activity reduce the risk of disorders of cognitive dysfunction?
- What are the physical activity mechanisms by which satellite cells are activated, proliferate, and fuse into muscle fibers?

A MILESTONE OF DISCOVERY

What are the molecular pathways regulating the activation of specific genes in response to exercise? This question has intrigued muscle biologists since the discovery that endurance training increases the activity and content of mitochondrial enzymes. One can imagine that any number of signaling events initiated by contractile activity (e.g., factors originating from the motor nerve, sympathetic stimulation, growth factors, or disturbances to ratios of intracellular ATP to ADP and NADH to NAD⁺) may ultimately lead to the transcriptional activation of exercise-responsive genes (49). Although a true milestone must stand the test of time, a recent body of research testing the hypothesis that Ca⁺⁺ transients evoked during dynamic exercise may represent an initiating signal leading to adaptive changes in chronically exercised skeletal muscle was selected as the milestone for this chapter. In 1998, while working with C2C12 muscle cells in the laboratory of Sanders Williams, Eva Chin found that overexpression of a constitutively active form of calcineurin, a calcium-activated protein phosphatase, induced the expression of metabolic genes normally expressed in oxidative fiber types (types I and IIa). She also discovered that these effects appeared to be mediated at least in part by the MEF2 transcription factor family (50). To test for the importance of MEF2 *in vivo*, Wu et al. (51), also in Williams's group, used a mouse with a transgene consisting of multiple MEF2 DNA binding sites driving the lacZ reporter gene. The lacZ gene produces the protein β-galactosidase, which can be detected histochemically by an enzymatic reaction that produces a blue color. Thus, expression of the reporter gene depends on the presence and functional activity of the MEF2 transcription factor. Despite the fact that MEF2 protein is present and able to bind to the MEF2-lacZ construct, the authors were unable to detect anything but a very low level of expression in the soleus muscle of sedentary mice.

However, when mice were given free access to running wheels, MEF2-mediated activation of transcription, as assessed by β-galactosidase blue staining, increased dramatically in hindlimb muscles recruited by running activity (that is, soleus, plantaris, and white vastus lateralis muscle). Interestingly, crossing these mice with a second line of mice engineered to express the myocyte-enriched calcineurin interacting protein 1, a calcineurin inhibitory protein, nearly completely abrogated the activation of the MEF2-driven reporter gene in mice allowed to run voluntarily for 3 days. This and subsequent studies from Williams's laboratory led to the working model suggesting that sustained increases in intracellular calcium brought on by dynamic exercise activates calcineurin and other calcium-activated events (not depicted). The result is the dephosphorylation or activation of MEF2 and together with other transcription factors and coactivators (coenzyme A), the transcriptional activation of target metabolic genes. Given that many oxidative metabolism genes are regulated by MEF2 promoter elements, this body of research provides exciting new evidence that intracellular Ca⁺⁺ transients evoked during dynamic exercise activate molecular pathways that ultimately lead to improvements in oxidative metabolic capacity associated with dynamic exercise training in skeletal muscle.

Wu H, Rothermel B, Kanatous S, et al. *Activation of MEF2 by muscle activity is mediated through a calcineurin-dependent pathway. EMBO J 2001;20:6414–6423.*

- Are there genes whose expression produces sedentary behavior?
- What are the connecting pathways by which the lack of food drives increased physical activity?

ACKNOWLEDGMENTS

J. Scott Pattison assisted in writing the section on genomic methodology. The chapter was written while the authors were supported by AR19393 (FWB) and AR45372 (PDN).

REFERENCES

1. Booth FW, Baldwin KM. Muscle plasticity: energy demand and supply processes. In Rowell LB, Shepherd JT, eds. The Handbook of physiology. Exercise: regulation and Integration of Multiple Systems. New York: Oxford University, 1996;1075–1123.
2. Hanis CL, Boerwinkle E, Chakraborty R, et al. A genome-wide search for human non-insulin-dependent (type 2) diabetes genes reveals a major susceptibility locus on chromosome 2. Nat Genet 1996;13:161–166.
3. Fitzpatrick DR, Wilson CB. Methylation and demethylation in the regulation of genes, cells, and responses in the immune system. Clin Immunol 2003;109:37–45.
4. Zhang CL, McKinsey TA, Olson EN. Association of class II histone deacetylases with heterochromatin protein 1: potential role for histone methylation in control of muscle differentiation. Mol Cell Biol 2002;22:7302–7312.
5. Pattison JS, Folk LC, Madsen RW, et al. Transcriptional profiling identifies extensive downregulation of extracellular matrix gene expression in sarcopenic rat soleus muscle. Physiol Genom 2003;15:34–43.
6. Curtis RK, Brand MD. Control analysis of DNA microarray expression data. Mol Biol Rep 2002;29:67–71.
7. Pattison JS, Folk LC, Madsen RW, et al. Expression profiling identifies dysregulation of myosin heavy chains IIb and IIx during limb immobilization in the soleus muscles of old rats. J Physiol (Lond) 2003;553:357–368.
8. Merrill GF, Kurth EJ, Hardie DG, et al. AICA riboside increases AMP-activated protein kinase, fatty acid oxidation, and glucose uptake in rat muscle. Am J Physiol 1997;273:E1107–E1112.

9. Mu J, Brozinick JT Jr, Valladares O, et al. A role for AMP-activated protein kinase in contraction- and hypoxia-regulated glucose transport in skeletal muscle. Mol Cell 2001;7:1085–1094.

10. Chakravarthy MV, Booth FW. Eating, exercise, and "thrifty" genotypes: connecting the dots toward an evolutionary understanding of modern chronic diseases. J Appl Physiol 2004;96:3–10.

11. Hawley JA, Zierath JR. Integration of metabolic and mitogenic signal transduction in skeletal muscle. Exerc Sport Sci Rev 2004;32:4–8.

12. van der Neut R. Targeted gene disruption: applications in neurobiology. J Neurosci Methods 1997;71:19–27.

13. Williams RS, Wagner PD. Transgenic animals in integrative biology: approaches and interpretations of outcome. J Appl Physiol 2000;88:1119–1126.

14. Fazio S, Linton MF. Mouse models of hyperlipidemia and atherosclerosis. Front Biosci 2001;6:D515–525.

15. Cotman CW, Berchtold NC. Exercise: a behavioral intervention to enhance brain health and plasticity. Trends Neurosci 2002;25:295–301.

16. Kitamura T, Mishina M, Sugiyama H. Enhancement of neurogenesis by running wheel exercises is suppressed in mice lacking NMDA receptor epsilon 1 subunit. Neurosci Res 2003;47:55–63.

17. Chang PY, Jensen J, Printz RL, et al. Overexpression of hexokinase II in transgenic mice. Evidence that increased phosphorylation augments muscle glucose uptake. J Biol Chem 1996;271:14834–14839.

18. Halseth AE, Bracy DP, Wasserman DH. Overexpression of hexokinase II increases insulin- and exercise-stimulated muscle glucose uptake in vivo. Am J Physiol 1999;276:E70–77.

19. Grobet L, Pirottin D, Farnir F, et al. Modulating skeletal muscle mass by postnatal, muscle-specific inactivation of the myostatin gene. Genesis 2003;35:227–238.

20. Ryding AD, Sharp MG, Mullins JJ. Conditional transgenic technologies. J Endocrinol 2001;171:1–14.

21. Carson JA, Schwartz RJ, Booth FW. SRF and TEF-1 control of chicken skeletal alpha-actin gene during slow-muscle hypertrophy. Am J Physiol 1996;270:C1624–C1633.

22. Fattori E, La Monica N, Ciliberto G, et al. Electro-gene-transfer: a new approach for muscle gene delivery. Somat Cell Mol Genet 2002;27:75–83.

23. Barton-Davis ER, Shoturma DI, Musaro A, et al. Viral mediated expression of insulin-like growth factor I blocks the aging-related loss of skeletal muscle function. Proc Natl Acad Sci USA 1998;95:15603–15607.

24. Molkentin JD, Lu JR, Antos CL, et al. A calcineurin-dependent transcriptional pathway for cardiac hypertrophy. Cell 1998;93:215–228.

25. Eto Y, Yonekura K, Sonoda M, et al. Calcineurin is activated in rat hearts with physiological left ventricular hypertrophy induced by voluntary exercise training. Circulation 2000;101:2134–2137.

26. Rothermel BA, McKinsey TA, Vega RB, et al. Myocyte-enriched calcineurin-interacting protein, MCIP1, inhibits cardiac hypertrophy in vivo. Proc Natl Acad Sci USA 2001;98:3328–3333.

27. Pette D, Vrbova G. Adaptation of mammalian skeletal muscle fibers to chronic electrical stimulation. Rev Physiol Biochem Pharmacol 1992;120:115–202.

28. Haggmark T, Eriksson E, Jansson E. Muscle fiber type changes in human skeletal muscle after injuries and immobilization. Orthopedics 1986;9:181–185.

29. Richter EA, Derave W, Wojtaszewski JF. Glucose, exercise and insulin: emerging concepts. J Physiol (Lond) 2001;535:313–322.

30. Booth FW, Thomason DB. Molecular and cellular adaptation of muscle in response to exercise: perspectives of various models. Physiol Rev 1991;71:541–585.

31. Terjung RL, Hood DA. Biochemical adaptations in skeletal muscle induced by exercise training. In Layman DK, ed. Nutrition and Aerobic Exercise. Washington: American Chemical Society, 1986;8–27.

32. Hildebrandt AL, Pilegaard H, Neufer PD. Differential transcriptional activation of select metabolic genes in response to variations in exercise intensity and duration. Am J Physiol 2003;285:E1021–E1027.

33. Booth F. Effects of endurance exercise on cytochrome C turnover in skeletal muscle. Ann NY Acad Sci 1977;301:431–439.

34. Hickson RC. Skeletal muscle cytochrome c and myoglobin, endurance, and frequency of training. J Appl Physiol 1981;51:746–749.

35. Keller C, Steensberg A, Pilegaard H, et al. Transcriptional activation of the IL-6 gene in human contracting skeletal muscle: influence of muscle glycogen content. FASEB J 2001;15:2748–2750.

36. Pilegaard H, Ordway GA, Saltin B, et al. Transcriptional regulation of gene expression in human skeletal muscle during recovery from exercise. Am J Physiol 2000;279:E806–E814.

37. Dudley GA, Tullson PC, Terjung RL. Influence of mitochondrial content on the sensitivity of respiratory control. J Biol Chem 1987;262:9109–9114.

38. Costill DL. A scientific approach to distance running. Track & Field News 1979;99.

39. McPherron AC, Lawler M, Lee SJ. Regulation of skeletal muscle mass in mice by a new TGF-beta superfamily member. Nature 1997;387:83–90.

40. Holloszy JO. Biochemical adaptations in muscle. Effects of exercise on mitochondrial oxygen uptake and respiratory enzyme activity in skeletal muscle. J Biol Chem 1967;242:2278–2282.

41. Laurin D, Verreault R, Lindsay J, et al. Physical activity and risk of cognitive impairment and dementia in elderly persons. Arch Neurol 2001;58:498–504.

42. Neel JV. Diabetes mellitus: a "thrifty" genotype rendered detrimental by "progress"? Am J Hum Genet 1962;14:353–362.

43. Åstrand PO, Rodahl K. Textbook of Work Physiology. 3rd ed. New York: McGraw-Hill, 1986.

44. Sugden MC, Holness MJ. Recent advances in mechanisms regulating glucose oxidation at the level of the pyruvate dehydrogenase complex by PDKs. Am J Physiol 2003;284:E855–E862.

45. Wu P, Sato J, Zhao Y, et al. Starvation and diabetes increase the amount of pyruvate dehydrogenase kinase isoenzyme 4 in rat heart. Biochem J 1998;329:197–201.

46. Pilegaard H, Keller C, Steensberg A, et al. Influence of pre-exercise muscle glycogen content on exercise-induced transcriptional regulation of metabolic genes. J Physiol (Lond) 2002;541:261–271.

47. Crow MT, Kushmerick MJ. Chemical energetics of slow- and fast-twitch muscles of the mouse. J Gen Physiol 1982;79:147–166.

48. Bouchard C, Malina R, Perusse L. Genetics of Fitness and Physical Performance. Champaign, IL: Human Kinetics, 1997.

49. Williams RS, Neufer PD. Regulation of gene expression in skeletal muscle by contractile activity. In Rowell LB, Shepherd JT, eds. Handbook of Physiology, Section 12: Exercise: Regulation and Integration of Multiple Systems. New York: Oxford University, 1996; 1124–1150.

50. Chin ER, Olson EN, Richardson JA, et al. A calcineurin-dependent transcriptional pathway controls skeletal muscle fiber type. Genes Dev 1998;12:2499–2509.

51. Wu H, Rothermel B, Kanatous S, et al. Activation of MEF2 by muscle activity is mediated through a calcineurin-dependent pathway. Embo J 2001;20: 6414–6423.

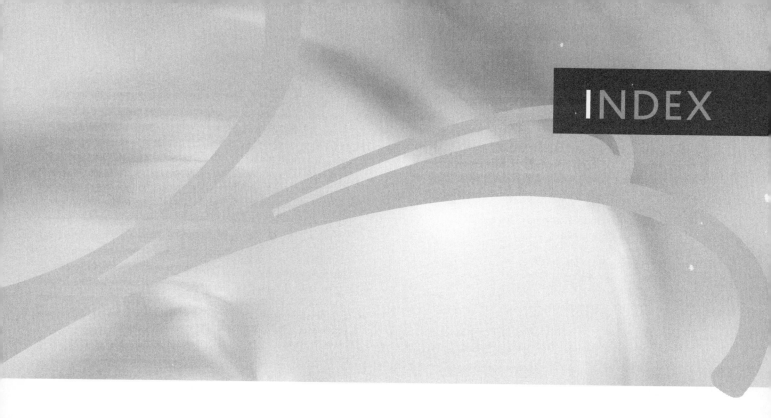

INDEX